Textbook of Neural Repair and Rehabilitation

In two freestanding volumes, Textbook of Neural Repair and Rehabilitation provides comprehensive coverage of the science and practice of neurologic rehabilitation. This volume, Neural Repair and Plasticity covers the basic sciences relevant to recovery of function following injury to the nervous system, reviewing anatomical and physiologic plasticity in the normal central nervous system, mechanisms of neuronal death, axonal regeneration, stem cell biology, and research strategies targeted at axon regeneration and neuron replacement. Edited and written by leading international authorities, it is an essential resource for neuroscientists and provides a foundation for the work of clinical rehabilitation professionals.

Michael E. Selzer is Professor of Neurology at the University of Pennsylvania and Research Director in the Department of Physical Medicine Rehabilitation. He is editor-in-chief of Neurorehabilitation and Neural Repair, the official Journal of the American Society of Neurorehabilitation and the World Federation of Neurorehabilitation.

Leonardo G. Cohen is Chief of the Human Cortical Physiology Section and the Stroke Rehabilitation Clinic at the National Institute of Neurologic Disorders and Stroke, National Institutes of Health, Bethesda.

Stephanie Clarke is Professor and Head of Neuropsychology at the University Hospital, Lausanne and President of the Swiss Society of Neurorehabilitation.

Pamela W. Duncan is Professor of Health Services Administration and Physical Therapy, and Director of the Brooks Center for Rehabilitation Studies, University of Florida.

Fred H. Gage is Professor in the Laboratory of Genetics at the Salk Institute, and served as President of the Society for Neuroscience, 2001–2002. He is a fellow of the American Association for the Advancement of Science and a member of the National Academy of Sciences and the Institute of Medicine.

Textbook of Neural Repair and Rehabilitation

Volume I
Neural Repair and Plasticity

EDITED BY

Michael E. Selzer
University of Pennsylvania

Stephanie Clarke
University of Lausanne

Leonardo G. Cohen
National Institutes of Health

Pamela W. Duncan
University of Florida

Fred H. Gage
The Salk Institute

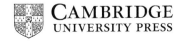
CAMBRIDGE UNIVERSITY PRESS

CAMBRIDGE UNIVERSITY PRESS
Cambridge, New York, Melbourne, Madrid, Cape Town, Singapore, São Paulo

CAMBRIDGE UNIVERSITY PRESS
The Edinburgh Building, Cambridge CB2 2RU, UK

Published in the United States of America by Cambridge University Press, New York

www.cambridge.org
Formation on this title: www.cambridge.org/9780521856416

© Cambridge University Press 2006

First published 2006

Printed in the United Kingdom at the University Press, Cambridge

A catalog record for this book is available from the British Library

Volume I:
ISBN-10 0-521-85641-8
ISBN-13 978-0-521-85641-6

Volume II:
ISBN-10 0-521-85642-6
ISBN-13 978-0-521-85642-3

2 volume set:
ISBN-10 0-521-83639-5
ISBN-13 978-0-521-83639-5

Contents (contents of Volume I)

Contents (contents of Volume II)

Preface

Neurorehabilitation is a medical specialty that is growing rapidly because medical advances have extended life expectancy and saved the lives of persons who previously would not have survived neurological injury. It is now urgent to develop a rigorous scientific basis for the field. The basic science relevant to functional recovery from neural injury is perhaps the most exciting and compelling of all the medical sciences. It encompasses areas of plasticity, regeneration and transplantation in the nervous system that individually have been the subjects of many monographs. With the *Textbook of Neural Repair and Rehabilitation*, these areas are integrated with each other and with the clinical topics to which they apply.

The *Textbook of Neural Repair and Rehabilitation* is organized into two volumes. *Volume I: Neural Repair and Plasticity* can stand alone as a textbook for graduate- or advanced undergraduate-level courses on recovery from neural injury. It is subdivided into two sections: *A: Neural Plasticity* and *B: Neural Repair*. Following an injury to the nervous system, most patients partially regain function. *Section A: Neural Plasticity*, addresses the mechanisms that underlie spontaneous recovery as well as the added recovery induced by therapies based on use, retraining and pharmacologic manipulations. The chapters cover the anatomical and physiologic responses of neurons to injury, mechanisms of learning and memory, and plasticity in specific areas of the nervous system consequent to intense use, disuse and injury. Ultimately, interventions aimed at repairing the damaged neural circuitry will be required if full function is to be restored. Thus *Section B: Neural Repair*, covers topics on neuronal death, trophic factors, axonal regeneration and the molecules that inhibit it, stem cell biology, and cell transplantation. *Section B* builds on *Section A* because the mechanisms of plasticity will have to be invoked to translate restored neuronal connections into useful function.

Volume II: Medical Neurorehabilitation can stand alone as a clinical handbook for physicians, therapists, rehabilitation nurses, and other neurorehabilitation professionals. It is organized into three sections. *Section C: The Technology of Neurorehabilitation* is a direct transition from *Volume I*, emphasizing the applications of basic scientific principles to the practice of neurorehabilitation. This section includes material on cell transplantation therapy, functional imaging, motor control, gait and balance assessment,

electrodiagnosis, virtual reality, and bioengineering and robotic applications to prosthetics and orthotics. *Section D: Symptom-Specific Neurorehabilitation* provides guidelines to managing spasticity, gait disorders, autonomic and sexual dysfunction, cognitive deficits and other disabling neurologic symptoms that are common to many disorders. *Section E: Disease-Specific Neurorehabilitation* describes comprehensive approaches to the rehabilitation of persons suffering from the major categories of disabling neurologic disorders, such as spinal cord injury, multiple sclerosis, stroke and neurodegenerative diseases.

Wherever possible, the chapters in this book refer the reader back to chapters that deal with relevant material at a different level. It is hoped that by stressing the integration of clinical and basic scientific knowledge, this book will help to advance the quality and scientific rigor of neurorehabilitation.

Contributors (contributors of Volume I)

Evangelos G. Antzoulatos
Department of Neurobiology and Anatomy
University of Texas Health Science Center at Houston
Houston, TX, USA

Zafar I. Bashir, PhD
Department of Anatomy
MRC Centre for Synaptic Plasticity
University of Bristol
Bristol, UK

Niels Birbaumer, PhD
Institute of Behavioural Neurosciences
Eberhard-Karls-University
Tubingen, Germany

Cesar E. Blanco, PhD
Department of Biomedical Engineering
A.E. Mann Institute for Biomedical Engineering
University of Southern California
Los Angeles, CA, USA

Mary Bartlett Bunge, PhD
The Miami Project to Cure Paralysis
University of Miami School of Medicine
Miami, FL, USA

John H. Byrne, PhD
Department of Neurobiology and Anatomy
University of Texas Health Science Center
at Houston
Houston, TX, USA

Huaibin Cai, PhD
Computational Biology Section
Laboratory of Neurogenetics, NIA
National Institutes of Health
Bethesda, MD, USA

Kimberly M. Christian
Neuroscience Program
University of Southern California
Los Angeles, CA, USA

Hollis T. Cline, PhD
Cold Spring Harbor Laboratory
Cold Spring Harbor, NY, USA

Leonardo G. Cohen, MD
Human Cortical Physiology Section
National Institute of Neurological Disorders and
Stroke
National Institutes of Health
Bethesda, MD, USA

Matthew B. Dalva, PhD
Department of Neuroscience
University of Pennsylvania School of Medicine
Philadelphia, PA, USA

Marco Domeniconi
Department of Biological Sciences
Hunter College
City University of New York
New York, NY, USA

John P. Donoghue, PhD
Department of Neuroscience
Brown University
Providence, RI, USA

V. Reggie Edgerton, PhD
Department of Physiological Science and
Neurobiology
University of California, Los Angeles
Los Angeles, CA, USA

Ines Eisner-Janowicz
Department of Molecular and
Integrative Physiology
University of Kansas Medical Center
Kansas City, KS, USA

Marie T. Filbin, PhD
Department of Biology
Hunter College
City University of New York
New York, NY, USA

Diasinou Fioravante
Department of Neurobiology and
Anatomy
University of Texas Health Science Center
at Houston
Houston, TX, USA

Itzhak Fischer, PhD
Department of Neurobiology and Anatomy
Drexel University College of Medicine
Philadelphia, PA, USA

Agnes Floel, MD
Human Cortical Physiology Section
National Institute of Neurological
Disorders and Stroke
National Institutes of Health
Bethesda, MD, USA

Thomas W. Gould
Department of Neurobiology and Anatomy and the
Neuroscience Program
Wake Forest University School of Medicine
Winston-Salem, NC, USA

John W. Griffin, MD
Departments of Neurology and Neuroscience
Johns Hopkins University School of Medicine
Baltimore, MD, USA

Kurt Haas, PhD
Department of Anatomy and Cell Biology
University of British Columbia
Vancouver, British Columbia, Canada

Peter Hagell, RN PhD
Department of Nursing
Faculty of Medicine
Lund University
Lund, Sweden

Steve Sang Woo Han, MD, PhD
Department of Neurobiology and Anatomy
Drexel University College of Medicine
Philadelphia, PA, USA

Ahmet Höke, MD, PhD
Department of Neurology
Johns Hopkins University School of Medicine
Baltimore, MD, USA

Ronaldo M. Ichiyama, PhD
Department of Physiological Science
University of California, Los Angeles
Los Angeles, CA, USA

Bharathi Jagadeesh, PhD
Department of Physiology and Biophysics
University of Washington
Seattle, WA, USA

Jon H. Kaas, PhD
Department of Psychology
Vanderbilt University
Nashville, TN, USA

Un Jung Kang, MD
Department of Neurology
University of Chicago
Chicago, IL, USA

Matthew S. Kayser
Department of Neuroscience
University of Pennsylvania School
of Medicine
Philadelphia, PA, USA

Gerd Kempermann, MD
Max Delbruck Center for Molecular
Medicine (MDC)
Berlin-Buch, Germany

Timothy E. Kennedy, PhD
Department of Neurology and Neurosurgery
Montreal Neurological Institute
McGill University
Montreal, Quebec, Canada

Angelo C. Lepore
Department of Neurobiology and Anatomy
Drexel University College of Medicine
Philadelphia, PA, USA

Joel M. Levine, PhD
Department of Neurobiology and Behavior
State University of New York at Stony Brook
Stony Brook, NY, USA

Tong Li
Department of Pathology
Johns Hopkins University School of Medicine
Baltimore, MD, USA

Olle F. Lindvall, MD, PhD
Section of Restorative Neurology
Wallenberg Neuroscience Center/BMC A11
Lund University Hospital
Lund, Sweden

Gerald E. Loeb, MD
Department of Biomedical Engineering
A.E. Mann Institute for Biomedical Engineering
University of Southern California
Los Angeles, CA, USA

Jeffrey D. Macklis, MD, DHST
Department of Neurology
MGH–HMS Center for Nervous System Repair
Harvard Medical School
Boston, MA, USA

Peter V. Massey, PhD
Department of Anatomy
MRC Centre for Synaptic Plasticity
University of Bristol
Bristol, UK

Lisa J. McKerracher, PhD
Départment de Pathologie et Biologie Cellulaire
Université de Montreal
Montreal, Quebec, Canada

Lorne M. Mendell, PhD
Department of Neurobiology and Behavior
State University of New York at Stony Brook
Stony Brook, NY, USA

Jared H. Miller
Department of Neurosciences
Case Western Reserve University
School of Medicine
Cleveland, OH, USA

Simon W. Moore
Department of Neurology and Neurosurgery
Center for Neuronal Survival
Montreal Neurological Institute
McGill University
Montreal, Quebec, Canada

Ken Nakamura, MD, PhD
Department of Neurology
University of California, San Francisco
San Francisco, CA, USA

Thien Nguyen, MD, PhD
Departments of Neurology and Neuroscience
Johns Hopkins University, School of Medicine
Baltimore, MD, USA

Randolph J. Nudo, PhD
Department of Molecular and Integrative Physiology
University of Kansas Medical Center
Kansas City, KS, USA

Catherine L. Ojakangas, PhD
Department of Neuroscience
Brown University
Providence, RI, USA

Ronald W. Oppenheim, MD, PhD
Department of Neurobiology and Anatomy
Wake Forest University
Winston-Salem, NC, USA

Tim P. Pons, PhD
Department of Neurosurgery
Wake Forest University School of Medicine
Winston-Salem, NC, USA

Andrew M. Poulos
Neuroscience Program
University of Southern California
Los Angeles, CA, USA

Donald L. Price, MD
Division of Neuropathology
Johns Hopkins University School of Medicine
Baltimore, MD, USA

Josef P. Rauschecker, PhD
Department of Physiology and Biophysics
Georgetown Institute for Cognitive and
Computational Sciences
Georgetown University Medical Center
Washington, DC, USA

Serge Rossignol, MD, PhD
du centre de rechercher en sciences
University de Montreal
Montreal, Quebec, Canada

Roland R. Roy, PhD
Brain Research Institute
University of California, Los Angeles
Los Angeles, CA, USA

Krishnankutty (Krish) Sathian, MD, PhD
Department of Neurology
Emory University
Atlanta, GA, USA

Ralf Schneggenburger, PhD
Abteilung Membranbiophysik and AG synaptische
Max-Planck Institut für Biophysikalische Chemie
Gottingen, Germany

Michael E. Selzer, MD, PhD
Department of Neurology
University of Pennsylvania School of Medicine
Philadelphia, PA, USA

Jerry Silver, PhD
Department of Neurosciences
School of Medicine
Case Western Reserve University
Cleveland, OH, USA

Tim Spencer
Department of Biological Sciences
Hunter College
City University of New York
New York, NY, USA

Oswald Steward, PhD
Departments of Anatomy and Neurobiology,
Neurobiology and Behavior, and Neurosurgery
Reeve-Irvine Research Center
College of Medicine
University of California, Irvine
Irvine, CA, USA

Ann M. Stowe
Department of Molecular and Integrative
Physiology
University of Kansas Medical Center
Kansas City, KS, USA

Alan R. Tessler, MD
Department of Neurobiology and Anatomy
Drexel University College of Medicine
Philadelphia, PA, USA

Richard F. Thompson, PhD
Department fo Psychology and Biological
Sciences
University of Southern California
Keck School of Medicine
Los Angeles, CA, USA

Wesley J. Thompson, PhD
Section of Neurobiology
University of Texas
Austin, TX, USA

Stephen G. Waxman, MD, PhD
Department of Neurology
Yale University School of Medicine
New Haven, CT, USA

Jonathan R. Wolpaw, MD
Laboratory of Nervous System Disorders
Wadsworth Center, NYS Department of Health
Department of Biomedical Sciences,
State University of New York at Albany
Albany, NY, USA

Philip C. Wong, PhD
Department of Pathology
Johns Hopkins University School of Medicine
Baltimore, MD, USA

Patrick M. Wood, PhD
The Miami Project to Cure Paralysis
Department of Neurological Surgery
University of Miami School of Medicine
Miami, FL, USA

Contributors (contributors of Volume II)

Mindy L. Aisen, MD
United Cerebral Palsy Research and Education
Foundation
Department of Neurology and Neuroscience,
Georgetown University

Gad Alon, PT, PhD
Department of Physical Therapy and
Rehabilitation Science
University of Maryland School of Medicine
Baltimore, MD, USA

Frank Andrasik, PhD
Institute for Human and Machine Cognition
University of West Florida
Pensacola, FL, USA

Antoaneta Balabanov, MD
Department of Neurological Sciences
Rush Medical College
Chicago, IL, USA

Michael P. Barnes, MD, FRCP
Department of Neurological Rehabilitation
Hunters Moor Regional Neurological
Rehabilitation Centre
Newcastle upon Tyne, UK

Serafin Beer, MD
Department of Neurology and Neurorehabilitation
Rehabilitation Centre
Valens, Switzerland

Claire Bindschaedler, PhD
Division de Neuropsychologie
Centre Hospitalier Universitaire Vaudois
Lausanne, Switzerland

Sarah Blanton, DPT, NCS
Department of Rehabilitation Medicine
Emory University
Atlanta, GA, USA

Michael L. Boninger, MD
Department of Rehabilitation
Science & Technology
University of Pittsburgh School of
Health and Rehabilitation Sciences
Pittsburgh, PA, USA

Carole W. Brown, EdD
Department of Education
The Catholic University of America
Washington, DC, USA

Stefano F. Cappa, MD
Department of Neuroscience
Vita-Salute University and San Raffaele
Scientific Institute
Milano, Italy

Diana D. Cardenas, MD, MHA
Department of Rehabilitation Medicine
University of Washington
Seattle, WA, USA

Leeanne Carey, BAppSc(OT), PhD
School of Occupational Therapy
Faculty of Health Sciences
LaTrobe University
Bundoora, Victoria, Australia

Stephanie Clarke, MD
Division de Neuropsychologie
Centre Hospitalier Universitaire Vaudois
Lausanne, Switzerland

Rory A. Cooper, PhD
Department of Rehabilitation
Science & Technology
University of Pittsburgh School of
Health and Rehabilitation Sciences
Pittsburgh, PA, USA

Rosemarie Cooper, MPT, ATP
Department of Rehabilitation
Science & Technology
University of Pittsburgh School of
Health and Rehabilitation Sciences
Pittsburgh, PA, USA

Mark D'Esposito, MD
Departments of Neuroscience and Psychology
Helen Wills Neuroscience Institute
University of California, Berkeley
Berkeley, CA, USA

Volker Dietz, MD, FRCP
Spinal Cord Injury Center
University Hospital Balgrist
Forchstr, Zurich, Switzerland

Bruce H. Dobkin, MD, FRCP
Department of Neurology
David Geffen School of Medicine, UCLA
Los Angeles, CA, USA

Neila J. Donovan, MA
Department of Communicative Disorders
VA RR&D Brain Rehabilitation Research Center
University of Florida
Gainesville, FL, USA

William K. Durfee, PhD
Department of Mechanical Engineering
University of Minnesota
Minneapolis, MN, USA

Gammon M. Earhart, PT, PhD
Program in Physical Therapy
Washington University School of Medicine
St. Louis, MO, USA

Georg Ebersbach, MD
Neurologisches Fachkrankenhaus
für Bewegungsstörungen/Parkinson
Beelitz-Heilstätten, Germany

Jonathan Evans, PhD
Section of Psychological Medicine
Gartnavel Royal Hospital
Glasgow, UK

Uri Feintuch, PhD
School of Occupational Therapy
Hadassah-Hebrew University
Jerusalem, Israel
Caesarea-Rothschild Institute for Interdisciplinary
Applications of Computer Science, University of
Haifa
Haifa, Israel

Peter J. Flett, MD
Department of Child and Adolescent Development,
Neurology and Rehabilitation, Women's and
Children's Hospital
North Adelaide
Melbourne, Victoria, Australia
Present Address:
Paediatric Rehabilitation,
Calvary Rehabilitation Services,
Hobart, Tasmania

Herta Flor, PhD
Department of Clinical and Cognitive
Neuroscience
University of Heidelberg
Central Institute of Mental Health
Mannheim, Germany

Richard S.J. Frackowiak, MD, PhD
Wellcome Department of Imaging Neuroscience
Institute of Neurology
University College London
London, UK

Adam Gazzaley
Helen Wills Neuroscience Institute and
Department of Psychology

University of California, Berkeley
Berkeley, CA, USA

David A. Gelber, MD
Springfield Clinic Neuroscience Institute
Springfield, IL, USA

Peter H. Gorman, MD
Department of Neurology and Rehabilitation
The James Lawrence Kernan Hospital
Baltimore, MD, USA

H. Kerr Graham, MD
Department of Orthopaedics,
University of Melbourne
The Royal Children's Hospital
Parkville, Victoria, Australia

Murray Grossman, MD, EdD
Department of Neurology
University of Pennsylvania School of Medicine,
Philadelphia, PA, USA

Amparo Gutierrez, MD
Department of Neurology
Louisiana State University Medical Center
New Orleans, LA, USA

Courtney D. Hall, PT, PhD
Atlanta Veterans Administration
Rehabilitation Research and Development, Decatur
Department of Rehabilitation Medicine
Emory University
Atlanta, GA, USA

Hans-Peter Hartung, MD
Department of Neurology
Heinrich-Heine-University
Düsseldorf, Germany

Susan J. Herdman, PhD, PT FAPTA
Atlanta Veterans Administration
Rehabilitation Research and Development, Decatur

Departments of Rehabilitation Medicine and
Otolaryngology-Head and Neck Surgery
Emory University
Atlanta, GA, USA

Hugh M. Herr, PhD
The Media Laboratory and The Harvard/MIT
Division of Health Sciences and Technology
Cambridge, MA, USA

Neville Hogan, PhD
Departments of Mechanical Engineering,
and Brain and Cognitive Sciences
Massachusetts Institute of Technology
Cambridge, MA, USA

Fay B. Horak, PhD, PT
Neurological Sciences Institute
Oregon Health & Science University
Beaverton, OR, USA

Jessica Johnson, OTR
Department of Occupational Therapy
University of Florida
Gainesville, FL, USA

Andres M. Kanner, MD
Department of Neurological Sciences
Rush Medical College
Chicago, IL, USA

Noomi Katz, MD
School of Occupational Therapy
Hadassah-Hebrew University,
Jerusalem, Israel

Danielle M. Kerkovich, PhD
Rehabilitation Research and Development Service
Department of Veterans Affairs
Washington, DC, USA

Jürg Kesselring, MD
Department of Neurology and
Neurorehabilitation
Rehabilitation Centre
Valens, Switzerland

Rachel Kizony, MSc
School of Occupational Therapy
Hadassah-Hebrew University, Jerusalem, Israel
Department of Occupational Therapy
University of Haifa
Haifa, Israel

Hubertus Köller, MD
Department of Neurology
Heinrich-Heine-University
Düsseldorf, Germany

Hermano Igo Krebs, PhD
Department of Mechanical Engineering
Massachusetts Institute of Technology,
Cambridge, MA, USA
Department of Neuroscience
The Winifred Masterson Burke Medical
Research Institute
Weill Medical College of Cornell University
New York, NY, USA

Catherine E. Lang, PT, PhD
Program in Physical Therapy
Washington University School of Medicine
St. Louis, MO, USA

James S. Lieberman, MD
Department of Rehabilitation Medicine
Columbia University College of Physicians and
Surgeons
New York, NY, USA

Francesco Lombardi, MD
Riabilitazione Intensiva Neurologica
Ospedale di Correggio
Correggio, Reggio, Emilia, Italy

Marilyn MacKay-Lyons, PhD
School of Physiotherapy
Dalhousie University
Halifax, Nova Scotia, Canada

Brenda S. Mallory, MD
Department of Rehabilitation Medicine
Columbia University College of Physicians &
Surgeons
New York, NY, USA

Francine Malouin, PhD, PT
Department of Rehabilitation and Centre for
Interdisciplinary Research in Rehabilitation and
Social Integration
Laval University
Quebec City, Quebec, Canada

William C. Mann, OTR, PhD
Department of Occupational Therapy
University of Florida
Gainesville, FL, USA

Beth Mineo Mollica, PhD
Center for Applied Science & Engineering and
Department of Linguistics
University of Delaware
Wilimington, DE, USA

C. Warren Olanow, MD
Departments of Neurology
Mount Sinai School of Medicine
New York, NY, USA

P. Hunter Peckham, PhD
Department of Biomedical Engineering
Case Western Reserve University and FES Center of
Excellence
Cleveland VA Medical Center
Cleveland, OH, USA

Thomas Platz, MD
Department of Neurological Rehabilitation
Free University Berlin
Berlin, Germany

Werner Poewe, MD
Department of Neurology
Medical University Innsbruck
Innsbruck, Germany

Karen T. Reilly, PhD
Department of Neurobiology and Anatomy
University of Rochester School of Medicine &
Dentistry
Rochester, NY, USA

Carol L. Richards, PhD
Department of Rehabilitation and Centre for
Interdisciplinary Research in Rehabilitation and
Social Integration
Laval University
Quebec City, Quebec, Canada

Keith M. Robinson, MD
Department of Physical Medicine and
Rehabilitation
University of Pennsylvania School of Medicine
Philadelphia, PA, USA

John C. Rosenbek, PhD
Department of Communicative Disorders
VA RR&D Brain Rehabilitation Research Center
University of Florida
Gainesville, FL, USA

Marc H. Schieber, MD, PhD
Department of Neurology
University of Rochester School of Medicine &
Dentistry
Rochester, NY, USA

Brian J. Snyder, MD
Department of Neurosurgery
Mount Sinai School of Medicine
New York, NY, USA

Jill Campbell Stewart, MS, PT, NCS
Department of Biokinesiology and Physical
Therapy
University of Southern California
Los Angeles, CA, USA

Nancy E. Strauss, MD
Department of Rehabilitation Medicine
Columbia University College of Physicians and
Surgeons
New York, NY, USA

Sheela Stuart, PhD
Children's Hearing and Speech Center
Children's National Medical Center
Washington, DC, USA

Austin J. Sumner, MD
Department of Neurology
Louisiana State University Medical Center
New Orleans, LA, USA

Antonio De Tanti, MD
Responsabile U.O. Gravi Cerebrolesioni e Disturbi
Cognitivi
Centro Riabilitativo "Villa Beretta"
Costamasnaga, Lecco, Italy

Cheryl Y. Trepagnier, PhD
Department of Psychology
The Catholic University of America
Washington, DC, USA

Nick S. Ward, MD, MRCP
Wellcome Department of Imaging Neuroscience
Institute of Neurology
University College London
London, UK

Catherine Warms, PhD, RN, ARNP, CRRN
Department of Rehabilitation Medicine
University of Washington
Seattle, WA, USA

Patrice L. Weiss, PhD
Department of Occupational Therapy
University of Haifa
Haifa, Israel

Carolee J. Winstein, PhD, PT, FAPTA
Department of Biokinesiology and Physical
Therapy
University of Southern California
Los Angeles, CA, USA

Jörg Wissel, MD
Neurologische Rehabilitationsklinik
Kliniken Beelitz GmbH
Beelitz-Heilstätten, Germany

Steven L. Wolf, PhD, PT, FAPTA
Department of Rehabilitation Medicine
Emory University
Atlanta, GA, USA

Sharon Wood-Dauphinee, PhD, PT
School of Physical and Occupational Therapy
McGill University
Montreal, Quebec, Canada

Richard D. Zorowitz, MD
Department of Physical Medicine
and Rehabilitation
University of Pennsylvania School of
Medicine
Philadelphia, PA, USA

Neural repair and rehabilitation: an introduction

Michael E. Selzer[1], Stephanie Clarke[2], Leonardo G. Cohen[3], Pamela W. Duncan[4] and Fred H. Gage[5]

University of Pennsylvania, Philadelphia, PA, USA; [2]University of Lausanne, Lausanne, Switzerland; [3]National Institutes of Health, Bethesda, MD, USA; [4]University of Florida, Gainesville, FL, USA; [5]The Salk Institute, La Jolla, CA, USA

Among medical specialties, rehabilitation has been one of the slowest to develop a basic science framework and to establish evidence-based practices as its norms. The reasons for this relate in part to the urgent need for clinical service and the dearth of experienced practitioners in the field during its formative years. It is imperative now, that the perceived lack of a scientific basis be reversed in order for rehabilitation medicine to achieve its full academic recognition and fulfill its great potential for relieving human suffering. This book represents an attempt to place the practice of neurorehabilitation in a rigorous scientific framework. Precisely because the need and the potential are so great, the editors have devoted equal space and emphasis to the clinical practice of neurorehabilitation and to its basic science underpinnings. In particular, two areas of basic science are highlighted – neuroplasticity and neural repair. In this respect, the book differs from most clinical textbooks. However, the professional neurorehabilitation community has been especially supportive of this direction and has taken very active steps to further the development of a basic scientific underpinning for its field. Similarly, the field of rehabilitation medicine, and in particular neurorehabilitation, has begun to put great emphasis on the development of evidence-based medical practices (DeLisa et al., 1999; Ottenbacher and Maas, 1999; Practice PPoE-B, 2001). The chapters in the clinical sections of this book stress those therapies for which evidence exists based on controlled clinical trials.

1 Definitions

Neurorehabilitation

Neurorehabilitation is the clinical subspecialty that is devoted to the restoration and maximization of functions that have been lost due to impairments caused by injury or disease of the nervous system. According to the social model of disability adopted by the World Health Organization (WHO), "' impairment' refers to an individual's biological condition …," whereas "… 'disability' denotes the collective economic, political, cultural, and social disadvantage encountered by people with impairments" (Barnes, 2001). These definitions have collapsed older distinctions of the WHOs 1980 International Classification of Impairments, Disabilities and Handicap (ICIDH) (Thuriaux, 1995). In that classification, "impairment" referred to a biological condition: for example, spinal cord injury; "disability" referred to the loss of a specific function: for example, loss of locomotor ability consequent to the impairment; and "handicap" referred to the loss of functioning in society: for example, inability to work as a postman, consequent to the disability. In order to improve healthcare data reporting by the nations of the world, the WHO replaced ICIDH with an International Classification of Functioning, Disability and Health (ICF) in 2001. ICF has two *parts*, each with two *components*:

- Part 1: Functioning and disability:
  - (a) body functions and structures,
  - (b) activities and participation.

- Part 2: Contextual factors:
    (c) environmental factors,
    (d) personal factors.

It is not possible to review the entire classification here, but because of its widespread use, including some of the chapters in this book, a brief summary is presented in Chapter 32 of volume II. The complete version can be found at http://www3.who.int/icf/icftemplate. cfm. By focusing on components of health, ICF can be used to describe both healthy and disabled populations, whereas the ICIDH focused on consequences of disease and thus had a narrower usefulness. However, the older classification is more useful in understanding the level of interventions and research performed by the rehabilitation community. Traditionally, rehabilitation medicine has concerned itself with disabilities and handicaps but very little with the level of impairment and even less with the molecular and cellular mechanisms that underlie impairments. In recent years, this state of affairs has begun to change as rehabilitation professionals have come to recognize the continuity that exists from molecular pathophysiology to impairments to disabilities and handicaps. Neurorehabilitation has come to represent the application of this continuum to neurologically impaired individuals.

Over the last 30 years, interest in understanding the mechanisms underlying recovery of function has increased. An expression of this interest has been the substantial increment in basic science and trans-lational studies geared to characterize the extent to which the central nervous system (CNS) can reorganize to sustain clinical rehabilitation.

Neuroplasticity

The term "neuroplasticity" is used to describe the ability of neurons and neuron aggregates to adjust their activity and even their morphology to alterations in their environment or patterns of use. The term encompasses diverse processes, as from learning and memory in the execution of normal activities of life, to dendritic pruning and axonal sprouting in response to injury. Once considered overused and trite, the term "neuroplasticity" has regained currency in the neurorehabilitation community as a concise way to refer to hypothetical mechanisms that may underlie spontaneous or coaxed functional recovery after neural injury and can now be studied in humans through such techniques as functional imaging (including positron-emission tomography (PET) and functional magnetic resonance imaging (fMRI)), electrical and magnetic event-related potentials (including electroencephalogram (EEG), evoked potentials (Eps), and magneto-encephalography (MEG)) and non-invasive brain stimulation in the form of transcranial magnetic or electrical stimulation (TMS and trancranial direct current stimulation, tDCS).

Neural repair

The term "neural repair" has been introduced in the past several years to describe the range of interventions by which neuronal circuits lost to injury or disease can be restored. Included in this term are means to enhance axonal regeneration, the transplantation of a variety of tissues and cells to replace lost neurons, and the use of prosthetic neuronal circuits to bridge parts of the nervous system that have become functionally separated by injury or disease. Although there is overlap with aspects of "neuroplasticity," the term "neural repair" generally refers to processes that do not occur spontaneously in humans to a degree sufficient to result in functional recovery. Thus therapeutic intervention is necessary to promote repair. The term is useful as part of the basic science of neurorehabilitation because it encompasses more than "regeneration" or "transplantation" alone. In recent years, concepts of neural plasticity have been accepted as important elements in the scientific understanding of functional recovery. The rehabilitation community has been slower to embrace repair as a relevant therapeutic goal. "Neural repair" has been used in the title of this textbook in order to convey the breadth of subject matter that it covers and is now considered relevant to neurorehabilitation.

2 History of neurorehabilitation as a medical subspecialty

Origins of rehabilitation medicine

In late 19th century America, interest developed in the possibility that then exotic forms of energy, that is, electricity, could help to heal patients with diseases and disabilities. In particular, high-frequency electrical stimuli were applied to generate deep heat in tissues (diathermy) and some physicians adopted this treatment modality as a specialty. In the early days, X-ray treatments and radiology were closely linked to electrotherapy (Nelson, 1973) and in 1923, the American College of Radiology and Physiotherapy was formed, changing its name to the American Congress of Physical Therapy in 1925. This organization merged with the American Physical Therapy Association in 1933 and in 1945, it adopted the name American Congress of Physical Medicine, then American Congress of Physical Medicine and Rehabilitation, and finally in 1966, the American Congress of Rehabilitation Medicine (ACRM). This is a multidisciplinary organization with membership open to physicians from many specialties and to non-physician rehabilitation specialists. With the large number of injuries to soldiers in World War I, the need for therapists to attend to their retraining and reintroduction to productive life created a new specialty that was based on physical modalities of treatment, including physical and occupational therapy, diathermy, electro-stimulation, heat and massage. These modalities were expanded during World War II. Training programs for physical therapy technicians were started in the 1920s and an American Medical Association (AMA) Council on Physical Therapy (later the Council on Physical Medicine) was started in 1926. By 1938, a medical specialty organization, the American Academy of Physical Medicine and Rehabilitation (AAPM&R) was formed and in 1947, the Academy sponsored a specialty board with a residency requirement and qualifying examination (Krusen, 1969). Gradually, the focus of rehabilitation has broadened to include the social and psychological adjustment to disability, treatment of medical complications such as bedsores, autonomic instability and urinary tract infections, management of pain syndromes and other medical aspects of the treatment of chronically ill patients. As with the name of the ACRM, the term "Rehabilitation Medicine" has replaced "Physical Medicine and Rehabilitation" in the naming of some hospital and university departments, since the latter term is associated with limitations to specific therapeutic modalities, such as physical therapy, rather than to a target patient population or therapeutic goal, i.e., restoration of function. With variations, parallel developments have occurred in many countries throughout the world.

A concomitant of the broadening of the focus of rehabilitation has been a trend toward specialization, including organ system-specific specialization. Previously, the tendency was to approach disabilities generically, based on their symptoms (e.g., gait disorder) and signs (e.g., spasticity), regardless of the cause. But with a growing conviction that the rehabilitation of patients requires knowledge of the pathophysiological basis of their disorders, medical specialists outside of physical medicine and rehabilitation (PM&R) became more interested in the rehabilitation of patients whom they might have treated during the acute phase of their illness. This was especially true among neurologists. The American Academy of Neurology formed a section on rehabilitation and in 1990, members of that section formed the American Society for Neurorehabilitation. National societies of neurorehabilitation were also formed in Europe and more recently in other parts of the world. In 2003, these national societies confederated officially as the World Federation of Neurorehabilitation, designating *Neurorehabilitation and Neural Repair* as its official journal.

Epidemiology of neurological disabilities

For many years, and especially during the two world wars, the practice of rehabilitation medicine was dominated by orthopedic problems, such as bone fractures and limb amputations. More recently, progress in keeping severely neurologically injured patients alive has shifted the emphasis toward rehabilitation of patients with developmental neurological disorders, stroke, traumatic injuries of the brain and spinal cord, and other chronic disabling diseases. It is estimated that in the USA, chronic health conditions cause activity limitations 61,047,000 times each year (Kraus et al., 1996). The five conditions causing the most limitations are: heart disease (7,932,000); back problems (7,672,000); arthritis (5,721,000); asthma (2,592,000); and diabetes (2,569,000). However, the conditions causing people to have major activity limitations most often are: mental retardation (87.5% of people with the condition have a limitation); multiple sclerosis (69.4%); malignant neoplasm of the stomach, intestine, colon, and rectum (62.1%); complete and partial paralysis of extremities (60.7%); malignant neoplasm of the lung, bronchus, and other respiratory sites (60.6%); and blindness in both eyes (60.3%). The WHO estimates that more than 300 million people worldwide are physically disabled, of whom over 70% live in the developing countries. In the USA, approximately 300,000 people are admitted to inpatient rehabilitation facilities each year. In a recent survey, orthopedic conditions (hip and limb fractures, amputations, hip replacements) accounted for 20% of rehabilitation admissions, while neurological conditions (stroke, traumatic brain injury, spinal cord injury, polyneuropathy, and other neurological conditions) accounted for 80% (Deutsch et al., 2000). The survey excluded Guillain–Barré syndrome, so the prevalence of neurological disabilities may have been underestimated. Thus disorders of the nervous system are those most often requiring intensive rehabilitation interventions.

3 Outcomes measurement in rehabilitation medicine

The complex medical, emotional, and social problems of the medically disabled patient population, and the complexity of the treatment regimens, has made assessing outcomes difficult. As practiced in most countries, rehabilitation is a multidisciplinary process, involving combinations of treatment modalities administered by multiple therapists. Moreover, the most important outcome of the rehabilitation process is the degree of reintegration of the patient in society, in terms of roles in work, family, and community. This also was difficult to assess with the limited instruments available only one generation ago. In order to catch up to other fields in the practice of evidence-based medicine, the rehabilitation field has been forced to become extremely resourceful in designing outcomes measures to evaluate the efficacy of its treatments (Stineman, 2001). The resulting sophistication of outcomes measurement has had an important impact on all of medicine, which now routinely considers quality of life in the evaluation of effectiveness in clinical trials.

4 Impact of evidence-based medicine on neurorehabilitation

Ironically, while outcomes measurement has begun to have an important impact on the evaluation of systems of rehabilitation, and on complex aspects of rehabilitation outcomes, the evaluation of outcomes for specific physical therapy treatments has lagged. A consensus conference was held in 2002, which developed a structured and rigorous methodology to improve formulation of evidence-based clinical practice guidelines (EBCPGs; Practice PPoE-B, 2001). This was used to develop EBCPGs based on the literature for selected rehabilitation interventions in the management of low back, neck, knee, and shoulder pain, and to make recommendations for randomized clinical trials. To date, only two large-scale, prospective, multicenter, randomized clinical trials have been carried out to test-specific physical therapy treatments. These are the trial of body weight-supported treadmill training for spinal cord injury (Dobkin et al., 2003; see Chapter 3 of volume II) and the trial of constraint-induced movement therapy for upper extremity dysfunction after stroke (Winstein et al., 2003; see Chapter 18 Volume II). Evidence that amphetamines combined with physical therapy can enhance recovery in several animal models of stroke and traumatic brain injury has led to several small-scale randomized clinical trials. These have suggested a tendency toward effect in human patients with ischemic stroke (Long and Young, 2003). A larger clinical trial is underway.

5 Impact of the revolution in the science of neuroplasticity and regeneration on neurorehabilitation

Between 1980 and 2003, there was a relatively constant 3.8-fold increase in annual publications in the field of rehabilitation medicine (best searched on Medline using the term "physical rehabilitation"). A Medline search using the terms "neuroplasticity" or "nerve regeneration" showed a steady or slightly accelerating 7.8-fold increase during the same time (Fig. 1). However, the combination of "rehabilitation" and either "neuroplasticity" or "regeneration" did not appear until after the term "neurorehabilitation" became current.

As indicated in Fig. 2, the term "neurorehabilitation" was used less than 10 times/year in Medline-indexed articles until 1994. From then until 2003, the annual number of articles on "neurorehabilitation" increased 9.4-fold. During that same period, the number of articles on ("neuroplasticity" or "regeneration") and "physical rehabilitation" increased 7.6-fold. Similarly, the terms "rehabilitation" and "evidence-based medicine" did not appear in the same article until 1994. From then until 2003, their coincidence increased 25.5-fold. Thus there is a correlation between the use of the term "neurorehabilitation" and acceleration in the application of basic science and evidence-based medicine to rehabilitation research. This can be ascribed to the accelerated interest in organ-specific rehabilitation, and in particular, to interest in the rehabilitation of patients disabled by neurological disorders. As in other fields of medicine, the trend toward specialization in the field of rehabilitation medicine carried with it recognition of the need to develop a basic science research underpinning and to become more rigorous in the evaluation of its therapies and clinical practices.

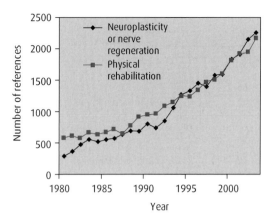

Figure 1. Parallel growth of research in medical rehabilitation and in neural plasticity and repair over the past 25 years. In order to estimate research in medical rehabilitation, a PubMed search was conducted using the term "physical rehabilitation," which yielded the highest combination of sensitivity and specificity among such terms as "medical rehabilitation," "rehabilitation," and "rehabilitation medicine." In order to estimate research on neuroplasticity, the term "neuroplasticity" was sufficient. In order to estimate research on regeneration in the nervous system, the best combination of specificity and sensitivity was achieved by searching for the term "nerve regeneration."

From the above, it can be seen that the maturation of neurorehabilitation as a clinical specialty has experienced two phases, which replicates the pattern seen in other specialties. In the first phase, the enormous need for clinical service was met by reliance on the experience and a priori reasoning of medical clinicians and therapists in devising methods to maximize function. In the second phase, scientific exploration in animal models was used to buttress the rationale for these therapies, while the rigors of prospective, controlled clinical trials were applied to test the effectiveness of those treatments in patients. This second phase is still very active, but we are already witnessing the beginning of a third phase, in which therapy is directed not only at maximizing function based on the post-injury residual anatomical substrate, but incorporates attempts at repairing that substrate. As with clinical trials of neuroprotective agents in human stroke and trauma, early results of cell and gene therapies for

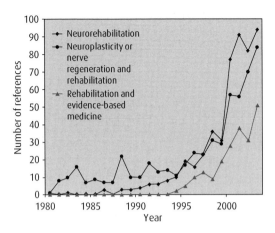

Figure 2. The subspecialization represented by the term "neurorehabilitation" has followed closely the application to rehabilitation medicine of basic research on neural plasticity and repair, and has closely led evidence-based clinical research. In order to estimate the frequency with which research on neuroplasticity and neural repair is applied to rehabilitation medicine, the best combination of sensitivity and specificity was obtained with the terms "rehabilitation," "neuroplasticity," and "nerve regeneration." Similarly the term "evidence-based medicine" was best paired with "rehabilitation" rather than other terms pairing "rehabilitation" with modifiers.

human injuries and diseases of the CNS have highlighted the need for caution in translating animal studies into human therapies. The most notable example is Parkinson's disease. Based on results in animal models, attempts to replace dopaminergic cells in human patients have been carried out for more than a decade. Yet despite promising results in small-scale studies on special populations (Lindvall, 1998; Chapter 34 of Volume I), larger double-blind, sham operated controlled clinical trials have not suggested major benefits in idiopathic Parkinson's disease (Olanow et al., 2003; Chapter 6 of Volume II). Despite favorable results in animals, intraventricular infusions of glial cell line-derived neurotrophic factor (GDNF) also failed to provide improvement in human Parkinson's disease. It turns out that because of the large size of the human brain, the GDNF failed to penetrate far enough into the brain parenchyma.

Thus a small-scale clinical trial of intraputamenal GDNF injections has been reported (Gill et al., 2003). A multicenter trial of *in vivo* gene therapy, using an adeno-associated virus vector containing the gene for neurturin, a GDNF-related peptide that has similar biological activity, is planned. A multicenter clinical trial of autologous macrophages activated by exposure to skin and injected into the spinal cord (Bomstein et al., 2003) is currently under way. The US Food and Drug Administration has approved small-scale clinical trials of intracerebral transplantation of tumor-derived neuronal progenitors for stroke, nerve growth factor-secreting fibroblasts for Alzheimer's disease, and epidural injection of a rho-A antagonist for spinal cord injury. In countries where clinical research is less stringently regulated, many patients have received transplants of stem cells and other highly invasive treatments for a variety of disabling neurological disorders, in the absence of evidence for effectiveness or experimental controls. The technical difficulties of carrying out controlled trials of these novel, highly invasive therapies are matched by ethical concerns. How do you convince patients to undergo a neurosurgical procedure that might be a sham operation? Should a clinical trial be performed on only the most severely disabled patients, who may have less to lose? Or should they be done on less disabled patients, who might have a better chance of responding favorably to an effective treatment, knowing that a failed trial might make it difficult to mount a subsequent one on a more favorable patient population? These and other questions are under intensive discussion and guidelines for the application of these advanced therapies to human patients are needed.

6 Rehabilitation of cognitive functions

Although rehabilitation is commonly thought of as relating primarily to motor retraining, the most disabling aspects of injury to the nervous system often relate to impairments in other domains, such as autonomic, sensory, and especially cognitive functions. Most major neuropsychological syndromes,

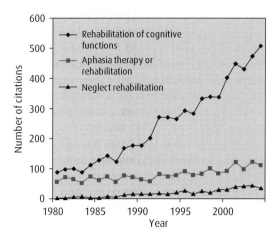

Figure 3. Increase in publications on neuropsychological rehabilitation. A PubMed search was conducted to identify articles published between 1980 and 2004 on rehabilitation of cognitive functions (key words: (neuropsychological OR aphasia) AND (rehabilitation OR therapy); aphasia (therapy OR rehabilitation); and neglect rehabilitation. The titles of the included publications were then checked for appropriateness.

such as aphasia, apraxia, visual agnosia, or neglect, have been identified in the second half of the 19th and the first half of the 20th century. Many of the original reports described the course of spontaneous recovery and proposed specific rehabilitative measures. During the last 25 years the field of rehabilitation of cognitive functions has expanded rapidly. The annual number of publications concerning neuropsychological rehabilitation, including aphasia therapy, has increased from about 100 in 1980 to over 500 in 2004, with a steep increase beginning around 1987 (Fig. 3). A small but important part of this increase can be accounted for by studies of specific neuropsychological syndromes. Most of the studies published in the early 1980s concerned aphasia, which continued to be investigated and experienced a 2-fold increase between 1980 and 2004. In recent years, research in other cognitive syndromes has grown even faster. Unilateral neglect, very little investigated in the 1980s, witnessed a 10-fold increase by 2004. This current expansion of rehabilitation studies of specific syndromes is linked to the application of cognitive models to rehabilitation and

to a better understanding of post-lesional plasticity as apparent in functional imaging studies.

However, most of the impressive increase in studies of neuropsychological rehabilitation was due to studies of disease-specific rehabilitation. Thus, rehabilitation of traumatic brain injury, stroke, tumors, degenerative diseases such as Parkison's disease or progressive diseases such as multiple sclerosis are increasingly investigated in their own rights. This type of research requires more than ever a multidisciplinary approach to neuropsychological rehabilitation, with close interactions between physicians, neuropsychologists, speech therapists, and physiotherapists and occupational therapists.

The chapters on rehabilitation of cognitive functions and on disease-specific rehabilitation demonstrate the necessity and the putative strength of evidence-based approaches. Although we need to understand the mechanisms underlying recovery from cognitive deficits, we also must have proof of the efficacy of our interventions. Specific fields, such as aphasia and neglect rehabilitation, have started accumulating this type of evidence. However, many more studies, and in particular large-scale multicenter investigations, are needed and should be carried out during the next decade.

7 Purpose and organization of this book

If most severely disabling disorders are neurological, why write a separate textbook of neurorehabilitation rather than incorporating it with the rest of rehabilitation medicine into a general rehabilitation textbook? The editors believe that it is time for rehabilitation medicine to go beyond optimizing function based on what is left to the body after an injury or illness. Rather, the goal should be full restoration of function by any means necessary, including actual repair of the injured tissues and organs. By focusing on the nervous system, we can present a cogent and intellectually rigorous approach to restoration of function, based on principles and professional interactions that have a deep vertical penetration. This requires two additions to the traditional rehabilitation approach, which had considered disabilities and handicaps in the abstract, apart from the specific disease processes that underlay them. First, there is a need to understand the pathophysiological bases of disabling neurological disorders. Second, there is a need to apply basic scientific knowledge about the plastic properties of the nervous system in order to effect anatomical repair and physiological restoration of lost functions.

This book is presented in two volumes, designed to be used either separately or as an integrated whole. *Volume I, Neural Plasticity and Repair*, explores the basic science underpinnings of neurorehabilitation and can be used as a textbook for graduate level courses in recovery of function after neural injury. It is divided into two sections. *Section A, Neural plasticity*, includes chapters on the morphological and physiological plasticity of neurons that underlie the ability of the nervous system to learn, accommodate to altered patterns of use, and adapt to injury. *Section B, Neural repair*, includes chapters on the neuronal responses to injury, stem cells and neurogenesis in the adult CNS, the molecular mechanisms inhibiting and promoting axon regeneration in the CNS, and strategies to promote cell replacement and axon regeneration after injury, the design of prosthetic neural circuitry, and translational research, applying animal experimental results to human patients. *Volume II, Medical Neurorehabilitation*, will be of greatest interest to clinical rehabilitation specialists, but will be useful to basic scientists who need to understand the clinical implications of their work. The volume is divided into three sections. *Section A, Technology of neurorehabilitation*, contains chapters on outcomes measurement, diagnostic techniques such as functional imaging and clinical electrophysiology, rehabilitation engineering and prosthetics design, and special therapeutic techniques. *Section B, Symptom-specific rehabilitation*, considers rehabilitation approaches to neurological symptoms that are common to many types of neurological disorders; for example, spasticity and other motor dysfunctions, autonomic, and sexual dysfunctions,

sensory disturbances including chronic pain, and cognitive dysfunctions. *Section C, Disease-specific neurorehabilitation systems*, considers the integrated approaches that have been developed to address the rehabilitation of patients with specific diseases and disease categories; multiple sclerosis, stroke, traumatic brain injury, neurodegenerative diseases, etc.

Throughout the two volumes, efforts have been made to relate the basic science to the clinical material, and to cross-reference relevant chapters where the integration is supported. In this way, we hope to stimulate basic scientists to broaden their understanding of the clinical relevance of their work. At the same time clinicians and clinical scientists in the various fields of rehabilitation medicine will be encouraged to enhance their curiosity and understanding of the mechanisms underlying their practice. Ultimately, we hope that encouraging communication between basic and clinical scientists in relevant areas of research will help to accelerate the translation of basic research into effective clinical treatments that will expand the degree of functional recovery of neurologically disabled persons.

REFERENCES

Barnes, C. (2001). World Health Organization – Disability and Rehabilitation Team Conference Report and Recommendations. In: *Rethinking Care from the Perspective of Disabled People*. WHO, Oslo, Norway.

Bomstein, Y., Marder, J.B., Vitner, K., Smirnov, I., Lisaey, G., Butovsky, O., Fulga, V. and Yoles, E. (2003). Features of skin-coincubated macrophages that promote recovery from spinal cord injury. *J Neuroimmunol*, **142**, 10–16.

DeLisa, J.A., Jain, S.S., Kirshblum, S. and Christodoulou, C. (1999). Evidence-based medicine in physiatry: the experience of one department's faculty and trainees. *Am J Phys Med Rehabil*, **78**, 228–232.

Deutsch, A., Fiedler, R.C., Granger, C.V. and Russell, C.F. (2000). The uniform data system for medical rehabilitation report of patients discharged from comprehensive medical rehabilitation programs in 1999. *Am J Phys Med Rehabil*, **81**, 133–142.

Dobkin, B.H., Apple, D., Barbeau, H., Basso, M., Behrman, A., Deforge, D., Ditunno, J., Dudley, G., Elashoff, R., Fugate, L., Harkema, S., Saulino, M. and Scott, M. (2003). Methods for a randomized trial of weight-supported treadmill training versus conventional training for walking during inpatient rehabilitation after incomplete traumatic spinal cord injury. *Neurorehabil Neural Repair*, **17**, 153–167.

Gill, S.S., Patel, N.K., Hotton, G.R., O'Sullivan, K., McCarter, R., Bunnage, M., Brooks, D.J., Svendsen, C.N. and Heywood, P. (2003). Direct brain infusion of glial cell line-derived neurotrophic factor in Parkinson disease. *Nat Med*, 9, 589–595.

Kraus, L., Stoddard, S. and Gilmartin, D. (1996). Section 3: Causes of disabilities. In: *Chartbook on Disability in the United States. An InfoUse Report*. U.S. National Institute on Disability and Rehabilitation Research, Washington, DC.

Krusen, F.H. (1969). Historical development in physical medicine and rehabilitation during the last forty years. Walter J. Zeiter Lecture. *Arch Phys Med Rehabil*, **50**, 1–5.

Lindvall, O. (1998). Update on fetal transplantation: the Swedish experience. *Mov Disord*, **13**, 83–87.

Long, D. and Young. J. (2003). Dexamphetamine treatment in stroke. *Quart J Nuclear Med*, **96**, 673–685.

Nelson, P.A. (1973). History of the once close relationship between electrotherapeutics and radiology. *Arch Phys Med Rehabil*, **54**(**Suppl.**), 608–640.

Olanow, C.W., Goetz, C.G., Kordower, J.H., Stoessl, A.J., Sossi, V., Brin, M.F., Shannon, K.M., Nauert, G.M., Perl, D.P., Godbold, J. and Freeman, T.B. (2003). A double-blind controlled trial of bilateral fetal nigral transplantation in Parkinson's disease. *Ann Neurol*, **54**, 403–414.

Ottenbacher, K.J. and Maas, F. (1999). How to detect effects: statistical power and evidence-based practice in occupational therapy research. *Am J Occup Ther*, **53**, 181–188.

Practice PPoE-B (2001). Philadelphia panel evidence-based clinical practice guidelines on selected rehabilitation interventions: overview and methodology. *Phys Ther*, **81**, 1629–1640.

Stineman, M.G. (2001). Defining the population, treatments, and outcomes of interest: reconciling the rules of biology with meaningfulness. *Am J Phys Med Rehabil*, **80**, 147–159.

Thuriaux, M.C. (1995). The ICIDH: evolution, status, and prospects. *Disabil Rehabil*, **17**, 112–118.

Winstein, C.J., Miller, J.P., Blanton, S., Taub, E., Uswatte, G., Morris, D., Nichols, D. and Wolf, S. (2003). Methods for a multisite randomized trial to investigate the effect of constraint-induced movement therapy in improving upper extremity function among adults recovering from a cerebrovascular stroke. *Neurorehabil Neural Repair*, **17**, 137–152.

Neural plasticity

CONTENTS

Cellular and molecular mechanisms of neural plasticity

CONTENTS

Anatomical and biochemical plasticity of neurons: regenerative growth of axons, sprouting, pruning, and denervation supersensitivity

Oswald Steward

Departments of Anatomy and Neurobiology, Neurobiology and Behavior, and Neurosurgery, Reeve-Irvine Research Center, University of California, Irvine, CA, USA

1.1 Introduction

Today, we tend to think of the nervous system as a highly plastic structure in which the structure and function of synapses is continually being modified. With this view, we are not surprised by reports of neuronal growth following injury, and indeed, are perhaps surprised that it does not occur more extensively. This is in stark contrast to the view during the first half of the 20th century, based on the extensive work of Ramon y Cajal (1959), that the nervous system was "fixed and immutable", and that neurons of the adult mammalian central nervous system (CNS) were incapable of any more than very limited and abortive growth. The origins of the shift in viewpoint can be traced to reports in the late 1960s and early 1970s that documented the formation of novel synaptic connections following CNS injury, especially the landmark study (Raisman, 1969) that provided the first electron microscopic evidence that neurons in the septal nucleus were reinnervated after their normal connections had been disrupted by lesions. Similar evidence was then obtained in studies of the superior colliculus (Lund and Lund, 1971) and olfactory bulb (Westrum and Black, 1971). What made these reports noteworthy was the demonstration of novel synaptic connections that had the potential of modifying circuit function.

Initially, these reports of neuronal growth in the mature nervous system were viewed with skepticism, and many felt that the growth occurred only in special circumstances, or was very limited in extent. Indeed, some opined that there was no growth at all – that the images suggestive of reinnervation reflected nothing more than a passive shift of presynaptic terminals from one postsynaptic site to another that had been left un-occupied by the removal of a degenerating synapse. There was also uncertainty about whether the apparent synapses were physiologically functional. Nevertheless, these reports motivated subsequent studies that provided more and more examples of synaptic reorganization following injury. Now, as a consequence of hundreds of studies over the past 35 years, we know that reorganization of circuitry after CNS injury is the norm rather than the exception, that new connections are capable of synaptic transmission, and that reorganization of circuitry can contribute to functional recovery (Steward, 1982).

We also now know that there is ongoing neurogenesis in the mature nervous system, and that newly-formed neurons extend axons for long distances and form synaptic connections (see Volume I, Chapter 18 by Maclis and Kempermann). These examples of growth potential raise the question of why growth and repair following injury is not more extensive, and why the prognosis following CNS injury still remains rather bleak.

This chapter will describe the reactive changes that CNS neurons do exhibit following injury – both degenerative responses that occur following denervation and axotomy, and reactive growth that may contribute to recovery of function. Other chapters consider the many new approaches to enhance regeneration or replace tissue destroyed by trauma through molecular manipulations, transplants, stem cell technologies, and by harnessing the potential for cell replacement that exists in the mature nervous system.

1.2 How injuries affect neurons and their connections

Damage to the CNS affects all cell populations in the brain including neurons, glia, ependymal cells, vascular elements, etc. In addition to directly damaging neurons, traumatic injuries disrupt blood flow, disrupt the blood–brain barrier, interfere with the manufacture, distribution, or re-absorption of cerebrospinal fluid (CSF), produce widespread changes in metabolism, and damage myelin-forming oligodendrocytes. In addition, injuries trigger delayed death of neurons and glia through apoptotic and other mechanisms (Volume I, Chapter 16). While all of these may lead directly or indirectly to alterations in neuronal function, we will focus here on what happens to neurons and their interconnections.

In this light, CNS trauma affects neuronal circuitry by:

1 interrupting axonal projections,
2 denervating certain populations of neurons,
3 removing some neurons entirely.

Indeed, most CNS injuries produce all of these effects. Due to the loss of some neurons, even if CNS neurons were capable of axonal regeneration, some regenerating axons would find nothing to innervate on reaching the area of damage. Thus, when considering repair mechanisms following CNS trauma, the important issues concern the fate of the tissue that survives and the mechanisms that contribute to the salvage of neurons that have either lost their normal targets or their normal inputs.

1.3 The fate of neurons that lose their normal inputs

The consequences of synapse loss for CNS neurons range from subtle changes in specific receptive elements (increased sensitivity to neurotransmitters, disappearance of dendritic spines, etc.) to changes that culminate in the disappearance of entire dendrites or even in the death of the denervated neurons (transneuronal atrophy or degeneration, respectively).

Denervation supersensitivity

Denervation supersensitivity is a phenomenon in which the postsynaptic cell becomes more sensitive to a neurotransmitter following denervation. The phenomenon was first described in muscle and peripheral ganglia (Cannon and Rosenbleuth, 1949). In muscle, denervation supersensitivity results from an increase in the number and a change in the distribution of acetylcholine (Ach) receptors (Fambrough, 1981). In normally innervated muscle, receptors are localized at the end plate beneath the motor nerve terminal. Following denervation, there is a dramatic induction of Ach receptor expression, and the newly-synthesized receptors are inserted all along the muscle fiber, making the muscle fiber sensitive to Ach all along its length. These changes are associated with overall atrophy of the muscle fibers, and other major changes in gene expression and muscle morphology. The alterations in receptor expression and distribution as well as the other changes are reversed if the muscle fiber is reinnervated either as a result of regeneration of the original axon or collateral sprouting of nearby axons that innervate nearby muscle fibers.

Neurons in peripheral ganglia also exhibit denervation supersensitivity, and if denervated cells survive and some projections are spared, the supersensitivity makes existing synapses more powerful (Zigmond et al., 1986). In this way, denervation supersensitivity may be a homeostatic mechanism that contributes to the maintenance of transmission when there is a partial loss of connections. Interestingly, loss of input from a particular neurotransmitter system does not necessarily lead to supersensitivity of all the receptor subtypes activated by that neurotransmitter. For example, removal of cholinergic input to neurons in the superior cervical ganglion (which normally transmit via both nicotinic and muscarinic mechanisms) leads to increased sensitivity to muscarinic agonists, but not nicotinic (Dun et al., 1976). In fact, the response to nicotinic agents is diminished.

The best-characterized example of denervation supersensitivity in the CNS is the increase in dopamine sensitivity in the striatum after the destruction of dopaminergic nigrostriatal projections (Creese et al., 1977; Zigmond et al., 1986). Early studies using ligand binding techniques did not revealed increases in dopamine receptors (Bennett and Wooten, 1986), suggesting that the mechanisms of the functional supersensitivity appear to be different than in muscle. More recent studies, however, have revealed that this example of functional supersensitivity involves both increases in the number of D(2) receptors, and increases in the coupling of D(1) and D(2) receptors to their respective G protein signaling partners (Cai et al., 2002).

There has been considerable speculation that the spasticity that develops in the chronic period after spinal cord injury reflects, in part, a supersensitivity phenomenon in which neurons that lose descending input become more sensitive to neurotransmitters. For example, in the chronic period following spinal cord injury, activation of sensory afferents to segments caudal to the injury elicits long-duration muscle spasms indicating enhanced excitability of segmental reflex circuitry. Recently, an *in vitro* model has been developed to explore the cellular mechanisms of this spasticity, in which the sacral spinal cord of rats that had received full transactions at S2 one month previously are maintained in recording chambers (Li et al., 2004). In these preparations, stimulation of dorsal roots elicits prolonged discharges of ventral root axons, mimicking the prolonged muscle spasms elicited by afferent stimulation *in vivo*. These chronically-denervated sacral segments also exhibited prolonged discharges in response to application of the neuromodulators, norepinephrine and seratonin, indicating supersensitivity to the neuromodulators.

Most of the well-characterized examples of denervation supersensitivity in the CNS involve neuromodulators like dopamine, norepinephrine, and seratonin, and there are few examples of denervation supersensitivity in the glutamatergic systems in the CNS (i.e. increases in glutamate receptor expression or sensitivity to glutamatergic agonists following loss of glutamatergic inputs). One interesting example, however, involves the nucleus tractus solitarius, which becomes supersensitive to glutamate after the extensive denervation produced by removal of the nodose ganglion (Colombari and Talman, 1995). It is noteworthy that the NTS receives a substantial proportion of its innervation from the nodose ganglion, and so the degree of denervation would be extensive. The fact that classical denervation supersensitivity is not seen in other systems may be because most CNS neurons receive tens of thousands, sometimes hundreds of thousands of synapses, and it is hard to imagine an experimental paradigm in which it would be possible to cause the degeneration of even a majority of the glutamatergic inputs to an individual neuron. Thus, with lesions that induce partial denervation, surviving glutamatergic inputs may be sufficient to maintain a sufficient level of postsynaptic activity to prevent compensatory changes in glutamate receptor expression. Alternatively, the very fact that CNS neurons receive a multitude of individual synapses may indicate that fundamentally different mechanisms exist than in muscle fibers and neurons in peripheral ganglia.

Transneuronal atrophy

Transneuronal atrophy refers to the phenomenon in which denervation leads to a decrease in the size of the postsynaptic cell or the disappearance of the part of the postsynaptic cell that has been denervated. The phenomenon was studied extensively in sensory relay nuclei of the visual and auditory systems, where the incoming afferents provide a substantial proportion of the input to the relay neurons. For example, destruction of the projections from the eye results in atrophy of neurons in the lateral geniculate nucleus

(Matthews et al., 1960), and interruption of the eighth nerve leads to atrophy of neurons in the cochlear nucleus (see below).

Transneuronal atrophy can involve only part of the postsynaptic cell's receptive surface. For example, if a given projection system terminates on dendritic spines, then the removal of that input will often lead to the disappearance of the denervated spines (Colonnier, 1964; White and Westrum, 1964; Parnavelas et al., 1974; Caceres and Steward, 1983). This usually involves a collapse of the spine into the parent dendrite (Caceres and Steward, 1983; Steward and Vinsant, 1983). Postsynaptic membrane specializations may also disappear, although some cells may retain un-innervated membrane specializations for a time (Pinching, 1969; Pinching and Powell, 1972).

Extensive denervation of a dendrite can result in atrophy of the entire dendrite. This phenomenon has been particularly well documented in the auditory pathways of the chick (Benes et al., 1977; Deitch and Rubel, 1989). For example, neurons of the avian homolog of the medial superior olive have bipolar dendritic trees that receive most of their innervation from the cochlear nucleus. One side of the bipolar dendritic arbor is innervated by the ipsilateral cochlear nucleus, while the opposite arbor receives contralateral input. When the inputs to one dendritic arbor are damaged, the denervated dendrites on one side of the cell body undergo substantial atrophy whereas the normally-innervated dendrites extending from the opposite pole are unaffected. When the denervation is partial, there is a partial preservation of the denervated dendrite (Rubel et al., 1981). Thus, in this system, the degree of dendritic atrophy is related to the degree of denervation.

The atrophy of denervated portions of postsynaptic cells can be a transient phenomenon, in that dendrites and their spines can be reconstructed if the dendrite is reinnervated. For example, denervation of the granule cells of the hippocampal formation results in a loss of spines and atrophy of affected dendrites at early post-lesion intervals, but these changes are reversed as synapses are replaced (Parnavelas et al., 1974; Caceres and Steward, 1983). In the auditory system, however, rapid dendritic atrophy may

prevent reinnervation that could otherwise occur. For example, dendrites are preserved when denervation occurs gradually over a prolonged period of time, and in this case, the dendrites are partially reinnervated (Rubel et al., 1981). Thus, the final extent of transneuronal atrophy may depend on the relationship between the timing of atrophy and the timing of reinnervation.

Transneuronal degeneration

When denervation results in the death of the affected neuron, the process is called transneuronal degeneration (Cowan, 1970). The best examples of transneuronal degeneration come from studies in sensory systems. For example, in addition to causing transneuronal atrophy, destruction of the projections from one eye results in the death of some neurons in the lateral geniculate nucleus (Matthews et al., 1960). In the olfactory system, removal of the olfactory epithelium results in transneuronal degeneration of cells in the olfactory bulb (Matthews and Powell, 1962), and interruption of the lateral olfactory tract leads to transneuronal degeneration of neurons in the pyriform cortex (Heimer and Kalil, 1978).

Transneuronal degeneration has been particularly well characterized in the auditory system. For example, neurons in the cochlear nucleus exhibit rapid transneuronal degeneration when input from the cochlea is disrupted in young animals (Levi-Montalcini, 1949; Powell and Erulkar, 1962). In mature animals, the same lesion causes transneuronal atrophy, but minimal degeneration. Thus, the extent of transneuronal degeneration depends critically on developmental age. Indeed, in chicks and mice, neurons become resistant to transneuronal degeneration over the interval of a few days. The mechanisms underlying the development of resistance remain to be defined.

Probably the most extensive studies of the mechanisms underlying transneuronal degeneration have been carried out in the auditory system of the chicken (Born and Rubel, 1985; Steward and Rubel, 1985; Born and Rubel, 1988). Removal of the cochlea in young chicks leads to the death of about 30% of the neurons in nucleus magnocellularis (the avian homolog of the cochlear nucleus). In this system, transneuronal degeneration is triggered by the cessation of synaptic activity. For example, transneuronal degeneration can be induced by infusing tetrodotoxin into the cochlea, which silences activity in the eighth nerve (Born and Rubel, 1988).

An interesting feature about this example of transneuronal degeneration is that it occurs very rapidly. Within hours after removal of the cochlea, neurons in nucleus magnocellularis cease producing protein (Steward and Rubel, 1985). The cessation of protein synthesis is one of the earliest signs of the impending degeneration, and occurs as a result of the virtually complete destruction of ribosomes within the affected cells (Canady and Rubel, 1992).

Transneuronal degeneration is not invariably observed, even when the denervation is substantial. For example, in mammals, the dorsal cochlear nucleus receives a substantial projection from the cochlea, but does not degenerate along with the ventral cochlear nucleus following interruption of cochlear input (Powell and Cowan, 1962). It may be that other inputs sustain these cells, or that elimination of eighth nerve activity does not affect postsynaptic activity to the same degree as in the ventral cochlear nucleus. Alternatively, it may be that certain neuron types are inherently more able to survive the loss of inputs than others.

1.4 Fate of neurons following axotomy and target loss

Trauma can cause physical transection of axons (axotomy), causing the portion distal to the injury to degenerate (Wallerian Degeneration). The affected neurons are thus both physically damaged and disconnected from the targets that the damaged axon normally contacts. Neurons exhibit a range of responses following axotomy ranging from atrophy and death (retrograde atrophy and degeneration, respectively) to survival with minimal obvious consequences (Cowan, 1970; Lieberman, 1971; Torvik, 1976). Obviously, neurons that die cannot regenerate

their axons or establish new connections that might contribute to recovery of function, and so protection from retrograde degeneration is a potential target for therapeutic interventions to preserve or improve recovery after trauma.

Retrograde atrophy and degeneration

Three factors appear to influence the degree of retrograde atrophy and degeneration following axotomy. First, the degree of atrophy and degeneration is greatest if axons are damaged proximal to the cell body than if the injury occurs more distally. Second, retrograde atrophy and degeneration is more likely if a substantial proportion of the projections to target cells are interrupted. This is thought to reflect the fact that retrograde atrophy and degeneration occur because neurons depend on trophic factors supplied by the target (the topics of neuronal death and rescue and the role of target-derived trophic factors are considered elsewhere in this volume, see Volume I, Chapter 16 by Gould and Oppenheim). For example, the degree of retrograde degeneration of a population of neurons is usually more or less directly related to the degree of target loss. Also, neurons with collateral projections to a number of different targets are more likely to survive the loss of one of these targets than neurons that project predominantly or exclusively to one site. This is the "principle of sustaining collaterals" (Rose and Woolsey, 1958). Third, retrograde degeneration is usually more severe in young animals.

Although retrograde atrophy and degeneration are most likely in young animals and following proximal axonal injury, recent studies have revealed that a surprising degree of retrograde degeneration can occur in mature animals following distal axonal injury. For example, it has recently been shown that a substantial number of cortical motoneurons exhibit signs of ongoing apoptosis following damage to the corticospinal tract (CST) in the thoracic spinal cord (Haines et al., 2003). Careful quantitative studies of CST neurons that had been labeled prior to the injury by retrograde tracing with fluorogold documented that CST neurons actually did die. This important study demonstrates that retrograde degeneration may be one of the key reasons that upper motoneurons fail to regenerate their axons following spinal cord injury.

One CNS that has served as a model for studies of retrograde atrophy and degeneration is the red nucleus following damage to rubrospinal axons in the spinal cord. Following interruption of the rubrospinal tract in the spinal cord, there is a dramatic decrease in the number of red nucleus neurons that can be seen in histological preparations.

Red nucleus neurons can be rescued by transplanting fetal spinal cord tissue into the injury site in the spinal cord (Bregman and Reier, 1986), and the neurons that are rescued are ones that have axon collaterals to rostral CNS areas, exemplifying the principal of sustaining collaterals (Bernstein-Goral and Bregman, 1997). In keeping with the idea that retrograde atrophy and degeneration are due to the loss of target-derived trophic support, the atrophy and degeneration can be reduced by delivering brain-derived neurotrophic factors (BDNF or NT3) into the cisterna magna (Novikova et al., 2000), or by transplanting fibroblasts that have been genetically modified to secrete BDNF (Tobias et al., 2003).

Although it was initially thought that many neurons in the red nucleus died after axotomy, recent studies indicate that the neurons actually undergo extreme retrograde atrophy, and that there is little or no actual cell death. Remarkably, following delivery of BDNF to the area of the brainstem containing the red nucleus 1 year after injury, red nucleus neurons again became visible in Nissl stains, indicating that the neurons had atrophied to the extent that they were un-detectable in routine histological preparations (Kwon et al., 2002). It remains to be seen how many other examples of apparent retrograde degeneration will turn out to involve extreme atrophy rather than actual neuronal death.

Synapse stripping

One interesting manifestation of the retrograde response to axotomy is synapse stripping, also called bouton shedding, in which presynaptic inputs to axotomized neurons disconnect and withdraw (Sumner and Sutherland, 1973; Purves, 1975; Sumner, 1977). Often, glial processes are interposed between presynaptic profiles and their former site of termination (Sumner and Sutherland, 1973). Synapse stripping can cause a substantial disruption of synaptic transmission along pathways that are otherwise intact (Purves, 1975). Nevertheless, disconnected synapses can re-establish contact with the axotomized neuron if the axotomized neuron successfully regenerates its axon, restoring synaptic communication (Sumner and Sutherland, 1973; Purves, 1975). The disconnection persists, however, if the axotomized neuron is prevented from re-connecting (Sumner, 1977).

Cascading degeneration

Both retrograde and transneuronal degeneration are not necessarily limited to one synaptic relay. If denervated neurons die, then their targets are denervated, and depending on the circumstances, the next neuron in the relay may also die. Furthermore, retrograde degeneration will remove the target of axons that normally terminate on the degenerating cells. This may then induce a secondary retrograde degeneration of the cells that normally innervate the neurons actually damaged by the trauma. For example damage to the limbic cortex results in retrograde degeneration in the anterior thalamic nucleus and secondary retrograde degeneration in the mammillary nucleus (Bleier, 1969; Cowan, 1970). This sort of cascading degeneration seems to occur predominantly when lesions occur during development, and in projection systems that are "closed" in that they receive and provide limited connections to other brain regions (Cowan, 1970). This is consistent with the concept of sustaining collaterals.

Delayed neuronal death following ischemia

An important form of delayed degeneration occurs in some neuronal populations that have suffered transient ischemia (Klatzo, 1975). Neurons that are susceptible to this form of degeneration survive the immediate ischemic period, but then die hours or days later. Certain populations of neurons in the cortex and hippocampus are particularly susceptible (Schmidt-Kastner and Freund, 1991). This form of degeneration is due in part to excitotoxic injury caused by massive release of glutamate during and after the ischemic insult (Rothman, 1984; Simon et al., 1984; Gill et al., 1987), and occurs via apoptosis (see Gould and Oppenheim in this volume for further discussion of excitotoxic and apoptotic processes).

Trauma-induced death of oligodendrocytes and de-myelination

Another form of degeneration that is related to axonal damage is a delayed degeneration of oligodendrocytes leading to demyelination of axons. This has been especially well-documented following spinal cord injury, where it has been shown that injuries at a particular segmental level cause the death of oligodendrocytes over many segments (Blight, 1985). The oligodendrocytes die days and even weeks after the injury through apoptotic mechanisms (Crowe et al., 1997). The loss of myelin segments from surviving axons (de-myelination) is thought to disrupt action potential propagation by the de-myelinated axons (see Volume I, Chapter 26 by Waxman for a further discussion of the consequences of de-myelination on axonal function).

If injury leads to extensive death of oligodendrocytes causing de-myelination of large numbers of axons, this points to several possible strategies for repair, including transplanting myelin-forming cells. Nevertheless, predicting the relationship between the death of oligodendrocytes and de-myelination of surviving axons is not straightforward. Consider for example the extensive death of oligodendrocytes that occurs following spinal cord injury. This death is seen in white matter tracts that contain degenerating axons, and one interpretation is that oligodendrocytes die as a consequence of Wallerian degeneration of the axons that they ensheath (Abe et al., 1999). It is important to recall that oligodendrocytes ensheath more than one axon (Fig. 1.1). Thus, at one extreme, it could be that oligodendrocytes dies only if all of the axons that they ensheath degenerate. In this case, there would be *no* demyelination. At the other extreme, it

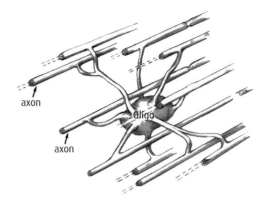

Figure 1.1. Oligodendrocytes in the CNS form myelin around multiple axons (from Steward, 2000).

may be that oligodendrocytes die in response to some signal that is not directly related to the Wallerian Degeneration of the axons they ensheath, in which case *all* of the axons ensheathed by a particular oligodendrocyte would be de-myelinated if that oligodendrocyte died. The answer is probably somewhere in-between these two extremes. The oligodendrocytes that die in white matter tracts probably ensheath both degenerating and non-degenerating axons, so that the surviving axons would in fact be de-myelinated over the segment supplied by the dead oligodendrocyte. These considerations point to the need for detailed studies to assess the relationship between oligodendrocyte death and the loss of myelin from surviving axons.

Recent studies in rats have revealed considerable numbers of un-myelinated axons more than 1 year after spinal cord injury in rats, and demonstrated that the number increases during the chronic injury period (Totoiu and Keirstead, in press). This is consistent with the idea that the death of oligodendrocytes is an ongoing process, and does cause significant de-myelination. As we look forward to the development of new strategies to restore myelin, it is now critical to assess the extent to which de-myelination is an important component of the pathology following spinal cord injury in human beings. The answer to this question will provide an indication of the degree of functional improvement that might be possible as a result of improving conduction in de-myelinated axons or restoring myelin through cell transplantation therapies.

1.5 Reorganization of neuronal connections following trauma

Axon regeneration and the restoration of normal circuitry

When the axon of a neuron is interrupted, the most functionally beneficial response would be the regeneration of the damaged axon back to its normal target (assuming that the target is still present). Accordingly, we reserve the term "specific regeneration" to indicate a specific re-growth of an interrupted axon to its normal target. If a projection system is normally highly specified (e.g. if the pattern of connectivity is specific between two single cells) then specific regeneration would involve the re-connection of a particular axon with its normal target cell.

However, in most neural circuits, connectivity is probably not specified on a cell-by-cell basis. For example, in the case of neuromuscular connections, specificity may be in terms of a muscle, not individual muscle fibers. The same is true of peripheral sensory axons, where sensory representation depends on an appropriate topographic pattern of innervation of the skin. In systems like this, re-connection of an axonal projection system with its normal target *region* in an appropriate topographic fashion may restore the degree of specificity that is normally present. We call this "region-specific regeneration". If region-specific regeneration occurs in a normal topographic order, we term this "orderly regeneration". If re-growing axons re-grow into the appropriate target area, but with a disrupted topographic order, we term this "disorderly regeneration".

In mammals, true regeneration of axonal projections rarely occurs, except in the peripheral nervous system (Guth, 1974; 1975; Puchala and Windle, 1977). Even in the peripheral nervous system, however, the regeneration that does occur is usually limited in scope, disorganized, and often of minimal functionality. This is especially true following peripheral nerve injury in human beings.

When CNS axons are transected during early development, some systems can grow to their normal targets (Kalil and Reh, 1979; 1982), sometimes via abnormal routes (Bregman and Goldberger, 1982; 1983; Xu and Martin, 1991). Whether this is "regeneration" (a response to injury) or a continuation of development is a matter of some debate.

It is thought that the lack of regeneration in the mature CNS is due to:

1 The presence of inhibitory molecules in the mature CNS, including molecules present in myelin (like Nogo, see Volume I, Chapter 21 by Spencer et al.) and molecules expressed by reactive astrocytes at the site of an injury (see Volume I, Chapter 22 by Miller and Silver).
2 A limited capability of mature CNS neurons to re-launch a program of gene expression that is sufficient to support axon growth (see Volume I, Chapters 23 and 24 by Levine and Mendell and McKerracher and Selzer).

Pitfalls for studies of axon regeneration

A steady stream of new studies report that axon regeneration can be induced in the mature mammalian nervous system by novel treatments or genetic manipulations. In assessing these reports, it is important to be mindful of the history of regeneration research, which is littered with the corpses of studies that reported regeneration that later proved incorrect. The main reason is the "spared axon conundrum", in which axons that survive a lesion are mistakenly identified as having regenerated. Accordingly, it is important to establish rigorous criteria that may be used to identify regenerated versus spared axons in the injured CNS.

On the face of it, a study of axon regeneration in the CNS would seem simple to perform. One simply cuts or otherwise damages a population of axons, and then evaluates whether those axons re-grow. In a typical experiment involving spinal cord injury, for example, one would produce a lesion in the spinal cord, wait for some period of time to allow for possible axon regeneration, and then trace particular spinal tracts using tract-tracing techniques. Numerous studies indicate that there is minimal axon regeneration in normal animals. The axons that had been cut retract for some distance from the injury, and persist as retraction balls, perhaps exhibiting regenerative sprouting into nearby territory. In contrast, several recent studies report that in animals that receive some treatment or that carry a mutation in a gene that presumably encodes an inhibitor of axon growth, the axons that had been cut regenerate around, beyond, or sometimes even through the lesion site.

What could possibly go wrong in such a simple experiment? The answer is that axons are remarkably resilient, and can survive displacement and stretch (for further discussion and documentation, see Steward et al. (2003)). As a result of this resiliency, axons that are revealed by tract tracing at some time point after a lesion may not have been cut in the first place, and treatments or genetic manipulations may result in an increased number of spared axons in the experimental group. This potential problem is exacerbated by the fact that many recent studies have adopted surgical approaches that are designed to minimize physical damage, in order to lower the bar for successful axon regeneration through the lesion site.

Based on these considerations, we have put forward a set of criteria that can be used to distinguish regenerated from spared axons (Steward et al., 2003). These criteria were developed based on studies of regeneration of corticospinal tract axons following spinal cord injury, but the criteria could also apply to other sites in the CNS. The proposed criteria to identify a regenerating or regenerated axon are:

1 the axon extends from the CNS into a non-CNS environment, specifically, the tissue environment of the scar that develops at the injury site;
2 the axon extends from the host CNS into a non-host graft or transplant;
3 the axon originates at or near a site of amputation;
4 the axon takes an unusual course through the tissue environment of the CNS;
5 the axon extends no further than could be accounted for by plausible regeneration rates;

6 the axon has a morphology that is not characteristic of normal axons of its type (e.g. exhibiting unusual branching patterns);
7 the axon is tipped with a growth cone.

Some of these criteria represent definitive evidence of regeneration (I and II). The other criteria are weaker, but support the decision that given axons are regenerated rather than spared. The more criteria that can be met, the more secure the interpretation can be. Importantly, some of the criteria require detailed reconstructions of axon trajectory, especially as the axon passes the lesion site (IV and V), which require a detailed anatomical analysis, including analyses of axons in serial sections. Other criteria require an analysis of the time course of regenerative growth (V and VII), which requires that animals be evaluated at different times after the injury. Hopefully, adoption of these and perhaps other rigorous criteria will help to avoid the problem of "false resurrections" that has plagued the study of axon regeneration, especially following spinal cord injury.

Abortive regeneration: dystrophic growth cones and tortuous axon arbors

Even Cajal in his pessimistic view of neuronal growth capabilities concluded that some axon growth does occur following injury, calling the growth "abortive" because the axons did not re-grow to a target. Nevertheless, even "abortive" growth involving the formation of axonal extensions does indicate that neurons possess some growth capacity. Thus, abortive growth provides indirect support for the concept that regeneration is blocked by inhibitors that are present in the tissue environment (like myelin-derived inhibitors and molecules that are expressed by reactive astrocytes). Two morphological forms are recognized that suggest an abortive growth response:

1 dystrophic growth cones;
2 tortuous (tangled) axonal arbors.

When an axon in a long tract (like the corticospinal tract) is cut, the distal portion undergoes Wallerian Degeneration, and the proximal portion dies back over a period of days or weeks. At the distal tip of the amputated axon, there is often an enlarged ball-shaped collection of cytoplasm termed a "retraction ball". Disconnected ball-shaped structures are often seen distal to the tip of the axon, suggesting that retraction balls become physically separated as axons die back.

Amputated axons may also be tipped by structures that resemble growth cones, however, and it is thought that these are "dystrophic", in the sense that their extension is impeded (see Volume I, Chapter 22, by Silver and Miller for further discussion of dystrophic growth cones). Structures resembling growth cones are evident even months after an injury, suggesting that there may be a continuous low-level attempt of the axon to re-grow (or at least a capacity for re-growth if growth inhibition could be removed). Indeed, these ideas form the basis for the optimistic view that it may be possible to stimulate axon regeneration even in the chronic post-injury period.

It should be noted that there are no definitive criteria for distinguishing between retraction balls and growth cones, especially at the light microscopic level. Using electron microscopy, certain characteristic features can be identified to bolster the interpretation that a given structure is a growth cone, but even then, differential identification of retraction balls and growth cones is a matter of some interpretation. In addition, electron microscopy is a very inefficient analytical tool. Some have used immunocytochemical markers (e.g. the presence of the growth-associated protein, GAP-43) as a marker for growth cones, but the general validity of GAP-43 as a marker for growth cones has not been established.

Another structure suggestive of abortive growth is a branched arbor at the end of an amputated axon. An example of one of these can be seen in Fig. 1.3 (double arrow). As axons in long tracts are un-branched, highly branched arbors at the end of an axon that has been cut clearly indicate some sort of growth response involving a sprouting at the damaged tip of the axon. It should be noted that the example shown in Fig. 1.3 may be at the tip of a regenerative sprout (i.e. from a collateral that has branched off the main axon, see regenerative sprouting section below). This can be determined with certainty only by reconstructing the axon in serial sections. It is noteworthy that similar structures are seen in areas in which there is collateral sprouting following denervation (see below).

Forms of axonal growth that would be most appropriate for long-tract regeneration

It is worth considering whether there are different modes of axon growth depending on the circumstances. For example, when growing for long distances in tracts, axons extend with little branching (what might be termed a "tract mode"). In contrast, on reaching the target region, axons often exhibit a branching form of growth involving the formation of complex and sometimes highly characteristic terminal arbors. This arborizing form of growth may reflect the axons response to cues presented in the target region (including cues that trigger synapse formation on target neurons). It is worth emphasizing that efficient long-distance regeneration will probably require a re-initiation of the tract mode of growth.

Other regenerative responses following injury to CNS axons

Although neurons in the mammalian CNS rarely if ever exhibit true regeneration as defined above (especially long-distance regeneration along appropriate tracts), axons do exhibit a number of growth responses that may lead to the formation of new connections, and may contribute to restoration of function. In addition, there are now promising strategies to induce regenerative growth (see elsewhere in this volume). In interpreting and evaluating axonal growth responses, it is important to use a standard terminology for the different growth events that can occur. For example, the term "axon regeneration" is often used imprecisely to refer to any regenerative growth of axons that have been transected. However, as noted above, and following Moore (1974), we prefer to use terms that distinguish between true regeneration as defined above, and other growth responses of damaged axons that do not lead to reconnection with normal targets and that probably have different functional consequences.

Regenerative sprouting

We use the term "regenerative sprouting" to refer to the formation of new axonal branches by axotomized axons. Regenerative sprouting would be distinguished from bona fide axon regeneration by the fact that regeneration involves the elongation of the cut axon without branching (tract mode) whereas regenerative sprouting would involve the formation of new axonal branches that do not necessarily follow the normal tract. Regenerative sprouts can arise at or near the site of transection, or as the result of the formation of new collateral branches at locations proximal to the site of an injury (see Figs 1.2 and 1.3).

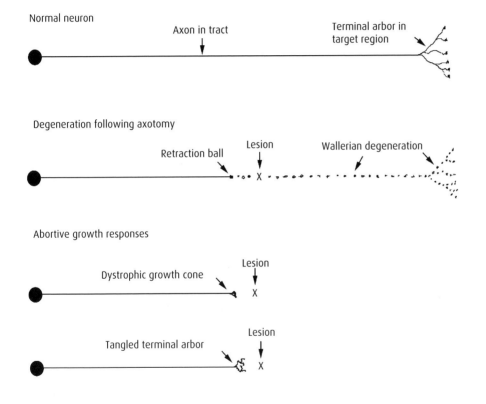

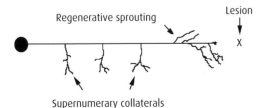

Figure 1.2. Responses of axons following axotomy. When axons are cut at a particular location, the distal segment degenerates (Wallerian Degeneration), and the proximal segment retracts forming retraction balls. Abortive growth is reflected by the presence of dystrophic growth cones and tangled arbors. Bona fide regeneration would involve the re-growth of the axon without branching (tract mode). Regenerative sprouting involves the formation of new branches at or near the point of injury. Axons may also grow new collaterals from proximal segments.

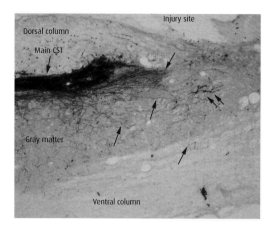

Figure 1.3. Regenerative sprouting of CST axons after spinal cord injury. The figure illustrates an experiment in which CST axons are traced by injecting BDA into the sensorimotor cortex after a dorsal hemisection at the thoracic level. The spinal cord injury and BDA injections were made during the same operation, and mice were allowed to survive for 18 days. In mice and rats, the CST is localized in the ventral portion of the dorsal column (main CST). This is a sagittal section that contains the labeled CST; dorsal is above, rostral is to the left. Note the sprays of axons extending ventrally and caudally from the labeled CST (unlabeled arrows). The double arrow indicates one of the tangled arbors that are also found in areas of collateral sprouting.

Recent studies have provided particularly striking examples of both types of growth following spinal cord injury. For example, tract-tracing studies following surgical transection of corticospinal tract (CST) axons in the spinal cord reveal sprays of axonal arbors emerging from CST axons near the point of transection (see Fig. 1.3). These have a different trajectory than the CST arbors that extend into the gray matter at segmental levels in un-injured animals, and are thus interpreted as lesion-induced growth. As noted above, unusual-looking highly branched arbors are also seen (double arrow), which may indicate an abortive axonal growth response. It should be noted, however, that there is no definitive way to identify any single axon here as a newly-formed sprout. It is the picture in aggregate, especially the presence of many axons with an unusual form and trajectory that suggests that these are sprouted axons.

Another form of growth has been documented by quantitative studies that have revealed higher numbers of CST collaterals extending into the gray matter in segments proximal to an injury, implying the formation of additional axon collaterals in response to distal axotomy (Fouad et al., 2001, and see Fig. 1.2). These supernumary collaterals are found many segments rostral to an injury. For example, new collaterals are seen at cervical levels following injuries at the thoracic level (Fouad et al., 2001). This form of growth may be related to the pruning-related sprouting described below, but we include it as a form of "regenerative sprouting" because supernumary collaterals are formed in areas in which few, if any, collaterals of the axon normally terminate (implying the formation of ectopic connections). It has been suggested that the formation of ectopic connections as a result of this form of growth actually removes a stimulus for growth (because the axon does re-connect with a target), and may be part of the reason that axons do grow for long distances (Bernstein and Bernstein, 1973). It is of considerable interest that recent studies suggest that this form of growth may result in the formation of novel intra-spinal relays involving connections between damaged CST axons and propriospinal neurons, which then provide an alternate route for CST input to segments caudal to an injury (Bareyre et al., 2004).

Pruning-related sprouting

In some cases, neurons that lose some of their normal targets elaborate additional connections in other areas that they normally innervate. For example, if a cell projects to two locations via collaterals, the removal of the target of one collateral may result in an increased projection by the other collateral. This represents what has been called the *principle of conservation of axon arbor*. The term derives from the fact that axons respond as if they seek to maintain a minimum quantity of terminal arborization (Schneider, 1973; Schneider and Jhaveri, 1974; Schneider et al., 1985). The phenomenon of conservation of axon arbor has also been termed the "pruning effect" by analogy with similar phenomena in plants (Schneider, 1973; Schneider and Jhaveri, 1974).

Growing axons may also be directed to some other site than they would normally innervate. For example, following destruction of one side of the superior colliculus of the developing hamster, some retinal axons that would normally terminate on that side are re-directed into the opposite colliculus via a re-crossing projection (Schneider, 1973). Such growth to an ectopic location is termed axonal re-direction if the lesions are made early in development while axons are still growing.

Factors that determine the extent of growth by axotomized and/or target-deprived neurons

Developmental age

Neurons that are still developing are already expressing genes that are necessary for axon growth, whereas in adult animals, it is thought that growth-related genes are down-regulated, and that growth requires the neuron to alter its gene expression. Thus, everything else being equal, developing neurons will probably exhibit more regenerative sprouting and pruning-related sprouting than their mature counterparts.

Target availability

New axonal arbors induced as a result of regenerative sprouting, pruning-related sprouting, or axonal redirection are not likely to be maintained unless targets are available that can accept innervation. Indeed, the targets may provide critical signals that enhance growth, especially the arborizing form of growth that is characteristic of axons when they reach their target structures. This may explain in part why pruning-related sprouting and the formation of ectopic projections are more likely to occur in developing animals. Developing neurons that have not received their full complement of innervation would be available to the aberrant axons. In mature animals, the prediction is that regenerative sprouting and pruning-related sprouting might not result in the formation of new connections unless sites were made available by denervation.

Reinnervation of denervated neurons

At least two types of neuronal growth can restore input to neurons that lose their normal connections. Perhaps the most common type of reinnervation involves local growth of afferents that terminate near the denervated sites. This type of growth can theoretically occur without significant axonal elongation, for example as a result of the formation of a new presynaptic specialization on an existing axon. This type of very local response is termed *reactive synaptogenesis* (Cotman and Nadler, 1978). Reinnervation may also occur as a result of *axonal sprouting* followed by the formation of new connections. The difference is the extent of presynaptic axon growth. Axonal sprouting is distinguished from regenerative sprouting in that axonal sprouting involves growth by an un-damaged axon rather than a response to axonal injury.

Reactive synaptogenesis

Reactive synaptogenesis has been documented in a number of regions, most often through the use of quantitative electron microscopy. The typical strategy is to count the number of synapses or presynaptic terminals in a neuropil region in normal animals and at various times after an injury. Synapse replacement is revealed by increases in the number of synapses over time (Raisman and Field, 1973; Matthews et al., 1976a, b; Lee et al., 1977; McWilliams and Lynch, 1983; Steward and Vinsant, 1983). Complicating factors include:

1 Shrinkage and/or collapse of the neuropil resulting in a compression in the remaining synapses.
2 The death of denervated neurons, and/or atrophy of the affected dendrites.
3 Alterations in the volume of pre- and postsynaptic components which affect the probability that they will be counted.

It is possible to control all of these confounding variables, allowing precise estimates of both the extent and the time course of synapse turnover on denervated cells.

Axonal sprouting

Axonal sprouting differs conceptually from reactive synaptogenesis in that axon sprouting involves the formation of additional axon arbors. The true nature of axonal sprouting can only be defined when individual axons are traced. For example, until the advent of tract-tracing techniques, it was not possible to determine exactly how much axonal growth actually occurred, and in most situations, it could not be excluded that reinnervation occurred via reactive synaptogenesis. However, the development of techniques to label individual axons made it possible to directly visualize the nature of the sprouting response. For example, using techniques that allow the tracing of individual axons and their terminal arbors, it was shown that sprouting in the denervated dentate gyrus after entorhinal cortex lesions involved the formation of collaterals, axonal extensions, and highly characteristic tangled terminal arbors (Deller and Frotscher, 1997). Indeed, some of the tangled terminal arbors are so unusual looking that they may be diagnostic of a sprouting response.

It is not yet known how far a sprouting axon may grow, but growth over several hundreds of microns has been documented. For example, following partial lesions of the inferior olive, surviving climbing fibers gave off new axonal sprouts that grew from one Purkinje cell to nearby denervated neurons (Rossi et al., 1991). On reaching the new target, the climbing fiber grew along the dendrite of the Purkinje cell in typical climbing fiber fashion. All told, the lesion-induced axon growth occurred over hundreds of microns.

The signals that trigger the sprouting of undamaged axons are not completely defined. One possibility is that sprouting is induced by signals from denervated neurons (e.g. diffusible molecules like trophic factors). Alternatively, it may be the presence of denervated synaptic sites that represents the key signal, so that the formation of additional terminal arbors and synapses occurs as the growing axons establish synapses.

Factors that determine the extent of reinnervation of denervated neurons

Local proliferation of neuronal processes versus axonal ingrowth: the proximity principle

Reactive synaptogenesis is a common response to denervation in mature animals, but there are few examples of sprouting involving growth into ectopic locations except following lesions in developing animals. One principle that seems to be a good predictor of which systems will participate in reinnervating neurons in the mature CNS is the proximity principle (Goodman and Horel, 1966; Raisman, 1969). Stated simply, reinnervating synapses are more likely to arise from afferent systems that are near the denervated zones. The greater the proximity and/or overlap of surviving afferents and denervated sites, the greater the probability of growth of those surviving afferents, all other things being equal.

Diffuse versus concentrated denervation

The fact that sprouting most often involves systems that are near denervated sites has important implications for understanding the optimal conditions for reinnervation. The proximity principle predicts that the effects of the removal of a given number of synapses will depend on whether degenerating synapses are distributed amongst intact synapses, or are concentrated within a discrete area.

As schematically illustrated in Fig. 1.4, even if reactive growth is spatially limited, one can remove a substantial portion of normal afferents and still have virtually complete reinnervation if surviving afferents are distributed the denervated zone. If, however, the same amount of denervation is concentrated, so that there are few intact fibers within the denervated zone, an equivalent amount of sprouting by intact afferents on each side of the region of denervation would not be capable of restoring the normal density of innervation. Thus, one would expect much more complete reinnervation in the case of diffuse injury

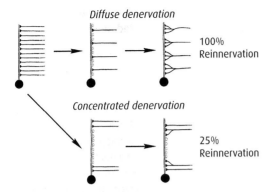

Figure 1.4. Hypothetical consequences of diffuse and concentrated denervation assuming a limitation on the distance over which sprouting will occur. If sprouting takes place only when there are intact fiber systems close to denervated sites, and if the extent of the growth is spatially limited, then reinnervation should be much more complete following diffuse denervation. For example, for a neuron that is innervated by a large number of afferent synapses (the left side of the figure) diffuse denervation might remove a substantial number of the normal contacts, but if the surviving synapses were distributed throughout the denervated zone, each could give rise to local connections that would fully restore normal synaptic density on the denervated neuron. Alternatively, the same amount of overall denervation would induce growth only in the surviving axons that were positioned near the denervated sites (lower portion of the figure). Since these would grow only into nearby regions, a substantial number of sites would be left uninnervated (from Steward et al., 1991).

than in the case of injury which results in a focus of denervation.

The fact that reinnervation is likely to be more complete following diffuse denervation is important for understanding the probable sequellae of CNS trauma. Many types of naturally-occurring CNS trauma involve diffuse injuries that produce diffuse denervation. Even in cases of focal injury, some sites are likely to be affected in a diffuse manner. For example, diffuse denervation would be expected in virtually all injuries that partially damage particular systems. Thus, naturally-occurring CNS trauma may produce injuries that are optimal for inducing naturally occurring repair processes.

Specificity and competition: the principle of hierarchical substitution

In the normal brain, different afferents terminate with highly specific patterns on postsynaptic cells. In addition, the numerical contribution of various afferents to certain cell types is reproducible. When normal patterns of connectivity are disrupted by lesions, reactive growth of surviving afferents results in a loss of normal specificity.

One measure of the specificity of post-lesion growth is that certain lesions result in the selective growth of only one of the systems that would seem eligible to grow based on proximity. For example, in the spinal cord, complete destruction of the dorsal roots to given segments induces a sprouting of descending projections. However, sprouting of descending projections is not observed if one root is spared (Goldberger and Murray, 1982). Instead, the spared root sprouts extensively within its normal zone of termination. Thus, the presence of one surviving root appears to limit the sprouting of other projections. Similarly, in the case of reinnervation of the septum following fimbria lesions, fibers from the contralateral fimbria appear to have a competitive advantage over other fibers following unilateral lesions (Field et al., 1980). These results suggest some sort of competitive interaction between potentially available afferent systems, and suggest that there are hierarchical preferences determining which afferent system will successfully re-occupy a denervated zone.

Another example hierarchical substitution comes from the work in the hippocampus. In normal rats, afferents from the ipsilateral entorhinal cortex terminate on the distal dendrites of dentate granule cells. Damage to the perforant path triggers a sprouting response that involves several systems that leads to a new but still highly specific pattern of connectivity (Cotman and Nadler, 1978). This is due in part to the fact that the sprouting is layer-specific, so that the normal pattern of afferent lamination is maintained

(Deller and Frotscher, 1997). Removal of the commissural portion of the commissural/associational projection system induces no detectable growth of entorhinal or septal afferents. Instead, the zone is reinnervated exclusively by the surviving associational projections (McWilliams and Lynch, 1978; 1979). If the commissural and associational projections are completely destroyed (by injecting kainic acid into the hippocampal formation), septal but not entorhinal afferents grow into the commissural/associational terminal zone (Cotman, 1979; Nadler et al., 1980).

The responses of the different afferent systems in different situations demonstrate that reactive changes set into motion by lesions are governed by principles of selectivity. If two homologous systems co-occupy a zone, removal of one usually leads to preferential sprouting of the other. When a zone is completely deprived of its "preferred" inputs, other afferents from nearby synaptic fields may grow in. However, some of the potential replacements are more likely to grow than in others (the principle of hierarchical substitution). If present, preferred afferents out-compete non-preferred afferents in occupying the denervated sites.

Developmental age: the principle of dynamic turnover

In general, post-lesion growth is more extensive in developing animals. Moreover, aged animals seem to have even less capacity for post-lesion growth than young adults, in that the extent of the lesion-induced growth is less. (Cotman and Scheff, 1979; Hoff et al., 1982). The time course of synapse replacement also varies across developmental age. For example, synapse replacement in the dentate gyrus after entorhinal cortical lesions occurs within 1–2 days after lesions in developing animals (Gall and Lynch, 1978; 1980; 1981). The same response does not begin until 5–6 days post-lesion in mature animals, and continues for several weeks (Steward and Vinsant, 1983). Synapse replacement is even slower in aged animals (Hoff et al., 1982).

Some types of reactive growth are more extensive and/or more rapid if the damage is preceded by a "priming" lesion. This applies both to reinnervation in the CNS (Scheff et al., 1978) and to regeneration of axotomized neurons. For example, prior axotomy of dorsal root ganglion neurons enhances subsequent axon regeneration in culture and *in vivo* (McQuarrie et al., 1977; McQuarrie, 1978; McQuarrie and Grafstein, 1981; Neumann and Woolf, 1999). It is thought that the priming lesions induce some growth process so that the responses to the later trauma are more extensive than would otherwise be the case. In the case of the priming of regeneration of dorsal root ganglion cells, it is thought that the priming lesion induces the expression of critical growth-associated genes that are critical for regeneration (Neumann and Woolf, 1999). It is noteworthy that axon regeneration can also be enhanced by injecting cyclic adenosine monophosphate (cAMP) into the dorsal root ganglion, which is thought to induce the expression of growth-associated genes (Neumann et al., 2002; Qiu et al., 2002). A process of this sort may account for the well-known "serial lesion effect" where deficits resulting from gradual damage are less severe than the deficits following similar damage produced in a single stage (Stein, 1974), and may account for the fact that slowly evolving lesions generally have less severe functional consequences than rapidly evolving ones (Finger, 1978).

The effects of age on neuronal reorganization and the effects of a priming lesion suggest that reorganization is likely to be more extensive in systems that are in a state of change. This represents the *principle of dynamic turnover*. Thus developing neuronal systems respond more quickly and more extensively to trauma than mature ones because they are growing already; the same is true of systems that are responding to previous trauma.

While injury may induce distinct growth responses in neurons, it is also possible that synaptic connections in the mature nervous system are constantly turning over (for a discussion of this concept, and a review of supporting evidence, see Cotman et al. (1981)). Thus, lesion-induced growth could be an accentuation of the normal dynamic synapse turnover that is constantly taking place.

Differences in the time course of lesion-induced growth across species: what might be expected in human beings?

The evidence that the time course of growth is different across species comes from studies of one type of sprouting (the sprouting of AChE containing septo-hippocampal fibers after destruction of the entorhinal cortex). This sprouting can be evaluated histochemically by measuring the increase in AChE staining in the denervated zone. In rats, the increase in AChE staining can first be observed at about 5 days post-lesion, and appears fully developed by 12 days (Nadler et al., 1977). In cats, the same type of growth does not begin until about 10 days post-lesion, and does not reach completion until about 20 days (Steward and Messenheimer, 1978). There is evidence that the same response occurs over a longer post-lesion interval in primates (Moss et al., 1982).

There is a critical need for further studies comparing the time course of different types of growth across species, particularly in higher primates, to give some hints about the probable time course of post-lesion growth in man.

What changes in gene expression occur during regenerative sprouting and other forms of naturally-occurring post-lesion growth?

One common explanation of why regeneration is so limited in the mammalian CNS is that the genes required for axon regeneration are down-regulated in mature neurons, and are not re-induced following injury. In this regard, it is noteworthy that the formation of additional axon arbors and synaptic connections during sprouting occurs without large-scale changes in expression of various growth-associated genes (see Steward (1995) and references therein). This is consistent with previous ideas that synapse turnover is an ongoing process in the normal brain (Cotman and Nieto-Sampedro, 1982), and that the reorganization of circuitry following injury may be the result of processes that are ongoing rather than being induced. These findings are consistent with the idea that CNS regeneration is limited in part because

neuronal genes are not up-regulated by signals that result from injury (see Volume I, Chapter 24). Thus, the lack of increases in neuronal gene expression may be part of the cause rather than simply the effect of abortive axonal regeneration. In this regard, new strategies to induce the expression of critical growth-associated genes are of particular interest (see Volume I, Chapter 29 by Nakmara and Kang).

REFERENCES

Abe, Y., Yamamoto, T., Sugiyama, Y., Watanabe, T., Saito, N., Kayama, H. and Kumagai, T. (1999). Apoptotic cells associated with Wallerian degeneration after experimental spinal cord injury: a possible mechanism of oligodendroglial death. *J Neurotrauma*, **16**, 945–952.

Bareyre, F.M., Kerschensteiner, M., Raineteau, O., Mettenleiter, T.C., Weinmann, O. and Schwab, M.E. (2004). The injured spinal cord spontaneously forms a new intraspinal circuit in adult rats. *Nat Neurosci*, **7**, 269–277.

Benes, F.M., Parks, T.N. and Rubel, E.W. (1977). Rapid dendritic atrophy following deafferentation: an EM morphometric analysis. *Brain Res*, **122**, 1–13.

Bennett, J.P. and Wooten, G.F. (1986). Dopamine denervation does not alter *in vivo* 3H-spiperone binding in rat striatum: implications for external imaging of dopamine receptors in Parkinson's disease. *Ann Neurol*, **19**, 378–383.

Bernstein, M.E. and Bernstein, J.J. (1973). Regeneration of axons and synaptic complex formation rostral to the site of hemisection in the spinal cord of the monkey. *Int J Neurosci*, **5**, 15–36.

Bernstein-Goral, H. and Bregman, B.S. (1997). Axotomized rubrospinal neurons rescued by fetal spinal cord transplants maintain axon collaterals to rostral CNS targets. *Exp Neurol*, **148**, 13–25.

Bleier, R. (1969). Retrograde transsynaptic cellular degeneration in mammillary and ventral tegmental nuclei following limbic decortication in rabbits of various ages. *Brain Res*, **15**, 365–393.

Blight, A.R. (1985). Delayed demyelination and macrophage invasion: a candidate for secondary cell damage in spinal cord injury. *CNS Trauma*, **2**, 299–315.

Born, D.E. and Rubel, E.W. (1985). Afferent influences on brain stem auditory nuclei of the chicken: neuron number and size following cochlea removal. *J Comp Neurol*, **231**, 435–445.

Born, D.E. and Rubel, E.W. (1988). Afferent influences on brain stem auditory nuclei of the chicken: presynaptic action potentials regulate protein synthesis in nucleus magnocellularis neurons. *J Neurosci*, **8**, 901–919.

Bregman, B.S. and Goldberger, M.E. (1982). Anatomical plasticity and sparing of function after spinal cord damage in neonatal cats. *Science*, **217**, 553–555.

Bregman, B.S. and Goldberger, M.E. (1983). Infant lesion effect. III. Anatomical correlates of sparing and recovery of function after spinal cord damage in newborn and adult cats. *Dev Brain Res*, **9**, 137–154.

Bregman, B.S. and Reier, P.J. (1986). Neural tissue transplants rescue axotomized rubrospinal cells from retrograde death. *J Comp Neurol*, **244**, 86–95.

Caceres, A. and Steward, O. (1983). Dendritic reorganization in the denervated dentate gyrus of the rat following entorhinal cortical lesions: a Golgi and electron microscopic analysis. *J Comp Neurol*, **214**, 387–403.

Cai, G., Wang, H.Y. and Friedman, E. (2002). Increased dopamine receptor signaling and dopamine receptor-G protein coupling in denervated striatum. *J Pharmacol Exp Ther*, **302**, 1105–1112.

Canady, K.S. and Rubel, E.W. (1992). Rapid and reversible astrocytic reaction to afferent activity blockade in chick cochlear nucleus. *J Neurosci*, **12**, 1001–1009.

Cannon, W.B. and Rosenbleuth, A. (1949). *The Supersensitivity of Denervated Structures: A Law of Denervation*, MacMillan, New York.

Colombari, E. and Talman, W.T. (1995). Denervation supersensitivity to glutamate in the nucleus tractus solitarii after removal of the nodose ganglion. *Brain Res*, **677**, 110–116.

Colonnier, M. (1964). Experimental degeneration in the cerebral cortex. *J Anat (Lond)*, **98**, 47–53.

Cotman, C.W. (1979). Specificity of synaptic growth in brain: remodeling induced by kainic acid lesions. *Prog Brain Res*, **51**, 203–215.

Cotman, C.W. and Nadler, J.V. (1978). Reactive synaptogenesis in the hippocampus. *Neuronal Plast*, 227–271.

Cotman, C.W. and Nieto-Sampedro, M. (1982). Brain function, synapse renewal and plasticity. *Annu Rev Psychol*, **33**, 371–401.

Cotman, C.W., Nieto-Sampedro, M. and Harris, E.W. (1981). Synapse replacement in the nervous system of adult vertebrates. *Physiol Rev*, **61**, 684–784.

Cotman, C.W. and Scheff, S.W. (1979). Compensatory synapse growth in aged animals after neuronal death. *Mech Aging and Dev*, **9**, 103–117.

Cowan, W.M. (1970). Anterograde and retrograde transneuronal degeneration in the central and peripheral nervous system. In: *Contemporary Research Methods in Neuroanatomy* (eds Nauta, W.J.H. and Ebbesson, S.O.E.), Springer-Verlag, New York.

Creese, I., Burt, D.R. and Snyder, S.H. (1977). Dopamine receptor binding enhancement accompanied lesion-induced behavioral supersensitivity. *Science*, **197**, 596–597.

Crowe, M.J., Bresnahan, J.C., Shuman, S.L., Masters, J.N. and Beattie, M.S. (1997). Apoptosis and delayed degeneration after spinal cord injury in rats and monkeys. *Nat Med*, **3**, 73–76.

Deitch, J.S. and Rubel, E.W. (1989). Rapid changes in ultrastructure during deafferentation-induced dendritic atrophy. *J Comp Neurol*, **281**, 234–258.

Deller, T. and Frotscher, M. (1997). Lesion-induced plasticity of central neurons: sprouting of single fibers in the rat hippocampus after unilateral entorhinal cortex lesion. *Prog Neurobiol*, **53**, 687–727.

Dun, N., Nishi, S. and Karczmar, A.G. (1976). Alteration in nicotinic and muscarinic responses of rabbit superior cervical ganglion cells after chronic preganglionic denervation. *Neuropharmacology*, **15**, 211–218.

Fambrough, D.M. (1981). Denervation: cholinergic receptors of skeletal muscle. In: *Receptors and Recognition Series* (ed. Lefkowitz, R.J.), Chapman and Hall, London, pp. 125–142.

Field, P.M., Coldham, D.E. and Raisman, G. (1980). Synapse formation after injury in the adult rat brain: preferential reinnervation of denervated fimbrial sites by axons of the contralateral fimbria. *Brain Res*, **189**, 103–113.

Finger, S. (1978). Lesion momentum and behavior. In: *Recovery from Brain Damage* (ed. Finger, S.), Plenum, New York, pp. 135–164.

Fouad, K., Pedersen, V., Schwab, M.E. and Brosamle, C. (2001). Cervical sprouting of corticospinal fibers after thoracic spinal cord injury accompanies shifts in evoked motor responses. *Current Biol*, **11**, 1766–1770.

Gall, C. and Lynch, G. (1978). Rapid axon sprouting in the neonatal rat hippocampus. *Brain Res*, **153**, 357–362.

Gall, C. and Lynch, G. (1980). The regulation of fiber growth and synaptogenesis in the developing hippocampus. *Curr Top Dev Biol*, **15**, 159–180.

Gall, C. and Lynch, G. (1981). Fiber architecture of the dentate gyrus following ablation of the entorhinal cortex in rats of different ages: evidence for two forms of axon sprouting in the immature brain. *Neuroscience*, **6**, 903–910.

Gill, R., Foster, A.C. and Woodruff, G.N. (1987). Systemic administration of MK-801 protects against ischemia-induced hippocampal neurodegeneration in the gerbil. *J Neurosci*, **7**, 3343–3349.

Goldberger, M.E. and Murray, M. (1982). Lack of sprouting and its presence after lesions of the cat spinal cord. *Brain Res*, **241**, 227–239.

Goodman, D.C. and Horel, J.A. (1966). Sprouting of optic tract projections in the brain stem of the rat. *J Comp Neurol*, **127**, 71–88.

Guth, L. (1974). Axonal regeneration and functional plasticity in the central nervous system. *Exp Neurol*, **45**, 606–654.

Guth, L. (1975). History of central nervous system regeneration research. *Exp Neurol*, **48**, 3–15.

Haines, B.C., Black, J.A. and Waxman, S.G. (2003). Primary cortical motor neurons undergo apoptosis after axotomizing spinal cord injury. *J Comp Neurol*, **462**, 328–341.

Heimer, L. and Kalil, R. (1978). Rapid transneuronal degeneration and death of cortical neurons following removal of the olfactory bulb in adult rats. *J Comp Neurol*, **178**, 559–609.

Hoff, S.F., Scheff, S.W., Bernardo, L.S. and Cotman, C.W. (1982). Lesion-induced synaptogenesis in the dentate gyrus of aged rats. I. Loss and reacquisition of normal synaptic density. *J Comp Neurol*, **205**, 246–252.

Kalil, K. and Reh, T. (1979). Regrowth of severed axons in the neonatal CNS. *Science*, **205**, 1158–1161.

Kalil, K. and Reh, T. (1982). Light and electron microscopic study of regrowing pyramidal tract fibers. *J Comp Neurol*, **211**, 265–275.

Klatzo, I. (1975). Pathophysiologic aspects of cerebral ischemia. In: *The Basic Neurosciences* (ed. Tower, D.B.), Raven Press, New York, pp. 313–322.

Kwon, B.K., Liu, J., Messerer, C., Kobayashi, N.R., McGraw, J. and Oschipok, L. (2002). Survival and regeneration of rubrospinal neurons 1 year after spinal cord injury. *Proc Nat Acad Sci*, **99**, 3246–3251.

Lee, K.S., Stanford, E.J., Cotman, C.W. and Lynch, G.S. (1977). Ultrastructural evidence for bouton proliferation in the partially deafferented dentate gyrus of the adult rat. *Exp Brain Res*, **29**, 475–485.

Levi-Montalcini, R. (1949). The development of the acoustico-vestibular centers in the chick embryo in the absence of the afferent root fibers and of descending fiber tracts. *J Comp Neurol*, **91**, 209–242.

Li, Y., Harvey, P.J., Li, X. and Bennett, D.J. (2004). Spastic long-lasting reflexes of the chronic spinal rat studied *in vitro*. *J Neurophysiol*, **91**, 2236–2246.

Lieberman, A.R. (1971). The axon reaction: a review of the principal features of perikaryal responses to axon injury. *Int Rev Neurobiol*, **14**, 49–124.

Lund, R.D. and Lund, J.S. (1971). Synaptic adjustment after deafferentation of the superior colliculus of the rat. *Science*, **171**, 804–807.

Matthews, M.R., Cowan, W.M. and Powell, T.P.S. (1960). Transneuronal cell degeneration in the lateral geniculate nucleus of the macaque monkey. *J Anat*, **94**, 145–169.

Matthews, M.R. and Powell, T.P.S. (1962). Some observations on transneuronal cell degeneration in the olfactory bulb of the rabbit. *Brain Res*, **115**, 23–41.

Matthews, D.A., Cotman, C. and Lynch, G. (1976a). An electron microscopic study of lesion-induced synaptogenesis in the dentate gyrus of the adult rat. I. Magnitude and time course of degeneration. *Brain Res*, **115**, 1–21.

Matthews, D.A., Cotman, C. and Lynch, G. (1976b). An electron microscopic study of lesion-induced synaptogenesis in the dentate gyrus of the adult rat. II. Reappearance of morphologically normal synaptic contacts. *Brain Res*, **115**, 23–41.

McQuarrie, I.G. (1978). The effect of a conditioning lesion on the regeneration of motor axons. *Brain Res*, **152**, 597–602.

McQuarrie, I.G. and Grafstein, B. (1981). The effect of a conditioning lesion on optic nerve regeneration in goldfish. *Brain Res*, **216**, 253–264.

McQuarrie, I.G., Grafstein, B. and Gershon, M.D. (1977). Axon regeneration in the rat sciatic nerve: effect of a conditioning lesion and of dbcAMP. *Brain Res*, **132**, 443–453.

McWilliams, J.R. and Lynch, G. (1983). Rate of synaptic replacement in denervated rat hippocampus declines precipitously from the juvenile period to adulthood. *Science*, **221**, 572–574.

McWilliams, R. and Lynch, G. (1978). Terminal proliferation and synaptogenesis following partial deafferentation: the reinnervation of the inner molecular layer of the dentate gyrus following removal of its commissural afferents. *J Comp Neurol*, **180**, 581–616.

McWilliams, R. and Lynch, G. (1979). Terminal proliferation in the partially deafferented dentate gyrus: time courses for the appearance and removal of degeneration and the replacement of lost terminals. *J Comp Neurol*, **187**, 191–198.

Moore, R.Y. (1974). Central regeneration and recovery of function: the problem of collateral reinnervation. In: *Plasticity and Recovery of Function in the Central Nervous System* (eds Stein, D.G., Rosen, J.J. and Butters, N.), Academic Press, New York, pp. 111–128.

Moss, M., Rosene, D.L. and Van Hoesen, G.W. (1982). Neuronal plasticity in the hippocampal formation of the adult monkey following lesions of the entorhinal area. Society for Neuroscience, Abstract 8, 746.

Nadler, J.V., Cotman, C.W. and Lynch, G.S. (1977). Histochemical evidence of altered development of cholinergic fibers in the rat dentate gyrus following lesions I. Time course after complete unilateral entorhinal lesions at various ages. *J Comp Neurol*, **171**, 561–588.

Nadler, J.V., Perry, B.W. and Cotman, C.W. (1980). Selective reinnervation of hippocampal area CA1 and the fascia dentata after destruction of CA3–CA4 afferents with kainic acid. *Brain Res*, **182**, 1–9.

Neumann, S., Bradke, F., Tessier-Lavigne, M. and Basbaum, A.I. (2002). Regeneration of sensory axons within the injured spinal cord induced by intraganglionic cAMP elevation. *Neuron*, **34**, 885–893.

Neumann, S. and Woolf, C.J. (1999). Regeneration of dorsal column fibers into and beyond the lesion site following adult spinal cord injury. *Neuron*, **23**, 83–91.

Novikova, L.N., Novikov, L.N. and Kellerth, J.O. (2000). Survival effects of BDNF and NT-3 on axotomized rubrospinal neurons depend on the temporal pattern of neurotrophin administration. *Eur J Neurosci*, **12**, 776–780.

Parnavelas, J., Lynch, G., Brecha, N., Cotman, C. and Globus, A. (1974). Spine loss and regrowth in the hippocampus following deafferentation. *Nature*, **248**, 71–73.

Pinching, A.J. (1969). Persistence of post-synaptic membrane thickening after degeneration of olfactory nerves. *Brain Res*, **16**, 277–281.

Pinching, A.J. and Powell, T.P.S. (1972). A study of terminal degeneration in the olfactory bulb of the rat. *J Cell Sci*, **10**, 585–619.

Powell, T.P.S. and Cowan, W.M. (1962). An experimental study of the projection of the cochlea. *J Anat (Lond)*, **96**, 269–284.

Powell, T.P.S. and Erulkar, S.D. (1962). Transneuronal cell degeneration in the auditory relay nuclei of the cat. *J Anat (Lond)*, **96**, 249–268.

Puchala, E. and Windle, W.F. (1977). The possibility of structural and functional restitution after spinal cord injury: a review. *Exp Neurol*, **55**, 1–42.

Purves, D. (1975). Functional and structural changes in mammalian sympathetic neurons following interruption of their axons. *J Physiol*, **252**, 429–463.

Qiu, J., Cai, D., Dai, H., McAtee, M., Hoffman, P.N., Bregman, B.S. and Filbin, M.T. (2002). Spinal axon regeneration induced by elevation of cyclic AMP. *Neuron*, **34**, 895–903.

Raisman, G. (1969). Neuronal plasticity in the septal nuclei of the adult rat. *Brain Res*, **14**, 25–48.

Raisman, G. and Field, P.M. (1973). A quantitative investigation of the development of collateral reinnervation after partial deafferentation of the septal nuclei. *Brain Res*, **50**, 241–264.

Ramon y Cajal, S. (1959). *Degeneration and Regeneration of the Nervous System*, Hafner, New York.

Rose, J.E. and Woolsey, C.N. (1958). *Biological and Biochemical Bases of Behavior*, University of Wisconsin Press, Madison, pp. 127–150.

Rossi, F., Wiklund, L., van der Want, J.J. and Strata, P. (1991). Reinnervation of cerebellar Purkinje cells by climbing fibres surviving a subtotal lesion of the inferior olive in the adult rat. I. Development of new collateral branches and terminal plexuses. *J Comp Neurol*, **308**, 513–535.

Rothman, S. (1984). Synaptic release of excitatory amino acid neurotransmitter mediates anoxic neuronal death. *J Neurosci*, **4**, 1884–1891.

Rubel, E.W., Smith, Z.D.G. and Steward, O. (1981). Sprouting in the avian brainstem auditory pathway: dependence on dendritic integrity. *J Comp Neurol*, **202**, 397–414.

Scheff, S.W., Bernardo, L.S. and Cotman, C.W. (1978). Effect of serial lesions on sprouting in the dentate gyrus: onset and decline of catalytic effect. *Brain Res*, **150**, 45–53.

Schmidt-Kastner, R. and Freund, T.F. (1991). Selective vulnerability of the hippocampus in brain ischemia. *Neuroscience*, **40**, 599–636.

Schneider, G.D. (1973). Early lesions of superior colliculus: factors affecting the formation of abnormal retinal projections. *Brain Behav Evol*, **8**, 73–109.

Schneider, G.E. and Jhaveri, J.R. (1974). Neuroanatomical correlates of spared or altered function after brain lesions in the newborn hamster. In: *Plasticity and Recovery of Function in the Central Nervous System* (eds Stein, D.G., Rosen, J.J. and Butters, N.), Academic Press, New York, pp. 65–109.

Schneider, G.E., Jhaveri, S., Edwards, M.A. and So, K.-F. (1985). Regeneration, re-routing and redistribution of axons after early lesions: changes with age and functional impact. In: *Recent Advances in Restorative Neurology I: Upper Motor Neuron Functions and Dysfunctions* (eds Eccles, J.C. and Dimitrijevic, M.), Karger, Basel, pp. 291–310.

Simon, R.P., Swan, J.H., Griffith, T. and Meldrum, B.S. (1984). Blockade of *N*-methyl-D-aspartate receptors may protect against ischaemic damage in the brain. *Science*, **226**, 850–852.

Stein, D.G. (1974). Some variables affecting recovery of function after central nervous system lesions in the rat. In: *Plasticity and Recovery of Function in the Central Nervous System* (eds Stein, D.G., Rosen, J.J. and Butters, N.), Academic Press, New York, pp. 373–427.

Steward, O. (1982). Assessing the functional significance of lesion-induced neuronal plasticity. *Int Rev Neurobiol*, **23**, 197–254.

Steward, O. (1995). The process of reinnervation in the dentate gyrus of adult rats: gene expression by neuron during the period of lesion-induced growth. *J Comp Neurol*, **359**, 391–411.

Steward, O. (2000). *Functional Neuroscience*, Springer-Verlag, New York.

Steward, O. and Messenheimer, J.A. (1978). Histochemical evidence for a postlesion reorganization of cholinergic afferents in the hippocampal formation of the mature cat. *J Comp Neurol*, **178**, 697–710.

Steward, O. and Rubel, E.W. (1985). Afferent influences on brain stem auditory nuclei of the chicken: cessation of amino acid incorporation as an antecedent to age-dependent transneuronal degeneration. *J Comp Neurol*, **231**, 385–395.

Steward, O. and Vinsant, S.L. (1983). The process of reinnervation in the dentate of the adult rat: a quantitative electron microscopic analysis of terminal proliferation and reactive synaptogenesis. *J Comp Neurol*, **214**, 370–386.

Steward, O., Tomasulo, R., Torre, E. and Trimmer, P. (1991). Reorganization of neural connections following CNS injury: is synaptic reorganization initiated by the changes in neuronal activity which occur following injury? *Brain Dysfunct*, **5**, 27–49.

Steward, O., Zheng, B. and Tessier-Lavigne, M. (2003). False resurrections: distinguishing regenerated from spared axons in the injured CNS. *J Comp Neurol*, **459**, 1–8.

Sumner, B.E.H. (1977). Responses in the hypoglossal nucleus to delayed regeneration of the transected hypoglossal nerve, a quantitative ultrastructural study. *Exp Brain Res*, **29**, 219–231.

Sumner, B.E.H. and Sutherland, F.I. (1973). Quantitative electron microscopy on the injured hypoglossal nucleus in the rat. *J Neurocytol*, **2**, 315–328.

Tobias, C.A., Shumsky, J.S., Shibata, M., Tuszynski, M.H., Fischer, I., Tessler, A. and Murray, M. (2003). Delayed grafting of BDNF and NT-3 producing fibroblasts into the injured spinal cord stimulates sprouting, partially rescues axotomized red

nucleus neurons from loss and atrophy, and provides limited regeneration. *Exp Neurol*, **184**, 97–113.

Torvik, A. (1976). Central chromatolysis and the axon reaction: a reappraisal. *Neuropathol App Neurobiol*, **2**, 423–432.

Totoiu, M.O. and Keirstead, H.S. (2005). Spinal cord injury is accompanied by chronic progressive demyelination. *J Comp Neurol*, **486**, 373–383.

Westrum, L.E. and Black, R.G. (1971). Fine structural aspects of the synaptic organization of the spinal trigeminal nucleus (pars interpolaris) of the cat. *Brain Res*, **25**, 265–287.

White, L.E. and Westrum, L.E. (1964). Dendritic spine changes in prepyriform cortex following olfactory bulb lesions. *Anat Rec*, **148**, 410–411.

Xu, X.M. and Martin, G.F. (1991). Evidence for new growth and regeneration of cut axons in developmental plasticity of the rubrospinal tract in the North American oppossum. *J Comp Neurol*, **313**, 103–112.

Zigmond, M.J., Stachowiak, M.K. and Stricker, E.M. (1986). Neurochemical events underlying continued function despite injury to monoaminergic systems. *Exp Brain Res (Suppl)*, **13**, 119–128.

Learning and memory: basic principles and model systems

Kimberly M. Christian, Andrew M. Poulos and Richard F. Thompson

Neuroscience Program, University of Southern California, Los Angeles, CA, USA

2.1 Introduction

If the ultimate aim of neural repair and rehabilitation is to restore functions vital to an individual's ability to live independently, then restoration of the capacity to learn and remember is of tremendous importance. The ability to learn, including the acquisition of novel information, relationships and strategies, and the ability to remember and act upon what has been learned, are essential for successful negotiation of our dynamic environment. While many behaviors are reflexive, stereotyped and innate, experience and memory shape much of our behavioral repertoire and allow us to perform basic tasks essential to our daily life by recognizing familiar faces, locating our homes, etc. Understanding how new information is encoded at the neural level and made accessible for later recall is a central goal of neuroscience. How are constellations of sensory input transformed into usable information, interpreted within a context, and remembered? Clearly, there must be causally relevant neural correlates of learning and memory that once identified should provide insight into the fundamental mechanics of brain organization and function. If we can understand how the brain changes in response to experience and thus how it is that we can learn and remember, then we will be well equipped to address many of the most devastating deficits resulting from brain injury.

By investigating how the brain changes to reflect learning in the absence of injury, researchers hope to characterize functional properties of neural structures and basic mechanisms of plasticity, both of which can ultimately be exploited to design targeted rehabilitation strategies. While some forms of plasticity (i.e., structural, physiological) would seem to be critical to the acquisition and storage of all memories, it appears unlikely that there is a single set of molecular or cellular markers necessary and sufficient for memory formation. We do know that there are qualitatively different forms of learning and memory that can be distinguished at the behavioral level and that these different forms often engage different neural systems. If the goal is to ameliorate deficits resulting from brain injury, an important first step is to classify learned behavior and memory in a manner that will reveal meaningful distinctions at the neural level and then to identify the critical neural circuitry involved. With this knowledge, cognitive deficits of patients may be more easily diagnosed using behavioral tests appropriate to the site(s) of neural damage. Restoration of function will require a more mechanistic understanding of the neural basis of learning and memory but will depend on this initial characterization of the behavior and its neural substrates. This chapter will provide a taxonomic overview of different forms of learning and memory at the behavioral and neural system levels. It will also include a discussion of how clinical observations, psychophysical investigations and animal experiments are integrated to answer some of the most basic questions in neuroscience: how do we learn and what is memory?

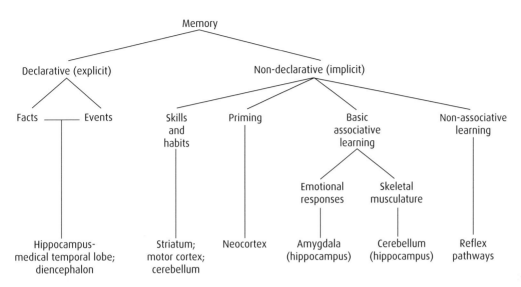

Figure 2.1. Taxonomy of long-term memory and the putative associated neural structures. Adapted from Squire and Knowlton (1994).

In the most general terms, long-term memory can be divided roughly into two categories, namely, declarative and non-declarative memory as seen in Fig. 2.1 (see Squire et al., 1993; Squire and Knowlton, 1994; Thompson and Kim, 1996; Gabrieli, 1998 for reviews). Non-declarative, or implicit, memories are those that can be expressed without awareness or conscious recollection. Declarative, or explicit, memories are subject to conscious recall and generally involve awareness that the memory is being invoked during expression. Declarative memories include direct experiential knowledge that you remember acquiring (i.e., what you had for breakfast, where you went to high school), referred to as episodic memory, as well as knowledge of facts about the world (i.e., the name of the President of the US, the sum of two plus two), referred to as semantic memory. Non-declarative memories encompass a wide range of phenomena from priming to skill learning. It is important to recognize that while declarative and non-declarative memories generally can be distinguished according to the criterion mentioned above and further delineated through dependence on distinct neural systems, these two types of memory are not mutually exclusive and are often formed in parallel.

2.2 Non-declarative memory

Non-associative

Some of the most basic forms of memory result from non-associative learning processes. Habituation and sensitization are two such processes that will be discussed at length in Chapter 5. Briefly, habituation is a decreased response to a stimulus that results from repetitive presentations of that stimulus. While you may initially look in the direction of a novel sound, a bird chirping outside, for instance, you will probably not continue to reorient yourself with each new chirp. Sensitization is a supranormal response to a given stimulus induced by a preceding strong stimulus. If you awake in the middle of the night due to a loud unexpected sound, your state of increased vigilance will lead you to react more strongly than you would normally to any subsequent sounds. Habituation and sensitization are adaptive behaviors that appear to belong to all animals with nervous systems, albeit in the absence of the modulatory influence of attention in the lowest animals.

Studies of habituation and sensitization in invertebrates reveal neural mechanisms of plasticity that can often be mapped to mammalian systems. In particular, the research of Eric Kandel on invertebrates and Richard Thompson on vertebrate preparations has shown a remarkable degree of similarity in the mechanisms underlying each form of learning (Thompson and Spencer, 1966; Carew and Sahley, 1986; Pittenger and Kandel, 2003). Habituation depends on synaptic depression due to a decrease in neurotransmitter release while sensitization involves a facilitation of neurotransmitter release and involves sensory, motor, and interneurons. Utilizing these two processes, it was possible to develop a "dual-process theory of habituation" that could account for a wide range of behavioral phenomena of habituation (Groves and Thompson, 1970). Invertebrate research has focused primarily on the gill-siphon withdrawal reflex in *Aplysia* while in mammals similar non-associative plasticity occurs in appropriately stimulated spinal reflexes. Study of these learning phenomena in the relatively tractable invertebrate preparation has led to critical insights into the nature of synaptic plasticity and its temporal characteristics. Habituation and sensitization may last for a few minutes or several weeks depending on the induction protocol and cellular response (Sutton et al., 2002). The morphological changes and de novo protein synthesis that accompany long-term expression of this non-associative memory have proven to be general properties of many forms of long-term memory in mammals. This evolutionary conservation in both the behavior and the underlying mechanisms provides evidence to support the use of animal models to study learning and memory in human beings.

Procedural

Another subset of non-declarative memory is procedural memory, the learning of sensorimotor or cognitive skills. This type of memory is capable of being formed and expressed without awareness of the learning context and can persist even if it is not accessible to conscious recall. This is not to say that the learning itself must be done in the absence of awareness, only that awareness is not necessary. Examples of motor skill learning identified in human amnesics include such tasks as mirror tracing (tracing a figure reflection in the mirror) and rotary pursuit (tracking a moving target). Several studies report intact learning of these tasks in amnesic patients and Alzheimer disease patients that have impaired declarative memory (see Gabrieli, 1998 for review). Brain damage in other regions (i.e., basal ganglia, cerebellum) can disrupt acquisition of these skills yet leave declarative memory formation intact suggesting a double dissociation and differentiated neural substrates for these different memories. Probabilistic learning in human beings involves a task in which subjects feel as though they are merely guessing in response to a request to predict outcomes but actually improve their performance based on hidden probabilities. This type of learning also shows a double dissociation in Parkinson's patients in which damage to the basal ganglia prevents the patients from acquiring this skill although they can report details related to the training session. Amnesics with medial temporal lobe damage appear to acquire this skill normally (Knowlton et al., 1994; Reber et al., 1996). Imaging studies suggest that the medial temporal lobe may be active during the early stages of classification learning but that the striatum of the basal ganglia becomes active in later stages. The negative correlation in activity levels in these structures suggests a competitive interaction between systems involved in declarative and non-declarative learning (Poldrack et al., 2001; Poldrack and Packard, 2003). The basal ganglia have been suggested to mediate stimulus–response (S–R) learning in non-human animals as well (see Packard and Knowlton, 2002 for review). S–R learning or habit learning is another form of non-declarative memory and can be impaired with pretraining lesions of the basal ganglia.

Priming

Non-declarative priming memory is a form of memory that results from exposure to stimuli prior to a testing session (Schacter et al., 1993). For example, if people are given a list of words to memorize quickly and then given another list of words with only the first two letters present and asked to complete the words with the first word that occurs to them, they will very likely use a word from the first list. This can occur even in the absence of awareness. Amnesics are not impaired in the acquisition or expression of this type of memory (Keane et al., 1994, 1995). Brain substrates underlying this form of memory appear to involve visual association areas of the cortex as damage to these regions impairs memory and imaging studies in normal subjects show changes in activation in these areas during expression of this memory (Squire et al., 1992; Samuelsson et al., 2000).

Non-declarative associative memory

Associative memory is essentially the learned relationship between two previously unrelated stimuli, responses or actions. While much of our declarative memory involves such learned associations, there is a class of basic associative memories that do not rely on our awareness of the learning process. These basic associative memories are formed through classical conditioning, a learning process first described by Ivan Pavlov in the early 20th century (Pavlov, 1927). Pavlov observed that dogs could be trained to salivate at the sound of a bell if it was presented repeatedly just prior to feeding time. Salivation at the sight of food is an unconditioned response (UR). The bell was a neutral stimulus prior to training, not eliciting any overt response, but after training, the bell could induce salivation as a conditioned response (CR). The bell and the food were the conditioned and unconditioned stimuli (CS, US), respectively. In addition to the solicitation of a CR to an appetitive CS, such as food, Pavlovian conditioning can also result from the cued presentation of an aversive stimulus, as in fear conditioning.

The concept of associative memory is ancient; the classical Greek philosophers observed it and the British school of associationist philosophers in the 18th and 19th centuries elaborated it. The basic notion is very simple: events that tend to occur together in time become associated with one another in the brain. If you place your finger in a flame the immediate consequence is pain and finger withdrawal. Association of events in time is termed *contiguity* and is an essential requirement for associative learning.

Important studies by Robert Rescorla (1988) showed that in many associative learning situations, contiguity by itself is not sufficient to yield good learning. Suppose you are studying learned fear in a group of rats. The animals are given several trials of a tone followed by a mild shock, a shock that is aversive or unpleasant but not necessarily painful. If you then measure a fear response in the rats, you will find that the tone now elicits a vigorous fear response. Contiguity was enough to establish learning. But suppose that you give another group of rats a number of experiences of the shock without the tone, as well as the same number of paired tone-shock trials as in the previous group of animals, you will find that in this group of rats the tone elicits much less fear response than in the original group. This seems counterintuitive; animals in the second group received *more* shocks than animals in the first group, yet they developed much *less* learned fear.

Rescorla showed that the degree of learning in this sort of situation depended on the proportion of trials where the tone and shock were paired. Indeed, if enough shock-alone trials are given, animals that are also given the same number of paired tone-shock trials as the original group will not learn any fear at all. Rescorla stressed that the key underlying requirement for associative learning is *contingency*. The degree of learning that occurs depends on the probability or contingency that two events will occur together, it is contingent on the proportion of times they are associated. Simple contiguity, although necessary, is not sufficient to account for learning.

Pavlovian conditioning is perhaps the most basic aspect of associative learning. In general terms it is a process by which an organism benefits from experience so that its future behavior is better adapted to its environment. In more specific terms, it is the way organisms, including human beings, learn about causal relationships in the world. It results from exposure to relations among events in the environment. To quote Rescorla, "Such learning is a primary means by which the organism represents the structure of its world" (1988, p. 152). Viewed in this way, Pavlovian conditioning is a basic aspect of complex, cognitive learning. For both modern Pavlovian and cognitive views of learning and memory (see below), the individual learns a representation of the causal structure of the world and adjusts this representation through experience to bring it into tune with the real causal structure of the world, striving to reduce any discrepancies or errors between its internal representation and external reality.

Much of the learning that birds and mammals do is associative. Learning occurs most readily when it has adaptive consequences, such as obtaining food or avoiding injury. This is often termed "ecological validity". There are clear biological constraints on what can be learned. In the wild, a rat's world resembles mazes, and rats learn a maze very well in the laboratory, especially if it leads to food or away from punishment. Pigeons readily learn to peck a key to obtain grain, a behavior very much like pecking grain itself. Rats cannot learn to peck and pigeons are poor maze learners. Human beings learn language naturally but no other species does so.

A striking example of biologically adaptive learning is *taste aversion learning*. This phenomenon was well known to sheep farmers. They would leave a poisoned sheep carcass out for the wolves to eat. Wolves that did not die became violently ill and thereafter would never attack sheep. Taste aversion learning was first brought into the laboratory by John Garcia (e.g., Garcia and Brett, 1977). He allowed rats to taste a distinctive solution they normally like, such as saccharin, and then induced sickness, either by radiation or by injecting lithium chloride. After this experience the animals avoided saccharin as though it were poison. The most remarkable aspect of this phenomenon is that the CS (taste of saccharin) can precede the US (sickness) by over an hour or more. Somehow, this association is formed over a very long period.

Another form of classical conditioning using an aversive stimulus can lead to the adaptation of a discrete movement or a motor reflex into a precisely timed, conditioned motor response to a CS. The most widely studied example is delay conditioning of the eye-blink reflex which results from the presentation of a neutral stimulus, such as a tone or light, that precedes and co-terminates with a reflex-eliciting stimulus such as a puff of air to the cornea. Extensive investigation into the neural substrates of this associative memory has resulted in perhaps the most complete description of mammalian memory formation to date (see Thompson and Kim, 1996; Kim and Thompson, 1997; Stanton, 2000; Steinmetz, 2000; Christian and Thompson, 2003 for reviews).

Recording neuronal action potentials actually implicated two brain systems in eye-blink conditioning: hippocampus and cerebellum. In each structure, learning induced an increased pattern of spike discharges that preceded the CR in time and formed a predictive amplitude-time course model of the behavioral CR (Berger et al., 1976; McCormick and Thompson, 1984). In the standard delay procedure, lesions of the hippocampus do not impair the learned response whereas lesions of the cerebellar interpositus (IP) nucleus do. However, in the trace conditioning procedure, where a period of no stimulation intervenes between CS offset and US onset, both hippocampal and cerebellar lesions are critical. We treat trace conditioning later in this chapter.

Regardless of the training procedure, the cerebellum and its associated circuitry is essential for both learning and memory of the eyeblink-CR, and to the extent tested, other discrete responses like limb flexion as well, learned with an aversive US. The well-delineated circuitry, as shown in Fig. 2.2, includes the afferent sensory pathways, efferent motor pathways, and the sites of memory formation and storage within the cerebellum. Sensory information related to the CS (tone, light, etc.) is relayed to the cerebellum via mossy fibers from the pontine nuclei. Information related to the aversive US (corneal airpuff, extraorbital shock, etc.) is relayed via climbing fibers, axons of inferior olivary neurons. Mossy fibers and climbing fibers converge on the IP nucleus (IP), one of the deep nuclei within the cerebellum (and on neurons in cerebellar cortex). If the IP is lesioned prior

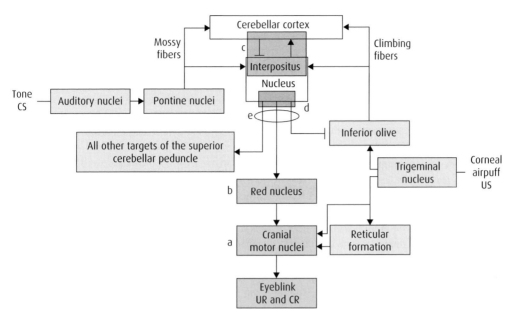

Figure 2.2. Highly simplified schematic of the cerebellar memory circuit. Shaded regions (a)–(e) indicate areas that have been inactivated during training. Only inactivation of the dorsal IP (c) blocks learning. Inactivation of other regions, including the ventral IP (d) block expression of the CR but not acquisition, demonstrating a highly localized region critical for learning the association between the CS and US. Modified from Thompson and Krupa (1994).

to training, the animal will be unable to form the association between the two stimuli and conditioning will not occur. If the IP is lesioned after training, the animal will no longer be able to express CRs, nor is there any recovery of the memory, even with extensive postlesion training. Stimulation of the appropriate region of the IP will result in an eyeblink, illustrating a hard-wired path from appropriate cerebellar activation to the overt behavioral response.

Reversible inactivation of the IP during training completely prevents learning, demonstrating that structures afferent to the cerebellum do not contain any behaviorally significant portion of the memory trace. Inactivation of structures efferent to the cerebellum prevent expression of learning but once the inactivation is removed, the memory trace appears intact suggesting that the critical brain regions in the formation of this associative memory are restricted to the cerebellum.

Important direct evidence for a strengthening of the mossy fiber – IP neuron synapses has been presented by Kleim et al. (2002), using eyeblink conditioning in the rat. They demonstrated a highly significant increase in the number of excitatory synapses in the IP nucleus but no change in inhibitory synapses following eyeblink conditioning, compared to unpaired stimulation control animals.

In sum, the evidence is now very strong from behavioral, physiological, pharmacological, and anatomical studies that the basic associative memory trace in eyeblink conditioning is established in the IP nucleus. The next step is to elucidate the causal chain from behavioral training to increased synaptic efficacy and synapse formation.

CS and US information also converge on Purkinje cells of the cerebellar cortex. Purkinje cells constitute the sole output of the cerebellar cortex and exert tonic inhibition on the deep nuclei, including the IP. Cerebellar learning theories (Marr, 1969; Albus, 1971) proposed plasticity, in the form of either long-term depression (LTD) or facilitation, at the synapses onto the Purkinje cells from parallel fibers that carry the

CS-related information from the pontine mossy fibers. A reduction in synaptic efficacy would result in a transient disinhibition of the IP, leading to a well-timed CR. Theoretical predictions of such plasticity received empirical support following identification of LTD produced by conjunctive activation of Purkinje cells by climbing and parallel fibers (Ito and Kano, 1982). While the extent and nature of the contribution of the cerebellar cortex to the formation of the memory trace have yet to be fully described, it appears that this plasticity complements plasticity in the IP to facilitate the acquisition of this associative memory (Chen et al., 1996; Bao et al., 2002).

Classical eyeblink conditioning is perhaps the best understood example of memory formation in a mammalian system. And while much work remains to be done to understand the cellular and molecular mechanisms that drive this cerebellar circuit, the investigative strategy that resulted in the methodical mapping of the neural structures and systems responsible for a simple form of non-declarative associative memory makes it a model for the exploration of the neural basis for more complex forms of learning and memory. Insights gleaned from this research, initially conducted in rabbits, appear to be applicable to all species thus far studied, including mice, rats and human beings. Patients with damage to the critical regions of the cerebellum have difficulty learning this association (Solomon et al., 1989; Daum et al., 1993; McGlinchey-Berroth et al., 1995). Imaging studies of healthy subjects show activation of the IP and cerebellar cortex during expression of this associative memory consistent with results from the animal experimental literature (Molchan et al., 1994; Logan and Grafton, 1995; Lemieux and Woodruff-Pak, 2000).

In a revealing series of studies by Diana Woodruff-Pak, performance on a classical eyeblink-conditioning task was significantly impaired in Alzheimer's patients compared to that of age-matched controls, a result that may involve the hippocampus (see below). Interestingly, several control subjects that showed impaired learning developed symptoms of Alzheimer's within a few years of the initial study suggesting that performance on this learning task

may have diagnostic properties and provide one of the first indications of cognitive decline associated with the onset of Alzheimer's disease (Woodruff-Pak, 2001). It is clear that the understanding gained through properly controlled experiments in animals can result in a viable model of memory formation that has direct parallels in human beings and may lead to significant clinical applications.

Fear conditioning

As just described, some of the clearest evidence for the neural localization of an essential memory trace has come from studies involving classical eyeblink conditioning. Another extensively investigated form of Pavlovian learning utilizes fear conditioning in the rat as a model system of aversive emotional memory. Fear in most cases represents the perception and recognition of danger, the learning and remembering of a dangerous experience and the coordination of defensive behaviors to an environmental threat (Fanselow and Gale, 2003). The expression of fear in the rat involves the synchronization of the defensive reactions which include autonomic increases in blood pressure, respiration and heart rate, neuroendocrine glucocorticoid release, behavioral immobilization or freezing and potentiated startle. Here, we will focus on studies measuring fear as freezing in response to discrete stimuli.

In a typical delay fear-conditioning procedure a rat is presented with a tone CS of several seconds during which a footshock US is administered. Following repeated pairings the tone comes to elicit conditioned freezing. Interestingly, as will be discussed later in more detail, re-exposure to the original training context alone is sufficient to trigger conditioned fear. Work in a number of laboratories (Michael Davis, Joseph LeDoux, Michael Fanselow and Stephen Maren) using lesioning, pharmacological and electrophysiological techniques demonstrates that the amygdala is essential for the acquisition, storage, and expression of conditioned fear.

Anatomical evidence reveals that both CS and US afferents converge on the amygdala. Lesions of the amygdala prevent the acquisition of conditioned fear to all CS modalities (tone, light and odor) (Davis, 1992; LeDoux et al., 1990; Maren and Fanselow, 1996). Lesions limited to medial geniculate nucleus, an afferent of the amygdala, block the acquisition of conditioned fear to a tone, but leave conditioning to light intact, suggesting that the amygdala is not part of the sensory pathway in the formation of a memory trace (LeDoux et al., 1986). Furthermore, in untrained animals, amygdala specific infusions of N-methyl-D-aspartate (NMDA) receptor antagonist AP5 prevent the acquisition of conditioned fear, whereas similar infusions in a well-trained animal show little effect (Maren et al., 1996). Alternatively, appropriate lesions of the amygdala in the well-trained animal completely and permanently abolish the expression of all forms of conditioned fear (freezing, tachycardia, respiration and blood pressure) (Maren, 2001).

Lesions of the periaqueductal gray, an amygdala efferent, selectively abolish the expression of conditioned freezing while leaving conditioned increases in blood pressure unaffected, whereas lesions in the hypothalamus abolish conditioned cardiovascular responses but do not prevent learned freezing, suggesting that the amygdala is not part of the motor output for the expression of a memory trace (LeDoux et al., 1988). Further, evidence using electrophysiological recordings of single amygdalar neurons reveals enhanced spike activity to acoustic stimuli following learning (Quirk et al., 1995). Together these studies strongly suggest that memory traces for conditioned fear are established and maintained in the amygdala.

Instrumental learning

The field concerned with possible brain substrates of instrumental learning is vast; there have been many thousands of studies over the 75 years since Karl Lashley began his search for the engram. A wide variety of different tasks have been used, ranging from one-trial passive avoidance to the operant procedures developed by B. F. Skinner at Harvard to maze learning and puzzle boxes.

The basic distinction between classical and instrumental conditioning is that in the latter, the animal or human controls the outcome. In instrumental avoidance learning, say a rat learning to press a lever in response to a tone CS, pressing the lever prior to the occurrence of the paw shock US prevents the US from occurring (in classical conditioning the shock US always occurs, regardless of what the animal does). In reward learning, for example, the rat learns to press a lever to obtain a food reward. The process of operant conditioning, developed by Skinner, simply involves the animal learning to make a response to obtain a reward. Skinner varied the schedules of reward and showed this had profoundly important effects on behavior. Indeed, operant techniques are very effective in dealing with severely disturbed patients.

Beginning with the extraordinary discovery by James Olds that animals would self-stimulate the reward circuit in the brain, we have learned a good deal about this circuitry (Kelley, 2004; Schultz, 2000). In brief, a system called the medial forebrain bundle projects dopamine containing neuron axons from the midbrain to forebrain structures, particularly the nucleus accumbens, the striatum and the prefrontal cortex. This system is activated by all types of rewarding stimuli, from food and water to sex. Importantly, this circuit, particularly the accumbens nucleus, is activated by all drugs of addiction. These drugs cause release of dopamine in the accumbens. Analysis of this reward-memory circuitry is a major field of research today. The dopamine projection to the striatum is of course essentially involved in Parkinson's disease and the projections to the prefrontal cortex and other higher brain regions are thought to be critically involved in schizophrenia.

Memory consolidation

The most interesting aspect of instrumental learning is the consolidation of memory. The consolidation story has two origins. In the 1940s Carl Duncan, working at Northwestern University, first made use of electroconvulsive shock (ECS) to impair memory (see Thompson, 2000). He trained rats in an instrumental avoidance task. The animals were on one side of a shuttle box, a box with a grid floor, two compartments and a connecting alley. When a light came on they had 10 s to cross to the other compartment or receive a foot shock from the grid floor. They were given one trial a day for 18 days. Control rats quickly learned the task, avoiding the shock on all but the first few days. Duncan ran a number of groups of experimental rats that received ECS (delivered through ear clips) at intervals ranging from 20 s to 14 h after each day's trial. The results were striking. Animals receiving ECS 20 s after each learning trial learned nothing at all. As the time between learning trials and ECS increased, the animals learned better and better, showing no memory impairment if the ECS came an hour or more after the training trial.

Duncan's result paralleled work in the field of psychiatry where patients with various forms of mental illness were given ECS treatments. ECS induces retrograde amnesia: events just prior to the ECS are forgotten. It has a gradient, the older the memory the better it is retained. But the gradient can be long. After a series of ECS treatments, patients may not be able to remember any of their experiences for a period of a year or more. Fortunately, most of these memories usually return, although the events immediately surrounding the ECS are usually not remembered. As with humans, so with rats.

Duncan's experiment began a large field of research. A number of possible explanations for the memory impairment were explored. Among the possibilities that were ruled out were that the ECS was strongly aversive (conditioned fear); that the ECS became conditioned to the apparatus (context-conditioned fear); that the body seizures were necessary. The fact that the ECS memory impairment also occurred when the ECS was given to anesthetized animals and humans seemed to rule out these possibilities. James McGaugh and his co-workers at the University of California at Irvine showed that the critical memory impairment could be obtained by disruptive electrical stimulation of the amygdala; seizures of the entire brain are not necessary.

The other origin of the memory consolidation story occurred early in the century in independent studies by Karl Lashley and Clark Hull, who showed that administration of strychnine or caffeine markedly improved maze-learning performance. Since they gave these substances before training, the effects could be more on the animals' performance than on memory. But McGaugh and others showed that the same memory facilitation occurred if the drugs were given shortly after training rather than before training. Possible rewarding effects of the drugs were also ruled out (see McGaugh, 2000).

Most recent work on memory facilitation has used simple one-trial learning procedures. Passive avoidance is a favorite. The animal is placed in a lighted compartment and allowed to step into a dark compartment (rats like the dark). But the grid in the dark compartment is electrified. After the animal receives a shock, it is removed. The next day it is placed in the lighted compartment and the time before it goes into the dark is measured: the longer the time, the better memory is presumed to be. This test by itself can be misinterpreted. For example, a sedative drug like a barbiturate that makes the animal inactive would produce a spurious memory. But other tests are also used, for example, active avoidance, the test Duncan used in his ECS study. Tasks involving food reward have also been used.

The bottom line in this work is that a wide range of drugs given after the learning experience can facilitate or impair subsequent memory performance in all these tasks, depending on the type of drug and the dose used. Earlier, it was thought that both ECS impairment and drug facilitation or impairment of memory acted on a specific brain process of consolidation, for example, circulating electrical activity in the brain that gradually stamped in memories. If this is so, then there ought to be a gradient of consolidation, a relatively fixed time period. However, there is no gradient, or rather there are many gradients, depending very much on the details of the procedure used in a particular experiment. This and other problems with the simple consolidation notion have led scientists to stress *modulation* rather than consolidation. Most workers in the field believe that ECS or drug administration modulates how well recent memories are stored in long-term memory.

Epinephrine (E) is among the most effective substances for memory facilitation, and it is of course an autonomic neurotransmitter and a critical hormone, released along with norepinephrine by the adrenal medulla in response to stress. In other words, in the real world we and other mammals tend to remember best those experiences that occur at times of arousal and moderate stress. This has been termed the "flashbulb" phenomenon – older readers will remember where they were and what they were doing when they learned that President Kennedy had been assassinated; younger readers will remember where they were when they experienced September 11, 2001 (actually, such memories are somewhat less than perfect). But we do remember best those events associated with a state of moderate arousal and stress.

2.3 Declarative memory

Human memory

Perhaps the most seminal work in advancing our understanding of human memory formation has been the striking clinical observations pioneered by Brenda Milner in the late 1950s (Scoville and Milner, 1957). A now famous patient, HM, had portions of his medial temporal lobe, including the hippocampus, removed bilaterally in an attempt to cure his severe epilepsy. While the epileptic foci were successfully removed, HM displayed a profound deficit in his ability to form new memories. Most of his long-term memories acquired previously – up to a period of about a year before the surgery – were intact but HM was completely incapable of creating new long-term memories both of his own experiences and facts about the world. In other words, he suffers from anterograde amnesia and an inability to form declarative memories. He has no conscious recollection of any experience from day to day. Each day, his doctors would introduce themselves and HM would report that he had not met them previously. Facts told to him are likewise inaccessible within a few minutes. HM's ability to form new non-declarative memories, however, was not compromised. He shows evidence

of priming effects and can learn motor skills and probability tasks at rates comparable to control subjects with no damage to the medial temporal lobe. The significance of this observation lies in the demonstrated dissociation of these two forms of memory at both the behavioral and anatomical levels. It is clear evidence that memory formation is not a unitary phenomenon but rather a collection of abilities that engage distinct neural systems, as we noted earlier.

The other profound implication of this observation results from the temporal dissociation of memory formation and storage. That HM's memories, formed before his surgery, were largely intact suggests that brain regions critical to memory formation may not be necessary for the later retrieval and expression of the memory. HM's memory in the year preceding the surgery was greatly affected, though, so the hippocampus and associated medial temporal lobe structures are likely to play a significant role for some period of time following initial acquisition of declarative memories but long-term storage may involve other brain structures. This temporally graded retrograde amnesia that leaves early memories intact has been observed in many patients (Zola-Morgan et al., 1986; Rempel-Clower et al., 1996; Reed and Squire, 1998; Bayley et al., 2003) but see Nadel and Moscovitch, 1997; Viskontas et al., 2000; Rosenbaum et al., 2001 for alternative views on the time-limited role of the hippocampus in memory formation.

Hippocampus: animal studies

In the years since the discovery of H M's dramatic and tragic memory impairment, there have been literally hundreds of animal studies attempting to produce HM's symptoms. The first seemingly successfully animal model of HM's amnesia was reported by Mishkin using monkeys in 1979. We will describe his work below. However, it is now clear that hippocampal damage in lower mammals does produce a number of deficits in memory-related performance and that neurons in the hippocampus show memory-related activity.

Rats are able to learn long sequences of odor discriminations. Work by Gary Lynch (1987) and his associates showed that rats can learn a very large number of odor discriminations in sequence, a possible example of semantic memory? Although hippocampal lesions do not prevent the rats from learning odor discrimination, their ability to learn a long sequence is impaired, as is their ability to reverse discriminations (i.e., learn to respond to odors they first learned not to respond to).

Howard Eichenbaum and his associates (e.g., Dusek and Eichenbaum, 1997) asked rats to master even more difficult aspects of odor learning where they had to infer an association between the two odors. Hippocampal lesions did not prevent the animal from learning the series of odor associations but completely prevented the animals from inferring associations they had not directly learned. Eichenbaum likens this type of impairment to human amnesia in that the rats with hippocampal damage do not show flexible associations. These studies, incidentally, show that the humble rat is capable of very complex associative learning.

John O'Keefe and John Dostrovsky (1971) at the University College, London made a startling discovery while recording from single pyramidal neurons of the hippocampus of freely moving rats. They noted that when the animal traveled down a runway, a given neuron would start firing only when the rat moved passed a specific "place" in the runway. These "place" cells, further identified in experiments recording from a large number of neurons, could encode the entire environment of the rat. Perhaps most striking were experiment by Bruce McNaughton and Carol Barnes and collaborators at the University of Arizona recording from up to 120 pyramidal neurons at a single time demonstrating place fields for each cell overlapped in a given environment providing a robust and stable map of animals environment (Barnes et al., 1990). This organization was so reliable that they were able to predict solely on firing pattern of specific "place" cells the spatial location of the rat. But, what role if any do "place" cell of hippocampus have in learning and memory. It is clear that lesions of the hippocampus disrupt spatial memory tasks such as learning to navigate a maze or water maze (Morris et al., 1982). In the water maze task a rat must swim in a circular pool of milk and water, and find the location of a hidden platform, situated just below the surface of liquid. Positioned around the perimeter of the pool are specific stimuli, which the rat can use to get their bearings. To test the rat's memory for the hidden platform the rat is placed back in the pool again to find the position of the platform. Rats with hippocampal lesions spend more time swimming aimlessly.

Trace conditioning

Trace-conditioning procedures provide interesting examples of "simple" procedural learning that also engage the declarative memory system. In eyeblink conditioning, introduction of a 500–1000-ms trace between the CS offset and US onset is more difficult to learn than a delay paradigm with a comparable interstimulus interval, as evidenced by a slower rate and lower level of CR acquisition in the trace paradigm (Solomon and Groccia-Ellison, 1996). Damage to medial temporal structures including the hippocampus in human studies is associated with marked impairments in trace eyeblink conditioning (McGlinchey-Berroth et al., 1997, 1999). As noted earlier, in rabbits lesions specific to the hippocampus prevent the acquisition and expression of trace-conditioned eyeblink responses, without affecting delay CRs (Solomon et al., 1986; Moyer et al., 1990).

If animals are first trained in the trace procedure, large bilateral hippocampal lesions made immediately after training completely abolish the trace eyeblink CR (such lesions have little effect on the delay CR). However, if the same lesions are made a month after training they do not impair the trace CR at all (Kim et al., 1995).

Hippocampal lesions thus impair subsequent trace conditioning (anterograde amnesia) and show time-limited impairment of prior trace conditioning (retrograde amnesia), the hallmarks of damage to the hippocampal-medial temporal lobe declarative memory system. In recent human studies performance on long trace interval eyeblink conditioning is correlated with the subjects' awareness of the training procedure (Clark and Squire, 1998; Manns et al., 2000a, b; see Clark et al., 2000 for review). Thus trace conditioning may provide an elementary animal model of declarative memory.

In a most interesting series of morphological studies, Geinisman and associates (2000, 2001) reported learning-induced changes in hippocampal synapses in rabbit CA1 stratum radiation following trace eyeblink conditioning. Using unbiased stereological methods, they compared tissue from trace versus control animals and found that:

1 The total number of synapses did not change.
2 The area of postsynaptic density was increased in axospinous non-perforated synapses.
3 The number of multiple-synapse boutons was increased.

In remarkable recent work, Shors, Gould and associates explored the fate of new adult-generated neurons in the hippocampal dentate gyrus in trace and delay eyeblink conditioning in the rat (Gould et al., 1999a, b; Shors et al., 2001). New neurons were labeled with a thymidine analog injection 1 week before training; delay and trace groups were given the same number of trials and both learned in the same number of trials and both learned in the same asymptote. The trace procedure resulted in a significantly and substantially higher number of new neurons in the dentate gyrus compared to the delay and control conditions. Similar results were found for Morris watermaze: an increase in number of neurons in spatial versus visual cue tasks. Further, injection of a toxin for proliferating cells (methylazoxy methanol acetate, MAM) markedly impaired trace but not delay eyeblink acquisition. These results raise the possibility that new adult-generated neurons may play a role in trace memory formation in the hippocampus.

Another example of a hippocampal-dependent trace paradigm is trace fear conditioning where a tone is separated for several seconds from the presentation of an aversive footshock. McEchron and colleagues (1998) demonstrated that appropriate lesions of the hippocampus prevent the acquisition of trace-conditioned fear. Further, mutant mice completely void of hippocampal NMDA receptors are impaired in learning trace fear responses (Heurta et al., 2000).

Conversely, if lesions are made specifically to the dorsal hippocampus following conditioning the expression of trace-conditioned fear is severely attenuated (Quinn et al., 2002). Similarly, fear conditioning to specific places or contexts, just as with a trace paradigm, is critically dependent upon the hippocampus. Contextual fear-conditioning procedures typically involve placing a rat in a novel training box for a fixed period of time then delivering a series of spaced footshocks. The following day the rat is returned to the original context (without shocks) and the total amount of time the rat freezes is recorded as an index of contextual fear conditioning. Lesions of the amygdala abolish all forms of conditioned fear including Pavlovian fear conditioning to context. However, unlike delay-conditioned fear, lesions of the hippocampus prevent the acquisition and expression of contextual-fear conditioning, as is true for trace conditioning. Lesions of the hippocampus made a day after conditioning completely abolished conditioned fear to context, whereas lesions made 28 days later had no effect on this conditioned fear (Kim and Fanselow, 1992).

A primate model

Mortimer Mishkin at the National Institute of Mental Health, reported in 1978 that bilateral removal of the hippocampus and related structures in the temporal lobe in the monkey caused amnesia that resembled HM's syndrome. Mishkin trained monkeys to perform a simple short-term visual recognition memory task. A monkey is first presented with a single small block or toy covering a food well that contains a peanut. The monkey reaches out and displaces the object and gets the peanut. After a delay period a screen is placed in front of the monkey so that it cannot see the objects, another tray is presented to the monkey with the old object and a new object each covering a food well, but only the well under the new object has a peanut. In the following trials with different objects, the monkey must learn the principle of always selecting the new object; of course the monkey must remember which was the old object. Monkeys learn this task well. It is called the *delayed*

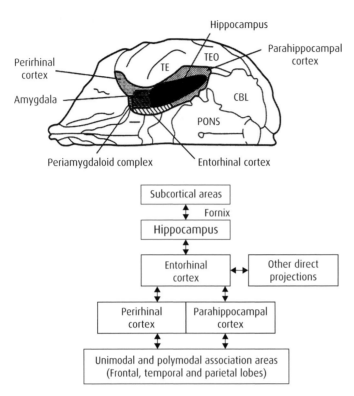

Figure 2.3. The primate declarative memory system. A ventral view of the monkey brain hemisphere showing regions critical for declarative memory. The hippocampus is solid black. The amygdala is represented by the square-shaped plaid region and does not appear to be involved in this form of memory. Other shaded regions and the hippocampus proper are integral to declarative memory. Destruction of these regions impairs declarative memory (e.g., delayed non-matching to sample) in proportion to the amount of tissue destroyed. CBL: cerebellum; TE, TEO: temporal lobe visual association areas. Adapted from Squire and Zola-Morgan (1988).

non-matching to sample task (interestingly, the *delayed matching to sample task*, where the animals are required each time to choose the old object, is more difficult). Delayed non-matching to sample was much impaired, particularly with long delays, by lesions of the temporal lobe.

The effective bilateral lesion in Mishkin's study included the hippocampus, the amygdala and cortical areas of the medial temporal lobe (see Fig. 2.3). In subsequent studies done by Mishkin's group, and by Larry Squire and Stuart Zola it became clear that the amygdala is not involved in object recognition but that the cortical areas adjacent to the hippocampus (Fig. 2.3) are very important, as is the hippocampus (Squire, 1987; Zola-Morgan and Squire, 1993). The more of these structures removed, the worse the impairment in object recognition memory. The same is true in humans with medial temporal lobe damage; the more damage to the structures, the worse the

amnesia, a remarkable agreement of the human and monkey brain functions in memory.

Neocortex

Many researchers have looked to the neocortex as the prime candidate for the permanent storage of declarative memories but there is limited evidence at this point to demonstrate this with certainty. It is important to contrast the proposed time-limited involvement of medial temporal lobe structures in the formation of declarative memories with structures such as the cerebellum, which is required for the formation, expression, and long-term permanent retention of associative non-declarative memories resulting from classical delay conditioning of reflexes. Following initial acquisition, neural substrates must be investigated throughout the temporal extent of the resultant memory.

Evidence to support neocortical storage of semantic memory (memory for facts about the world) has come from reports of remarkably specific deficits in some patients with frontal and temporal lobe damage to identify particular categories of objects. The most commonly observed deficits are for living versus non-living things (Warrington and Shallice, 1984; Hart et al., 1985). Selective deficits for non-living things (Warrington and McCarthy, 1987; Hillis and Caramazza, 1991; Moss and Tyler, 2000) have also been observed suggesting a double dissociation and a broad categorical distinction that may have a physical basis. This phenomenon is complicated by even more specific deficits that are seen in patients unable to identify manufactured items such as tools (Tranel et al., 1997) or the inability to name most living things but retention of the ability to name body parts (Gainotti et al., 1995), or a selective deficit in naming living things and musical instruments (Dixon et al., 2000).

This fascinating area of research has important implications for the study of memory storage in the neocortex. It is still not clear how category-specific deficits occur and whether an anatomical basis for broad categorical semantic distinctions can even be identified. Furthermore, it is unknown whether the proposed categories can be generalized across subjects or whether repositories of semantic knowledge depend critically on individual experience and familiarity with the objects. Mode of interaction with the object and modality specific sensory acquisition of knowledge about objects may also mediate the ultimate storage sites. In other words, if the primary means of attaining information about an object is through the visual system, then cortical visual areas may be preferentially involved in either the retrieval or expression of memory about that object.

Specificity of neocortical sites for memory storage and retrieval has been observed in imaging studies of healthy patients. Some studies report the categorical dissociations as discussed above (Damasio et al., 1996). Other reports describe specificity in terms of the form of memory being encoded or recalled. Most evidence demonstrates prefrontal and parietal (and cerebellar) activation during working memory tasks,

prefrontal and temporal cortical activation correlated with semantic memory, prefrontal, frontal and medial temporal region activity associated with episodic memory encoding and retrieval, parietal and motor cortex and basal ganglia involvement in non-declarative skill learning, and visual association cortex activity during priming memory tasks (Gabrieli 1998; Schacter et al., 1998). There is ongoing debate about the degree of lateralization in these proposed centers of activity and the exact substrates of these memory processes. Much ambiguity exists due to a lack of consistency in the tasks performed by the subjects and the lack of standardization in data analysis but some of these issues should be resolved as the field of functional brain imaging matures.

2.4 Conclusion

The collaborative efforts of many investigators concerned with understanding learning and memory has led to remarkable progress in describing the neural substrates of these most important abilities. However, the critical neural circuitry has yet to be described for most forms of memory nor is there a complete understanding of the mechanisms involved. Nevertheless, we know that the brain undergoes tremendous plasticity in adult mammals and that the differentiation of new neurons may be functionally relevant to the acquisition of some learned behaviors. The brain can compensate for the loss of individual neurons and some of the modest physical effects of aging but there appear to be critical thresholds of damage beyond which the neural systems cannot recover. Strategies for clinical rehabilitation are designed on many levels, from the complete replacement of damaged structures through silicon-based implants to pharmaceutical remedies targeting key molecular events. All of these approaches will benefit from, and will likely require, a deeper understanding of the compromised behavior, the associated circuitry, systems-level information processing, and the cellular and molecular mechanisms. Clinical observations have led to the development of animal models in which many of these processes can be explored systematically. Relevant findings can then be used to revise current models of memory formation, and predictions can be tested through imaging and behavioral studies in human beings, providing the essential foundation for neural rehabilitation efforts.

ACKNOWLEDGEMENTS

Work described in this chapter was supported in part by National Science Foundation Grant IBN-9215069 and funds from the University of Southern California.

REFERENCES

Albus, J.S. (1971). A theory of cerebellar function. *Math Biosci*, **10**, 25–61.

Bao, S., Chen, L., et al. (2002). Cerebellar cortical inhibition and classical eyeblink conditioning. *Proc Natl Acad Sci USA*, **99**(3), 1592–1597.

Barnes, C.A., McNaughton, B.L., et al. (1990). Comparison of spatial and temporal characteristics of neuronal activity in sequential stages of hippocampal processing. *Prog Brain Res*, **83**, 287–300.

Bayley, P.J., Hopkins, R.O., et al. (2003). Successful recollection of remote autobiographical memories by amnesic patients with medial temporal lobe lesions. *Neuron*, **38**(1), 135–144.

Berger, T.W., Alger, B., et al. (1976). Neuronal substrate of classical conditioning in the hippocampus. *Science*, **192**(4238), 483–485.

Carew, T.J. and Sahley, C.L. (1986). Invertebrate learning and memory: from behavior to molecules. *Annu Rev Neurosci*, **9**, 435–487.

Chen, L., Bao, S., et al. (1996). Impaired classical eyeblink conditioning in cerebellar-lesioned and Purkinje cell degeneration (pcd) mutant mice. *J Neurosci*, **16**(8), 2829–2838.

Christian, K.M. and Thompson, R.F. (2003). Neural substrates of eyeblink conditioning: acquisition and retention. *Learn Mem*, **10**(6), 427–455.

Clark, R.E., Manns, J.R., et al. (2002). Classical conditioning, awareness, and brain systems. *Trend Cogn Sci*, **6**(12), 524–531.

Clark, R.E. and Squire, L.R. (1998). Classical conditioning and brain systems: the role of awareness. *Science*, **280**(5360), 77–81.

Damasio, H., Grabowski, T.J., et al. (1996). A neural basis for lexical retrieval. *Nature*, **380**(6574), 499–505.

Daum, I., Schugens, M.M., et al. (1993). Classical conditioning after cerebellar lesions in humans. *Behav Neurosci*, **107**(5), 748–756.

Davis, M. (1992). The role of the amygdala in fear and anxiety. *Annu Rev Neurosci*, **15**, 353–375.

Dixon, M.J., Piskopos, M., et al. (2000). Musical instrument naming impairments: the crucial exception to the living/nonliving dichotomy in category-specific agnosia. *Brain Cogn*, **43**(1–3), 158–164.

Dusek, J.A. and Eichenbaum, H. (1997). The hippocampus and memory for orderly stimulus relations. *Proc Natl Acad Sci USA*, **94**(13), 7109–7114.

Fanselow, M.S. and Gale, G.D. (2003). The amygdala, fear, and memory. *Ann N Y Acad Sci*, **985**, 125–134.

Gabrieli, J.D. (1998). Cognitive neuroscience of human memory. *Annu Rev Psychol*, **49**, 87–115.

Gainotti, G., Silveri, M.C., et al. (1995). Neuroanatomical correlates of category-specific semantic disorders: a critical survey. *Memory*, **3**(3–4), 247–264.

Garcia, J. and Brett, L.P. (1977). Conditioned responses to food odor and taste in rats and wild predators. *The Chemical Senses and Nutrition* (ed. Kare, M.), Academic Press, New York, pp. 277–289.

Geinisman, Y. (2000). Structural synaptic modifications associated with hippocampal LTP and behavioral learning. *Cereb Cortex*, **10**(10), 952–962.

Geinisman, Y., Berry, R.W., et al. (2001). Associative learning elicits the formation of multiple-synapse boutons. *J Neurosci*, **21**(15), 5568–5573.

Geinisman, Y., Disterhoft, J.F., et al. (2000). Remodeling of hippocampal synapses after hippocampus-dependent associative learning. *J Comp Neurol*, **417**(1), 49–59.

Gould, E., Beylin, A., et al. (1999). Learning enhances adult neurogenesis in the hippocampal formation. *Nat Neurosci*, **2**(3), 260–265.

Gould, E., Tanapat, P., et al. (1999). Neurogenesis in adulthood: a possible role in learning. *Trend Cogn Sci*, **3**(5), 186–192.

Groves, P.M. and Thompson, R.F. (1970). Habituation: a dual-process theory. *Psychol Rev*, **77**(5), 419–450.

Hart Jr. J., Berndt, R.S., et al. (1985). Category-specific naming deficit following cerebral infarction. *Nature*, **316**(6027), 439–440.

Hillis, A.E. and Caramazza, A. (1991). Category-specific naming and comprehension impairment: a double dissociation. *Brain*, **114**(Pt 5), 2081–2094.

Ito, M. and Kano, M. (1982). Long-lasting depression of parallel fiber-Purkinje cell transmission induced by conjunctive stimulation of parallel fibers and climbing fibers in the cerebellar cortex. *Neurosci Lett*, **33**(3), 253–258.

Keane, M.M., Gabrieli, J.D., et al. (1994). Priming in perceptual identification of pseudowords is normal in Alzheimer's disease. *Neuropsychologia*, **32**(**3**), 343–356.

Keane, M.M., Gabrieli, J.D., et al. (1995). Double dissociation of memory capacities after bilateral occipital-lobe or medial temporal-lobe lesions. *Brain*, **118** (**Pt 5**), 1129–1148.

Kelley, A.E. (2004). Ventral striatal control of appetitive motivation: role in ingestive behavior and reward-related learning. *Neurosci Biobehav Rev*, **27**, 765–776.

Kim, J.J. and Fanselow, M.S. (1992). Modality-specific retrograde amnesia of fear. *Science*, **256**(**5057**), 675–677.

Kim, J.J. and Thompson, R.F. (1997). Cerebellar circuits and synaptic mechanisms involved in classical eyeblink conditioning. *Trend Neurosci*, **20**(**4**), 177–181.

Kim, J.J., Clark, R.E., et al. (1995). Hippocampectomy impairs the memory of recently, but not remotely, acquired trace eyeblink conditioned responses. *Behav Neurosci*, **109**(**2**), 195–203.

Kleim, J.A., Freeman Jr., J.H., et al. (2002). Synapse formation is associated with memory storage in the cerebellum. *Proc Natl Acad Sci USA*, **99**(**20**), 13228–13231.

Knowlton, B.J., Squire, L.R., et al. (1994). Probabilistic category learning in amnesia. *Learn Mem*, **1**, 106–120.

LeDoux, J.E., Cicchetti, P., et al. (1990). The lateral amygdaloid nucleus: sensory interface of the amygdala in fear conditioning. *J Neurosci*, **10**(**4**), 1062–1069.

LeDoux, J.E., Iwata, J., et al. (1988). Different projections of the central amygdaloid nucleus mediate autonomic and behavioral correlates of conditioned fear. *J Neurosci*, **8**(**7**), 2517–2529.

LeDoux, J.E., Sakaguchi, A., et al. (1986). Interruption of projections from the medial geniculate body to an archineostriatal field disrupts the classical conditioning of emotional responses to acoustic stimuli. *Neuroscience*, **17**(**3**), 615–627.

Lemieux, S.K. and Woodruff-Pak, D.S. (2000). Functional MRI studies of eyeblink classical conditioning. *Eyeblink Classical Conditioning: Applications in Humans* (eds Woodruff-Pak, D.S. and Steinmetz, J.E.), Vol. 1. Kluwer Academic Publishers, Boston, pp. 71–93.

Logan, C.G. and Grafton, S.T. (1995). Functional anatomy of human eyeblink conditioning determined with regional cerebral glucose metabolism and positron-emission tomography. *Proc Natl Acad Sci USA*, **92**(**16**), 7500–7504.

Lynch, G. (1987). *Synapses, Circuits, and the Beginnings of Memory*, MIT Press, Cambridge, MA.

Manns, J.R., Clark, R.E., et al. (2000a). Awareness predicts the magnitude of single-cue trace eyeblink conditioning. *Hippocampus*, **10**(**2**), 181–186.

Manns, J.R., Clark, R.E., et al. (2000b). Parallel acquisition of awareness and trace eyeblink classical conditioning. *Learn Mem*, **7**(**5**), 267–272.

Maren, S. (2001). Neurobiology of Pavlovian fear conditioning. *Annu Rev Neurosci*, **24**, 897–931.

Maren, S., Aharonov, G., et al. (1996). *N*-methyl-D-aspartate receptors in the basolateral amygdala are required for both acquisition and expression of conditional fear in rats. *Behav Neurosci*, **110**(**6**), 1365–1374.

Maren, S. and Fanselow, M.S. (1996). The amygdala and fear conditioning: has the nut been cracked? *Neuron*, **16**(**2**), 237–240.

Marr, D. (1969). A theory of cerebellar cortex. *J Physiol*, **202**(**2**), 437–470.

McCormick, D.A. and Thompson, R.F. (1984). Cerebellum: essential involvement in the classically conditioned eyelid response. *Science*, **223**(**4633**), 296–299.

McEchron, M.D., Bouwmeester, H., et al. (1998). Hippocampectomy disrupts auditory trace fear conditioning and contextual fear conditioning in the rat. *Hippocampus*, **8**(**6**), 638–646.

McGaugh, J.L. (2000). Memory – a century of consolidation. *Science*, **287**(**5451**), 248–251.

McGlinchey-Berroth, R., Cermak, L.S., et al. (1995). Impaired delay eyeblink conditioning in amnesic Korsakoff's patients and recovered alcoholics. *Alcohol Clin Exp Res*, **19**(**5**), 1127–1132.

McGlinchey-Berroth, R., Carrillo, M.C., et al. (1997). Impaired trace eyeblink conditioning in bilateral, medial-temporal lobe amnesia. *Behav Neurosci*, **111**(**5**), 873–882.

McGlinchey-Berroth, R., Brawn, C., et al. (1999). Temporal discrimination learning in severe amnesic patients reveals an alteration in the timing of eyeblink conditioned responses. *Behav Neurosci*, **113**(**1**), 10–18.

Mishkin, M. (1978). Memory in monkeys severely impaired by combined but not by separate removal of amygdala and hippocampus. *Nature*, **273**(**5660**), 297–298.

Molchan, S.E., Sunderland, T., et al. (1994). A functional anatomical study of associative learning in humans. *Proc Natl Acad Sci USA*, **91**(**17**), 8122–8126.

Morris, R.G., Garrud, P., et al. (1982). Place navigation impaired in rats with hippocampal lesions. *Nature*, **297**(**5868**), 681–683.

Moss, H.E. and Tyler, L.K. (2000). A progressive category-specific semantic deficit for non-living things. *Neuropsychologia*, **38**(**1**), 60–82.

Moyer Jr., J.R., Deyo, R.A., et al. (1990). Hippocampectomy disrupts trace eye-blink conditioning in rabbits. *Behav Neurosci*, **104**(**2**), 243–252.

Nadel, L. and Moscovitch, M. (1997). Memory consolidation, retrograde amnesia and the hippocampal complex. *Curr Opin Neurobiol*, **7**(**2**), 217–227.

O'Keefe, J. and Dostrovsky, J. (1971). The hippocampus as a spatial map. Preliminary evidence from unit activity in the freely-moving rat. *Brain Res*, **34**(**1**), 171–175.

Packard, M.G. and Knowlton, B.J. (2002). Learning and memory functions of the basal ganglia. *Annu Rev Neurosci*, **25**, 563–593.

Pavlov, I.P. (1927). *Conditioned Reflexes: An Investigation of the Physiological Activity of the Cerebral Cortex*, Oxford University Press, London.

Pittenger, C. and Kandel, E.R. (2003). In search of general mechanisms for long-lasting plasticity: aplysia and the hippocampus. *Philos Trans R Soc Lond B Biol Sci*, **358**(**1432**), 757–763.

Poldrack, R.A. and Packard, M.G. (2003). Competition among multiple memory systems: converging evidence from animal and human brain studies. *Neuropsychologia*, **41**(**3**), 245–251.

Poldrack, R.A., Clark, J., et al. (2001). Interactive memory systems in the human brain. *Nature*, **414**(**6863**), 546–550.

Quinn, J.J., Oommen, S.S., et al. (2002). Post-training excitotoxic lesions of the dorsal hippocampus attenuate forward trace, backward trace, and delay fear conditioning in a temporally specific manner. *Hippocampus*, **12**(**4**), 495–504.

Quirk, G.J., Repa, C., et al. (1995). Fear conditioning enhances short-latency auditory responses of lateral amygdala neurons: parallel recordings in the freely behaving rat. *Neuron*, **15**(**5**), 1029–1039.

Reber, P.J., Knowlton, B.J., et al. (1996). Dissociable properties of memory systems: differences in the flexibility of declarative and nondeclarative knowledge. *Behav Neurosci*, **110**(**5**), 861–871.

Reed, J.M. and Squire, L.R. (1998). Retrograde amnesia for facts and events: findings from four new cases. *J Neurosci*, **18**(**10**), 3943–3954.

Rempel-Clower, N.L., Zola, S.M., et al. (1996). Three cases of enduring memory impairment after bilateral damage limited to the hippocampal formation. *J Neurosci*, **16**(**16**), 5233–5255.

Rescorla, R.A. (1988). Pavlovian conditioning. It's not what you think it is. *Am Psychol*, **43**(**3**), 151–160.

Rosenbaum, R.S., Winocur, G., et al. (2001). New views on old memories: re-evaluating the role of the hippocampal complex. *Behav Brain Res*, **127**(**1–2**), 183–197.

Samuelsson, S., Bogges, T.R., et al. (2000). Visual implicit memory deficit and developmental surface dyslexia: a case of early occipital damage. *Cortex*, **36**(**3**), 365–376.

Schacter, D.L., Buckner, R.L., et al. (1998). Memory, consciousness and neuroimaging. *Philos Trans R Soc Lond B Biol Sci*, **353**(**1377**), 1861–1878.

Schacter, D.L., Chiu, C.Y., et al. (1993). Implicit memory: a selective review. *Annu Rev Neurosci*, **16**, 159–182.

Schultz, W. (2000). Multiple reward signals in the brain. *Nat Rev Neurosci*, **1**(**3**), 199–207.

Scoville, W.B. and Milner, B. (1957). Loss of recent memory after bilateral hippocampal lesions. *J Neurochem*, **20**(**1**), 11–21.

Shors, T.J., Miesegaes, G., et al. (2001). Neurogenesis in the adult is involved in the formation of trace memories. *Nature*, **410**(**6826**), 372–376.

Solomon, P.R. and Groccia-Ellison, M.E. (1996). Classic conditioning in aged rabbits: delay, trace, and long-delay conditioning. *Behav Neurosci*, **110**(**3**), 427–435.

Solomon, P.R., Vander Schaaf, E.R., et al. (1986). Hippocampus and trace conditioning of the rabbit's classically conditioned nictitating membrane response. *Behav Neurosci*, **100**(**5**), 729–744.

Solomon, P.R., Stowe, G.T., et al. (1989). Disrupted eyelid conditioning in a patient with damage to cerebellar afferents. *Behav Neurosci*, **103**(**4**), 898–902.

Squire, L.R. (1987). *Memory and Brain*, Oxford University Press, New York.

Squire, L.R. and Knowlton, B.J. (1994). Memory, hippocampus, and brain systems. *The Cognitive Neurosciences* (ed. Gazzaniga, M.), MIT Press, Cambridge, MA, pp. 825–837.

Squire, L.R. and Zola-Morgan, S. (1988). Memory: brain systems and behavior. *Trend Neurosci*, **11**(**4**), 170–175.

Squire, L.R., Ojemann, J.G., et al. (1992). Activation of the hippocampus in normal humans: a functional anatomical study of memory. *Proc Natl Acad Sci USA*, **89**(**5**), 1837–1841.

Squire, L.R., Knowlton, B., et al. (1993). The structure and organization of memory. *Annu Rev Psychol*, **44**, 453–495.

Stanton, M.E. (2000). Multiple memory systems, development and conditioning. *Behav Brain Res*, **110**(**1–2**), 25–37.

Steinmetz, J.E. (2000). Brain substrates of classical eyeblink conditioning: a highly localized but also distributed system. *Behav Brain Res*, **110**(**1–2**), 13–24.

Sutton, M.A., Ide, J., et al. (2002). Interaction between amount and pattern of training in the induction of intermediate- and long-term memory for sensitization in aplysia. *Learn Mem*, **9**(**1**), 29–40.

Thompson, R.F. (2000). *The Brain: A Neuroscience Primer*, Worth Publishers, New York.

Thompson, R.F. and Kim, J.J. (1996). Memory systems in the brain and localization of a memory. *Proc Natl Acad Sci USA*, **93**(**24**), 13438–13444.

Thompson, R.F. and Krupa, D.J. (1994). Organization of memory traces in the mammalian brain. *Annu Rev Neurosci*, **17**, 519–549.

Thompson, R.F. and Spencer, W.A. (1966). Habituation: a model phenomenon for the study of neuronal substrates of behavior. *Psychol Rev*, **73**(**1**), 16–43.

Tranel, D., Damasio, H., et al. (1997). A neural basis for the retrieval of conceptual knowledge. *Neuropsychologia*, **35**(**10**), 1319–1327.

Viskontas, I.V., McAndrews, M.P., et al. (2000). Remote episodic memory deficits in patients with unilateral temporal lobe epilepsy and excisions. *J Neurosci*, **20**(**15**), 5853–5857.

Warrington, E.K. and McCarthy, R.A. (1987). Categories of knowledge. Further fractionations and an attempted integration. *Brain*, **110**(**Pt 5**), 1273–1296.

Warrington, E.K. and Shallice, T. (1984). Category specific semantic impairments. *Brain*, **107**(**Pt 3**), 829–854.

Woodruff-Pak, D.S. (2001). Eyeblink classical conditioning differentiates normal aging from Alzheimer's disease. *Integr Physiol Behav Sci*, **36**(**2**), 87–108.

Zola-Morgan, S. and Squire, L.R. (1993). Neuroanatomy of memory. *Annu Rev Neurosci*, **16**, 547–563.

Zola-Morgan, S., Squire, L.R., et al. (1986). Human amnesia and the medial temporal region: enduring memory impairment following a bilateral lesion limited to field CA1 of the hippocampus. *J Neurosci*, **6**(**10**), 2950–2967.

3

Short-term plasticity: facilitation and post-tetanic potentiation

Ralf Schneggenburger

AG Synaptische Dynamik und Modulation, Abteilung Membranbiophysik, Max-Planck-Institut für Biophysikalische Chemie, Göttingen, Germany and Laboratory of Synaptic Mechanisms, Ecole Polytechnique Fédérale de Lausanne, Brain Mind Institute, 1015 Lausanne, Switzerland

Summary

Fast point-to-point communication between neurons in the brain is mediated by chemical synaptic transmission. During brief trains of action potentials (APs) in a presynaptic neuron, the response in the postsynaptic cell will not follow with equal strength. Rather, processes of short-term plasticity will decrease the amplitude of postsynaptic potentials (PSPs) during short-term depression, or increase PSP amplitudes, as occurs during short-term enhancement (STE) of synaptic transmission. Various phases of STE can be distinguished based on their kinetics of decay after brief trains of presynaptic activity: Facilitation, augmentation and post-tetanic potentiation. STE of synaptic transmission is induced by a rise of Ca^{2+} in presynaptic nerve terminals, and represents an increased number of vesicles which fuse in response to a presynaptic AP. Facilitation, which decays within less than half a second, is the shortest form of Ca^{2+}-induced plasticity identified so far. STE and synaptic depression can be expressed simultaneously at a synapse, but the degree, and the direction of short-term plasticity is specifically regulated at a given type of synapse, and subject to modulation during postnatal development. This chapter discusses the presynaptic, Ca^{2+}-dependent mechanisms of STE of synaptic transmission.

3.1 Overview of chemical synaptic transmission

Synaptic transmission takes place at specialized contact sites, at which the active zone of the presynaptic neuron approaches the postsynaptic density of a postsynaptic neuron (Fig. 3.1). Transmission is initiated when an action potential (AP) arrives at the nerve terminal, where it opens voltage-gated Ca^{2+} channels. The ensuing influx of Ca^{2+} ions into the presynaptic cytoplasm rapidly increases in the intracellular Ca^{2+} concentration at and near the presynaptic active zones (see Section 3.4). The elevation of intracellular Ca^{2+} concentration triggers neurotransmitter release, by enhancing the probability that docked, and fusion-competent vesicles fuse with the plasma membrane. A neurotransmitter, stored in the presynaptic vesicles, is released upon vesicle fusion, diffuses over the synaptic cleft, and activates transmitter-gated ion channels on the postsynaptic neuron (Fig. 3.1). At excitatory synapses, like glutamatergic synapses in the central nervous system (CNS), transmitter-gated ion channels permeable to cations generate an excitatory postsynaptic potential (EPSP), which depolarizes the neuron and drives it closer to the threshold for AP generation. At inhibitory synapses, like GABAergic or glycinergic synapses, transmitter-gated channels permeable to anions (mainly Cl^-) generate an

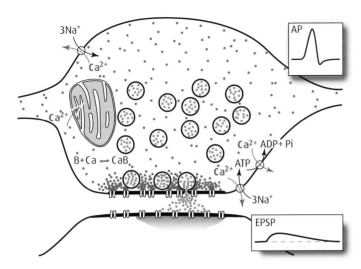

Figure 3.1. A schematic view of an axo-dendritic, or axo-somatic excitatory synapse formed by an hypothetical en passant bouton with a single active zone. An AP in the presynaptic terminal opens voltage-gated Ca^{2+} channels, which allow Ca^{2+} influx into the nerve terminal. After a brief period of a few milliseconds in small nerve terminals (Atluri and Regehr, 1996), Ca^{2+} will be spatially equilibrated, and most of the previously entered Ca^{2+} ions will be bound to endogenous Ca^{2+} buffers (B). Vesicles fusing with the plasma membrane (Jahn et al., 2003) release neurotransmitter, which acts on receptor-gated ion channels in the postsynaptic neuron to generate an EPSP. For further details, see text.

inhibitory postsynaptic potential (IPSP), which stabilizes, or hyperpolarizes, the postsynaptic membrane potential.

The strength of synaptic transmission, as measured by the amplitude of successive PSPs, is not constant with repetitive APs in the presynaptic neuron. During short bursts of presynaptic activity, synaptic strength either increases in a process referred to as synaptic facilitation, or it decreases in a process called synaptic depression. During prolonged AP trains, short-term enhancement of synaptic transmission, like augmentation, and post-tetanic potentiation (PTP) are also observed at many synapses (see Section 5).

3.2 Synapse-specificity of short-term plasticity

The two opposing forms of short-term plasticity, STE and depression, are observed at many types of synapses in the brain, but their relative strength varies from one type of synapse to another, and during development of the nervous system. Whole-cell recording from neurons in brain slices has been used to characterize the transmission properties, and the short-term plasticity of specific synaptic connections in different CNS regions. For most of the following discussion, we will concentrate on glutamatergic excitatory synapses in the CNS, as these have been studied in considerable detail.

Synapses with strong depression are, for example, the climbing fiber synapse onto cerebellar Purkinje cells (Konnerth et al., 1990; Silver et al., 1998) or the giant excitatory synapses in the auditory system, like the calyx of Held (Schneggenburger et al., 2002; von Gersdorff and Borst, 2002) and the endbulb of Held synapses (Zhang and Trussell, 1994; Bellingham and Walmsley, 1999). Other synapses, like hippocampal CA3–CA1 synapses (Dittman et al., 2000), show a mixed behavior of initial facilitation, giving way to depression during short bursts of presynaptic activity. On the other end of the spectrum of short-term plasticity behavior are strongly facilitating synapses, like the hippocampal mossy-fiber – CA3 cell synapse (Salin et al., 1996), or corticothalamic synapses in the visual system (Granseth et al., 2002). At these synapses, prolonged presynaptic activity also induces longer-lasting forms of STE like synaptic augmentation. The direction and the magnitude of short-term plasticity will influence the temporal integration of information flow in neuronal circuits (Abbott et al., 1997; Nadim et al., 1999; Chung et al., 2002; Cook et al., 2003). Short-term plasticity adds a dynamic component to synaptic information flow, which depends on the frequency of presynaptic action potential firing (Tsodyks and Markram, 1997).

Short-term plasticity can be different for synapses made by a single neuron onto different target neurons. This target-cell specificity has been observed in cortex and hippocampus (Maccaferri et al., 1998; Markram et al., 1998; Reyes et al., 1998; Scanziani et al., 1998). Pyramidal neurons in layer 2/3 of the cortex, for example, make excitatory synapses with two classes of inhibitory neurons, the bitufted cells, and the multipolar cells. EPSPs generated by a pyramidal neuron in a bitufted cell facilitate, whereas EPSPs in a multipolar cell generated by the *same* layer 2/3 pyramidal neuron showed depression (Reyes et al., 1998). A similar situation exists in layer 4 of the somatosensory cortex, where excitatory synapses made by regularly spiking stellate cells (regular spiking (RS) in Fig. 3.2) onto one class of inhibitory interneurons, the fast spiking (FS) cells, show depression (Fig. 3.2a), whereas synapses onto another type of layer 4 interneurons, the low-threshold spiking (LTS) interneurons, show strong facilitation (Fig. 3.2b) (Beierlein et al., 2003). At these facilitating synapses, transmission is very unreliable at low frequencies, but literally "wakes up" at higher frequencies of presynaptic action potential firing (Fig. 3.2b, lower panel). Thus, different networks of cortical inhibitory interneurons might be recruited differentially at low- versus high-frequency activity states (Gibson et al., 1999).

Target-cell specificity in the direction of short-term plasticity (Fig. 3.2) implies that short-term plasticity is tightly, and specifically regulated for each type of synapse. Target-cell specificity shows that the postsynaptic neuron influences the dynamic

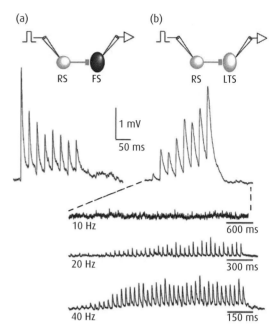

Figure 3.2. Short-term plasticity is synapse-specific. An example from the rat somatosensory cortex is shown. RS, excitatory neurons in layer 4 make synapses onto two types of interneurons: FS and LTS interneurons. Upon repetitive stimulation of the RS neuron, EPSPs recorded in an FS neuron depressed (a). Conversely, EPSPs generated at the contact sites between RS neurons and LTS neurons showed strong synaptic facilitation upon repetitive use (b). With permission by the American Physiological Society.

behavior of synaptic transmission at a given synaptic contact. This might be a more general principle. An individual neuron may contact hundreds of postsynaptic target neurons in various CNS regions, and it is likely, and functionally relevant, that synapses onto one class of target neurons have different short-term plasticity than synapses formed by different axon branches onto other types of target neurons.

3.3 Quantal mechanisms of short-term plasticity

A framework for understanding in which ways synaptic strength can be modified is the quantal hypothesis of transmitter release, which originated from electrophysiological studies at the neuromuscular junction (Fatt and Katz, 1952; del Castillo and Katz, 1954a, b). Combined with a binomial model of quantal availability (Johnson and Wernig, 1971; Quastel, 1997), it states that the PSP evoked by the activity of a given synapse depends on the number of release sites, N; the probability that a release event occurs at a given site, P; and the quantal amplitude, q:

$$PSP = N \times P \times q$$

Here, N is a number, P is a probability (ranging from 0 to 1), and q is a measure of the average amplitude of a PSP induced by the release of a single "quantum". At many synapses, spontaneous miniature PSPs (or miniature postsynaptic current (PSC) in case of voltage-clamp measurements) can be resolved in whole-cell recordings of the postsynaptic cell. It is thus possible to estimate, within certain limits, the value of q from amplitude distributions of miniature PSPs or PSCs. The quantal parameters during the evoked PSP, however, are not immediately evident from PSP amplitude measurements, because at many synapses, evoked PSPs are generated by multiple release sites. However, information on the quantal properties of transmitter release can be inferred from the trial-to-trial variability of the PSP amplitudes (Silver et al., 1998; Meyer et al., 2001; Scheuss et al., 2002), or from methods of quantal analysis based on amplitude histograms of evoked PSPs (del Castillo and Katz, 1954a, b; Redman, 1990).

The interpretation of the binomial parameter N derived from quantal analysis is still controversial. Studies combining fluctuation analysis of PSPs to measure the quantal parameters P and N with a subsequent morphological analysis have found a good correlation of N with the number of morphologically identified contact sites (Korn et al., 1981; Silver et al., 2003). This has led to the view that zero, or maximally one quantum can be released during a presynaptic AP at a given active zone (univesicular release constraint). Ultrastructural analysis by electron microscopy (EM) has shown, however, that individual active zones typically contain 3–10

"morphologically" docked vesicles (Schikorski and Stevens, 1997; Xu-Friedman et al., 2001; Sätzler et al., 2002). This number of morphologically docked vesicles is thought to correspond to the number of immediately fusion-competent vesicles (Schikorski and Stevens, 2001). Studies at the calyx of Held (Meyer et al., 2001; Sun and Wu, 2001; Wölfel and Schneggenburger, 2003) and at the climbing fiber synapse in the cerebellum (Wadiche and Jahr, 2001) indicate that during strong, pool-depleting stimuli, or with action potentials under conditions of elevated release probability, more than one vesicle is released at each active zone (multi-vesicular release). In this case, one expects the binomial parameter N to be larger than the number of active zones, approaching the number of releasable vesicles. However, with multi-vesicular release, the degree of postsynaptic receptor saturation upon the release of a single vesicle (Silver et al., 1996; Liu et al., 1999; Ishikawa et al., 2002) also becomes an issue in the interpretation of N (Meyer et al., 2001).

According to the quantal hypothesis, synaptic plasticity can arise either from a change in the postsynaptic quantal size q. Alternatively, changes in the presynaptic parameters P (release probability) or N (number of readily releasable vesicles, or number of release sites) can cause synaptic plasticity. It is generally agreed that facilitation is presynaptic, that is that facilitation is caused by an increased number of released quanta (del Castillo and Katz, 1954a, b; Dudel and Kuffler, 1961). The number of released quanta at a synaptic connection is often called the "quantal content", m, and is given by the product of the number of release sites N, and the average release probability P ($m = N \times P$). At many synapses, an increase in the release probability P was found responsible for the increased quantal content (Zucker, 1973), without an increase in the size of the pool of readily releasable vesicles (Felmy et al., 2003). Some studies, however, have indicated that an increase of N, seen as the number of active release sites, contributes to facilitation (Wojtowicz et al., 1994; Worden et al., 1997).

At many synapses which show depression under conditions of normal release probability P, lowering the extracellular Ca^{2+} concentration (thereby lowering P, see below) converts depression into facilitation. This shows, first, that processes of depression and facilitation are simultaneously present at most synapses. The net short-term behavior depends on the exact superimposition of both processes. Second, at high P, depression prevails, and depression observed at many synapses is use dependent. This is often interpreted as the consequence of the depletion of some synaptic resource(s) during the first few stimuli (Liley and North, 1953). The depleted resources most likely are a decrease in the number of readily releasable vesicles (von Gersdorff et al., 1997; Scheuss et al., 2002), or else, a decrease in the postsynaptic quantal amplitude the postsynaptic quantal size q due to desensitization or saturation of postsynaptic receptors (Otis et al., 1996; Scheuss et al., 2002).

A postsynaptic mechanism of facilitation has been observed at glutamatergic synapses which contain a molecular variant of postsynaptic α-amino-3-hydroxy-5-methyl-isoxazole-4-propionic acid (AMPA)-type glutamate receptors sensitive to block by intracellular polyamines (Rozov and Burnashev, 1999). At these synapses, the multiple use of AMPA receptors relieves the polyamine block for a short time period, and this is expected to increase the postsynaptic quantal size q. This process, however, is only relevant at rather high P, when the net short-term behavior is depression rather than facilitation. Unblock by polyamines of AMPA receptors thus counterbalances the effects of synaptic depression (Rozov and Burnashev, 1999).

3.4 Ca^{2+}-dependent mechanisms of short-term enhancement

We will now discuss in more detail the presynaptic mechanisms causing STE of transmitter release. The three forms of STE, facilitation, augmentation and PTP represent an increase in the number of released quanta. Another common feature of these forms of STE is that they are caused by the accumulation of "residual" Ca^{2+} in the presynaptic nerve terminal, and the decay kinetics of the various forms of STE is

probably dictated by the decay of residual Ca^{2+} in the nerve terminal. Thus, understanding presynaptic Ca^{2+} signaling, and the way in which Ca^{2+} triggers transmitter release are important prerequisites for understanding the mechanisms of STE.

Presynaptic Ca^{2+} signaling

The shortest form of Ca^{2+} signaling in the nerve terminal is the Ca^{2+} signal for transmitter release. In response to a presynaptic AP, transmitter is released only during a brief period of a few milliseconds or less (Barrett and Stevens, 1972; Borst and Sakmann, 1996; Schneggenburger and Neher, 2000) during which the rate of transmitter release is strongly increased. The intracellular $[Ca^{2+}]_i$ signal for this "phasic" transmitter release is a highly localized, microdomain signal. Theoretical work has shown that the fast rise and decay of transmitter release is best explained by a close spatial co-localization of release-ready vesicles, and Ca^{2+} channels (Chad and Eckert, 1984; Simon and Llinás, 1985; Augustine et al., 1991; Yamada and Zucker, 1992; Roberts 1994; Meinrenken et al., 2002; see Neher, 1998a, b for a review). Tight spatial co-localization ensures that $[Ca^{2+}]_i$ builds up rapidly near the vesicles, and, when the presynaptic Ca^{2+} channels close after less than 1 ms (Borst and Sakmann, 1998; Bischofberger et al., 2002), that $[Ca^{2+}]_i$ near the vesicles drops rapidly, mainly because Ca^{2+} diffuses into the bulk volume of the presynaptic cytosol (see Fig. 3.1). The Ca^{2+} signal at the sites of docked, and readily releasable vesicles will be called the "local $[Ca^{2+}]_i$" signal. As this signal is fast (~1 ms), and limited to a small area (an estimated volume of less than $300 \times 300 \times 30$ nm for a single active zone), the amplitude and the kinetics of the local Ca^{2+} signal cannot be quantified directly with current imaging technology.

If the intracellular free Ca^{2+} concentration, $[Ca^{2+}]_i$, is measured with Ca^{2+}-sensitive fluorescent dyes introduced into the bulk of the presynaptic cytosol (Delaney et al., 1989; Swandulla et al., 1991; Regehr et al., 1994; Helmchen et al., 1997), then the measured Ca^{2+} signal reflects the $[Ca^{2+}]_i$ signal after spatial equilibration in the presynaptic terminal, and after equilibration with endogenous Ca^{2+}-binding substances (see Fig. 3.1). After equilibration with endogeneous Ca^{2+} buffers, roughly one Ca^{2+} ion out of 30 remains free – it is said that the intracellular Ca^{2+}-binding ratio is 30 (Neher and Augustine, 1992; Helmchen et al., 1997). In cells expressing high concentrations of Ca^{2+}-binding proteins, the Ca^{2+}-binding ratio can be higher, up to a few hundred or more (Fierro and Llano, 1996; Maeda et al., 1999).

It is likely that the measured, spatially averaged Ca^{2+} signal is similar to the "residual" free $[Ca^{2+}]_i$ that remains in a nerve terminal after stimulation with an AP. The amplitude of this Ca^{2+} signal has been estimated to be $\sim 0.5\,\mu M$ in glutamatergic synapses of the CNS (Helmchen et al., 1997), as compared to a baseline $[Ca^{2+}]_i$ value of $\sim 50\,nM$. Residual $[Ca^{2+}]_i$ is removed from the presynaptic cytosol via a plasma membrane Ca^{2+} – ATPase, via plasma membrane Na^+/Ca^{2+} exchangers, and into mitochondria (Fig. 3.1). These processes are often collectively referred to as Ca^{2+} extrusion. After a single AP, Ca^{2+} is extruded from presynaptic terminals with a time constant of 100–200 ms (Regehr and Atluri, 1995; Helmchen et al., 1997).

How high does $[Ca^{2+}]_i$ rise near the docked and readily releasable vesicles, and how long does this local $[Ca^{2+}]_i$ signal persist? As the local $[Ca^{2+}]_i$ signal is not accessible to direct measurements (see above), a "reverse approach" employing Ca^{2+} uncaging in presynaptic nerve terminals has been used to estimate its amplitude and kinetics. Ca^{2+} uncaging (Delaney and Zucker, 1990; Heidelberger et al., 1994; Heinemann et al., 1994; Beutner et al., 2001) produces a spatially homogenous $[Ca^{2+}]_i$ signal in the cytoplasm of the nerve terminal. Thus, with Ca^{2+} uncaging, the fluorescent Ca^{2+} indicators present in the bulk of the presynaptic cytosol, and the Ca^{2+} sensors for vesicle fusion at docked vesicles close to the membrane (Fig. 3.1) will "see" the same $[Ca^{2+}]_i$ signal. In this case, the Ca^{2+} signal measured by the Ca^{2+} indicators is immediately relevant for vesicle fusion and transmitter release, and a relationship between transmitter release and $[Ca^{2+}]_i$ can be obtained, and fitted with a kinetic model of Ca^{2+} binding and vesicle fusion. Knowing the Ca^{2+} sensitivity of

vesicle fusion, the local $[Ca^{2+}]_i$ signal which drives the phasic transmitter release during the presynaptic AP can then be back-calculated in a "reverse approach" (Chow et al., 1994; Bollmann et al., 2000; Schneggenburger and Neher, 2000), under certain limiting assumptions.

This approach has been used at a large CNS glutamatergic brainstem synapse, the calyx of Held. At this synapse, whole-cell recordings can be made directly from the presynaptic terminal due to its unusually large size (~ 10–$15\,\mu m$ in perimeter (Forsythe, 1994; Borst et al., 1995)), and Ca^{2+} indicators and photolyzable Ca^{2+} chelators can be introduced into the presynaptic cytoplasm with a whole-cell patch-clamp pipette. Ca^{2+} uncaging in these large presynaptic terminals has shown that transmitter release depends steeply on the intracellular Ca^{2+} concentration attained by Ca^{2+} uncaging, following a power relation with exponent of ~ 4–5 (Bollmann et al., 2000; Schneggenburger and Neher, 2000; Felmy et al., 2003). This indicates that 4–5 Ca^{2+} ions bind co-operatively to a Ca^{2+} sensor for vesicle fusion before release can take place. This is in agreement with earlier findings at the neuromuscular junction, where a steep, 4th power relationship was found between transmitter release rates and *extracellular* Ca^{2+} concentration (Dodge and Rahamimoff, 1967). At the calyx of Held, fast transmitter release rates were observed when Ca^{2+} uncaging produced $[Ca^{2+}]_i$ steps of $10\,\mu M$ or higher (Bollmann et al., 2000; Schneggenburger and Neher, 2000; Wölfel and Schneggenburger, 2003). Using the "reverse approach", the measured Ca^{2+} sensitivity of synaptic vesicle fusion indicates that a local $[Ca^{2+}]_i$ signal of 10–$20\,\mu M$ amplitude, and half-width of less than 1 ms is sufficient to explain phasic transmitter release during a presynaptic AP (Bollmann et al., 2000; Schneggenburger and Neher, 2000). At the calyx of Held, quantitative estimates are thus available for both the local $[Ca^{2+}]_i$ signal relevant for transmitter release (amplitude, 10–$20\,\mu M$) and the residual $[Ca^{2+}]_i$ signal after spatial equilibration (amplitude, $0.5\,\mu M$; Helmchen et al., 1997). It is seen that the residual $[Ca^{2+}]_i$ is about 20–40 times smaller than the local $[Ca^{2+}]_i$ signal.

Ways of increasing the synaptic release probability, *P*

Facilitation, augmentation and PTP are thought to result from an increase in *P*, the probability that docked, and fusion-competent vesicles are released, with relatively small influences by changes in *N* (Zucker, 1973; Stevens and Wesseling, 1999; but see Wojtowicz et al., 1994). A change in *P* can, in principle, be induced by different presynaptic mechanisms (Fig. 3.3). First, activity-dependent broadening of the presynaptic AP occurs at some presynaptic terminals as a consequence of cumulative K^+ current inactivation (Jackson et al., 1991; Geiger and Jonas, 2000). AP broadening will cause an increased integral Ca^{2+} influx (Augustine, 1990; Geiger and Jonas, 2000), although the peak Ca^{2+} current is reduced at some synapses (Geiger and Jonas, 2000). The increased overall Ca^{2+} influx causes an increased transmitter release probability *P*.

In many synapses, AP broadening has been found not to contribute to the shortest form of STE, namely facilitation as studied with paired-pulse protocols (see Zucker (1989) for a review). However, even when two subsequent APs are identical in shape, the Ca^{2+} influx in response to the second AP can be slightly enhanced (~10%) (Borst and Sakmann, 1998a, b; Cuttle et al., 1998; Tsujimoto et al., 2002). This "Ca^{2+} current facilitation", caused by an increased open probability of Ca^{2+} channels, is expected to lead to a proportional increase in local $[Ca^{2+}]_i$, and will thereby contribute to facilitation of transmitter release. However, in simultaneous voltage-clamp experiments of presynaptic terminals and their postsynaptic partner cells, it was shown that transmitter release in response to a pair of identical Ca^{2+} currents still showed substantial facilitation (Charlton et al., 1982; Wright et al., 1996; Felmy et al., 2003). Thus, there must be a component of transmitter release facilitation which is *independent* of changes in the amount of Ca^{2+} influx during the presynaptic AP, and it is generally agreed that this component accounts for most of the observed paired-pulse facilitation (Zucker and Regehr, 2002). Residual $[Ca^{2+}]_i$ remaining from the

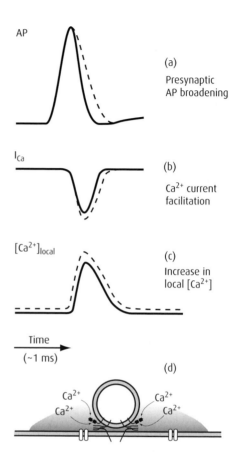

Figure 3.3. Possible ways to increase the transmitter release probability *P*. In (a)–(c), the time-course of presynaptic signals is depicted, and the arrow in (c) corresponds to roughly 1 ms. (a) In some synapses, repetitive use leads to an activity-dependent broadening of the AP recorded in the presynaptic terminal, caused by cumulative inactivation of presynaptic K^+ channels. AP broadening will increase the integral Ca^{2+} influx with each AP, and thereby increase *P*. (b) Ca^{2+} current facilitation can also lead to an increased Ca^{2+} influx with each AP, even for unchanged AP-waveforms. (c) The local $[Ca^{2+}]_i$ signal can be enhanced by elevated residual $[Ca^{2+}]_i$ in the nerve terminal (broken line). (d) The local $[Ca^{2+}]_i$ signal near the sites of vesicles fusion. For references and further explanations, see text.

first stimulus will add to the local $[Ca^{2+}]_i$ signal created by the subsequent opening of Ca^{2+} channels (see dashed line in Fig. 3.3c). Whether the resulting increase in the local $[Ca^{2+}]_i$ is sufficient to explain transmitter release facilitation, or whether residual Ca^{2+} has additional signaling targets in the presynaptic terminal will be discussed below.

Residual Ca^{2+} causes facilitation of transmitter release

Evidence for a role of Ca^{2+} in facilitation became available more than 30 years ago, in now classical electrophysiological studies on the neuromuscular junction by Katz and colleagues. Using local and temporally restricted iontophoretic application of extracellular Ca^{2+} in a preparation otherwise bathed in Ca^{2+} free solution, Katz and Miledi (1968) showed that paired-pulse facilitation depended on the presence of Ca^{2+} during the first pulse. They proposed that a "residue" of the Ca^{2+} which entered the nerve terminal during the first pulse caused facilitation during the second pulse. They realized that it is difficult to explain transmitter release and facilitation, two processes with widely differing decay kinetics

(~1 ms for release and ~100 ms for facilitation) with one mechanism, namely with "the presence and gradual subsistence of Ca^{2+}". However, they pointed out that the steep relationship between transmitter release and Ca^{2+} (Dodge and Rahamimoff, 1967), and a biphasic decay of $[Ca^{2+}]$ at the sites of vesicle fusion would help to resolve this difficulty. Assuming a power relation between release and $[Ca^{2+}]$ with exponent $n = 4$, they concluded (Katz and Miledi, 1968):

Take $n = 4$ and suppose the first impulse raises Ca^{2+} to a maximum value a which declines rapidly to, say, 20%, and much more slowly thereafter. When Ca^{2+} has fallen to $0.2\,a$, the release will be reduced to 0.2^4, i.e. 0.16% of its peak value. But a second nerve impulse raises $[Ca^{2+}]$ to $1.2\,a$, and the release by a factor which is 1.2^4 times, i.e. more than twice as large as that due to the first impulse.

Since then, various models have been proposed to explain the action of residual Ca^{2+} in facilitation (Table 3.1). The *linear summation model* is attractive because of its simplicity: It assumes that Ca^{2+} acts co-operatively on a single class of Ca^{2+} sensor with

Table 3.1. Properties of four models of residual Ca^{2+} in synaptic facilitation. *Linear Ca^{2+} summation* and the *Ca^{2+}-buffer saturation* model both assume that the release probability P is increased during facilitation because of an enhanced local $[Ca^{2+}]_i$ signal for vesicle fusion. In contrast, the *bound Ca^{2+} model*, and the *facilitation site model* assume that the local $[Ca^{2+}]_i$ signal is essentially unchanged, and that the increased release probability results from Ca^{2+} binding to special high-affinity sites, which are either part of the Ca^{2+} sensor for vesicle fusion (*bound Ca^{2+} model*), or a separate Ca^{2+} site for facilitation (*facilitation site model*).

	Linear Ca^{2+} summation	Bound Ca^{2+} model	Facilitation site model	Ca^{2+} buffer saturation
Ca^{2+} sensor for vesicle fusion	• High – to intermediate affinity • Positive co-operativity	• Intermediate affinity • Negative co-operativity	• Low affinity	• Intermediate affinity • Positive co-operativity
Local $[Ca^{2+}]_i$ signal	↑during facilitation	No significant change during facilitation		↑during facilitation
Facilitation site?	–	–	Yes, $K_d \sim 1\,\mu M$	–
Saturable Ca^{2+} buffer?	–	–	–	Yes, $K_d \sim 1\,\mu M$
Apparent Ca^{2+} sensitivity of vesicle fusion	Unchanged during facilitation	↑during facilitation	↑during facilitation	Unchanged during facilitation

intermediate – to high affinity to induce release (see Table 3.1). This model uses the same rationale as first stated by Katz and Miledi (1968) (see above): The high co-operativity of Ca^{2+} in inducing transmitter release makes a relatively small increment of the local $[Ca^{2+}]_i$ highly efficient in increasing the transmitter output.

It is now generally accepted that linear summation of residual Ca^{2+} to local $[Ca^{2+}]_i$ cannot explain the full amount of facilitation, because of the relatively large difference between the estimates for the local $[Ca^{2+}]_i$ signal (10–20 µM) and the residual $[Ca^{2+}]_i$ signal (~0.5 µM; see above). Nevertheless, it has been shown at the calyx of Held that elevating the basal $[Ca^{2+}]_i$ by about 1 µM causes a threefold facilitation of transmitter release, and that roughly one-third of this facilitation can be explained by linear summation of residual free $[Ca^{2+}]_i$ on top of the local $[Ca^{2+}]_i$ signal inferred from the "reverse approach" (Felmy et al., 2003). Thus, the contribution of linear Ca^{2+} summation to facilitation is not negligible.

The *bound Ca^{2+} model* (Table 3.1) (Stanley, 1986; Yamada and Zucker, 1992; Bertram et al., 1996) explains facilitation by assuming that Ca^{2+} remains bound to one or several high-affinity site(s) with slow unbinding kinetics, which are part of a multisite Ca^{2+} sensor for vesicle fusion. This explanation effectively introduces some negative co-operativity to the Ca^{2+} binding to the Ca^{2+} sensor for vesicle fusion (see Table 3.1). In this model, it is not the decay of free residual $[Ca^{2+}]_i$ which determines the decay of facilitation, but rather the unbinding rate of Ca^{2+} from a high-affinity site. Therefore, this model predicts that a faster decay of residual free $[Ca^{2+}]_i$ in the nerve terminal should not affect the decay of facilitation; a prediction that was not confirmed experimentally (Kamiya and Zucker, 1994; Atluri and Regehr, 1996). Rapidly lowering the residual free $[Ca^{2+}]_i$ by well-timed photolytic activation of a caged Ca^{2+} chelator speeded the decay of facilitation (Kamiya and Zucker, 1994), opposite to the prediction of the bound Ca^{2+} model.

With these difficulties in mind, *facilitation site models* were developed (Atluri and Regehr, 1996;

Tang et al., 2000). These assume that vesicle fusion is triggered by a low-affinity Ca^{2+} sensor, and that an additional high-affinity site with rapid equilibration kinetics (facilitation site; K_d, ~1 µM) senses the residual free $[Ca^{2+}]_i$. These models are two-sensor models, with physically separate Ca^{2+} sensors for vesicle fusion and facilitation. The model is attractive, because the expression level of genes coding for such a facilitation site would then determine the degree of facilitation at a given synaptic connection. However, the molecular nature of the proposed facilitation site has not been determined unambiguously. Thus, whereas it is generally agreed that the C2 domains of Synaptotagmin 1/2 mediate the highly co-operative, intermediate affinity Ca^{2+} binding necessary for phasic transmitter release (Littleton et al., 1993; Geppert et al., 1994; Fernández-Chacón et al., 2001), various proteins have been implicated as potential facilitation sites, among them Ca^{2+}/calmodulin kinase II (CamK II) (Chapman et al., 1995) and the C2 domain containing active zone protein piccolo (Gerber et al., 2001). It is also possible that Synaptotagmin isoforms with higher Ca^{2+} affinities (Südhof, 2002) represent candidate Ca^{2+} sensors for facilitation. Recently, it was reported that overexpression of the EF-hand Ca^{2+}-binding protein neuronal Ca^{2+} sensor-1 (NCS-1; also known as frequenin), increases the amount of synaptic facilitation in hippocampal neurons, without a concomitant decrease in synaptic strength (Sippy et al., 2003). However, frequenin also mediates facilitation of P/Q-type Ca^{2+} channels upon double-pulse stimulation in presynaptic terminals (Tsujimoto et al., 2002); therefore, part of its effect might be mediated by increased Ca^{2+} current facilitation (see Fig. 3.3b). Thus, the exact mechanism of frequenin action in facilitation remains to be determined.

The *buffer saturation model*, finally, stems from the idea that saturable cellular Ca^{2+} buffers can introduce a supra-linearity in the summation of intracellular Ca^{2+} signals (Neher, 1998a, b; Maeda et al., 1999). A Ca^{2+} buffer with rapid binding kinetics can bind some fraction of the incoming Ca^{2+} before it reaches the Ca^{2+} sensor for vesicle fusion, even when the vesicles are quite closely co-localized with the

Ca^{2+} channels (and therefore, when the diffusion time between Ca^{2+} channels and vesicles is short). The Ca^{2+} buffer would thus effectively decrease the local $[Ca^{2+}]_i$, and thereby reduce the release probability P during a first pulse. Assuming that the Ca^{2+} buffer has a sufficiently high affinity (K_d 1 μM or less), residual free $[Ca^{2+}]_i$ remaining after the first pulse (partially) saturates the buffer. Therefore, the Ca^{2+} influx during a second pulse would meet with less intracellular Ca^{2+} buffering capacity, and the local $[Ca^{2+}]_i$ rises somewhat higher than the algebraic sum of residual $[Ca^{2+}]_i$, and the local $[Ca^{2+}]_i$ signal under control conditions (Felmy et al., 2003). Even a small supra-linearity in Ca^{2+} summation should boost facilitation significantly (Felmy et al., 2003), because small differences in $[Ca^{2+}]_i$ are strongly amplified by the highly supra-linear relationship between transmitter release and $[Ca^{2+}]_i$ (see Section on "Ca^{2+}-dependent mechanisms of short-term enhancement).

Evidence for the buffer saturation model comes from the finding that sub-millimolar concentrations of the rapidly binding, high-affinity Ca^{2+} buffer 1,2-bis (2-aminophenoxy) ethane-N,N,N',N' tetraacetic acid (BAPTA) leads to a decrease of transmitter release in cortical nerve terminals, with a concomitant increase in paired-pulse facilitation. Since this facilitation was induced by an exogenously added buffer, it was termed "pseudofacilitation" (Rozov et al., 2001). At other synapses, however, intracellularly added BAPTA, or BAPTA-like Ca^{2+} buffers reduce the amount of facilitation (Bain and Quastel, 1992; Tang et al., 2000), an effect which is not, at first sight, compatible with the buffer saturation model. In agreement with Ca^{2+} buffer saturation, it has been found that paired-pulse facilitation at the hippocampal mossy fiber to CA3 cell synapse was reduced in knock-out mice lacking Calbindin (Blatow et al., 2003), an EF-hand Ca^{2+}-binding protein with relatively rapid Ca^{2+} binding (Nägerl et al., 2000). This suggests that Calbindin, which is expressed in hippocampal mossy-fiber terminals, normally buffers some of the Ca^{2+} which would otherwise contribute to the free local $[Ca^{2+}]_i$ signal triggering transmitter release. Partial saturation of Calbindin by residual free $[Ca^{2+}]_i$ then reduces its buffering capacity, and

contributes to facilitation. Ca^{2+} uncaging at the calyx of Held showed that the intracellular Ca^{2+} sensitivity of transmitter release was unchanged during facilitation (Felmy et al., 2003), as opposed to the predictions of the *bound Ca^{2+} model*, and the *facilitation site model* (see Table 3.1). Since linear Ca^{2+} summation could not account for the entire magnitude of facilitation, Ca^{2+} buffer saturation was proposed to mediate part of the facilitation at this synapse. However, a presynaptic endogenous Ca^{2+}-binding protein which might function as a saturable buffer during facilitation has not been identified at the calyx of Held.

Comparison of the residual Ca^{2+} models

There is quite general agreement that the residual Ca^{2+} model in its simplest form, the linear summation of residual and local $[Ca^{2+}]_i$, cannot account for the entire amount of facilitation (Zucker and Regehr, 2002), and there is experimental evidence against bound Ca^{2+} models for facilitation (Kamiya and Zucker, 1994; Atluri and Regehr, 1996; Felmy et al., 2003). Up to date, it seems difficult to distinguish experimentally between the two remaining models, the *facilitation site model* and the *buffer saturation model* (Felmy et al., 2003). Although the two models make quite different assumptions about the underlying mechanisms of facilitation (see Table 3.1), they are kinetically similar, because they both propose Ca^{2+}-binding site(s) with (i) high affinity and (ii) rapid equilibration kinetics. In the buffer saturation model, it is the mass action of Ca^{2+} binding to a buffer and the subsequent reduction in buffering power which matters, whereas in the facilitation site model, Ca^{2+} binding to a rapid site induces a downstream signaling step, which increases P. This difference is reminiscent of the two functions of different classes of EF-hand Ca^{2+}-binding proteins: Ca^{2+} buffering in proteins like Calbindin and Calretinin versus Ca^{2+} signaling mediated by, for example, Calmodulin or Frequenin (Ikura, 1996). Future work will have to determine whether a Ca^{2+}-signalling step, or else the reduction of presynaptic Ca^{2+}-buffering power, mediates the action of residual Ca^{2+} in facilitation of transmitters release.

3.5 Longer-lasting forms of STE

Following longer-lasting trains of presynaptic APs, other forms of STE besides facilitation occur. These can be separated from one another by their time course of decay following the trains (Magleby, 1987). Facilitation has the shortest decay time (<0.5 s) followed by augmentation, which has been identified in some synapses based on decay time constants in the range of 5–10 s (Magleby and Zengel, 1976; Stevens and Wesseling, 1999). PTP usually decays within several tens of seconds up to over 1 min. Augmentation and PTP can be present at the same synapse (Magleby and Zengel, 1976), but their kinetic properties are different. The decay of PTP is prolonged when the strength of the induction trains was increased by increasing the number, or the frequency of presynaptic APs. Augmentation, on the other hand, shows a fixed decay rate independent of the strength of the induction, as originally shown at the frog neuromuscular junction (Magleby and Zengel, 1976).

Augmentation and PTP are both caused by an increase in the number of released quanta, and presynaptic Ca^{2+} elevations are thought to induce these longer-lasting forms of STE (Delaney et al., 1989; Swandulla et al., 1991; Delaney and Tank, 1994; Kamiya and Zucker, 1994; Stevens and Wesseling, 1999; Rosenmund et al., 2002). During augmentation at hippocampal synapses, the size of the readily releasable pool of vesicles was not enhanced (Stevens and Wesseling, 1999), thus augmentation at these synapses is caused by an increased release probability P. At other synapses, however, an increase in the number of functional active zones (Wojtowicz et al., 1994) or an increase in the size of the readily releasable vesicle pool (Rosenmund et al., 2002) contributed to augmentation/PTP.

During long trains of presynaptic APs, residual Ca^{2+} builds up, and the longer presence of elevated $[Ca^{2+}]_i$ probably activates various Ca^{2+}-dependent signaling pathways, distinct from the brief action of the high local $[Ca^{2+}]_i$ at the Ca^{2+} sensor for vesicle fusion. Thus, evidence for a role of Ca^{2+}/calmodulin-activated kinase II (CaMK II) in PTP has been obtained, possibly via phosphorylating Synapsin 1 (Llinás et al., 1991).

However, PTP was normal in Synapsin 1 KO mice (Rosahl et al., 1993), as well as in CaMK II KO mice (Stevens et al., 1994). More recently, evidence for a role of protein kinase C (PKC) in PTP was obtained at hippocampal synapses, based on experiments with PKC-selective inhibitors (Alle et al., 2001; Brager et al., 2003). Excitatory synapses in hippocampal cultures from munc-13-1 KO mice showed augmentation, whereas synapses from wild-type animals underwent depression with the same protocol. Munc-13-1 is a presynaptic vesicle priming factor (Augustin et al., 1999), and hippocampal neurons express both munc-13-1 and munc-13-2. The direction of short-term plasticity therefore depended on whether synapses primarily used munc-13-1 (as in wild-type mice) or munc-13-2 (as in munc-13-1 KO mice) as their priming factor. Augmentation seen in munc-13-2 driven synapses was sensitive to phospholipase C (PL-C) inhibitors, but it was unaffected by various protein kinase inhibitors (Rosenmund et al., 2002). This indicates a role of the PL-C product diacylglycerol, which might directly activate munc-13-2 via binding to its C1 domain.

The fact that various Ca^{2+}-dependent signaling pathways have been proposed in PTP and augmentation (see above) might indicate that the signaling pathways mediating STE differ between synapses. Synapses vary greatly among each other, both in their morphology and their ultrastructural organization (Walmsley et al., 1998; Atwood and Karunanithi, 2002), as well as in their molecular composition. Differences between synapses might also explain some of the difficulty in finding a generally accepted model of how residual Ca^{2+} acts to cause facilitation (see above and Table 3.1). Various factors determine the signaling properties and the short-term plasticity of a synapse. First, the ultrastructural organization, like the exact co-localization of Ca^{2+} channels and vesicles (Rozov et al., 2001; Atwood and Karunanithi, 2002), and the size, number and density of active zones (Walmsley et al., 1998) will exert an influence on short-term plasticity. Second, molecules which mediate Ca^{2+}-regulated membrane fusion, that is soluble NSF (*N*-ethylmaleimide-sensitive factor) attachment protein receptor (SNARE) proteins, synaptotagmins and other proteins associated with the SNARE complex (Rettig and Neher, 2002; Jahn et al., 2003) might exert influences on the kinetics, and on the Ca^{2+} sensitivity of vesicle fusion. Third, modulatory proteins like Ca^{2+}-binding proteins acting as Ca^{2+} buffers (Caillard et al., 2000; Blatow et al., 2003), or as signaling molecules (Tsujimoto et al., 2002; Sippy et al., 2003) will influence synaptic facilitation (see Table 3.1), and specific phospholipases and protein kinases induce longer-lasting forms of STE, or presynaptic forms of long-term changes in synaptic strength (see Chapter 4). Thus, synapses have a wide range of possibilities to fine-tune their signaling properties and short-term plasticity, according to the needs of the neuronal networks in which they operate.

REFERENCES

Abbott, L.F., Varela, J.A., Sen, K. and Nelson, S.B. (1997). Synaptic depression and cortical gain control. *Science*, **275**, 220–224.

Alle, H., Jonas, P. and Geiger, J.R.P. (2001). PTP and LTP at a hippocampal mossy fiber-interneuron synapse. *Proc Natl Acad Sci USA*, **98**, 14708–14713.

Atluri, P.P. and Regehr, W.G. (1996). Determinants of the time course of facilitation at the granule cell to Purkinje cell synapse. *J Neurosci*, **16**, 5661–5671.

Atwood, H.L. and Karunanithi, S. (2002). Diversification of synaptic strength: presynaptic elements. *Nat Rev Neurosci*, **3**, 497–516.

Augustine, G.J. (1990). Regulation of transmitter release at the squid giant synapse by presynaptic delayed rectifier potassium current. *J Physiol*, **431**, 343–364.

Augustine, G.J., Adler, E.M. and Charlton, M.P. (1991). The calcium signal for transmitter secretion from presynaptic nerve terminals. *Ann NY Acad Sci*, **635**, 365–381.

Augustin, I., Rosenmund, C., Südhof, T.C. and Brose, N. (1999). Munc13-1 is essential for fusion competence of glutamatergic synaptic vesicles. *Nature*, **400**, 457–461.

Bain, A.I. and Quastel, D.M.J. (1992). Multiplicative and additive Ca^{2+}-dependent components of facilitation at mouse endplates. *J Physiol*, **455**, 383–405.

Barrett, E.F. and Stevens, C.F. (1972). The kinetics of transmitter release at the frog neuromuscular junction. *J Physiol*, **227**, 691–708.

Beierlein, M., Gibson, J.R. and Connors, B.W. (2003). Two dynamically different inhibitory networks in layer 4 of the neocortex. *J Neurophysiol*, **90**, 2987–3000.

Bellingham, M.C. and Walmsley, B. (1999). A novel presynaptic inhibitory mechanism underlies paired pulse depression at a fast central synapse. *Neuron*, **23**, 159–170.

Bertram, R., Sherman, A. and Stanley, E.F. (1996). Single-domain/bound calcium hypothesis of transmitter release and facilitation. *J Neurophysiol*, **75**, 1919–1931.

Beutner, D., Voets, T., Neher, E. and Moser, T. (2001). Calcium dependence of exocytosis and endocytosis at the cochlear inner hair cell afferent synapse. *Neuron*, **29**, 681–690.

Bischofberger, J., Geiger, J.R. and Jonas, P. (2002). Timing and efficacy of Ca^{2+} channel activation in hippocampal mossy fiber boutons. *J Neurosci*, **22**, 10593–10602.

Blatow, M., Caputi, A., Burnashev, N., Monyer, H. and Rozov, A. (2003). Ca^{2+} buffer saturation underlies paired pulse facilitation in Calbindinh-D28k-containing terminals. *Neuron*, **38**, 79–88.

Bollmann, J., Sakmann, B. and Borst, J. (2000). Calcium sensitivity of glutamate release in a calyx-type terminal. *Science*, **289**, 953–957.

Borst, J.G.G. and Sakmann, B. (1996). Calcium influx and transmitter release in a fast CNS synapse. *Nature*, **383**, 431–434.

Borst, J.G.G. and Sakmann, B. (1998a). Calcium current during a single action potential in a large presynaptic terminal of the rat brainstem. *J Physiol*, **506**, 143–157.

Borst, J.G.G. and Sakmann, B. (1998b). Facilitation of presynaptic calcium currents in the rat brainstem. *J Physiol*, **513**, 149–155.

Borst, J.G.G., Helmchen, F. and Sakmann, B. (1995). Pre- and postsynaptic whole-cell recordings in the medial nucleus of the trapezoid body of the rat. *J Physiol*, **489**, 825–840.

Brager, D.H., Cai, X. and Thompson, S.M. (2003). Activity-dependent activation of presynaptic protein kinase C mediates post-tetanic potentiation. *Nat Neurosci*, **6**, 551–552.

Caillard, O., Moreno, H., Schwaller, B., Llano, I., Celio, M.R. and Marty, A. (2000). Role of the calcium-binding protein parvalbumin in short-term synaptic plasticity. *Proc Natl Acad Sci USA*, **97**, 13372–13377.

Chad, J.E. and Eckert, R. (1984). Calcium domains associated with individual channels can account for anomalous voltage relations of Ca-dependent responses. *Biophys J*, **45**, 993–999.

Chapman, P.F., Frenguelli, B.G., Smith, A., Chen, C.M. and Silva, A.J. (1995). The alpha-Ca^{2+}/calmodulin kinase II: a bidirectional modulator of presynaptic plasticity. *Neuron*, **14**, 591–597.

Charlton, M.P., Smith, S.J. and Zucker, R.S. (1982). Role of presynaptic calcium ions and channels in synaptic facilitation and depression at the squid giant synapse. *J Physiol*, **323**, 173–193.

Chow, R.H., Klingauf, J. and Neher, E. (1994). Time course of Ca^{2+} concentration triggering exocytosis in neuroendocrine cells. *Proc Natl Acad Sci USA*, **91**, 12765–12769.

Chung, S., Li, X. and Nelson, S.B. (2002). Short-term depression at thalamocortical synapses contributes to rapid adaptation of cortical sensory responses *in vivo*. *Neuron*, **34**, 437–446.

Cook, D.L., Schwindt, P.C., Grande, L.A. and Spain, W.J. (2003). Synaptic depression in the localization of sound. *Nature*, **421**, 66–70.

Cuttle, M.F., Tsujimoto, T., Forsythe, I.D. and Takahashi, T. (1998). Facilitation of the presynaptic calcium current at an auditory synapse in rat brainstem. *J Physiol*, **512**, 723–729.

del Castillo, J. and Katz, B. (1954a). Quantal components of the end-plate potential. *J Physiol*, **124**, 560–573.

del Castillo, J. and Katz, B. (1954b). Statistical factors involved in neuromuscular facilitation and depression. *J Physiol*, **124**, 574–585.

Delaney, K.R. and Tank, D.W. (1994). A quantitative measurement of the dependence of short-term synaptic enhancement on presynaptic residual calcium. *J Neurosci*, **14**, 5885–5902.

Delaney, K.R. and Zucker, R.S. (1990). Calcium released by photolysis of DM-nitrophen stimulates transmitter release at squid giant synapse. *J Physiol*, **426**, 473–498.

Delaney, K.R., Zucker, R.S. and Tank, D.W. (1989). Calcium in motor nerve terminals associated with posttetanic potentiation. *J Neurosci*, **9**, 3558–3567.

Dittman, J.S., Kreitzer, A.C. and Regehr, W.G. (2000). Interplay between facilitation, depression, and residual calcium at three presynaptic terminals. *J Neurosci*, **20**, 1374–1385.

Dodge, F.A. and Rahamimoff, R. (1967). Co-operative action of calcium ions in transmitter release at the neuromuscular junction. *J Physiol*, **193**, 419–432.

Dudel, J. and Kuffler, S.W. (1961). Mechanism of facilitation at the crayfish neuromuscular junction. *J Physiol*, **155**, 530–542.

Fatt, P. and Katz, B. (1952). Spontaneous subthreshold activity at motor nerve endings. *J Physiol*, **117**, 109–128.

Felmy, F., Neher, E. and Schneggenburger, R. (2003). Probing the intracellular calcium sensitivity of transmitter release during synaptic facilitation. *Neuron*, **37**, 801–811.

Fernández-Chacón, R., et al. (2001). Synaptotagmin I functions as a calcium regulator of release probability. *Nature*, **410**, 41–49.

Fierro, L. and Llano, I. (1996). High endogenous calcium buffering in Purkinje cells from rat cerebellar slices. *J Physiol*, **496**, 617–625.

Forsythe, I.D. (1994). Direct patch recording from identified presynaptic terminals mediating glutamatergic EPSCs in the rat CNS, *in vitro*. *J Physiol*, **479**, 381–387.

Geiger, J.R. and Jonas, P. (2000). Dynamic control of presynaptic Ca^{2+} inflow by fast-inactivating K^+ channels in hippocampal mossy fiber boutons. *Neuron*, **28**, 927–939.

Geppert, M., Goda, Y., Hammer, R.E., Li, C., Rosahl, T.W., Stevens, C.F. and Südhof, T.C. (1994). Synaptotagmin I: a major Ca^{2+} sensor for transmitter release at a central synapse. *Cell*, **79**, 717–727.

Gerber, S.H., Garcia, J., Rizo, J. and Südhof, T.C. (2001). An unusual C_2-domain in the active-zone protein piccolo: implications for Ca^{2+} regulation of neurotransmitter release. *EMBO J*, **20**, 1605–1619.

Gibson, J.R., Beierlein, M. and Connors, B.W. (1999). Two networks of electrically coupled inhibitory neurons in neocortex. *Nature*, **402**, 75–79.

Granseth, B., Ahlstrand, E. and Lindström, S. (2002). Paired pulse facilitation of corticogeniculate EPSCs in the dorsal lateral geniculate nucleus of the rat investigated *in vitro*. *J Physiology*, **544**, 477–486.

Heidelberger, R., Heinemann, C., Neher, E. and Matthews, G. (1994). Calcium dependence of the rate of exocytosis in a synaptic terminal. *Nature*, **371**, 513–515.

Heinemann, C., Chow, R.H., Neher, E. and Zucker, R.S. (1994). Kinetics of the secretory response in bovine chromaffin cells following flash photolysis of caged Ca^{2+}. *Biophys J*, **67**, 2546–2557.

Helmchen, F., Borst, J.G.G. and Sakmann, B. (1997). Calcium dynamics associated with a single action potential in a CNS presynaptic terminal. *Biophys J*, **72**, 1458–1471.

Ikura, M. (1996). Calcium binding and conformational response in EF-hand proteins. *Trend Biochem*, **21**, 14–17.

Ishikawa, T., Sahara, Y. and Takahashi, T. (2002). A single packet of transmitter does not saturate postsynaptic glutamate receptors. *Neuron*, **34**, 613–621.

Jackson, M., Konnerth, A. and Augustine, G. (1991). Action potential broadening and frequency-dependent facilitation of calcium signals in pituitary nerve terminals. *Proc Natl Acad Sci USA*, **88**, 380–384.

Jahn, R., Lang, T. and Südhof, T.C. (2003). Membrane fusion. *Cell*, **112**, 519–533.

Johnson, E.W. and Wernig, A. (1971). The binomial nature of transmitter release at the crayfish neuromuscular junction. *J Physiol*, **218**, 757–767.

Kamiya, H. and Zucker, R.S. (1994). Residual Ca^{2+} and short-term synaptic plasticity. *Nature*, **371**, 603–606.

Katz, B. and Miledi, R. (1968). The role of calcium in neuromuscular facilitation. *J Physiol*, **195**, 481–492.

Konnerth, A., Llano, I. and Armstrong, C. (1990). Synaptic currents in cerebellar Purkinje cells. *Proc Natl Acad Sci USA*, **87**, 2662–2665.

Korn, H., Triller, A., Mallet, A. and Faber, D.S. (1981). Fluctuating responses at a central synapse: n of binomial fit predicts number of stained presynaptic boutons. *Science*, **213**, 898–901.

Liley, A.W. and North, K.A.K. (1953). An electrical investigation of effects of repetitive stimulation on mammalian neuromuscular junction. *J Neurophysiol*, **16**, 509–527.

Littleton, J.T., Stern, M., Schulze, K., Perin, M. and Bellen, H.J. (1993). Mutational analysis of drosophila *synaptotagmin* demonstrates its essential role in Ca^{2+}-activated neurotransmitter release. *Cell*, **74**, 1125–1134.

Liu, G., Choi, S. and Tsien, R.W. (1999). Variability of neurotransmitter concentration and nonsaturation of postsynaptic AMPA receptors at synapses in hippocampal cultures and slices. *Neuron*, **22**, 395–409.

Llinás, R., Gruner, J.A., Sugimori, M., McGuinness, T.L. and Greengard, P. (1991). Regulation by synapsin I and Ca^{2+}-calmodulin-dependent protein kinase II of transmitter release in squid giant synapse. *J Physiol*, **436**, 257–282.

Maccaferri, G., Tóth, K. and McBain, C.J. (1998). Target-specific expression of presynaptic mossy fiber plasticity. *Science*, **279**, 1368–1370.

Maeda, H., Ellis-Davies, G.C.R., Ito, K., Miyashita, Y. and Kasai, H. (1999). Supralinear Ca^{2+} signaling by cooperative and mobile Ca^{2+} buffering in Purkinje neurons. *Neuron*, **24**, 989–1002.

Magleby, K.L. (1987). Short-term changes in synaptic efficacy. In: *Synaptic Function* (eds Edelman, G.M., Gall, W.E. and Cowan, W.M.), Wiley, New York, pp. 21–56.

Magleby, K.L. and Zengel, J.E. (1976). Augmentation: a process that acts to increase transmitter release at the frog neuromuscular junction. *J Physiol*, **257**, 449–470.

Markram, H., Wang, Y. and Tsodyks, M. (1998). Differential signaling via the same axon of neocortical pyramidal neurons. *Proc Natl Acad Sci USA*, **95**, 5323–5328.

Meinrenken, C., Borst, J.G.G. and Sakmann, B. (2002). Calcium secretion coupling at calyx of Held governed by nonuniform channel-vesicle topography. *J Neurosci*, **22**, 1648–1667.

Meyer, A.C., Neher, E. and Schneggenburger, R. (2001). Estimation of quantal size and number of functional active zones at the calyx of Held synapse by nonstationary EPSC variance analysis. *J Neurosci*, **21**, 7889–7900.

Nadim, F., Manor, Y., Kopell, N. and Marder, E. (1999). Synaptic depression creates a switch that controls the frequency of an oscillatory circuit. *Proc Natl Acad Sci USA*, **96**, 8206–8211.

Nägerl, U.V., Novo, D., Mody, I. and Vergara, J.L. (2000). Binding kinetics of calbindin-D_{28k} determined by flash photolysis of caged Ca^{2+}. *Biophys J*, **79**, 3009–3018.

Neher, E. (1998a). Usefulness and limitations of linear approximations to the understanding of Ca^{++} signals. *Cell Calcium*, **24**, 345–357.

Neher, E. (1998b). Vesicle pools and Ca^{2+} microdomains: new tools for understanding their roles in neurotransmitter release. *Neuron*, **20**, 389–399.

Neher, E. and Augustine, G.J. (1992). Calcium gradients and buffers in bovine chromaffin cells. *J Physiol*, **450**, 273–301.

Otis, T., Zhang, S. and Trussell, L.O. (1996). Direct measurement of AMPA receptor desensitization induced by glutamatergic synaptic transmission. *J Neurosci*, **16**, 7496–7504.

Quastel, D.M.J. (1997). The binomial model in fluctuation analysis of quantal neurotransmitter release. *Biophys J*, **72**, 728–753.

Redman, S. (1990). Quantal analysis of synaptic potentials in neurons of the central nervous system. *Physiol Rev*, **70**, 165–198.

Regehr, W.G. and Atluri, P.P. (1995). Calcium transients in cerebellar granule cell presynaptic terminals. *Biophys J*, **68**, 2156–2170.

Regehr, W.G., Delaney, K.R. and Tank, D.W. (1994). The role of presynaptic calcium in short-term enhancement at the hippocampal mossy fiber synapse. *J Neurosci*, **14**, 523–537.

Rettig, J. and Neher, E. (2002). Emerging roles of presynaptic proteins in Ca^{++}-triggered exocytosis. *Science*, **298**, 781–785.

Reyes, A., Lujan, R., Rozov, A., Burnashev, N., Somogyi, P. and Sakmann, B. (1998). Target-cell-specific facilitation and depression in neocortical circuits. *Nat Neurosci*, **1**, 279–285.

Roberts, W.M. (1994). Localization of calcium signals by a mobile calcium buffer in frog saccular hair cells. *J Neurosci*, **14**, 3246–3262.

Rosahl, T.W., Geppert, M., Spillane, D., Herz, J., Hammer, R.E., Malenka, R.C. and Südhof, T.C. (1993). Short-term synaptic plasticity is altered in mice lacking synapsin I. *Cell*, **75**, 661–670.

Rosenmund, C., Sigler, A., Augustin, I., Reim, K., Brose, N. and Rhee, J.-S. (2002). Differential control of vesicle priming and short-term plasticity by munc13 isoforms. *Neuron*, **33**, 411–424.

Rozov, A. and Burnashev, N. (1999). Polyamine-dependent facilitation of postsynaptic AMPA receptors counteracts paired-pulse depression. *Nature*, **401**, 594–598.

Rozov, A., Burnashev, N., Sakmann, B. and Neher, E. (2001). Transmitter release modulation by intracellular Ca^{2+} buffers in facilitating and depressing nerve terminals of pyramidal cells in layer 2/3 of the rat neocortex indicates a target cell-specific difference in presynaptic calcium dynamics. *J Physiol*, **531**, 807–826.

Salin, P.A., Scanziani, M., Malenka, R.C. and Nicoll, R.A. (1996). Distinct short-term plasticity at two excitatory synapses in the hippocampus. *Proc Natl Acad Sci USA*, **93**, 13304–13309.

Sätzler, K., Söhl, L.F., Bollmann, J.H., Borst, J.G.G., Frotscher, M., Sakmann, B. and Lübke, J.H. (2002). Three-dimensional reconstruction of a calyx of Held and its postsynaptic principal neuron in the medial nucleus of the trapezoid body. *J Neurosci*, **22**, 10567–10579.

Scanziani, M., Gähwiler, B.H. and Charpark, S. (1998). Target cell-specific modulation of transmitter release at terminals from a single axon. *Proc Natl Acad Sci USA*, **95**, 12004–12009.

Scheuss, V., Schneggenburger, R. and Neher, E. (2002). Separation of presynaptic and postsynaptic contributions to depression by covariance analysis of successive EPCSs at the calyx of Held synapse. *J Neurosci*, **22**, 728–739.

Schikorski, T. and Stevens, C.F. (1997). Quantitative ultrastructural analysis of hippocampal excitatory synapses. *J Neurosci*, **17**, 5858–5867.

Schikorski, T. and Stevens, C.F. (2001). Morphological correlates of functionally defined synaptic vesicle populations. *Nat Neurosci*, **4**, 391–395.

Schneggenburger, R. and Neher, E. (2000). Intracellular calcium dependence of transmitter release rates at a fast central synapse. *Nature*, **406**, 889–893.

Schneggenburger, R., Sakaba, T. and Neher, E. (2002). Vesicle pools and short-term synaptic depression: lessons from a large synapse. *Trend Neurosci*, **25**, 206–212.

Silver, R.A., Cull-Candy, S.G. and Takahashi, T. (1996). Non-NMDA glutamate receptor occupancy and open probability at a rat cerebellar synapse with single and multiple release sites. *J Physiol*, **494**, 231–250.

Silver, R.A., Momiyama, A. and Cull-Candy, S.G. (1998). Locus of frequency-dependent depression identified with multiple-probability fluctuation analysis at rat climbing fibre-Purkinje cell synapses. *J Physiol*, **510**, 881–902.

Silver, R.A., Lübke, J., Sakmann, B. and Feldmeyer, D. (2003). High-probability uniquantal transmission at excitatory synapses in the barrel cortex. *Science*, **302**, 1981–1984.

Simon, S.M. and Llinás, R.R. (1985). Compartmentalization of the submembrane calcium activity during calcium influx and its significance in transmitter release. *Biophys J*, **48**, 485–498.

Sippy, T., Cruz-Martin, A., Jeromin, A. and Schweizer, F.E. (2003). Acute changes in short-term plasticity at synapses with elevated levels of neuronal calcium sensor-1. *Nat Neurosci*, **6**, 1031–1038.

Stanley, E.F. (1986). Decline in calcium cooperativity as the basis of facilitation at the squid giant synapse. *J Neurosci*, **6**, 782–789.

Stevens, C.F. and Wesseling, J.F. (1999). Augmentation is a potentiation of the exocytotic process. *Neuron*, **22**, 139–146.

Stevens, C.F., Tonegawa, S. and Wang, Y. (1994). The role of calcium–calmodulin kinase II in three forms of synaptic plasticity. *Curr Biol*, **4**, 687–693.

Südhof, T.C. (2002). Synaptotagmins: why so many? *J Biol Chem*, **277**, 7629–7632.

Sun, J.-Y. and Wu, L.-G. (2001). Fast kinetics of exocytosis revealed by simultaneous measurements of presynaptic capacitance and postsynaptic currents at a central synapse. *Neuron*, **30**, 171–182.

Swandulla, D., Hans, M., Zipser, K. and Augustine, G.J. (1991). Role of residual calcium in synaptic depression and posttetanic potentiation: fast and slow calcium signaling in nerve terminals. *Neuron*, **7**, 915–926.

Tang, Y., Schlumpberger, T., Kim, T., Lueker, M. and Zucker, R.S. (2000). Effects of mobile buffers on facilitation: experimental and computational studies. *Biophys J*, **78**, 2735–2751.

Tsodyks, M.V. and Markram, H. (1997). The neural code between neocortical pyramidal neurons depends on neurotransmitter release probability. *Proc Natl Acad Sci USA*, **94**, 719–723.

Tsujimoto, T., Jeromin, A., Saitoh, N., Roder, J.C. and Takahashi, T. (2002). Neuronal calcium sensor 1 and activity-dependent facilitation of P/Q-type calcium currents at presynaptic nerve terminals. *Science*, **295**, 2276–2279.

von Gersdorff, H. and Borst, J.G.G. (2002). Short-term plasticity at the calyx of Held. *Nat Rev Neurosci*, **3**, 53–64.

von Gersdorff, H., Schneggenburger, R., Weis, S. and Neher, E. (1997). Presynaptic depression at a calyx synapse: the small contribution of metabotropic glutamate receptors. *J Neurosci*, **17**, 8137–8146.

Wadiche, J.I. and Jahr, C.E. (2001). Multivesicular release at climbing fiber-Purkinje cell synapses. *Neuron*, **32**, 301–313.

Walmsley, B., Alvarez, F.J. and Fyffe, R.E.W. (1998). Diversity of structure and function at mammalian central synapses. *Trend Neurosci*, **21**, 81–88.

Wojtowicz, J.M., Marin, L. and Atwood, H.L. (1994). Activity-dependent changes in synaptic release sites at the crayfish neuromuscular junction. *J Neurosci*, **14**, 3688–3703.

Wölfel, M. and Schneggenburger, R. (2003). Presynaptic capacitance measurements and Ca^{2+} uncaging reveal submillisecond exocytosis kinetics and characterize the Ca^{2+} sensitivity of vesicle pool depletion at a fast CNS synapse. *J Neurosci*, **23**, 7059–7068.

Worden, M.K., Bykhovskaja, M. and Hackett, J.T. (1997). Facilitation at the lobster neuromuscular junction: a stimulus-dependent mobilization model. *J Neurophysiol*, **78**, 417–428.

Wright, S.N., Brodwick, M.S. and Bittner, G.D. (1996). Calcium currents, transmitter release and facilitation of release at voltage-clamped crayfish nerve terminals. *J Physiol*, **496**, 363–378.

Xu-Friedman, M.A., Harris, K.M. and Regehr, W.G. (2001). Three-dimensional comparison of ultrastructural characteristics at depressing and facilitating synapses onto cerebellar Purkinje cells. *J Neurosci*, **21**, 6666–6672.

Yamada, W.M. and Zucker, R.S. (1992). Time course of transmitter release calculated from simulations of a calcium diffusion model. *Biophys J*, **61**, 671–682.

Zhang, S. and Trussell, L. (1994). Voltage clamp analysis of excitatory synaptic transmission in the avian nucleus magnocellularis. *J Physiol*, **480**, 123–136.

Zucker, R. (1973). Changes in the statistics of transmitter release during facilitation. *J Physiol*, **229**, 787–810.

Zucker, R. (1989). Short-term synaptic plasticity. *Ann Rev Neurosci*, **12**, 13–31.

Zucker, R.S. and Regehr, W.G. (2002). Short-term synaptic plasticity. *Annu Rev Physiol*, **64**, 355–405.

4

Long-term potentiation and long-term depression

Zafir I. Bashir and Peter V. Massey

Department of Anatomy, MRC Centre for Synaptic Plasticity, University of Bristol, Bristol, UK

4.1 Introduction

In 1949, Donald Hebb (Hebb, 1949) introduced an important model for the encoding of information in the brain. It stated that the repetitive activation of a presynaptic neuron together with the simultaneous activation of its postsynaptic counterpart would lead to a change in one or both neurons so as to produce an increase in the synaptic strength between them. Some 20 years after the introduction of this theory Lømo (1966), studying evoked responses in the hippocampus of anaesthetised rabbits, discovered that high-intensity stimulation (tetanus) resulted in a form of frequency-dependent potentiation. Further detailed investigation confirmed that brief high-frequency stimulation (HFS) induced long-lasting (several hours) enhancement of the magnitude of recorded extracellular field potentials (Bliss and Gardner-Medwin, 1973; Bliss and Lømo, 1973). These initial investigations were of major importance, because for the first time they provided a potential substrate for Hebb's theory of memory formation. Furthermore, this type of sustained synaptic strengthening was later demonstrated to possess properties consistent with Hebb's model. Long-term potentiation (LTP) and long-term depression (LTD) are long-lasting alterations in synaptic strength that have been demonstrated at glutamatergic synapses throughout the central nervous system (CNS) and are used as a model for the biochemical and cellular processes that may underlie learning and memory (Volume I, Chapter 2).

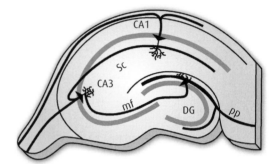

Figure 4.1. Schematic diagram of the *in vitro* hippocampal slice preparation showing the main regions: CA1, CA3, dentate gyrus (DG), and excitatory pathways: perforant path (pp), mossy fibres (mf) and Schaffer collaterals (Sc).

Since those early studies, synaptic plasticity has continued to be studied intensively in the rodent hippocampus both *in vivo* and *in vitro* following the development of the hippocampal slice preparation. Its large cells and well-defined circuitry make the *in vitro* hippocampal slice a particularly useful system for studying synaptic physiology. A schematic figure of the slice preparation is shown in Fig. 4.1. The hippocampus is a bilateral structure divided into three principal areas CA1, 2 and 3 (*cornu ammonis*) and together with the dentate gyrus make up the *hippocampal formation*. Hippocampus afferents arising from neighbouring layer II entorhinal cortex pass via the perforant path and synapse on the dendrites of granule cells in the dentate gyrus. From here, mossy fibres pass to and synapse in area CA3 and the CA3

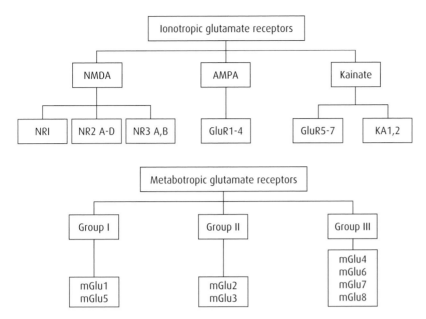

Figure 4.2. Glutamate receptors in the CNS. See main text for details.

neurones then synapse with the apical dendrites of CA1 neurones via the Schaffer collateral/commissural pathway.

Brain slices can be maintained in artificial cerebrospinal fluid (aCSF) and synaptic plasticity studied by recording excitatory responses from neuronal populations (extracellular excitatory postsynaptic potentials; field EPSPs (fEPSPs)) or individual cells (excitatory postsynaptic currents (EPSCs)). Measuring the response amplitude prior to and after the conditioning stimulation allows changes in synaptic transmission to be monitored. It can be seen from Fig. 4.1 that the hippocampus possesses three major sets of excitatory synapses: in the dentate gyrus (entorhinal cortex to granule cells of the dentate gyrus); at mossy fibre to CA3 pyramidal cells and from CA3 to CA1 cells (the Schaffer collateral/commissural pathway). The majority of investigations into synaptic plasticity have focussed on the latter area, which will henceforth be referred to as CA1 synapses.

L-glutamate mediates the majority of excitatory neurotransmission in the CNS and acts on two classes of receptor-ionotropic and metabotropic glutamate receptors, illustrated in Fig. 4.2.

The ionotropic glutamate receptors are ligand-gated cationic-selective channels classified into three groups based on pharmacology and structural similarity: N-methyl-D-aspartate receptors (NMDARs), α-amino-3-hydroxy-5-methyl-4-isoxazole propionic acid receptors (AMPARs) and kainate receptors (KARs); for a review see Dingledine et al. (1999). The ionotropic glutamate receptors are multimeric assemblies of four or five subunits, each encoded by a separate gene. Different subunit combinations and post-transcriptional modifications confer a vast degree of functional diversity to these receptors. Each subunit has three transmembrane domains, an extracellular N-terminus and an intracellular C-terminus domain.

There are three NMDAR subunit gene families containing one or more members: NR1, NR2A-D and NR3A-B. The NR1 subunits determine Ca^{2+} permeability and are essential for a functional NMDAR and the NR2 subunits form heteromeric receptors with NR1 and determine many of the biophysical and pharmacological properties of the receptor

(Dingledine et al., 1999). Little is currently known about NR3 subunits but coexpression of NR3A with NR1 and NR2 subunits may form a type of excitatory glycine receptor (Chatterton et al., 2002). NR2A and NR2B subunit expression predominates in adult rat forebrain (Sun et al., 2000). AMPARs are composed of four possible subunits (GluR1-4). Hippocampal neurones are assembled of predominantly GluR1/GluR2 or GluR3/GluR2 (Wenthold et al., 1996). Five KAR subunits have been cloned and classified as GluR5, 6, 7 (low affinity) KA1 and KA2 (high affinity) of which there exist multiple splice variants. AMPA and KARs principally mediate the fast synaptic transmission in the CNS whilst NMDARs contribute little to excitatory synaptic transmission under normal conditions owing to an Mg^{2+}-dependent block; NMDAR activation requires prolonged depolarisation. Postsynaptic potentials elicited by AMPA/KA receptor activation are due to increased cation conductance (Na^+, K^+, and to a smaller extent, Ca^{2+}) whereas, NMDARs once activated are highly permeable to Ca^{2+} as well as to Na^+ and K^+.

4.2 Long-term potentiation

LTP can be defined as a long-lasting (>1 h) increase in synaptic strength following the delivery of brief HFS (typically 50–200 Hz). Brief forms of potentiation that occur on a timescale from milliseconds to minutes after delivery of HFS such as those discussed in the previous chapter (*facilitation* and *post-tetanic potentiation*) are distinct from LTP and rely on transitory [Ca^{2+}] changes in the presynaptic terminal. A further temporal division can be made based on observations that the potentiation induced by HFS decays over about 1 h in the presence of certain protein kinase inhibitors (see later); this mechanistically distinct period is termed *short-term potentiation* (STP). There are now known to be different forms of LTP at different synapses, and the mechanisms of LTP induction may differ with regard to cell type, stimulation protocol and even dendritic subfield (Sanes and Lichtman, 1999). LTP has been demonstrated at all of the major synapses in the hippocampus, and

although this chapter will concentrate mainly on experiments from the hippocampus, it should be noted that activity-dependent LTP is a commonly observed feature of the neocortex and generally does not differ greatly from the hippocampus in its induction or expression mechanisms (see Tsumoto, 1992; Kirkwood and Bear, 1994; Bear and Kirkwood, 1993). Although controversial, there is compelling evidence linking LTP to learning and memory. For example, blockade or prior saturation of hippocampal LTP impairs hippocampus-dependent spatial learning in rats (Morris, 2003), and one group have convincingly demonstrated the occurrence of LTP processes in the motor cortex of rats after the learning of motor tasks (Rioult-Pedotti et al., 2000).

Properties of LTP

LTP has been shown to possess Hebbian properties: *cooperativity, synapse-specificity and associativity*. These properties are considered important in simple models of associative learning. First, for LTP to occur the postsynaptic membrane must be sufficiently depolarised. This requires the simultaneous stimulation of a minimum number of presynaptic fibres that act cooperatively to depolarise the postsynaptic cell (*cooperativity*). As stimulus intensity is increased more presynaptic fibres are "recruited" and an inverse relationship exists between stimulus frequency and intensity in that as one increases the need for the other diminishes. Secondly, LTP also exhibits *synapse-specificity*, which means that LTP occurs only at those synapses subjected to HFS, whilst neighbouring synapses do not undergo LTP (Kelso and Brown, 1986). This property relies on the spatial restriction of Ca^{2+} influx through NMDARs and is known as *homosynaptic* LTP. In contrast, *heterosynaptic* LTP is induced at one set of synapses following stimulation of a separate group of synapses. Heterosynaptic LTP is infrequently observed, but has been demonstrated in CA3 (Bradler and Barrioneuvo, 1989) and may play an important role in early development (Chen, 2001). Thirdly, and very important if it is to be used as a model for memory, LTP exhibits *associativity*. Experiments demonstrating the associative properties of LTP have exploited the existence of separate, well-defined pathways that converge onto the same neurons (McNaughton et al., 1978). Levy and Steward (1983) and Barrionuevo and Brown (1983) both demonstrated, in the dentate gyrus *in vivo* and CA1 *in vitro*, respectively, that a weak tetanus delivered to one pathway that alone is unable to produce LTP becomes able to do so if a strong tetanus is applied concurrently to the other. Associativity provides a cellular analogue of Pavlovian Classical Conditioning (see Chapter 5), where in these experiments the weak pathway is analogous to the conditioned stimulus and the strong pathway to the unconditioned stimulus (Bliss and Collingridge, 1993).

Role of glutamate receptors in LTP

A number of early studies identified a critical role for the NMDAR in hippocampal LTP (Collingridge, 2003). Induction of LTP most often requires NMDAR activation, although a notable NMDAR-independent form of LTP has been characterised at the mossy fibre-CA3 synapse (Harris and Cotman, 1986; Nicoll and Malenka, 1995) and involves other types of glutamate receptor (see later). The NMDAR antagonist D-2-amino-5-phosphonovalerate (AP5) has no effect on low-frequency-evoked responses, but blocks the induction of LTP if applied during HFS. Furthermore, NMDAR antagonists applied after LTP induction have no effect on potentiated synaptic transmission. Therefore, NMDARs play a critical role for the induction of LTP with HFS but not before or after LTP (Collingridge, 2003). Crucially, once activated, the NMDAR is highly permeable to Ca^{2+}, a key ion for triggering multiple biochemical pathways.

NMDARs are localised on postsynaptic dendritic spines and the unique biophysical properties of this receptor make it a prime candidate for involvement in LTP. At resting membrane potentials (normally between -60 and -75 mV) Mg^{2+} ions block the NMDAR, preventing the passage of ions. However, once the membrane is sufficiently depolarised, such as occurs during HFS, Mg^{2+} is rapidly removed from the channel allowing Na^+, K^+, and crucially, Ca^{2+} influx (Nowak et al., 1984). Thus at a low-stimulation rate (<0.01 Hz) fast EPSPs are mediated predominantly by glutamate activating AMPARs and KARs. NMDAR activation requires the temporal conjunction of coincident glutamate binding to NMDARs with prolonged postsynaptic depolarisation, thereby fulfilling the criterion of Hebbs' conjunctive pre- and postsynaptic activity. HFS *per se* is not required for LTP; thus low-frequency stimulation (LFS) is sufficient to induce LTP when paired with depolarising pulses (Wigstrom et al., 1986), whilst on the other hand HFS fails to induce LTP when postsynaptic depolarisation is limited (Malinow and Miller, 1986). Those properties of LTP outlined earlier can now be understood in terms of the properties of the NMDAR. Cooperativity relies on the collective activation of sufficient fibres to enhance the spread of depolarisation and consequent unblocking of NMDARs. Associativity can be understood in similar terms except that the required depolarisation can be transmitted to activated synapses by adjacent, simultaneously activated synapses. Synapse specificity can be understood as a requirement for sufficient NMDARs to be activated. NMDARs are concentrated in dendritic spines and allow a fairly localised Ca^{2+} signal.

L-glutamate can also mediate slow postsynaptic potentials and modulate ion channels through metabotropic glutamate receptors (mGluRs). These can be pre- or postsynaptically located. The eight known mGluR subtypes (mGluR1–8) are divided into three groups on the basis of sequence homology, transduction mechanisms and pharmacology (Fig. 4.2; see Anwyl (1999) for review). Group I mGluRs (mGluR1, 5) are positively coupled to phospholipase C (PLC) and stimulate production of diacylglycerol (DAG) and inositol-(1,4,5)-triphosphate (IP_3). DAG activates protein kinase C (PKC), and IP_3 triggers the release of intracellular Ca^{2+} from endoplasmic reticulum stores (Berridge, 1998). The remaining mGluRs-Group II (mGluR2, 3) and Group III (mGluR4, 6, 7, 8) are negatively coupled to adenylyl cyclase (AC), and inhibit the turnover of cyclic 3′, 5′-adenosine monophosphate (cAMP), thus attenuating the activity of protein kinase A (PKA).

MGluRs are considered to be located perisynaptically (Baude et al., 1993) and therefore may only contribute to the EPSP at relatively high levels of glutamate release. Evidence suggests that mGluRs are involved in hippocampal LTP (see Bortolotto et al., 1999a for review). The first report of a role for Group I mGluRs in LTP showed that NMDAR-independent LTP at mossy fibre synapses and NMDAR-dependent LTP in CA1 is blocked by the mGluR antagonist (RS)-α-methyl-4-carboxyphenylglycine (MCPG) (Bashir et al., 1993). A number of subsequent investigations into mGluRs and hippocampal LTP produced conflicting results, ultimately leading to the proposal by Bortolotto et al. (1994) of a putative "molecular switch". In this model, prior mGluR activation initiates a long-lasting intracellular cascade, or "molecular switch" that allows LTP to be induced with NMDAR activation. Therefore, this helps to explain why MCPG fails to block LTP at conditioned synapses (at which activation of mGluRs has occurred) but does block LTP at unconditioned synapses (Bortolotto et al., 1994). Further work has identified the mGluR5 subtype as responsible for setting the switch (Bortolotto et al., 1999a). In summary, therefore, these findings highlight the interplay that can exist between NMDA and mGluRs, and that the involvement of mGluRs in LTP depends on the prior experience of synapses tested.

In the hippocampus KARs elicit an excitatory postsynaptic current and presynaptically modulate glutamate release (Lerma, 2003). It has been proposed that presynaptic KARs may act to facilitate excitatory transmission during moderate synaptic activation, but suppress it during strong or sustained activity (Huettner, 2001). Research into KARs is at an early stage, but evidence suggests that they may be required for LTP at the mossy fibre synapse. The GluR5-selective antagonist LY382884 reduces frequency facilitation of AMPAR-mediated synaptic transmission and blocks LTP induction at the mossy fibre synapse (Bortolotto et al., 1999b; Lauri et al., 2001a, b).

Importantly, non-glutamatergic, inhibitory γ-aminobutyric acid receptors (GABARs) also act to influence LTP induction. Postsynaptic $GABA_A$ and $GABA_B$Rs mediate hyperpolarising inhibitory postsynaptic potentials (IPSPs) that under normal conditions restrict depolarisation and hence NMDAR activation. $GABA_B$Rs also exist as autoreceptors on GABAergic terminals so that GABA can inhibit its own release during HFS. Therefore during HFS, presynaptic $GABA_B$Rs indirectly contribute to postsynaptic depolarisation. Thus $GABA_A$R and $GABA_B$R antagonists, respectively, facilitate and inhibit LTP induction (Davies et al., 1991; Collingridge, 2003).

It is possible at this point to summarise the generally accepted model of LTP induction in CA1 (Fig. 4.3). A single stimulus applied to the Schaffer Collateral-Commissural pathway will evoke an AMPA/KAR-mediated EPSP (Fig. 4.3(a)). NMDARs are not activated due to a voltage-dependent Mg^{2+} block and mGluRs are only weakly activated due to their perisynaptic location. A biphasic IPSP mediated by postsynaptic $GABA_A$ (fast) and $GABA_B$Rs (slow) constrains postsynaptic depolarisation and hence NMDAR activation, which has slow activation kinetics. During HFS (Fig. 4.3(b)), AMPA/kainate EPSPs summate, and IPSPs are inhibited due to the autoinhibition through $GABA_B$ autoreceptors. Prolonged depolarisation allows strong activation of NMDAR activation and influx of Ca^{2+}. Furthermore, mGluRs are also likely activated during high levels of glutamate, resulting in the production of intracellular second messengers, such as IP_3 and PKC.

Induction mechanisms of LTP

LTP induction is triggered by, and depends upon a postsynaptic Ca^{2+} increase (Lynch et al., 1983; Malenka et al., 1988). Whilst NMDARs are an important trigger for increasing $[Ca^{2+}]_i$, the signal may be amplified through activation of voltage-gated calcium channels and from release from internal stores (through activation of metabotropic receptors) (Fitzjohn and Collingridge, 2002). Increased $[Ca^{2+}]_i$ can activate various protein kinases that phosphorylate and therefore activate proteins involved in LTP. Known Ca^{2+}-dependent, LTP-related protein kinases include Ca^{2+}/calmodulin-dependent kinase II (CaMKII), the Ca^{2+}/phospholipid-dependent PKC and mitogen-activated protein kinases (MAPKs) (Bliss and Collingridge, 1993; Lisman, 2003).

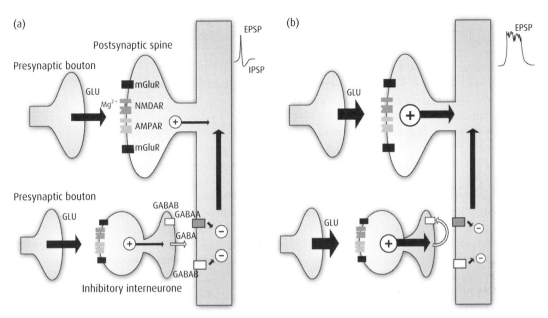

Figure 4.3. A schematic diagram showing the receptors involved in mediating excitatory synaptic transmission at (a) low frequency and (b) at high frequency in CA1. See main text (after Collingridge and Bliss, 1993).

PKC, a Ca^{2+}/phospholipid-dependent protein kinase was the first protein kinase to be studied for its role in LTP. Selective activation of PKC by phorbol esters potentiates synaptic transmission that occludes the induction of further LTP (Malenka et al., 1986; Hu et al., 1987; Malinow et al., 1989) and in the presence of PKC inhibitors HFS elicits only an initial STP that decays within 1 h. Furthermore, when applied after established LTP, PKC inhibitors may reduce LTP back to baseline levels but within a time limit (around 3 h) (Lovinger et al., 1987). Therefore, overall it seems that PKC is critical for the induction of LTP. Furthermore, its activity may outlast the initial induction signal and thus be involved in the conversion of STP into LTP (Bliss and Collingridge, 1993).

CaMKII is concentrated in postsynaptic spines and pharmacological experiments have explicitly demonstrated that it is required for LTP (Malenka et al., 1989; Malinow et al., 1989). Furthermore, mice lacking the most common CaMKII isoform αCaMKII exhibit impaired hippocampal LTP (Silva et al., 1992). CaMKII requires the formation of Ca^{2+}-calmodulin complex, after which it becomes autophosphorylated

and, therefore, remains independent of further Ca^{2+} to remain phosphorylated and therefore activated. There is evidence that the AC and cAMP-dependent PKA pathway is involved in LTP. LTP induction results in activation of PKA (Roberson and Sweatt, 1996) and PKA is required for both early and late-phase LTP (Otmakhova et al., 2000). The cAMP/PKA pathway contributes to LTP in one way by suppressing serine/threonine protein phosphatase PP1, thus swinging the balance in favour of greater stimulus-evoked kinase activity (see Section 4.3). Protein phosphatases are involved in LTP (see Winder and Sweatt, 2001 for review) and collectively, evidence suggests that PP2B (calcineurin) inhibits LTP induction in CA1 and that persistent PP2A inhibition contributes to its maintenance.

In addition to the post-translational modification of existing proteins, the synthesis of new proteins is to be important for the maintenance of LTP. Frey et al. (1988) and Frey and Morris (1997) divided LTP into two mechanistically distinct phases: "early" LTP (E-LTP; up to 3 h) and "late" LTP (L-LTP; 3–6 h). L-LTP requires transcription and translation processes that may play a role in structural modifications. It is known that L-LTP involves activation of AC and cAMP-dependent PKA (Frey et al., 1993).

Two members of the MAPK family, namely ERKI and ERKII, have also been shown to be critically important for LTP. ERKs are activated by a number of neurotransmitters that are coupled to PKC and PKA, including NMDARs and muscarinic acetylcholine receptors (mAChRs). MAPK is rapidly phosphorylated after LTP and ERK inhibition blocks L-LTP and attenuates E-LTP in CA1. This is perhaps not surprising, as ERKs play a major role in regulating gene transcription. MAPK translocates to the nucleus and can regulate the transcription of genes, one target being the transcription factor CREB (cAMP response element binding protein). ERKs can be activated by

both PKC and PKA and the interaction between these kinases is potentially complex. See Sweatt (2001).

LTP expression mechanisms

So how and where is LTP expressed? LTP can theoretically be expressed by the following:

1 Postsynaptic modifications, for example an increase in the number of excitatory receptors, or change in kinetics.
2 Presynaptic modifications resulting in an increase in L-glutamate release.
3 Morphological changes in synapse number, or spine size, density or number (Fig. 4.4(a–c)). In reality a combination of these most likely occur

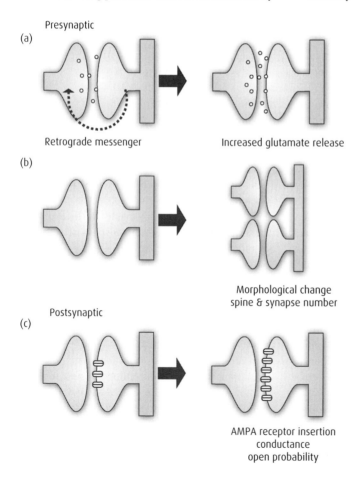

Figure 4.4. Potential LTP expression mechanisms. There is evidence that LTP can be expressed by one of three or a combination of (a) a presynaptic increase in the release, or probability of release of glutamate; (b) an increase in the number of dendritic spines and (c) a change in the conductance, open channel probability or increased number of postsynaptic AMPA receptors. See text for details.

with different time courses (Bliss and Collingridge, 1993).

As AMPARs mediate the greater part of fast excitatory transmission in the CNS, changes in AMPAR distribution, number, unitary conductance or kinetics represent potential mechanisms by which long-lasting changes in synaptic strength may take place. AMPAR trafficking is increasingly gaining acceptance as a prime expression mechanism for LTP. The potential importance of AMPAR trafficking in synaptic plasticity initially emerged following a report describing "silent synapses". Silent synapses are so called because they contain NMDARs but lack AMPARs and so are effectively silent during LFS. Isaac et al. (1995) showed that LTP-inducing stimuli act to "unsilence" these synapses as expressed by the subsequent appearance of AMPAR currents. It has only fairly recently been recognised that AMPARs are highly mobile and are internalised and inserted surprisingly rapidly, and that a variety of external stimuli can affect this process (see Carroll et al., 2001; Malinow and Malenka, 2002 for review). It seems that the phosphorylation state of AMPAR subunits controls the AMPAR trafficking process. Target sites for phosphorylation reside on AMPA receptor subunit C-termini. For example, the GluR1 AMPA receptor subunit is phosphorylated on Serine residue 845 (Ser 845) by a number of kinases and may underlie potentiation of AMPAR function (Roche et al., 1996). Phosphorylation of this site results in surface insertion of receptors and mutations of the Ser845 site prevent delivery of GluR1 to synapses by active CaMKII or LTP (Malinow and Malenka, 2002). AMPAR trafficking will be discussed further in Section 4.3.

Whilst LTP certainly involves postsynaptic modification, quantal analysis supports evidence for persistent increases in glutamate release *and* an increase in postsynaptic efficacy (Kullmann and Siegelbaum, 1995). This has led to the idea of diffusible "retrograde messengers" that originate postsynaptically and diffuse back to the presynaptic terminal. Several candidate retrograde messengers have been proposed: these include nitric oxide (O'Dell et al., 1991), carbon monoxide (Stevens and Wang, 1993), arachidonic acid (Williams and Bliss, 1988), platelet-activating factor (Kato et al., 1994) and brain-derived neurotrophic factor (BDNF) (Zakharenko et al., 2003).

"Late" LTP in some cases may also involve morphological modifications in synapse number, or/and spine size, and number. This appears to be particularly true in tissue from young animals or slice cultures, whereas in adult preparations, the data is not strongly supportive of substantial morphological changes following LTP. This perhaps serves to underline the fact that synapses possess more than one mechanism by which they can express LTP (see Gazzaley et al. (2002)).

Other neurotransmitters in LTP

Neurotransmitters of the ascending modulatory systems (acetylcholine (ACh) and the monoamines 5-hydroxytryptamine (5-HT), dopamine and noradrenaline) are known to modulate LTP, but the extent to which they do so is often a complex issue depending on the brain region studied, its circuitry and receptor subtype profile. These neurotransmitters may influence LTP in a number of ways: by modulating cortical excitability, enhancing the signal-to-noise ratio of cortical responses, or modifying the threshold for activity-dependent synaptic plasticity (Gu, 2002). For example, there is a substantial amount of literature supporting an involvement of muscarimic acetylcholine receptors (mAChRs) in LTP throughout numerous cortical areas where LTP is often blocked or at least attenuated by atropine or other similar muscarinic antagonists (Ramusson, 2000). The two prominent consequences of muscarinic acetylcholine receptor (mAChR) activation: namely pyramidal cell depolarisation and inhibition of GABA release could theoretically promote LTP. MAChRs are metabotropic receptors and are linked to similar intracellular pathways as those described for mGluRs. An important link between ACh and synaptic plasticity is in the facilitating interaction between mAChR and NMDAR activity (Harvey et al., 1993). ACh may simply facilitate LTP induction by lowering the threshold for NMDAR activation or act as an independently by activating numerous intracellular mechanisms

(Ramusson, 2000). ACh has long been implicated in learning and memory, since the discovery that death of cholinergic neurones in the "cholinergic basal forebrain" is one of the consequences of Alzheimer's disease (Bartus, 2000; Volume I, Chapter 31) and loss of cholinergic modulation may contribute to the cognitive impairments associated with this condition.

4.3 LTD

Synapses should be able to undergo decreases as well as increases in strength, otherwise network saturation would occur. LTD is defined as a long-lasting decrease in synaptic strength and has been demonstrated in the hippocampus, neocortex and cerebellum where it is thought to play a role in motor learning. In contrast to LTP, LTD induction typically requires prolonged, LFS (1–5 Hz) (Bliss and Collingridge, 1993).

Two forms of LTD have received particular attention: homosynaptic LTD at hippocampal and neocortical synapses, and associative LTD at cerebellar parallel fibre-purkinje cell synapses. LTD in the cerebellum was initially reported by Ito and colleagues (Ito et al., 1982). A hypothetical role for the cerebellum in motor learning had been formalised by Marr (1969) and Albus (1971) who predicted that the repeated coincident activation of two excitatory inputs (climbing and parallel fibres) would lead to LTD of synaptic strength at parallel fibre inputs. Ito et al. (1982) provided direct experimental evidence to support the existence of this form of associative LTD. The mechanisms of cerebellar LTD have now been fairly well established, but whether cerebellar LTD provides the cellular mechanisms that underlie the physiological role of the cerebellum in motor learning is still a question that is hotly debated (see Mauk et al., 1998). There is little doubt that cerebellar efferents drive the conditioned response that is an integral component of simple Pavlovian conditioning, such as the conditioned eyeblink response. However, whether LTD mechanisms *per se* are responsible for Pavlovian conditioning is the million-dollar question. As with studies involving similar questions in other parts of the brain much of the data has arisen through correlation studies. Whilst studies such as this suggest that LTD may be required for the physiological function of cerebellum there are still many caveats that need to be resolved before the link between plasticity and learning is sufficiently strong (see Mauk et al., 1998).

Properties of LTD

The first report of activity-dependent LTD was demonstrated in hippocampal CA1 slices *in vitro* (Lynch et al., 1977) and then subsequently in the dentate gyrus *in vivo* (Levy and Steward, 1979). In these studies, LTP-inducing stimuli delivered to one pathway resulted in long-lasting synaptic depression in a separate, non-tetanised pathway and therefore this type of LTD was *heterosynaptic*. Not long after this discovery, it was found that prolonged low-frequency patterns of stimulation (LFS; 1–5 Hz) if delivered after induction of stable LTP in the hippocampus *in vivo* reversed LTP back to pre-tetanic levels (Barrionuevo et al., 1980; Staubli and Lynch, 1990). This type of LTD is known as *depotentiation*, is optimally induced by prolonged LFS, and requires activation of NMDARs (Fujii et al., 1991) or mGluRs (Bashir et al., 1993). Input-specific (*homosynaptic*), de novo LTD (meaning LTD of naïve inputs without requirement for prior LTP) was eventually demonstrated in CA1 *in vitro* using a similar low-frequency protocol to that which produces depotentiation (LFS; 600–900 pulses, 1–3 Hz), and is NMDAR dependent (Dudek and Bear, 1992; Mulkey and Malenka, 1992). Both homosynaptic LTD and depotentiation have been demonstrated in hippocampus and neocortex (Kemp and Bashir, 2001).

Induction mechanisms of LTD

In the hippocampus and other brain regions LTD induction is developmentally downregulated, and thus whilst prolonged LFS may readily induce LTD in very young animals, the same stimulus protocol is often ineffective in adult preparations (Dudek and Bear, 1993; Wagner and Alger, 1995; Kemp et al., 2000).

This developmental switch does not simply reflect a loss of plasticity, since LTD can still be induced if the protocol is adjusted. For example, in adult CA1, where standard LFS (1 Hz, 15 min) is ineffective, 1 Hz trains of 900 paired pulses (50 ms interpulse interval), or 5–10 Hz for 15 min can induce LTD (Kemp and Bashir, 1997; Beretta and Cherubini, 1998). Alternatively, pharmacological manipulations such as antagonism of $GABA_A$ receptors can facilitate LTD (Kerr and Abraham, 1995). Furthermore, it should be noted that standard LFS can again induce LTD in aged (20–24 months) rats (Norris et al., 1996). Taken together, these reports suggest that the stimulation parameters for LTD induction change during development and old age. It is not yet established how those changes take place, but there is reason to believe that a developmental change in NMDAR subunit composition may be responsible (Paupard et al., 1997). In general, LTD induction follows the same rules *in vivo* as *in vitro* (Kemp and Bashir, 2001).

Hippocampal LTD and depotentiation appear to require either NMDAR (Fujii et al., 1991; Dudek and Bear, 1992; Mulkey and Malenka, 1992) or mGluR activation (Bashir et al., 1993; Otani and Connor, 1998). Furthermore, brief application of the agonist NMDA to hippocampal slices results in robust LTD in CA1 that is occluded by activity-dependent LTD suggesting that they share a common mechanism (Lee et al., 1998). NMDAR-dependent LTD and depotentiation has also been demonstrated outside the hippocampus, in many brain regions, for example in visual cortex (Kirkwood and Bear, 1994), at thalamo-cortical synapses in somatosensory cortex (Feldman et al., 1998), and perirhinal cortex (Ziakopoulos et al., 1999).

MGluRs also play a crucial role in LTD (see Bortolotto et al., 1999a; Kemp and Bashir, 2001, for review). The development of mGluR antagonists, for example the Group I/II mGluR antagonist αMCPG, has facilitated investigation into the role of mGluRs in LTD. A clear role for mGluRs in LTD first emerged when it was shown that MCPG blocks depotentiation in CA1 *in vitro* (Bashir et al., 1993; Bashir and Collingridge, 1994). It has been subsequently shown using MCPG that mGluRs can also play a role in de novo LTD in CA1 under certain conditions, although there have been reports showing that in some instances MCPG does not block LTD (e.g. Berretta and Cherubini, 1998). However, MCPG blocks LTD in neonatal CA1 (Bolshakov and Siegelbaum, 1994; Oliet et al., 1997), in adult CA1 *in vitro* (Otani and Connor, 1998) and *in vivo* (Manahan-Vaughan, 1997). Furthermore, modified stimulation protocols can uncover mGluR involvement. Thus, 1 Hz trains of 900 paired pulses (50 ms interpulse interval) has been used to induce mGluR-dependent LTD in adult hippocampus (Kemp and Bashir, 1999; Huber et al., 2000). The roles of different groups of mGluRs in LTD can depend on the induction parameters used or on the particular brain region under investigation. For example, in the dentate gyrus *in vitro*, each of the Group I mGluR antagonist aminoindan-1,5-dicarboxylic acid (AIDA) (Camodeca et al., 1999), MCPG and Group II mGluR antagonists (O'Mara et al., 1995a; Huang et al., 1997) have been shown to block LTD. In CA3, as in CA1, the role of mGluRs in LTD is not clear-cut and different forms of LTD exist that rely on different mechanisms (Kemp and Bashir, 2001). However, MCPG blocks LTD at mossy fibre synapses in CA3 (Bashir et al., 1993; Kobayashi et al., 1996). LTD in the cerebellum requires activation of mGluRs – most likely mGlu1 (Kano and Kato, 1987; Linden et al., 1991; Conquet et al., 1994; Shigemoto et al., 1994). In addition, there is a requirement for the activation of the AMPARs (Linden et al., 1991; Hemart et al., 1995) and for the activation of voltage-gated (most likely L-type) calcium channels (Linden et al., 1991; Konnerth et al., 1992). LTD and depotentiation requiring mGluR activation have also been demonstrated in other brain regions such as prefrontal cortex (Group I, II and dopamine) (Otani et al., 1999), perirhinal cortex (Cho et al., 2000) and striatum (Gubellini et al., 2001).

The requirement for NMDARs or mGluRs in LTD is almost invariably mutually exclusive, but one notable exception is in perirhinal cortex (Cho et al., 2000). Here, NMDARs, Group I and II mGluRs are required for LTD at resting (−70 mV) membrane potentials, whereas at more depolarised (−40 mV) membrane potentials Group II mGluR involvement became unnecessary. This suggests synergy between Group I and II mGluRs, most likely through an enhancement of intracellular Ca^{2+} release at hyperpolarised potentials (Cho et al., 2000).

In addition to activity-dependent LTD induced by LFS, a well-characterised form of LTD has also been observed following direct application of the mGluR Group I agonist (RS)-3,5-dihydroxyphenylglycine (DHPG) (Palmer et al., 1997; Fitzjohn et al., 1999; Schnabel et al., 1999a, b; Huber et al., 2000; Moult et al., 2002). DHPG-LTD is mediated through the mGlu5 subtype and does not require afferent stimulation (Palmer et al., 1997; Fitzjohn et al., 1999).

The role of other neurotransmitters in LTD

Non-glutamatergic receptors may be involved in the regulation of LTD induction. As in the case of LTP, the role of different neurotransmitters on modulating LTD is potentially complex. There are far fewer reports of a role for non-glutamatergic receptors in LTD than for LTP. However, beta-adrenergic receptors play a role in CA1 LTD (Katsuki et al., 1997) and in prefrontal cortex LTD requires coactivation of dopamine and mGluRs (Otani et al., 1999). Also, in a similar way to the previously described agonist-induced mGluR-LTD in CA1, pharmacological activation of mAChRs (Kirkwood et al., 1999; Massey et al., 2001) or noradrenergic receptors (Kirkwood et al., 1999) induces a form of NMDAR-independent and stimulation-independent LTD in visual and perirhinal cortex. A topic of current investigation is that of cannabinoids in synaptic plasticity and memory; cannabinoid receptors have been shown to be essential for certain types of synaptic depression (Ronesi et al., 2004).

Second messenger pathways involved in LTD

Like LTP, LTD is dependent upon a rise in postsynaptic Ca^{2+} and in CA1 LTD is blocked by postsynaptic infusion of Ca^{2+} buffering agents (Mulkey and Malenka, 1992). Ca^{2+} can be derived from NMDARs, mGluRs and voltage-gated Ca^{2+} channels (Fitzjohn

and Collingridge, 2002). Pharmacological agents that deplete IP_3-mediated release of Ca^{2+} from internal stores have also been shown to block LTD (O'Mara et al., 1995b; Reyes and Stanton, 1996). Additionally, NMDAR-mediated increases in Ca^{2+} are reduced by these agents (Alford et al., 1993), indicating that release from internal stores can be important for LTD mediated by NMDARs or mGluRs.

If Ca^{2+} is critical for both LTP *and* LTD, an explanation is required to explain how the same single messenger is able to achieve this. The results of many studies are consistent with the notion proposed in the Bienenstock–Cooper–Munro (BCM) model (Bienenstock et al., 1982) that the bi-directional control of synaptic strength depends on a combined function of pre- and postsynaptic activity. Therefore, progressive increases in activity will initially result in LTD and then in LTP. Experimental evidence is consistent with there being different thresholds for the induction of LTD and LTP. Artola and Singer (1993) provided evidence that these thresholds depend on postsynaptic membrane potential whilst others (Lisman, 1989) have suggested that the thresholds rely on some function of postsynaptic Ca^{2+} levels. Thus partial buffering of postsynaptic Ca^{2+} by intracellular Ca^{2+} buffers can result in the conversion of LTP to LTD (Kimura et al., 1990). There is also evidence for there being a U-shaped relationship between Ca^{2+} levels and the induction of LTD. Thus stimulation at frequencies between 0.01 and 10 Hz can produce increasing and then decreasing levels of LTD (Dudek and Bear, 1993). Furthermore, increasing the concentration of the NMDA receptor antagonist AP5 results in initially increasing and then decreasing levels of LTD (Cummings et al., 1996). Finally, a more direct approach to this question came with the findings that altering the concentration of intracellular Ca^{2+} buffer could produce the full range of plasticity from LTP through to LTD induced by the same induction protocol (Cho et al., 2001). Thus it is quite likely that both the magnitude and the direction (i.e., LTD or LTP) of plasticity is very tightly regulated by the magnitude of the postsynaptic rise in Ca^{2+}.

Lisman (1989) proposed that the magnitude of the Ca^{2+} signal could result in either LTP or LTD by selectively activating protein kinases or phosphatases, respectively. An important step in the biochemical cascade leading to LTD is the binding of Ca^{2+} to calmodulin to form a complex that can activate Ca^{2+}-calmodulin-dependent protein kinase (CaMKII) and Ca^{2+}-calmodulin-dependent protein phosphatase (PP2B/calcineurin). Lisman (1989) suggested that high $[Ca^{2+}]_i$ influx (such as would occur during HFS), would trigger the formation of the Ca^{2+}-calmodulin complex and hence CaMKII activation, leading to the phosphorylation of AMPA receptors or perhaps other substrates proteins involved in synaptic plasticity. Alternatively prolonged, moderate $[Ca^{2+}]_i$ influx by weak NMDAR activation (such as would occur during LFS) would lead to the Ca^{2+}-calmodulin complex selectively activating protein phosphatase PP2B (calcineurin) over CaMKII. An important aspect of this model is that PP2B is activated by nanomolar $[Ca^{2+}]_i$ and has a greater affinity for Ca^{2+} than CaMKII and PKC. Lisman's model was validated by Mulkey et al. (1993) who blocked LTD in CA1 with inhibitors of serine–threonine phosphatases PP1 and PP2A. Furthermore, LTD can also be blocked by calcineurin inhibitors (Mulkey et al., 1993). An increase in phosphatase activity is also observed in association with LTD (Thiels et al., 1998). The generally accepted pathway for this event is that calcineurin inactivates inhibitor-1 (I-1), thereby relieving the inhibition of PP1 and/or PP2, leading to LTD via dephosphorylation of AMPARs. Furthermore, in addition to AMPA receptor phosphorylation, phosphatases can dephosphorylate and thereby inhibit CaMKII, thus facilitating LTD and inhibiting LTP (Kemp and Bashir, 2001).

LTD and depotentiation are similar in that they are NMDAR dependent and involve phosphatase activity, but there is accumulating evidence that they are mediated by different mechanisms. For example, in adult rats depotentiation can be induced when LTD cannot (Bashir and Collingridge, 1994). Further, the Aα isoform of calcineurin has been shown to be crucial for induction of depotentiation (but not LTD or LTP) in the hippocampus (Zhuo et al., 1999). Depotentiation probably involves additional processes that act to reverse LTP-associated events, for example dephosphorylation of CAMKII (Winder and Sweatt, 2001).

LTD expression mechanisms

Potential expression mechanisms for LTP were discussed and summarised in Fig. 4.3. LTD has been associated with AMPAR endocytosis and there is also reason to believe that in some cases LTD is expressed presynaptically (Oliet et al., 1997).

Postsynaptic AMPAR internalisation is thought to be important in the expression of LTD and involves the endocytic pathway that relies on dynamin-dependent formation of clathrin-coated pits. Predictably, NMDAR-mediated AMPAR endocytosis requires Ca^{2+} and protein phosphatase activity (Carroll et al., 2001; Malinow and Malenka, 2002). AMPARs undergo rapid endocytosis in response to glutamate receptor activation, and LTD results in a decrease in the expression of detectable surface AMPARs at synapses in hippocampal cultures. Furthermore, LTD is blocked by inhibition of clathrin-mediated endocytosis. Similarly, the expression of cerebellar LTD is most likely due to a decrease in postsynaptic AMPA receptors since interfering with the mechanisms that result in endocytosis of AMPA receptors blocks LTD (Wang and Linden, 2000). However, in the cerebellum it is considered that mGlu-dependent activation of PKC is essential for phosphorylation of the C-terminal of the GluR2 subunit of AMPA receptors, recruitment of PICK1 and endocytosis of AMPA receptors (Xia et al., 2000; Chung et al., 2003). The involvement of PKC rather than protein phosphatases in the cerebellum serves to highlight the possibility that AMPAR endocytosis may be cell-type specific, perhaps depending on the constituent AMPA subunits and their associated proteins (Malinow and Malenka, 2002).

There is intense interest in how AMPARs are directed to the membrane surface and how these process regulate LTP and LTD. A number of key proteins that interact with AMPAR subunits and are though to be important in AMPA receptor trafficking have been identified. A detailed discussion of these candidate proteins is beyond the scope of this review, but more information can be obtained from Henley (2003).

4.4 Metaplasticity

In the preceding sections we have concentrated on mechanisms of induction of LTP and LTD. However it is now well established that the induction and/or the magnitude of LTP and LTD can be affected by prior activity that in itself does not produce observable changes in synaptic efficacy. Thus there is some "plastic" change of a different, or "meta", form that influences traditional synaptic plasticity – this phenomenon is known as *metaplasticity* (see Abraham and Tate, 1997 for review).

Numerous forms of metaplasticity have been described (Abraham and Tate, 1997), the differences of which relate mainly to the stimulation protocols or drug applications used and the different brain regions studied. Essentially each of these protocols "primes" (produces the metaplasticity in) the synapses in order that there is subsequently a change in the induction of LTP or LTD that would not have occurred otherwise. For example, short bursts of priming stimulation that do not cause any long-lasting change in synaptic strength have been reported to facilitate subsequent LTD induction (Wexler and Stanton, 1993; Wagner and Alger, 1995). Similarly, various forms of priming stimulation have also been described to inhibit or to facilitate the induction of LTP (Christie et al., 1995; Abraham and Tate, 1997). Proposed candidate mechanisms underlying metaplasticity include a change in the function of glutamate receptors. NMDAR-mediated synaptic transmission can undergo potentiation (Bashir et al., 1991) and depression (Selig et al., 1995), and given the critical role for NMDARs in LTP and LTD induction it is readily apparent that any change in NMDAR synaptic transmission brought about by a "priming" stimulus could have dramatic consequences for subsequent induction of LTP and LTD. Therefore, it is not surprising that both the metaplastic facilitation of LTD and the inhibition of LTP are reported

to rely on activation of NMDARs. In addition to a role for NMDARs in metaplasticity, there is also evidence that priming stimulation can produce changes in mGluR function. Again, given the role of mGluRs in synaptic plasticity it is not surprising that this might have profound effects on subsequent induction of synaptic plasticity (Abraham and Tate, 1997). Indeed, the induction and persistence of LTP can be facilitated by prior pharmacological activation of mGluRs as demonstrated by the "molecular switch hypothesis" of Bortolotto et al. (1994) and reported by Cohen and Abraham (1996). In summary, the data is supportive of a role for NMDARs in metaplasticity in one direction (in the facilitation of LTD or inhibition of LTP) and for mGluRs in the other (facilitation of LTP) (Abraham and Tate, 1997).

The BCM model (Bienenstock et al., 1982), which was based on experience-dependent modification in the visual cortex, proposes that low levels of afferent activity will result in the induction of LTD, whilst higher levels of afferent activity produce LTP. Furthermore, it also postulated that the modification threshold (crossover between LTD and LTP) is not fixed but dynamic, being determined at any time by afferent prior activity (Bear, 1995). Thus the "sliding" threshold can be considered to represent the phenomenon of "metaplasticity" (and vice versa) in that this threshold regulates the plastic outcome (induction or magnitude of LTP/LTD) of a given bout of afferent activity.

4.5 Conclusions

In this chapter, we have concentrated on the basic mechanisms that are thought to underlie induction and expression of long-term plasticity (LTP and LTD). These mechanisms of plasticity have been postulated to underlie a variety of physiological and pathophysiological processes.

For example, the activity-dependent development of the visual and somatosensory cerebral cortex is considered to rely on the same or similar processes that underlie LTP and LTD. Therefore, it is possible that remapping of the cerebral cortex that occurs, for example, following limb amputation (see

Volume I, Chapter 6) is akin to the activity-dependent development of the cortex and therefore may rely on similar underlying processes. Understanding these processes may provide strategies for remapping lost functions to undamaged brain regions Volume I, Chapters 8, 9, 11, 14 and 15. Similarly, other forms of neural recovery following injury may rely on, or be aided by, underlying processes that are akin to those that control cortical development.

In this same vein if LTP/LTD mechanisms truly are the cellular correlates of learning and memory then understanding these mechanisms may be crucial in preventing loss of such function that occurs during various brain disorders. Furthermore, if such loss of function is not preventable, then it may be possible to construct strategies to reverse loss of learning and memory once a more complete understanding of the cellular and molecular mechanisms of these processes has been achieved. Finally, it may turn out that understanding the mechanisms of "metaplasticity", that regulate the induction and or magnitude of subsequent LTP and LTP, may prove to be of equal or even greater value when considering potential strategies to prevent or overcome loss of synaptic function.

REFERENCES

Abraham, W.C. and Tate, W.P. (1997). Metaplasticity: a new vista across the field of synaptic plasticity. *Prog Neurobiol*, **52**, 303–323.

Albus, J.S. (1971). A theory of cerebellar function. *Math Biosci*, **10**, 25–61.

Alford, S., Frenguelli, B.G., Schofield, J.G. and Collingridge, G.L. (1993). Characterization of Ca2+ signals induced in hippocampal CA1 neurones by the synaptic activation of NMDA receptors. *J Physiol*, **469**, 693–716.

Anwyl, R. (1999). Metabotropic glutamate receptors: electrophysiological properties and roles in plasticity. *Brain Res Rev*, **29**(1), 83–120.

Artola, A. and Singer, W. (1993). Long-term depression of excitatory synaptic transmission and its relationship to long-term potentiation. *TiNs*, **16**, 480–487.

Barrionuevo, G. and Brown, T.H. (1983). Associative long-term potentiation in hippocampal slices. *Proc Natl Acad Sci USA*, **80**, 7374–7351.

Barrionuevo, G., Schottler, F. and Lynch, G. (1980). The effects of repetitive low frequency stimulation on control and "potentiatied" synaptic responses in the hippocampus. *Life Sci*, **27**, 2385–2391.

Bartus, R.T. (2000). On neurodegenerative diseases, models, and treatment strategies: lessons learned and lessons forgotten a generation following the cholinergic hypothesis. *Exp Neurol*, **163**, 495–529.

Bashir, Z.I. and Collingridge, G.L. (1994). An investigation of depotentiation of long-term potentiation in the CA1 region of the hippocampus. *Exp Brain Res*, **100**(3), 437–443.

Bashir, Z.I., Alford, S., Davies, S.N., Randall, A.D. and Collingridge, G.L. (1991). Long-term potentiation of NMDA receptor-mediated synaptic transmission in the hippocampus. *Nature*, **349**, 156–158.

Bashir, Z.I., Bortolotto, Z.A., Davies, C.H., Beretta, N., Irving, A.J., Seal, A.J., Henley, J.M., Jane, D.E., Watkins, J.C. and Collingridge, G.L. (1993). Induction of LTP in the hippocampus needs synaptic activation of glutamate metabotropic receptors. *Nature*, **363**, 347–350.

Bashir, Z.I., Jane, D.E., Sunter, D.C., Watkins, J.C. and Collingridge, G.L. (1993). Metabotropic glutamate receptors contribute to the induction of long-term depression in the CA1 region of the hippocampus. *Eur J Pharmacol*, **239**(1–3), 265–266.

Baude, A., Nusser, Z., Roberts, J.D., Mulvihill, E., McIlhinney, R.A. and Somogyi, P. (1993). The metabotropic glutamate receptor (mGluR1 alpha) is concentrated at perisynaptic membrane of neuronal subpopulations as detected by immunogold reaction. *Neuron*, **11**(4), 771–787.

Bear, M.F. (1995). Mechanism for a sliding synaptic modification threshold. *Neuron*, **15**, 1–4.

Bear, M.F. and Kirkwood, A. (1993). Neocortical long-term potentiation. *Curr Opin Neurobiol*, **2**, 197–202.

Beattie, E.C., Carroll, R.C., Yu, X., Morishita, W., Yasuda, H., Von Zastrow, M. and Malenka, R.C. (2000). Regulation of AMPA receptor endocytosis by a signalling mechanism shared with LTD. *Nat Neurosci*, **3**, 1291–1300.

Berretta, N. and Cherubini, E. (1998). A novel form of long-term depression in the CA1 area of the adult rat hippocampus independent of glutamate receptors activation. *Eur J Neurosci*, **9**, 2957–2963.

Berridge, M. (1998). Neuronal calcium signalling. *Neuron*, **21**, 13–26.

Bienenstock, E., Cooper, L. and Munro, P. (1982). Theory for the development of neuron selectivity: orientation specificity and binocular interaction in visual cortex. *J Neurosci*, **2**, 32–48.

Bliss, T.V.P. and Collingridge, G.L. (1993). A synaptic model of memory: long-term potentiation in the hippocampus. *Nature*, **361**, 31–39.

Bliss, T.V. and Gardner-Medwin, A.R. (1973). Long-lasting potentiation of synaptic transmission in the dentate area of the unanaesthetized rabbit following stimulation of the perforant path. *J Physiol (Lond)*, **232**, 357–374.

Bliss, T.V. and Lømo, T. (1973). Long-lasting potentiation of synaptic transmission in the dentate area of the anaesthetized rabbit following stimulation of the perforant path. *J Physiol*, **232**, 331–356.

Bolshakov, V.Y. and Siegelbaum, S.A. (1994). Postsynaptic induction and presynaptic expression of hippocampal long-term depression. *Science*, **264**(**5162**), 1148–1152.

Bortolotto, Z.A., Bashir, Z.I., Davies, C.H. and Collingridge, G.L. (1994). A molecular switch activated by metabotropic glutamate receptors regulates induction of long-term potentiation. *Nature*, **368**, 740–743.

Bortolotto, Z.A., Fitzjohn, S.M. and Collingridge, G.L. (1999a). Roles of metabotropic glutamate receptors in LTP and LTD in the hippocampus. *Curr Opin Neurobiol*, **9**, 299–304.

Bortolotto, Z.A., Clarke, V.R., Delany, C.M., Parry, M.C., Smolders, I., Vignes, M., Ho, K.H., Miu, P., Brinton, B.T., Fantaske, R., Ogden, A., Gates, M., Ornstein, P.L., Lodge, D., Bleakman, D. and Collingridge, G.L. (1999b). Kainate receptors are involved in synaptic plasticity. *Nature*, **402**, 297–301.

Bradler, J.E. and Barrioneuvo, G. (1989). Long-term potentiation in hippocampal CA3 neurons: tetanized input regulates heterosynaptic efficacy. *Synapse*, **4**, 132–142.

Camodeca, N., Breakwell, N.A., Rowan, M.J. and Anwyl, R. (1999). Induction of LTD by activation of group I mGluR in the dentate gyrus *in vitro*. *Neuropharmacology*, **38**(**10**), 1597–1606.

Carroll, R.C., Beattie, E.C., von Zastrow, M. and Malenka, R.C. (2001). Role of AMPA receptor endocytosis in synaptic plasticity. *Nat Rev Neurosci*, **2**, 315–324.

Chatterton, J., Awobuluyi, M., Premkumar, L.S., Takahashi, H., Talantova, M., Shin, Y., Cui, J., Tu, S., Sevarino, K.A., Nakanishi, N., Tong, G., Lipton, S.A., Zhang, D. (2002). Excitatory glycine receptors containing the NR3 family of NMDA receptor subunits. *Nature*, **415**, 793–798.

Chen, C. (2001). Heterosynaptic LTP in early development. *Neuron*, **31**, 510–512.

Cho, K., Kemp, N., Noel, J., Aggleton, J.P., Brown, M.W. and Bashir, Z.I. (2000). A new form of long-term depression in the perirhinal cortex. *Nat Neurosci*, **2**, 150–156.

Cho, K., Aggleton, J.P., Brown, M.W. and Bashir, Z.I. (2001). An experimental test of the role of postsynaptic calcium levels in determining synaptic strength using perirhinal cortex of rat. *J Physiol*, **532**(**Pt 2**), 459–466.

Christie, B.R., Stellwagen, D. and Abraham, W.C. (1995). Evidence of common expression mechanisms underlying hetero-synaptic and associative long-term depression in the dentate gyrus. *J Neurophysiol*, **74**, 1244–1247.

Chung, H.J., Steinberg, J.P., Huganir, R.L. and Linden, D.J. (2003). Requirement of AMPA receptor GluR2 phosphorylation for cerebellar long-term depression. *Science*, **300**(**5626**), 1751–1755.

Cohen, A. and Abraham, W.C. (1996). Facilitation of long-term potentiation by prior activation of metabotropic glutamate receptors. *J Neurophysiol*, **76**, 953–962.

Collingridge, G.L. (2003). The induction of *N*-methyl-D-aspartate receptor-dependent long-term potentiation. *Philos Trans R Soc Lond B Biol Sci*, **358**, 635–641.

Conquet, F., Bashir, Z.I., Davies, C.H., Daniel, H., Ferraguti, F., Bordi, F., Franz-Bacon, K., Reggiani, A., Matarese, V., Condé, F., Collingridge, G.L. and Crépel, F. (1994). Motor deficit and impairment of synaptic plasticity in mice lacking mGluR1. *Nature*, **372**, 218–219.

Cummings, J.A., Mulkey, R.M., Nicoll, R.A. and Malenka, R.C. (1996). Ca^{2+} signaling requirements for long-term depression in the hippocampus. *Neuron*, **16**(**4**), 825–833.

Davies, C.H., Starkey, S.J., Pozza, M.F. and Collingridge, G.L. (1991). GABA autoreceptors regulate the induction of LTP. *Nature*, **349**, 609–611.

Dingledine, R., Borges, K., Bowie, D. and Traynellis, S.F. (1999). The glutamate receptor ion channels. *Pharmacol Rev*, **51**, 7–61.

Dudek, S.M. and Bear, M.F. (1992). Homosynaptic long-term depression in area CA1 of hippocampus and effects of *N*-methyl-D-aspartate receptor blockade. *Proc Natl Acad Sci USA*, **89**, 4363–4367.

Dudek, S.M. and Bear, M.F. (1993). Bidirectional long-term modification of synaptic effectiveness in the adult and immature hippocampus. *J Neurosci*, **13**(**7**), 2910–2918.

Feldman, D.E., Nicoll, R.A., Malenka, R.C. and Isaac, J.T. (1998). Long-term depression at thalamocortical synapses in developing rat somatosensory cortex. *Neuron*, **21**(**2**), 347–357.

Fitzjohn, S.M. and Collingridge, G.L. (2002). Calcium stores and synaptic plasticity. *Cell Calcium*, **32**(**5–6**), 405–411.

Fitzjohn, S.M., Kingston, A.E., Lodge, D. and Collingridge, G.L. (1999). DHPG-induced LTD in area CA1 of juvenile rat hippocampus; characterisation and sensitivity to novel mGlu receptor antagonists. *Neuropharmacology*, **38**(**10**), 1577–1583.

Frey, U., Huang, Y.Y. and Kandel, E.R. (1993). Effects of cAMP simulate a late stage of LTP in hippocampal CA1 neurons. *Science*, **260**(**5114**), 1661–1664.

Frey, U., Krug, M., Reymann, K.G., Matthies, H. (1998). Anisomycin, an inhibitor of protein synthesis, blocks late phases of LTP phenomena in the hippocampal CA1 region *in vitro*. *Brain Res*, **452**, 57–65.

Frey, U. and Morris, R.G. (1997). Synaptic tagging and long-term potentiation. *Nature*, **385**, 533–536.

Fujii, S., Saito, K., Miyakawa, H., Ito, K. and Kato, H. (1991). Reversal of long-term potentiation (depotentiation) induced by tetanus stimulation of the input to CA1 neurons of guinea pig hippocampal slices. *Brain Res*, **555(1)**, 112–122.

Gazzaley, A., Kay, S. and Benson, D.L. (2002). Dendritic spine plasticity in hippocampus. *Neuroscience*, **111(4)**, 853–862.

Gu, Q. (2002). Neuromodulatory transmitter systems in the cortex and their role in cortical plasticity. *Neuroscience*, **111**, 815–835.

Gubellini, P., Saulle, E., Centonze, D., Bonsi, P., Pisani, A., Bernardi, G., Conquet, F. and Calabresi, P.(2001). Selective involvement of mGlu1 receptors in corticostriatal LTD. *Neuropharmacology*, **40(7)**, 839–846.

Harris, E.W. and Cotman, C.W. (1986). Long-term potentiation of guinea pig mossy fiber responses is not blocked by *N*-methyl D-aspartate antagonists. *Neurosci Lett*, **70**, 132–137.

Harvey, J. and Collingridge, G.L. (1992). Thapsigargin blocks the induction of long-term potentiation in rat hippocampal slices. *Neurosci Lett*, **139**, 197–200.

Harvey, J., Balasubramaniam, R. and Collingridge, G.L. (1993). Carbachol can potentiate *N*-methyl-D-aspartate responses in the rat hippocampus by a staurosporine and thapsigargin-insensitive mechanism. *Neurosci Lett*, **162**, 165–168.

Hebb, D.O. (1949). *The Organization of Behavior*. New York, Wiley (Interscience).

Hemart, N., Daniel, H., Jaillard, D. and Crepel, F. (1995). Receptors and second messengers involved in long-term depression in rat cerebellar slices *in vitro*: a reappraisal. *Eur J Neurosci*, **7**, 45–53.

Henley, J.M. (2003). Proteins interactions implicated in AMPA receptor trafficking: a clear destination and an improving route map. *Neurosci Res*, **45**, 243–254.

Hu, G.Y., Hvalby, O., Walaas, S.I., Albert, K.A., Skjeflo, P., Andersen, P. and Greengard, P. (1987). Protein kinase C injection into hippocampal pyramidal cells elicits features of long term potentiation. *Nature*, **328**, 426–429.

Huang, L.Q., Rowan, M.J. and Anwyl, R. (1997). mGluR II agonist inhibition of LTP induction, and mGluR II antagonist inhibition of LTD induction, in the dentate gyrus *in vitro*. *Neuroreport*, **8(3)**, 687–693.

Huber, K.M., Kayser, M.S. and Bear, M.F. (2000). Role for rapid dendritic protein synthesis in hippocampal mGluR-dependent long-term depression. *Science*, **288**, 1254–1257.

Huettner, J.E. (2001). Kainate receptors: knocking out plasticity. *TiNs*, **24**, 365–366.

Issac, J.T., Nicoll, R.A. and Malenka, R.C. (1995). Evidence for silent synapses: implications for the expression of LTP. *Neuron*, **15**, 427–434.

Ito, M. (1996). Cerebellar long-term depression. *TiNs*, **19**, 11–12.

Ito, M., Sakurai, M. and Tongroach, P. (1982). Climbing fibre induced depression of both mossy fiber responsiveness and glutamate sensitivity of cerebellar Purkinje cells. *J Physiol Lond*, **234**, 113–134.

Kamal, A., Ramakers, G.M.J., Urban, I.J.A., De Graan, P.N.E. and Gispen, W.H. (1999). Chemical LTD in the CA1 field of the hippocampus from young and mature rats. *Eur J Neurosci*, **11**, 3512–3516.

Kano, M. and Kato, M. (1987). Quisqualate receptors are specifically involved in cerebellar synaptic plasticity. *Nature*, **325**, 276–279.

Kato, K., Clark, G.D., Bazan, N.G. and Zorumski, C.F. (1994). Platelet-activating factor as a potential retrograde messenger in CA1 hippocampal long-term potentiation. *Nature*, **367**, 175–179.

Katsuki, H., Izumi, Y. and Zorumski, C.F. (1997). Noradrenergic regulation of synaptic plasticity in the hippocampal CA1 region. *J Neurophysiol*, **77**, 3013–3020.

Kelso, S.R. and Brown, T.H. (1986). Differential conditioning of associative synaptic enhancement in hippocampal brain slices. *Science*, **232**, 85–87.

Kemp, N. and Bashir, Z.I. (1997). NMDA receptor-dependent and -independent long-term depression in the CA1 region of the adult rat hippocampus *in vitro*. *Neuropharmacology*, **36(3)**, 397–399.

Kemp, N. and Bashir, Z.I. (1999). Induction of LTD in the adult hippocampus by the synaptic activation of AMPA/kainate and metabotropic glutamate receptors. *Neuropharmacology*, **38(4)**, 495–504.

Kemp, N. and Bashir, Z.I. (2001). Long-term depression: a cascade of induction and expression mechanisms. *Progr Neurobiol*, **65**, 339–365.

Kemp, N., McQueen, J., Faulkes, S. and Bashir, Z.I. (2000). Different forms of LTD in the CA1 region of the hippocampus: role of age and stimulus protocol. *Eur J Neurosci*, **12(1)**, 360–366.

Kerr, D.S. and Abraham, W.C. (1995). Cooperative interactions among afferents govern the induction of homosynaptic long-term depression in the hippocampus. *Proc Natl Acad Sci USA*, **92(25)**, 11637–11641.

Kimura, F., Tsumoto, T., Nighigori, A. and Yoshimura, Y. (1990). Long-term depression but not potentiation is induced in calcium-chelated visual cortex neurons. *NeuroReport*, **1**, 65–68.

Kirkwood, A. and Bear, M.F. (1994). Homosynaptic long-term depression in the visual cortex. *J Neurosci*, **14(5 Pt 2)**, 3404–3412.

Kirkwood, A., Rozas, C., Kirkwood, J., Perez, F. and Bear, M.F. (1999). Modulation of long-term depression in visual cortex by acetylcholine and norepinephrine. *J Neurosci*, **19**, 1599–1609.

Kobayashi, K., Manabe, T. and Takahashi, T. (1996). Presynaptic long-term depression at the hippocampal mossy fiber-CA3 synapse. *Science*, **273**(**5275**), 648–650.

Konnerth, A., Dreesen, J. and Augustine, G.J. (1992). Brief dendritic calcium signals initiate long-lasting synaptic depression in cerebellar Purkinje cells. *Proc Natl Acad Sci USA*, **89**, 7051–7055.

Kullmann, D.M. and Siegelbaum, S.A. (1995). The site of expression of NMDA receptor-dependent LTP: new fuel for an old fire. *Neuron*, **15**, 997–1002.

Lauri, S.E., Bortolotto, Z.A., Bleakman, D., Ornstein, P.L., Lodge, D., Isaac, J.T.R. and Collingridge, G.L. (2001a). Critical role of a facilitatory presynaptic kainate receptor in mossy fiber LTP. *Neuron*, **32**, 697–709.

Lauri, S.E., Delany, C.J., Clarke, V.R., Bortolotto, Z.A., Ornstein, P.L., Isaac, J.T.R. and Collingridge, G.L. (2001b). Synaptic activation of a presynaptic kainate receptor facilitates AMPA receptor-mediated synaptic transmission at hippocampal mossy fibre synapses. *Neuropharmacology*, **41**, 907–915.

Lee, H.-K., Kameyama, K., Huganir, R.L. and Bear, M.F. (1998). NMDA induces long-term synaptic depression and dephosphorylation of the GluR1 subunit of AMPA receptors in hippocampus. *Neuron*, **21**, 1151–1162.

Lerma, J. (2003). Roles and rules of kainite receptors in synaptic transmission. *Nat Rev Neurosci*, **4**, 481–489.

Levy, W.B. and Steward, O. (1979). Synapses as associative memory elements in the hippocampal formation. *Brain Res*, **175**(**2**), 233–245.

Levy, W.B. and Steward, O. (1983). Temporal contiguity requirements for long-term associative potentiation/depression in the hippocampus. *Neuroscience*, **8**(**4**), 791–797.

Linden, D.J. and Connor, J.A. (1991). Participation of postsynaptic PKC in cerebellar long-term depression in culture. *Science*, **254**, 1656–1659.

Linden, D.J., Dickinson, M.H., Smeyne, M. and Connor, J.A. (1991). A long-term depression of AMPA currents in cultured cerebellar Purkinje cells. *Neuron*, **7**, 81–89.

Lisman, J. (1989). A mechanism for the Hebb and the anti-Hebb processes underlying learning and memory. *Proc Natl Acad Sci USA*, **86**(**23**), 9574–9578.

Lisman, J. (2003). Long-term potentiation: outstanding questions and attempted synthesis. *Philos Trans R Soc Lond B Biol Sci*, **358**, 829–842.

Lomo, T. (1966). Frequency potentiation of excitatory synaptic activity in the dentate area of the hippocampal formation.

Acta Physiologica Scandinavia (**Suppl. 277**), *Scandinavian Congress of Physiology*, p. 128.

Lovinger, D.M., Wong, K.L., Murakami, K. and Routtenberg, A. (1987). Protein kinase C inhibitors eliminate hippocampal long-term potentiation. *Brain Res*, **436**(**1**), 177–183.

Lynch, G.S., Dunwiddie, T. and Gribkoff, V. (1977). Heterosynaptic depression: a post-synaptic correlate of long-term potentiation. *Nature*, **266**, 737–739.

Lynch, G.S., Larson, J., Kelso, S., Barrionuevo, G. and Schottler, F. (1983). Intracellular injections of EGTA block the induction of hippocampal long-term potentiation. *Nature*, **305**, 719–721.

Malenka, R.C., Madison, D.V. and Nicoll, R.A. (1986). Potentiation of synaptic transmission in the hippocampus by phorbol esters. *Nature*, **321**, 175–177.

Malenka, R., Kauer, J.A., Zucker, R.S. and Nicoll, R.A. (1988). Postsynaptic calcium is sufficient for potentiation of hippocampal synaptic transmission. *Science*, **242**, 81–84.

Malenka, R., Kauer, J.A., Perkel, D., Mauk, M., Kelly, P., Nicoll, R. and Waxham, M. (1989). An essential role for postsynaptic calmodulin and protein kinase activity in long-term potentiation. *Nature*, **340**, 554–557.

Malinow, R. and Malenka, R.C. (2002). AMPA receptor trafficking and synaptic plasticity. *Annu Rev Neurosci*, **25**, 103–126.

Malinow, R. and Miller, J.P. (1986). Postsynaptic hyperpolarization during conditioning reversibly blocks induction of long-term potentiation. *Nature*, **320**(**6062**), 529–530.

Malinow, R., Schulman, H. and Tsien, R.W. (1989). Inhibition of postsynaptic PKC or CaMKII blocks induction but not expression of LTP. *Nature*, **245**, 862–865.

Manahan-Vaughan, D. (1997). Group 1 and 2 metabotropic glutamate receptors play differential roles in hippocampal long-term depression and long-term potentiation in freely moving rats. *J Neurosci*, **17**(**9**), 3303–3311.

Marr, D. (1969). A theory of cerebellar cortex. *J Physiol*, **202**, 437–470.

Massey, P.V., Bhabra, G., Cho, K., Brown, M.W. and Bashir, Z.I. (2001). Activation of muscarinic receptors induces protein synthesis-dependent long-lasting depression in the perirhinal cortex. *Eur J Neurosci*, **14**, 1–9.

Mauk, M.D., Garcia, K.S., Medina. J.F. and Steele, P.M. (1998). Does cerebellar LTD mediate motor learning? Toward a resolution without a smoking gun. *Neuron*, **20**, 359–362.

McNaughton, B.L. (2003). Long-term potentiation, cooperativity and Hebb's cell assemblies: a personal history. *Philos Trans R Soc Lond B Biol Sci*, **358**(**1432**), 629–634.

McNaughton, B.L., Douglas, R.M. and Goddard, G.V. (1978). Synaptic enhancement in fascia dentata: cooperativity among coactive afferents. *Brain Res*, **157**(**2**), 277–293.

Morris, R.G.M. (2003). Long-term potentiation and memory. *Philos Trans R Soc Lond B Biol Sci*, **358**, 643–647.

Moult, P.R., Schnabel, R., Kilpatrick, I.C., Bashir, Z.I. and Collingridge, G.L. (2002). Tyrosine phosphorylation underlies DHPG-induced LTD. *Neuropharmacology*, **43**, 175–180.

Mulkey, R.M. and Malenka, R.C. (1992). Mechanisms underlying induction of homosynaptic long-term depression in area CA1 of the hippocampus. *Neuron*, **9**, 967–975.

Mulkey, R.M., Herron, C.E. and Malenka, R.C. (1993). An essential role for protein phosphatases in hippocampal long-term depression. *Science*, **261**, 1051–1055.

Nicoll, R.A. and Malenka, R.C. (1995). Contrasting properties of two forms of long-term potentiation in the hippocampus. *Nature*, **377**, 115–118.

Norris, C.M., Korol, D.L. and Foster, T.C. (1996). Increased susceptibility to induction of long-term depression and long-term potentiation reversal during aging. *J Neurosci*, **16(17)**, 5382–5392.

Nowak, L., Bregestovski, P., Ascher, P., Herbert, A. and Prochiantz, A. (1984). Magnesium gates glutamate-activated channels in mouse central neurones. *Nature*, **307**, 462–465.

O'Dell, T.J., Hawkins, R.D., Kandel, E.R. and Arancio, O. (1991). Tests of the roles of two diffusible substances in long-term potentiation: evidence for nitric oxide as a possible early retrograde messenger. *Proc Natl Acad Sci USA*, **88**, 11285–11289.

Oliet, S.H.R., Malemka, R.C. and Nicoll, R.A. (1997). Two distinct forms of long-term depression coexist in CA1 hippocampal pyramidal cells. *Neuron*, **18**, 969–982.

O'Mara, S.M., Rowan, M.J. and Anwyl, R. (1995a). Dantrolene inhibits long-term depression and depotentiation of synaptic transmission in the rat dentate gyrus. *Neuroscience*, **68(3)**, 621–624.

O'Mara, S.M., Rowan, M.J. and Anwyl, R. (1995b). Metabotropic glutamate receptor-induced homosynaptic long-term depression and depotentiation in the dentate gyrus of the rat hippocampus *in vitro*. *Neuropharmacology*, **34(8)**, 983–989.

Otani, S. and Connor, J.A. (1998). Requirement of rapid Ca2+ entry and synaptic activation of metabotropic glutamate receptors for the induction of long-term depression in adult rat hippocampus. *J Physiol*, **511(Pt 3)**, 761–770.

Otani, S., Auclair, N., Desce, J.M., Roisin, M-P. and Crépel, F. (1999). Dopamine receptors and groups I and II mGluRs cooperate for long-term depression induction in rat prefrontal cortex through converging postsynaptic activation of MAP kinases. *J Neurosci*, **19(22)**, 9788–9802.

Otmakhova, N.A., Otmakhov, N., Mortenson, L.H. and Lisman, J.E. (2000). Inhibition of the cAMP pathway decreases early long-term potentiation at CA1 hippocampal synapses. *J Neurosci*, **20(12)**, 4446–4451.

Palmer, M.J., Irving, A.J., Seabrook, G.R., Jane, D.E. and Collingridge, G.L. (1997). The group I mGlu receptor agonist DHPG induces a novel form of LTD in the CA1 region of the hippocampus. *Neuropharmacology*, **36**, 1517–1532.

Paupard, M.C., Friedman, L.K. and Zukin, R.S. (1997). Developmental regulation and cell-specific expression on *N*-methyl-D-aspartate receptor splice variants in rat hippocampus. *Neuroscience*, **79**, 399–409.

Ramusson, D.D. (2000). The role of acetylcholine in cortical synaptic plasticity. *Behav Brain Res*, **115**, 205–218.

Reyes, M. and Stanton, P.K. (1996). Induction of hippocampal long-term depression requires release of Ca^{2+} from separate presynaptic and postsynaptic intracellular stores. *J Neurosci*, **16(19)**, 5951–5960.

Rioult-Pedotti, M.-S., Friedman, D. and Donoghue, J.P. (2000). Learning-induced LTP in neocortex. *Science*, **290**, 533–536.

Roberson, E.D. and Sweatt, J.D.(1996). Transient activation of cyclic AMP-dependent protein kinase during hippocampal long-term potentiation. *J Biol Chem*, **271(48)**, 30436–30441.

Roche, K.W., O'Brien, R.J., Mammen, A.L., Bernhardt, J. and Huganir, R.L. (1996). Characterization of multiple phosphorylation sites on the AMPA receptor GluR1 subunit. *Neuron*, **16**, 1179–1188.

Ronesi, J., Gerdeman, G.L. and Lovinger, D.M. (2004). Disruption of endocannabinoid release and striatal long-term depression by postsynaptic blockade of endocannabinoid membrane transport. *J Neurosci*, **24(7)**, 1673–1679.

Sanes, J.R. and Lichtman, J.W. (1999). Can molecules explain long-term potentiation? *Nat Neurosci*, **2**, 597–604.

Schnabel, R., Palmer, M.J., Kilpatrick, I.C. and Collingridge, G.L. (1999a). A CaMKII inhibitor, KN-62, facilitates DHPG-induced LTD in the CA1 region of the hippocampus. *Neuropharmacology*, **38**, 605–608.

Schnabel, R., Kilpatrick, I.C. and Collingridge, G.L. (1999b). An investigation into signal transduction mechanisms involved in DHPG-induced LTD in the CA1 region of the hippocampus. *Neuropharmacology*, **38**, 1585–1596.

Selig, D.K., Hjelmstad, G.O., Herron, C., Nicoll, R.A. and Malenka, R.C. (1995). Independent mechanisms for long-term depression of AMPA and NMDA responses. *Neuron*, **15**, 417–426.

Shigemoto, R., Abe, T., Numura, S., Nakanishi, S. and Hirano, T. (1994). Antibodies inactivating mGluR1 metabotropic glutamate receptors block long-term depression in cultured Purkinje cells. *Neuron*, **12**, 1245–1255.

Silva, A.J., Stevens, C.F., Tonegawa, S. and Wang, Y. (1992). Deficient hippocampal long-term potentiation in alpha-calcium-calmodulin kinase II mutanat mice. *Science*, **257**, 201–206.

Staubli, U. and Lynch, G. (1990). Stable depression of potentiated synaptic responses in the hippocampus with 1–5 Hz stimulation. *Brain Res*, **513**, 113–118.

Stevens, C.F. and Wang, Y. (1993). Reversal of long-term potentiation by inhibitors of haem oxygenase. *Nature*, **364**, 147–149.

Sun, L., Shipley, M.T. and Lidow, M. (2000). Expression of NR1, NR2A-D, and NR3 subunits of the NMDA receptor in the cerebral cortex and olfactory bulb of adult rat. *Synapse*, **35**, 212–221.

Sweatt, D.J. (2001). The neuronal MAP kinase cascade: a biochemical signal integration system subserving synaptic plasticity and memory. *J Neurochem*, **76**, 1–10.

Thiels, E., Norman, E.D., Barrionuevo, G. and Klann, E. (1998). Transient and persistent increases in protein phosphatase activity during long-term depression in the adult hippocampus *in vivo*. *Neuroscience*, **86**(**4**), 1023–1029.

Tsumoto, T. (1992). Long-term potentiation and long-term depression in the neocortex. *Prog Neurobiol*, **39**, 209–228.

Wagner, J.J. and Alger, B.E. (1995). GABAergic and developmental influences on homosynaptic LTD and depotentiation in rat hippocampus. *J Neurosci*, **15**, 1577–1586.

Wang, Y.T. and Linden, D.J. (2000). Expression of cerebellar long-term depression requires postsynaptic clathrin-mediated endocytosis. *Neuron*, **25**(**3**), 635–647.

Wang, Y., Rowan, M.J. and Anwyl, R. (1977). Induction of LTD in the dentate gyrus *in vitro* is NMDA receptor independent, but dependent on Ca^{2+} influx via low-voltage-activated Ca^{2+} channels and release of Ca^{2+} from intracellular stores. *J Neurophysiol*, **77**(**2**), 812–825.

Wang, Y., Wu, J., Rowan, M.J. and Anwyl, R. (1998). Role of protein kinase C in the induction of homosynaptic long-term depression by brief low frequency stimulation in the dentate gyrus of the rat hippocampus *in vitro*. *J Physiol*, **513**(**Pt 2**), 467–475.

Wenthold, R.J., Petralia, R.S., Blahos, J. and Niedzielski, A.S. (1996). Evidence for multiple AMPA receptor complexes in hippocampal CA1/CA2 neurons. *J Neurosci*, **16**, 1982–1989.

Wexler, E.M. and Stanton, P.K. (1993). Priming of homoynaptic long-term depression in hippocampus by previous synaptic activity. *NeuroReport*, **4**, 591–594.

Wigstrom, H., Gustafsson, B., Huang, Y.Y. and Abraham, W.C. (1986). Hippocampal long-term potentiation is induced by pairing single afferent volleys with intracellularly injected depolarizing current pulses. *Acta Physiol Scand*, **126**(**2**), 317–319.

Williams, J.H. and Bliss, T.V. (1988). Induction but not maintenance of calcium-induced long-term potentiation in dentate gyrus and area CA1 of the hippocampal slice is blocked by nordihydroguaiaretic acid. *Neurosci Lett*, **88**, 81–85.

Winder, D.G. and Sweatt, J.D. (2001). Roles of serine/threonine phosphatases in hippocampal synaptic plasticity. *Nat Neurosci Rev*, **2**, 461–474.

Xia, J., Chung, H.J., Wihler, C., Huganir, R.L. and Linden, D.J. (2000). Cerebellar long-term depression requires PKC-regulated interactions between GluR2/3 and PDZ domain-containing proteins. *Neuron*, **28**(**2**), 499–510.

Zakharenko, S.S., Patterson, S.L., Dragatsis, I., Zeitlin, S.O., Siegelbaum, S.A., Kandel, E.R. and Morozov, A. (2003). Presynaptic BDNF required for a presynaptic but not postsynaptic component of LTP at hippocampal CA1–CA3 synapses. *Neuron*, **39**(**6**), 975–990.

Zhuo, M., Zhang, W., Son, H., Mansuy, I., Sobel, R., Seidman, J. and Kandel, E. (1999). A selective role of calcineurin Aα in synaptic depotentiation in hippocampus. *Proc Natl Acad Sci USA*, **96**, 4650–4655.

Ziakopoulos, Z., Tillett, C.W., Brown, M.W. and Bashir, Z.I. (1999). Input- and layer-dependent synaptic plasticity in the rat perirhinal cortex *in vitro*. *Neuroscience*, **92**, 459–472.

Cellular and molecular mechanisms of associative and nonassociative learning

John H. Byrne, Diasinou Fioravante and Evangelos G. Antzoulatos

Department of Neurobiology and Anatomy, University of Texas Health Science Center at Houston, Houston, TX, USA

5.1 Introduction

All animals have the capacity to adapt to environmental changes by modifying their behaviors. The experience-dependent modification of behavior is a manifestation of learning (which generally refers to the process of acquiring new information), whereas memory is the retention of learning over time. The neural mechanisms that contribute to the adaptation of an organism to environmental changes through learning are also likely to contribute to the adaptation of the organism to physical changes (e.g., trauma) through repair and rehabilitation. Some molecular mechanisms, such as neurotrophin signaling, second messenger cascades, transcription factor-mediated gene regulation, structural remodeling and growth, are likely sites of convergence between memory, development, and rehabilitation. Therefore, delineating the mechanisms that govern learning and memory could facilitate both the understanding of mechanisms that govern repair and rehabilitation, and the development of therapeutic pharmacological agents.

Four elementary forms of learning: habituation, sensitization, classical, and operant conditioning

Learning can be distinguished depending on whether it is associative or nonassociative. Nonassociative forms of learning include habituation and sensitization. Habituation is defined as the gradual waning of a behavioral response to a weak or moderate stimulus that is presented repeatedly. Following habituation, the response may be restored to its initial state either passively with time (i.e., spontaneous recovery), or with the presentation of a novel stimulus (i.e., dishabituation). Sensitization is defined as the enhancement of a behavioral response, either the response elicited by the repeated presentation of a moderate to strong intensity stimulus (operationally the opposite phenomenon of habituation), or the response elicited by a weak stimulus following a noxious stimulus to another part of the animal (also known as pseudo-conditioning).

Associative learning includes classical and operant conditioning and involves the formation of an association either between two stimuli (i.e., classical conditioning), or between a behavior and its outcomes (i.e., operant conditioning). In classical (or Pavlovian) conditioning, a benign stimulus (conditional stimulus; CS) is paired with a stimulus that elicits a reflexive response (unconditional stimulus and response, respectively; US and UR). After sufficient training with contingent CS-US presentations (which may be a single trial), the CS comes to elicit a learned response (conditional response; CR), which often resembles the UR (or some aspect of it). The emergence of the anticipatory CR reveals that the US has become predictable. Operant (or instrumental) conditioning is an experimental procedure based on Thorndike's Law of Effect, which states that behaviors followed by desirable effects will tend to be repeated, whereas behaviors followed by aversive effects will tend to be

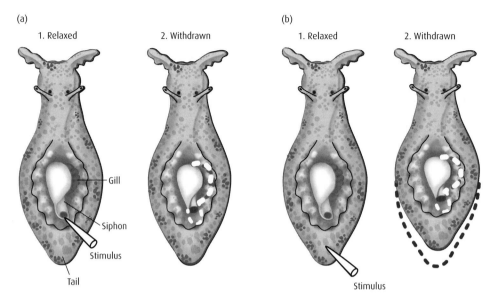

Figure 5.1. Siphon-gill and tail-siphon withdrawal reflexes of *Aplysia*. (a) Siphon-gill withdrawal, dorsal view of *Aplysia*: (1) relaxed position and (2) a stimulus (e.g., a water jet, brief touch, or weak electric shock) applied to the siphon causes the siphon and the gill to withdraw into the mantle cavity. (b) Tail-siphon withdrawal reflex: (1) relaxed position and (2) a stimulus applied to the tail elicits a reflex withdrawal of the tail and siphon.

suppressed. Similarly, in the experimental procedure of operant conditioning the behavior of an animal may be followed by either a positive or a negative stimulus arranged by the experimenter. The positive stimulus (e.g., food) will typically increase the future occurrence of this behavior (a process called *reinforcement*). A negative stimulus (e.g., a painful electric shock) will tend to decrease the future probability of this behavior (a process called *punishment*).

Humans and other animals are capable of displaying more complex forms of learning than the four associative and nonassociative types outlined above (see Volume I, Chapter 2). However, the basic processes underlying these simpler forms of learning are likely to constitute the building blocks for more complex forms of learning. Thus, a major goal of neurobiologists is to explain the neural processes that underlie elementary forms of learning, at anatomical, biophysical, and molecular levels of analysis. To that end, the examination of learning in simple model systems, such as the marine mollusc *Aplysia californica*, has proven to be very fruitful.

Aplysia behaviors and underlying neural circuits

The marine invertebrate *A. californica* is well suited for the examination of molecular, cellular, morphological, and network mechanisms underlying neuronal plasticity, learning, and memory. A major advantage of this animal is the simplicity of its nervous system and the large size of its neurons. In addition, *Aplysia* displays reflexive withdrawal responses, which support associative and nonassociative learning. These features make the neural circuits that underlie withdrawal reflexes amenable to the molecular dissection of neural plasticity that accompanies learning and memory.

Two well-studied behaviors in *Aplysia* are the tail-siphon and siphon-gill withdrawal reflexes. Tactile or electrical stimulation of the siphon elicits reflexive withdrawal of the siphon and gill, the respiratory organ of *Aplysia* (siphon-gill withdrawal reflex; Fig. 5.1(a)), whereas stimulation of the tail elicits withdrawal of the tail and the siphon (tail-siphon withdrawal reflex; Fig. 5.1(b)). The circuitry underlying

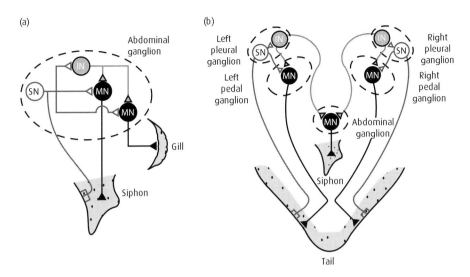

Figure 5.2. Simplified circuit diagrams of the (a) siphon-gill and (b) tail-siphon withdrawal reflexes. Stimuli activate the afferent terminals of mechanoreceptor SNs whose somata are located in central ganglia. The SNs make excitatory synaptic connections (triangles) with INs and MNs. The excitatory INs provide a parallel pathway for excitation of the MNs. Action potentials elicited in the MNs, triggered by the combined input from the SNs and INs, propagate out peripheral nerves to activate muscle cells and produce the subsequent reflex withdrawal of the organs. Modulatory MNs not shown here but see Fig. 5.3(a1), such as those containing serotonin (5-HT), regulate the properties of the circuit elements, and, consequently, the strength of the behavioral responses.

these reflexes has been described in detail (Fig. 5.2). The afferent limb of the siphon-gill withdrawal reflex consists of sensory neurons (SNs) with cell bodies in the abdominal ganglion (Fig. 5.2(a)). The siphon SNs monosynaptically excite gill and siphon motor neurons (MNs), also located in the abdominal ganglion, leading to contraction of the gill and siphon. Excitatory, inhibitory, and modulatory interneurons (INs) have also been identified as integral components in mediating the reflex and its modification through learning (Frost et al., 1988; Frost and Kandel, 1995). The afferent limb of the tail-siphon withdrawal reflex consists of a bilaterally symmetric cluster of SNs that are located in the left and right pleural ganglia (Fig. 5.2(b)). These SNs make monosynaptic excitatory connections with MNs in the adjacent pedal ganglion, which produce withdrawal of the tail (Walters et al., 1983a). In addition, the tail SNs form synapses with various identified excitatory and inhibitory INs (Cleary and Byrne, 1993; White et al., 1993), some of which activate MNs in the abdominal

ganglion, thus causing reflex withdrawal of the siphon. Moreover, several additional neurons modulate the tail-siphon withdrawal reflex. In both circuits the SNs and their glutamatergic synapses appear to have similar functional properties and to be modified as a function of the animal's training history. As will be discussed below, plasticity in the SN, resulting in changes in sensorimotor synaptic efficacy, contributes to several forms of learning and memory.

5.2 Nonassociative learning in *Aplysia*

Neural mechanisms of habituation

Habituation, perhaps the simplest form of nonassociative learning, refers to the decrement of a response due to the repetitive presentation of a weak stimulus. It is distinguished from simple fatigue in that the response can be restored (dishabituated) by the presentation of a novel stimulus to the animal (Thompson and Spencer, 1966).

Upon repetitive stimulation, withdrawal reflexes of *Aplysia* undergo short- and long-term habituation (Pinsker et al., 1970; Carew and Kandel, 1973). Habituation of the withdrawal reflexes has historically been attributed to depression of the sensorimotor synapse, leading to decreased recruitment of MNs (Castellucci et al., 1970; Phares et al., 2003; see however Stopfer and Carew, 1996; Ezzeddine and Glanzman, 2003). Thus, since the early 1970s, understanding behavioral habituation in *Aplysia* has rested almost exclusively on understanding the mechanisms of depression that is induced by intrinsic activity (i.e., homosynaptic depression) in the sensorimotor synapse. Most studies of short-term homosynaptic depression in *Aplysia* sensorimotor synapse suggest it is mediated by presynaptic changes in transmitter release (e.g., Castellucci and Kandel, 1974), whereas long-term depression and habituation have been attributed to structural changes in SNs (Bailey and Chen, 1983).

Experimental and computational studies of the sensorimotor synapse have suggested that short-term activity-dependent changes in transmitter release are in part determined by the dynamics of vesicle mobilization in presynaptic terminals and are limited by the gradual depletion of available vesicles (Gingrich and Byrne, 1985; Bailey and Chen, 1988). Recent studies provided evidence for the involvement of the protein synapsin in the regulation of synaptic vesicle availability and release in *Aplysia* (Humeau et al., 2001; Angers et al., 2002). Under basal conditions, synapsin is associated both with synaptic vesicles and with the cytoskeleton, forming a proteinaceous meshwork that limits vesicle mobilization. Upon activity-dependent phosphorylation, synapsin dissociates from vesicles, thus rendering them free to mobilize to release sites and sustain transmission.

In addition to presynaptic mechanisms of depression, postsynaptic mechanisms have also been implicated. For example, challenging the sensorimotor synapse with physiological bursts of activity results in its depression, partly due to desensitization of postsynaptic receptors (Antzoulatos et al., 2003; Phares et al., 2003). In addition, more prolonged depression of the sensorimotor synapse (i.e., around 2 h) relies

on activation of postsynaptic *N*-methyl-D-aspartate (NMDA) like receptors and a rise in postsynaptic Ca^{2+} (Lin and Glanzman, 1996). Thus, despite the apparent operational simplicity of habituation and synaptic depression, the underlying mechanisms appear to be complex and to involve multiple targets.

Neural mechanisms of sensitization

Short-term sensitization

Delivery of brief but strong electric shocks to a region of the animal's body can enhance the withdrawal reflexes elicited by weak stimuli delivered to other regions (Carew et al., 1971). This form of experience-dependent behavioral modification is termed sensitization. Weak stimuli elicit enhanced withdrawal reflexes when these stimuli come to generate, after training, increased activity in MNs (e.g., Walters et al., 1983b). The increase in the activity of MNs likely results from enhanced sensory input, partially due to two mechanisms (Byrne and Kandel, 1996). First, the same peripheral stimulus can evoke a greater number of action potentials in the presynaptic SN (i.e., enhanced excitability). Second, each action potential fired by an SN produces a stronger synaptic response in the MN (i.e., synaptic facilitation). Because both of these mechanisms are mimicked by application of the neuromodulator serotonin (5-HT) and release of 5-HT from modulatory INs during training is strongly suggested to mediate sensitization (Brunelli et al., 1976; Walters et al., 1983b; Glanzman et al., 1989; Levenson et al., 1999; Marinesco and Carew, 2002), 5-HT-induced facilitation is frequently used as an *in vitro* analog of behavioral sensitization.

Serotonin binds to multiple types of G-protein-coupled receptors localized in the membrane of SNs (Fig. 5.3). Activation of these receptors and their coupled G-proteins has been suggested to recruit at least two signaling cascades in the SNs: The cyclic adenosine monophosphate/protein kinase A (cAMP/PKA) and the diacylglycerol/protein kinase C (DAG/PKC) cascades (Byrne and Kandel, 1996). PKA and PKC target membrane ion channels, thus affecting the spike waveform and the excitability of the SN. Specifically,

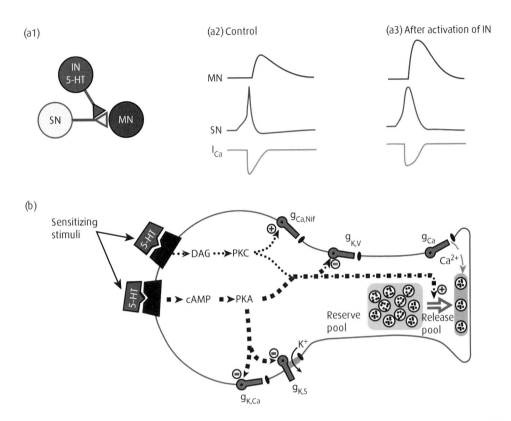

Figure 5.3. Model of heterosynaptic facilitation of the sensorimotor connection that contributes to short-term sensitization in *Aplysia*. (a1) Sensitizing stimuli activate facilitatory INs that release modulatory transmitters, such as 5-HT. The modulator leads to an alteration of the properties of the SN. (a2, a3) An action potential in an SN after the sensitizing stimulus results in greater transmitter release and hence larger postsynaptic potential in the MN than an action potential prior to the sensitizing stimulus. For short-term sensitization the enhancement of transmitter release is due, at least in part, to broadening of the action potential and an enhanced flow of Ca^{2+} into the SN. (b) Molecular events in the SN. 5-HT released from the facilitatory IN (a1) binds to at least two distinct classes of receptors on the outer surface of the membrane of the SN, which leads to the transient activation of two intracellular second messengers DAG and cAMP. These second messengers, acting through their respective protein kinases, PKC and PKA, affect multiple cellular processes, the combined effects of which lead to enhanced transmitter release when a subsequent action potential is fired in the SN.

activation of the PKA/PKC cascades modifies various K$^+$ channels, leading to depolarization of the SN, decrease in spike threshold, enhanced spiking activity, and broadening of the action potential (Klein et al., 1982; Baxter and Byrne, 1989). Spike broadening leads to enhanced Ca^{2+} influx in presynaptic terminals and facilitates transmitter release (i.e., heterosynaptic facilitation; Klein and Kandel, 1980). In addition to spike broadening, a spike-duration-independent

mechanism of enhanced transmitter release has been implicated in 5-HT-induced heterosynaptic facilitation (Gingrich and Byrne, 1985; Hochner et al., 1986; Dale and Kandel, 1990; Klein, 1994; Sugita et al., 1997). This mechanism presumably involves an increase in the number of transmitter-containing synaptic vesicles that become available for release, possibly through synapsin-regulated vesicle mobilization (Fig. 5.3; Byrne and Kandel, 1996; Angers et al., 2002).

Long-term sensitization

In addition to short-term sensitization, withdrawal reflexes can also display long-term sensitization, lasting from several hours to weeks (Pinsker et al., 1973). Whereas short-term sensitization (or its *in vitro* analog called short-term synaptic facilitation) can be induced by brief treatments (lasting a few seconds to minutes), long-term sensitization and 5-HT-induced long-term facilitation require more extensive training, involving multiple trials, preferably spaced over hours or days. One hypothesis that has driven the research on long-term sensitization in *Aplysia* is that the same molecular mechanisms that are employed for short-term memory are also used for long-term memory, only extended in time. This hypothesis has been partially confirmed, as the mechanisms of short-term and long-term memory have been shown to overlap. However, they are not identical, as will be discussed below.

One similarity between the two temporal forms of sensitization is the critical role played by the cAMP/PKA signaling cascade (Fig. 5.4). Whereas in short-term facilitation this cascade leads to phosphorylation-dependent modification of membrane ion channels and release machinery (Fig. 5.3(b)), in long-term facilitation the cAMP/PKA cascade leads to phosphorylation of cAMP response element-binding protein 1 (CREB1) by PKA, and possibly CREB2 by mitogen-activated protein kinase (MAPK; Kandel, 2001; Pittenger and Kandel, 2003). Both CREB1 and CREB2 are transcription factors, and can be activated by kinases that translocate to the nucleus. Whereas CREB1 acts as an *initiator* of gene transcription and it is *activated* by PKA phosphorylation, CREB2 acts constitutively as a *repressor* of gene transcription and it is *suppressed* by MAPK phosphorylation (Bartsch et al., 1998; Guan et al., 2002). The coordinated activation of CREB1 and suppression of CREB2 lead to the transcription of immediate early genes (i.e., genes whose transcription does not rely on new protein synthesis). Therefore, the emerging theme is that the formation of long-term memory

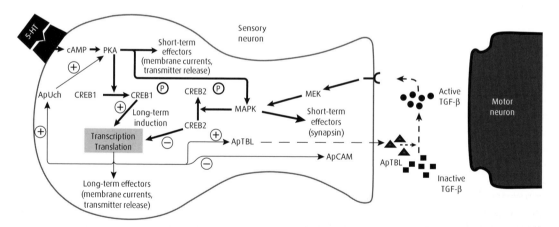

Figure 5.4. Simplified scheme of the mechanisms in SNs that contribute to long-term sensitization and some aspects of short-term sensitization. Sensitization training leads to cAMP-dependent regulation of short-term effectors (see Fig. 5.3(b) for details) and CREB1. cAMP also activates MAPK, which regulates CREB2 (however, there is also evidence that 5-HT can activate MAPK independently of cAMP). Whereas CREB1 acts as an initiator of gene transcription, CREB2 acts as a repressor of gene transcription. The combined effects of activation of CREB1 and de-repression of CREB2 lead to regulation of the synthesis of at least 10 proteins, only three of which (ApTBL, ApUch, and ApCAM) are shown (for more details on ApUch and ApCAM, see text). ApTBL is believed to activate latent forms of TGF-β, which can then bind to receptors on the SN. TGF-β activates MAPK, which can have both acute and long-term actions. One of its acute effects is the regulation of transmitter release. MAPK may also act by initiating a second round of gene regulation by affecting CREB2-dependent pathways.

depends on the modulation of transcription-initiating and repressing elements.

The neural basis of long-term memory is typically examined from two perspectives: induction and expression. If the cAMP/PKA and MAPK signaling cascades are responsible for the *induction* of long-term facilitation, what are the mechanisms that underlie the *expression* of long-term facilitation and sensitization? Two approaches have been followed to answer that question in *Aplysia*, and both have been fruitful. One approach is to identify cellular correlates of long-term behavioral sensitization and the second is to identify proteins that are regulated by long-term sensitization-inducing treatments.

The prototypical procedure in studies of cellular correlates of long-term memory in *Aplysia* is to train animals until behavioral memory is displayed (in this case, 24 h sensitization of the withdrawal reflexes), and then isolate certain critical parts of the underlying neural circuit to identify differences from controls. Such studies have indicated that the mechanisms that correlate with long-term sensitization resemble the mechanisms supporting short-term sensitization, including changes in SN excitability and facilitation of sensorimotor synapses (Frost et al., 1985; Scholz and Byrne, 1987; Cleary et al., 1998). Although identification of all the mechanisms supporting long-term facilitation is still in progress, some of these involve structural modifications of SNs, namely outgrowth of neurites and remodeling of active zones. These data suggest that enhanced transmission is mediated by an increase in transmitter release and in number of synapses (Bailey and Chen, 1983; Wainwright et al., 2002). Long-term behavioral sensitization and long-term synaptic facilitation also correlate with enhanced uptake of glutamate (Levenson et al., 2000), the endogenous transmitter of SNs (Dale and Kandel, 1993). The exact role of the upregulation of glutamate uptake is unknown and several hypotheses are currently under investigation. Long-term sensitization has also been correlated with changes in the properties of MNs (Cleary et al., 1998), and long-term facilitation has been accompanied by increased synthesis of postsynaptic receptors (Trudeau and Castellucci, 1995; Zhu et al., 1997). Thus, there is accumulating evidence to suggest that expression of long-term memory in this simple system does not rely on a unitary mechanism, but on multiple mechanisms at multiple sites.

The second approach that has been employed to identify expression mechanisms of long-term facilitation in *Aplysia* involves identification and characterization of target proteins. Of the several proteins that are involved in expression of long-term facilitation, three appear to be particularly important and will be discussed here (Fig. 5.4). First, ApCAM, an *Aplysia* homolog of neuronal cell adhesion molecule (NCAM), is downregulated following prolonged 5-HT treatment. This downregulation is believed to be a necessary step for remodeling of preexisting structures to occur (Mayford et al., 1992; Bailey et al., 1997). Second, transcription of the gene coding for the *Aplysia* tolloid/bone morphogenic-like protein-1 (ApTBL-1) is enhanced following long-term sensitization treatments (Liu et al., 1997). The proposed function of ApTBL-1 involves the activation of the transforming growth factor β (TGF-β), which has been related to long-term facilitation and excitability increases in *Aplysia* (Zhang et al., 1997; Chin et al., 1999, 2002). TGF-β induces activation of MAPK and its translocation to the nucleus (where MAPK could phosphorylate and suppress CREB2, as noted above). Therefore, it appears that, in response to sensitization training, upregulation of ApTBL-1 can lead to activation of TGF-β, which may in turn initiate an extracellular feedback loop that sustains further gene transcription and long-term facilitation. Since TGF-β is a cytokine that has been implicated in normal development, its recent implication in learning and memory supports the notion that pre-programmed developmental plasticity and experience-driven plasticity may share common molecular mechanisms; the same mechanisms are possibly involved in neural repair. Finally, *Aplysia* ubiquitin C-terminal hydrolase (ApUch), a molecule involved in protein degradation through the proteasome, is upregulated following long-term facilitation (Hegde et al., 1997). This 5-HT-induced increase in ApUch could serve to enhance the degradative function of the proteasome, whose targets include the regulatory subunit of PKA (Hegde et al., 1993). Degradation of the regulatory subunit of PKA allows for the persistent activation of the free catalytic subunit of the kinase, which in turn would sustain gene transcription (through CREB1 phosphorylation) and long-term facilitation (Chain et al., 1999). This persistent activation of PKA suggests that the kinase is important not only for the induction but also for the maintenance of long-term facilitation.

Intermediate-term sensitization

Memory has been traditionally divided in short-term and long-term domains. Short-term memory lasts up to several minutes and relies on modification of pre-existing proteins, whereas long-term memory can last up to a lifetime and relies on synthesis of new proteins. Studies of sensitization in *Aplysia* have revealed the existence of intermediate-term memory, which is distinct from the other two forms both temporally and mechanistically (Ghirardi et al., 1995; Sutton and Carew, 2000). Intermediate-term facilitation and sensitization last from 30 min to 3 h after training (depending on the training protocol), and, similar to long-term memory, they are blocked by inhibitors of protein synthesis. However, in contrast to long-term memory, the intermediate forms of memory are resilient to inhibitors of gene transcription. Therefore, intermediate-term memory relies on translation (protein synthesis), but not on transcription (mRNA synthesis). In addition, intermediate-term synaptic facilitation, induced by repeated 5-HT exposures, requires persistent activity of key enzymatic proteins, such as PKA and/or PKC (e.g., Sutton et al., 2004). Intermediate-term facilitation has recently been correlated with activation of previously "silent" release sites by the recruitment of synaptic vesicles to preexisting varicosities (Kim et al., 2003).

5.3 Associative learning in *Aplysia*

Neural mechanisms of classical conditioning of withdrawal reflexes

In classical conditioning of *Aplysia* withdrawal reflexes, a weak stimulus (CS) that originally elicits a weak response becomes more effective in eliciting a response (CR) after training (Carew et al., 1981). Training typically involves repeated presentations of the CS followed at a short interval by a strong stimulus (US), which reliably elicits the unconditioned withdrawal reflex (UR). In the differential conditioning variant of the procedure, there are two CSs presented to the animal (CS+ and CS−), only one of which (CS+) is paired with the US. After training, only the CS+ acquires the ability to elicit the CR (Carew et al., 1983). *Aplysia* withdrawal reflexes exhibit differential classical conditioning, and the underlying neurobiological mechanism was suggested in the early 1980s to be activity-dependent neuromodulation, an elaboration of the 5-HT-induced modulation that underlies sensitization (Hawkins et al., 1983; Walters and Byrne, 1983).

One key distinction between sensitization, a nonassociative form of learning, from the associative learning exemplified by classical conditioning, is that the enhancement must be dependent on the temporal association (contiguity) of the CS+ and US. Responses evoked by unpaired stimuli (e.g., the CS−) should not be enhanced to the same extent. Any enhancement of the responses evoked by CS− would likely be due to the underlying sensitizing (nonassociative) effects of the US. To achieve this pairing-specificity, the coincident activity in the pathways processing CS+ and US must be detected. Since only the synapses processing the CS+ are active at the time of US presentation, activity-dependent mechanisms of plasticity will preferentially strengthen these, and only these synapses (Fig. 5.5). As in sensitization training, presentation of the strong US leads to activation of modulatory INs and diffuse release of 5-HT. 5-HT will bind its G-protein-coupled receptors at the SN membrane and activate adenylyl cyclase (AC) to synthesize cAMP, which will in turn activate PKA, leading to the known modifications in membrane excitability and transmitter release described for sensitization above (Fig. 5.6). In SNs that were recently activated by the CS+, the recent activity-induced rise in intracellular Ca^{2+} primes AC, leading to an enhanced 5-HT-induced activity of AC. As the cAMP/PKA cascade is particularly enhanced by the coincidence of intrinsic

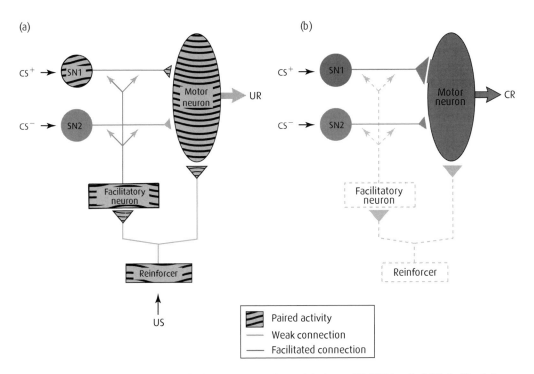

Figure 5.5. General scheme of associative facilitation. (a) *Learning*: Activity in one SN (SN1) is paired (CS+) with reinforcement (US), whereas activity in another SN (SN2) is not paired (CS−) with the US. The US itself activates the MN to produce the UR. The US also activates a modulatory system (facilitatory neuron) that increases the synaptic strength of both SN1 and SN2 nonspecifically. This nonspecific (nonassociative) facilitation contributes to behavioral sensitization. The paired activity in SN1 results in specific (associative) enhancement of the US-induced facilitation. (b) *Memory*: As a result of paired activity, the synapse between SN1 and MN is strengthened, increasing the probability of activating the MN and eliciting the CR. Because the activity in SN2 was not paired with the US, the synapse between SN2 and MN is not strengthened to the same extent. (Reprinted from Lechner and Byrne, 1998; copyright (1998), with permission from Elsevier.)

SN activity (CS+) and extracellular presence of 5-HT (US), the modulatory effects will be augmented, resulting in enhanced SN activity and sensorimotor transmission upon the subsequent CS+ presentation (Hawkins et al., 1983; Walters and Byrne, 1983; Lechner and Byrne, 1998).

Apart from activity-dependent presynaptic modulation, another mechanism that has been implicated in classical conditioning resembles long-term potentiation between neurons of areas CA1–CA3 of the mammalian hippocampus. Intense activity of the MNs during performance of UR depolarizes the MN postsynaptic membrane and this depolarization is hypothesized to release the NMDA-type receptors from their constitutive Mg^{2+} block (Fig. 5.6). If the NMDA receptor is released from the Mg^{2+} block while presynaptically released glutamate is bound, the NMDA receptor is activated. This activation allows influx of Ca^{2+} in the postsynaptic MN and subsequent induction of synapse-specific long-term potentiation (Murphy and Glanzman, 1997, 1999). Recent studies in semi-intact *Aplysia* preparations have suggested that classical conditioning of the siphon withdrawal reflex relies on the interaction of

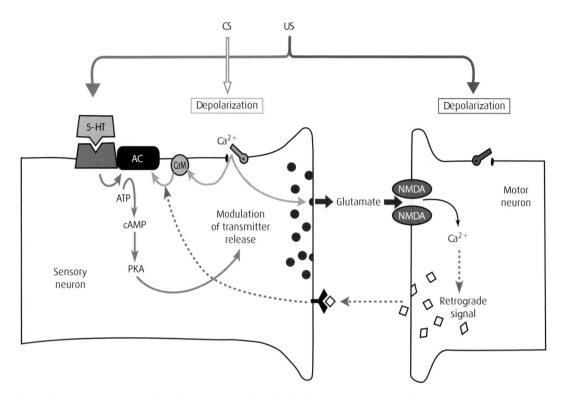

Figure 5.6. Molecular processes believed to mediate associative facilitation in *Aplysia*. A retrograde signal and two sites of coincidence detection are hypothesized. Spike activity in the SNs (CS) leads to Ca^{2+} influx and activation of Ca^{2+}/calmodulin (CAM). AC serves as the presynaptic coincidence detector, being activated by CAM and 5-HT receptors (US). In addition, NMDA receptors detect coincidence of release of glutamate (CS) and postsynaptic depolarization (US). NMDA-mediated Ca^{2+} influx leads to release of a retrograde signal. The hypothetical retrograde signal acts presynaptically to enhance synaptic transmission. (Reprinted from Lechner and Byrne (1998); copyright (1998), with permission from Elsevier.)

activity-dependent presynaptic modulation and postsynaptically induced long-term potentiation (Antonov et al., 2003).

Regardless of the locus of induction, activity-dependent plasticity appears to be expressed presynaptically (i.e., changes in SN excitability and sensorimotor synaptic efficacy), although postsynaptic expression mechanisms cannot be ruled out. These mechanisms of plasticity are reminiscent of mammalian forms of long-lasting synaptic plasticity (see Volume I, Chapter 4). They also suggest the existence of retrograde messengers, which have not been identified yet.

Neural mechanisms of operant conditioning of feeding behavior

Ingestive or biting movements that are components of the feeding behavior of *Aplysia* have recently been shown to display operant conditioning (Brembs et al., 2002). In operant conditioning of feeding behavior the reinforcer is a stimulus to the esophageal nerve (En), which is enriched in dopamine processes. En activity signals presence of food in the mouth, and when En is artificially stimulated contingent upon a spontaneous biting movement, this activity results in an increase in the number of spontaneous bites

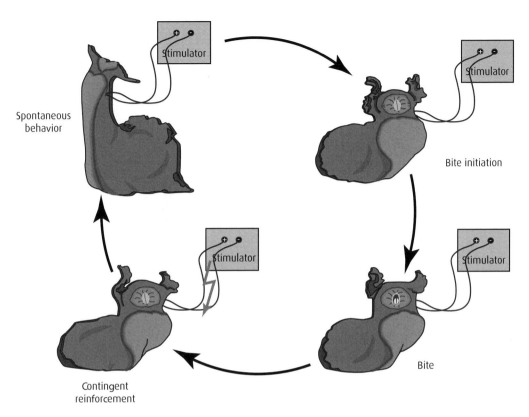

Spontaneous behavior

Bite initiation

Bite

Contingent reinforcement

Figure 5.7. Operant conditioning of feeding behavior in *Aplysia*. While unrestrained in the experimental chamber, an animal moves about freely and engages in spontaneous behaviors. Throughout the experiment, the animal is observed and all bites recorded. Bite is a stereotypic movement, defined as opening of the jaws and protraction of the radula (a tongue-like organ). Animals are assigned to one of three groups: (i) A contingent reinforcement group, which receives En stimulation (reinforcer) whenever the jaws close after a bite during training, (ii) a yoked control group, which receives the same sequence of stimulations as the contingent group, but the stimulation occurs uncorrelated with their behavior, or (iii) a control group, which does not receive any stimulation at all. Both 1 and 24 h after training, the contingent reinforcement group of animals displays significantly higher probability of spontaneous bites than the other two groups. Therefore, activity in En can reinforce the biting component of feeding behavior in *Aplysia*. (Adapted from Brembs et al. (2002).)

(Fig. 5.7). This conditioning is apparent both 1 and 24 h after training, compared to control animals.

The central pattern generator that gives rise to the stereotyped biting movements during feeding is located in the buccal ganglia. Ingestive movements are accompanied by ingestive-like buccal motor programs, the generation of which critically relies on activity on a buccal IN, B51 (Nargeot et al., 1999a, b). Operant conditioning correlates with changes in the biophysical properties of B51, namely an increase in input resistance and a decrease in burst threshold

(Brembs et al., 2002). These biophysical changes serve to increase the probability of spontaneous activation of B51 and the consequent expression of ingestive movements. These results suggest that intrinsic cell-wide plasticity may be one important mechanism underlying operant conditioning. Interestingly, pairing spike activity in cultured B51 with a puff of exogenous dopamine leads to the same biophysical changes in B51 as those produced by operant conditioning *in vivo* (Brembs et al., 2002). Thus, activity-dependent enhancement of diffuse neuromodulation may be a general mechanism that renders some behavioral modifications to be stimulus- or response-specific in classical and operant conditioning, respectively.

Aplysia feeding behavior also displays classical conditioning, both *in vivo* and *in vitro* (an analog in reduced preparation; Lechner et al., 2000a, b; Mozzachiodi et al., 2003). Similar to classical conditioning of withdrawal reflexes, classical conditioning of feeding behavior also involves long-lasting plasticity of the critical synapses. Interestingly, whereas classical conditioning is mediated by enhanced synaptic input to key INs, thus rendering this form of learning CS-specific, operant conditioning is mediated by enhanced excitability of another key IN, thus augmenting the frequency of the behavior in a stimulus-independent way.

5.4 Emerging principles for associative and nonassociative learning

The simplicity and tractability of the neural circuits mediating some behaviors in *Aplysia* have allowed the cellular/molecular dissection of the underlying neural mechanisms. Indeed a number of critical cells, synapses, and molecules have been identified in *Aplysia* to mediate basic forms of learning. At a more general level, the research of learning and memory in *Aplysia* has illuminated several basic principles. These principles can be summarized as follows:

- Learning and memory rely on multiple mechanisms of plasticity at multiple physical sites.
- The intracellular signaling cascades that induce short-term, transient modifications in synaptic transmission can also be used to induce long-term changes. However, the target proteins are different.
- Whereas short-term memory relies on modifications of preexisting proteins, long-term memory also requires upregulation and downregulation of critical molecules, through regulated gene transcription and translation.
- The induction of long-term memory requires not only the generation of positive signals, but also the suppression of constitutive, inhibitory signals.

- Maintenance of long-term cellular memory involves both intracellular and extracellular feedback loops, which sustain the regulation of gene expression and the modification of targeted molecules.
- Associative forms of learning and memory can arise from the neural mechanisms that are used for nonassociative learning, provided that these mechanisms are specifically enhanced by coincident intrinsic activity.

5.5 Relation of learning to rehabilitation

The processes of neuronal development, rehabilitation, and memory formation are likely to share similar mechanisms of neural plasticity. For example, the cytokine TGF-β is involved not only in neural development and survival but also in certain forms of plasticity in *Aplysia*. Therefore, understanding the basic principles of neural plasticity will likely contribute to delineating the mechanisms of repair and rehabilitation. Identification and characterization of the molecular pathways that are involved in long-term memory can also help generate pharmacological agents to regulate genes and induce functional and structural changes in central and/or peripheral neurons.

In addition, one way to recruit the processes of neuronal plasticity in repair and rehabilitation is through behavioral learning paradigms, which provide the basis for current therapeutic strategies. These strategies exploit the plastic properties of the nervous system in order to aid recovery of function (Taub et al., 2002, see Volume II, Chapter 18). Following injury, the initial deficit is frequently followed by spontaneous functional recovery. This recovery can be accelerated and improved through behavioral training (see Volume I, Chapters 13 and 14), which may result in dramatic remapping of the brain as adjacent, healthy cells take over the functions of damaged cells. This functional remapping of the brain following injury has been observed not only in animals but also in humans. Classical and operant conditioning paradigms have been employed to "train" neural circuits in the spinal cord, promoting recovery of locomotion. The range of disorders for which behavioral training might be an effective treatment encompasses conditions such as aphasia, cerebral palsy, phantom limb pain, and dyslexia.

5.6 Conclusions

Since the 1960s research on neural mechanisms of learning and memory in *Aplysia* has provided a wealth of information concerning simple forms of nonassociative and associative learning. The cellular and molecular modifications of the neural circuits that underlie behavioral plasticity in *Aplysia* have generated important principles that can be extended to all animals. These principles include the role played by second messenger systems and regulated gene expression in neural plasticity and memory formation. The knowledge obtained from the work in *Aplysia* can lead to understanding the mechanisms not only of more complex forms of learning and memory, but also of neuronal repair and rehabilitation.

REFERENCES

Angers, A., Fioravante, D., Chin, J., Cleary, L.J., Bean, A.J. and Byrne, J.H. (2002). Serotonin stimulates phosphorylation of *Aplysia* synapsin and alters its subcellular distribution in sensory neurons. *J Neurosci*, **22**, 5412–5422.

Antonov, I., Antonova, I., Kandel, E.R. and Hawkins, R.D. (2003). Activity-dependent presynaptic facilitation and Hebbian LTP are both required and interact during classical conditioning in *Aplysia*. *Neuron*, **37**, 135–147.

Antzoulatos, E.G., Cleary, L.J., Eskin, A., Baxter, D.A. and Byrne, J.H. (2003). Desensitization of postsynaptic glutamate receptors contributes to high-frequency homosynaptic depression of *Aplysia* sensorimotor connections. *Learn Mem*, **10**, 309–313.

Bailey, C.H. and Chen, M. (1983). Morphological basis of long-term habituation and sensitization in *Aplysia*. *Science*, **220**, 91–93.

Bailey, C.H. and Chen, M. (1988). Morphological basis of short-term habituation in *Aplysia*. *J Neurosci*, **8**, 2452–2459.

Bailey, C.H., Kaang, B.K., Chen, M., Martin, K.C., Lim, C.S., Casadio, A. and Kandel, E.R. (1997). Mutation in the phosphorylation sites of MAP kinase blocks learning-related internalization of apCAM in *Aplysia* sensory neurons. *Neuron*, **18**, 913–924.

Bartsch, D., Casadio, A., Karl, K.A., Serodio, P. and Kandel, E.R. (1998). CREB1 encodes a nuclear activator, a repressor, and a cytoplasmic modulator that form a regulatory unit critical for long-term facilitation. *Cell*, **95**, 211–223.

Baxter, D.A. and Byrne, J.H. (1989). Serotonergic modulation of two potassium currents in the pleural sensory neurons of *Aplysia*. *J Neurophysiol*, **62**, 665–679.

Brembs, B., Lorenzetti, F.D., Reyes, F.D., Baxter, D.A. and Byrne, J.H. (2002). Operant reward learning in *Aplysia*: neuronal correlates and mechanisms. *Science*, **296**, 1706–1709.

Brunelli, M., Castellucci, V. and Kandel, E.R. (1976). Synaptic facilitation and behavioral sensitization in *Aplysia*: possible role of serotonin and cyclic AMP. *Science*, **194**, 1178–1181.

Byrne, J.H. and Kandel, E.R. (1996). Presynaptic facilitation revisited: state and time dependence. *J Neurosci*, **16**, 425–435.

Carew, T.J. and Kandel, E.R. (1973). Acquisition and retention of long-term habituation in *Aplysia*: correlation of behavioral and cellular processes. *Science*, **182**, 1158–1160.

Carew, T.J., Castellucci, V.F. and Kandel, E.R. (1971). An analysis of dishabituation and sensitization of the gill-withdrawal reflex in *Aplysia*. *Int J Neurosci*, **2**, 79–98.

Carew, T.J., Walters, E.T. and Kandel, E.R. (1981). Classical conditioning in a simple withdrawal reflex in *Aplysia californica*. *J Neurosci*, **1**, 1426–1437.

Carew, T.J., Hawkins, R.D. and Kandel, E.R. (1983). Differential classical conditioning of a defensive withdrawal reflex in *Aplysia californica*. *Science*, **219**, 397–400.

Castellucci, V.F. and Kandel, E.R. (1974). A quantal analysis of the synaptic depression underlying habituation of the gill-withdrawal reflex in *Aplysia*. *Proc Natl Acad Sci USA*, **71**, 5004–5008.

Castellucci, V., Pinsker, H., Kupfermann, I. and Kandel, E.R. (1970). Neuronal mechanisms of habituation and dishabituation of the gill-withdrawal reflex in *Aplysia*. *Science*, **167**, 1745–1748.

Chain, D.G., Casadio, A., Schacher, S., Hegde, A.N., Valbrun, M., Yamamoto, N., Goldberg, A.L., Bartsch, D., Kandel, E.R. and Schwartz, J.H. (1999). Mechanisms for generating the autonomous cAMP-dependent protein kinase required for long-term facilitation in *Aplysia*. *Neuron*, **22**, 147–156.

Chin, J., Angers, A., Cleary, L.J., Eskin, A. and Byrne, J.H. (1999). TGF-beta1 in *Aplysia*: role in long-term changes in the excitability of sensory neurons and distribution of TbetaR-II-like immunoreactivity. *Learn Mem*, **6**, 317–330.

Chin, J., Angers, A., Cleary, L.J., Eskin, A. and Byrne, J.H. (2002). Transforming growth factor beta1 alters synapsin distribution and modulates synaptic depression in *Aplysia*. *J Neurosci*, **22**, RC220.

Cleary, L.J. and Byrne, J.H. (1993). Identification and characterization of a multifunction neuron contributing to defensive arousal in *Aplysia*. *J Neurophysiol*, **70**, 1767–1776.

Cleary, L.J., Lee, W.L. and Byrne, J.H. (1998). Cellular correlates of long-term sensitization in *Aplysia*. *J Neurosci*, **18**, 5988–5998.

Dale, N. and Kandel, E.R. (1990). Facilitatory and inhibitory transmitters modulate spontaneous transmitter release at cultured *Aplysia* sensorimotor synapses. *J Physiol*, **421**, 203–222.

Dale, N. and Kandel, E.R. (1993). L-glutamate may be the fast excitatory transmitter of *Aplysia* sensory neurons. *Proc Natl Acad Sci USA*, **90**, 7163–7167.

Ezzeddine, Y. and Glanzman, D.L. (2003). Prolonged habituation of the gill-withdrawal reflex in *Aplysia* depends on protein synthesis, protein phosphatase activity, and postsynaptic glutamate receptors. *J Neurosci*, **23**, 9585–9594.

Frost, W.N. and Kandel, E.R. (1995). Structure of the network mediating siphon-elicited siphon withdrawal in *Aplysia*. *J Neurophysiol*, **73**, 2413–2427.

Frost, W.N., Castellucci, V.F., Hawkins, R.D. and Kandel, E.R. (1985). Mono-synaptic connections made by the sensory neurons of the gill-withdrawal and siphon-withdrawal reflex in *Aplysia* participate in the storage of long-term-memory for sensitization. *Proc Nat Acad Sci USA*, **82**, 8266–8269.

Frost, W.N., Clark, G.A. and Kandel, E.R. (1988). Parallel processing of short-term memory for sensitization in *Aplysia*. *J Neurobiol*, **19**, 297–334.

Ghirardi, M., Montarolo, P.G. and Kandel, E.R. (1995). A novel intermediate stage in the transition between short- and long-term facilitation in the sensory to motor neuron synapse of *Aplysia*. *Neuron*, **14**, 413–420.

Gingrich, K.J. and Byrne, J.H. (1985). Simulation of synaptic depression, posttetanic potentiation, and presynaptic facilitation of synaptic potentials from sensory neurons mediating gill-withdrawal reflex in *Aplysia*. *J Neurophysiol*, **53**, 652–669.

Glanzman, D.L., Mackey, S.L., Hawkins, R.D., Dyke, A.M., Lloyd, P.E. and Kandel, E.R. (1989). Depletion of serotonin in the nervous system of *Aplysia* reduces the behavioral enhancement of gill withdrawal as well as the heterosynaptic facilitation produced by tail shock. *J Neurosci*, **9**, 4200–4213.

Guan, Z., Giustetto, M., Lomvardas, S., Kim, J.H., Miniaci, M.C., Schwartz, J.H., Thanos, D. and Kandel, E.R. (2002). Integration of long-term-memory-related synaptic plasticity involves bidirectional regulation of gene expression and chromatin structure. *Cell*, **111**, 483–493.

Hawkins, R.D., Abrams, T.W., Carew, T.J. and Kandel, E.R. (1983). A cellular mechanism of classical conditioning in *Aplysia*: activity-dependent amplification of presynaptic facilitation. *Science*, **219**, 400–405.

Hegde, A.N., Goldberg, A.L. and Schwartz, J.H. (1993). Regulatory subunits of cAMP-dependent protein kinases are degraded after conjugation to ubiquitin: a molecular mechanism underlying long-term synaptic plasticity. *Proc Natl Acad Sci USA*, **90**, 7436–7440.

Hegde, A.N., Inokuchi, K., Pei, W., Casadio, A., Ghirardi, M., Chain, D.G., Martin, K.C., Kandel, E.R. and Schwartz, J.H. (1997). Ubiquitin C-terminal hydrolase is an immediate-early gene essential for long-term facilitation in *Aplysia*. *Cell*, **89**, 115–126.

Hochner, B., Klein, M., Schacher, S. and Kandel, E.R. (1986). Additional component in the cellular mechanism of presynaptic facilitation contributes to behavioral dishabituation in *Aplysia*. *Proc Natl Acad Sci USA*, **83**, 8794–8798.

Humeau, Y., Doussau, F., Vitiello, F., Greengard, P., Benfenati, F. and Poulain, B. (2001). Synapsin controls both reserve and releasable synaptic vesicle pools during neuronal activity and short-term plasticity in *Aplysia*. *J Neurosci*, **21**, 4195–4206.

Kandel, E.R. (2001). The molecular biology of memory storage: a dialogue between genes and synapses. *Science*, **294**, 1030–1038.

Kim, J.H., Udo, H., Li, H.L., Youn, T.Y., Chen, M., Kandel, E.R. and Bailey, C.H. (2003). Presynaptic activation of silent synapses and growth of new synapses contribute to intermediate and long-term facilitation in *Aplysia*. *Neuron*, **40**, 151–165.

Klein, M. (1994). Synaptic augmentation by 5-HT at rested *Aplysia* sensorimotor synapses: independence of action potential prolongation. *Neuron*, **13**, 159–166.

Klein, M. and Kandel, E.R. (1980). Mechanism of calcium current modulation underlying presynaptic facilitation and behavioral sensitization in *Aplysia*. *Proc Natl Acad Sci USA*, **77**, 6912–6916.

Klein, M., Camardo, J. and Kandel, E.R. (1982). Serotonin modulates a specific potassium current in the sensory neurons that show presynaptic facilitation in *Aplysia*. *Proc Natl Acad Sci USA*, **79**, 5713–5717.

Lechner, H.A. and Byrne, J.H. (1998). New perspectives on classical conditioning: a synthesis of Hebbian and non-Hebbian mechanisms. *Neuron*, **20**, 355–358.

Lechner, H.A., Baxter, D.A. and Byrne, J.H. (2000a). Classical conditioning of feeding in *Aplysia*. I. Behavioral analysis. *J Neurosci*, **20**, 3369–3376.

Lechner, H.A., Baxter, D.A. and Byrne, J.H. (2000b). Classical conditioning of feeding in *Aplysia*. II. Neurophysiological correlates. *J Neurosci*, **20**, 3377–3386.

Levenson, J., Byrne, J.H. and Eskin, A. (1999). Levels of serotonin in the hemolymph of *Aplysia* are modulated by light/dark cycles and sensitization training. *J Neurosci*, **19**, 8094–8103.

Levenson, J., Endo, S., Kategaya, L.S., Fernandez, R.I., Brabham, D.G., Chin, J., Byrne, J.H. and Eskin, A. (2000). Long-term regulation of neuronal high-affinity glutamate and glutamine uptake in *Aplysia*. *Proc Natl Acad Sci USA*, **97**, 12858–12863.

Lin, X.Y. and Glanzman, D.L. (1996). Long-term depression of *Aplysia* sensorimotor synapses in cell culture: inductive role of a rise in postsynaptic calcium. *J Neurophysiol*, **76**, 2111–2114.

Liu, Q.R., Hattar, S., Endo, S., MacPhee, K., Zhang, H., Cleary, L.J., Byrne, J.H. and Eskin, A. (1997). A developmental gene (Tolloid/BMP-1) is regulated in *Aplysia* neurons by treatments that induce long-term sensitization. *J Neurosci*, **17**, 755–764.

Marinesco, S. and Carew, T.J. (2002). Serotonin release evoked by tail nerve stimulation in the CNS of *Aplysia*: characterization and relationship to heterosynaptic plasticity. *J Neurosci*, **22**, 2299–2312.

Mayford, M., Barzilai, A., Keller, F., Schacher, S. and Kandel, E.R. (1992). Modulation of an NCAM-related adhesion molecule with long-term synaptic plasticity in *Aplysia*. *Science*, **256**, 638–644.

Mozzachiodi, R., Lechner, H.A., Baxter, D.A. and Byrne, J.H. (2003). *In vitro* analog of classical conditioning of feeding behavior in *Aplysia*. *Learn Mem*, **10**, 478–494.

Murphy, G.G. and Glanzman, D.L. (1997). Mediation of classical conditioning in *Aplysia californica* by long-term potentiation of sensorimotor synapses. *Science*, **278**, 467–471.

Murphy, G.G. and Glanzman, D.L. (1999). Cellular analog of differential classical conditioning in *Aplysia*: disruption by the NMDA receptor antagonist DL-2-amino-5-phosphonovalerate. *J Neurosci*, **19**, 10595–10602.

Nargeot, R., Baxter, D.A. and Byrne, J.H. (1999a). *In vitro* analog of operant conditioning in *Aplysia*. I. Contingent reinforcement modifies the functional dynamics of an identified neuron. *J Neurosci*, **19**, 2247–2260.

Nargeot, R., Baxter, D.A. and Byrne, J.H. (1999b). *In vitro* analog of operant conditioning in *Aplysia*. II. Modifications of the functional dynamics of an identified neuron contribute to motor pattern selection. *J Neurosci*, **19**, 2261–2272.

Phares, G.A., Antzoulatos, E.G., Baxter, D.A. and Byrne, J.H. (2003). Burst-induced synaptic depression and its modulation contribute to information transfer at *Aplysia* sensorimotor synapses: empirical and computational analyses. *J Neurosci*, **23**, 8392–8401.

Pinsker, H., Kupfermann, I., Castellucci, V. and Kandel, E. (1970). Habituation and dishabituation of the gill-withdrawal reflex in *Aplysia*. *Science*, **167**, 1740–1742.

Pinsker, H.M., Hening, W.A., Carew, T.J. and Kandel, E.R. (1973). Long-term sensitization of a defensive withdrawal reflex in *Aplysia*. *Science*, **182**, 1039–1042.

Pittenger, C. and Kandel, E.R. (2003). In search of general mechanisms for long-lasting plasticity: *Aplysia* and the hippocampus. *Philos Trans Roy Soc Lond B Biol Sci*, **358**, 757–763.

Scholz, K.P. and Byrne, J.H. (1987). Long-term sensitization in *Aplysia*: biophysical correlates in tail sensory neurons. *Science*, **235**, 685–687.

Stopfer, M. and Carew, T.J. (1996). Heterosynaptic facilitation of tail sensory neuron synaptic transmission during habituation in tail-induced tail and siphon withdrawal reflexes of *Aplysia*. *J Neurosci*, **16**, 4933–4948.

Sugita, S., Baxter, D.A. and Byrne, J.H. (1997). Differential effects of 4-aminopyridine, serotonin, and phorbol esters on facilitation of sensorimotor connections in *Aplysia*. *J Neurophysiol*, **77**, 177–185.

Sutton, M.A. and Carew, T.J. (2000). Parallel molecular pathways mediate expression of distinct forms of intermediate-term facilitation at tail sensory-motor synapses in *Aplysia*. *Neuron*, **26**, 219–231.

Sutton, M.A., Bagnall, M.W., Sharma, S.K., Shobe, J. and Carew, T.J. (2004). Intermediate-term memory for site-specific sensitization in *Aplysia* is maintained by persistent activation of protein kinase C. *J Neurosci*, **24**, 3600–3609.

Taub, E., Uswatte, G. and Elbert, T. (2002). New treatments in neurorehabilitation founded on basic research. *Nat Rev Neurosci*, **3**, 228–236.

Thompson, R.F. and Spencer, W.A. (1966). Habituation: a model phenomenon for the study of neuronal substrates of behavior. *Psychol Rev*, **73**, 16–43.

Trudeau, L.E. and Castellucci, V.F. (1995). Postsynaptic modifications in long-term facilitation in *Aplysia*: upregulation of excitatory amino acid receptors. *J Neurosci*, **15**, 1275–1284.

Wainwright, M.L., Zhang, H., Byrne, J.H. and Cleary, L.J. (2002). Localized neuronal outgrowth induced by long-term sensitization training in *Aplysia*. *J Neurosci*, **22**, 4132–4141.

Walters, E.T. and Byrne, J.H. (1983). Associative conditioning of single sensory neurons suggests a cellular mechanism for learning. *Science*, **219**, 405–408.

Walters, E.T., Byrne, J.H., Carew, T.J. and Kandel, E.R. (1983a). Mechanoafferent neurons innervating tail of *Aplysia*.

I. Response properties and synaptic connections. *J Neurophysiol*, **50**, 1522–1542.

Walters, E.T., Byrne, J.H., Carew, T.J. and Kandel, E.R. (1983b). Mechanoafferent neurons innervating tail of *Aplysia*. II. Modulation by sensitizing stimulation. *J Neurophysiol*, **50**, 1543–1559.

White, J.A., Ziv, I., Cleary, L.J., Baxter, D.A. and Byrne, J.H. (1993). The role of interneurons in controlling the tail-withdrawal reflex in *Aplysia*: a network model. *J Neurophysiol*, **70**, 1777–1786.

Zhang, F., Endo, S., Cleary, L.J., Eskin, A. and Byrne, J.H. (1997). Role of transforming growth factor-beta in long-term synaptic facilitation in *Aplysia*. *Science*, **275**, 1318–1320.

Zhu, H., Wu, F. and Schacher, S. (1997). Site-specific and sensory neuron-dependent increases in postsynaptic glutamate sensitivity accompany serotonin-induced long-term facilitation at *Aplysia* sensorimotor synapses. *J Neurosci*, **17**, 4976–4986.

Functional plasticity in CNS system

CONTENTS

Plasticity of mature and developing somatosensory systems

Jon H. Kaas[1] and Tim P. Pons[2]

[1]Department of Psychology, Vanderbilt University, Nashville, TN and [2]Department of Neurosurgery, Wake Forest University School of Medicine, Winston-Salem, NC, USA

6.1 Introduction

The somatosensory system of humans and other primates includes spinal cord and brain stem circuits and nuclei, several thalamic nuclei, and an array of cortical areas that are complexly interconnected to form an impressive network of functionally distinct, interacting parts (Kaas, 2004). The early stages of processing can be summarized in a highly simplified schematic that emphasizes serial steps in the system (Fig. 6.1). Due to nerve and brain injuries, strokes and degeneration, any component of this system can be damaged and partially or fully inactivated. The question we address in this review is what happens to the rest of the system when part of the system is damaged. The answer, of course, is that the system adjusts to the damage, and reorganizes. Components of this reorganization can be adaptive, and help compensate for the loss, but other components can be disruptive and lead to misperceptions, misguided motor control, and sometimes "thalamic" pain (e.g. Doetsch, 1998; Ramachandran and Hirstein, 1998; see Volume II, Chapter 15). Here we review what happens when damage occurs at each of four levels of the system: (a) the receptor or primary afferent level, (b) the level of the brain stem relay to the dorsal column-trigeminal complex, (c) the thalamic ventroposterior nucleus, and (d) primary somatosensory cortex. The effects of lesions of higher-order areas (e) have not been adequately studied yet. However, the consequence of damage not only depends on the level of the injury, but also on the extent and completeness of the injury. Another factor is the age at the time of injury. The consequences of damage to the developing system can be quite different from those to the fully developed system.

Although our interest is in the plasticity of the human somatosensory system (see Volume II, Chapter 16), most of the relevant experimental evidence comes from invasive studies on monkeys, and this evidence is the focus of this review. We also briefly include results from relevant studies on other mammals, such as rats and raccoons, but we do so with caution as these mammals have different, and less complex somatosensory systems. While the early stages of processing of Fig. 6.1 are present in these mammals, they are not identical in detail, and the consequences of damage sometimes differ in significant ways. The somatosensory systems of monkeys are much more similar to those of humans, so that results from monkeys more likely apply to humans. However, this assumption should be made with caution, and evaluated relative to observable results from humans.

6.2 The complexity of the somatosensory system provides a rich framework for plasticity

The simplified somatosensory system in Fig. 6.1 portrays several relevant levels of study, and suggests an important consequence of damage; sensory losses and reorganization that occur at one

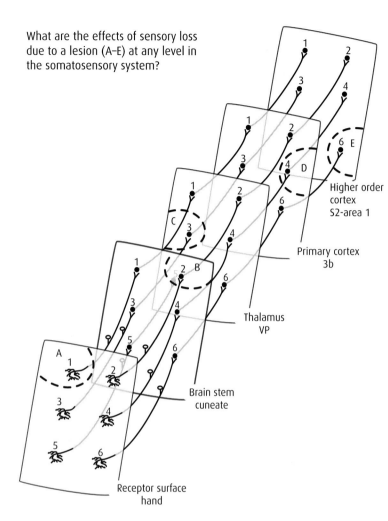

What are the effects of sensory loss due to a lesion (A–E) at any level in the somatosensory system?

Higher order cortex
S2-area 1

Primary cortex
3b

Thalamus
VP

Brain stem
cuneate

Receptor surface
hand

Figure 6.1. A schematic of (a) the topographic relay of cutaneous information from the skin to (b) the brain stem dorsal column nuclei; (c) the ventroposterior nucleus of the thalamus; (d) area 3b of primary somatosensory cortex; (e) then higher-order somatosensory areas such as area 1 and the second somatosensory area, S2. At each stage, a lesion may remove part of the topographic pattern, disrupt function, and be followed by sequences of adjustments that reorganize the topography of parts of the system. The dashed line outlines the lesion at each level.

level will be relayed to subsequent levels. For example, changes in cortical organization have often been described as a result of damage to peripheral nerve afferents (e.g. Merzenich et al., 1983a, b). This is a convenient way of assessing whether or not reorganization occurs in the early stages of the system, but it does not distinguish between changes in the system at cortical and subcortical levels. If only the cortex is examined, investigators may be misled into attributing subcortical reorganizations to cortical changes. While useful, the diagram does not reflect the great complexity of the anatomy of the early stages of processing, and the many

possibilities for reorganization at each level that in turn affect processing at other levels.

Some of the relevant complexity of the early stages of the somatosensory system in primates is included in Fig. 6.2. There are several important features that relate to plasticity (Kaas and Florence, 2001) that are as follows:

1 While sensory afferents project topographically to second order neurons in the spinal cord and brain stem, their terminal axon arbors contact groups of neurons, and contacts from afferents subserving nearby regions of skin overlap. Thus, nearby

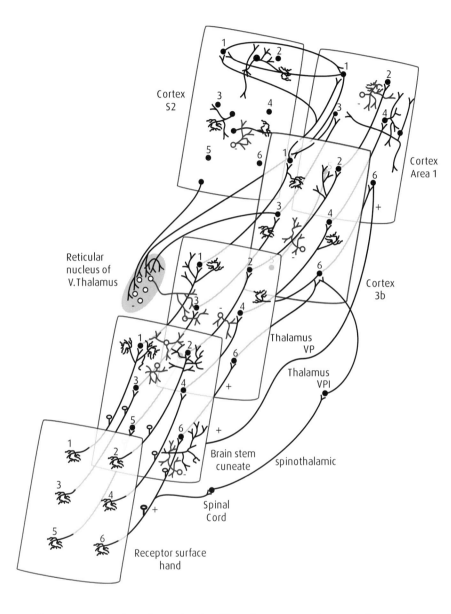

Figure 6.2. A schematic of the somatosensory system that more realistically reflects the complexity of the system than the serial model in Fig. 6.1. This complexity provides a rich number of possibilities for synaptic and connectional modifications that would reorganize topography after damage to part of the system. Excitatory (+) and inhibitory (−) connections are indicated. RT, reticular nucleus of the ventral thalamus.

afferents can substitute for each other if overlapping but weak inputs are potentiated. In addition, new synaptic contacts would depend on only local axonal growth. A similar divergence and convergence of axon terminations occurs at each subsequent level of processing.

2 There are parallel paths to the brain stem, thalamus, and cortex (dorsal columns, spinothalamics, and spinocervical tract) that are functionally distinct, but they may partially substitute for each other.

3 Axon terminations are on both relay (projection) neurons, which are excitatory, and local circuit inhibitory neurons. The inhibitory neurons constrain the sizes of receptive fields of the relay neurons by producing an "iceburg effect" so that many of the excitatory inputs on the relay

neurons are below the threshold for activation. Any loss of excitatory input at any level removes the drive to inhibitory neurons, allowing some relay neurons to be disinhibited enough that previously "silent" synapses are expressed. Inhibition is also rapidly reduced after sensory loss by activity-dependent mechanisms that alter the expression of inhibitory neurotransmitters and receptors (Garraghty et al., 1991; Jones, 1993).

4 Cortical areas have extensive, but short-range, intrinsic connections that spread information across the topographic map. The excitatory effects of these horizontal or lateral connections can be enhanced in many ways: new synapses may form, and new axon growth may lengthen or increase the number of these horizontal connections.

5 Cortical areas provide extensive numbers of feedback connections to the somatosensory thalamus and brain stem. These connections contact both excitatory and inhibitory neurons, possibly potentiating and suppressing different parts of the representation (Ergenzinger et al., 1998). Cortical areas also project to the thalamic reticular nucleus, containing solely inhibitory neurons that project in turn to the somatosensory thalamus (see Kaas and Ebner, 1998).

6 Cortical areas feedforward to activate neurons in several higher-order areas, and these areas send feedback connections. Thus, each area is under the direct influence of several higher-order areas. In addition, each area has callosal connections with its homolog and 2–3 other areas of the other hemisphere.

7 Finally, somatosensory areas project to the anterior pulvinar, which in turn distributes to cortical somatosensory areas (not shown). Thus, there is a connection network with multiple possibilities for effective substitution.

6.3 What happens after damage to peripheral neurons?

Peripheral sensory loss can occur in humans and other mammals as a result of accidents. Here we briefly discuss the consequences of a nerve crush with regeneration, a nerve cut and repair with regeneration, a nerve cut without regeneration, and transplanting and regenerating a nerve to a new skin location.

When a nerve (Wall et al., 1986; Florence et al., 1994, 2001) or nerves (Paul et al., 1972) of the hand of a monkey are cut, approximated, and sutured, the subsequent regeneration into the former skin territory of that nerve is often disorderly and nearly random (Fig. 6.3, see Thompson, Volume I, Chapter 27). During the process of regeneration, the deprived portions of primary somatosensory cortex, those representing the skin subserved by the cut nerve or nerves, likely becomes responsive to inputs from other parts of the hand (see below), but this cortical territory is recaptured by the inputs from the cut nerve as it functionally reinnervates the hand. In adult monkeys, the topographic consequences of the disordered regeneration are not corrected in the relay via the cuneate nucleus of the brain stem and the ventroposterior nucleus of the thalamus to area 3b (primary somatosensory cortex) or even to area 1 (which depends on area 3b inputs for activation, see Garraghty et al., 1990b). Instead of the normal topographic maps of the hand in these areas, somatotopy is jumbled so that neurons at various locations have similar, overlapping receptive fields, and many neurons have several receptive fields in different locations or unusually large receptive fields with indistinct borders. In humans, the disordered regeneration of cut nerves results in perceptual errors including mislocating sensations produced by punctate probes on the skin and poor tactile acuity (see Wall and Kaas, 1986). Performance can be improved with experience (e.g. Dellon, 1981; Van Boven and Johnson, 1994), but the neural basis of this recovery is not well understood.

One mechanism of improved performance may be the suppression of multiple receptive fields and weak receptive field fringes, as there is evidence that these abnormalities are more expressed at the thalamic level in the ventroposterior nucleus than in area 3b of cortex (Florence et al., 2001). In monkeys with early postnatal nerve sections, extensive use of

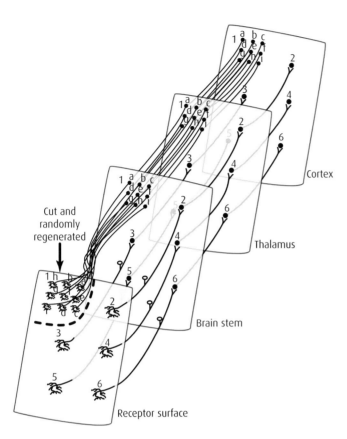

Cut and randomly regenerated

Receptor surface

Brain stem

Thalamus

Cortex

Figure 6.3. The major effects of nerve section and regeneration in the somatosensory system. The surviving proximal ends of cut afferents from skin region 1 regenerate randomly into skin region 1 so that they no longer activate neurons in a topographical pattern in the brain stem relay. Subsequent projections to the thalamus and then to cortex remain topographic and thus the scrambled input from the skin is not rearranged to form a topographic representation of skin region 1. Small sections of skin region 1, corresponding to the receptive fields of individual afferents, are lettered as a–i.

the reinnervated hand appeared to enhance the reduction of receptive field sizes and multiple receptive fields of neurons in area 3b compared to neurons in the ventroposterior nucleus (Florence et al., 2001). Also, nerve section and regeneration in late prenatal and early postnatal life results in a more normal cortical organization, but considerable somatotopic disorder persists (Florence et al., 1996). Perhaps the most dramatic demonstration of the usefulness of even disordered nerve regeneration is the recovery of some sensation and motor control of the hand in a unique patient with bilateral hand transplantation (Giraux et al., 2001). Peripheral nerves regenerated into the new hand, and these inputs activated the hand regions of somatosensory cortex.

Nerve crush produces a different outcome. The crushed nerve regenerates in a normal somatotopic pattern, and normal peripheral nerve function is restored (Dykes and Terzis, 1979), although new spinal cord terminations grow during regeneration and they may persist (Florence et al., 1993). In monkeys with a crushed and regenerated median nerve, the restored inputs reactivate hand cortex, and a normal somatotopic map is re-established in area 3b (Wall et al., 1983).

In some instances of sensory loss, one treatment has been to translocate a peripheral nerve so that it innervates a foreign skin territory (e.g. Terzis and Papakonstantinou, 2000). As expected from such procedures, regeneration of a nerve into foreign skin can lead to false localization. In an early and dramatic example of such mislocalized sensation, Sperry (1943) transposed peripheral nerves innervating the skin of the right and left hind limbs of rats and found that after the crossed nerves had regenerated, the rats persisted in withdrawing the wrong foot to mild electric shock to the sole of the foot. In unpublished experiments by Wunderlich, Wall, and Kaas, similar behavioral results in rats were obtained after the proximal end of the sciatic nerve of one hind limb was cut and sutured to the distal end of the sciatic nerve of the other leg and allowed to regenerate. Micro-electrode recordings from primary somatosensory cortex indicated that the representation of the foot was altered. The intact saphenous nerve represented part of the contralateral hind paw in a normal man-ner, but the skin territory of the sciatic nerve was activated by touch on the ipsilateral foot; and the rep-resentation due to the translocated and regenerated sciatic nerve was topographically disordered. These rats would withdraw either the pinched hindfoot or the other hindfoot, depending on whether the skin territory of the normal saphenous nerve or the crossed and regenerated sciatic nerve was pinched. In related experiments in monkeys, the ulnar nerve to the D5–D3 side of the glabrous hand and the median nerve to the D3–D1 side were transected and the proximal stump of the ulnar nerve was cross-sutured to the distal end of the median nerve where it regenerated into median nerve skin territory (Wall and Kaas, 1986). When these monkeys were trained to reach blindly through a screen to grasp a food reward touched on the D3–D1 side of the hand, they incorrectly grasped toward the D5–D3 side of the hand, indicating a perceptual error that was not cor-rected over weeks of experience. As expected, the misdirected ulnar nerve produced a disordered map of digits 5–3 and adjoining palm in the cortical terri-tory for the median nerve. These results indicate cortical maps in primary cortex do not reorganize to create a systematic somatotopic representation that incorporates the new source of input from the translo-cated nerve. Such inputs are persistently mislocated. Nevertheless, they may guide behavior in a useful way for humans after experience. Possibly, higher-order representations reorganize.

An injured and transected nerve may fail to recon-nect and regenerate into its former skin territory. This situation can be created experimentally by cut-ting a peripheral nerve and tying a suture around the cut end to prevent regeneration. When this was done to the median nerve in monkeys (which subserves the D1–D3 side of the glabrous hand), the deprived portion of the hand representation in area 3b of somatosensory cortex became reactivated by the remaining inputs from the hand over a period of days to weeks (Merzenich et al., 1983a, b; Garraghty and Kaas, 1991b; Wall et al., 1992a, b; Kolarick et al., 1994; Silva et al., 1996). The major source of the reactivation was by afferents from the dorsal hairy surface of the hand. In a similar manner, afferents from the dorsal surface of D3–D5 and adjoining dorsal hand reacti-vate the deprived part of area 3b when the ulnar nerve to the D3–D5 side of the glabrous hand is cut (Garraghty and Kaas, 1991b). The rapid replacement of glabrous hand inputs by dorsal hand inputs appears to be a result of a close approximation of these two inputs in their normal terminations in the cuneate nucleus of the brain stem (see Kaas and Collins, 2003). A rapid substitution of preserved for missing inputs does not occur when afferents from both surfaces of the hand are missing (Garraghty et al., 1994). However, a filling-in by the palm and other fingers may occur for missing fingers over longer recoveries (Merzenich et al., 1984; Jain et al., 1998). The hypothesis that dorsal skin inputs rapidly and easily substitute for glabrous skin inputs is supported, not only by the conjunction of inputs from dorsal and ventral fingers in the cuneate nucleus (Florence et al., 1991), but also by the electrophysiological evi-dence for partial substitution of dorsal hand affer-ents from missing ventral hand afferents at the level of the cuneate nucleus (Xu and Wall, 1999a, b; Churchill et al., 2001). A much more extensive sub-stitution occurs at the level of the ventroposterior nucleus (Garraghty and Kaas, 1991a).

6.4 Reorganization after a major loss of inputs from a hand or forelimb

Until recently, there was little appreciation of the extensive reorganization of the fully developed somatosensory system that is possible after massive sensory loss. The first clear evidence for extensive reorganization came with the opportunity to study the somatosensory cortex of monkeys with a long-standing loss of all afferents from a forelimb. Due to the interest in rehabilitating individuals who have suffered damage to the dorsal roots of the peripheral nerves of the arm while leaving motor output intact, a small number of macaque monkeys received training on the use of an arm deafferented by cutting the dorsal roots subserving the arm (see Taub, 1980 for review). When it became possible to study several of these monkeys some 12–20 years after the deafferentation, the complete forelimb region of somatosensory cortex was found to be activated by light touch on various parts of the face (Pons et al., 1991). The reorganization included not only area 3b, but also the adjoining representations in areas 3a, 1, and 2. Altogether, this involved the reactivation of a region of cortex some 10–14 mm in mediolateral length and a similar width across the four somatosensory areas. As expected, the long-standing loss of afferents also caused some transneuronal degeneration of parts of the cuneate nucleus and the ventroposterior nucleus (Woods et al., 2000).

Similar results were soon obtained from monkeys studied years after accidental injuries to a limb that required a therapeutic amputation of part or most of the limb. These few monkeys came from the various primate facilities where they were maintained after injury, but they all demonstrated an extensive reactivation of deprived regions of somatosensory cortex. In brief, after the long-standing loss of a forelimb, the deprived portions of areas 3b and 1 responded to touch on the stump of the amputated limb, and to the face; often many neurons responded to both the stump and face (Florence and Kaas, 1995; Florence et al., 1998, 2000). After hind-limb amputations, deprived regions of somatosensory cortex were largely activated by touch on the hip stump and adjoining trunk. Similar changes in the somatotopy of somatosensory cortex as a result of limb amputations have been reported in humans. The usual, non-invasive approach has been to use magnetoencephalography (MEG) to localize equivalent current dipoles on magnetic resonance images of the brains of subjects with amputations. The dipoles

are produced by electrically stimulating locations on the lip, face, and intact limb, producing a spatial resolution of the dipole in the range of 2–3 mm. The results suggest that the center of the lip representation shifted medially in the cortex of patients with forelimb amputations to the normal location of the hand representation (Elbert et al., 1994, 1997; Yang et al., 1994; Flor et al., 1995, 1998). Thus, given a long recovery time, major reactivation of deprived regions of somatosensory cortex is likely to occur in both monkeys and humans.

A further demonstration of the potential for extensive reorganization of somatosensory cortex after a major sensory loss came from monkeys studied after return of ascending branches of peripheral nerve afferents in the dorsal columns of the spinal cord (Jain et al., 1997, 2000). Cutting these afferents at a high cervical level deprives somatosensory cortex of activating inputs from all but a narrow strip of the skin of the anterior arm, and those from the face. Yet terminations of peripheral nerve afferents persist in the spinal cord, and locomotion and considerable limb use remains, although skilled use of the hand is impaired. Initially, the deprived zone of somatosensory cortex is unresponsive to tactile stimulation, but 6–8 months later, the deprived zone is activated by touch on the face and on the anterior arm. These experiments demonstrate extensive reorganization takes as long as 6–8 months to emerge.

One mechanism for the extensive reactivation appears to be the growth of new connections (see Moore and Kennedy, Volume I, Chapter 19) in the brain stem. After a cervical dorsal column section, afferents from the face grow into the cuneate nucleus of the brain stem; with arm amputations, other afferents from the stump grow into the part of the cuneate nucleus that represents the hand (Jain et al., 2000; Wu and Kaas, 2002). The growth of new afferents in the brain stem is sparse, but this growth could activate a small population of neurons, and the relay of this activation could be amplified in the thalamus and cortex. The growth of new connections has also been demonstrated in deprived cortex (Florence et al., 1998), and axon growth may also occur in the thalamus. However, much of the reactivation appears to be complete at the level of the ventroposterior nucleus, both in monkeys (Jones and Pons, 1998; Florence et al., 2000) and in humans (Davis et al., 1998). The dependence on the growth of axons over considerable distances may be the main factor in the lengthy time course of the reactivation (6–8 months) (Jain et al., 1997).

Surprisingly, other ascending pathways, especially the spinothalamic pathways, do not substitute for the dorsal columns after they are cut in adult monkeys. Inputs from the hand that are relayed over the spinothalamic pathway never activated the hand cortex after a dorsal column section. However, the effects of dorsal column section on the developing system may be different, as preliminary studies in monkeys reared after dorsal column section as infants resulted in activation in hand cortex by stimulating the hand. However, neurons responded poorly and had very large receptive fields. Thus, it appears likely that spinothalamic pathways can substitute for dorsal column pathways if the loss occurs early in postnatal development.

In both newborn and adult rats, high cervical dorsal column section is followed by some reactivation of forepaw cortex by preserved anterior arm inputs, but face cortex does not activate forepaw cortex even after months of recovery (Jain et al., 1995, 2003). Thus, sensory loss in rats is not followed by the extensive reorganization of the somatosensory system that is seen in monkeys and humans.

The major behavioral consequence of activating hand cortex by inputs from the face in humans is that stimuli on the face or shoulder may also be felt on the hand (Ramachandran et al., 1992; Davis et al., 1998; Doetsch, 1998; Ramachandran and Hirstein, 1998). Thus, the somatosensory system does not appear to reinterpret the major changes in sources of cortical activation so that they can correctly guide behavior.

6.5 The significance of preserving some of the afferents from the hand

When afferents from the hand are extensively damaged, the preservation of only a few afferents can have great impact on the activation of somatosensory

cortex, and on the usefulness of the hand. Ascending branches of afferents from the hand can be completely lost due to damage to the dorsal columns at a high cervical level, but it can be difficult to determine if the lesion is complete and if some afferents remain. If only a few afferents survive dorsal column section in monkeys, initially there may be too few to activate cortex, or they may only activate their normal territory in the hand representation in area 3b (Jain et al., 1997). However, over a period of days to weeks, the sparse inputs are potentiated and much or all of the hand representation becomes responsive to these inputs. In such monkeys, hand use appears to be nearly normal, suggesting that the preservation of only a few afferents has significant behavioral as well as physiological import. The importance of these afferents in behavior is further suggested by the previous conclusions that dorsal column damage in humans has little effect on sensory capacity (Wall and Noordenbos, 1977) and that nearly complete dorsal column sections in monkeys leave sensory abilities largely intact (Schwartz et al., 1972). More recently, Darian-Smith and Brown (2000) cut most of the afferents subserving the hand by sectioning dorsal roots. Initially, stimuli on the hand failed to activate cortex even though a few afferents remained. However, after 2–4 months of recovery, these remaining afferents effectively activated cortex and guided behavior. As another example, Jones et al. (1997; see Fig. 6.4) placed lesions in the ventroposterior nucleus of the thalamus, and found that a loss of 30% of the inputs to cortex had no appreciable effect on the responsiveness of cortex.

6.6 Thalamic and cortical plasticity after lesion of somatosensory cortex

Lesions of somatosensory cortex have been used to address three important questions about the impact of such lesions on the somatosensory system. First, if part of an orderly representation is removed, what happens to the rest of the representation? The apparent answer is that if the lesion is small, neurons in the

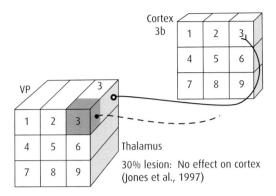

Figure 6.4. A partial loss of afferents as central connections devoted to a limited skin region has little or no noticeable effect on the responsiveness of neurons at the next stage of processing, or causes only a temporary loss of responsiveness. In this case, thalamic lesions of 30% or less of the representation of a given skin region produced no detectable change in the responsiveness of neurons in area 3b of macaque monkeys.

cortex of the immediate surround of the lesion may acquire new receptive fields so that they create new representations of the missing information. When parts of the hand representation in monkeys (Jenkins and Merzenich, 1987; Xerri et al., 1998) and raccoons (Doetsch et al., 1990) are ablated, neurons in tissue around the lesions became responsive to skin surfaces formerly represented in the lesioned cortex. However, recovery after lesions within the representation appears to be quite limited in extent (see Nudo et al., Volume I, Chapter 14) and it likely depends on the potentiation of preserved off-focus thalamocortical connections that formerly produced subthreshold responses. Due to the reorganization of cortex paralleled behavioral recovery of hand use, the recovery of lost parts of the hand representation seems to be responsible for behavioral improvement.

A second important question that has been addressed by cortical lesions and inactivation is what happens at the level of the thalamus after the feedback inputs from the cortex have been removed. In monkeys, chemically blocking the activity of neurons in the hand representation in area 3b resulted in greatly enlarged receptive fields for neurons in the ventroposterior nucleus of the thalamus (Ergenzinger et al., 1998). Similar results have been obtained in rats (Krupa et al., 1999). Thus, one of the consequences of a cortical lesion is the removal of feedback inputs to subcortical inhibitory neurons, thus allowing previously subthreshold activations of thalamic neurons to be relayed to cortex. This reduction in thalamic inhibition may be the source of much of the local reorganization of somatosensory cortex that follows focal cortical lesions.

The third question addressed in such experiments is what happens to higher-order cortical areas after a cortical source of activating inputs have been removed. In monkeys, lesions of areas 3b and 3a deactivate the second somatosensory area, S2 (Pons et al., 1992), as well as other higher-order areas such as the parietal ventral somatosensory area, PV (Garraghty et al., 1990a). When the cortical lesion completely removed the hand representations in areas 3a, 3b, 1 and 2, and monkeys were allowed 6–8 weeks to recover, the portion of S2 that is normally responsive to the hand was found to be responsive to touch on other body parts, largely the foot (Pons et al., 1988). Thus, higher-order sensory representations are capable of reorganization by using preserved inputs to activate deprived neurons.

6.7 Summary and conclusions

The somatosensory system of adult primates is capable of considerable reactivation after the loss of some of the activating connections. The reactivation depends on the expanded effectiveness of local preserved inputs only, which results in somatotopic reorganization. Some reactivations might depend only on changes in synaptic strength, but they often involve axonal growth and the formation of new connections. If the reactivations depend on the potentiation of previously existing connections, or the formation of new connections and synapses over short distances, reactivations can be rapid, and occur over hours to weeks. Immediate changes in activation patterns result from reduced drive on inhibitory neurons that suppress weaker excitatory synaptic influences, and this can occur with the disruption of either feedforward or feedback excitatory connections. Reactivations that depend on the growth of axons over long distances require longer times to emerge, perhaps 6–8 months. Similar deprivations in newborn monkeys can result in different types of reorganization, based on different substitutions, and similar deprivations in rats and monkeys may have different outcomes. The more limited reactivations involving inputs from nearby skin regions appear to contribute to sensory and motor performance, while the more extensive reactivations may lead to perceptual errors.

REFERENCES

Churchill, J.D., Arnald, L.L. and Garraghty, P.E. (2001). Somatotopic reorganization in the brainstem and thalamus following peripheral nerve inquiry in adult primates. *Brain Res*, **910**, 142–152.

Darian-Smith, C. and Brown, S. (2000). Functional changes at periphery and cortex following dorsal root lesions in adult monkeys. *Nat Neurosci*, **3**, 476–481.

Davis, K.D., Kiss, Z.H., Lou, L., Tasker, R.R., Lozano, A.M. and Dostrovsky, J.O. (1998). Phantom sensations generated by thalamic microstimulation. *Nature*, **391**, 385–387.

Dellon, A.L. (1981). *Evaluation of Sensibility and Re-education of Sensation in the Hand.* Williams and Wilkins, Baltimore, MD.

Doetsch, G.S. (1998). Perceptual significance of somatosensory cortical reorganization following peripheral denervation. *NeuroReport*, **9**, R29–R35.

Doetsch, G.S., Johnston, K.W. and Hannan, C.J. (1990). Physiological changes in the somatosensory forepaw cerebral cortex of adult raccoons following lesions of a single cortical digit representation. *Exp Neurol*, **108**, 162–175.

Dykes, R.W. and Terzis, J.K. (1979). Reinnervation of glabrous skin in baboons: properties of cutaneous mechanoreceptors subsequent to nerve crush. *J Neurophysiol*, **42**, 1461–1478.

Elbert, T., Flor, H., Birbaumer, N., Knecht, S., Hampson, S., Larbig, W. and Taub, E. (1994). Extensive reorganization of the somatosensory cortex in adult humans after nervous system injury. *NeuroReport*, **5**, 2593–2597.

Elbert, T., Sterr, A., Flor, H., Rockstroh, B., Knecht, S., Pantev, C., Wienbruch, C. and Taub, E. (1997). Input-increase and input-decrease types of cortical reorganization after upper extremity amputation in humans. *Exp Brain Res*, **117**, 161–164.

Ergenzinger, E.R., Glasier, M.M., Hahn, J.O. and Pons, T.P. (1998). Cortically induced thalamic plasticity in the primate somatosensory system. *Nat Neurosci*, **1**, 226–229.

Flor, H., Elbert, T., Knecht, S., Wienbruch, C., Pantev, C., Birbaumer, N., Larbig, W. and Taub, E. (1995). Phantom-limb pain as perceptual correlate of cortical reorganization following arm amputation. *Nature*, **375**, 482–484.

Flor, H., Elbert, T., Muhlnickel, W., Pantev, C., Wienbruch, C. and Taub, E. (1998). Cortical reorganization and phantom phenomena in congenital and traumatic upper-extremity amputees. *Exp Brain Res*, **119**, 205–212.

Florence, S.L. and Kaas, J.H. (1995). Large-scale reorganization at multiple levels of the somatosensory pathway follows therapeutic amputation of the hand in monkeys. *J Neurosci*, **15**, 8083–8095.

Florence, S.L., Wall, J.T. and Kaas, J.H. (1991). Central projections from the skin of the hand in squirrel monkeys. *J Comp Neurol*, **311**, 563–578.

Florence, S.L., Garraghty, P.E., Carlson, M. and Kaas, J.H. (1993). Sprouting of peripheral nerve axons in the spinal cord of monkeys. *Brain Res*, **601**, 343–348.

Florence, S.L., Garraghty, P.E., Wall, J.T. and Kaas, J.H. (1994). Sensory afferent projections and area 3b somatotopy following median nerve cut and repair in macaque monkeys. *Cereb Cortex*, **4**, 391–407.

Florence, S.L., Jain, N., Pospichal, M.W., Beck, P.D., Sly, D.L. and Kaas, J.H. (1996). Central reorganization of sensory pathways following peripheral nerve regeneration in fetal monkeys. *Nature*, **381**, 69–71.

Florence, S.L., Taub, H.B. and Kaas, J.H. (1998). Large-scale sprouting of cortical connections after peripheral injury in adult macaque monkeys. *Science*, **282**, 1117–1121.

Florence, S.L, Hackett, T.A. and Strata, F. (2000). Thalamic and cortical contributions to neural plasticity after limb amputation. *J Neurophysiol*, **83**, 3154–3159.

Florence, S.L., Boydston, L.A., Hackett, T.A., Lachoff, H.T., Strata, F. and Niblock, M.M. (2001). Sensory enrichment after peripheral nerve injury restores cortical, not thalamic, receptive field organization. *Eur J Neurosci*, **13**, 1755–1766.

Garraghty, P.E. and Kaas, J.H. (1991a). Functional reorganization in adult monkey thalamus after peripheral nerve injury. *NeuroReport*, **2**, 747–750.

Garraghty, P.E. and Kaas, J.H. (1991b). Large-scale functional reorganization in adult monkey cortex after peripheral nerve injury. *Proc Natl Acad Sci USA*, **88**, 6976–6980.

Garraghty, P.E., Pons, T.P. and Kaas, J.H. (1990a). Ablations of areas 3b (S-I proper) and 3a of somatosensory cortex in marmosets deactivate the second and parietal ventral somatosensory areas. *Somatosens Mot Res*, **7**, 125–135.

Garraghty, P.E., Florence, S.L. and Kaas, J.H. (1990b). Ablations of areas 3a and 3b of monkey somatosensory cortex abolish cutaneous responsivity in area 1. *Brain Res*, **528**, 165–169.

Garraghty, P.E., La Chica, E.A. and Kaas, J.H. (1991). Injury-induced reorganization of somatosensory cortex is accompanied by reductions in GABA staining. *Somatosens Mot Res*, **8**, 347–354.

Garraghty, P.E., Hanes, D.P., Florence, S.L. and Kaas, J.H. (1994). Pattern of peripheral deafferentation predicts reorganizational limits in adult primate somatosensory cortex. *Somatosen Mot Res*, **11**, 109–117.

Giraux, P., Sirigu, A., Schneider, F. and Dubernard, J.-M. (2001). Cortical reorganization in motor cortex after graft of both hands. *Nat Neurosci*, **4**(7), 691–692.

Jain, N., Florence, S.L. and Kaas, J.H. (1995). Limits on plasticity in somatosensory cortex of adult rats: hindlimb cortex is not reactivated after dorsal column section. *J Neurophysiol*, **73**, 1537–1546.

Jain, N., Catania, K.C. and Kaas, J.H. (1997). Deactivation and reactivation of somatosensory cortex after dorsal spinal cord injury. *Nature*, **386**, 495–498.

Jain, N., Catania, K.C. and Kaas, J.H. (1998). A historically visible representation of the fingers and palm in primate area 3b and its immutability following long-term deafferentations. *Cereb Cortex*, **8**, 227–236.

Jain, N., Florence, S.L., Qi, H.-X. and Kaas, J.H. (2000). Growth of new brainstem connections in adult monkeys with massive sensory loss. *Proc Natl Acad Sci USA*, **97**, 5546–5550.

Jain, N., Diener, P.S., Cog, J.O. and Kaas, J.H. (2003). Patterned activity via spinal dorsal quadrant inputs is necessary for the formation of organized somatosensory maps. *J Neurosci*, **23**, 10321–10330.

Jenkins, W.M. and Merzenich, M.M. (1987). Reorganization of neocortical representations after brain injury: a neuropsychological model of the basis of recovery from stroke. *Prog Brain Res*, **71**, 249–266.

Jones, E.G. (1993). GABAergic neurons and their role in cortical plasticity in primates. *Cereb Cortex*, **3**, 361–372.

Jones, E.G. and Pons, T.P. (1998). Thalamic and brainstem contributions to large-scale plasticity of primate somatosensory cortex. *Science*, **282**, 1121–1125.

Jones, E.G., Manger, P.R. and Woods, T.M. (1997). Maintenance of a somatotopic cortical map in the face of diminishing thalamocortical inputs. *Proc Natl Acad Sci USA*, **94**, 11003–11007.

Kaas, J.H. (2004). Somatosensory system. In: *The Human Nervous System* (eds Paxinos, G. and Mai, J.K.), 2nd edn., Elsevier Academic Press, New York, pp. 1059–1092.

Kaas, J.H. and Collins, C.E. (2003). Anatomical and functional reorganization of somatosensory cortex in mature primates

after peripheral nerve and spinal cord injury. In: *Advances in Neurology* (eds Siegel, A.M., Andersen, R.A., Feund, H.J. and Spencer, D.), Vol. 93, Lippincott, Williams, & Wilkins Philadelphia, PA, pp. 87–95.

Kaas, J.H. and Ebner, F. (1998). Intrathalmic connections: a new way to modulate cortical plasticity? *Nat Neurosci*, **1**, 341–342.

Kaas, J.H. and Florence, S.L. (2001). Reorganization of sensory and motor systems in adult mammals after injury. In: *The Mutable Brain* (ed. Kaas, J.H.), Harwood Academic Publishers, New York, pp. 165–242.

Kolarick, R.C., Rasey, S.K. and Wall, J.T. (1994). The consistency, extent, and locations of early-onset changes in cortical nerve dominance aggregates following injury of nerves to primate hands. *J Neurosci*, **14**, 4269–4288.

Krupa, D.J., Ghazanfar, A.A. and Nicolelis, M.A.L. (1999). Immediate thalamic sensory plasticity depends on corticothalamic feedback. *Proc Natl Acad Sci USA*, **96**, 8200–8205.

Merzenich, M.M., Kaas, J.H., Wall, J.T., Sur, M., Nelson, R.J. and Felleman, D.J. (1983a). Topographic reorganization of somatosensory cortical areas 3b and 1 in adult monkeys following restricted deafferentation. *J Neurosci*, **8**, 33–55.

Merzenich, M.M., Kaas, J.H., Wall, J.T., Sur, M., Nelson, R.J. and Felleman, D.J. (1983b). Progression of change following median nerve section in the cortical representation of the hand in areas 3b and 1 in adult owl and squirrel monkeys. *J Neurosci*, **10**, 639–665.

Merzenich, M.M., Nelson, R.J., Stryker, M.P., Cynader, M.S., Schoppmann, A. and Zook, J.M. (1984). Somatosensory cortical map changes following digit amputation in adult monkeys. *J Comp Neurol*, **224**, 591–605.

Paul, R.L., Goodman, H. and Merzenich, M.M. (1972). Alterations in mechanoreceptor input to Broadmann's areas 1 and 3 of the postcentral hand area of *Macaca mulatta* after nerve section and regeneration. *Brain Res*, **39**, 1–19.

Pons, T.P., Garraghty, P.E. and Mishkin, M. (1988). Lesion-induced plasticity in the second somatosensory cortex of adult macaques. *Proc Natl Acad Sci USA*, **85**, 5279–5281.

Pons, T.P., Garraghty, P.E. and Ommaya, A.K., Kaas, J.H., Taub, E. and Mishkin, M. (1991). Massive cortical reorganization after sensory deafferentation in adult macaques. *Science*, **252**, 1857–1860.

Pons, T.P., Garraghty, P.E. and Mishkin, M. (1992). Serial and parallel processing of tactual information in somatosensory cortex of rhesus monkeys. *J Neurophysiol*, **68**, 518–527.

Ramachandran, V.S. and Hirstein, W. (1998). The perception of phantom limbs. The D.O. Hebb Lecture. *Brain*, **121**, 1603–1630.

Ramachandran, V.S., Rogers-Ramachandran, D. and Stewart, M. (1992). Perceptual correlates of massive cortical reorganization. *Science*, **258**, 1159–1160.

Schwartz, A.S., Eidelberg, E., Marchok, P. and Azulary, A. (1972). Tactile discrimination in the monkey after section of the dorsal funiculus and lateral lemniscus. *Exp Neurol*, **37**, 582–596.

Silva, A.C., Rasey, S.K., Wu, X. and Wall, J.T. (1996). Initial cortical reactions to injury of the median and radial nerves to the hands of adult primates. *J Comp Neurol*, **366**, 700–716.

Sperry, R.W. (1943). Functional results of crossing sensory nerves in rats. *J Comp Neurol*, **78**, 59–90.

Taub, E. (1980). Somatosensory deafferentation research in monkeys: implications for rehabilitation medicine. In: *Behavioral Psychology in Rehabilitation Medicine: Clinical Applications* (ed. Ince, L.P.), Williams & Wilkins, Baltimore, MD, pp. 371–401.

Terzis, J.K. and Papakonstantinou, K.C. (2000). The surgical treatment of brachial plexus injuries in adults. *Plast Reconstr Surg*, **106**, 1097–1122.

Van Boven, R.W. and Johnson, K.O. (1994). A psychophysical study of the mechanisms of sensory recovery following nerve injury in humans. *Brain*, **117**, 149–167.

Wall, J.T. and Kaas, J.H. (1986). Long-term cortical consequences of reinnervation errors after nerve regeneration in monkeys. *Brain Res*, **372**, 400–404.

Wall, J.T., Felleman, D.J. and Kaas, J.H. (1983). Recovery of normal topography in the somatosensory cortex of monkeys after nerve crush and regeneration. *Science*, **221**, 771–773.

Wall, J.T., Kaas, J.H., Sur, M., Nelson, R.J., Felleman, D.J. and Merzenich, M.M. (1986). Functional reorganization in somatosensory cortical areas 3b and 1 of adult monkeys after median nerve repair: possible relationships to sensory recovery in humans. *J Neurosci*, **6**, 218–233.

Wall, J.T., Huerta, M.F. and Kaas, J.H. (1992a). Changes in the cortical map of the hand following postnatal median nerve injury in monkeys: I. Modification of somatotopic aggregates. *J Neurosci*, **12**, 3445–3455.

Wall, J.T., Huerta, M.F. and Kaas, J.H. (1992b). Changes in the cortical map of the hand following postnatal ulnar and radial nerve injury in monkeys: II. Organization and modification of nerve dominance aggregates. *J Neurosci*, **12**, 3457–3465.

Wall, P.D. and Noordenbos, W. (1977). Sensory functions which remain in man after complete transaction of dorsal columns. *Brain*, **100**, 641–653.

Woods, T.M., Cusick, C.G., Pons, T.P., Taub, E. and Jones, E.G. (2000). Progressive transneuronal changes in the brainstem and thalamus after long-term dorsal rhizotomies in adult macaque monkeys. *J Neurosci*, **20**, 3884–3899.

Wu, C.W.H. and Kaas, J.H. (2002). The effects of long-standing limb loss on anatomical reorganization of somatosensory afferents in the brainstem and spinal cord. *Somatosens Mot Res*, **19**, 153–163.

Xerri, C., Merzenich, M.M., Peterson, B.E. and Jenkins, W. (1998). Plasticity of primary somatosensory cortex paralleling sensorimotor skill recovery from stroke in adult monkeys. *J Neurophysiol*, **79**, 2119–2148.

Xu, J. and Wall, J.T. (1999a). Rapid changes in brainstem maps of adult primates after peripheral injury. *Brain Res*, **774**, 211–215.

Xu, J. and Wall, J.T. (1999b). Evidence for brainstem and suprabrainstem contributions to rapid cortical plasticity in adult monkeys. *J Neurosci*, **19**, 7578–7590.

Yang, T.T., Gallen, C.C., Ramachandran, V.S., Cobb, S., Schwartz, B.J. and Bloom, F.E. (1994). Noninvasive detection of cerebral plasticity in adult human somatosensory cortex. *NeuroReport*, **5**, 701–704.

Activity-dependent plasticity in the intact spinal cord

Jonathan R. Wolpaw

Laboratory of Nervous System Disorders, Wadsworth Center, NYS Department of Health, Albany, NY, USA

"… the learning of motor skills may be as much task of the spinal cord as of the cortex."

A. Brodal,
Neurological Anatomy in Relation to Clinical Medicine, 3rd edn,
Oxford University Press, New York, p. 246, 1981.

7.1 Introduction

The traditional view of the spinal cord

A major feature of neuroscience over the past 30 years has been the steadily growing recognition of the ubiquity of activity-dependent plasticity in the central nervous system (CNS). Recognition of the multiple mechanisms of synaptic and neuronal plasticity, of their existence in many different regions, and of the frequency with which they are activated, has wholly overturned the traditional view of a hard-wired CNS that stores the effects of past experience by a limited set of mechanisms and only in a few specialized places. This new understanding, however, still focuses mainly on the brain, and excludes, intentionally or otherwise, the spinal cord. As late as the 18th century, the spinal cord was seen as simply a big well-protected nerve through which the brain interacts with the world; and it is still commonly assumed to be merely a stable way station between the brain and the periphery, the repository of nothing more than a few fixed reflexes. The original rationale for this 19th-century assumption was as much theological as scientific (reviewed in Wolpaw and Tennissen, 2001). Nevertheless, it remains embedded in neuroscientific theory and research. Activity-dependent plasticity, or persistent CNS modification that results from past experience and affects future behavior, is still considered by many neuroscientists to be a purely supraspinal capacity.

The recognition of spinal cord plasticity

It is now abundantly clear that the spinal cord possesses capacities for activity-dependent plasticity comparable to those found elsewhere in the CNS. During development as well as later in life, the spinal cord changes in response to activity reaching it from the periphery and/or from the brain. Like plasticity elsewhere, this spinal cord plasticity appears to involve both synaptic and neuronal mechanisms (e.g., long-term potentiation (LTP), changes in neuronal morphology and electrical properties), to be influenced by growth factors, and to be associated with gene activation (e.g., Liu and Sandkühler, 1997; Eyre et al., 2000; Gibson et al., 2000; Inglis et al., 2000; Mendell et al., 2001; Wolpaw and Tennissen, 2001; Tillakaratne et al., 2002; Dupont-Versteegden et al., 2004).

Numerous laboratory and clinical studies have explored the functional effects of such activity-dependent plasticity in health and disease. The principal measures of spinal cord function have been two major categories of spinal cord responses to peripheral inputs: *flexion-withdrawal reflexes* (mediated by oligosynaptic nociceptive pathways to spinal motoneurons from unmyelinated C fibers and small myelinated A-delta fibers) and *proprioceptive reflexes* (mediated by mono- and oligosynaptic pathways to spinal motoneurons from larger afferents that innervate the muscle spindles, the Golgi tendon organs, and the other receptors that reflect muscle length and tension, and limb position) (Matthews, 1972;

Baldissera et al., 1981; Burke, 1998; Kandel et al., 2000; Zehr, 2002; Misiaszek, 2003).

Flexion-withdrawal reflexes in the isolated spinal cord show habituation and sensitization with a variety of stimulation protocols (Mendell, 1984). Most work has addressed pain mechanisms and sensitization of spinal cord responses to C and A fiber input. This activity-dependent spinal cord plasticity is covered in Volume II, Chapter 15 and in numerous recent reviews (e.g., Herrero et al., 2000; Zimmermann, 2001; Ji et al., 2003; Melzack et al., 2004). Furthermore, these reflexes can display both classical and operant conditioning phenomena (reviewed in Patterson, 1976; Kandel, 1977; Thompson, 2001). Activity in proprioceptive afferents can also change the spinal cord (Lloyd, 1949; Kandel, 1977).

The spinal locomotor pattern generator (LPG), which is normally activated and influenced by descending activity, is capable of functioning autonomously in the isolated spinal cord. Most apparent in lower vertebrates, this is evident also in higher vertebrates such as the cat; and a spinal LPG appears to exist in humans as well (Holmes, 1915; Kuhn, 1950; Bussel et al., 1988; Calancie et al., 1994; Dietz et al., 1995; Dobkin et al., 1995; Rossignol, 1996, 2000; Dimitrijevic et al., 1998; Kiehn et al., 1998; Orlovsky et al., 1999; Rossignol, 2000). Studies first begun 50 years ago and resumed over the past 20 years show that locomotion controlled by the isolated spinal cord improves with training and that this improvement depends on spinal cord plasticity (Shurrager and Dykman, 1951; Lovely et al., 1986; Barbeau and Rossignol, 1987; Barbeau et al., 2002; Rossignol et al., 2002; Tillakaratne et al., 2002). This work (addressed in Volume I, Chapter 13; Volume II, Chapters 3 and 19) suggests that the operation of a human LPG might be encouraged and guided in people with spinal cord injuries so as to restore useful locomotion. Similar techniques for inducing and guiding activity-dependent spinal cord plasticity might help to restore bladder, bowel, and other autonomic functions after spinal cord injury.

Destruction or severe impairment of descending spinal cord pathways initiates gradual changes in spinal cord function (Riddoch, 1917; Kuhn, 1950;

Mountcastle, 1980; Ronthal, 1998; Hiersemenzel et al., 2000). The final result is typically characterized by increased resistance to passive muscle stretch, particularly in antigravity muscles (i.e., leg extensors and arm flexors), hyperactive tendon jerks, and increased flexion-withdrawal responses. These effects comprise the syndrome of spasticity, and their gradual development reflects spinal cord plasticity caused by the destruction of supraspinal connections, by the accompanying loss of descending input, and by the associated changes in peripheral input. This plasticity includes changes in motoneuron and motor unit properties, in motoneuron synaptic coverage, in primary afferent excitatory postsynaptic potentials (EPSPs), and in interneuronal pathways (Nelson and Mendell, 1979; Cope et al., 1986; Munson et al., 1986; Boorman et al., 1991; Shefner et al., 1992; Thompson et al., 1992; Hochman and McCrea, 1994a–c; Tai and Goshgarian, 1996; Tai et al., 1997). Rapid activity-dependent spinal cord plasticity in response to the more specific and limited change in descending input caused by a cerebellar lesion was first demonstrated 80 years ago (DiGiorgio, 1929; 1942; Manni, 1950; Gerard, 1961; Chamberlain et al., 1963). This phenomenon, called "spinal fixation", was considered by Gerard and others to be a good model for the fixation or consolidation of memory. Comparable phenomena occur in the spinal cord with a variety of supraspinal lesions and can also follow manipulation of labyrinthian sensory inputs (Giulio, 1952; Straka and Dieringer, 1995). Clearly, altered descending input that lasts for sufficient time produces spinal cord plasticity that persists after the input stops.

The importance of spinal cord plasticity

Recent appreciation of these data and their implications have coincided with and been encouraged by great interest and optimism now centered on possibilities for restoring spinal cord structure and function after spinal cord injury (addressed in numerous other chapters in this volume). The exciting prospects for regenerating damaged pathways and lost neurons lead inevitably to the question of how newly regenerated tissue is to become capable of supporting useful function. A properly functioning adult spinal cord is the product of appropriate activity-dependent plasticity in early development and throughout later life. Thus, a newly (and probably imperfectly) regenerated spinal cord will almost certainly not support useful function very well (Muir and Steeves, 1997); it is likely to display diffuse infantile reflexes and/or other disordered and dysfunctional behaviors. Thus, as methods for producing spinal cord regeneration are developed, methods for properly educating the regenerated spinal cord will become essential.

This future need is directing attention to activity-dependent spinal cord plasticity, to the mechanisms which shape spinal cord neurons and pathways to support both basic and specialized behaviors as varied as locomotion, urination, ballet, and playing a musical instrument. In addition, recent appreciation of the latent capacities for plasticity of the injured unregenerated spinal cord provides additional incentive for exploring activity-dependent plasticity in the spinal cord (e.g., see Volume I, Chapter 13). Understanding this plasticity is essential for understanding both the changes that follow injury and the processes that could be accessed and guided to restore useful function.

Interest in activity-dependent spinal cord plasticity is increasing further with the growing recognition that the acquisition and maintenance of normal motor performances reflect activity-dependent plasticity at multiple sites throughout the CNS, including the spinal cord. The peripheral and descending inputs occurring during practice change the spinal cord, and these changes combine with changes elsewhere to modify behavior. Thus, understanding of the processes of spinal cord plasticity and its interactions with plasticity elsewhere is essential for understanding normal behaviors as well as the complex motor disabilities associated with disorders such as spinal cord injury.

7.2 Activity-dependent spinal cord plasticity in normal life

In the intact CNS, descending and peripheral inputs to the spinal cord are a continual barrage of activity in a variety of pathways. The immediate short-term products of this activity (e.g., voluntary movements, responses to peripheral disturbances, locomotion, respiration, urination, task-specific adjustments in spinal reflexes) are readily apparent. In contrast, the gradual long-term effects of these inputs on the spinal cord are not as obvious. Nevertheless, while the immediate effects are easily seen and conveniently studied, the gradual long-term effects are also important. They help establish and maintain spinal cord function in a state that supports effective performance. Such gradual activity-dependent plasticity, driven by descending input and associated peripheral input, shapes spinal cord function during early development and continues to adjust it throughout life. The next sections address the range of activity-dependent plasticity during normal life, and the accompanying Table 7.1 provides a variety of examples.

Table 7.1. Examples of activity-dependent spinal cord plasticity in normal life.

Development

Focusing of proprioceptive reflexes (Myklebust et al., 1986; O'Sullivan et al., 1991)

Directionality of nociceptive-withdrawal responses (Levinsson et al., 1999; Waldenström et al., 2003)

Lateralization of descending cortical control (Eyre et al., 2001; Martin et al., 2004)

Maturation of bladder reflex pathways (de Groat, 2002)

Motoneuron morphology (Inglis et al., 2000)

Skill acquisition and other experiences later in life

Ballet (Goode and Van Hoven, 1982; Koceja et al., 1991; Nielsen et al., 1993)

Athletic training (Rochcongar et al., 1979; Casabona et al., 1990)

Activity level (Yamanaka et al., 1999; Gomez-Pinilla et al., 2002)

Hopping (Voigt et al., 1998)

Backward locomotion (Schneider and Capaday, 2003)

Limb trajectory maintenance (Meyer-Lohmann et al., 1986)

Age-related changes in proprioceptive reflexes (Morita et al., 1995; Koceja and Mynark, 2000)

Operant conditioning of proprioceptive reflexes (Wolpaw et al., 1983; Segal, 1997)

Plasticity during development

Early in life, both descending and peripheral inputs play critical roles in the plasticity that leads to a normally functioning adult spinal cord, a spinal cord that displays characteristic adult reflex patterns, that supports standard motor skills such as locomotion and urination, and that permits the acquisition of more specialized skills.

The rapid withdrawal from painful stimuli is a basic and important function of spinal cord pathways, and this function is acquired early in life. In the newborn rat, focal nociceptive stimulation produces diffuse and often inappropriate muscle contractions and limb movements. In contrast, in the normal adult such stimulation excites the appropriate muscles, that is, the muscles that withdraw the limb from the painful stimulus. Schouenborg and his colleagues have demonstrated the importance of descending influence in producing these properly focused adult flexion-withdrawal reflexes (e.g., Levinsson et al., 1999). When neonatal spinal cord transection abolishes descending input, the adult pattern does not develop, and non-specific and inappropriate flexion-withdrawal reflexes persist into adulthood (Fig. 7.1(a)).

Spinal cord proprioceptive reflex pathways contribute to locomotion and other important motor functions (Rossignol, 1996). In human infants, muscle stretch produces very short-latency spinally-mediated stretch reflexes in both the stretched muscles and in their antagonists (Myklebust et al., 1986; O'Sullivan et al., 1998). Normally, the antagonist-stretch reflexes gradually disappear during childhood, leaving the adult with standard, the so-called knee-jerk reflexes limited to the stretched muscles. In people with cerebral palsy in whom perinatal supraspinal damage distorts activity in descending pathways, this normal evolution can fail to occur, and antagonist-stretch reflexes can persist into adulthood and contribute to motor disability. In Fig. 7.1(b) are agonist- and antagonist-stretch reflexes from a normal infant and a normal adult, and from an adult with cerebral palsy. Like the normal infant and unlike the normal adult, the adult with cerebral palsy has short-latency responses in both the agonist and antagonist muscles. In such individuals, the original damage is supraspinal. Thus, the likely explanation for the abnormal persistence of infantile spinal reflexes into adulthood is the absence or distortion of the long-term descending input that gradually eliminates or suppresses these reflexes in the first years of life.

Descending pathways are also important for the development of normal urinary function. In newborn animals and humans, voiding is readily elicited by peripheral stimuli via a purely spinal reflex pathway. During normal postnatal development, this reflex voiding is suppressed and supraspinal mediation of voiding becomes dominant. The change appears to result from change in the relative strengths of peripheral and descending excitatory connections to the spinal cord preganglionic neurons that produce micturition (de Groot, 2002). The decrease in response to peripheral input is probably due to a presynaptic decrease in glutamic acid release, rather than to a post-synaptic change. Neonatal spinal cord transection prevents this evolution, so that the infantile pattern of reflex voiding is retained into adulthood. The primitive pattern can also re-emerge in adulthood following spinal cord injury.

During development, corticospinal pathways change so as to produce the normal adult pattern of predominantly contralateral innervation (Eyre et al., 2001; Eyre, 2003). Perinatal damage to sensorimotor cortex of one hemisphere may prevent this normal evolution, and lead to abnormal adult innervation in which the undamaged hemisphere has strong ipsilateral as well as contralateral spinal cord projections. This abnormal innervation appears to result from absence of normal activity-dependent competition between ipsilateral and contralateral connections. Figure 7.1(c) illustrates this abnormality by comparing responses to transcranial magnetic stimulation in a normal adult and in an adult with cerebral palsy (Eyre et al., 2001). While the normal adult has a large contralateral response and a minimal ipsilateral response, the adult with cerebral palsy has large responses on both sides. Such lesions also affect muscle afferent innervation in spinal

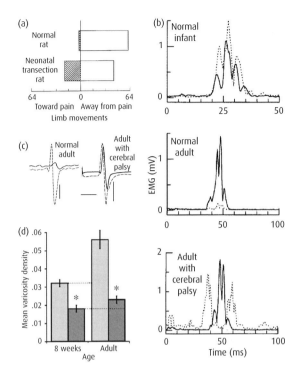

Figure 7.1. Activity-dependent spinal cord plasticity during development. (a) Direction of limb movement produced by flexion-withdrawal responses to a nociceptive stimulus in normal adult rats and in adult rats which had undergone spinal cord transection just after birth. Direction is almost always appropriate, i.e., away from the stimulus, in normal adults, but is often inappropriate in transected adults. Neonatal transection prevents normal shaping of flexion-withdrawal reflexes by descending input (modified from Levinsson et al. (1999)). (b) Short-latency electromyographic (EMG) responses of soleus (solid) and tibialis anterior (dotted) muscles to sudden foot dorsiflexion, which stretches the soleus and shortens the tibialis anterior, in a normal infant, a normal adult, and an adult with cerebral palsy. In the normal infant, spinal stretch reflexes (SSRs) occur in both muscles. In the normal adult, a reflex occurs only in the stretched muscle, i.e., the soleus, and little or no response occurs in the tibialis anterior. In contrast, in the adult with cerebral palsy, in whom perinatal supraspinal injury has impaired descending input, the infantile pattern persists: reflexes occur in both muscles (from Myklebust, B., unpublished data (Myklebust et al., 1982; Myklebust et al., 1986, for comparable data)). (c) Ipsilateral (solid) and contralateral (dashed) EMG responses (first dorsal interosseus muscle) to transcranial magnetic stimulation over motor cortex in a normal adult (left) and a subject with cerebral palsy (right). Horizontal scale bar is 20 ms, vertical bar is 200 μV. The large ipsilateral response seen in the subject with cerebral palsy indicates abnormal preservation of the strong ipsilateral corticospinal connections that normally disappear early in life (modified from Eyre et al. (2001)). (d) Densities in 8-week-old and adult cats of putative corticospinal tract boutons (varicosities) in cervical spinal cord ipsilateral (dark gray) and contralateral (light gray) to forelimb muscle paralyzed from age 3 to 7 weeks. Muscle paralysis during development reduces corticospinal tract innervation and this deficit persists into adulthood. Asterixes indicate significant differences from the contralateral data (modified from Martin et al. (2004)).

cord, and in addition appear to affect spinal neuronal properties (e.g., expression of parvalbumin and the early immediate gene c-Jun) (Gibson et al., 2000). The functional impact of the abnormal innervation is particularly severe in humans, in whom corticospinal connections become prominent early in development and eventually play important roles in motor control (Eyre et al., 2000). Indeed, the movement disorders produced by a perinatal hemispheric lesion may be minimal in the infant and only become prominent over months or years as complex skills fail to develop properly.

Peripheral as well as descending inputs play important roles in development of a normally functional adult spinal cord. The evolution of normal flexion-withdrawal responses in rats depends not only on descending pathways (e.g., Fig. 7.1(a)) but on peripheral input also. Peripheral anesthesia during development prevents development of normal adult reflexes (Waldenström et al., 2003). Interestingly, painful input is not essential. Tactile input alone is sufficient to support normal development. Abnormal peripheral input during development due to paralysis of a specific muscle can also lead to adult abnormalities in corticospinal motoneuronal connections (Fig. 7.1(d)) and in motor function as well (Martin et al., 2004).

Plasticity with acquisition and maintenance of motor skills

The acquisition of motor skills later in life is associated with changes in spinal cord circuitry. These changes have been detected in animals and humans primarily by measuring the spinal stretch reflex (SSR) (produced mainly by a monosynaptic pathway consisting of the Ia afferent from the muscle spindle, its synapse on the motoneuron, and the motoneuron itself), and its electrical analog, the H-reflex, which is elicited by direct electrical stimulation of the Ia afferents (Magladery et al., 1951; Matthews, 1972; Henneman and Mendell, 1981; Brown, 1984; Zehr, 2002). The simple spinal pathways assessed by these reflexes contribute to both simple and complex behaviors, and thus changes in them change multiple behaviors and/or change the CNS activity responsible for these behaviors. Numerous studies in normal adults show that these spinal reflexes are affected by the nature, intensity, and duration of past physical activity and by specialized training regimens.

Reflexes differ between athletes and non-athletes, and among different groups of athletes (Rochcongar et al., 1979; Goode and Van Hoven, 1982; Casabona et al., 1990; Koceja et al., 1991; Nielsen et al., 1993; Augé and Morrison, 2000). Nielsen et al. (1993) studied H-reflexes in soleus muscles of people who were

sedentary, moderately active, or extremely active, or were professional ballet dancers. Both H-reflexes and disynaptic reciprocal inhibition were larger in moderately active people than in sedentary people, and still larger in very active people. As the human soleus muscle consists mainly of slow (i.e., type I) fibers, exercise-induced change in motor unit properties cannot easily account for the reflex increase associated with activity. The most striking finding, illustrated in Fig. 7.2(a), was that the H-reflex and disynaptic reciprocal inhibition as well, were weakest in the professional dancers, even though the dancers were far more active than the other groups. Their values were lower than those of sedentary people, and far lower than those of active people. Starting from the fact that muscle co-contraction is associated with increased presynaptic inhibition and decreased reciprocal inhibition, the authors hypothesized that the prolonged co-contractions required by the classical ballet postures eventually lead to lasting decreases in synaptic transmission at the Ia synapses, and thereby account for the weak H-reflexes and the weak reciprocal inhibition. From the perspective of performance, the decreased direct peripheral influence on motoneurons underlying the smaller reflexes may augment cortical control and thereby facilitate more precise movement.

In such studies of humans with different athletic histories, it is difficult to eliminate the potential confounding effects of differences in original genetic endowments (e.g., between dancers and other people, or between dancers and runners). Controlled studies of the effects of specialized training regimens, which do not face this difficulty, provide further evidence of activity-dependent spinal cord plasticity. In an early study, monkeys were trained to make smooth repetitive flexion and extension movements at the elbow, and random brief perturbations were superimposed (Meyer-Lohmann et al., 1986). Over months and years, the SSR elicited by the perturbation gradually grew larger and took over the task of responding to the perturbation, and longer-latency reflex responses gradually disappeared. As illustrated in Fig. 7.2(b), the larger SSR was adaptive: it was associated with faster recovery from the

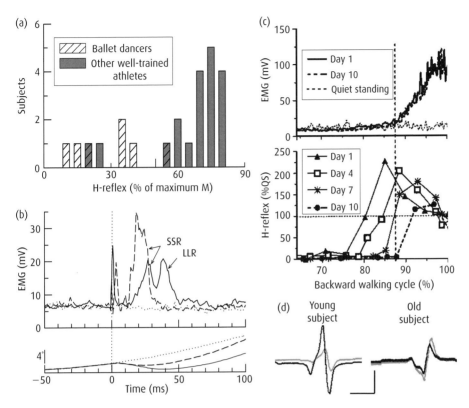

Figure 7.2. Activity-dependent spinal cord plasticity associated with skill acquisition and with aging. (a) Soleus H-reflexes are much smaller in professional ballet dancers than in other well-trained athletes (e.g., runners, swimmers, cyclists) (H-reflexes of sedentary subjects fall in between) (modified from Nielsen et al. (1993)). (b) Working for reward, monkeys performed an elbow flexion–extension task on which brief perturbations were randomly superimposed. Biceps EMG and elbow angle (flexion upward) for an unperturbed trial (dotted), a perturbed trial early in training (solid), and a perturbed trial late in training (dashed) are shown. Early in training, perturbation elicits both a SSR and a long-latency polysynaptic response (LLR). After intermittent training over several years, the SSR is much larger and the LLR has disappeared. The SSR has gradually taken over the role of opposing the perturbation. This improves performance: the disturbance in the smooth course of elbow flexion is smaller and briefer (modified from Meyer-Lohmann et al. (1986)). (c) Change in soleus H-reflex size as a function of time in the backward-walking step cycle as a person masters backward walking over 10 days. (Top) Soleus EMG of Day 1 and Day 10 just before and after onset of the soleus burst associated with the stance phase of the step cycle. Dotted line shows soleus EMG for quiet standing. (Bottom) H-reflex size (as % of size during quiet standing) versus time in the backward-walking step cycle for Days 1, 4, 7, and 10 of training. Soleus EMG does not change with training. In contrast, the marked increase in H-reflex size prior to the soleus burst that is seen on Day 1 disappears by Day 10. (d) Soleus H-reflexes in prone (black) and standing (gray) positions from a young person and an old person. In old subjects, the H-reflex tends to be smaller and to be less affected by body position (modified from Koceja et al. (1995)).

disturbance in limb trajectory caused by the perturbation. The investigators concluded (p. 398) that the results "demonstrate a growing role for fast segmental mechanisms in the reaction to external disturbances as motor learning progresses."

More recent human studies have revealed reflex changes produced over days and weeks by specialized training regimens (Pérot et al., 1991; Voigt et al., 1998; Yamanaka et al., 1999; Schneider and Capaday, 2003). For example, 15 min/day of training in a backward-walking task produced a gradual shift in the relationship between H-reflex size and the time in the step cycle at which the reflex was elicited. On Day 1 of backward-walking training, the soleus H-reflex became large well before the onset of the soleus burst associated with the stance phase of the cycle. By Day 10, the H-reflex did not become detectable until the onset of the burst. This effect of training is shown in Fig. 7.2(c). The early increase in H-reflex size on Day 1 may represent compensation for uncertainty as to when the stance phase of the step cycle, with its need for increased soleus activity, will begin. The increased sensitivity of the reflex arc helps ensure a rapid excitatory response to foot contact. As training proceeds, and the time of contact becomes predictable, such compensation becomes less necessary.

Additional evidence for adaptive spinal cord plasticity during adult life and in response to specific demands comes from studies of reflex changes in humans associated with aging (Sabbahi and Sedgwick, 1982; DeVries et al., 1985; Koceja et al., 1995; Morita et al., 1995; Angulo-Kinzler et al., 1998; Koceja and Mynark, 2000; Zheng et al., 2000). The age-related changes in reflex strength and in task-related reflex modulation that are described in these studies and illustrated in Fig. 7.2(d) are likely to reflect both direct and indirect effects of aging, that is, direct effects on the neuronal circuitry responsible for the reflexes and indirect effects secondary to the effects of aging elsewhere in the CNS or on the muscles, joints, and peripheral nerves that implement motor behaviors.

7.3 Activity-dependent spinal cord plasticity and behavioral change

The data reviewed in the previous section indicate that activity-dependent changes in spinal cord function are associated with the acquisition and maintenance of motor skills throughout life. At the same time, they do not distinguish clearly the respective contributions to changing spinal cord function of: plasticity in the spinal cord itself; modifications in

descending influence on the spinal cord due to supraspinal plasticity; and peripheral neuromuscular modifications that change sensory inputs and/or the effects of spinal cord outputs. Current progress in making these distinctions, in beginning to understand how plasticity of specific kinds at specific sites can contribute to the acquisition and maintenance of specific behaviors, depends on the same spinal cord reflexes that have been used to detect this plasticity.

While these simple spinal cord reflexes (stretch reflexes, H-reflexes, flexion-withdrawal reflexes) normally function as parts of complex behaviors, they are themselves simple behaviors, the simplest behaviors of which the mammalian nervous system is capable, and adaptive changes in them are essentially simple skills that can be used as laboratory models for the plasticity underlying skill acquisition. Operant conditioning of the SSR, or its electrical analog the H-reflex, which has been demonstrated in monkeys, rats, and humans, has furnished direct evidence of activity-dependent plasticity at specific sites in the spinal cord, and is giving insights into its mechanisms (Wolpaw et al., 1983; Wolpaw, 1987; Evatt et al., 1989; Wolf and Segal, 1996; Segal, 1997; Wolpaw and Tennissen, 2001).

In the standard protocol, used in monkeys, rats, and humans, SSR or H-reflex size is measured as electromyographic (EMG) activity, and reward occurs when the size is above (for up-conditioning) or below (for down-conditioning) a criterion value. The fundamental observation is that, after imposition of the reward criterion, reflex size changes appropriately over days and weeks (Fig. 7.3(a)). This adaptive change appears to occur in two phases: a small rapid phase-1 change in the first few hours or days (thought to reflect rapid mode-appropriate change in descending influence over the spinal arc of the reflex) and a much slower phase-2 change that continues to grow for weeks (and probably reflects gradual spinal cord plasticity produced by the chronic continuation of the descending input responsible for phase 1) (Wolpaw and O'Keefe, 1984). This descending input is conveyed by the corticospinal tract; other major descending pathways are not required (Chen and Wolpaw, 1997; 2002).

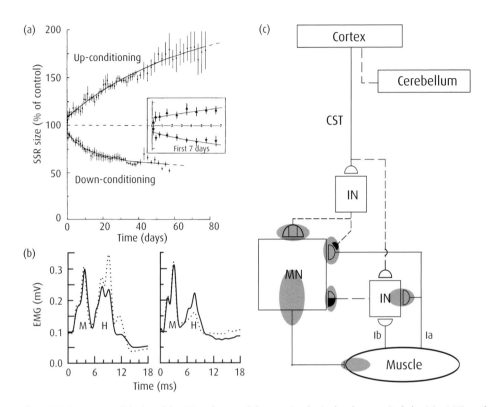

Figure 7.3. Operant conditioning of the SSR pathway and the associated spinal and supraspinal plasticity. (a) Two-phase courses of SSR up- or down-conditioning in monkeys. Rapid phase-1 change, reflecting appropriate change in descending corticospinal influence over the spinal reflex arc, occurs within 6 h (inset). Gradual phase-2 change, reflecting spinal cord plasticity produced by the continuation of the altered descending input, develops over at least 40 days (modified from Wolpaw and O'Keefe (1984)). (b) Average poststimulus EMG for representative days from two rats before (solid lines) or near the end of (dashed lines) a 50-day exposure to up- (rat on left) or down-conditioning (rat on right) of the H-reflex, the electrical analog of the SSR. The H-reflex is much larger after up-conditioning and much smaller after down-conditioning, while background EMG (indicated here by EMG at zero time) and M responses (direct muscle responses) are unchanged (modified from Wolpaw (1997)). (c) Sites (shaded ovals) of plasticity associated with operant conditioning of the SSR or its electrical analog, the H-reflex. "MN" is the motoneuron, "CST" is the main corticospinal tract, and each "IN" is one or more spinal interneuron types. Open synaptic terminals are excitatory, solid ones are inhibitory, half-open ones could be either, and the subdivided one is a cluster of C terminals. Dashed pathways imply the possibility of intervening spinal interneurons. The monosynaptic and probably oligosynaptic SSR/H-reflex pathway from Ia and Ib afferents to the motoneuron is shown. Definite or highly probable sites of plasticity include: the motoneuron membrane (i.e., firing threshold and axonal conduction velocity), motor unit properties, C terminals on the motoneuron, the Ia afferent synaptic connection, and terminals conveying disynaptic group I inhibition or excitation to the motoneuron. The essential roles of the corticospinal tract (originating in sensorimotor cortex) and of cerebellar output to cortex are indicated (updated from Wolpaw (1997)).

Training is possible in humans or rats with partial spinal cord injuries, but does not occur in people with strokes involving sensorimotor cortex or in rats in which sensorimotor cortex has been ablated (Segal and Wolf, 1994; Segal, 1997; Chen et al., 2002).

This spinal cord plasticity includes changes in motoneuron properties (Carp and Wolpaw, 1994; Halter et al., 1995; Carp et al., 2001). Down-training is accompanied by a positive shift in motoneuron firing threshold and a reduction in axonal conduction velocity. Both changes suggest a positive shift in sodium channel activation voltage, and the change in threshold could account in large part for the smaller reflex. While activity-dependent synaptic plasticity has received the most attention up to the present, the occurrence and importance of plasticity in neuronal properties (e.g., in neuronal voltage-gated ion channels) is now drawing interest (Spitzer, 1999; Cantrell and Catterall, 2001). This shift in motoneuron firing threshold provides an example of such plasticity, and illustrates its behavioral significance. Additional physiological and anatomical studies suggest that SSR or H-reflex training also affects the Ia afferent-motoneuron synapse, other synaptic terminals on the motoneuron, and interneurons that convey oligosynaptic Group 1 input to the motoneuron (Carp and Wolpaw, 1995; Feng-Chen and Wolpaw, 1996). Figure 7.3(c) summarizes the current understanding of this multi-site plasticity. Furthermore, acquisition and maintenance of H-reflex change appear to reflect the continuing interaction of spinal and supraspinal plasticity (reviewed in Wolpaw and Tennissen, 2001).

7.4 Principles underlying activity-dependent plasticity

The evidence that activity-dependent plasticity can occur at multiple sites in the spinal cord and is associated with supraspinal plasticity, and that multi-site plasticity occurs with acquisition of even the simplest skill, is consistent with the growing evidence that activity-dependent plasticity is ubiquitous in the CNS and is a characteristic feature of even the simplest learning both in invertebrates and vertebrates (Carrier et al., 1997; Cohen et al., 1997; Lieb and Frost, 1997; Thompson et al., 1997; Whelan and Pearson, 1997; Wolpaw and Lee, 1989; Lisberger, 1998; Garcia et al., 1999; Hansel et al., 2001; King et al., 2001; Wolpaw and Tennissen, 2001; van Alphen and De Zeeuw, 2002; Medina et al., 2002). Consideration of the main function of the CNS (i.e., to produce appropriate behaviors) and of the ubiquity of activity-dependent plasticity in the CNS) suggests

that such multi-site plasticity is both necessary and inevitable, particularly in the spinal cord.

Together with its homologous brainstem nuclei, the spinal cord is the final assembly point for all neuromuscular behaviors, both simple and complex. It is, in Sherrington's phrase, "the final common path" (Clarke and O'Malley, 1996), creating and conveying the end product of activity elsewhere in the CNS. Thus, the motoneurons, interneurons, and synapses of the lumbosacral spinal cord execute all the various forms of locomotion and postural maintenance, withdraw the legs from painful stimuli, participate properly in actions involving all four limbs, support bladder and bowel function, produce many different specialized movements and complex performances, and so forth. That the normal spinal cord is able to support these many behaviors satisfactorily, as well as to incorporate new behaviors throughout life, implies that its neuronal and synaptic function is continually adjusted and readjusted to serve the current behavioral repertoire. That such adjustments occur in the short term as the CNS shifts from one behavior to another, or cycles through the different phases of a single behavior is known from studies like those showing the differences in presynaptic inhibition among standing, walking, and running, and the changes that occur in responses to group I afferent input over the step cycle (Capaday and Stein, 1987; Stein, 1995; Faist et al., 1996; Rossignol, 1996; Pearson and Ramirez, 1997; Zehr, 2002).

As the data summarized in the preceding sections show, adjustments occur in the long term as well as in the short term. Gradual activity-dependent plasticity, driven by descending and peripheral inputs, is presumably responsible for maintaining spinal cord circuitry in a functional state suitable to its current roster of behaviors. This long-term control, a consensus arising from the different patterns of activity associated with these different behaviors, appears to function as a coarse adjustment, defining ranges over which the fine adjustments specific to each behavior are made. Thus, for example, at any given time, the possible strength of primary afferent input to soleus motoneurons has a range that encompasses values appropriate to standing, walking, and running (Zehr, 2002).

In this setting, the neural activity that adds a new behavior to the repertoire (whether the activity is produced by daily practice and the behavior is an athletic skill or the activity results from a peripheral or central lesion and the behavior represents or compensates for a functional deficit) is likely to cause plasticity that accommodates the new behavior as well as plasticity that maintains the old behaviors. For example, the stronger motoneuron response to Ia afferent input that underlies a new behavior (e.g., up-conditioning in Fig. 7.3(a)) is likely to affect many other behaviors that involve such input to the motoneuron. As a result, these effects may trigger additional activity-dependent plasticity that restores the other behaviors. The as yet mysterious additional plasticity that maintains a normal contralateral H-reflex in the monkey that has undergone H-reflex down-conditioning (Wolpaw and Lee, 1989; Wolpaw et al., 1993) may be compensatory, serving to maintain normal contralateral function. Furthermore, as activity-dependent plasticity can occur at numerous sites in the spinal cord, the changes in activity caused by plasticity that supports a new behavior or maintains old behaviors are likely to trigger additional plasticity at other sites. For example, the smaller stretch reflexes found in the apparently normal arm contralateral to an arm paralyzed by a hemispheric stroke (Thilmann et al., 1990), may reflect reactive plasticity caused by change in activity in segmental pathways connecting the right and left sides of the spinal cord.

Such considerations imply that acquisition of any new behavior is likely to involve three categories of plasticity: primary plasticity responsible for the new behavior, compensatory plasticity that maintains previous behaviors despite the impact of the primary plasticity, and reactive plasticity caused by the changes in activity resulting from primary and compensatory plasticity. This etiological categorization helps explain the multi-site plasticity associated with even the simplest behavioral change by indicating that multi-site plasticity is both necessary (to maintain the full repertoire of behaviors) and

inevitable (due to the widespread capacity for activity-dependent plasticity). It also helps explain why some examples of plasticity (such as the contralateral spinal cord plasticity with H-reflex training (Wolpaw and Lee, 1989)) may bear no apparent relationship to the behavioral changes with which they are associated. Furthermore, recognition of these different etiological categories of plasticity can help define factors controlling the effectiveness of new therapeutic methods, and thus help guide research.

The normal activity-dependent spinal cord plasticity reviewed here – those occurring during development, during skill acquisition later in life, or induced in the laboratory – is largely created and directed by descending activity from the brain, sometimes with and sometimes without associated activity in peripheral afferent pathways. This supraspinal influence is likely to be accompanied by, and may often depend for its induction and maintenance on, supraspinal plasticity in cortex, cerebellum, and/or elsewhere. Furthermore, the behavioral effects associated with spinal cord plasticity appear to reflect the interaction of plasticity at both spinal and supraspinal sites (Carrier et al., 1997; Whelan and Pearson, 1997; Wolpaw and Tennissen, 2001).

7.5 Theoretical and practical significance of activity-dependent spinal cord plasticity

The substantial capacity for activity-dependent plasticity in the spinal cord has important theoretical and practical implications. It suggests that most motor skills that are acquired gradually through prolonged practice involve spinal cord plasticity. That this is the case is consistent on the one hand with the extensive evidence that activity does gradually change the spinal cord and on the other hand with the lengthy periods and intensive practice required for acquisition and maintenance of athletic skills and other motor skills such as playing a musical instrument. In sum, these skills probably cannot be understood or explained simply by studying the changes that occur in cortex, cerebellum, or other supraspinal areas. The changes in the spinal cord need to be defined as well. This reality has rarely received adequate, or even minimal recognition in studies focused on the role of cortical plasticity in modifying motor behaviors. That spinal cord plasticity can, and probably often does, contribute to normal as well as pathological behavioral changes certainly complicates explorations of the mechanisms of such changes. Nevertheless, without proper attention to spinal cord plasticity, attempts to understand how CNS plasticity accounts for behavioral change may often yield only incomplete or misleading insights.

Furthermore, the fact that gradually acquired motor skills depend on multi-site and multi-level (i.e., spinal and supraspinal) plasticity suggests that gradually acquired intellectual skills, such as language mastery or mathematical facility, may also depend on widely distributed plasticity. The rapid changes in behavior that have traditionally engaged most research attention, such as the one-trial acquisition of a new word, may merely reflect minor adjustments in patterns of plasticity gradually acquired through prolonged practice, adjustments analogous to the change in presynaptic inhibition that accompanies the transition from standing to running, or the alteration in descending influence responsible for phase-1 change in the SSR (Fig. 7.3(a)). Thus, adequate understanding of most skilled behaviors may require exploration of gradually acquired activity-dependent plasticity comparable to that found in the spinal cord. Indeed, such exploration might best begin with simple motor skills and with the spinal cord, for its relative simplicity and accessibility, and its connections to the brain by well-defined pathways facilitate location and study of activity-dependent plasticity and delineation of how multiple sites of plasticity, spinal and supraspinal, interact to produce behavioral changes.

In developing effective rehabilitation methods for chronic neuromuscular disorders such as spinal cord injury (see Volume II, Chapter 37) or cerebral palsy (see Volume II, Chapter 39), the spinal cord's capacities for activity-dependent plasticity are both a challenge and an opportunity. On the one hand, these capacities contribute to the disabilities that follow spinal cord injury and will certainly affect the outcomes of new therapeutic methods that promote regeneration. On the other hand, they offer the opportunity to guide restoration of neuronal and synaptic function, and should allow imperfect regeneration to support significant functional improvements. For both these reasons, the productive engagement of activity-dependent plasticity in the spinal cord is likely to be a key component of new therapeutic programs for spinal cord injury and other chronic neuromuscular disorders. Therapeutic induction and guidance of activity-dependent spinal cord plasticity will require training protocols that induce appropriate patterns of peripheral and descending inputs to the spinal cord. Development of such methods has just begun for locomotion (see Volume I, Chapter 13 and Volume II, Chapters 3 and 19); other equally important behaviors, such as urination, are yet to be addressed.

This work will be greatly affected by the complexity of the activity-dependent plasticity associated with even apparently simple training protocols (e.g., Fig. 7.3(c)), and will also be affected by what is perhaps the most distinctive feature of activity-dependent spinal cord plasticity as it functions in normal life and in the presence of disease: the slow rate of its effect on behavior. Despite the rapidity of activity-dependent processes, such as LTP that are known to occur in the spinal cord, the changes in behavior that result from activity-dependent spinal cord plasticity occur gradually, probably because each is the end product of multiple activity-dependent processes. Reflex changes during normal development and those associated with skills, such as ballet, develop over months and years; and those produced by H-reflex operant conditioning or other specialized training regimens occur over days and weeks. While reflexes, such as the H-reflex, can differ markedly across established behaviors (e.g., standing and running (Zehr, 2002)), or even between different phases of one behavior (e.g., stance and swing phases of locomotion (Faist et al., 1996)), the establishment of the reflex strengths associated with a particular behavior occurs slowly. This characteristic is probably fortunate – rapid large changes in the pathways underlying specific reflexes independent of the contexts of specific behaviors could wreak havoc with movement control and require prodigious supraspinal compensations. At the same time, the characteristically gradual effect of activity-dependent spinal cord plasticity on behavior implies that laboratory studies and clinical applications need to extend over sufficient time periods. Furthermore, the ubiquity of activity-dependent plasticity and the inevitable interaction between primary, compensatory, and reactive types, implies that functional effects may change over time. Early gains will not always evolve into long-term improvements, while deleterious early effects may give way to long-term benefits.

7.6 Summary

During normal life, activity-dependent plasticity occurs in the spinal cord as well as in brain. Like plasticity elsewhere in the CNS, this spinal cord plasticity can occur at many different neuronal and synaptic sites, and through a variety of mechanisms. Spinal cord plasticity is prominent during development and contributes to acquisition of basic behaviors, such as locomotion and rapid withdrawal from painful stimuli. Later in life, spinal cord plasticity contributes to acquisition and maintenance of specialized motor skills, and to compensation for peripheral and central changes associated with aging. Acquisition of even the simplest behaviors is associated with a complex pattern of spinal and supraspinal plasticity. This complexity is both necessary, to preserve the entire roster of behaviors, and inevitable, due to the ubiquity of activity-dependent plasticity in the CNS. Exploration of spinal cord plasticity is essential for adequate understanding of motor skills; and, due to the relative simplicity and accessibility of the spinal cord, may be a convenient starting point for describing skill development. Appropriate induction and guidance of activity-dependent spinal cord plasticity is also likely to be a key component of the development of new rehabilitation methods for chronic motor disorders, such as spinal cord injury and cerebral palsy.

ACKNOWLEDGMENTS

Drs. Jonathan S. Carp and Elizabeth Winter Wolpaw provided valuable comments on the manuscript. Work in the author's laboratory has been supported by NIH (NS22189 and HD36020), the International Spinal Research Trust, and the Christopher Reeve Paralysis Foundation.

REFERENCES

Angulo-Kinzler, R.M., Mynark, R.G. and Koceja, D.M. (1998). Soleus H-reflex gain in elderly and young adults: modulation due to body position. *J Gerontol A: Biol Sci Med Sci*, **53**(2), M120–M125.

Augé II, W.K. and Morrison, D.S. (2000). Assessment of the infraspinatus spinal stretch reflex in the normal, athletic, and multidirectionally unstable shoulder. *Am J Sport Med*, **28**(2), 206–213.

Baldissera, F., Hultborn, H. and Illert, M. (1981). Integration in spinal neuronal systems. In: *Handbook of Physiology, Section I: The Nervous System, Vol. 2, Motor Control, Part I* (ed. Brooks, V.B.), Williams and Wilkins Company, Baltimore, Maryland, pp. 509–595.

Barbeau, H. and Rossignol, S. (1987). Recovery of locomotion after chronic spinalization in the adult cat. *Brain Res*, **412**, 84–95.

Barbeau, H., Ladouceur, M., Mirbagheri, M.M. and Kearney, R.E. (2002). The effect of locomotor training combined with functional electrical stimulation in chronic spinal cord injured subjects: walking and reflex studies. *Brain Res Rev*, **40**, 274–291.

Boorman, G., Hulliger, M., Lee, R.G., Tako, K. and Tanaka, R. (1991). Reciprocal Ia inhibition in patients with spinal spasticity. *Neurosci Lett*, **127**, 57–60.

Brown, W.F. (1984). *The Physiological and Technical Basis of Electromyography*. Butterworths, Boston, MA.

Burke, R.E. (1998). Spinal cord: ventral horn. In: *The Synaptic Organization of the Brain* (ed. Shepherd G.M.), Vol. 3. Oxford University Press, New York, pp. 77–120.

Bussel, B., Roby-Brami, A., Azouvi, P., Biraben, A., Yakovleff, A. and Held, J.P. (1988). Myoclonus in a patient with spinal cord transection: possible involvement of the spinal stepping generator. *Brain*, **111**, 1235–1245.

Calancie, B., Needham-Shropshire, B., Jacobs, P., Willer, K., Zych, G. and Green, B.A. (1994). Involuntary stepping after chronic spinal cord injury: evidence for a central rhythm generator for locomotion in man. *Brain*, **117**, 1143–1159.

Cantrell, A.R. and Catterall, W.A. (2001). Neuromodulation of Na⁺ channels: an unexpected form of cellular plasticity. *Nat Rev Neurosci*, **2**(6), 397–407.

Capaday, C. and Stein, R.B. (1987). A method for stimulating the reflex output of a motoneuron pool. *J Neurosci Meth*, **21**, 91–104.

Carp, J.S. and Wolpaw, J.R. (1994). Motoneuron plasticity underlying operantly conditioned decrease in primate H-reflex. *J Neurophysiol*, **72**, 431–442.

Carp, J.S. and Wolpaw, J.R. (1995). Motoneuron properties after operantly conditioned increase in primate H-reflex. *J Neurophysiol*, **73**, 1365–1373.

Carp, J.S., Chen, X.Y., Sheikh, H. and Wolpaw, J.R. (2001). Operant conditioning of rat H-reflexes affects motoneuronal axonal conduction velocity. *Experimental Brain Res*, **136**, 69–73.

Carrier, L., Brustein, E. and Rossignol, S. (1997). Locomotion of the hindlimbs after neurectomy of ankle flexors in intact and spinal cats: model for the study of locomotor plasticity. *J Neurophysiol*, **77**, 1979–1993.

Casabona, A., Polizzi, M.C. and Perciavalle, V. (1990). Differences in H-reflex between athletes trained for explosive contraction and non-trained subjects. *Eur J Appl Physiol*, **61**(1–2), 26–32.

Chamberlain, T., Halick, P. and Gerard, R.W. (1963). Fixation of experience in the rat spinal cord. *J Neurophysiol*, **22**, 662–673.

Chen, L., Wolpaw, J.R., Smith, B. and Chen, X.Y. (2002). Sensorimotor cortex ablation prevents H-reflex down conditioning. Program No. 66.15 2002 Abstract Viewer/Itinerary Planner, Society for Neuroscience, Washington, DC, CD-ROM.

Chen, X.Y. and Wolpaw, J.R. (1997). Dorsal column but not lateral column transection prevents down conditioning of H-reflex in rats. *J Neurophysiol*, **78**(3), 1730–1734.

Chen, X.Y. and Wolpaw, J.R. (2002). Probable corticospinal tract control of spinal cord plasticity in rats. *J Neurophysiol*, **87**, 645–652.

Chen, X.Y. and Wolpaw, J.R. (2005). Ablation of cerebellar nuclei prevents H-reflex down-conditioning in rats. *Learn Mem*, **12**, 248–254.

Clarke, E. and O'Malley, C.D. (1996). *The Human Brain and Spinal Cord*, Norman Publishing, San Francisco.

Cohen, T.E., Kaplan, S.W., Kandel, E.R. and Hawkins, R.D. (1997). A simplified preparation for relating cellular events to behavior: mechanisms contributing to habituation, dishabituation, and sensitization of the *Aplysia* gill-withdrawal reflex. *J Neurosci*, **17**(8), 2886–2899.

Cope, T.C., Bodine, S.C, Fournier, M. and Edgerton, V.R. (1986). Soleus motor units in chronic spinal transected cats: physiological and morphological alterations. *J Neurophysiol*, **55**, 1202–1220.

de Groat, W.C. (2002). Plasticity of bladder reflex pathways during postnatal development. *Physiol Behav*, **77**, 689–692.

DeVries, H.A., Wiswell, R.A., Romero, G.T. and Heckathorne, E. (1985). Changes with age in monosynaptic reflexes elicited by mechanical and electrical stimulation. *Am J Phys Med Rehabil*, **64**, 71–81.

Dietz, V., Colombo, G., Jensen, L. and Baumgartner, L. (1995). Locomotor capacity of spinal cord in paraplegic patients. *Ann Neurol*, **37**, 574–586.

DiGiorgio, A.M. (1929). Persistenza nell'animale spinale, di asymmetrie posturali e motorie di origine cerebellare: I, II, III. *Arch Fisiol*, **27**, 518–580.

DiGiorgio, A.M. (1942). Azione del cervelletto-neocerebellum-sul tono posturale degli arti e localizzazioni cerebellari nell'-animale rombencefalico. *Arch Fisiol*, **42**, 25–79.

Dimitrijevic, M.R., Gerasimenko, Y. and Pinter, M.M. (1998). Evidence for a spinal central pattern generator in humans. *Ann NY Acad Sci*, **860**, 360–376.

Dobkin, B., Harkema, S., Requejo, P.S. and Edgerton, V.R. (1995). Modulation of locomotor-like EMG activity in subjects with complete and incomplete spinal cord injury. *J Neurol Rehabil*, **9**, 183–190.

Dupont-Versteegden, E.E., Houlé, J.D., Dennis, R.A., Zhang, J., Knox, B.S., Wagoner, G. and Peterson, C.A. (2004). Exercise-induced gene expression in soleus muscle is dependent on time after spinal cord injury in rats. *Muscle Nerve*, **29**, 73–81.

Evatt, M.L., Wolf, S.L. and Segal, R.L. (1989). Modification of human spinal stretch reflexes: preliminary studies. *Neurosci Lett*, **105**, 350–355.

Eyre, J.A. (2003). Development and plasticity of the corticospinal system in man. *Neural Plasticity*, **10**(1–2), 93–106.

Eyre, J.A., Miller, S., Clowry, G.J., Conway, E.A. and Watts, C. (2000). Functional corticospinal projections are established prenatally in the human foetus permitting involvement in the development of spinal motor centres. *Brain*, **123**, 51–64.

Eyre, J.A., Taylor, J.P., Villagra, F., Smith, M. and Miller, S. (2001). Evidence of activity-dependent withdrawal of corticospinal projections during human development. *Neurology*, **57**, 1543–1554.

Faist, M., Dietz, V. and Pierrot-Deseilligny, E. (1996). Modulation, probably presynaptic in origin, of monosynaptic Ia excitation during human gait. *Exp Brain Res*, **109**, 441–449.

Feng-Chen, K.C. and Wolpaw, J.R. (1996). Operant conditioning of H-reflex changes synaptic terminals on primate motoneurons. *Proc Natl Acad Sci USA*, **93**, 9206–9211.

Garcia, K.S., Steele, P.M. and Mauk, M.D. (1999). Cerebellar cortex lesions prevent acquisition of conditioned eyelid responses. *J Neurosci*, **19**(**24**), 10940–10947.

Gerard, R.W. (1961). The fixation of experience. In: *Brain Mechanisms and Learning* (eds Gerard, R.W. and Konorski, J.), Blackwell, Oxford, pp. 21–32.

Gibson, C.L., Arnott, G.A. and Clowry, G.J. (2000). Plasticity in the rat spinal cord seen in response to lesions to the motor cortex during development but not to lesions in maturity. *Exp Neurobiol*, **166**, 422–434.

Giulio, L. (1952). Sulla funzione del midollo spinale. Persistenza di asimmetrie da eccitamento labirintico. *Bollet Soc Ital Biol Sper*, **28**, 1651–1652.

Gomez-Pinilla, F., Ying, Z., Roy, R.R., Molteni, R. and Edgerton, V.R. (2002). Voluntary exercise induces a BDNF-mediated mechanism that promotes neuroplasticity. *J Neurophysiol*, **88**, 2187–2195.

Goode, D.J. and Van Hoven, J. (1982). Loss of patellar and achilles tendon reflex in classical ballet dancers. *Arch Neurol*, **39**, 323.

Halter, J.A., Carp, J.S. and Wolpaw, J.R. (1995). Operantly conditioned motoneuron plasticity: possible role of sodium channels. *J Neurophysiol*, **74**, 867–871.

Hansel, C., Linden, D.J. and D'Angelo, E. (2001). Beyond parallel fiber LTD: the diversity of synaptic and non-synaptic plasticity in the cerebellum. *Nat Neurosci*, **4**, 467–475.

Henneman, E. and Mendell, L.M. (1981). Functional organization of motoneuron pool and inputs. In: *Handbook of Physiology, Section I: The Nervous System, Vol. 2, Motor Control, Part I* (ed. Brooks, V.B.), Williams & Wilkins, Baltimore, Maryland, pp. 423–507.

Herrero, J.F., Laird, J.M. and Lopez-Garcia, J.A. (2000). Wind-up of spinal cord neurones and pain sensation: much ado about something? *Prog Neurobiol*, **61**, 169–203.

Hiersemenzel, L.P., Curt, A. and Dietz, V. (2000). From spinal shock to spasticity: neuronal adaptations to a spinal cord injury. *Neurology*, **54**(**8**), 1574–1582.

Hochman, S. and McCrea, D.A. (1994a). Effects of chronic spinalization on ankle extensor motoneurons. II. Motoneuron electrical properties. *J Neurophysiol*, **71**(**4**), 1468–1479.

Hochman, S. and McCrea, D.A. (1994b). Effects of chronic spinalization on ankle extensor motoneurons I. Composite monosynaptic Ia EPSPs in four motoneuron pools. *J Neurophysiol*, **71**(**4**), 1452–1467.

Hochman, S. and McCrea, D.A. (1994c). Effects of chronic spinalization on ankle extensor motoneurons. III. Composite Ia EPSPs in motoneurons separated into motor unit types. *J Neurophysiol*, **71**(**4**), 1480–1490.

Holmes, G. (1915). Spinal injuries of warfare. *Br Med J*, **2**, 815–821.

Inglis, F.M., Zuckerman, K.E. and Kalb, R.G. (2000). Experience-dependent development of spinal motor neurons. *Neuron*, **26**, 299–305.

Ji, R., Kohno, T., Moore, K.A. and Woolf, C.J. (2003). Central sensitization and LTP: do pain and memory share similar mechanisms? *Trends Neurosci*, **26**(**12**), 696–705.

Kandel, E.R. (1977). Neuronal plasticity and the modification of behavior. In: *Handbook of Physiology, Section I: The Nervous System, Vol. 1, Cellular Biology of Neurons* (eds Brookhart, J.M. and Mountcastle, V.B.), Williams & Wilkins, Bethesda, Maryland, pp. 1137–1382.

Kandel, E.R., Schwartz, J.H. and Jessell, T.M. (2000). *Principles of Neural Science*, McGraw-Hill, New York.

Kiehn, O., Harris-Warrick, R.M., Jordan, L.M., Hultborn, H. and Kudo, N. (eds) (1998). *Neuronal Mechanisms for Generating Locomotor Activity*, New York Academy of Sciences, New York.

King, D.A.T, Krupa, D.J., Foy, M.R. and Thompson, R.F. (2001). Mechanisms of neuronal conditioning. *Int Rev Neurobiol*, **45**, 313–337.

Koceja, D.M. and Mynark, R.G. (2000). Comparison of heteronymous monosynaptic Ia facilitation in young and elderly subjects in supine and standing positions. *Int J Neurosci*, **103**, 1–17.

Koceja, D.M., Burke, J.R. and Kamen, G. (1991). Organization of segmental reflexes in trained dancers. *Int J Sports Med*, **12**(**3**), 285–289.

Koceja, D.M., Markus, C.A. and Trimble, M.H. (1995). Postural modulation of the soleus H reflex in young and old subjects. *Electroenceph Clin Neurophysiol*, **97**, 387–393.

Kuhn, R.A. (1950). Functional capacity of the isolated human spinal cord. *Brain*, **1**, 1–51.

Levinsson, A., Luo, X.L., Holmberg, H. and Schouenborg, J. (1999). Developmental tuning in a spinal nociceptive system: effects of neonatal spinalization. *J Neurosci*, **19**(**23**), 10397–10403.

Lieb, J.R. and Frost, W.N. (1997). Realistic simulation of the *Aplysia* siphon-withdrawal reflex circuit: roles of circuit elements in producing motor output. *J Neurophysiol*, **77**(**3**), 1249–1268.

Lisberger, S.G. (1998). Physiologic basis for motor learning in the vestibulo-ocular reflex. *Otolaryngol Head Neck Surg*, **119**(**1**), 43–48.

Liu, X. and Sandkühler, J. (1997). Characterization of long-term potentiation of C-fiber-evoked potentials in spinal dorsal horn of adult rat: essential role of NK1 and NK2 receptors. *J Neurophysiol*, **78**(**4**), 1973–1982.

Lloyd, D.P.C. (1949). Post-tetanic potentiation of response in monosynaptic reflex pathways of the spinal cord. *J Gen Physiol*, **33**, 147–170.

Lovely, R.G., Gregor, R.J., Roy, R.R. and Edgerton, V.R. (1986). Effects of training on the recovery of full-weight-bearing stepping in the adult spinal cat. *Exp Neurol*, **92**, 421–435.

Magladery, J.W., Porter, W.E., Park, A.M. and Teasdall, R.D. (1951). Electrophysiological studies of nerve and reflex activity in normal man. IV. The two-neuron reflex and identification of certain action potentials from spinal roots and cord. *Bull Johns Hopkins Hosp*, **88**, 499–519.

Manni, E. (1950). Localizzazoni cerebellari corticali nella cavia, Nota 1: II Corpus cerebelli. *Arch Fisiol*, **49**, 213–237.

Martin, J.H., Choy, M., Pullman, S. and Meng, Z. (2004). Corticospinal system development depends on motor experience. *J Neurosci*, **24**(9), 2122–2132.

Matthews, P.B.C. (1972). *Mammalian Muscle Receptors and Their Central Actions*, Williams & Wilkins, Baltimore, Maryland.

Medina, J.F., Repa, J.C., Mauk, M.D. and LeDoux, J.E. (2002). Parallels between cerebellum- and amygdala-dependent conditioning. *Nat Rev Neurosci*, **3**, 122–131.

Melzack, R., Coderre, T.J., Katz, J. and Vaccarino, A.L. (2004). Central neuroplasticity and pathological pain. *Ann NY Acad Sci*, **933**, 157–174.

Mendell, L.M. (1984). Modifiability of spinal synapses. *Physiol Rev*, **64**, 260–324.

Mendell, L.M., Munson, J.B. and Arvanian, V.L. (2001). Neurotrophins and synaptic plasticity in the mammalian spinal cord. *J Physiol*, **533**(1), 91–97.

Meyer-Lohmann, J., Christakos, C.N. and Wolf, H. (1986). Dominance of the short-latency component in perturbation induced electromyographic responses of long-trained monkeys. *Exp Brain Res*, **64**, 393–399.

Misiaszek, J.E. (2003). The H-reflex as a tool in neurophysiology: its limitations and uses in understanding nervous system function. *Muscle Nerve*, **28**, 144–160.

Morita, H., Shindo, M., Yanagawa, S., Yoshida, T., Momoi, H. and Yanagisawa, N. (1995). Progressive decrease in heteronymous monosynaptic Ia facilitation with human ageing. *Exp Brain Res*, **104**, 167–170.

Mountcastle, V.B. (ed.) (1980). Effects of spinal cord transection. In: *Medical Physiology*, Vol. 1, Mosby, St. Louis, pp. 781–786.

Muir, G.D. and Steeves, J.D. (1997). Sensorimotor stimulation to improve locomotor recovery after spinal cord injury. *Trend Neurosci*, **20**(2), 72–77.

Munson, J.B., Foehring, R.C., Lofton, S.A., Zengel, J.E. and Sypert, G.W. (1986). Plasticity of medial gastrocnemius motor units following cordotomy in the cat. *J Neurophysiol*, **55**, 619–634.

Myklebust, B.M., Gottlieb, G.L., Penn, R.L. and Agarwal, G.C. (1982). Reciprocal excitation of antagonistic muscles as a differentiating feature in spasticity. *Ann Neurol*, **12**, 367–374.

Myklebust, B.M., Gottlieb, G.L. and Agarwal, G.C. (1986). Stretch reflexes of the normal human infant. *Dev Med Child Neurol*, **28**, 440–449.

Nelson, S.G. and Mendell, L.M. (1979). Enhancement in Iamotoneuron synaptic transmission caudal to chronic spinal cord transection. *J Neurophysiol*, **42**, 642–654.

Nielsen, J., Crone, C. and Hultborn, H. (1993). H-reflexes are smaller in dancers from the Royal Danish Ballet than in well-trained athletes. *Eur J Appl Physiol*, **66**, 116–121.

O'Sullivan, M.C., Eyre, J.A., Miller, S. (1991). Radiation of phasic stretch reflex in biceps brachii to muscles of the arm in man and its restriction during development. *J Physiol*, **439**, 529–543.

O'Sullivan, M.C., Miller, S., Ramesh, V., Conway, E., Gilfillan, K., McDonough, S. and Eyre, J.A. (1998). Abnormal development of biceps brachii phasic stretch reflex and persistence of short latency heteronymous reflexes from biceps to triceps brachii in spastic cerebral palsy. *Brain*, **121**, 2381–2395.

Orlovsky, G.N., Deliagina, T.G. and Grillner, S. (1999). *Neuronal Control of Locomotion from Mollusc to Man*, Oxford University Press, New York.

Patterson, M.M. (1976). Mechanisms of classical conditioning and fixation in spinal mammals. *Adv Psychobiol*, **3**, 381–436.

Pearson, K.G. and Ramirez, J.M. (1997). Sensory modulation of pattern-generating circuits. In: *Neurons, Networks and Motor Behavior* (eds Stein, P.S.G., et al.), MIT Press, Cambridge, MA, pp. 225–235.

Pérot, C., Goubel, F. and Mora, I. (1991). Quantification of T- and H-responses before and after a period of endurance training. *Eur J Appl Physiol*, **63**, 368–375.

Riddoch, G. (1917). The reflex functions of the completely divided spinal cord in man, compared with those associated with less severe lesions. *Brain*, **40**, 264–402.

Rochcongar, P., Dassonville, J. and Le Bars, R. (1979). Modifications du reflexe de Hoffmann en fonktion de l'entraînement chez le sportif. *Eur J Appl Physiol*, **40**, 165–170.

Ronthal, M. (1998). Spinal cord injury. In: *Clinical Neurology* (eds Joynt, R.J. and Griggs, R.C.), Vol. 47, Lippincott Williams & Wilkins, Hagerstown, Maryland, pp. 1–28.

Rossignol, S. (1996). Neural control of stereotypic limb movements. In: *Handbook of Physiology* (eds Rowell, L.B. and Sheperd, J.T.), Oxford University Press, New York, pp. 173–216.

Rossignol, S. (2000). Locomotion and its recovery after spinal injury. *Curr Opin Neurol*, **10**, 708–716.

Rossignol, S., Bouyer, L., Barthélemy, D., Langlet, C. and Leblond, H. (2002). Recovery of locomotion in the cat following spinal cord lesions. *Brain Res Rev*, **40**, 257–266.

Sabbahi, M.A. and Sedgwick, E.M. (1982). Age-related changes in monosynaptic reflex excitability. *J Gerontol*, **37**(1), 24–32.

Schneider, C. and Capaday, C. (2003). Progressive adaptation of the soleus H-reflex with daily training at walking backward. *J Neurophysiol*, **89**, 648–656.

Segal, R.L. (1997). Plasticity in the central nervous system: operant conditioning of the spinal stretch reflex. *Top Stroke Rehabil*, **3**(4), 76–87.

Segal, R.L. and Wolf, S.L. (1994). Operant conditioning of spinal stretch reflex in patients with spinal cord injuries. *Exp Neurol*, **130**, 202–213.

Shefner, J.M., Berman, S.A., Sarkarati, M. and Young, R.R. (1992). Recurrent inhibition is increased in patients with spinal cord injury. *Neurology*, **42**, 2162–2168.

Shurrager, P.S. and Dykman, R.A. (1951). Walking spinal carnivores. *J Comp Physiol Psychol*, **44**, 252–262.

Spitzer, N.C. (1999). New dimensions of neuronal plasticity. *Nat Neurosci*, **2**(6), 489–491.

Stein, R.B. (1995). Presynaptic inhibition in humans. *Prog Neurobiol*, **47**, 533–544.

Straka, H. and Dieringer, N. (1995). Spinal plasticity after hemilabyrinthectomy and its relation to postural recovery in the frog. *J Neurophysiol*, **73**, 1617–1631.

Tai, Q. and Goshgarian, H.G. (1996). Ultrastructural quantitative analysis of glutamatergic and GABAergic synaptic terminals in the phrenic nucleus after spinal cord injury. *J Comp Neurol*, **372**(3), 343–355.

Tai, Q., Palazzolo, K.L. and Goshgarian, H.G. (1997). Synaptic plasticity of 5-hydroxytrypamine-immunoreactive terminals in the phrenic nucleus following spinal cord injury: a quantitative electron microscopic analysis. *J Comp Neurol*, **386**(4), 613–624.

Thilmann, A., Fellows, S. and Garms E. (1990). Pathological stretch reflexes on the "good" side of hemiparetic patients. *J Neurol, Neurosurg Psychiat*, **53**(3), 208–214.

Thompson, R.F. (2001). Spinal plasticity. In: *Spinal Cord Plasticity: Alterations in Reflex Function* (eds Patterson, M.M. and Grau, J.W.), Kluwer Academic, Boston, MA.

Thompson, F.J., Reier, P.J., Lucas, C.C. and Parmer, R. (1992). Altered patterns of reflex excitability subsequent to contusion injury of the rat spinal cord. *J Neurophysiol*, **68**, 1473–1486.

Thompson, R.F., Bao, S., Chen, L., Cipriano, B.D., Grethe, J.S., Kim, J.J., Thompson, J.K., Tracy, J.A., Weninger, M.S. and Krupa, D.J. (1997). Associative learning. *Int Rev Neurobiol*, **41**, 151–189.

Tillakaratne, N.J.K., de Leon, R.D., Hoang, T.X., Roy, R.R., Edgerton, V.R. and Tobin, A.J. (2002). Use-dependent

modulation of inhibitory capacity in the feline lumbar spinal cord. *J Neurosci*, **22**(8), 3130–3143.

van Alphen, A.M. and De Zeeuw, C.I. (2002). Cerebellar LTD facilitates but is not essential for long-term adaptation of the vestibulo-ocular reflex. *Eur J Neurosci*, **16**, 486–490.

Voigt, M., Chelli, F. and Frigo, C. (1998). Changes in the excitability of soleus muscle short latency stretch reflexes during human hopping after 4 weeks of hopping training. *Eur J Appl Physiol*, **78**, 522–532.

Waldenström, A., Thelin, J., Thimansson, E., Levinsson, A. and Schouenborg, J. (2003). Developmental learning in a pain-related system: evidence for a cross-modality mechanism. *J Neurosci*, **23**(20), 7719–7725.

Whelan, P.J. and Pearson, K.G. (1997). Plasticity in reflex pathways controlling stepping in the cat. *J Neurophysiol*, **78**(3), 1643–1650.

Wolf, S.L. and Segal, R.L. (1996). Reducing human biceps brachii spinal stretch reflex magnitude. *J Neurophysiol*, **75**(4), 1637–1646.

Wolpaw, J.R. (1987). Operant conditioning of primate spinal reflexes: the H-reflex. *J Neurophysiol*, **57**, 443–459.

Wolpaw, J.R. (1997). The complex structure of a simple memory. *Trends Neurosci*, **20**, 588–594.

Wolpaw, J.R. and Lee, C.L. (1989). Memory traces in primate spinal cord produced by operant conditioning of H-reflex. *J Neurophysiol*, **61**, 563–572.

Wolpaw, J.R. and O'Keefe, J.A. (1984). Adaptive plasticity in the primate spinal stretch reflex: evidence for a two-phase process. *J Neurosci*, **4**, 2718–2724.

Wolpaw, J.R. and Tennissen, A.M. (2001). Activity-dependent spinal cord plasticity in health and disease. *Annu Rev Neurosci*, **24**, 807–843.

Wolpaw, J.R., Braitman D.J. and Seegal R.F. (1983). Adaptive plasticity in the primate spinal stretch reflex: initial development. *J Neurophysiol*, **50**, 1296–1311.

Wolpaw, J.R., Herchenroder, P.A. and Carp, J.S. (1993). Operant conditioning of the primate H-reflex: factors affecting the magnitude of change. *Exp Brain Res*, **97**, 31–39.

Yamanaka, K., Yamamoto, S., Nakazawa, K., Yano, H., Suzuki, Y. and Fukunaga, T. (1999). The effects of long-term bed rest on H-reflex and motor evoked potential in the human soleus muscle during standing. *Neurosci Lett*, **266**, 101–104.

Zehr, E.P. (2002). Considerations for use of the Hoffman reflex in exercise studies. *Eur J Appl Physiol*, **86**, 455–468.

Zheng, Z., Gibson, S.J., Khalil, Z., Helme, R. and McMeeken, J.M. (2000). Age-related differences in the time course of capsaicin-induced hyperalgesia. *Pain*, **85**, 51–58.

Zimmermann, M. (2001). Pathobiology of neuropathic pain. *Eur J Pharmacol*, **429**, 23–37.

Plasticity of cerebral motor functions: implications for repair and rehabilitation

Catherine L. Ojakangas and John P. Donoghue

Department of Neuroscience, Brown University, RI, USA

8.1 Introduction

Neurobiologists have only recently been discovering the extent to which injured, adult nervous systems can undergo remarkable functional and structural rearrangement, commonly termed neural plasticity. Neuronal processes, including axons, dendrites, and the synaptic contacts between them are capable of reorganization (see Volume I, Chapter 1) and evidence of neurogenesis has been uncovered in adult primate brains (see Volume I, Chapter 18). Observations of neural plasticity spanning sensory, motor, and association systems at all levels of the neuroaxis have lead to the conclusion that neural plasticity is a general phenomenon of the nervous system including the adult central nervous system (CNS). Forms of plasticity have been suggested as mechanisms for recovery of function, as well as for learning and memory, as described in Chapters 2–5 of this volume. Understanding the form and mechanisms of neural plasticity induced by injury or during learning may lead to the development of better means of neurological rehabilitation through physical, therapeutic and pharmacological manipulations, or neuroprostheses development.

This chapter will focus on the plasticity now known to be possible in the motor regions of the brain. Motor behavior is particularly well suited for studies in plasticity. The overtness of movement lends itself well to documentation of learning, and the sensorimotor cortex has received considerable attention by basic scientists and clinicians alike because of its frequent damage by disease and its relative ease of access for experiment investigation in comparison to deeper lying structures. We will conclude the chapter with an overview of the development in a new field of rehabilitation, neural prostheses, also called "brain–machine interfaces (BMIs)." The functioning of neural prostheses shows the ultimate ability of the brain to adapt in a plastic manner. Neurons must change their biologically given function to fit the requirements of the computer-controlled output device.

Functional organization of the motor cortex

Over 100 years ago early German neuroscientists, Gustav Fritsch and Edouard Hitzig, first came to the notion that a "motor cortex" existed, based on stimulation experiments on dogs with minute amounts of current. These two observed that contralateral motor activity could be disrupted with lesions while preserving sensation, and they were the first to propose that discrete areas of the cortex might control small groups of muscles (Fritsch and Hitzig, 1870). Hughlings Jackson (1835–1911) and David Ferrier (1843–1928) continued and expanded the knowledge of somatotopy in the motor cortex of epileptic patients and monkeys, respectively (Jackson, 1863; Ferrier, 1873/1874). Finally, Victor Horsley (1857–1916) elucidated pre-central gyrus as being purely motor and the post-central gyrus sensory (Beevor and Horsley, 1887; 1890; 1894). Subsequently, pioneer neuroscientists discovered that the relationship between muscles and the area of primary motor cortex (M1) that connects to those muscles is not fixed, but flexible (Graham Brown and Sherrington, 1912; Leyton and Sherrington, 1917; Lashley, 1923). The M1 contains a topography of movement representations which can be differentiated by brief (50 ms) electrical stimulation. Focal stimulation of distant regions of the motor cortex surface or deep in layer V near cortical spinal neurons reveals an organization in which contralateral face, arm and leg movements can be elicited from distinct regions, although the internal organization of each of these areas may be complex. The overall somatotopy has been described as "the little man in the brain," the "homunculus" (Penfield and Boldrey, 1937). Penfield described both a motor and a somatosensory homunculus. An homunculus lays on each hemisphere, the foot and leg regions most medial (toes touching deep in the longitudinal cerebral fissure), and the arm and hand and face regions progressively more lateral. Regions of the body with more innervation and dexterity (e.g., the hand for the precentral gyrus) or more innervation and sensation (e.g., the tongue for post-central gyrus) are allotted more space in the cortex. While the homunculus has been described primarily in the primary sensorimotor cortex, M1, somatotopy is a prevailing characteristic across many brain regions. The somatotopic organization can be changed by injury, both peripheral and central, electrical stimulation, pharmacological experience, and learning or experience. Reorganization of M1 output maps occurs with shifting of borders between areas that represent different body parts.

The organizational plans for cortical areas controlling higher-order processing are less clear than for the primary cortical sensory-motor fields. The topographic organization of sensory and motor areas has frequently been exploited to investigate the potential for plasticity in other systems, since distortions of these maps are more readily recognized than in non-primary areas. Although it has become apparent that output maps in M1 can be reorganized, how and under what circumstances are not yet fully understood. This chapter will explore the most recent findings regarding motor cortex plasticity and reorganization.

While the somatotopic regions of M1 are readily differentiable, micro-organization of the motor cortex and its connections to individual muscles is less segregated than the somatotopy suggests. Individual pyramidal tract neurons, originating from layers II/III and V, innervate many muscles peripherally (divergence), and an individual muscle receives input from a large area of cortex (convergence). Additionally, cortical areas representing muscles overlap with one another (Donoghue et al., 1992). Lastly, a vast network of horizontal axon collaterals extends across M1, spanning several mm and connecting regions controlling analogous as well as proximal and distal musculature.

8.2 Plasticity of motor maps

Cortical motor representations are not static but fluid and regulated by use. The most common approach taken to investigate the potential for cortical plasticity has been to evaluate the reorganization of sensory and motor maps following peripheral or central lesions and compare them to normal animals. In these studies either the receptive field properties or the kinds of movements evoked by electrical stimulation are examined over a large set of sites in the cortex. The data collected from these sites can be used to construct maps of the cortical representation pattern. The expansion or reduction in the size of an area of representation and the time course of these events are then compared. An important principle of reorganization is Use It Or Lose It. If a limb is amputated and hence, not used, the cortical representation shrinks. If limb use is increased, for example, in learning a new motor skill, the representation increases. Research has increasingly become focused on the synaptic mechanisms underlying this plasticity in order to apply the findings to rehabilitation of stroke and neurological disorders. Recent experimental research is elucidating the synaptic mechanisms underlying cortical reorganization (Kaas and Qi,

2004) and the effect of therapy on this process (Nelles, 2004).

Lesion-induced changes

Peripheral lesions

When peripheral nerves are lesioned, whether sensory or motor, or if a limb is amputated, the motor cortical area to or from which those nerves project is reorganized. Studies in the primary somatosensory cortex have shown striking cortical reorganization when sensory input to the cortex is modified either by amputating or deafferenting digits or limbs (Merzenich et al., 1983a, b; 1984) by surgically connecting the skin of two fingers (syndactyly) or by grafting skin from one region of a limb to another in the monkey. With time somatotopic boundaries change during cortical mapping to reflect the reconfigured skin surfaces (Clark et al., 1988; Allard et al., 1991) and representations of intact inputs expand to fill areas previously representing the deafferentated digits (Merzenich et al., 1983a, b; 1984). After human subjects underwent surgical correction of congenital syndactyly, S1 mapping revealed similar cortical reorganization to reflect anatomy (Mogilner et al., 1993). Imaging of paraplegic patients has revealed that motor cortical representation of non-affected limbs increases with practice (Curt et al., 2002). For a more extensive discussion of plasticity after somatosensory cortex lesions, see Volume I, Chapters 6 and 14.

Reorganization of motor representation patterns in M1 following nerve transection has been investigated systematically in the rat. The rat motor cortex (M1) has a simpler (less specialized) organization than that of primates and the variety of movements that can be evoked from each body part appears to be more limited (see Wise and Donoghue, 1984). Nevertheless, the major body parts have distinct cortical representations in this and in all other mammals examined. The forelimb, vibrissa, and periocular representations of a normal rat revealed with intracortical electrical stimulation methods form successive rostrocaudally elongated zones, with the forelimb zone located most laterally in M1.

Other body parts are also represented within M1, including the hindlimb, jaw, trunk, and neck, but they form only a small proportion of the rat motor cortex.

When the peripheral facial motor nerve controlling the whiskers is cut, forelimb movements are induced with stimulation to the area of the motor cortex which previously controlled the whiskers (Donoghue et al., 1990). Similar changes in the motor cortex representation pattern occur after either injury to neonatal or adult animals (Donoghue and Sanes, 1988; Sanes et al., 1990), although mechanisms may be different. Considerably more subtle manipulations can also reorganize the motor representation. Simple maintenance of the limb in a position which stretches the muscles most activated from the cortex expands the representation of those muscles in M1 (see next section). This strongly suggests that sensory feedback (in this case probably via muscle spindles) has a profound influence on cortical organization.

The form of M1 reorganization appears to generalize across body parts, since injury separately to either forelimb or vibrissa nerves yielded qualitatively similar results (Donoghue and Sanes, 1988; Sanes et al., 1990). However, a level of specificity to reorganization exists since novel sites of hindlimb or neck movements did not appear after forelimb or vibrissa movements; the reason for this is not clear, but may be related to intracortical connection patterns. In terms of their role in movement, the reorganized M1 areas appear to be functionally similar to their normal adjacent counterparts. For example, the types of movements and amounts and patterns of electromyogram (EMG) evoked from stimulation of sites within normal and "expanded" regions of M1 are indistinguishable. Further, stimulation thresholds required to elicit movements in expanded representations are either equivalent to or lower than normal (Sanes et al., 1990). These results tentatively suggest that reorganized areas of cortex may subsume a role similar to normal representation.

Subsequent to the demonstration of changes in motor cortical representation patterns in experimental animals, similar findings were observed in humans in association with amputation or nerve blocks. In these studies either transcranial electrical or magnetic stimulation was used; these non-invasive stimulation methods activate relatively large areas of cortex compared to intracortical microstimulation (ICMS). Despite the coarseness of resolution, the results closely follow that found earlier in the rat. Muscles proximal to the amputation could be activated from a larger than normal cortical area, based on a comparison of the motor representations of the two hemispheres of individual patients. Motor-evoked potential amplitudes from muscles proximal to the block were increased and those from distal muscles decreased (Cohen et al., 1991; Fuhr et al., 1992; Ziemann et al., 1998). Deafferentation using a blood pressure cuff produced a similar, rapidly reversible result (Brasil-Nieto et al., 1992; 1993). These studies further implicate sensory feedback in controlling motor representations.

Central lesions

Several investigations have indicated functional reorganization of cortical representations following CNS lesions, especially at the level of the cerebral cortex. Perhaps the earliest study of this type was done by Grünbaum and Sherrington (1903) in which the presumed arm area of the motor cortex of apes was ablated and subsequent motor function was analyzed. Grünbaum and Sherrington (1903) observed only a transient paralysis that was not impaired by additional ipsilateral or contralateral motor cortical lesions. The conclusion from this study was that redundant motor control substrates at subcortical sites took over the functions subsumed by motor cortex. Although these results generated much controversy over the coming decades (summarized by Cole and Glees, 1951), studies in the past two decades have come to similar, although not identical conclusions.

Motor cortical map plasticity is dependent on limb use, both after cortical ischemic damage (Nudo et al., 1996b) and in the intact monkey (Nudo et al., 1996a). In the intact monkey, representations increased in size for specific muscle groups if used in a skilled task, and movement combinations used

together in the learning of a task became spatially linked in the same cortical area. Interestingly, the repetitive motor movement alone, without the need for learning, does not change functional reorganization of the cortical map (Plautz et al., 2000).

Functional reorganization can involve other cortical regions, as well. Premotor cortex has been shown to be able to subsume control of injured M1 if needed (Liu and Rouiller, 1999; Frost et al., 2003). Reciprocal anatomical connections were proposed to be the anatomical substrate in this process. For a complete discussion of motor cortical reorganization after ischemic injury, the reader is referred to Volume I, Chapter 14 (Nudo et al.).

With the increasing use of functional imaging in the past few decades, motor cortical reorganization is now being examined in human subjects. With imaging, premotor cortex (Weiller et al., 1992; Miyai et al., 2002), supplementary motor cortex (Weiller et al., 1993), and the intact, contralateral primary motor cortex (Seitz et al., 1998; Nelles et al., 1999) have all been linked in a compensatory way to M1 injury and post-injury motor recovery. The differences seen in the exact regions activated (i.e., Nelles and colleagues saw contralateral sensorimotor cortex activation post stroke, while Seitz and colleagues did not) may be the result of the subcortical spared tissue available for recruitment as compensatory pathways. Areas best able to subsume M1 function may exhibit cortico-cortical connections with M1, direct spinal-cord projections, movement activations to cortical stimulation, and similar functional homologies. The ventral part of the premotor cortex satisfies all of these requirements (Stepniewska et al., 1993; He et al., 1998; Rizzolatti et al., 2002). Motor cortical reorganization may be the rule, not the exception, for the normal brain as well as for the impaired brain.

Experience-dependent changes

Environmental/positional changes

Motor cortical plasticity has recently been documented with experience, enabling the study of learning and memory and how the brain changes with experience. At the simplest end of the behavioral spectrum, changes in *environment* can alter cortical representations and improve behavioral recovery after injury. Rats exposed to an enriched environment after focal ischemic strokes improved more in sensorimotor tasks than did rats housed in a standard environment post injury (Ohlsson and Johansson, 1995; Johansson and Ohlsson, 1995). This behavioral improvement has been attributed to plasticity of surrounding, healthy tissue. If trained on tasks with the impaired limb while being housed in the enriched environment, behavioral improvement was even greater and layer V pyramidal cells in the unaffected hemisphere showed increased arborization of dendrites (Biernaskie and Corbett, 2001). In this study, rats which did not experience enrichment did not improve despite training and showed no dendritic changes. The authors attribute the enriched environment with enabling neuronal plasticity of the homologous non-injured hemisphere by way of cortico-cortical connections. Interestingly, therapy initiated too soon after injury can be counterproductive to long-term recovery of function and plasticity (Kozlowski et al., 1996; Humm et al., 1998).

Changes in *limb position* are able to modify cortical representations, as well, if they are prolonged (Sanes et al., 1992). In addition, if limbs are held immobile for long periods of time, for example with a splint or cast, motor cortical representations decrease in size compared to those of the opposite, healthy limb as measured with transcranial magnetic stimulation (TMS) methods (Liepert et al., 1995). These studies again implicate sensory feedback as important in modifying cortical representations.

Simple movement tasks

Movement repetition, even if involving no learning, has been documented to change cortical representations. Short-term repetition of isolated digit or paired movements can induce small changes in TMS-evoked movements in as quickly as 5–10 min, indicative of alteration in cortical representation (Classen et al., 1998). Functional magnetic imaging during and after repetition of previously-learned movement sequences has documented changes in M1 activation; activation in M1 is decreased within the initial practice session, but by the fourth week of training the activation area is increased (Karni et al., 1995). A pair of well-controlled studies by Nudo and colleagues indicated, however, that repetitive motor behavior without motor learning does not change primary motor cortex representations (Plautz et al., 2000). Monkeys retrieved pellets from large wells repeatedly, a task which did not require any adaptation to perform well. In contrast, when monkeys performed a task in which they were required to learn to retrieve pellets from small wells representation changed (Nudo et al., 1996a). As new patterns of digit coordination emerged, so did cortical reorganization as evidenced by ICMS of the primary motor cortex. The discrepancies between the length of movement repetition required to change cortical representation between these studies may be due to the methods used to measure the change, as well as the behavioral tasks. It is unclear with TMS and fMRI exactly which brain matter is activated; what is known is that both methods, while useful, appear to activate much larger groups of neurons than ICMS. An additional contributing factor may be subtle changes that take place with so-called "repetition of known sequences." Small kinematic adjustments may be occurring to enhance movement efficiency, such that even repetition of simple movements may involve learning of sorts. The take-home message is that, until we know exactly what movement variables or processes are coded in primary motor cortex, the most accurate statement about motor cortical plasticity and movement repetition, is that it can and does occur.

Motor learning, skilled movement training

While results are less than perfectly clear regarding the changes seen in motor cortical representation during practice of over-learned movements, evidence is abundant and ever accumulating that motor skill learning changes M1 representations. When rats learned a skilled reaching movement, wrist and digit

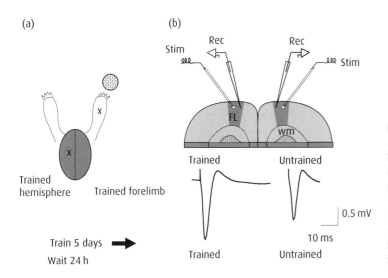

Figure 8.1. Motor skill learning changes synaptic excitability in layers II/III horizontal connections in M1: (a) experimental paradigm showing unilateral training on forelimb reaching task and (b) evoked-field potentials (below) from slice recording from trained and untrained hemispheres. Stim = stimulate, Rec = record. Adapted from Rioult-Pedotti et al., 1998.

representations in M1 increased and unused shoulder representations decreased in size, whereas no increase was seen with practice of an unskilled movement (Kleim et al., 1998; 2002). Likewise, strength training requiring no additional skill also did not increase movement representations (Remple et al., 2001).

Direct evidence of a link between motor skill learning, synaptic modification and long-term potentiation (LTP) mechanisms has been demonstrated (Fig. 8.1). Rats trained for several days to perform a novel reaching movement to grasp a food pellet showed increases in electrically-stimulated field potential amplitude in the forelimb but not in the hindlimb regions of the contralateral hemisphere as compared to the ipsilateral hemisphere (Rioult-Pedotti et al., 1998). After 5 days of training, rats were sacrificed and motor cortical slices examined electrophysiologically. Less LTP and more long-term depression (LTD) could be induced in the trained hemisphere (layer II/III intracortical connections) than in untrained, indicating LTP involvement in the changing efficacy of the horizontal cortical connections (Rioult-Pedotti et al., 2000). Skill learning has been associated with an increase in the overall cortical area of involved limbs (Remple et al., 2001) as well as the number of synapses in the region (Kleim et al., 2002) compared to controls.

Functional reorganization of the human sensorimotor cortex has been documented after the learning of many skills, including playing a string instrument (Elbert et al., 1995), playing a keyboard professionally (Gaser and Schlaug, 2003), piano exercises (Pascual-Leone et al., 1995), racquet ball (Pearce et al., 2000), or finger to thumb sequences (Karni et al., 1995). In another study, TMS came to evoke a recently practiced movement after initially evoking a movement to a different direction (Classen et al., 1998), suggesting the region stimulated had changed motor representations. Reorganization has appeared to be temporally variable, however. After learning a repetitive pinch task, movement evoked potential (MEP) amplitude increases seen during the training period in involved muscles decreased (Muellbacher et al., 2001), suggesting that cortical circuitry changes with skill learning may occur in stages. After extensive practice with the finger-thumb sequences mentioned above, increased motor cortical representations were documented in an imaging study over and above those after the skill was initially learned (Karni et al., 1998). Brain regions activated with a newly learned motor skill and detected with positron emission tomography (PET) imaging shift with consolidation of the motor skill from prefrontal regions initially to premotor to parietal and cerebellar regions (Shadmehr and Holcomb, 1997). In summary, motor representation changes in the cortex may be the road map for discovering how the brain creates and stores motor programs. In the next section we will explore what we know about the structure of the motor cortex and how it relates to plasticity.

8.3 Substrates and mechanisms for repair and plasticity

Connectional substrates: intrinsic

The motor cortex contains a neural circuitry conducive to motor plasticity, which includes both intrinsic and extrinsic components. Connections intrinsic to the primary motor cortex include both horizontal and vertical systems of neurons. The vertical system extends from the pyramidal cells of layers II and III to layer V. The horizontal system consists of long, widely-branching fibers, also arising from pyramidal cells, which form many synapses along their extent and appear to connect somatic motor representations of the same body part for the monkey (Huntley and Jones, 1991). One horizontal "web" lies in layers II and III, and another across layer V. These excitatory connections are mediated by glutamate (Hess et al., 1994) with some synapses linked to *N*-methyl-D-aspartate (NMDA) receptors, a receptor subtype associated with synaptic modification (Malenka and Nicoll, 1993). The pyramidal neuron collaterals can excite gamma aminobutyric acid (GABA)-ergic inhibitory neurons as well as other pyramidal cells (Keller and Asanuma, 1993). An oblique horizontal plexus extends from layer V to III and also distributes information in the horizontal direction. These fibers have been shown to extend 1.25 mm and more in the rat and are excitatory (Hess and Donoghue, 1994; 1996).

How intrinsic connections might underlie plasticity

An appealing idea is that the horizontal connections enable dynamic motor ensembles to form which

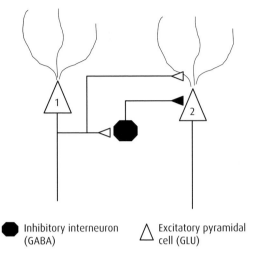

● Inhibitory interneuron (GABA)   △ Excitatory pyramidal cell (GLU)

Figure 8.2. M1 circuitry depicting feed-forward inhibition in horizontal connections. Disynaptic inhibition and monosynaptic excitation from Neuron 1 can change excitability of Neuron 2.

may be the basis of motor plasticity. When GABA-ergic inhibition in M1 is blocked, latent horizontal connections are unmasked which are usually blocked by feed-forward inhibition (Jacobs and Donoghue, 1991), as illustrated in Fig. 8.2. Feed-forward inhibition may play an important role, in that disynaptic inhibition and monosynaptic excitation in the horizontal layers could modulate reciprocally to dynamically change cortical excitation (Hess et al., 1994; 1996). Short- and long-term modifications may utilize this substrate, which can allow expression of various M1 motor maps, as depicted in cartoon-fashion in Fig. 8.3. Huntley found support for this type of mechanism *in vivo* in experiments in which the contralateral facial nerve was cut in adult rats, and forelimb and vibrissa movement representations were mapped with microelectrodes. After lesions, forelimb representations expanded into the territory previously held by vibrissae and labeled axons from forelimb representations extended horizontally, crossing the forelimb/vibrissae border (Huntley, 1997). Long-term synaptic modifications may occur through processes which result in LTP in

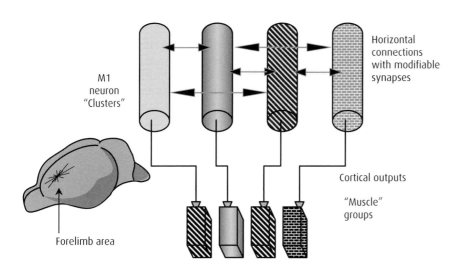

M1
neuron
"Clusters"

Horizontal
connections
with modifiable
synapses

Cortical outputs

"Muscle"
groups

Forelimb area

Figure 8.3. Reorganization of motor representations by horizontal connections in M1. Schematic showing how cortical output can be changed by horizontal network.

this same network of fibers (Hess and Donoghue, 1994). When peripheral stimulation of sensory afferents is coupled with TMS of the motor cortex, mimicking associative LTP protocols, quickly forming and long-lasting plasticity can be induced (Stefan et al., 2000). In addition, in the motor cortex, pharmacological manipulations which reduce the effectiveness of lateral inhibition reorganize the motor output map in a form similar to that produced by nerve lesions (Jacobs and Donoghue, 1991). Thus, inhibition may provide the means to regulate the horizontal intracortical system, and sensory input may be the means by which inhibition is imparted. It is important to be cautionary in interpretation of results utilizing TMS, as the site of stimulation with this method cannot be localized only to pyramidal tract neurons but also may include intra-, inter-, and subcortical circuitry.

Connectional substrates: extrinsic

Extrinsic connections of M1 include two important pathways. The first, the thalamic pathway, transmits movement-related information from the basal ganglia and the cerebellum through the ventrolateral thalamic complex to layer III in the motor cortex (Thach, 1987; Holsapple et al., 1991). Thalamic axons

arborize carrying sensory and motor information in the cortex beyond the range that would be predicted from functional measures (Landry and Deschennes, 1981; Zarzeki and Wiggin, 1982; Zarzecki et al., 1983). A second extrinsic pathway also enters vertically and transmits information from other cortical sites, such as the frontal and parietal lobes (Asanuma and Mackel, 1989; Andersen et al., 1990). Input from this pathway brings sensory information into the primary motor cortex.

How extrinsic connections might underlie plasticity

Although the function of extrinsic connections are poorly understood, several lines of evidence support an important role for their involvement in cortical plasticity. After amputation-induced reorganization of the raccoon somatic sensory cortex the cortico-cortical input from adjacent cortex to the deafferented cortex increased in efficacy; this input carried information from skin surfaces that came to be represented in the deafferented zone (Zarzecki et al., 1993). Secondly, thalamocortical neurons arborize widely in the cortex and plasticity of S1 representations have been related to changing efficacy of these fibers (Rausell and Jones, 1995). Reorganization of thalamocortical input may involve the long horizontal intracortical connections. Further, TMS of the contralateral primary motor cortex can induce long-lasting increased excitability in the ipsilateral motor cortex, evidence of intercortical interaction (Schambra et al., 2003). In conclusion, modifications of local inhibitory or extrinsic pathways by experience may transiently allow for long-term synaptic modification to occur via LTP or LTD which could structurally alter the M1 output map.

Mechanisms for change

Cortical plasticity in the motor cortex could rely on one or more of the following mechanisms: changes in balance of excitation and inhibition resulting in the unmasking of latent connections, strengthening or weakening of existing connections by LTP or LTD, generalized modulatory effects with pharmacological or state changes, or neurogenesis/synaptogenesis. LTP, which results in long-term changes in synaptic efficacy, is Hebbian in nature, resulting from exact temporal patterning of inputs to a target neuron (Bliss and Lomo, 1973). Conditional LTP especially has received much attention as a mechanism capable of reorganizing the motor cortical network. Pharmacological manipulations or activation of particular afferent pathways aimed at reducing inhibition paired with afferent pathway stimulation have been shown to modify motor cortical synapses. Activity-dependent synaptic plasticity is restricted to specific synapses activated by inputs and is, therefore, very restrictive and focal, an appealing mechanism for learning. It could explain how converging afferent inputs from disparate sources could interact in the cortex to induce plasticity.

Unmasking of existing connections

One possible mechanism for reorganization of cortical representations is unmasking of existing but functionally weak synaptic connections by intracortical facilitation or inhibition. The unmasking hypothesis is based on the assumption that there are a large number of hidden synaptic connections

in the cortex: these connections can be revealed, or strengthened upon an appropriate stimulus, such as a change in activity. In support of this hypothesis, it has been clearly demonstrated that inputs to single cortical neurons come from much wider areas than are normally observed. As described above there is a rich horizontal interconnection in the cortex that may serve as a substrate for intracortical routes of reorganization.

In the motor cortex, local blockade of cortical inhibition demonstrates that single sites in M1 have access to a wide variety of muscles that are not evident under normal mapping conditions (Jacobs and Donoghue, 1991). Further, unblocked latent connections are capable of participating in newly forming M1 representations. With inhibition blocked, LTP may be possible with increased potential for depolarization to occur. Similarly, after limb amputation or anesthesia, muscles proximal to the affected limb show increased excitability levels indicative of disinhibition of existing synaptic connections, perhaps in the cortex (Brasil-Neto et al., 1992). Using TMS and paired conditioning and test stimuli together with EMG, intracortical inhibition and facilitation have been demonstrated and shown to influence motor representations for different muscles differentially (Chen et al., 1998). Thus, the substrate upon which cortical plasticity acts is non-uniform in anatomy and/or function. Further, with ischemic nerve block mimicking deafferentation and the applications of GABA receptor agonists, Na^+- and Ca^{2+} blockers, and NMDA-receptor blockers, Ziemann and colleagues showed that the deafferentation induced plasticity in M1 was due to removing GABA-dependent intracortical inhibition and that this long-lasting disinhibition involved NMDA receptors and LTP-like mechanisms (Ziemann et al., 1998).

Excitability changes: generalized or by LTP/LTD

Long-lasting generalized changes in the excitability of neurons could increase the probability of firing in a neuron or groups of neurons. Such a phenomenon has been documented in the hippocampus during a classical conditioning paradigm (Aou et al., 1992), in which short- as well as long-latency responses of neurons were increased after rapid eye blink conditioning. This type of excitability change would be generalized to all inputs arriving at a specific neuron and is, therefore, less specific than LTP or LTD.

LTP has been the widely studied in relation to learning, mostly in the subcortical hippocampal region. This Hebbian synaptic modification as a basis for learning has been documented throughout the nervous system and is an appealing model for learning and plasticity. Efficacy changes occur in recently active synapses which then drive post-synaptic targets. With *in vivo* experiments electrical stimulation of synaptic strengths of horizontal connections in layers II and III have been shown to modify with LTP and LTD, thereby reorganizing motor maps (Hess and Donoghue, 1994; Hess et al., 1996; Hess and Donoghue, 1996). As described earlier in this chapter, by recording field potentials in layers II/III of M1 and inducing LTP and LTD as an assay of synaptic strength, Rioult-Pedotti and colleagues demonstrated in the rat that motor learning can change the synaptic strength of the horizontal connections in M1 by an LTP-like mechanism (Rioult-Pedotti et al., 2000).

Whether LTP-like and LTD-like plasticity could be induced in humans after motor learning was tested recently by Ziemann and colleagues. Repeated fast thumb abduction movements (which showed improvement over time) decreased LTP and increased the amount of LTD achievable in a subsequent Paired Association Stimulation Protocol (Stefan et al., 2000), which paired peripheral nerve stimulation with TMS (Ziemann et al., 2004). Slow thumb abduction (involving no learning) had no effect on this protocol, indicating that human motor learning may also involve LTP-like mechanisms.

Ziemann and colleagues showed that changes in motor cortical plasticity in humans induced by ischemic nerve blocks and low-frequency repetitive TMS were dependent on removal of GABA-induced cortical inhibition and that LTP-like mechanisms were involved in maintaining the inhibitory blockade

(Ziemann et al., 1998). Whether new synapses are added, existing synapses are increased in size, or the weighting of the existing synapses is rearranged all possibly underlie LTP. See Volume I, Chapter 4 for more a more comprehensive discussion of LTP and LTD.

Pharmacological changes or overall modulation of M1 plasticity

Several factors may impart a modulatory effect on motor cortical reorganization. Attention has been implicated in modulating the extent to which M1 reorganizes (Stefan et al., 2004). Neuromodulators such as acetylcholine (ACh) (Conner et al., 2003) and norepinephrine (Burgard et al., 1989) have been suggested to influence the site and incidence of synaptic plasticity, as well. Of the two modulators, most evidence is available for ACh, which has been connected both to LTP and plasticity of cortical circuits. The basal forebrain cholinergic system is involved in the acquisition but not the performance of learned tasks (Orsetti et al., 1996), and nucleus basalis ACh neurons projecting specifically to the cortex, when destroyed, disrupt motor learning, but not the performance of a skilled reaching task (Conner et al., 2003). Thus, the presence or absence of ACh could then alter the connectional organization of the cortex and affect many aspects of its information processing capacity.

Inhibitory, excitatory, and modulatory processes may act cooperatively to regulate the potential for synaptic modification. There may be many pharmacotherapeutic routes to the control of reorganization. Additionally, each of these mechanisms may be engaged by changes in sensory feedback, so that new approaches using physical therapeutic regimens may hold promise for promoting higher levels of functional recovery (Matthews et al., 2004).

Neurogenesis in the motor cortex

Traditionally, neurogenesis in the adult mammalian brain has been thought to be near if not non-existant, with the exception of the dentate gyrus of the hippocampus and subventricular zone olfactory bulb system of rodents, monkeys, and humans (Kaplan and Hinds, 1977; Eriksson et al., 1998; Kornack and Rakic, 1999). The debate continues on whether new neurons are formed in the cortex of the adult brain (see Fuchs and Gould, 2000; Nowakowski and Hayes, 2000; Koketsu et al., 2003; and see Bernier et al., 2002). Gould and colleagues have used a thymidine analog, bromodeoxyuridine labeling technique and asserted that neurogenesis is prolific and continual in the adult monkey and that new neurons are added to the association neocortex (Gould et al., 1999). If substantiated, this could have tremendous implications for rehabilitation of neurodegenerative diseases and brain injuries. Most recent evidence suggests, however, that in the primate motor cortex the majority of new cells are microglia or astrocytes, not neurons (Ehninger and Kempermann, 2003). In addition, these are more abundant in the young versus the old animal. In normal adult primates living in an enriched environment, evidence suggests that any new neurons generated are in the hippocampus or olfactory bulb not the neocortex (Kornack and Rakic, 2001; Koketsu et al., 2003). An excellent review of adult neurogenesis can be found in Emsley et al., 2005, and in Chapter 18 of this volume.

Synaptogenesis in the motor cortex

While neurogenesis in the adult mammalian cortex remains controversial, the forming or remodeling of new synapses (synaptogenesis) or collateral sprouting of axons is not questioned. More than 30 years ago, in the hippocampus and associated structures the seminal study of Raisman (1969) showed an increase in the number of synaptic contacts in the septal nucleus following the destruction of one of its inputs. Injury-induced synaptogenesis is well documented and can cause such peripheral syndromes as phantom limb, neuroma formation, allodynia (painful sensation elicited by non-noxious stimuli) and hypersensitivity. Centrally, neuronal sprouting has even been linked to epilepsy (Cavazos et al., 2004). Contralateral dendritic arborization of layer V

pyramidal cells and increased number of synapses are present after lesioning of the ipsilateral sensorimotor cortex in adult rats (Jones, 1999). For a more detailed discussion of synaptogenesis and neurogenesis following brain injury, see Volume I, Chapter 14. Chapters 18 and 20 in this volume discuss neurogenesis and synaptogenesis in greater detail, respectively.

In normal animals, synaptogenesis is an important process in development. Synaptic contacts increase with development of complex movement ability in the motor cortex in young rats (Markus and Petit, 1987). In the adult rat, synaptogenesis is a constant process and a constant synaptic density may be the result of equal rates of synapse creation and elimination, rather than the absence of synaptogenesis (Trachtenberg et al., 2002).

Experience, especially learning of skilled tasks, increases synaptic density in various regions of the adult brain. Purkinje cells in the cerebellar cortex of adult rats show increased synaptic contacts after learning complex acrobatic skills, but not after simple exercise (Black et al., 1990). The motor cortex of adult rats shows increased synaptogenesis after skilled learning, as well as an increased expression of an immediate early gene, c-FOS, which is related to protein synthesis (Kleim et al., 1996). In addition, the synaptogenesis occurs in the same region that shows motor map representation size increases (Kleim et al., 2002), giving powerful support to the idea that synaptogenesis is behind changes seen cortically during motor learning. Subsequently, this synaptogenesis was shown to occur during the late consolidation phase of motor learning, but before motor representation changes emerge (Kleim et al., 2004).

In addition to being linked to skill learning and motor representation enlargement, synaptogenesis is also associated with LTP formation, although this is controversial. Toni et al. (1999) used a hippocampal slice preparation and induced LTP with theta-burst stimulation, subsequently detecting new synapses with the two photon imaging technique between activated axons and dendrites. These synapses appeared functional, as they contained calcium precipitates, and pharmacological blockage of LTP prevented these changes. One group using similar techniques found similar results (Engert and Bonhoeffer, 1999), but another could not document increased synaptic density in hippocampal slices (Sorra and Harris, 1998).

8.4 Significance of cortical reorganization

Reorganization of cortical representations acting through the mechanisms described above may serve as an important route for recovery of function after damage to the nervous system and it may be possible to exploit such reorganization to enhance functional recovery. The current state of knowledge suggests that it is timely to begin a serious effort to develop a scientific basis for neurorehabilitation and that there is great promise in this endeavor. Although there is clearly an enormous amount still to be learned about the basic form and mechanism related to the potential for change to occur in the mature nervous system, the current evidence suggests that interventions can be designed to promote recovery of function by utilizing remaining neural circuitry. Neurorehabilitation may use pharmacological or physical intervention or both. Pharmacological therapies clearly have potential: we know that the balance of excitatory and inhibitory synaptic strength has important consequences upon cortical organization. Glutamatergic, GABAergic, and cholinergic systems all are likely targets for action and drugs that act at each of these sites are available. Major problems now are localizing the site of delivery of these agents (since they have many sites of action in the CNS) and determining the appropriate action (i.e. do we want to increase or decrease their levels). The understanding from basic experimental work concerning the way these agents might affect lesion- or experience-induced reorganization is still rather limited.

Physical intervention through experiential manipulation may also be important. Even simple limb position changes in rats can influence the amount of motor cortex related to a particular group of muscles. It could be useful to switch control to new sets of muscles. Thus, in an amputee it might be useful to engage cortical sites previously involved in distal control to control more proximal sites that remain. In addition, we know that the effectiveness of cortical synapses can be regulated through activity-dependent processes. Thus, therapeutic regimens which selectively activate specific intracortical pathways may promote a fuller or more rapid recovery. However, it remains equally possible that reorganization may be in part the cause of dysfunction and may indeed *prevent* recovery. Thus, we need to know not only how to regulate reorganization, but also the functional consequences of such reorganization. For example, switching of a cortical representation to the control of a set of muscles which have different biomechanical properties and different neural control architectures might contribute to spasticity. In this case one might want to suppress reorganization.

Incorporation of these data into rehabilitation strategies is just beginning. A number of therapies exist to improve motor function in stroke and other movement-disordered patients. The Bobath neurodevelopmental method (Bobath, 1977) has been used for many years in rehabilitation and involves maintenance of the limb in positions which resemble those used by Sanes and colleagues (Sanes et al., 1992) to shift the M1 map. This method is based on a design to overcome spastic synergies. For a recent study evaluating the effectiveness of the Bobath method (see Paci, 2003). By contrast, the Brunnstrom movement therapy method (Brunnstrom, 1966) utilizes the spastic synergies in its therapeutic approach. It is noteworthy that completely opposite strategies have been adopted. Other methods stress the importance of sensory feedback in rehabilitation (see Goff, 1969). This would fit well with the available evidence that sensory input plays a significant role in the maintenance of cortical organization both in sensory and motor areas. Constraint-induced movement therapy was recently developed for treatment of chronic hemiparesis and is related to the basic science discussed earlier in this chapter. In short, it involves constraining use of the non-affected limb for a period of weeks while intensely training the affected limb (Taub et al., 1999; Mark and Taub, 2002). For more detailed discussions of rehabilitation strategies related to movement, see Volume I, Chapter 15; Volume II, Chapters 2, 3, 7 and 18.

8.5 Neural prostheses

A completely different strategy for rehabilitation has experienced renewed interest within the past decade. Work by several researchers is underway to develop a neural prosthesis, or BMI to aid severely movement-disordered or paralyzed individuals regain increased control over the environment. While the BMI may seem compensatory upon initial reflection, it depends critically on brain plasticity to function. Users must actively learn to control their neuronal activity and mold this activity to the desired output. Neural prostheses will open an important window into plasticity by allowing detailed research into how the brain changes with practice and learning and the extent to which the brain is able to adapt.

Neural prostheses research has benefited tremendously by recent technological advances in the simultaneous recording of multiple neurons and the development of devices which can be implanted neurosurgically deep in the human brain to relieve movement disorders. Minute devices are implanted into the basal ganglia or other areas of movement-disordered individuals, which impart new patterns of activity to distinct brain nuclei (Benabid et al., 1989). The BMI, is amazingly science fiction-like, yet still in primitive stages of development. The BMI connects the living human brain with the external world in a novel manner. These devices attempt to decode the language of the brain with mathematical algorithms and use the decoded messages to act upon the environment, thereby establishing a new communication link. Meant to aid neurologically impaired individuals, such as those with spinal-cord injury, stroke, or degenerative muscular diseases, researchers hope these devices will improve the mobility, environmental control, and functional independence of persons with severe paralysis.

Components of a BMI

A BMI consists of three modules: input, interpretation and output.

Scientific development is progressing with each module. The Input module consists of the brain signal to be interpreted. BMIs (Fig. 8.4) have attempted to use many types of brain signals as input, varying in specificity and sensitivity (Donoghue, 2002; Friehs et al., 2004). Brain signals can range from external electroencephalograms (EEGs) recorded from outside the skull to multiple single cell recordings recorded from inside the brain. The Interpretation module is at the heart of the computer or "machine" used for BMIs. A mathematical algorithm(s) decodes the brain signals and calibrates the available neuronal signals with the desired output (perhaps a direction for a cursor to move, a click of a computer mouse, a scrolling across a list of choices, etc.). Then, while the algorithm decodes the ongoing neural activity, the subject attempts to control the output device using "brain control." Two interdependent factors contribute to the success of the interpretation module: (1) the algorithm; if reliable, it is able to convert complicated neuronal activity into useful commands, and, (2) the neuronal signals; if they are diverse and task-specific, one is able to successfully decode different states, that is, analog or binary (continuous or discrete commands) (Hatsopoulos et al., 2004). The extent to which both these conditions are met is the extent to which the individual has the highest chances of success. The individual's job is to learn to control his brain signals to operate some new functional output device. This could be a computer, a prosthetic limb, or even, someday, the individual's own paralyzed limb.

BMI's utilizing external brain signals

The least invasive brain interface input comes from EEGs, an electrical brain signal recorded from the

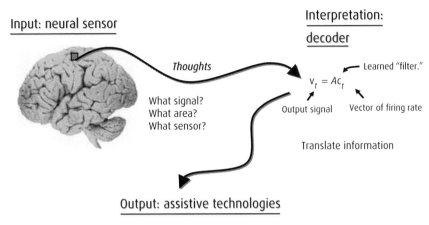

Input: neural sensor

Interpretation: decoder

Thoughts

What signal?
What area?
What sensor?

Learned "filter."

$$v_t = Ac_t$$

Output signal   Vector of firing rate

Translate information

Output: assistive technologies

What technology?

Figure 8.4. Components of a BMI.

surface of the scalp. The signal is relatively easy to obtain, but limited in its information content compared with action potentials from single neurons (Donoghue et al., 1998). With electrodes placed on the outside of the skull, changes in electrical potential of the brain can be measured. Various components of these signals have been used as input with some success. Individuals can modulate slow cortical potentials, mu/beta rhythms, or P300 with practice. So-called "indirect BMIs" use these crude signals as input. Although control has been achieved with these devices, they possess a number of negatives. First of all, the EEG signal reflects the summed activity of a large number of neurons. The signal quality is low as is signal-to-noise ratio. The signal is variable trial-by-trial and bandwidth is limited. Additionally, the information transfer rate in such a system is very low, at approximately 20–30 bit/min (i.e., 0.5 bit/s). BMIs require that signals be analyzed on the spot, in real time, and utilizing such a complex and variable signal presents quite a challenge. These devices also require an extended "learning" period; often it can take weeks to months for a patient to gain adequate control of his/her EEG signal.

Despite these limitations, however, several groups have developed BMIs using specific components of the EEG signal or slow cortical potentials with some success. Slow cortical potentials or components of the EEG move a cursor on a screen or open or close a prosthetic hand (Wolpaw et al., 1991; Pfurtscheller et al., 1996; Lauer et al., 1999). Movement is slow, however, and the information regarding intent encoded in the spiking of individual neurons is lost due to the averaging and filtering across the skull.

BMIs utilizing internal brain signals

With recent advancement of information technology, miniaturization and biological compatability of materials, it is now possible to implant recording electrodes inside the human skull, either on or within the brain and to record neural signals for use with BMIs. Ability to decode a behavioral intent from a group of neurons directly should greatly aid functionality of such a device. Pioneering work was done by Kennedy and colleagues with the implantation of a glass-cone electrode into the primary motor cortex of patients with locked-in syndrome. A uni-dimensional increase in neuronal signals from nearby axons together with one or more EMG signals was used to drive a cursor on a computer monitor for operating a simple communication system (Kennedy and Bakay, 1998; Kennedy et al.,

2000). Training was accomplished over weeks, and maximum rate reached three words per minute.

Recently, multi-electrode arrays implanted in the motor cortex of the monkey have recorded populations of neurons simultaneously and demonstrated on-line control of a cursor (Wessberg et al., 2000; Serruya et al., 2002; Taylor et al., 2002). With this degree of control achieved, exploration has begun to develop a more direct human BMI. On-line control in humans was demonstrated by Donoghue and colleagues using small groups of less than 10 neurons with a 5-microelectrode drive in Parkinson patients who were having a deep-brain stimulator implanted for treatment of their movement disorder (Donoghue et al., 2003). It is now common for neurosurgeons to record neural activity in the basal ganglia to aid in placement of deep-brain stimulating electrodes for the treatment of movement disorders (e.g., Parkinson's disease, essential tremor, dystonia and others). As these electrodes necessarily traverse a small portion of frontal (often premotor) cortex en route to the subcortical target, this surgery provides the (otherwise rare) opportunity to record human premotor neural activity intraoperatively, when the patient is awake (as he/she would be for a standard stimulator placement). In this study, with the microelectrodes recording single- and multi-unit neural activity from the premotor cortex, patients were able to move a cursor operated by "brain control" to large targets in a high percentage of trials after the neuronal activity was used to train mathematical filters during arm-controlled movement of the cursor to the targets. Ability to do this using these direct signals required only minutes of practice. Off-line decoding of movement intent and direction was successful in four data sets from three Parkinson patients using as few as four prefrontal/premotor neurons (Ojakangas et al., 2004). Small ensembles of neurons were able to predict movement intent with a high degree of accuracy in a task in which the patient was required to remember whether to move or not in the upcoming trial. Single neurons as well as small groups of neurons also predicted direction significantly in a four-direction movement task.

What is the optimum site for implantation of electrodes for BMIs? This is as yet unclear and may depend on type of output signal desired. Primary motor cortex has been viewed as the optimum area of implantation because of its direct connection to movement, although other areas could provide signals which require less effort to consciously modulate. Planning signals before movement begins seen in other areas may provide faster decoding. M1 is superior to dorsal premotor area (PMd) for continuous reconstruction of hand movement, as demonstrated by Hatsopoulos and colleagues in off-line decoding in monkeys. PMd, however, predicted discrete targets more accurately (Hatsopoulos et al., 2004). Shenoy showed recently that real-time prediction of discrete visual targets (state control) using PMd neurons in monkeys was much faster than monkey's real reaches with information transfer rates of over 5 bit/s (Ryu et al., 2004). Neuronal signals from non-motor areas related to other cognitive processes are also being explored. In non-human primates the posterior and lateral parietal cortex (Pesaran et al., 2002; Shenoy et al., 2003; Musallam et al., 2004), as well as many areas simultaneously (Carmena et al., 2003) are being examined.

Nicolelis and colleagues used movement-related neurons from subcortical structures to predict hand-force off-line to determine if such sites may be feasible for BMI implantation. Neuronal activity was recorded from the subthalamic nucleus and thalamus in the basal ganglia while patients squeezed a ball to drive a bar to a visual target. Off-line analysis showed groups of neurons predicted hand-gripping force modestly yet significantly, leading the authors to conclude that subcortical regions may provide useful control signals for BMIs (Patil et al., 2004). Ultimately, research may show that the site of implantation is less important than the degree to which a patient may be able to adapt neuronal signals consciously to suit particular BMI requirements.

Recently, Food and Drug Administration (FDA) investigational device exemption approval was given to a pilot study utilizing a 100-micro-electrode array (Bionics, Inc., Cyberkinetics Technologies,

Inc.). The first patient, a quadriplegic, was successfully implanted in the motor cortex. Initial results are very promising; the young man is able to play several simple video games, control his environment (i.e., turning his television on and off, switching channels), and interact with the world through his e-mail and Internet with "mind control" alone (Mukand et al., 2004; J.P. Donoghue, unpublished results). Several more patients are scheduled for this experimental implantation.

The development of BMIs, although still in its infancy, has made substantial progress in the last few years. Knowledge from plasticity research will be invaluable in designing future devices which will take into account how the brain adapts and learns with time. Ultimately, feasibility of a site for implantation, type of signal required for a particular output device, output desired (e.g., continuous or state control), decoding algorithm used, and quality, quantity, and diversity of neuronal signals available as well as a patient's ability to control them consciously will interact to determine the success of a particular BMI.

REFERENCES

Allard, T., Clark, S.A., Jenkins, W.M. and Merzenich, M.M. (1991). Reorganization of somatosensory area 3b representations in adult owl monkeys after digital syndactyly. *J Neurophysiol*, **66**, 1048–1058.

Andersen, R.A., Asanuma, C., Essick, G. and Siegel, R.M. (1990). Corticocortical connections of anatomically and physiologically defined subdivisions within the inferior parietal lobe. *J Comparat Neurol*, **296**, 65–113.

Aou, S., Woody, C.D. and Birt, D. (1992). Changes in the activity of units of the cat motor cortex with rapid conditioning and extinction of a compound eye blink movement. *J Neurosci*, **12**, 549–559.

Asanuma, H. and Mackel, R. (1989). Direct and indirect sensory input pathways to the motor cortex, its structure and function in relation to learning of motor skills. *Jpn J Physiol*, **39**, 1–19.

Beevor, C.E. and Horsley, V. (1887). A minute analysis (experimental) of the various movements produced by stimulating in the monkey different regions of the cortical centre for the upper limb, as defined by Professor Ferrier. *Philos Trans Roy Soc London*, **178**, 153–167.

Beevor, C.E. and Horsley, V. (1890). A record of the results obtained by electrical excitation of the so-called motor cortex and internal capsule in an orang-outang (*Simia satyrus*). *Philos Trans Roy Soc London*, **181**, 129–158.

Beevor, C.E. and Horsley, V. (1894). A further minute analysis by electrical stimulation of the so-called motor regions (facial area) of the cortex cerebri in the monkey, *Macacus sinicus*. *Philos Trans Roy Soc London*, **185**, 39–81.

Benabid, A.L., Pollak, P., Louveau, A., Henry, S. and de Rougemont, J. (1989). Combined (thalamotomy and stimulation) stereotactic surgery of the VIM thalamic nucleus for bilateral Parkinson disease. *Appl Neurophysiol*, **50**, 344–366.

Bernier, P.J., Bedard, A., Vinet, J., Levesque, M. and Parent, A. (2002). Newly generated neurons in the amygdale and adjoining cortex of adult primates. *Proc Natl Acad Sci*, **99**, 11464–11469.

Biernaskie, J. and Corbett, D. (2001). Enriched rehabilitative training promoters improved forelimb motor function and enhanced dendritic growth after focal ischemic injury. *J Neurosci*, **21**, 5272–5280.

Black, J.E., Isaacs, K.R., Anderson, B.J., Alcantara, A.A. and Greenough, W.T. (1990). Learning causes synaptogenesis, whereas motor activity causes angiogenesis, in cerebellar cortex of adult rats. *Proc Natl Acad Sci*, **87**, 5568–5572.

Bliss, T.V. and Lomo, T. (1973). Long-lasting potentiation of synaptic transmission in the dentate area of the anaesthetized rabbit following stimulation of the perforant path. *J Physiol*, **232**, 331–356.

Bobath, B. (1977). Treatment of adult hemiplegia. *Physiotherapy*, **63**, 310–313.

Brasil-Neto, J.P., Cohen, L.G., Pascual-Leone, A., Jabir, R.T., Wall, R.T. and Hallet, M. (1992). Rapid reversible modulation of human motor outputs after transient deafferentation of the forearm: a study with transcranial magnetic stimulation. *Neurology*, **42**, 1302–1306.

Brasil-Neto, J.P., Valls-Sole, J., Pascual-Leone, A., Cammarota, A., Amassian, V.E., Cracco, R., Maccabee, P., Cracco, J., Hallett, M. and Cohen, L.G. (1993). Rapid modulation of human cortical motor outputs following ischemic nerve block. *Brain*, **116**, 511–525.

Brunnstrom, S. (1966). Motor testing procedures in hemiplegia: based on sequential recovery stages. *Phys Ther*, **46**, 357–375.

Burgard, E.C., Decker, G. and Sarvey, J.M. (1989). NMDA receptor antagonists block norepinephrine-induced long-lasting potentiation and long-term potentiation in rat dentate gyrus. *Brain Res*, **482**, 351–355.

Carmena, J.M., Lebedev, M.A., Crist, R.E., O'Doherty, J.E., Santucci, D.M., Dimitrov, D.F., Patil, P.G., Henriquez, C.S. and Nicolelis, M.A.L. (2003). Learning to control a brain–machine interface for reaching and grasping by primates. *Publ Libr Sci Biol*, **1**, 193–208.

Cavazos, J.E., Jones, S.M. and Cross, D.J. (2004). Sprouting and synaptic reorganization in the subiculum and CA region of the hippocampus in acute and chronic models of partial onset epilepsy. *Neuroscience*, **126**, 677–688.

Chen, R., Tam, A., Buetefisch, C., Corwell, B., Ziemann, U., Rothwell, J.C. and Cohen, L.G. (1998). Intracortical inhibition and facilitation in different representations of the human motor cortex. *J Neurophysiol*, **80**, 2870–2881.

Clark, S.A., Allard, T., Jenkins, W.M. and Merzenich, M.M. (1988). Receptive fields in the body-surface map in adult cortex defined by temporally correlated inputs. *Advan Neurol*, **63**, 187–200.

Classen, J., Liepert, J., Wise, S.P., Hallett, M. and Cohen, L.G. (1998). Rapid plasticity of human cortical movement representation induced by practice. *J Neurophysiol*, **79**, 1117–1123.

Cohen, L.G., Roth, B.J., Wassermann, E.M., Topka, H., Fuhr, P., Schultz, J. and Hallet, M. (1991). Magnetic stimulation of the human cerebral cortex, an indicator or reorganization in motor pathways in certain pathological conditions. *J Clin Neurophysiol*, **8**, 56–65.

Cole, J. and Glees, P. (1951). The recovery of manual ability after lesions in the hanad area of the sensory cortex in monkeys. *J Physiol*, **115**, 1–15.

Conner, J.M., Culberson, A., Packowski, C., Chiba, A.A. and Tuszynski, M.H. (2003). Lesions of the basal forebrain cholinergic system impair task acquisition and abolish cortical plasticity associated with motor skill learning. *Neuron*, **38**, 819–829.

Curt, A., Alkadhi, H., Crelier, G.R., Boendermaker, S.H., Hepp-Reymond, M.C. and Kolliass, S.S. (2002). Changes of non-affected upper limb cortical representation in paraplegic patients as assessed by fMRI. *Brain*, **125**, 2567–2578.

Donoghue, J.P. (2002). Connecting cortex to machines: recent advances in brain interfaces. *Nat Neurosci Suppl*, **5**, 1085–1088.

Donoghue, J.P. and Sanes, J.N. (1988). Organization of adult motor cortex representation patterns following neonatal forelimb nerve injury in rats. *J Neurosci*, **8**, 3221–3232.

Donoghue, J.P., Suner, S. and Sanes, J.N. (1990). Dynamic organization of primary motor cortex output to target muscles in adult rats. II. Rapid reorganization following motor nerve lesions. *Exp Brain Res*, **79**, 492–503.

Donoghue, J.P., Hess, G. and Sanes, J.N. (1996). Substrates and mechanisms for learning in motor cortex. In: *The Acquisition of Motor Behavior in Vertebrates* (eds Bloedel, J.R., Ebner, T.J. and Wise S.P.), The MIT Press, Cambridge, MA, London, England.

Donoghue, J.P., Sanes, J.N., Hatsopoulos, N.G. and Gaal, G. (1998). Neural discharge and local field potential oscillations in primate motor cortex during voluntary movements. *J Neurophysiol*, **79**, 159–173.

Donoghue, J.P., Leibovic, S. and Sanes, J.N. (2002). Organization of the forelimb area in squirrel monkey cortex: representation of digit, wrist, and elbow muscles. *Exp Brain Res*, **89**, 1–19.

Donoghue, J.P., Saleh, M., Caplan, A., Serruya, M.D., Morris, D.J., Ramchandani S., Ojakangas, C. and Friehs, G. (2003). Direct control of a computer cursor by frontal cortical ensembles in humans: prospects for neural prosthetic control. *Society for Neuroscience, Abstract* 607.9.

Ehninger, D. and Kempermann, G. (2003). Regional effects of wheel running and environmental enrichment on cell genesis and microglia proliferation in the adult murine neocortex. *Cerebr Cortex*, **13**, 845–851.

Elbert, T., Pantev, C., Wienbruch, C., Rockstroh, B. and Taub, E. (1995). Increased cortical representation of the fingers of the left hand in string players. *Science*, **270**, 305–307.

Emsley, J.G., Mitchell, B.D., Kempermann, G., Macklis, J.D. (2005). Adult neurogenesis and repair of the adult CNS with neural progenitors, precursors, and stem cells. *Prog Neurobiol* **75**, 321–341.

Engert, F. and Bonhoeffer, T. (1999). Dendritic spine changes associated with hippocampal long-term synaptic plasticity. *Nature*, **399**, 66–70.

Eriksson, P.S., Perfilieva, E., Bjork-Eriksson, T., Alborn, A., Nordborg, C., Peterson, D.A. and Gage, F.H. (1988). Neurogenesis in the adult human hippocampus. *Nat Med*, **4**, 1313–1317.

Ferrier, D. (1873/1874). The localization of function in the brain. *Proc Roy Soci London*, **22**, 228–232.

Friehs, G.M., Zerris, V.A., Ojakangas, C.L., Fellows, M.R. and Donoghue, J.P. (2004). Brain–machine and brain computer interfaces. *Stroke*, **35**(**11 Suppl. 1**), 2702–2705.

Fritsch, G. and Hitzig, E. (1870). Ueber die elektrische Erregbarkeit des Grosshirns. *Arch Anatom Physiol Wissenschaft Med Leipzig*, **37**, 300–332.

Frost, S.B., Barbay, S., Friel, K.M., Plautz, E.J. and Nudo, R.J. (2003). Reorganization of remote cortical regions after ischemic brain injury: a potential substrate for stroke recovery. *J Neurophysiol*, **89**, 3205–3214.

Fuchs, E. and Gould, E. (2000). *In vivo* neurogenesis in the adult brain: regulation and functional implications. *Eur J Neurosci*, **12**, 2211–2214.

Fuhr, P., Cohen, L.G., Dang, N., Findley, T.W., Haghighi, S., Oro, J. and Hallett, M. (1992). Physiological analysis of motor reorganization following lower limb amputation. *Electroencephalogr Clin Neurophysiol*, **85**, 53–60.

Gaser, C. and Schlaug, G. (2003). Brain structures differ between musicians and non-musicians. *J Neurosci*, **23**, 9240–9245.

Goff, B. (1969). Appropriate afferent stimulation. *Physiotherapy*, **55**, 9–17.

Gould, E., Reeves, A.J., Graziano, M.S. and Gross, C.G. (1999). Neurogenesis in the neocortex of adult primates. *Science*, **286**, 548–552.

Graham Brown, T. and Sherrington, C.S. (1912). On the instability of a cortical point. *Proc Roy Soci London*, **85**, 250–277.

Grünbaum, A.S.F. and Sherrington, C. (1903). Observations on physiology of the cerebral cortex of some of the higher apes. *Proc Roy Soc London*, **72**, 152–209.

Hatsopoulos, N., Joshi, J. and O'Leary, J.G. (2004). Decoding continuous and discrete motor behaviors using motor and premotor cortical ensembles. *J Neurophysiol*, **92**, 1165–1174.

He, Y., Janssen, W.G.M. and Morrison, J.H. (1998). Synaptic coexistence of AMPA and NMDA receptors in the rat hippocampus: a postembedding immunogol study. *J Neurosci Res*, **54**, 444–449.

Hess, G. and Donoghue, J.P. (1994). Long-term potentiation of horizontal connections provides a mechanism to reorganize cortical motor maps. *J Neurophysiol*, **71**, 2543–2547.

Hess, G. and Donoghue, J.P. (1996). Long-term depression of horizontal connections in rat motor cortex. *Eur J Neurosci*, **8**, 658–665.

Hess, G., Jacobs, K.M. and Donoghue, J.P. (1994). *N*-methyl-D-aspartate receptor mediated component of field potentials evoked in horizontal pathways of rat motor cortex. *Neuroscience*, **61**, 225–235.

Hess, G., Aizenman, C.D. and Donoghue, J.P. (1996). Conditions for the induction of long-term potentiation in layer II/III horizontal connections of the rat motor cortex. *J Neurophysiol*, **75**, 1765–1778.

Holsapple, J.W., Preston, J.B. and Strick, P.L. (1991). The origin of thalamic inputs to the "hand" representation in the primary motor cortex. *J Neurosci*, **11**, 2644–2654.

Humm, J.L., Kozlowski, D.A., Bland, S.T., James, D.C. and Schallert, T. (1998). Use-dependent exaggeration of brain injury: is glutamate involved? *Exp Neurol*, **157**, 349–358.

Huntley, G.W. (1997). Correlation between patterns of horizontal connectivity and the extent of short-term representational plasticity in rat motor cortex. *Cerebral Cortex*, **7**, 143–156.

Huntley, G.W. and Jones, E.G. (1991). Relationship of intrinsic connections to forelimb movement representations in monkey motor cortex: a correlative anatomic and physiological study. *J Neurophysiol*, **66**, 390–413.

Jackson, J.H. (1863). Convulsive spasms of the right hand and arm preceding epileptic seizures. *Med Time Gazette*, **2**, 110–111.

Jacobs, K.M. and Donoghue, J.P. (1991). Reshaping the cortical motor map by unmasking latent intracortical connections. *Science*, **251**, 944–947.

Johansson, B.B. and Ohlsson, A.L. (1996). Environment, social interaction, and physical activity as determinants of functional outcome after cerebral infarction in the rat. *Exp Neurol*, **139**, 322–327.

Jones, T.A. (1999). Multiple synapse formation in the motor cortex opposite unilateral sensorimotor cortex lesions in adult rats. *J Comp Neurol*, **414**, 57–66.

Kaas, J.H. and Qi, H.-K. (2004). The reorganization of the motor system in primates after the loss of a limb. *Restor Neurol Neurosci*, **22**, 145–152.

Kaplan, M.S. and Hinds, J.W. (1977). Neurogenesis in the adult rat: electron microscopic analysis of light radioautographs. *Science*, **197**, 1092–1094.

Karni, A., Meyer, G., Jezzard, P., Adams, M.M., Turner, R. and Ungerleider, L.G. (1995). Functional MRI evidence for adult motor cortex plasticity during motor skill learning. *Nature*, **377**, 155–158.

Karni, A., Meyer, G., Rey-Hipolito, C., Jezzard, P., Adams, M.M., Turner, R. and Ungerleider, L.G. (1998). The acquisition of skilled motor performance: fast and slow experience-driven changes in primary motor cortex. *Proc Natl Acad Sci*, **95**, 861–868.

Keller, A. and Asanuma, H. (1993). Synaptic relationships involving local axon collaterals of pyramidal neurons in the cat motor cortex. *J Comparat Neurol*, **336**, 229–242.

Kennedy, P.R. and Bakay, R.A.E. (1998). Restoration of neural output from a paralyzed patient by a direct brain connection. *NeuroReport*, **9**, 193–208.

Kennedy, P.R., Bakay, R.A.E., Moore, M.M., Adams, K. and Goldwaithe, J. (2000). Direct control of a computer from the human central nervous system. *IEEE Trans Rehabil Eng*, **8**, 198–202.

Kleim, J.A., Lussnig, E., Schwarz, E.R., Comery, T.A. and Greeough, W.R. (1996). Synaptogenesis and FOS expression in the motor cortex of the adult rat after motor skill learning. *J Neurosci*, **16**, 4529–4535.

Kleim, J.A., Barbay S. and Nudo R.J. (1998). Functional reorganization of the rat motor cortex following motor skill learning. *J Neurophysiol*, **80**, 3321–3325.

Kleim, J.A., Barbay, S., Cooper, N.R., Hogg, T.M., Reidel, C.N., Remple, M.S. and Nudo, R.J. (2002). Motor learning-dependent synaptogenesis is localized to functionally reorganized motor cortex. *Neurobiol Learn Memory*, **77**, 63–77.

Kleim, J.A., Hogg, T.M., VandenBerg, P.M., Cooper, N.R., Bruneau, R. and Remple, M.S. (2004). Cortical synaptogenesis and motor map reorganization occur during late, but not early, phase of motor skill learning. *J Neurosci*, **24**, 628–633.

Koketsu, D., Mikami, A., Miyamoto, Y. and Hisatsune, T. (2003). Nonrenewal of neurons in the cerebral neocortex of adult macaque monkeys. *J Neurosci*, **23**, 937–942.

Kornack, D.R. and Rakic, P. (1999). Continuation of neurogenesis in the hippocampus of the adult macaque monkey. *Proc Natl Acad Sci USA*, **96**, 5768–5773.

Kornack, D.R. and Rakic, P. (2001). Cell proliferation without neurogenesis in adult primate neocortex. *Science*, **294**, 2127–2130.

Kozlowski, D.A., James, D.C. and Schallert, T. (1996). Use-dependent exaggeration of neuronal injury after unilateral sensorimotor cortex lesions. *J Neurosci*, **16**, 4776–4786.

Landry, P. and Deschennes, M. (1981). Intracortical arborizations and receptive fields of identified ventrobasl thalamo-cortical afferents to the primary somatic sensory cortex in the cat. *J Comparat Neurol*, **199**, 345–371.

Lashley, K.S. (1923). Cerebral organization and behavior. *Res Publ Assoc Res Nerv Ment Dis*, **36**, 1–4.

Lauer, R.T., Peckham, P.H. and Kilgore, K.L. (1999). EEG-based control of a hand grasp neuroprosthesis. *NeuroReport*, **10**, 1767–1771.

Leyton, A.S.F. and Sherrington, C.S. (1917). Observation on the excitable cortex of the chimpanzee, orangutan and gorilla. *Quart J Exp Physiol*, **11**, 135–222.

Liepert, J., Tenenthoff, M. and Malin, J.-P. (1995). Changes of cortical motor area size during immobilization. *Electroencephalogr Clin Neurophysiol*, **97**, 382–386.

Liu, Y. and Rouiller, E.M. (1999). Mechanisms of recovery of dexterity following unilateral lesion of the sensorimotor cortex in adult monkeys. *Exp Brain Res*, **128**, 149–159.

Malenka, R.C. and Nicoll, R.A. (1993). NMDA-receptor-dependent synaptic plasticity: multiple forms and mechanisms. *Trend Neurosci*, **16**, 521–527.

Mark, V.W. and Taub, E. (2002). Constraint-induced movement therapy for chronic stroke hemiparesis and other disabilities. *Restor Neurol Neurosci*, **22**, 317–336.

Markus, E.J. and Petit, T.L. (1987). Neocortical synaptogenesis, aging, and behavior: lifespan development in the motor-sensory system of the rat. *Exp Neurol*, **96**, 262–268.

Matthews, P.M., Johansen-Berg, H. and Reddy, H. (2004). Non-invasive mapping of brain functions and brain recovery: applying lessons from cognitive neuroscience to neurorehabilitation. *Restor Neurol Neurosci*, **22**, 245–260.

Merzenich, M.M, Kaas, J.H., Wall, J., Nelson, R.J., Sur, M. and Felleman, D. (1983a). Topographic reorganization of somatosensory cortical areas 3b and 1 in adult monkeys following restricted deafferentation. *Neuroscience*, **8**, 33–55.

Merzenich, M.M., Kaas, J.H., Wall, J.T., Sur, M., Nelson, R.J. and Felleman, D.J. (1983b). Progression of change following median nerve section in the cortical representation of the hand in areas 3b and 1 in adult owl and squirrel monkeys. *Neuroscience*, **10**, 639–655.

Merzenich, M.M., Nelson, R.J., Stryker, M.P., Cynader M.S., Schoppmann, A. and Zook, J.M. (1984). Somatosensory cortical map changes following digit amputation in adult monkeys. *J Comparat Neurol*, **224**, 591–605.

Mogilner, A., Grossman, J.A., Ribary, U., Joliot, M., Volkmann, J., Rapaport, D., Beasley, R.W. and Llinas, R.R. (1993). Somatosensory cortical plasticity in adult humans revealed by magnetoencephalography. *Proc Natl Acad Sci USA*, **90**, 3593–3597.

Miyai, I., Yagura, H., Oda, I., Konishi, I., Eda, H., Suzuki, T. and Kubota, K. (2002). Premotor cortex is involved in restoration of gait in stroke. *Ann Neurol*, **52**, 188–194.

Muellbacher, W., Ziemann, U., Boroojerdi, B., Cohen, L. and Hallett, M. (2001). Role of the human motor cortex in rapid motor learning. *Exp Brain Res*, **136**, 431–438.

Mukand, J.A., Williams, S., Shaikhouni, Am., Morris, D., Serruya, M. and Donoghue, J.P. (2004). Feasibility study of a neural interface system for quadriplegic patients. *Archiv Phys Med Rehabil*, **85**, E48.

Musallam, S., Corneil, B.D., Greger, B., Scherberger, H. and Andersen, R.A. (2004). Cognitive control signals for neural prosthetics. *Science*, **305**, 258–262.

Nelles, G. (2004). Cortical reorganization – effects of intensive therapy. *Restor Neurol Neurosci*, **22**, 239–244.

Nelles, G., Spiekermann, G., Jueptner, M., Leonhardt, G., Mueller, S., Gerhard, H. and Diener, H.C. (1999). Evolution of functional reorganization in hemiplegic stroke: a serial positron emission tomographic activation study. *Ann Neurol*, **46**, 901–909.

Nowakowski, R.S. and Hayes, N.L. (2000). New neurons: extraordinary evidence or extraordinary conclusion? *Science*, **288**, 771a.

Nudo, R.J., Milliken, G.W., Jenkins, W.M. and Merzenich, M.M. (1996a). Use-dependent alterations of movement representations in primary motor cortex of adult squirrel monkeys. *J Neurosci*, **16**, 787–807.

Nudo, R.J., Wise, Bm., SiFuentes, F. and Milliken, G.W. (1996b). Neural substrates for the effects of rehabilitative training on motor recovery after ischemic infarct. *Science*, **272**, 1791–1794.

Ohlsson, A.-L. and Johansson, B.B. (1995). Environment influences functional outcome of cerebral infarction in rats. *Stroke*, **26**, 644–649.

Ojakangas, C.L., Shaikhouni, A., Friehs, G.M. and Donoghue, J.P. (2004). Decoding of movement intent from human premotor cortical neurons. *Soc Neurosci Abstr*, 421.12.

Orsetti, M., Casamenti, F., Pepeu, G. (1996). Enhanced acetylcholine release in the hippocampus and cortex during acquisition of an operant behavior. *Brain Res*, **724**, 89–96.

Paci, M. (2003). Physiotherapy based on the Bobath concept for adults with post-stroke hemiplegia: a review of effectiveness studies. *J Rehabil Med*, **35**, 2–7.

Pascual-Leone, A., Dang, N., Cohen, L.G., Brasil-Neto, J.P., Cammarota, A. and Hallett, M. (1995). Modulation of muscle responses evoked by transcranial magnetic stimulation during the acquisition of new fine motor skills. *J Neurophysiol*, **74**, 1037–1045.

Patil, P.G., Carmena, J.M., Nicolelis, M.A. and Turner, D.A. (2004). Ensemble recordings of human subcortical neurons as a source of motor control signals for a brain–machine interface. *Neurosurgery*, **55**, 27–35; discussion 35–38.

Pearce, A.J., Thickbroom, G.W., Byrnes, M.L. and Mastaglia, F.L. (2000). Functional reorganisation of the corticomotor projection to the hand in skilled racquet players. *Exp Brain Res*, **130**, 238–243.

Penfield, W. and Boldrey, E. (1937). Somatic motor and sensory representation in the cerebral cortex of man as studied by electrical stimulation. *Brain*, **60**, 389–443.

Pesaran, B., Pezaris, J.S., Sahani, M., Mitra, P.P. and Andersen, R.A. (2002). Temporal structure in neuronal activity during working memory in macaque parietal cortex. *Nat Neurosci*, **5**, 805–811.

Pfurtscheller, G., Kalcher, J., Neuper, C., Flotzinger, D. and Pregenzer, M. (1996). On-line EEG classification during externally-paced hand movements using a neural network-based classifier. *Electroencephalogr Clin Neurophysiol*, **99**, 416–425.

Plautz, E.J., Milliken, G.W. and Nudo, R.J. (2000). Effects of repetitive motor training on movement representations in adult squirrel monkeys: role of use versus learning. *Neurobiol Learn Memory*, **74**, 27–55.

Rausell, E. and Jones, E.G. (1995). Extent of intracortical arborization of thalamocortical axons as a determinant of representational plasticity in monkey somatic sensory cortex. *J Neurosci*, **15**, 4270–4288.

Remple, M.S., Bruneau, R.M., VandenBerg, P.M., Goertzen, C. and Kleim, J.A. (2001). Sensitivity of cortical movement representations to motor experience: evidence that skill learning but not strength training induces cortical reorganization. *Behav Brain Res*, **123**, 133–141.

Rioult-Pedotti, M.-S., Friedman, D., Hess, G. and Donoghue, J.P. (1998). Strengthening of horizontal cortical connections following skill learning. *Nat Neurosci*, **1**, 230–234.

Rioult-Pedotti, M.-S., Friedman, D. and Donoghue, J.P. (2000). Learning-induced LTP in neocortex. *Science*, **290**, 533–536.

Rizzolatti, G., Fogassi, L. and Gallese, V. (2002). Motor and cognitive functions of the ventral premotor cortex. *Curr Opin Neurobiol*, **12**, 149–154.

Ryu, S.I., Santhanam, G., Yu, B.M. and Shenoy, K.V. (2004). High speed neural prosthetic icon positioning. *Soc Neurosci Abstr*, 263.1.

Sanes, J.N., Suner, S., Donoghue, J.P. (1990). Dynamic organization of primary motor cortex output to target muscles in adult rats. I. Long-term patterns of reorganization following motor or mixed peripheral nerve lesions. *Exp Brain Res*, **79**, 479–491.

Sanes, J.N., Wang, J. and Donoghue, J.P. (1992). Immediate and delayed changes of rat motor cortical output representation with new forelimb configurations. *Cerebr Cortex*, **2**, 141–152.

Schambra, H.M., Sawaki, L. and Cohen, L.G. (2003). Modulation of excitability of human motor cortex (MI) by 1Hz transcranial magnetic stimulation of the contralateral MI. *Clin Neurophysiol*, **114**, 130–133.

Seitz, R.J., Hoeflich, P., Binkofski, F., Tellmann, L., Herzog, H. and Freund, H.-J. (1998). Role of the premotor cortex in recovery from middle cerebral artery infarction. *Archiv Neurol*, **55**, 1081–1088.

Serruya, M.D., Hatsopoulos, N.G., Paninski, L., Fellows, M.R. and Donoghue, J.P. (2002). Instant neural control of a movement signal. *Nature*, **416**, 141–142.

Shadmehr, R. and Holcomb, H.H. (1997). Neural correlates of motor memory consolidation. *Science*, **277**, 821–825.

Shenoy, K.V., Meeker, D., Cao, S, Kureshi, S.A., Pesaran B., Buneo, C.A., Batista, A.P., Mitra, P.P., Burdick, J.W. and Andersen, R.A. (2003). Neural prosthetic control signals from plan activity. *NeuroReport*, **14**, 591–596.

Sorra, K.E. and Harris, K.M. (1998). Stability in synapse number and size at 2 h after long-term potentiation in hippocampal area CA1. *J Neurosci*, **18**, 658–671.

Stefan, K., Kunesch, E., Cohen, L.G., Benecke, R. and Classen, J. (2000). Induction of plasticity in the human motor cortex by paired associative stimulation. *Brain*, **123**, 572–584.

Stefan, K., Wycislo, M. and Classen J. (2004). Modulation of associative human motor cortical plasticity by attention. *J Neurophysiol*, **92**, 66–72.

Stepniewska, I., Preuss, T.M. and Kaas, J.H. (1993). Architectonics, somatotopic organization, and ipsilateral cortical connections of the primary motor area (MI) of owl monkeys. *J Comparat Neurol*, **33**, 238–271.

Taub, E., Uswatte, G. and Pidikiti, R. (1999). Constraint-induced movement therapy: a new family of techniques with broad application to physical rehabilitation – a clinical review. *J Rehabil Res Develop*, **36**, 237–251.

Taylor, D.M., Tillery, S.I. and Schwartz, A.B. (2002). Direct cortical control of 3D neuroprosthetic devices. *Science*, **296**, 1829–1832.

Thach, W.T. (1987). Cerebellar inputs to motor cortex. *Ciba Found Symp*, **132**, 201–220.

Toni, M., Buchs, P.-A., Nikonenko, I., Bron, C.R. and Muller, D. (1999). LTP promotes formation of multiple spine synapses between a single axon terminal and a dendrite. *Nature*, **402**, 421–425.

Trachtenberg, J.T., Chen, B.E., Knott, G.W., Feng, G., Sanes, J.R., Welker, E. and Svoboda, K. (2002). Long-term *in vivo* imaging of experience-dependent synaptic plasticity in adult cortex. *Nature*, **420**, 788–894.

Weiller, C., Chollet, F., Friston, K.J., Wise, R.J. and Frackowiak, R.S. (1992). Functional reorganization of the brain in recovery from striatocapsular infarction in man. *Ann Neurol*, **31**(**5**), 463–472.

Weiller, C., Ramsey, S.C., Wise, R.J., Friston, K.J. and Frackowiak, R.S. (1993). Individual patterns of functional reorganization in the human cerebral cortex after capsular infarction. *Ann Neurol*, **33**, 181–189.

Wessberg, J., Stambaugh, C.R., Kralik, J.D., Beck, P.D., Laubach, M., et al. (2000). Real-time prediction of hand trajectory by ensembles of cortical neurons in primates. *Nature*, **408**, 361–365.

Wolpaw, J.R., McFarland, D.J., Neat, G.W. and Forneris, C.A. (1991). An EEG-based brain–computer interface for cursor control. *Electroencephalogr Clin Neurophysiol*, **78**, 252–259.

Zarzeki, P. and Wiggin, D.M. (1982). Convergence of sensory inputs upon projection neurons of somatosensory cortex. *Exp Brain Res*, **48**, 28–42.

Zarzecki, P., Blum, P.S., Bakker, D.A. and Herman, D. (1983). Convergence of sensory inputs upon projection neurons of somatosensory cortex: vestibular, neck, head, and forelimb inputs. *Exp Brain Res*, **50**, 408–414.

Zarzecki P., Witte, P., Smits, E., Gordon, D., Kirchberger, P. and Rasmussen, D. (1993). Synaptic mechanisms of cortical representational plasticity: somatosensory and corticocortical EPSPs in reorganized raccoon SI cortex. *J Neurophysiol*, **69**, 1422–1432.

Ziemann, U., Hallet, M. and Cohen, L.G. (1998). Mechanisms of deafferentation-induced plasticity in human motor cortex. *J Neurosci*, **18**, 7000–7007.

Ziemann, U., Iliac, T.V., Pauli, C., Meintzschel, F. and Ruge, D. (2004). Learning modifies subsequent induction of long-term potentiation-like and long-term depression-like plasticity in human motor cortex. *J Neurosci*, **24**, 1666–1672.

Plasticity in visual connections: retinal ganglion cell axonal development and regeneration

Kurt Haas[1] and Hollis T. Cline[2]

[1]*Department of Cellular and Physiological Sciences, Brain Research Centre, University of British Columbia, Vancouver, BC, Canada*
[2]*Cold Spring Harbor Laboratory, Cold Spring Harbor, NY, USA*

9.1 Introduction

One of the leading challenges facing neuroscience research today is how to promote functional regeneration after neuronal damage within the human central nervous system (CNS). Unlike neurons in the peripheral nervous system (PNS), or CNS neurons in lower vertebrates, damaged mammalian CNS axons fail to reinitiate growth to re-establish functioning circuits (Richardson et al., 1982; Davies et al., 1996). Careful optimism to this problem has risen due to advances in our understanding of factors controlling axonal growth and circuit formation during both development and regeneration. Importantly, it is now clear that damaged mammalian CNS neurons posses the ability to survive and sprout new axons, but this regenerative capacity is dependent on cell responses and molecular signals in their local environment (Schnell and Schwab, 1990; Huang et al., 1999; Stichel et al., 1999; Bahr, 2000; Behar et al., 2000; Goldberg and Barres, 2000; Dergham et al., 2002; Ellezam et al., 2002; Koeberle and Ball, 2002). Once barriers preventing axonal sprouting following injury are overcome, regenerating axons must often rediscover convoluted paths to distant targets. The mechanisms axons use to navigate through complex three-dimensional tissue have become clearer since the discovery of numerous extracellular guidance molecules that attract or repel axonal growth cones (Li and David, 1996; Nakamoto et al., 1996; Kolodkin and Ginty,

1997; Brose et al., 1999; Stuermer and Bastmeyer, 2000; Wilkinson, 2001). Even when challenges associated with promotion of new axonal sprouting and rediscover of pathways to denervated targets are solved, a final hurdle to regeneration remains. The ability to fully recapture the functionality of a severed neuronal circuit requires the re-establishment of the specific and highly complex patterns of synaptic connections between afferent and target neurons. In this chapter, we will discuss current knowledge of how precisely ordered afferent synaptogenesis occurs during development, and the potential for reforming functional circuits by correct rewiring during regeneration.

9.2 Development of retinotectal connections

Most of our knowledge of the mechanisms involved in establishing circuits between distant CNS neuronal populations comes from studies of the axonal projection from the eye to central brain targets (Sperry, 1943, 1963; Gaze, 1970; Horder and Martin, 1978; Jacobson, 1978). The output neurons of the eye are the retinal ganglion cells (RGCs), whose axons exit the eye as the optic nerve, cross the midline at the optic chiasm, and innervate central brain structures. This axonal tract has proven ideal for studies of axonal development and regeneration due to the accessibility of the optic nerve for discrete lesion, the compartmentalization of projection and target neuronal populations for restricted pharmacological treatment, and the highly ordered pattern of RGC axonal terminations (Sperry, 1943; Gaze and Jacobson, 1963; Fujisawa et al., 1982). The capacity of lower vertebrates to readily regenerate the optic nerve has allowed their use as model systems for examination and comparison of the formation of patterned afferent synaptogenesis during development and rewiring following axonal damage.

Visuotopic specificity of retinotectal innervation

The pattern of connections between RGCs and their target tissue, the optic tectum in lower vertebrates, is similar to many afferent projections in that it maintains the spatial properties of information from the afferent input to the retinorecipient target (Gaze, 1958). This order is accomplished in the retinotectal system by preserving the same spatial relationships between the positions of the soma of RGCs in the retina and the tectal neurons with which they form synapses. Maintaining such near-neighbor connections creates a topographic representation of the retinal input, and therefore visual space, in the tectum. Physically, the retina is mapped onto the tectum by axons of RGCs in dorsal retina terminating in the ventral tectum, ventral retina RGCs projecting to dorsal tectum, nasal RGCs projecting to caudal tectum, and temporal retina RGC axons terminating in rostral tectum (Sperry, 1963; Walter et al., 1987a, b; Godement and Bonhoeffer, 1989; Vielmetter and Stuermer, 1989; Roskies and O'Leary, 1994).

During early development of fish and frogs, the first RGC axons enter the optic tectum as simple projections that terminate in retinotopically appropriate regions (Holt and Harris, 1983; Holt, 1984; Sakaguchi and Murphey, 1985). Thus the retinotectal map is established at the earliest stages of RGC innervation. After reaching their target zones, RGC axons extend branches to form arborizations, which grow to cover relatively large regions of the tectum (Sakaguchi and Murphey, 1985). While the tectum

continues to grow, however, RGC axonal arbors do not expand their tangential extent. Therefore, the relative size of RGC axonal arbors compared to the entire tectum decreases throughout development (Gaze et al., 1974; Sretavan and Shatz, 1984; Sakaguchi and Murphey, 1985). This shift in the relative size of axon arbors compared to the tectal field is supported by electrophysiological recordings of tectal neurons demonstrating a progressive decrease in the area of tectum responding to a region of visual space with maturation. Thus, in normal development the retinotopic map goes through stages of initial highly ordered RGC axonal termination, followed by extensive axonal arborization, and subsequent refinement of the map through an increase in tectum size and a decrease in receptive field size.

Sperry's Chemoaffinity Hypothesis

Mechanisms underlying the development of topographic axonal terminations has been the center of much debate for more than 30 years (Cline, 2003). In the 1960s, Sperry put forth a model proposing that the retinotopic map is created by RGC axons detecting unique molecular cues on specific tectal neurons (Sperry, 1963). This system, however, would require a one-to-one chemical address system conferring preordered assignment of distinct tectal neuronal targets for each RGC axon. The tremendous amount of genetically encoded information for such an address system led Sperry to simplify his model. The new model, coined the Sperry Chemoaffinity Hypothesis, suggested that unique addresses can be conferred using a small number of chemical cues, distributed in gradients of different orientations. In the simplest case, the target tissue would express two chemical cues distributed in gradients orthogonal to each other. All RGC axons would express receptors to detect both cues, but individual RGCs would be uniquely sensitive to the concentration of each cue. Depending on its position in the retina, an RGC's axon would have unique receptor expression or responsivity to guidance molecules distributed in gradients in the target that promote axonal termination at a specific point within two dimensions of the target tissue.

Evidence supporting the Sperry Chemoaffinity Hypothesis has been found throughout the retinotectal pathway. Secreted and membrane-bound guidance cues provide both attractive and repulsive influence directing growth of RGC axons across the retina and into the optic nerve (Deiner et al., 1997), across the optic chiasm (Niclou et al., 2000; Plump et al., 2002), and towards the tectum. RGC axons from the same eye in developing frogs and fish, or homonymous hemiretina mammals, make similar decisions at choice points while growing from the eye to the tectum. However, once they reach the tectum, each axon must find an appropriate and unique termination zone. A role for the Sperry Chemoaffinity Hypothesis in the patterning of RGC axonal termination within the tectum is supported by the expression of members of the ephrin family of extracellular proteins in the tectum and corresponding expression of their receptors, the Eph receptors, in RGCs (Wilkinson, 2001) (Fig. 9.1). Ephrin-A (glycosylphosphatidylinositol (GPI) linked) and ephrin-B (transmembrane)

ligands bind to EphA and EphB tyrosine kinase receptors, respectively. As predicted by Sperry, Eph receptors and ephrin ligands are expressed in complimentary gradients in the retina and tectum during development (Frisen et al., 1998; Hornberger et al., 1999). Eph receptors are expressed on RGC axonal growth cones and ephrin/Eph guidance of RGC axonal growth cone motility has been shown to be a major contributor to the initial establishment of the retinotectal projection (Drescher et al., 1997; Flanagan and Vanderhaeghen, 1998; O'Leary and Wilkinson, 1999). Repulsion of RGC axonal growth cones by ephrin-As (Nakamoto et al., 1996) mediates ordering of the temporal/nasal retinal axis projection onto the anterior/posterior axis of the tectum (Feldheim et al., 2000; Sakurai et al., 2002; McLaughlin et al., 2003), while ephrin-Bs/Eph-B interactions control development of the dorsal/ventral retinal axis mapping to the lateral/medial tectal axis (Hindges et al., 2002; Mann et al., 2002).

The preponderance of evidence supporting the chemoaffinity model for controlling axonal growth and ordered termination has fueled speculation

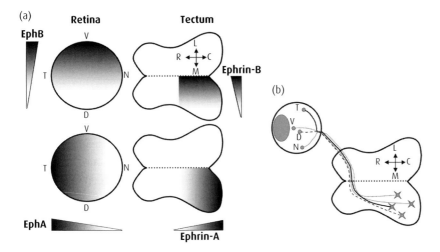

Figure 9.1. *Chemoaffinity in the development of retinotectal projections.* (a) Gradients of expression levels of Eph receptors in the retina and ephrin ligands in the tectum guide RGC axons to correct termination zones in the tectum. EphB receptors and ephrin-B ligands establish the dorsal (D)/ventral (V) retinal axis onto the medial (M)/lateral (L) tectum, and EphA receptors in the retina and ephrin-A ligands in tectum orientate the retinal temporal (T)/nasal (N) axis onto the rostral (R)/caudal (C) dimension of the tectum. (b) As predicted by the Sperry Chemoaffinity Hypothesis, Eph/ephrin gradients guide axons from RGCs at different positions in the retina to specific termination zones within the tectum.

that guidance molecules may be both necessary and sufficient to produce the complex synaptic patterning between afferent projections and their targets. However, an independent model for how neuronal populations wire together was concurrently developing and was also supported by convincing data. This model, based largely on the theoretical work of Hebb (1949) implicated patterned neuronal activity as a major influence for directing formation of ordered afferent-target maps (Hebb, 1949). Hebbian models state that correlated activity between afferent and target neurons mediates synapse strengthening and weakening. Furthermore, Hebbian models predict that the correlation of activity between pairs of projection neurons that synapse on the same target neurons dictates whether these synapses will be strengthened (by correlated activity), or weakened (by uncorrelated activity). Studies on the formation of ocular dominance columns in mammalian primary visual cortex found that the formation of eye-specific innervation to cortical neurons is sensitive to visual experience during a critical period in development (Wiesel and Hubel, 1963, 1965; Hubel and Wiesel, 1977). These results suggested that neuronal activity is necessary, if not sufficient for the development of organized afferent innervation (Katz and Shatz, 1996). Thus, two distinct models of how ordered networks form have competed for scientific acceptance.

Crucial findings that helped to reconcile these apparently conflicting models come from an elegant series of experiments designed to separate molecular guidance and activity cues in the same system. These studies forced duplicate, molecularly identical, RGC populations that received different neuronal activity to innervate the same tectal target tissue. In one version of this approach, an additional eye primordium was graphed onto the tadpole embryo's head (Constantine-Paton and Law, 1978). The implanted tissue developed into a functional ectopic eye projecting RGC axons to the optic tectum, forming dually innervated tecta. A similar experiment grafted duplicate portions of retina to one eye to create double-nasal or double-temporal retinae (Ide et al., 1983; Coletti et al., 1990). In each of these cases, duplicate populations of RGCs expressing the same receptors for guidance molecules innervated the optic tectum. Therefore, axons from pairs of spatially separated RGCs, receiving stimulation from different regions of visual space, were directed to the same tectal locations by identical chemoaffinity cues. If chemoaffinity cues were solely responsible for establishing the retinotopic map, it would be expected that the RGC axonal terminal arborizations from ectopic and endogenous populations would completely overlap. In general, chemoaffinity rules are followed, with the RGC axons from both endogenous and ectopic populations terminating according to a crude topography. However, in the case of three-eyed frogs the RGC axonal terminal arborizations of the two eyes do not intermingle, but segregate into eye-specific termination zones, or ocular dominance bands. Similar bands arise in double-nasal or double-temporal retinae and when both endogenous eyes are forced to innervate a single tectum by the early ablation of one tectum (Straznicky and Glastonbury, 1979; Law and Constantine-Paton, 1980; Ruthazer et al., 2003; Ruthazer and Cline, 2004). These similar results from three separate types of surgical manipulations demonstrate that RGC axons segregate from other RGC axons programmed to recognize identical tectal targets if these RGC somas are not physically located next to each other. It seemed unlikely that this segregation could be due to additional chemoaffinity cues since no distribution of guidance molecules corresponding to these bands has been found within the tectum, and would not be expected in a tissue that is normally innervated by a single afferent input. These results suggest that a force independent of chemoaffinity must exist.

The role of patterned neuronal activity and *N*-methyl-ᴅ-aspartate receptors

The origins of ocular dominance bands in dually innervated tectum was elucidated by the critical findings that their formation requires correlated neuronal activity (Meyer, 1982; Boss and Schmidt, 1984; Cline et al., 1987; Ruthazer et al., 2003). Intraocular injection of the sodium channel blocker, tetrodotoxin (TTX), which inhibits action potential firing, eliminates band formation (Knoll et al., 2001). Likewise, band formation is prevented by tectal exposure to N-methyl-D-aspartate (NMDA) receptor antagonists, which block the postsynaptic detection of correlated afferent activity (Cline et al., 1987; Ruthazer et al., 2003). Furthermore, since retinal (Reh and Constantine-Paton, 1985) or tectal (Cline et al., 1987) activity blockade cause dispersion of existing ocular dominance bands, activity is required to both establish and maintain ocular RGC axonal segregation. In normal animals, intraocular TTX injection during development of the retinotectal projection does not prevent the establishment of a crude retinotopic organization of RGC afferents in the tectum (Kobayashi et al., 1990; Kaethner and Stuermer, 1994). However, the resulting retinotopic maps are abnormal with enlarged RGC terminal fields. Blocking postsynaptic retinotectal activity by tectal exposure to NMDA receptor antagonists also decreases precision of the RGC retinotopic projection (Cline and Constantine-Paton, 1989; Simon and O'Leary, 1992), although it did not result in increased RGC axonal arbor size (Reh and Constantine-Paton, 1985). This indicates that NMDA receptor activity controls the topographic position of RGC axons in the tectum, but does not control their overall growth.

The requirement for NMDA receptor-mediated transmission supports Hebbian-type mechanisms underlying activity-dependent refinement, in which correlated presynaptic and postsynaptic activity promotes strengthening of synaptic connections. Likewise, synaptic activity that is uncorrelated to postsynaptic activity leads to weakening of those synapses (Hebb, 1949; Stent, 1973). NMDA receptors play an essential role in detecting correlated pre- and postsynaptic activity because they are opened by glutamate released from RGC axonal terminals, but only transmit ions when magnesium ions (Mg^{2+}) blocking their pores are removed by sufficient postsynaptic depolarization (Nowak et al., 1984). Once Mg^{2+} blockade is removed, NMDA receptors are permeable to Ca^{2+}, which activates second messenger cascades mediating synaptic plasticity. Pairing RGC and tectal neuronal activity produces strengthening,

or long-term potentiation (LTP) of retinotectal synapses (Zhang et al., 1998), while uncorrelated activity results in weakening, or long-term depression (LTD), of these synapses (Zhang et al., 1998, 2000; Tao et al., 2001). Morphological studies show that upon reaching appropriate target zones within the tectum, RGC axons extend large arbors that overlap with the arbors of many other RGC axons (Sakaguchi and Murphey, 1985). When the two RGCs with overlapping axonal arbors terminate on dendrites of the same tectal neurons, correlated activity between these RGCs will depolarize the tectal cell dendrite to a greater extent than when one fires alone. Excitation from converging axons is more likely to release postsynaptic Mg^{2+} blockade of NMDA receptors and promote strengthening of activated retinotectal synapses. When activity of two RGCs converging onto a single tectal dendrite is uncorrelated, their activity would not promote NMDA receptor-mediated synaptic strengthening. Rather, RGC activity uncorrelated to strong postsynaptic activity would be expected to lead to weakening of these synapses (Zhang et al., 1998). This model predicts that pairs of RGCs with axonal terminal that overlap onto the same tectal neuron dendritic arbors will promote strengthening of each others retinotectal synapses if these RGCs fire in close temporal proximity, and pairs not firing together will lead to weakening of their synapses.

Research from a number of studies suggests that neuronal activity is not simply permissive for ordered synaptogenesis. In fact, strong visual stimulation that excites the entire retina, created by bright strobe light illumination, actually prevents activity-dependent refinement of the retinotopic map (Meyer, 1983; Schmidt and Eisele, 1985; Cook and Rankin, 1986; Schmidt and Buzzard, 1993). Strobe light stimulation uniformly excites RGCs across the retina, inducing synchronous discharge of RGC axons. RGC axonal arbors and electrophysiologically measured tectal neuron receptive fields fail to refine normally following rearing under stroboscopic lighting conditions (Schmidt and Buzzard, 1993). These results indicate that activity itself is not critical, but that patterned activity that increases correlated firing between near RGCs, but not distant RGCs, is required for retinotopy refinement.

In mammalian systems, but not frogs or fish, the requirement for patterned activity to achieve map refinement raises theoretical challenges since refinement of the RGC projection occurs at developmental stages prior to photoreceptor function. How can RGCs express the spatially correlated patterns of activity required for axonal arbor refinement without visual stimuli? In fact, recordings of immature retina have found waves of activity propagating across the RGC layer (Meister et al., 1991; Wong et al., 1993; Feller et al., 1996; Mooney et al., 1996). These internally generated waves of activity create an ideal situation for activity-dependent, Hebbian type refinement. During wave propagation, RGCs from nearby locations in the retina fire patterns of action potentials with greater temporal correlation than RGCs from distant regions. Evidence that this early retinal activity contributes to retinotectal map formation comes from findings that retinal exposure to TTX (Shatz and Stryker, 1988; Sretavan et al., 1988) or cholinergic antagonists (Penn et al., 1998) block RGC wave activity and disrupt ordered RGC termination in the mammalian lateral geniculate nucleus. Similarly, knockout animals, lacking the β2 subunit of the acetylcholine receptor (AChR) in RGC, lack spontaneous waves of activity in the retina and demonstrate reduced ability to organize a topographic retino-geniculate projection (McLaughlin et al., 2003b). In this way, the CNS produces internally generated patterns of activity capable of promoting Hebbian activity-dependent refinement between projection and target neuronal populations when sensory organs are not yet functional. Once photoreceptor cells develop and the retinal circuit is able to process visual stimulation, evidence indicates that patterned light input drives activity-dependent retinotectal synaptic and morphologic plasticity (Katz and Shatz, 1996). Indeed, visual stimulation has been shown to rapidly alter tectal neuronal receptive field properties (Engert et al., 2002). The possibility that similar activity waves contribute to patterned synaptogenesis between distant loci in other regions of the CNS is supported by the discovery of activity waves in newborn rodent cortex (Garaschuk et al., 2000).

Results from these experiments have given rise to a model in which chemoaffinity cues direct RGC axons to appropriate regions within the tectum, producing a crude retinotopic map. Subsequent activity-dependent mechanisms driven by patterned retinal stimulation and correlated RGC/tectal neuron activity refine the retinotectal projection (O'Leary and Cowan, 1983; Shatz and Stryker, 1988). Therefore, the formation of highly orderly afferent innervation of target tissues in the CNS, such as the retinotopic maps, results from a collaboration of 'Sperry-type' chemoaffinity cues and 'Hebbian-type' activity-dependent synaptogenesis. Combining hard-wired patterning with variable sculpting by sensory input allows adaptation to an unpredictable environment (Fig. 9.2a, b).

9.3 Regeneration of retinotectal connections in mature animals

Initially imprecise reinnervation suggests reduced influence of chemoaffinity

Insights from these studies of the developing retinotectal projection lead to a series of questions associated with regeneration of this circuit following optic nerve damage. To what extent does regeneration recapitulate development? Do regenerating RGC axons use chemoaffinity cues and activity-dependent mechanisms to re-establish functional topographic maps? Are the gradients of guidance molecules and their receptors required for chemoaffinity orientation present during regeneration? Can complete recovery of function be achieved? These questions have been addressed by severing or crushing the optic nerve in animals capable of regeneration (Sperry, 1943, 1963; Attardi and Sperry, 1963; Gaze and Jacobson, 1963; Gaze and Keating, 1970; Fujisawa et al., 1982; Stuermer and Easter, 1984; Udin and Fawcett, 1988). RGCs in fish and frogs survive optic nerve lesion and sprout new axonal extensions that correctly navigate to the tectum, reform the retinotectal map, and demonstrate visual responsivity. Extensive experiments in these systems reveal

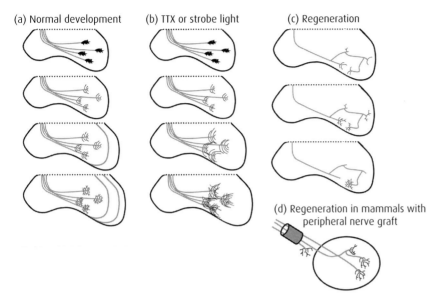

(a) Normal development   (b) TTX or strobe light   (c) Regeneration

(d) Regeneration in mammals with peripheral nerve graft

Figure 9.2. *Role of neuronal activity in refinement of retinotectal maps.* (a) During normal development of the retinotectal projection, RGC axons initially innervate the tectum as simple processes directed by growth cones to appropriate termination zones. Only after reaching target zones, do RGC axons arborize. With time, RGC arbors increase in complexity while the tectum grows. An important contribution to the process of map refinement with development is the relatively small increase in the tangential extent of the axon arbor compared to the vast increase in size of the tectal field. (b) When retinotectal activity is blocked by retinal exposure to TTX or synchronized by exposure to strobe illumination, RGC axonal arbors grow larger than normal and retinal topography is disrupted. When the tectum is exposed to NMDA receptor antagonists, retinal axon arbor size is normal but topography is disrupted because the arbors project to topographically incorrect sites. These results demonstrate involvement of Hebbian activity-dependent mechanisms for retinotectal map refinement. (c) During regeneration in lower vertebrates, RGC axons re-innervate the tectum in a disorganized fashion, extending branches into inappropriate regions and taking circuitous routes before locating appropriate termination zones. With time, retinotectal map refinement can be achieved. (d) Regeneration of the mammalian retino-collicular pathway is possible using a peripheral nerve graft creating a permissive environment for RGC axonal growth. However, these conditions are still not optimal for reinnervation since few RGC axons survive, some axons synapse indiscriminately upon exiting the graft and sparse innervation of the target appears to limit activity-dependent refinement.

similarities and differences between development and regeneration. In contrast to development, in which initial projections are fairly accurate, the regenerating retinotectal projection progresses in a stepwise fashion, initially forming a diffuse projection, which is then refined (Gaze and Jacobson, 1963; Westerman, 1965; Gaze and Keating, 1970; Meyer, 1980; Fujisawa et al., 1982; Humphrey and Beazley, 1982; Murray and Edwards, 1982; Schmidt et al., 1984; Stuermer and Easter, 1984). While RGC axons during development typically grow directly to appropriate termination zones before extending arbors, regenerating RGC axons initially innervate the tectum with

less order. Regenerating RGC axons take circuitous routes and extend branches to aberrant target zones before finding appropriate target zones (Meyer, 1980; Fujisawa, 1981; Adamson and Grobstein, 1982; Fujisawa et al., 1982; Humphrey and Beazley, 1982; Murray and Edwards, 1982; Schmidt et al., 1984; Stuermer and Easter, 1984; Rankin and Cook, 1986; Stuermer, 1988a, b). During early stages of regeneration, RGC axonal arbors show a high incidence of severely misguided RGC axons outside normal termination zones (Fujisawa et al., 1982; Schmidt et al., 1984; Johnson et al., 1999). Over time, mistargeted branches are selectively retracted (Schmidt et al.,

1988; Stuermer, 1988a, b). Ectopic axons and branches farthest from the center of the arbor have a higher rate of retraction, and this pruning results in condensation of the arbor (Schmidt et al., 1988; Stuermer, 1988a, b; Johnson et al., 1999 (Fig. 9.2c)). Pruning causes a shift from a retinotopic projection with widespread overlap of RGC axonal arbors to a more precise map with less overlap (Cook and Rankin, 1986). Electrophysiological recording from tectal neurons show a similar change towards increased visual resolution throughout regeneration (Northmore, 1989a, b). Importantly, both visually evoked electrophysiological responses in tectal neurons and visual behaviors can be evoked following retinotectal regeneration (Northmore and Masino, 1984; Northmore, 1989a, b; Oh and Northmore, 1998).

The failure of regenerating RGC axons to directly navigate to appropriate tectal zones suggests a decreased influence of chemoaffinity guidance and adoption of a strategy of trial and error to search for targets. Indeed, to a large extent, the molecular cues responsible for directing initial growth of the retinotectal pathway and RGC axonal termination zones are down-regulated following development. Tectal expression of ephrin ligands decreases with maturation (Schmidt and Eisele, 1985). However, the findings that crude retinotopy is achieved following regeneration while retinal activity is blocked by TTX demonstrates that activity-independent guidance is present during regeneration in the adult fish and frog tectum (Meyer, 1983; Schmidt, 1985a, b; Cook and Rankin, 1986; Schmidt and Buzzard, 1990). The source of this activity-independent guidance likely comes from the up-regulation and gradient expression of ephrins and Eph receptors, or other guidance molecules following optic nerve lesion (Wizenmann et al., 1993; Rodger et al., 2000; Rodger et al., 2001; King et al., 2003; King et al., 2004).

Importance of neuronal activity and NMDA receptors in refinement of regenerated retinotectal connections

Unlike early development when intrinsic retinal activity can be the source of RGC activity, the mature eye provides visual stimulation of RGCs during regeneration. Similar to its role in orchestrating retinotectal map refinement during development, evidence suggests a requirement for activity for increasing precision of the map during regeneration (Meyer, 1983; Schmidt and Edwards, 1983; Reh and Constantine-Paton, 1985; Schmidt, 1985a, b; Schmidt and Eisele, 1985; Cook and Rankin, 1986; Eisele and Schmidt, 1988; Cook and Becker, 1990; Schmidt and Buzzard, 1990; Olson and Meyer, 1991; Schmidt and Lemere, 1996; Johnson et al., 1999; Dunlop et al., 2003). Intraocular TTX prevents refinement of the regenerating retinotectal map, resulting in RGCs with enlarged terminal fields (Meyer, 1983; Schmidt and Edwards, 1983; Reh and Constantine-Paton, 1985; Schmidt and Buzzard, 1990; Olson and Meyer, 1991; Johnson et al., 1999). While blocking activity with TTX does not influence regenerative sprouting at the lesion or crude patterning of the retinotectal map, TTX prevents activity-dependent elimination of inappropriate ectopic axonal branches. There is a critical period (14–34 days post-lesion in fish) in which the regenerating map is sensitive to the effects of TTX (Schmidt and Edwards, 1983).

The importance of correlated activity in refinement of the regenerating retinotectal projection is also evident from studies showing that strobe light illumination and NMDA receptor blockade prevents refinement (Schmidt and Eisele, 1985; Eisele and Schmidt, 1988; Cook and Becker, 1990; Schmidt and Buzzard, 1990). Like the effects of intraocular TTX, strobe light prevents refinement only during a critical period corresponding to early synaptogenesis of regeneration (20–34 days post-optic nerve lesion) (Schmidt and Eisele, 1985). Subsequent exposure to normal visual stimulation is unable to promote pruning of inappropriate axonal collaterals to sharpen map refinement (Schmidt and Eisele, 1985). Tectal NMDA receptor blockade also prevents refinement of the regenerating retinotectal projection by preventing selective elimination of ectopic branches (Schmidt et al., 2000; Dunlop, 2003). The regenerating projection fails to sharpen and tectal neuronal receptive fields remain large, similar to the effects of intraocular TTX or strobe light exposure (Schmidt and

Buzzard, 1990). Interestingly, during the period of refinement the regenerating RGC projection has an increased capacity for LTP. This heightened capacity for synaptic plasticity may be related to activity-dependent sharpening since it follows the same time course of morphological refinement (Schmidt, 1990). Also surprising, exposing fish to complete darkness during regeneration does not interfere with map refinement, as might be expected by loss of correlated patterned visual stimuli (Cook and Rankin, 1986; Keating et al., 1986; Cook and Becker, 1990; Olson and Meyer, 1991). In darkness, the regenerating retino-tectal projection shows a similar time course and extent of refinement as growth in normal light sug-gesting that the spontaneous activity of RGCs in darkness is sufficient for these activity-dependent processes. It is not known to what extent RGC activ-ity in darkness is influenced by position within the retina or neighbor RGC activity. An unexpected find-ing is that retinotectal map refinement is not affected by the resolution of the visual stimulus since lens ablation, which blurs vision, has no discernable effect (Cook and Rankin, 1986).

These studies show that in animals with per-missive environments for RGC axonal regrowth, re-establishment of the retinotectal map can be achieved. While the failure of regenerating RGC axons to directly target appropriate termination zones and ectopic arborization suggests a decreased influence of chemoaffinity guidance, activity-independent cues do contribute. It also appears that, regeneration recapitulates a critical period of heightened plastic-ity during which activity-dependent mechanisms mediate map refinement through pruning of ectopic axonal branches.

Regeneration of retinotectal connections in mammals

While studies with lower vertebrates have allowed dissection of the essential components for regener-ation, primary goal is to promote regeneration in humans. Unfortunately, the retinotectal regenera-tion capacity demonstrated in fish and frogs (Attardi and Sperry, 1963; Gaze and Jacobson, 1963;

Stuermer and Easter, 1984; Udin and Fawcett, 1988) largely fails in reptiles and mammals. RGC axons in lizards will regenerate following optic nerve lesion, but ordered retinotectal maps fail to form and vision is not restored (Beazley et al., 1997; Dunlop et al., 2004). However, behavioral training to promote use of vision improves retinotectal map refinement and visual responses in lizards (Beazley et al., 2003), sug-gesting that functional activation of a damaged neuronal circuit may be essential for functional recovery. Limited regeneration of the optic nerve has been found in mammals including rodents (Inoue and Fukuda, 1998; Foerster and Holmes, 1999) and cats (Kawaguchi et al., 1986). While suc-cess is higher in early developmental stages, rein-nervation in neonatal rats yields poor topographic map formation (Galli et al., 1989). Critical initial limi-tations to regeneration of the mammal optic nerve are the lack of a permissive environment for RGC survival and sprouting of new axons, and difficulties rediscovering targets (Caroni and Schwab, 1988; McLoon et al., 1988; McKerracher et al., 1994; Smith-Thomas et al., 1995; Rager et al., 1996; Ghosh and David, 1997). An absence of guidance cues appears not to be a problem since ephrin expression that is reduced following development is increased following optic nerve lesion in the adult rat (Knoll et al., 2001; Rodger et al., 2001). Grafts of peripheral nerves have been shown to partly overcome problems of survival and pathfinding, allowing regenerating RGC axons to enter the superior colliculus (SC), the mammalian version of the optic tectum (Vidal-Sanz et al., 1987; Carter et al., 1989, 1994; Sauve et al., 1995, 2001) (Fig. 9.2d). The use of a peripheral nerve graft cre-ates a supportive environment and promotes regen-eration to the SC in adult hamsters. Regenerating RGC axons terminate in appropriate layers of the SC (Carter et al., 1989; Sauve et al., 1995) and visual responses can be recorded from collicular neurons postsynaptic to regenerated RGC axons (Sauve et al., 1995). Unfortunately, few RGC axons regenerate in mam-mals even with peripheral nerve grafts (Vidal-Sanz et al., 1987). Also, many RGC axons terminate directly after exiting the peripheral nerve graft (Aviles-Trigueros et al., 2000). While it is possible to evoke visually driven responses in re-innervated SC neurons (Keirstead et al., 1989; Sauve et al., 1995), the RGC projection is sparse with poor retinotopy. It is likely that the dispersed innervation of SC produces little opportunity for refinement of overlapping RGC arbors based on correlated activity.

9.4 Conclusions

Further advances are required to promote more extensive RGC survival and regeneration following lesion in mammals. In addition to increasing visual acuity, sufficient RGC axonal arbors are likely required to allow activity-dependent map refinement based on correlated activity of overlapping arbors. Another important difference between development and regeneration is the increased ability of the mature RGC axon to form synapses prior to reaching target sites. During development RGC axons enter the tectum and proceed to the correct termination zones as simple axons directed by growth cones, prior to exuberant arborization, and synaptogenesis. Regenerating RGC axons, however extend multiple termination arbors and synapses at ectopic locations in the fish, and often synapse indiscriminately directly after exiting peripheral nerve grafts in mammals. It appears that during development the stages of axonal growth, pathfinding, arborization and synaptogenesis are controlled in a temporal manner lost by mature regenerating neurons. Finding how to recapitulate this order of growth behavior may be an important step in promoting regeneration in mammals.

REFERENCES

Adamson, J.R. and Grobstein, P. (1982). Reestablishment of the ipsilateral oculotectal projection after optic nerve crush in the frog: evidence for synaptic remodeling during regeneration. *Soc Neurosci Abstr*, **8**, 514.

Attardi, D.G. and Sperry, R.W. (1963). Preferential selection of central pathways by regenerating optic fibers. *Exp Neurol*, **7**, 46–64.

Aviles-Trigueros, M., Sauve, Y., et al. (2000). Selective innervation of retinorecipient brainstem nuclei by retinal ganglion cell axons regenerating through peripheral nerve grafts in adult rats. *J Neurosci*, **20**(1), 361–374.

Bahr, M. (2000). Live or let die – retinal ganglion cell death and survival during development and in the lesioned adult CNS. *Trend Neurosci*, **23**(10), 483–490.

Beazley, L.D., Sheard, P.W., et al. (1997). Optic nerve regenerates but does not restore topographic projections in the lizard *Ctenophorus ornatus*. *J Comp Neurol*, **377**(1), 105–120.

Beazley, L.D., Rodger, J., et al. (2003). Training on a visual task improves the outcome of optic nerve regeneration. *J Neurotraum*, **20**(11), 1263–1270.

Behar, O., Mizuno, K., et al. (2000). Putting the spinal cord together again. *Neuron*, **26**(2), 291–293.

Boss, V.C. and Schmidt, J.T. (1984). Activity and the formation of ocular dominance patches in dually innervated tectum of goldfish. *J Neurosci*, **4**(12), 2891–2905.

Brose, K., Bland, K.S., et al. (1999). Slit proteins bind robo receptors and have an evolutionarily conserved role in repulsive axon guidance. *Cell*, **96**(6), 795–806.

Caroni, P. and Schwab, M.E. (1988). Two membrane protein fractions from rat central myelin with inhibitory properties for neurite growth and fibroblast spreading. *J Cell Biol*, **106**(4), 1281–1288.

Carter, D.A., Bray, G.M., et al. (1989). Regenerated retinal ganglion cell axons can form well-differentiated synapses in the superior colliculus of adult hamsters. *J Neurosci*, **9**(11), 4042–4050.

Carter, D.A., Bray, G.M., et al. (1994). Long-term growth and remodeling of regenerated retino-collicular connections in adult hamsters. *J Neurosci*, **14**(2), 590–598.

Cline, H. (2003). Sperry and Hebb: oil and vinegar? *Trend Neurosci*, **26**(12), 655–661.

Cline, H.T. and Constantine-Paton, M. (1989). NMDA receptor antagonists disrupt the retinotectal topographic map. *Neuron*, **3**(4), 413–426.

Cline, H.T., Debski, E.A., et al. (1987). *N*-methyl-D-aspartate receptor antagonist desegregates eye-specific stripes. *Proc Natl Acad Sci USA*, **84**(12), 4342–4345.

Coletti, S.M., Ide, C.F., et al. (1990). Ocular dominance stripe formation by regenerated isogenic double temporal retina in *Xenopus laevis*. *J Neurobiol*, **21**(2), 276–282.

Constantine-Paton, M. and Law, M.I. (1978). Eye-specific termination bands in tecta of three-eyed frogs. *Science*, **202**(4368), 639–641.

Cook, J.E. and Becker, D.L. (1990). Spontaneous activity as a determinant of axonal connections. *Eur J Neurosci*, **2**(2), 162–169.

Cook, J.E. and Rankin, E.C. (1986). Impaired refinement of the regenerated retinotectal projection of the goldfish in stroboscopic light: a quantitative WGA-HRP study. *Exp Brain Res*, **63**(**2**), 421–430.

Davies, S.J., Field, P.M., et al. (1996). Regeneration of cut adult axons fails even in the presence of continuous aligned glial pathways. *Exp Neurol*, **142**(**2**), 203–216.

Deiner, M.S., Kennedy, T.E., et al. (1997). Netrin-1 and DCC mediate axon guidance locally at the optic disc: loss of function leads to optic nerve hypoplasia. *Neuron*, **19**(**3**), 575–589.

Dergham, P., Ellezam, B., et al. (2002). Rho signaling pathway targeted to promote spinal cord repair. *J Neurosci*, **22**(**15**), 6570–6577.

Drescher, U., Bonhoeffer, F., et al. (1997). The Eph family in retinal axon guidance. *Curr Opin Neurobiol*, **7**(**1**), 75–80.

Dunlop, S.A. (2003). Axonal sprouting in the optic nerve is not a prerequisite for successful regeneration. *J Comp Neurol*, **465**(**3**), 319–334.

Dunlop, S.A., Stirling, R.V., et al. (2003). Failure to form a stable topographic map during optic nerve regeneration: abnormal activity-dependent mechanisms. *Exp Neurol*, **184**(**2**), 805–815.

Dunlop, S.A., Tee, L.B., et al. (2004). Failure to restore vision after optic nerve regeneration in reptiles: interspecies variation in response to axotomy. *J Comp Neurol*, **478**(**3**), 292–305.

Eisele, L.E. and Schmidt, J.T. (1988). Activity sharpens the regenerating retinotectal projection in goldfish: sensitive period for strobe illumination and lack of effect on synaptogenesis and on ganglion cell receptive field properties. *J Neurobiol*, **19**(**5**), 395–411.

Ellezam, B., Dubreuil, C., et al. (2002). Inactivation of intracellular rho to stimulate axon growth and regeneration. *Prog Brain Res*, **137**, 371–380.

Engert, F., Tao, H.W., et al. (2002). Moving visual stimuli rapidly induce direction sensitivity of developing tectal neurons. *Nature*, **419**(**6906**), 470–475.

Feldheim, D.A., Kim, Y.I., et al. (2000). Genetic analysis of ephrin-A2 and ephrin-A5 shows their requirement in multiple aspects of retinocollicular mapping. *Neuron*, **25**(**3**), 563–574.

Feller, M.B., Wellis, D.P., et al. (1996). Requirement for cholinergic synaptic transmission in the propagation of spontaneous retinal waves. *Science*, **272**(**5265**), 1182–1187.

Flanagan, J.G. and Vanderhaeghen, P. (1998). The ephrins and Eph receptors in neural development. *Annu Rev Neurosci*, **21**, 309–345.

Foerster, A.P. and Holmes, M.J. (1999). Spontaneous regeneration of severed optic axons restores mapped visual responses to the adult rat superior colliculus. *Eur J Neurosci*, **11**(**9**), 3151–3166.

Frisen, J., Yates, P.A., et al. (1998). Ephrin-A5 (AL-1/RAGS) is essential for proper retinal axon guidance and topographic mapping in the mammalian visual system. *Neuron*, **20**(**2**), 235–243.

Fujisawa, H. (1981). Persistence of disorganized pathways and tortuous trajectories of regenerating retinal fibers in the adult newt *Cynops pyrrhogaster*. *Dev Growth Differ*, **23**, 215–219.

Fujisawa, H., Tani, N., et al. (1982). Branching of regenerating retinal axons and preferential selection of appropriate branches for specific neuronal connection in the newt. *Dev Biol*, **90**(**1**), 43–57.

Galli, L., Rao, K., et al. (1989). Transplanted rat retinae do not project in a topographic fashion on the host tectum. *Exp Brain Res*, **74**(**2**), 427–430.

Garaschuk, O., Linn, J., et al. (2000). Large-scale oscillatory calcium waves in the immature cortex. *Nat Neurosci*, **3**(**5**), 452–459.

Gaze, R.M. (1958). The representation of the retina on the optic lobe of the frog. *Quart J Exp Physiol Cogn Med Sci*, **43**(**2**), 209–214.

Gaze, R.M. (1970). *The Formation of Nerve Connections*, Academic Press, New York.

Gaze, R.M. and Jacobson, M. (1963). A study of the retinotectal projection during regeneration of the optic nerve in the frog. *Proc Roy Soc London (Biol)*, **157**, 420–448.

Gaze, R.M. and Keating, M.J. (1970). The restoration of the ipsilateral visual projection following regeneration of the optic nerve in the frog. *Brain Res*, **21**(**2**), 207–216.

Gaze, R.M., Keating, M.J., et al. (1974). The evolution of the retinotectal map during development in *Xenopus*. *Proc Roy Soc London B Biol Sci*, **185**(**80**), 301–330.

Ghosh, A. and David, S. (1997). Neurite growth-inhibitory activity in the adult rat cerebral cortical gray matter. *J Neurobiol*, **32**(**7**), 671–683.

Godement, P. and Bonhoeffer, F (1989). Cross-species recognition of tectal cues by retinal fibers *in vitro*. *Development*, **106**(**2**), 313–320.

Goldberg, J.L. and Barres, B.A. (2000). The relationship between neuronal survival and regeneration. *Annu Rev Neurosci*, **23**, 579–612.

Hebb, D. (1949). *The Organization of Behavior*, John Wiley and Sons, New York.

Hindges, R., McLaughlin, T., et al. (2002). EphB forward signaling controls directional branch extension and arborization required for dorsal–ventral retinotopic mapping. *Neuron*, **35**(**3**), 475–487.

Holt, C.E. (1984). Does timing of axon outgrowth influence initial retinotectal topography in *Xenopus*? *J Neurosci*, **4**(**4**), 1130–1152.

Holt, C.E. and Harris, W.A. (1983). Order in the initial retinotectal map in *Xenopus*: a new technique for labelling growing nerve fibres. *Nature*, **301**(**5896**), 150–152.

Horder, T.J. and Martin, K.A. (1978). Morphogenetics as an alternative to chemospecificity in the formation of nerve connections. A review of literature, before 1978, concerning the control of growth of regenerating optic nerve fibres to specific locations in the optic tectum and a new interpretation based on contact guidance. *Symp Soc Exp Biol*, **32**, 275–358.

Hornberger, M.R., Dutting, D., et al. (1999). Modulation of EphA receptor function by coexpressed ephrinA ligands on retinal ganglion cell axons. *Neuron*, **22**(**4**), 731–742.

Huang, D.W., McKerracher, L., et al. (1999). A therapeutic vaccine approach to stimulate axon regeneration in the adult mammalian spinal cord. *Neuron*, **24**(**3**), 639–647.

Hubel, D.H. and Wiesel, T.N. (1977). Ferrier lecture. Functional architecture of macaque monkey visual cortex. *Proc Roy Soc London B Biol Sci*, **198**(**1130**), 1–59.

Humphrey, M.F. and Beazley, L.D. (1982). An electrophysiological study of early retinotectal projection patterns during optic nerve regeneration in *Hyla moorei*. *Brain Res*, **239**(**2**), 595–602.

Ide, C.F., Fraser, S.E., et al. (1983). Eye dominance columns from an isogenic double-nasal frog eye. *Science*, **221**(**4607**), 293–295.

Inoue, T. and Fukuda, Y. (1998). Optic nerve regeneration and functional recovery of vision following peripheral nerve transplant. *No To Shinkei*, **50**(**3**), 227–235.

Jacobson, M. (1978). *Developmental Neurobiology*, Holt, Rinehard and Winston Inc., New York.

Johnson, F.A., Dawson, A.J., et al. (1999). Activity-dependent refinement in the goldfish retinotectal system is mediated by the dynamic regulation of processes withdrawal: an *in vivo* imaging study. *J Comp Neurol*, **406**(**4**), 548–562.

Kaethner, R.J. and Stuermer, C.A. (1994). Growth behavior of retinotectal axons in live zebrafish embryos under TTX-induced neural impulse blockade. *J Neurobiol*, **25**(**7**), 781–796.

Katz, L.C. and Shatz, C.J. (1996). Synaptic activity and the construction of cortical circuits. *Science*, **274**(**5290**), 1133–1138.

Kawaguchi, S., Miyata, H., et al. (1986). Regeneration of the cerebellofugal projection after transection of the superior cerebellar peduncle in kittens: morphological and electrophysiological studies. *J Comp Neurol*, **245**(**2**), 258–273.

Keating, M.J., Grant, S., et al. (1986). Visual deprivation and the maturation of the retinotectal projection in *Xenopus laevis*. *J Embryol Exp Morphol*, **91**, 101–115.

Keirstead, S.A., Rasminsky, M., et al. (1989). Electrophysiologic responses in hamster superior colliculus evoked by regenerating retinal axons. *Science*, **246**(**4927**), 255–257.

King, C., Lacey, R., et al. (2004). Characterisation of tectal ephrin-A2 expression during optic nerve regeneration in goldfish: implications for restoration of topography. *Exp Neurol*, **187**(**2**), 380–387.

King, C.E., Wallace, A., et al. (2003). Transient up-regulation of retinal EphA3 and EphA5, but not ephrin-A2, coincides with re-establishment of a topographic map during optic nerve regeneration in goldfish. *Exp Neurol*, **183**(**2**), 593–599.

Knoll, B., Isenmann, S., et al. (2001). Graded expression patterns of ephrin-As in the superior colliculus after lesion of the adult mouse optic nerve. *Mech Dev*, **106**(**1–2**), 119–127.

Kobayashi, T., Nakamura, H., et al. (1990). Disturbance of refinement of retinotectal projection in chick embryos by tetrodotoxin and grayanotoxin. *Brain Res Dev Brain Res*, **57**(**1**), 29–35.

Koeberle, P.D. and Ball, A.K. (2002). Neurturin enhances the survival of axotomized retinal ganglion cells *in vivo*: combined effects with glial cell line-derived neurotrophic factor and brain-derived neurotrophic factor. *Neuroscience*, **110**(**3**), 555–567.

Kolodkin, A.L. and Ginty, D.D. (1997). Steering clear of semaphorins: neuropilins sound the retreat. *Neuron*, **19**(**6**), 1159–1162.

Law, M.I. and Constantine-Paton, M. (1980). Right and left eye bands in frogs with unilateral tectal ablations. *Proc Natl Acad Sci USA*, **77**(**4**), 2314–2318.

Li, M.S. and David, S. (1996). Topical glucocorticoids modulate the lesion interface after cerebral cortical stab wounds in adult rats. *Glia*, **18**(**4**), 306–318.

Mann, F., Ray, S., et al. (2002). Topographic mapping in dorsoventral axis of the *Xenopus* retinotectal system depends on signaling through ephrin-B ligands. *Neuron*, **35**(**3**), 461–473.

McKerracher, L., David, S., et al. (1994). Identification of myelin-associated glycoprotein as a major myelin-derived inhibitor of neurite growth. *Neuron*, **13**(**4**), 805–811.

McLaughlin, T., Hindges, R., et al. (2003a). Regulation of axial patterning of the retina and its topographic mapping in the brain. *Curr Opin Neurobiol*, **13**(**1**), 57–69.

McLaughlin, T., Torborg, C.L., et al. (2003b). Retinotopic map refinement requires spontaneous retinal waves during a brief critical period of development. *Neuron*, **40**, 1147–1160.

McLoon, S.C., McLoon, L.K., et al. (1988). Transient expression of laminin in the optic nerve of the developing rat. *J Neurosci*, **8**(**6**), 1981–1990.

Meister, M., Wong, R.O., et al. (1991). Synchronous bursts of action potentials in ganglion cells of the developing mammalian retina. *Science*, **252**(**5008**), 939–943.

Meyer, R.L. (1980). Mapping the normal and regenerating retinotectal projection of goldfish with autoradiographic methods. *J Comp Neurol*, **189**(**2**), 273–289.

Meyer, R.L. (1982). Tetrodotoxin blocks the formation of ocular dominance columns in goldfish. *Science*, **218**(**4572**), 589–591.

Meyer, R.L. (1983). Tetrodotoxin inhibits the formation of refined retinotopography in goldfish. *Brain Res*, **282**(**3**), 293–298.

Mooney, R., Penn, A.A., et al. (1996). Thalamic relay of spontaneous retinal activity prior to vision. *Neuron*, **17**(**5**), 863–874.

Murray, M. and Edwards, M.A. (1982). A quantitative study of the reinnervation of the goldfish optic tectum following optic nerve crush. *J Comp Neurol*, **209**(**4**), 363–373.

Nakamoto, M., Cheng, H.J., et al. (1996). Topographically specific effects of ELF-1 on retinal axon guidance *in vitro* and retinal axon mapping *in vivo*. *Cell*, **86**(**5**), 755–766.

Niclou, S.P., Jia, L., et al. (2000). Slit2 is a repellent for retinal ganglion cell axons. *J Neurosci*, **20**(**13**), 4962–4974.

Northmore, D.P. (1989a). Quantitative electrophysiological studies of regenerating visuotopic maps in goldfish. I. Early recovery of dimming sensitivity in tectum and torus longitudinalis. *Neuroscience*, **32**(**3**), 739–747.

Northmore, D.P. (1989b). Quantitative electrophysiological studies of regenerating visuotopic maps in goldfish. II. Delayed recovery of sensitivity to small light flashes. *Neuroscience*, **32**(**3**), 749–757.

Northmore, D.P. and Masino, T. (1984). Recovery of vision in fish after optic nerve crush: a behavioral and electrophysiological study. *Exp Neurol*, **84**(**1**), 109–125.

Nowak, L., Bregestovski, P., et al. (1984). Magnesium gates glutamate-activated channels in mouse central neurones. *Nature*, **307**(**5950**), 462–465.

O'Leary, D.D. and Cowan, W.M. (1983). Topographic organization of certain tectal afferent and efferent connections can develop normally in the absence of retinal input. *Proc Natl Acad Sci USA*, **80**(**19**), 6131–6135.

O'Leary, D.D. and Wilkinson, D.G. (1999). Eph receptors and ephrins in neural development. *Curr Opin Neurobiol*, **9**(**1**), 65–73.

Oh, D.J. and Northmore, D.P. (1998). Functional properties of retinal ganglion cells during optic nerve regeneration in the goldfish. *Vis Neurosci*, **15**(**6**), 1145–1155.

Olson, M.D. and Meyer, R.L. (1991). The effect of TTX-activity blockade and total darkness on the formation of retinotopy in the goldfish retinotectal projection. *J Comp Neurol*, **303**(**3**), 412–423.

Penn, A.A., Riquelme, P.A., et al. (1998). Competition in retinogeniculate patterning driven by spontaneous activity. *Science*, **279**(**5359**), 2108–2112.

Plump, A.S., Erskine, L., et al. (2002). Slit1 and Slit2 cooperate to prevent premature midline crossing of retinal axons in the mouse visual system. *Neuron*, **33**(**2**), 219–232.

Rager, G., Morino, P., et al. (1996). Expression of the axonal cell adhesion molecules axonin-1 and Ng-CAM during the development of the chick retinotectal system. *J Comp Neurol*, **365**(**4**), 594–609.

Rankin, E.C. and Cook, J.E. (1986). Topographic refinement of the regenerating retinotectal projection of the goldfish in standard laboratory conditions: a quantitative WGA–HRP study. *Exp Brain Res*, **63**(**2**), 409–420.

Reh, T.A. and Constantine-Paton, M. (1985). Eye-specific segregation requires neural activity in three-eyed *Rana pipiens*. *J Neurosci*, **5**(**5**), 1132–1143.

Richardson, P.M., Issa, V.M., et al. (1982). Regeneration and retrograde degeneration of axons in the rat optic nerve. *J Neurocytol*, **11**(**6**), 949–966.

Rodger, J., Bartlett, C.A., et al. (2000). Transient up-regulation of the rostrocaudal gradient of ephrin A2 in the tectum coincides with reestablishment of orderly projections during optic nerve regeneration in goldfish. *Exp Neurol*, **166**(**1**), 196–200.

Rodger, J., Lindsey, K.A., et al. (2001). Expression of ephrin-A2 in the superior colliculus and EphA5 in the retina following optic nerve section in adult rat. *Eur J Neurosci*, **14**(**12**), 1929–1936.

Roskies, A.L. and O'Leary, D.D. (1994). Control of topographic retinal axon branching by inhibitory membrane-bound molecules. *Science*, **265**(**5173**), 799–803.

Ruthazer, E.S. and Cline, H.T. (2004). Insights into activity-dependent map formation from the retinotectal system: a middle-of-the-brain perspective. *J Neurobiol*, **59**(**1**), 134–146.

Ruthazer, E.S., Akerman, C.J., et al. (2003). Control of axon branch dynamics by correlated activity *in vivo*. *Science*, **301**(**5629**), 66–70.

Sakaguchi, D.S. and Murphey, R.K. (1985). Map formation in the developing *Xenopus* retinotectal system: an examination of ganglion cell terminal arborizations. *J Neurosci*, **5**(**12**), 3228–3245.

Sakurai, T., Wong, E., et al. (2002). Ephrin-A5 restricts topographically specific arborization in the chick retinotectal projection *in vivo*. *Proc Natl Acad Sci USA*, **99**(**16**), 10795–10800.

Sauve, Y., Sawai, H., et al. (1995). Functional synaptic connections made by regenerated retinal ganglion cell axons in the superior colliculus of adult hamsters. *J Neurosci*, **15**(**1 Pt 2**), 665–675.

Sauve, Y., Sawai, H., et al. (2001). Topological specificity in reinnervation of the superior colliculus by regenerated retinal ganglion cell axons in adult hamsters. *J Neurosci*, **21**(3), 951–960.

Schmidt, J.T. (1985a). Formation of retinotopic connections: selective stabilization by an activity-dependent mechanism. *Cell Mol Neurobiol*, **5**(1–2), 65–84.

Schmidt, J.T. (1985b). Selective stabilization of retinotectal synapses by an activity-dependent mechanism. *Fed Proc*, **44**(12), 2767–2772.

Schmidt, J.T. (1990). Long-term potentiation and activity-dependent retinotopic sharpening in the regenerating retinotectal projection of goldfish: common sensitive period and sensitivity to NMDA blockers. *J Neurosci*, **10**(1), 233–246.

Schmidt, J.T. and Buzzard, M. (1990). Activity-driven sharpening of the regenerating retinotectal projection: effects of blocking or synchronizing activity on the morphology of individual regenerating arbors. *J Neurobiol*, **21**(6), 900–917.

Schmidt, J.T. and Buzzard, M. (1993). Activity-driven sharpening of the retinotectal projection in goldfish: development under stroboscopic illumination prevents sharpening. *J Neurobiol*, **24**(3), 384–399.

Schmidt, J.T. and Edwards, D.L. (1983). Activity sharpens the map during the regeneration of the retinotectal projection in goldfish. *Brain Res*, **269**(1), 29–39.

Schmidt, J.T. and Eisele, L.E. (1985). Stroboscopic illumination and dark rearing block the sharpening of the regenerated retinotectal map in goldfish. *Neuroscience*, **14**(2), 535–546.

Schmidt, J.T. and Lemere, C.A. (1996). Rapid activity-dependent sprouting of optic fibers into a local area denervated by application of beta-bungarotoxin in goldfish tectum. *J Neurobiol*, **29**(1), 75–90.

Schmidt, J.T., Buzzard, M.J., et al. (1984). Morphology of regenerated optic arbors in goldfish tectum. *Soc Neurosci Abstr*, **10**, 667.

Schmidt, J.T., Turcotte, J.C., et al. (1988). Staining of regenerated optic arbors in goldfish tectum: progressive changes in immature arbors and a comparison of mature regenerated arbors with normal arbors. *J Comp Neurol*, **269**(4), 565–591.

Schmidt, J.T., Buzzard, M., et al. (2000). MK801 increases retinotectal arbor size in developing zebrafish without affecting kinetics of branch elimination and addition. *J Neurobiol*, **42**(3), 303–314.

Schnell, L. and Schwab, M.E. (1990). Axonal regeneration in the rat spinal cord produced by an antibody against myelin-associated neurite growth inhibitors. *Nature*, **343**(6255), 269–272.

Shatz, C.J. and Stryker, M.P. (1988). Prenatal tetrodotoxin infusion blocks segregation of retinogeniculate afferents. *Science*, **242**(4875), 87–89.

Simon, D.K. and O'Leary, D.D. (1992). Development of topographic order in the mammalian retinocollicular projection. *J Neurosci*, **12**(4), 1212–1232.

Smith-Thomas, L.C., Stevens, J., et al. (1995). Increased axon regeneration in astrocytes grown in the presence of proteoglycan synthesis inhibitors. *J Cell Sci*, **108**(Pt 3), 1307–1315.

Sperry, R.W. (1943). Visuomotor coordination in the newt (*Triturus viridescens*) after regeneration of the optic nerves. *J Comp Neurol*, **79**, 33–55.

Sperry, R.W. (1963). Chemoaffinity in the orderly growth of nerve fiber patterns and connections. *Proc Natl Acad Sci USA*, **50**, 703–710.

Sretavan, D. and Shatz, C.J. (1984). Prenatal development of individual retinogeniculate axons during the period of segregation. *Nature*, **308**(5962), 845–848.

Sretavan, D.W., Shatz, C.J., et al. (1988). Modification of retinal ganglion cell axon morphology by prenatal infusion of tetrodotoxin. *Nature*, **336**(6198), 468–471.

Stent, G.S. (1973). A physiological mechanism for Hebb's postulate of learning. *Proc Natl Acad Sci USA*, **70**(4), 997–1001.

Stichel, C.C., Niermann, H., et al. (1999). Basal membrane-depleted scar in lesioned CNS: characteristics and relationships with regenerating axons. *Neuroscience*, **93**(1), 321–333.

Straznicky, C. and Glastonbury, J. (1979). Anomalous ipsilateral optic fibre projection in Xenopus induced by larval tectal ablation. *J Embryol Exp Morphol*, **50**, 111–122.

Stuermer, C.A. (1988a). Trajectories of regenerating retinal axons in the goldfish tectum. I. A comparison of normal and regenerated axons at late regeneration stages. *J Comp Neurol*, **267**(1), 55–68.

Stuermer, C.A. (1988b). Trajectories of regenerating retinal axons in the goldfish tectum. II. Exploratory branches and growth cones on axons at early regeneration stages. *J Comp Neurol*, **267**(1), 69–91.

Stuermer, C.A. and Bastmeyer, M. (2000). The retinal axon's pathfinding to the optic disk. *Prog Neurobiol*, **62**(2), 197–214.

Stuermer, C.A. and Easter Jr., S.S. (1984). A comparison of the normal and regenerated retinotectal pathways of goldfish. *J Comp Neurol*, **223**(1), 57–76.

Tao, H.W., Zhang, L.I., et al. (2001). Emergence of input specificity of ltp during development of retinotectal connections *in vivo*. *Neuron*, **31**(4), 569–580.

Udin, S.B. and Fawcett, J.W. (1988). Formation of topographic maps. *Annu Rev Neurosci*, **11**, 289–327.

Vidal-Sanz, M., Bray, G.M., et al. (1987). Axonal regeneration and synapse formation in the superior colliculus by retinal ganglion cells in the adult rat. *J Neurosci*, **7**(9), 2894–2909.

Vielmetter, J. and Stuermer, C.A. (1989). Goldfish retinal axons respond to position-specific properties of tectal cell membranes *in vitro*. *Neuron*, **2**(**4**), 1331–1339.

Walter, J., Henke-Fahle, S., et al. (1987a). Avoidance of posterior tectal membranes by temporal retinal axons. *Development*, **101**(**4**), 909–913.

Walter, J., Kern-Veits, B., et al. (1987b). Recognition of position-specific properties of tectal cell membranes by retinal axons *in vitro*. *Development*, **101**(**4**), 685–696.

Westerman, R.A. (1965). *Specificity of Optic and Olfactory Pathways in Teleost Fish*, Springer-Verlag, Berlin.

Wiesel, T.N. and Hubel, D.H. (1963). Effects of visual deprivation on morphology and physiology of cells in the cats lateral geniculate body. *J Neurophysiol*, **26**, 978–993.

Wiesel, T.N. and Hubel, D.H. (1965). Comparison of the effects of unilateral and bilateral eye closure on cortical unit responses in kittens. *J Neurophysiol*, **28**(**6**), 1029–1040.

Wilkinson, D.G. (2001). Multiple roles of EPH receptors and ephrins in neural development. *Nat Rev Neurosci*, **2**(**3**), 155–164.

Wizenmann, A., Thies, E., et al. (1993). Appearance of target-specific guidance information for regenerating axons after CNS lesions. *Neuron*, **11**(**5**), 975–983.

Wong, R.O., Meister, M., et al. (1993). Transient period of correlated bursting activity during development of the mammalian retina. *Neuron*, **11**(**5**), 923–938.

Zhang, L.I., Tao, H.W., et al. (1998). A critical window for cooperation and competition among developing retinotectal synapses. *Nature*, **395**(**6697**), 37–44.

Zhang, L.I., Tao, H.W., et al. (2000). Visual input induces long-term potentiation of developing retinotectal synapses. *Nat Neurosci*, **3**(**7**), 708–715.

10

Plasticity in auditory functions

Josef P. Rauschecker

Department of Physiology and Biophysics, Georgetown University School of Medicine, Washington, DC, USA

Summary

This chapter covers plasticity in the central auditory system, most notably in the auditory cortex, from a variety of viewpoints. Neuroanatomical and neurophysiological studies in animals as well as behavioral and functional imaging studies in humans will be considered. Plasticity in the auditory system will be compared to plasticity in other sensory systems, and the reorganization of the central auditory system during early blindness and deafness will be discussed. The findings from research in auditory cortical plasticity have important implications for the design of auditory prostheses, such as cochlear implants, in the deaf, and visual prostheses in the blind using nonvisual modalities. They also further the understanding and treatment of common ailments, including hearing loss and tinnitus in an aging population as well as the effects of otitis media in young children.

10.1 Introduction

Auditory cortex plays a crucial role in higher perceptual and cognitive functions, including those of speech and music, and in the processing of auditory space. Cortical plasticity, as in other sensory systems, is used to fine-tune these higher functions and plays an important role in reorganization after early injury. Auditory cortical plasticity can be demonstrated after lesions of the cochlea and appears to participate in generating tinnitus. Early musical training leads to an expansion of auditory cortex representing complex harmonic sounds. Similarly, the early phonetic environment has a strong influence on speech development and, presumably, cortical organization of speech. In auditory spatial perception, the spectral cues generated by the head and outer ears vary individually and have to be calibrated by learning. The neural mechanisms of plasticity are likely the same across cortical regions. It will be useful, therefore, to relate some of the findings and hypotheses in auditory cortical plasticity to previous studies of other sensory systems.

Research on the auditory system has been much slower to recognize the relevance of cortical self- and re-organization than research in the other major sensory systems, that is vision and touch. Although there have been a number of studies of auditory plasticity up to the level of the inferior colliculus, most work on plasticity of auditory cortex is comparatively recent. Many important functions of the auditory system, however, can only be fully understood with cortical plasticity in mind. For instance, even with an innate capacity for language, normal speech can hardly be acquired without auditory feedback and a capacity for learning. Likewise, a system capable of localizing sound at extraordinary precision, using various sets of cues, cannot accomplish this without resorting to tuning mechanisms that re-calibrate the system continually, especially during the growth phase of the head and outer ears. Spatial processing of sound and acoustic communication (speech perception in humans) epitomize the two major functions of hearing. The review will concentrate on auditory cortical plasticity from these two vantage points and,

in surveying some of the existing literature, will make suggestions for further study.

Finally, plasticity of the auditory system has an important function in the compensation of early loss of vision and hearing. When animals or humans are born or grow up blind, auditory functions expand into previously visual regions of the brain. This can be demonstrated with neurobiological and functional imaging techniques and confirms behavioral observations. Conversely, in deaf individuals auditory cortex also reorganizes to take on other functions that permit those individuals to use it for communication through other sensory modalities.

10.2 Plasticity of auditory spatial functions

Epigenetic adaptation of sound localization cues

One of the arguments for the adaptive value of cortical plasticity has long been that it helps the brain to cope with a changing environment. This is especially important during early postnatal development, when the organism itself is still growing and undergoing rapid physical change. The genome cannot possibly anticipate head size or interocular distance in its efforts to develop functional stereoscopic vision, or at the very least such a program would be highly costly to purely genetic resources. A much simpler solution is to build a brain under adaptive control by environmental stimuli, that is developmental plasticity of synaptic connections that mediate the corresponding function. Using this information, in addition to the genetic code, will also enhance the precision with which a system can respond to environmental needs and possibly compensate for drastic insults.

Similarly, in the developing auditory system head size plays a role for interaural comparisons that underlie binaural hearing. Interaural time and intensity differences are computed in the brain stem and are, one might assume, largely hard wired. This is, however, not the case: the map of auditory space, which is formed in the superior colliculus (SC) on the basis of these interaural cues, is highly dependent

on both auditory and visual experience (Knudsen, 1985). As auditory spatial information is sent up to the auditory cortex, the well-known malleability of thalamo-cortical and cortico-cortical connections enhances the plasticity of auditory space perception even further. Monaural spectral cues, which reflect the differences in filtering by the head and outer ear for different frequencies, are most likely integrated at the cortical level, where tonotopic maps exist and facilitate the combination of complex spectral information.

Sound localization based on spectral cues compares the incoming sound with stored templates of the head-related transfer function (HRTF) in each individual (Middlebrooks and Green, 1991; Blauert, 1996). Spectral cues are important not only as an additional cue in spatial processing along azimuth. They are indispensable for the disambiguation of front–back confusions, and they are essentially the only set of cues for spatial processing in elevation. The latter has been demonstrated to be especially dependent on learning and experience (Blauert, 1996). Recent studies on guinea pigs have found large interindividual differences in the shape and size of external ears and, consequently, their HRTFs (Sterbing et al., 2003). These differences, which can also be found in humans (Hofman et al., 1998; Wightman and Kistler, 1998), can hardly be anticipated by genetics. Assuming that monaural spectral cues are represented in the auditory cortex, spectral coding of sound location can be adjusted by means of cortical plasticity. Elevation judgments improve with experience, knowing the spectrum of complex sounds improves the accuracy of elevation processing, and filtering a sound in specific ways can bias its perceived elevation (Blauert, 1996). Evidence that the evaluation of monaural cues can change with experience comes also from studies on blind humans, whose sound localization abilities are improved (Lessard et al., 1998).

Sound localization in the blind

Cats that are binocularly lid sutured from birth for several months do not show any signs of overt behavioral impairments in spatial behavior, as one would predict if vision was needed for its development. Quantitative measurements of sound localization behavior confirm this impression. Sound localization error was measured in a task that required the cats to walk towards a sound source that varied randomly in azimuth location in order to get a food reward. The error was consistently smaller in visually deprived cats as compared to sighted controls (Rauschecker and Kniepert, 1994). The improvement was largest for lateral and rear positions of space, but even in straight-ahead positions, where the localization error is already small in normal controls, no deterioration by any means was found (Fig. 10.1).

Identical results have been described in visually deprived ferrets (King and Semple, 1996; King and Parsons, 1999), thus confirming the earlier cat studies. Similar findings have also been reported for blind humans (Muchnik et al., 1991; Lessard et al., 1998; Röder et al., 1999). The study by Röder et al. (1999) confirmed the animal studies even in quite specific detail in that it found the improvements to be most significant in lateral azimuth positions and no deterioration whatsoever in straight-ahead positions. These recent studies also fit extremely well with the classical findings by Rice and colleagues, who analyzed the echolocation abilities of blind humans and found them to be improved particularly in lateral positions of space (Rice et al., 1965; Rice, 1970).

Head motion contributes to the localization of sounds with longer duration (Middlebrooks and Green, 1991). Cats deprived of vision from birth develop conspicuous scanning movements of head and pinnae in the vertical dimension (Rauschecker and Henning, 2001). These movements are triggered only by sound, are never found in sighted cats (even in the dark), but occur in blind cats regardless of ambient light conditions (Fig. 10.2). One must assume, therefore, that vertical auditory scanning is part of the compensatory plasticity process in visually deprived cats (Rauschecker, 1995) and provides an advantage for these animals in terms of improved sound perception in elevation. In addition, scanning may also contribute to improving signal-to-noise ratio in auditory object recognition.

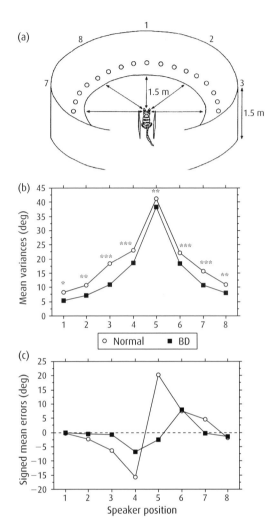

Figure 10.1. *Sound localization in visually deprived and normal cats.* The experimental setup is shown in (a) with azimuth positions 1 ... 8 in clockwise fashion. The middle and bottom panels display the results of the sound localization task at the eight positions in terms of (b) "precision" (= localization error or width of distribution) and (c) "accuracy" (= deviation from the mean). The results demonstrate that all cats are more precise in localizing straight ahead than rear positions (b) but blind cats are more precise than sighted cats at practically every position ($P < 0.002$; two-way ANOVA). Blind cats are also more accurate than normal cats (c) if the characteristic undershoot at lateral positions is taken into account ($P < 0.02$) (modified from Rauschecker (1995); data from Rauschecker and Kniepert (1994).

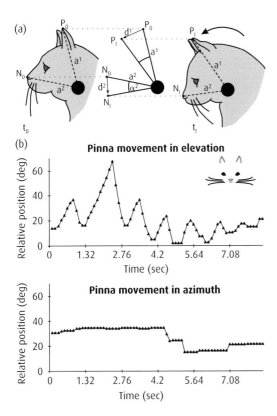

(a)

(b)

Pinna movement in elevation

Pinna movement in azimuth

Figure 10.2. *Vertical head and pinna scanning in visually deprived cats.* Cats that are deprived of vision from birth for extended periods develop characteristic scanning movements of the head and pinnae, which are presumed to improve the cats' sound localization in elevation but may also assist with auditory object recognition. Measurements were taken from video recordings using the scheme shown in (a). The panels in (b) demonstrate that scanning occurs only in elevation but not in azimuth (recordings performed by Peter Henning).

Neural basis of improved sound localization in blind animals

Neurophysiological recordings were undertaken in visually deprived cats to find the neural basis of the improved sound localization abilities in blind animals and humans. At first an involvement of the SC in the midbrain tectum, a pivotal structure for orienting behavior, was suspected. Indeed, an increased number of neurons responsive to auditory (and somatosensory) stimuli was found (Rauschecker and Harris, 1983). Later, attention turned to the cerebral

cortex: it was found on the basis of retrograde tracer experiments that the projection from visual cortex to the SC was impoverished, whereas that from association areas such as the anterior ectosylvian sulcus (AES) was preserved in at least the same strength as in normal animals (Fig. 10.3; Rauschecker and Aschoff, unpublished).

The AES region quickly moved into focus, as it is also the main source of auditory cortical input to the SC (Meredith and Clemo, 1989). In the AES region, visual responses of the anterior ectosylvian visual (AEV) area in the fundus of the AES (the probable homolog, for reasons of connectivity, of posterior parietal cortex in primates) virtually disappeared. Neurons in this region, however, did not become unresponsive, but were replaced by neurons with brisk responses to auditory and tactile stimuli. Apparently, auditory and somatosensory areas within the AES had expanded at the expense of formerly visual territory (Rauschecker and Korte, 1993).

The response properties of the expanded auditory ectosylvian area (AEA) and those of neighboring auditory fields in the AES region were homogeneous. Auditory spatial tuning (the tuning for the location of a sound source in free field) was significantly sharper in the whole AES region when compared to sighted controls. Visually deprived cats had close to 90% spatially tuned cells (with a spatial tuning ratio of better than 2 : 1 between best and worst location) (Fig. 10.4a). In addition, neurons with spatial tuning ratios of 10 : 1 or better were more abundant in blind cats (Korte and Rauschecker, 1993). The improvement of spatial tuning was independent of best frequency of the neurons (Fig. 10.4b).

The increased number of auditory cortical neurons, together with their sharpened spatial filtering characteristics, is likely to improve the sampling density of auditory space and provide the neural basis for the improved spatial abilities of early blind cats and ferrets (Fig. 10.5; Rauschecker, 1995, 2002).

Neuroimaging of auditory spatial functions in blind humans

How do the changes in visually deprived animals translate into compensation of early blindness

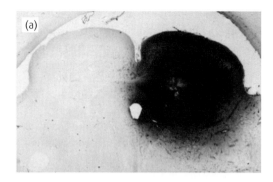

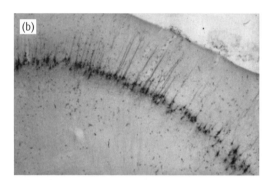

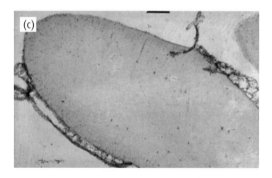

Figure 10.3. *Results of horseradish-peroxidase (HRP) injections into the SC of normal and visually deprived cats.* The SC on one side was completely filled with HRP (a), and retrogradely labeled cells in various cortical areas were displayed and counted. Cells were consistently encountered in layer 5, as expected. Visual cortex (as well as a number of other areas) was labeled at high density in normal cats (b), whereas it was only sparsely labeled in visually deprived cats (c). The AE region in visually deprived cats appeared to show denser label than in normal cats (Rauschecker and Aschoff, unpublished).

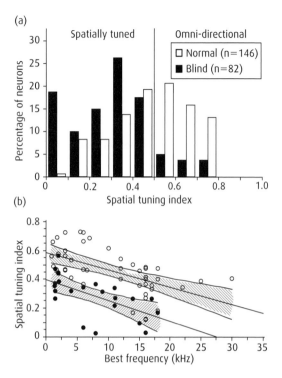

Figure 10.4. *Sharpening of spatial tuning in the AE cortical region of visually deprived cats.* (a) Responses of auditory neurons in the AE region were tested at different azimuth positions, and their spatial tuning index was determined by the ratio of least to best responses. Spatially tuned neurons were defined as having an index of <0.5. Blind cats had significantly more spatially tuned neurons ($P < 0.001$). In (b) the correlation of spatial tuning index with best frequency was plotted in each neuron. Although a clear correlation was found in a regression analysis between the two parameters, the normal and the blind group differed across the whole frequency spectrum. The hatched areas correspond to 95% confidence intervals (modified from Korte and Rauschecker, 1993).

in man? Apart from behavioral studies modern neuroimaging has contributed to a better understanding of these processes. One of the first imaging studies in the blind was performed by Veraart and colleagues, who found that visual cortex displayed cerebral blood flow that was actually higher, on average, than in sighted controls (Wanet-Defalque et al., 1988; see also Uhl et al., 1993). These results were later substantiated by a number of studies

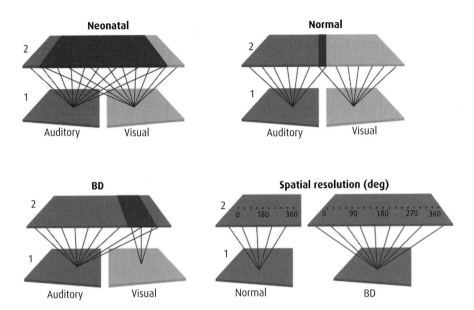

Figure 10.5. *Schematic display of crossmodal plasticity.* Developmental plasticity across sensory modalities is shown during normal development (top panels) and during binocular deprivation (BD; bottom panels). Expansion of auditory cortical regions in blind cats results in a simultaneous narrowing of spatial filters (after Rauschecker, 1995).

from several laboratories that showed specific activation of occipital cortex in the blind by nonvisual stimuli (Sadato et al., 1996; Büchel et al., 1998; De Volder et al., 1999; Weeks et al., 2000; Arno et al., 2001).

In the study by Weeks et al. (2000), congenitally blind and sighted subjects were tested in a virtual auditory space environment (simulating quasi-free-field sound with standardized HRTFs and headphones) and their relative cerebral blood flow (rCBF) was measured in a whole-head positron emission tomography (PET) scanner. The task was (a) to decide whether two subsequent sounds were coming from the same or a different azimuth position in space, or (b) to move a joystick into the presumed direction. Both tasks yielded similar results.

In all subjects (sighted or blind) posterior inferior parietal cortex was activated, which provides clear evidence for an involvement of this region in auditory spatial processing. It was confirmed by independent studies that this parietal region (presumably the human analog of the ventral intraparietal area (VIP) in monkeys) contains in fact a unimodal auditory area (Bushara et al., 1999; Weeks et al., 1999). It is part and parcel of a dorsal auditory processing stream (Rauschecker and Tian, 2000) and receives its input from auditory belt and parabelt cortex in the posterior superior temporal gyrus (STG) (Lewis and Van Essen, 2000). Both sighted and blind subjects also activated frontal areas, owing to the delayed matching task involving working memory, which are also part of the auditory "where" stream (Romanski et al., 1999).

In blind subjects, occipital cortex was activated in addition to the above areas (Fig. 10.6a). Activation zones originated in posterior parietal cortex and extended all the way into Brodmann areas 18 and 19, as determined on the basis of Talairach coordinates (Talairach and Tournoux, 1988). The expansion was most extensive in the right hemisphere, which testifies to its special involvement in spatial processes (Mesulam, 1999). Similar results of auditory activation in the occipital cortex of blind subjects were obtained using event-related potential (ERP) techniques (Kujala et al., 1992, 1995).

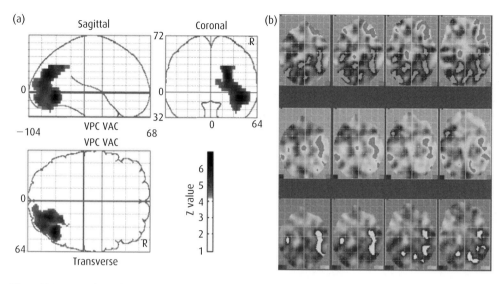

Figure 10.6. *PET evidence that in blind persons representation of sound localization is expanded into areas of cortex normally devoted to visual functions.* (a) Group comparison between blind and normal subjects is shown which demonstrates a massive increase of activation in occipital cortex, particularly in the right hemisphere (from Weeks et al., 2000). (b) Interregional analysis. Correlations of the right IPL with other parts of cortex are shown. Positive correlations are shown in **red**, negative correlations in **blue**. Auditory cortex in the superior temporal region is negatively correlated with the right IPL in sighted subjects (top panel) but positively in the blind (middle panel). Statistically significant differences are shown in the bottom panel with higher correlation in the blind in **yellow**. The increased correlation of the IPL with the superior temporal region is evident as is an increased correlation in prestriate cortex (Brodmann area 18). This amounts to a functional network for sound localization in the blind involving auditory, parietal and occipital regions.

The surprising activation of occipital, formerly visual cortical areas in blind subjects raises two fundamental questions: why was such activation not found in visually deprived cats? And is the auditory activation of occipital areas in the blind due to feedforward, bottom-up activation from auditory areas, or is it due to feedback input from higher-order, parietal cortical regions, homologous to the AES in cats? The answer to the first question is simple: occipital areas in visually deprived cats were never tested with auditory stimuli. It is, therefore, quite possible that auditory activity would also be found in binocularly deprived (BD) cats. Some earlier studies in fact reported auditory activation of visual cortex even in normal cats (Spinelli et al., 1968; Fishman and Michael, 1973), but these reports were never taken very seriously, because the activation was sparse and was generally attributed to unspecific

effects of anesthesia or arousal. Auditory projections to visual cortex had also been demonstrated in very young kittens (Innocenti and Clarke, 1984), but a stabilization of these transitory connections by visual deprivation has not been shown. Recent anatomical data with more sensitive tracers have demonstrated, however, that a direct projection from auditory to visual cortex does exist in adult rhesus monkeys (Falchier et al., 2002; Rockland and Ojima, 2003). These results may be interpreted in favor of a more metamodal organization of the brain (Pascual-Leone and Hamilton, 2001), which could be utilized for compensatory plasticity.

Interregional analysis of the PET imaging data by Weeks et al. (2000) suggests that feedback connections from the inferior parietal lobule (IPL) could also provide a stronger auditory signal in blind than in sighted individuals and perhaps be responsible for the auditory activation in the occipital lobe (Fig. 10.6b). Whereas auditory cortex in the superior temporal region is negatively correlated with the right IPL in sighted subjects, it shows strongly positive correlation with the IPL in blind subjects. In addition, IPL activation is strongly correlated with occipital regions. This indicates that the IPL region is dominated by auditory input in the blind, which is further carried into occipital cortex by a strengthened back projection from IPL.

10.3 Plasticity of auditory object recognition

It is uncontroversial that auditory cortex is involved in the identification and recognition of auditory objects including the decoding and interpretation of speech sounds and the appreciation of music. This general achievement, which is one of the most astounding capabilities of our whole brain, calls for a high degree of adaptive plasticity, especially in speech perception, where daily learning occurs from an early age. The ability to learn languages persists to a some extent into adulthood, but there are clearly sensitive or critical periods for the acquisition of some aspects of language (Lenneberg, 1967). Regional accents, for instance, necessitate the replication of precise auditory information and are acquired at a certain age. Findings on phonological development demonstrate that foreign accents in a second language invariably persist if the latter is acquired after the age of eight (Johnson and Newport, 1989).

Speech perception: influence of early phonetic environment

Communication sounds in animals sometimes appear to be hard wired. In particular, emotionally driven calls in nonhuman primates do not seem to be modulated much by the animal's auditory experience (Zoloth et al., 1979; Seyfarth et al., 1980; Hauser, 1996). Other vocalization classes, however, that have more sophisticated social functions are highly modifiable (Hauser, 1992). Similar differences seem to hold in

songbirds, where some species display hard-wired patterns, whereas others produce lengthy sequences of learned songs, often taught to young birds by a parent (Doupe and Kuhl, 1999). In these cases, experience clearly modifies the tuning properties of neurons during recognition learning, giving rise to plastic representations of behaviorally meaningful auditory objects (Gentner and Margoliash, 2003). Humans, though endowed with an innate capacity for language, acquire language in a process that takes the better part of their childhood (~12 years; Lenneberg, 1967). Human speech and language has almost exclusively social importance and is, therefore, almost entirely plastic in most of its components.

The most obvious demonstration of experiential factors in language acquisition is the fact that infants raised in different cultures or by different parents can acquire the language of their surrounding phonetic environment without impairment (Werker and Logan, 1985; Jusczyk, 1997). The inability to distinguish (and, therefore, to produce) the characteristic sounds for "r" and "l" by speakers of some Asian languages is thus owing to the absence of the distinguishing features in their early auditory environment (Lively et al., 1993). Once acquired through early exposure, such a predisposition can only be reversed through intensive training (Logan et al., 1991), which provides further evidence for the existence of a sensitive period of language acquisition.

Compelling studies to prove the influence of early auditory experience on speech development and phonetic perception have been designed by Kuhl and co-workers (Kuhl, 2000). Infants in different countries (Sweden, Russia, and USA) initially do not show a preference for phonemes unique to their own language. By about 6 months of age, however, they suddenly develop this preference (Kuhl et al., 1992). Work by Jusczyk and colleagues shows that language-specific preferences for prosodic cues, which are necessary for the segmentation of the speech stream into perceptual units, also develop between 6 and 9 months of age (Jusczyk, 1997).

Functional imaging studies point to an involvement of cortical areas in the anterior STG with the processing of speech as well as other auditory object information (Binder et al., 2000, 2004; Rauschecker and Tian, 2000; Scott et al., 2000; Zatorre et al., 2004). Neurophysiologically, one has to imagine that neurons specific for certain speech sounds are created by combining input from lower-order neurons in earlier regions, which contain feature detectors for elements of speech. How the invariance of speech perception against changes of pitch or naturally imposed distortions is guaranteed by neural mechanisms is one of the great challenges of auditory neuroscience. Some investigators postulate that invariance is not possible without learning to generalize from the multitude of experienced samples; in other words, neuronal plasticity in the best sense. Auditory cortical plasticity enables the formation of such combinations under the influence of an early phonetic environment. Such self-organization processes ultimately lead to the establishment of phonological representations in higher-order computational maps (Kohonen and Hari, 1999).

The study of bilingual subjects is particularly instructive with regard to self-organization of language representations in the brain. Pre-neurosurgical mapping in a group of epileptic patients has demonstrated that two languages occupy largely overlapping brain space in individuals with low proficiency in the second language (Ojemann and Whitaker, 1978). As the same patients were re-mapped several years later (before a second surgery had to be undertaken), after their proficiency in the second language had increased, the amount of separation of the two language representations had increased accordingly. This result is in perfect agreement with a functional imaging study on bilingual subjects, which demonstrates that the two languages show little overlap, as long as the subjects were fluent in the second language (Kim et al., 1997).

Effects of musical training

The conclusions that can be drawn from language acquisition studies apply also to the acquisition of musical abilities. While there is undoubtedly an inherited component in "musicality" and while the capacity to appreciate and make music is universal for the human species, early experience and training makes a significant difference in how much of the brain is engaged in music processing. Early musical training in children seems to be closely related to the development of absolute pitch and a concomitant expansion of auditory cortex (Schlaug et al., 1995; Gaab and Schlaug, 2003; Gaser and Schlaug, 2003). While a structural expansion could perhaps be ascribed to genetic factors as well as to experiential ones, specific and rapid functional changes are less readily explained by genetics (Pantev et al., 1998, 2003; Shahin et al., 2003; Trainor et al., 2003). Experience-dependent plasticity for the perception of harmonic sounds is greatest before the age of eight or nine (Pantev et al., 1998). The timing of this "sensitive period" corresponds strikingly to that of phonological development mentioned earlier (Johnson and Newport, 1989).

In search for a possible neurophysiological substrate, one is again confronted with the view that preferences of higher-order neurons for specific types of complex sounds are brought about by combining features of lower-order neurons. The binding of the lower-order features is dependent on coincident timing and, thus, co-activation of neurons, as postulated originally by Hebb (1949) (for review see Rauschecker, 1991). Activity-dependent mechanisms are also suggested by monkey studies that train the animals with particular combinations of tones and find an overrepresentation of these frequencies in the auditory cortex (Recanzone et al., 1993). Subsequent studies in monkeys have demonstrated that the map expansions can be facilitated by concomitant electrical stimulation of the basal forebrain, which leads to excretion of acetylcholine, a neurotransmitter that has been implicated in plasticity and learning in a number of systems (Kilgard and Merzenich, 1998; Weinberger, 2003).

Auditory object recognition in the blind

As mentioned earlier (see Section 10.2.2), blind individuals are able to use echoes very efficiently for spatial orientation (Rice et al., 1965). Other reports claim that biosonar-like abilities enable the blind to use sound also for object recognition and obstacle avoidance ("facial vision") (Cotzin and Dallenbach,

1950) and have prompted some authors to postulate the existence of a "sonar system in the blind" (Kellogg, 1962). Findings that visual cortex in the early blind is activated by speech and environmental sounds provide further evidence that auditory compensation for early blindness extends not only to spatial hearing but also to auditory object recognition (Röder et al., 2000, 2002; Röder and Rösler, 2003).

Attempts to build prostheses for the blind based on the fact that occipital cortex is innervated by auditory input appear promising. Most devices use a transformation of visual position into frequency (Meijer, 1992; Arno et al., 2001). Complex visual patterns are transformed into complex auditory stimuli, and subjects learn to interpret them readily. In fact, many of them are cited as "seeing" a visual scene through their ears. Meijer's "vOICe" technology (Meijer, 1992) uses real visual input from a PC camera or "web cam" (http://www.seeingwithsound.com). Through special software this enables blind people carrying a laptop and a PC camera to hear live views ("soundscapes") from their environment through stereo headphones, thus hearing the very same shapes and things that sighted individuals see with their eyes. The software translates images from the camera on-the-fly into closely corresponding sounds. Blind users of this technology seem to be able to use their visual cortex to interpret complex sound patterns in similar ways as sighted people do for visual scenes. Similar conclusions were drawn by the group of DeVolder and Veraart (Renier et al., 2005) using their own substitution device. To investigate how isomorphic this process really is requires controlled studies, possibly in animal models.

10.4 Auditory plasticity and hearing impairment

Cortical reorganization in congenital deafness

Processes analogous to the auditory compensation in the blind can be demonstrated in congenitally deaf subjects. Results from ERP as well as neuroimaging techniques have shown that the brain of deaf subjects is reorganized profoundly. Visual motion areas in the right parietal cortex thought to be involved in the initial decoding of visual motion cues in American sign language (ASL) are expanded (Neville and Lawson, 1987). At the same time, "auditory" cortex in the superior temporal cortex is also activated by visual sign language (Nishimura et al., 1999; Petitto et al., 2000) and other visual stimuli (Finney et al., 2001, 2003), but is not activated by the presentation of English words, as it normally is in hearing subjects (Neville et al., 1998).

In addition to visual inputs, vibrotactile somatosensory activation has also been found in the auditory cortex of congenitally deaf humans (Levänen et al., 1998; Levänen and Hamdorf, 2001). In these studies, the stimuli were applied to palm and fingers and were registered with magnetoencephalography (MEG).

In neurobiological terms, the mechanisms responsible for crossmodal reorganization during visual or auditory deprivation are bound to be quite similar. As has been argued above, the neural mechanisms are even likely the same for reorganization within and across modalities.

Auditory cortical plasticity during the life span

Otitis media is an infection of the middle ear, frequently occurring in infants and small children (repeatedly in nearly one-third of all infants before the age of three (Gravel et al., 1996)), whose long-term effect on hearing should not be underestimated. Infections typically lead to an attenuation of auditory input by 20 dB or more. This results in significant distortions of speech, especially at higher frequencies (Dobie and Berlin, 1979). It has been found that, as a result, masking thresholds are severely altered in children with a history of otitis media (Moore et al., 1991). The question arises, therefore, whether this very common disease is a major cause of perceptual and, ultimately, language deficits. This is plausible in view of the effects of visual deprivation on visual cortical development (Wiesel, 1982). Similarly, auditory deprivation resulting from peripheral causes, such as otitis media, could exert lasting effects on the development of auditory cortex, rendering cortical neurons unresponsive to sound, and should, therefore, be observed more carefully (Moore et al., 2003). Unfortunately, comparatively little animal experimentation has been done to establish sensitive periods in auditory cortex, as they have been known to exist in visual cortex for some time (Hubel and Wiesel, 1970; Blakemore, 1991). Although some of the effects of early hearing impairment may be reversible, if hearing is restored (Moore et al., 1999), we do not know enough about possible permanent damage to discount these risks.

Impairments of speech discrimination in noisy environments, especially in the presence of multiple speakers, are becoming increasingly apparent in the elderly population (Sommers, 1997). The solution of this "cocktail-party" situation probably involves top-down processing from higher areas of the auditory cortex (similar to the classic "figure-ground discrimination" in the visual domain (Rauschecker, 1998)). Backward masking is another function altered with increasing age (Gehr and Sommers, 1999). One can easily imagine that an auditory cortex deprived of the proper input would lead to impairment in just these functions. Clearly, much more research needs to be devoted to the plasticity of central auditory plasticity during the life span.

The success story of cochlear implants and auditory cortical plasticity

Profoundly deaf individuals that still have an intact auditory nerve have profited from the dramatic advances made over the past 30 years in the field of cochlear implants (CIs) (Loeb, 1985; Rauschecker, 1999b; Rauschecker and Shannon, 2002). The CI is a microelectrode array implanted in the cochlea that directly stimulates the auditory nerve. With more than 40,000 patients worldwide, the success of these devices is nothing short of miraculous: most adults are able to converse on the phone, and most children are able to be educated in mainstream classrooms. Despite the relatively crude CI signal, delivered by a discrete and limited number of stimulating electrodes, most implant listeners are capable of excellent language understanding. Processing by the auditory

cortex fills in much of the missing information, just as the visual cortex fills in the blanks left by our blind spot or by illusory contours. In other words, auditory cortex, by means of its adaptive plasticity, learns to interpret the impoverished signal.

Obviously, a difference exists between patients that become deaf before or after acquiring speech (pre- and postlingual deafness, respectively). Whereas the postlingually deaf "re-connect" almost immediately after receiving their CI, success in prelingually deaf individuals depends on the age of implantation. As with corrections of early visual defects, such as cataract or strabismus, the maxim is "the earlier the better" (Svirsky et al., 2000). Thus, another fundamental and encouraging lesson can be learned from CI research about the plasticity of neural representations of auditory information in the brains of young children, that is, in response to sound, the stimulated auditory cortex can recruit neurons from adjacent regions of the brain and can form new neuronal connections (Fig. 10.7).

Studies in congenitally deaf cats confirm the malleability of the auditory cortex, which is molded by auditory experience from an early age (Klinke et al., 1999). If environmental sounds transmitted via a microphone and CI are used to stimulate the central auditory pathways of young deaf cats, the animals soon begin to respond with appropriate behaviors to these sounds and their auditory cortex begins to develop normal activation patterns. Much less plasticity is observed in congenitally deaf animals that are exposed to sound at an older age (Klinke et al., 1999). These results are very much in tune with the visual deprivation literature (Rauschecker and Singer, 1981; Wiesel, 1982) and indicate the existence of a sensitive period during early postnatal development of the central auditory system, especially the auditory cortex (Rauschecker, 1999a; Kral et al., 2001).

Tinnitus: auditory phantom sensation due to cortical reorganization?

Tinnitus, the hearing of a disturbing tone or noise in the absence of a real sound source, is in many ways comparable to the experience of phantom pain, which

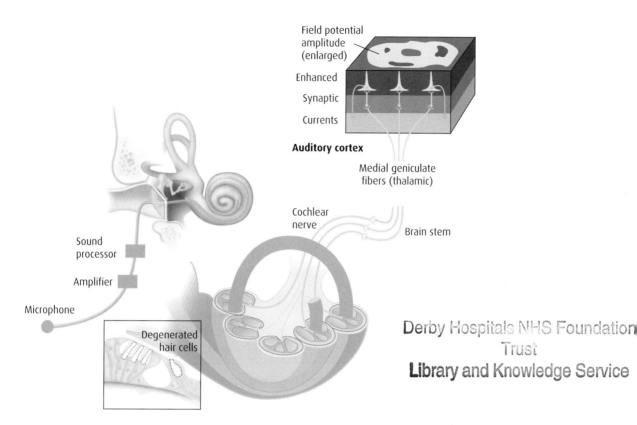

Field potential
amplitude
(enlarged)

Enhanced

Synaptic

Currents

Auditory cortex

Medial geniculate
fibers (thalamic)

Cochlear
nerve

Brain stem

Sound
processor

Amplifier

Microphone

Degenerated
hair cells

Figure 10.7. *CIs and auditory cortex.* CIs transform environmental sounds into electrical signals by means of a microphone and digital signal processing. Stimulation of auditory nerve fibers in a tonotopic fashion induces activity in the auditory cortex, which leads to a strengthening of synaptic connections in young kittens (Klinke et al., 1999). The same process of auditory cortical plasticity is assumed to lead to excellent speech understanding in CI patients despite a highly incomplete signal (from Rauschecker, 1999b).

can still be felt in an amputated limb. Tinnitus can be thought of as an auditory phantom phenomenon, in which the firing of central auditory neurons, quite possibly in the auditory cortex, still convey specific perceptual experiences, even though the corresponding sensory receptor cells that used to encode them have long been destroyed (Rauschecker, 1999a).

One of the most promising theories on the origin of tinnitus is that of a plastic reorganization in the auditory cortex following peripheral trauma caused, for instance, by loud noise exposure or aging (Jastreboff et al., 1988; Jastreboff, 1990; Rauschecker, 1999a). According to this hypothesis, the process leading to tinnitus begins with a sensorineural hearing loss in

the auditory periphery. This could be a cochlear lesion from loud noise exposure or age-related hair cell loss within a certain frequency range (often high frequencies). While the loss of hair cells causes elevated thresholds in that frequency range, neighboring frequency portions may actually be amplified because their central representation expands into the vacated frequency range (Fig. 10.8). Indeed, preliminary evidence exists from MEG and PET for an expansion of the frequency representation in auditory cortex around the tinnitus frequency (Mühlnickel et al., 1998; Lockwood et al., 1999, 2002). These results await confirmation with high-resolution functional magnetic resonance imaging (fMRI). Recent results from

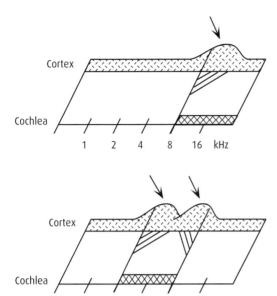

Figure 10.8. *Tinnitus model as a phantom sensation from cortical reorganization.* Loss of hair cells in parts of the cochlea (by loud noise exposure or aging) leads to an expansion of neighboring frequency regions into the vacated space and, accordingly, to their overrepresentation. In addition, these regions may lose intracortical inhibitory input from the deafferented cortex. Cortical neurons with input from frequency ranges next to the cut-off frequency thus display permanently elevated spontaneous activity levels (after Rauschecker, 1999a). Recent brain mapping studies in human patients provide evidence for an expansion of auditory cortex around the tinnitus frequency (Mühlnickel et al., 1998; Lockwood et al., 1999, 2002), but these findings await confirmation from fMRI studies at higher resolution.

high-resolution structural MRI studies using voxel-based morphometry indicate the medial geniculate nucleus as another central auditory site, alternative or in addition to auditory cortex, in which this reorganisation may occur (Mühlan et al., 2005).

The assumption that the ultimate origin of tinnitus must be central is underscored by the fact that tinnitus persists after transection of the auditory nerve, such as after acoustic neurinoma removal (Seidman and Jacobson, 1996; Matthies and Samii, 1997). Other recent findings compatible with a central origin of

tinnitus include a change in the firing pattern of auditory cortical neurons (Norena and Eggermont, 2003). Furthermore, studies using 2-deoxyglucose and c-fos autoradiography in gerbils treated with salicylate (which is known to generate tinnitus) demonstrate reduced activity in the inferior colliculus but increased activation in portions of auditory cortex (Wallhausser-Franke et al., 1996, 2003).

The origin of tinnitus according to the above hypotheses is based on the same mechanisms as cortical reorganization after lesions of the cochlea (Rajan et al., 1993; Irvine et al., 2001). As has been shown in animal studies, the resulting loss of hair cells in a specific part of the cochlea leads to a characteristic cortical reorganization of auditory cortex. Frequency regions neighboring to the lesioned part expand into the vacated space and become overrepresented. In addition, these regions lose intracortical inhibitory input from the deafferented cortical region. Cortical neurons with input from frequency ranges next to the cut-off frequency thus display permanently elevated spontaneous activity levels. Similar effects are observed after loud noise exposure or aging (the latter especially in the high-frequency region). It is assumed that the same synaptic mechanisms are responsible for reorganization after lesions and in tinnitus that lead to reorganization from experiential effects of auditory training (Calford et al., 1993; Edeline and Weinberger, 1993).

10.5 Conclusions

As in many other cortical regions, auditory cortex displays a high degree of plasticity, which has consequences for various forms of auditory function and behavior. The two main functions of hearing, spatial processing and auditory object recognition, are equally affected by auditory plasticity. Plasticity in most cases can be seen as an adaptive process (Rauschecker, 2005), but sometimes has consequences that expose the vulnerability of the brain for deprivation during critical periods of sensory development. Sensory deprivation in one modality, on the other hand, as studies of crossmodal plasticity have shown, can also have beneficial effects on other modalities. Early blindness leads to an expansion of auditory representations in the cerebral cortex; congenital deafness leads to a reassignment of auditory regions towards visual functions. Deleterious consequences of auditory plasticity are also revealed in phenomena such as tinnitus.

ACKNOWLEDGEMENTS

Portions of this manuscript are based on an updated version of an earlier review (Rauschecker, 1999a). The writing of this manuscript was partially supported by NIH grant DC003489 and a grant from the Tinnitus Research Consortium.

REFERENCES

Arno, P., De Volder, A.G., Vanlierde, A., Wanet-Defalque, M.C., Streel, E., Robert, A., Sanabria-Bohorquez, S. and Veraart, C. (2001). Occipital activation by pattern recognition in the early blind using auditory substitution for vision. *Neuroimage*, **13**, 632–645.

Binder, J.R., Frost, J.A., Hammeke, T.A., Bellgowan, P.S.F., Springer, J.A., Kaufman, J.N. and Possing, E.T. (2000). Human temporal lobe activation by speech and nonspeech sounds. *Cereb Cortex*, **10**, 512–528.

Binder, J.R., Liebenthal, E., Possing, E.T., Medler, D.A. and Ward, B.D. (2004). Neural correlates of sensory and decision processes in auditory object identification. *Nat Neurosci*, **7**, 295–301.

Blakemore, C. (1991). Sensitive and vulnerable periods in the development of the visual system. *Ciba Found Symp*, **156**, 129–147.

Blauert, J. (1996). *Spatial Hearing*, 2nd edn., MIT Press, Cambridge, MA.

Büchel, C., Price, C., Frackowiak, R.S. and Friston, K. (1998). Different activation patterns in the visual cortex of late and congenitally blind subjects. *Brain*, **121**, 409–419.

Bushara, K.O., Weeks, R.A., Ishii, K., Catalan, M.-J., Tian, B., Rauschecker, J.P. and Hallett, M. (1999). Modality-specific frontal and parietal areas for auditory and visual spatial localization in humans. *Nat Neurosci*, **2**, 759–766.

Calford, M.B., Rajan, R. and Irvine, D.R. (1993). Rapid changes in the frequency tuning of neurons in cat auditory cortex resulting from pure-tone-induced temporary threshold shift. *Neuroscience*, **55**, 953–964.

Cotzin, M. and Dallenbach, K.M. (1950). "Facial vision:" the role of pitch and loudness in the perception of obstacles by the blind. *Am J Psychol*, **63**, 485–515.

De Volder, A.G., Catalan-Ahumada, M., Robert, A., Bol, A., Labar, D., Coppens, A., Michel, C. and Veraart, C. (1999). Changes in occipital cortex activity in early blind humans using a sensory substitution device. *Brain Res*, **826**, 128–134.

Dobie, R.A. and Berlin, C.I. (1979). Influence of otitis media on hearing and development. *Ann Otol Rhinol Laryngol*, (**Suppl. 88**), 48–53.

Doupe, A.J. and Kuhl, P.K. (1999). Birdsong and human speech: common themes and mechanisms. *Annu Rev Neurosci*, **22**, 567–631.

Edeline, J.M. and Weinberger, N.M. (1993). Receptive field plasticity in the auditory cortex during frequency discrimination training: selective retuning independent of task difficulty. *Behav Neurosci*, **107**, 82–103.

Falchier, A., Clavagnier, S., Barone, P. and Kennedy, H. (2002). Anatomical evidence of multimodal integration in primate striate cortex. *J Neurosci*, **22**, 5749–5759.

Finney, E.M., Fine, I. and Dobkins, K.R. (2001). Visual stimuli activate auditory cortex in the deaf. *Nat Neurosci*, **4**, 1171–1173.

Finney, E.M., Clementz, B.A., Hickok, G., Dobkins, K.R. (2003). Visual stimuli activate auditory cortex in deaf subjects: evidence from MEG. *NeuroReport*, **14**, 1425–1427.

Fishman, M.C. and Michael, P. (1973). Integration of auditory information in the cat's visual cortex. *Vision Res*, **13**, 1415–1419.

Gaab, N. and Schlaug, G. (2003). Musicians differ from non-musicians in brain activation despite performance matching. *Ann NY Acad Sci*, **999**, 385–388.

Gaser, C. and Schlaug, G. (2003). Brain structures differ between musicians and non-musicians. *J Neurosci*, **23**, 9240–9245.

Gehr, S.E. and Sommers, M.S. (1999). Age differences in backward masking. *J Acoust Soc Am*, **106**, 2793–2799.

Gentner, T.Q. and Margoliash, D. (2003). Neuronal populations and single cells representing learned auditory objects. *Nature*, **424**, 669–674.

Gravel, J.S., Wallace, I.F. and Ruben, R.J. (1996). Auditory consequences of early mild hearing loss associated with otitis media. *Acta Otolaryngol*, **116**, 219–221.

Hauser, M.D. (1992). Articulatory and social factors influence the acoustic structure of rhesus monkey vocalizations: a learned mode of production? *J Acoust Soc Am*, **91**, 2175–2179.

Hauser, M.D. (1996). *The Evolution of Communication*, MIT Press, Cambridge, MA.

Hebb, D.O. (1949). *The Organization of Behavior*, Wiley, New York.

Hofman, P.M., Van Riswick, J.G. and Van Opstal, A.J. (1998). Relearning sound localization with new ears. *Nat Neurosci*, **1**, 417–421.

Hubel, D.H. and Wiesel, T.N. (1970). The period of susceptibility to the physiological effects of unilateral eye closure in kittens. *J Physiol*, **206**, 419–436.

Innocenti, G.M. and Clarke, S. (1984). Bilateral transitory projection from auditory cortex in kittens. *Dev Brain Res*, **14**, 143–148.

Irvine, D.R., Rajan, R. and Brown, M. (2001). Injury- and use-related plasticity in adult auditory cortex. *Audiol Neurootol*, **6**, 192–195.

Jastreboff, P.J. (1990). Phantom auditory perception (tinnitus): mechanisms of generation and perception. *Neurosci Res*, **8**, 221–254.

Jastreboff, P.J., Brennan, J.F., Coleman, J.K. and Sasaki, C.T. (1988). Phantom auditory sensation in rats: an animal model for tinnitus. *Behav Neurosci*, **102**, 811–822.

Johnson, J.S. and Newport, E.L. (1989). Critical period effects in second language learning: the influence of maturational state on the acquisition of English as a second language. *Cognit Psychol*, **21**, 60–99.

Jusczyk, P.W. (1997). *The Discovery of Spoken Language*, MIT Press, Cambridge, MA.

Kellogg, W.N. (1962). Sonar system of the blind. *Science*, **137**, 399–404.

Kilgard, M.P. and Merzenich, M.M. (1998). Cortical map reorganization enabled by nucleus basalis activity. *Science*, **279**, 1714–1718.

Kim, K.H., Relkin, N.R., Lee, K.M. and Hirsch, J. (1997). Distinct cortical areas associated with native and second languages. *Nature*, **388**, 171–174.

King, A.J. and Parsons, C. (1999). Improved auditory spatial acuity in visually deprived ferrets. *Eur J Neurosci*, **11**, 3945–3956.

King, A.J. and Semple, D.J. (1996). Improvement in auditory spatial acuity following early visual deprivation in ferrets. *Soc Neurosci Abstr*, **22**, 129.4.

Klinke, R., Kral, A., Heid, S., Tillein, J. and Hartmann, R. (1999). Recruitment of the auditory cortex in congenitally deaf cats by long-term cochlear electrostimulation. *Science*, **285**, 1729–1733.

Knudsen, E.I. (1985). Experience alters the spatial tuning of auditory units in the optic tectum during a sensitive period in the barn owl. *J Neurosci*, **5**, 3094–3109.

Kohonen, T. and Hari, R. (1999). Where the abstract feature maps of the brain might come from. *Trend Neurosci*, **22**, 135–139.

Korte, M. and Rauschecker, J.P. (1993). Auditory spatial tuning of cortical neurons is sharpened in cats with early blindness. *J Neurophysiol*, **70**, 1717–1721.

Kral, A., Hartmann, R., Tillein, J., Heid, S. and Klinke, R. (2001). Delayed maturation and sensitive periods in the auditory cortex. *Audiol Neurootol*, **6**, 346–362.

Kuhl, P.K. (2000). A new view of language acquisition. *Proc Natl Acad Sci USA*, **97**, 11850–11857.

Kuhl, P.K., Williams, K.A., Lacerda, F., Stevens, K.N. and Lindblom, B. (1992). Linguistic experience alters phonetic perception in infants by 6 months of age. *Science*, **255**, 606–608.

Kujala, T., Alho, K., Paavilainen, P., Summala, H. and Näätänen, R. (1992). Neural plasticity in processing sound location by the early blind: an event-related potential study. *Electroencephalogr Clin Neurophysiol*, **84**, 469–472.

Kujala, T., Huotilainen, M., Sinkkonen, J., Ahonen, A.I., Alho, K., Hamalainen, M.S., Ilmoniemi, R.J., Kajola, M., Knuutila, J.E. and Lavikainen, J. (1995). Visual cortex activation in blind humans during sound discrimination. *Neurosci Lett*, **183**, 143–146.

Lenneberg, E.H. (1967). *Biological Foundations of Language*, Wiley, New York.

Lessard, N., Pare, M., Lepore, F. and Lassonde, M. (1998). Early-blind human subjects localize sound sources better than sighted subjects. *Nature*, **395**, 278–280.

Levänen, S. and Hamdorf, D. (2001). Feeling vibrations: enhanced tactile sensitivity in congenitally deaf humans. *Neurosci Lett*, **301**, 75–77.

Levänen, S., Jousmaki, V. and Hari, R. (1998). Vibration-induced auditory-cortex activation in a congenitally deaf adult. *Curr Biol*, **8**, 869–872.

Lewis, J.W. and Van Essen, D.C. (2000). Corticocortical connections of visual, sensorimotor, and multimodal processing areas in the parietal lobe of the macaque monkey. *J Comp Neurol*, **428**, 112–137.

Lively, S.E., Logan, J.S. and Pisoni, D.B. (1993). Training Japanese listeners to identify English /r/ and /l/. II: the role of phonetic environment and talker variability in learning new perceptual categories. *J Acoust Soc Am*, **94**, 1242–1255.

Lockwood, A.H., Salvi, R.J., Burkard, R.F., Galantowicz, P.J., Coad, M.L. and Wack, D.S. (1999). Neuroanatomy of tinnitus. *Scand Audiol*, (**Suppl. 51**), 47–52.

Lockwood, A.H., Salvi, R.J. and Burkard, R.F. (2002). Tinnitus. *New Engl J Med*, **347**, 904–910.

Loeb, G.E. (1985). The functional replacement of the ear. *Sci Am*, **252**, 104–111.

Logan, J.S., Lively, S.E. and Pisoni, D.B. (1991). Training Japanese listeners to identify English /r/ and /l/: a first report. *J Acoust Soc Am*, **89**, 874–886.

Matthies, C. and Samii, M. (1997). Management of 1000 vestibular schwannomas (acoustic neuromas): clinical presentation. *Neurosurgery*, **40**, 1–9; discussion 9–10.

Meijer, P.B. (1992). An experimental system for auditory image representations. *IEEE Trans Biomed Eng*, **39**, 112–121.

Meredith, M.A. and Clemo, H.R. (1989). Auditory cortical projection from the anterior ectosylvian sulcus (Field AES) to the superior colliculus in the cat: an anatomical and electrophysiological study. *J Comp Neurol*, **289**, 687–707.

Mesulam, M.M. (1999). Spatial attention and neglect: parietal, frontal and cingulate contributions to the mental representation and attentional targeting of salient extrapersonal events. *Philos Trans Roy Soc Lond B Biol Sci*, **354**, 1325–1346.

Middlebrooks, J.C. and Green, D.M. (1991). Sound localization by human listeners. *Annu Rev Psychol*, **42**, 135–159.

Moore, D.R., Hutchings, M.E. and Meyer, S.E. (1991). Binaural masking level differences in children with a history of otitis media. *Audiology*, **30**, 91–101.

Moore, D.R., Hine, J.E., Jiang, Z.D., Matsuda, H., Parsons, C.H., King, A.J. (1999). Conductive hearing loss produces a reversible binaural hearing impairment. *J Neurosci*, **19**, 8704–8711.

Moore, D.R., Hartley, D.E. and Hogan, S.C. (2003). Effects of otitis media with effusion (OME) on central auditory function. *Int J Pediatr Otorhinolaryngol*, **67**(**Suppl. 1**), S63–S67.

Muchnik, C., Efrati, M., Nemeth, E., Malin, M. and Hildesheimer, M. (1991). Central auditory skills in blind and sighted subjects. *Scand Audiol*, **20**, 19–23.

Mühlau, M., Rauschecker, J.P., Oestreicher, E., Gaser, C., Röttinger, M., Simon, F., Etgen, T., Conrad, B. and Sander, D. (2005). Structural brain changes in tinnitus. Society for Neuroscience, Abstract 31, 282.11.

Mühlnickel, W., Elbert, T., Taub, E. and Flor, H. (1998). Reorganization of auditory cortex in tinnitus. *Proc Natl Acad Sci USA*, **95**, 10340–10343.

Neville, H.J. and Lawson, D. (1987). Attention to central and peripheral visual space in a movement detection task: an event-related potential and behavioral study. II. Congenitally deaf adults. *Brain Res*, **405**, 268–283.

Neville, H.J., Bavelier, D., Corina, D., Rauschecker, J.P., Karni, A., Lalwani, A., Braun, A., Clark, V., Jezzard, P. and Turner, R. (1998). Cerebral organization for language in deaf and hearing subjects: biological constraints and effects of experience. *Proc Natl Acad Sci USA*, **95**, 922–929.

Nishimura, H., Haskikawa, K., Doi, K., Iwaki, T., Watanabe, Y., Kusuoka, H., Nishimura, T. and Kubo, T. (1999). Sign language "heard" in the auditory cortex. *Nature*, **397**, 116.

Norena, A.J. and Eggermont, J.J. (2003). Changes in spontaneous neural activity immediately after an acoustic trauma: implications for neural correlates of tinnitus. *Hear Res*, **183**, 137–153.

Ojemann, G.A. and Whitaker, H.A. (1978). The bilingual brain. *Arch Neurol*, **35**, 409–412.

Pantev, C., Oostenveld, R., Engelien, A., Ross, B., Roberts, L.E. and Hoke, M. (1998). Increased auditory cortical representation in musicians. *Nature*, **392**, 811–814.

Pantev, C., Ross, B., Fujioka, T., Trainor, L.J., Schulte, M. and Schulz, M. (2003). Music and learning-induced cortical plasticity. *Ann NY Acad Sci*, **999**, 438–450.

Pascual-Leone, A. and Hamilton, R. (2001). The metamodal organization of the brain. *Prog Brain Res*, **134**, 427–445.

Petitto, L.A., Zatorre, R.J., Gauna, K., Nikelski, E.J., Dostie, D. and Evans, A.C. (2000). Speech-like cerebral activity in profoundly deaf people processing signed languages: implications for the neural basis of human language. *Proc Natl Acad Sci USA*, **97**, 13961–13966.

Rajan, R., Irvine, D.R., Wise, L.Z. and Heil, P. (1993). Effect of unilateral partial cochlear lesions in adult cats on the representation of lesioned and unlesioned cochleas in primary auditory cortex. *J Comp Neurol*, **338**, 17–49.

Rauschecker, J.P. (1991). Mechanisms of visual plasticity: Hebb synapses, NMDA receptors and beyond. *Physiol Rev*, **71**, 587–615.

Rauschecker, J.P. (1995). Compensatory plasticity and sensory substitution in the cerebral cortex. *Trend Neurosci*, **18**, 36–43.

Rauschecker, J.P. (1998). Cortical control of the thalamus: top-down processing and plasticity. *Nat Neurosci*, **1**, 179–180.

Rauschecker, J.P. (1999a). Auditory cortical plasticity: a comparison with other sensory systems. *Trend Neurosci*, **22**, 74–80.

Rauschecker, J.P. (1999b). Making brain circuits listen. *Science*, **285**, 1686–1687.

Rauschecker, J.P. (2002). Auditory reassignment. In: *Handbook of Neuropsychology, Plasticity and Rehabilitation* (eds Boller, F. and Grafman, J.), 2nd edn., Vol. 9. Elsevier, Amsterdam, pp. 167–176.

Rauschecker, J.P. (2005). Adaptive plasticity and sensory substitution in the cerebral cortex. In: *Reprogramming the Cerebral Cortex: Plasticity Following Central and Peripheral Lesion* (eds Lomber, S.G. and Eggermont, J.J.), Oxford University Press (in press), Oxford.

Rauschecker, J.P. and Harris, L.R. (1983). Auditory compensation of the effects of visual deprivation in the cat's superior colliculus. *Exp Brain Res*, **50**, 69–83.

Rauschecker, J.P. and Henning, P. (2001). Crossmodal expansion of cortical maps in early blindness. In: *The Mutable Brain* (ed. Kaas, J.), Harwood Academic Publishers, Singapore, pp. 243–259.

Rauschecker, J.P. and Kniepert, U. (1994). Enhanced precision of auditory localization behavior in visually deprived cats. *Eur J Neurosci*, **6**, 149–160.

Rauschecker, J.P. and Korte, M. (1993). Auditory compensation for early blindness in cat cerebral cortex. *J Neurosci*, **13**, 4538–4548.

Rauschecker, J.P. and Shannon, R.V. (2002). Sending sound to the brain. *Science*, **295**, 1025–1029.

Rauschecker, J.P. and Singer, W. (1981). The effects of early visual experience on the cat's visual cortex and their possible explanation by Hebb synapses. *J Physiol*, **310**, 215–239.

Rauschecker, J.P. and Tian, B. (2000). Mechanisms and streams for processing of "what" and "where" in auditory cortex. *Proc Natl Acad Sci USA*, **97**, 11800–11806.

Recanzone, G.H., Schreiner, C.E. and Merzenich, M.M. (1993). Plasticity in the frequency representation of primary auditory cortex following discrimination training in adult owl monkeys. *J Neurosci*, **13**, 87–103.

Renier, L., Collignon, O., Poirier, C., Tranduy, D., Vanlierde, A., Bol, A., Veraart, C. and De Volder, A.G. (2005). Cross-modal activation of visual cortex during depth perception using auditory substitution of vision. *Neuroimage*, **26(2)**, 573–580.

Rice, C.E. (1970). Early blindness, early experience, and perceptual enhancement. *Res Bull Am Found Blind*, **22**, 1–22.

Rice, C.E., Feinstein, S.H. and Schusterman, R.J. (1965). Echo-detection ability of the blind: size and distance factor. *J Exp Psychol*, **70**, 246–251.

Rockland, K.S. and Ojima, H. (2003). Multisensory convergence in calcarine visual areas in macaque monkey. *Int J Psychophysiol*, **50**, 19–26.

Röder, B. and Rösler, F. (2003). Memory for environmental sounds in sighted, congenitally blind and late blind adults: evidence for cross-modal compensation. *Int J Psychophysiol*, **50**, 27–39.

Röder, B., Rösler, F. and Neville, H.J. (2000). Event-related potentials during auditory language processing in congenitally blind and sighted people. *Neuropsychologia*, **38**, 1482–1502.

Röder, B., Stock, O., Bien, S., Neville, H. and Rösler, F. (2002). Speech processing activates visual cortex in congenitally blind humans. *Eur J Neurosci*, **16**, 930–936.

Röder, B., Teder-Salejarvi, W., Sterr, A., Rosler, F., Hillyard, S.A. and Neville, H.J. (1999). Improved auditory spatial tuning in blind humans. *Nature*, **400**, 162–166.

Romanski, L.M., Tian, B., Fritz, J., Mishkin, M., Goldman-Rakic, P.S. and Rauschecker, J.P. (1999). Dual streams of auditory afferents target multiple domains in the primate prefrontal cortex. *Nat Neurosci*, **2**, 1131–1136.

Sadato, N., Pascual-Leone, A., Grafman, J., Ibanez, V., Deiber, M.-P., Dold, G. and Hallett, M. (1996). Activation of the primary visual cortex by Braille reading in blind subjects. *Nature*, **380**, 526–528.

Schlaug, G., Jancke, L., Huang, Y. and Steinmetz, H. (1995). *In vivo* evidence of structural brain asymmetry in musicians. *Science*, **267**, 699–701.

Scott, S.K., Blank, C.C., Rosen, S. and Wise, R.J.S. (2000). Identification of a pathway for intelligible speech in the left temporal lobe. *Brain*, **123**, 2400–2406.

Seidman, M.D. and Jacobson, G.P. (1996). Update on tinnitus. *Otolaryngol Clin North Am*, **29**, 455–465.

Seyfarth, R.M., Cheney, D.L. and Marler, P. (1980). Monkey responses to three different alarm calls: evidence of predator classification and semantic communication. *Science*, **210**, 801–803.

Shahin, A., Bosnyak, D.J., Trainor, L.J. and Roberts, L.E. (2003). Enhancement of neuroplastic P2 and N1c auditory evoked potentials in musicians. *J Neurosci*, **23**, 5545–5552.

Sommers, M.S. (1997). Speech perception in older adults: the importance of speech-specific cognitive abilities. *J Am Geriatr Soc*, **45**, 633–637.

Spinelli, D.N., Starr, A. and Barrett, T.W. (1968). Auditory specificity in unit recordings from cat's visual cortex. *Exp Neurol*, **22**, 75–84.

Sterbing, S.J., Hartung, K. and Hoffmann, K.P. (2003). Spatial tuning to virtual sounds in the inferior colliculus of the guinea pig. *J Neurophysiol*, **90**, 2648–2659.

Svirsky, M.A., Robbins, A.M., Kirk, K.I., Pisoni, D.B. and Miyamoto, R.T. (2000). Language development in profoundly deaf children with cochlear implants. *Psychol Sci*, **11**, 153–158.

Talairach, J. and Tournoux, P. (1988). *A Coplanar Sterotaxic Atlas of the Human Brain*, Thieme Verlag, Stuttgart, Germany.

Trainor, L.J., Shahin, A. and Roberts, L.E. (2003). Effects of musical training on the auditory cortex in children. *Ann NY Acad Sci*, **999**, 506–513.

Uhl, F., Franzen, P., Podreka, I., Steiner, M. and Deecke, L. (1993). Increased regional cerebral blood flow in inferior occipital cortex and cerebellum of early blind humans. *Neurosci Lett*, **150**, 162–164.

Wallhausser-Franke, E., Braun, S. and Langner, G. (1996). Salicylate alters 2-DG uptake in the auditory system: a model for tinnitus? *NeuroReport*, **7**, 1585–1588.

Wallhausser-Franke, E., Mahlke, C., Oliva, R., Braun, S., Wenz, G. and Langner, G. (2003). Expression of c-fos in auditory and non-auditory brain regions of the gerbil after manipulations that induce tinnitus. *Exp Brain Res*, **153**, 649–654.

Wanet-Defalque, M.C., Veraart, C., De Volder, A., Metz, R., Michel, C., Dooms, G. and Goffinet, A. (1988). High metabolic activity in the visual cortex of early blind human subjects. *Brain Res*, **446**, 369–373.

Weeks, R., Horwitz, B., Aziz-Sultan, A., Tian, B., Wessinger, C.M., Cohen, L., Hallett, M. and Rauschecker, J.P. (2000). A positron emission tomographic study of auditory localisation in the congenitally blind. *J Neurosci*, **20**, 2664–2672.

Weeks, R.A., Aziz-Sultan, A., Bushara, K.O., Tian, B., Wessinger, C.M., Dang, N., Rauschecker, J.P. and Hallett, M. (1999). A PET study of human auditory spatial processing. *Neurosci Lett*, **262**, 155–158.

Weinberger, N.M. (2003). The nucleus basalis and memory codes: auditory cortical plasticity and the induction of specific, associative behavioral memory. *Neurobiol Learn Mem*, **80**, 268–284.

Werker, J.F. and Logan, J.S. (1985). Cross-language evidence for three factors in speech perception. *Percept Psychophys*, **37**, 35–44.

Wiesel, T.N. (1982). Postnatal development of the visual cortex and the influence of environment. *Nature*, **299**, 583–591.

Wightman, F. and Kistler, D. (1998). Of vulcan ears, human ears and "earprints". *Nat Neurosci*, **1**, 337–339.

Zatorre, R.J., Bouffard, M. and Belin, P. (2004). Sensitivity to auditory object features in human temporal neocortex. *J Neurosci*, **24**, 3637–3642.

Zoloth, S.R., Petersen, M.R., Beecher, M.D., Green, S., Marler, P., Moody, D.B. and Stebbins, W. (1979). Species-specific perceptual processing of vocal sounds by monkeys. *Science*, **204**, 870–873.

11

Cross-modal plasticity in sensory systems

Krishnankutty Sathian

Departments of Neurology and Rehabilitation Medicine, Emory University School of Medicine, Atlanta, GA, USA

This chapter reviews studies of cross-modal interactions from two perspectives. One is the issue of cross-modal plasticity resulting from sensory deprivation, which is considered in terms of the twin questions: does deprivation of inputs in one sensory modality (1) improve perception in the remaining modalities? and (2) alter neural processing of the remaining inputs? With respect to this issue, plasticity of sensory-perceptual processing is distinguished from that of linguistic processing. Further, the effects of short-term versus long-term sensory deprivation, and of the age of onset of deprivation are addressed, to the extent that they have been studied. A complementary perspective is offered by investigations of cross-modal involvement and multisensory processing in cortical regions that have traditionally been associated with a single sensory modality. The focus in this chapter is on studies of cross-modal interactions that affect the visual system. Similar interactions affecting the auditory system are reviewed in the previous chapter (this volume) by Rauschecker. The interested reader is referred to a review of the phenomena, neural correlates and possible mechanisms of cross-modal plasticity (Bavelier and Neville, 2002).

11.1 Superior non-visual perception in the blind

According to common belief, blindness is associated with superior non-visual perception. However, the empirical literature offers mixed support for this idea, despite over a century of investigation (Griesbach,

1899; Hollins, 1989). For instance, studies of haptic perception of three-dimensional shape have yielded conflicting results, ranging from better performance in the blind (Heller, 1989a), through equal performance in sighted and blind individuals (Morrongiello et al., 1994), to better performance in the sighted (Hollins, 1985; Bailes and Lambert, 1986; Lederman et al., 1990). One view is that any advantage of the blind on haptic tasks is not due to heightened sensitivity, but rather to practice in attending to cues that normally are ignored by the sighted (Hollins, 1989), or the use of efficient sensorimotor strategies (Davidson, 1972; Shimizu et al., 1993; D'Angiulli et al., 1998).

The situation appears to be different for tactile perception of two-dimensional patterns presented to a fingerpad. The results of studies using such patterns have been interpreted in the light of Braille-reading experience. Braille is a spatial code, with each character comprising raised dots arranged in a 3×2 matrix: a dot may be present or absent at each of the six positions in the matrix. An early study found that blind Braille readers out-performed their sighted counterparts on tactile recognition of dot patterns resembling Braille, when such patterns were presented in 3×3 and 4×4 matrices but not 5×5 or 6×6 matrices (Foulke and Warm, 1967). These findings were explained in terms of carry-over of Braille-reading experience to the smaller patterns, which could be entirely covered by the fingerpad, whereas the larger patterns required sequential exploration.

More recently, a number of studies have extended these observations to other kinds of two-dimensionally varying patterns. In one of these studies, blind Braille readers could detect smaller gaps in bar stimuli, and judge the orientation of shorter bars, compared to sighted controls (Stevens et al., 1996). A popular test of tactile spatial acuity uses discrimination of grating orientation, which involves applying gratings of alternating ridges and grooves to the pad of the immobilized finger, and requiring subjects to report whether the grating is oriented along or across the long axis of the finger (van Boven and Johnson, 1994). Performance in this task is an increasing function of groove width, and an acuity threshold can be computed in terms of the minimal groove width required to permit reliable discrimination of grating orientation. Two studies employing this test found that the blind performed superiorly (van Boven et al., 2000; Goldreich and Kanics, 2003). Although our laboratory failed to find a significant difference between blind and sighted subjects on this test, we showed that blind subjects excel at a task requiring the detection of a minute spatial change (Grant et al., 2000). This latter task, which yielded the largest reported difference between blind and sighted subjects on a tactile perceptual task, involved distinguishing whether or not the central dot in a linear three-dot array was offset laterally. The magnitude of offset was less than 1 mm, which corresponds to the limit of tactile spatial acuity; thus, this task was in the hyperacuity range. Not all tasks, however, are associated with superior performance in the blind, who do not differ significantly from the sighted on discriminating bar length (Stevens et al., 1996), laboratory textures such as gratings (Grant et al., 2000) or real-world textures like sandpapers or abrasive stones (Heller, 1989b).

Is superior tactile spatial performance a consequence of practice? Some evidence supports this idea. For instance, practiced sighted subjects can match the blind on the hyperacuity task (Grant et al., 2000) and the Optacon (Craig, 1988), a vibrotactile reading aid for the blind. They can also do as well as the deaf–blind in decoding speech by the Tadoma method, feeling the speaker's face and neck (Reed et al., 1978, 1982). Interestingly, blind subjects showed no improvement in hyperacuity over the 3–4 day period of practice that benefited the sighted

(Grant et al., 2000), suggesting that the blind were already operating at maximal capability. The role of specific practice with reading Braille is another factor that has been investigated, with mixed results. One study reported a lower grating orientation discrimination threshold on the Braille-reading finger than on other fingers tested (van Boven et al., 2000), while another study found no significant difference on the same test between blind subjects who read Braille and those who did not (Goldreich and Kanics, 2003), and our study did not reveal superior hyperacuity on the hand used for reading Braille (Grant et al., 2000).

Is the age at onset of blindness important? If tactile performance is different in the congenitally blind and late blind, this would imply that plasticity during the critical period of visual development is an additional factor influencing cross-modal perception. Two of the studies cited above (Grant et al., 2000; Goldreich and Kanics, 2003) included both early blind and late blind subjects. In neither study was there a significant performance difference between the early and late blind, although there were trends for the early blind to be better. Thus, there is currently no definite evidence that visual deprivation during a critical period in early life, compared to that in later life, results in enhanced tactile capabilities.

What about other sensory domains? Although their absolute olfactory sensitivity appears to be poorer, the blind outperform the sighted on identification of odors (Murphy and Cain, 1986). A similar situation may pertain to auditory perception. Tests of elementary auditory sensitivity, such as sound intensity discrimination, demonstrated no significant differences between blind and sighted human subjects, although the blind did seem to be slightly better at discriminating tone frequency (Starlinger and Niemeyer, 1981). On more complex auditory tasks, however, blind subjects were found to be superior to sighted controls at speech discrimination and at discriminating the intensity of a tone presented to one ear in the presence of masking sounds in the other ear (Niemeyer and Starlinger, 1981). It appears that the blind also differ from the sighted in their ability to localize auditory stimuli, as reviewed by Rauschecker in the preceding chapter. Along the horizontal plane, the blind are reported to do better at peripheral locations (70°–90° eccentricity) while both groups perform similarly at central locations (Röder et al., 1999). In contrast, the blind seem to be worse along the vertical axis (Zwiers et al., 2001). These findings may reflect, on the one hand, practice-related effects that confer superiority in certain domains and on the other hand, a deficit in domains that depend on visual input for optimal calibration. Further research into these intriguing cross-modal questions is warranted.

11.2 Somatosensory cortical plasticity following visual deprivation

Rats deprived of vision at birth are able to navigate a maze for a food reward faster than normal, and also show altered somatosensory receptive fields in the whisker barrel representation in somatosensory cortex (Toldi et al., 1994a). Following neonatal visual deprivation, mice demonstrate expansion of the whisker representation in somatosensory cortex, in association with longer facial vibrissae (Rauschecker et al., 1992). Incidentally, the longer vibrissae appear to be the only evidence for any effect of sensory deprivation on peripheral sensory structures. In humans, somatosensory evoked potentials and transcranial magnetic stimulation (TMS) in blind Braille readers demonstrate an expanded cortical sensory representation of the Braille-reading finger (Pascual-Leone and Torres, 1993), motor output maps of which expand and contract dynamically as a function of the amount of Braille reading in the hours prior to derivation of the maps by TMS (Pascual-Leone et al., 1995). Blind subjects who use multiple fingers in concert to read Braille demonstrate both disordered cortical somatotopy, as revealed by magnetoencephalography (MEG), and mislocalizations of touch on the reading fingers (Sterr et al., 1998). These plastic changes are probably a consequence of increased use as a result of visual deprivation.

11.3 Involvement of visual cortical areas in non-visual perception in the blind

Paralleling the changes in performance and somatosensory cortex noted above, neonatal visual deprivation in rats results in the appearance of somatosensory responsiveness in the anterior parts of occipital cortex, as shown by both electrophysiology and autoradiography (Toldi et al., 1994b). Monkeys whose eyelids were sutured shut in the first year of life and opened thereafter were found to show somatosensory responses (absent in controls) in neuronal recordings in dorsal extrastriate visual cortex, while visual responsiveness was decreased compared to controls (Hyvärinen et al., 1981). This procedure, however, had no effect on haptic discrimination ability, albeit in a different cohort of monkeys (Carlson et al., 1989).

An early indication of cross-modal plasticity in blind humans was provided by a report that used positron emission tomographic (PET) scanning to show that occipital cortical areas, generally considered to be visual in function, were more metabolically active in early blind individuals than in the late blind or sighted (Veraart et al., 1990). This was interpreted as evidence of greater synaptic activity in the early blind, possibly reflecting incomplete developmental pruning of synapses. Subsequently, event-related potentials (ERPs) and MEG recordings were used to demonstrate occipital cortical recruitment in the blind during auditory discrimination of tones (Alho et al., 1993; Kujala et al., 1995). However, because occipital activity was evoked in another ERP study during both tactile discrimination of line orientation and auditory tone discrimination, it has been considered to result from non-specific attentional effects (Röder et al., 1996). Occipital cortical activity in the blind also occurs during sound localization, as first shown by ERP (Kujala et al., 1992). As detailed in the preceding chapter by Rauschecker, a recent PET study showed that this activity was mainly in right dorsal extrastriate cortex, which exhibited higher functional connectivity with right posterior parietal cortex than in sighted subjects (Weeks et al., 2000).

Considerable excitement has been generated by the observations that visual cortical regions of blind subjects are involved in reading Braille. One line of evidence for this comes from activation of neuroimaging studies. In interpreting these functional imaging studies, it is important to note that the underlying experimental design relies on measurement of a difference in the local hemodynamic response between an experimental condition of interest and a control condition. In the first article of this series, a swath of medial occipital cortex including the anatomic region corresponding to primary visual cortex (V1) was shown by PET scanning to be activated in the blind, relative to a rest control, during reading Braille to discriminate words from non-words (Sadato et al., 1996). Similar, but less intense, activation was found in this study when blind subjects performed other non-Braille discrimination tasks that included discrimination of angles or the width of grooves cut in homogeneous Braille fields or of Roman letters composed of Braille dots. However, no activation occurred when subjects simply swept the finger over a Braille field. In contrast, sighted subjects showed decreased activation of these visual cortical areas during the non-Braille discrimination tasks. Following this up, it was reported that, in the blind, the same non-Braille discriminative tasks activated ventral occipital cortex but deactivated a region presumed to correspond to second somatosensory cortex (S2), with the reverse pattern in sighted subjects (Sadato et al., 1998). In these two studies, subjects actively moved the finger over Braille fields. That the observed effects were due to finger movement was excluded by a functional magnetic resonance imaging (fMRI) study of Braille character discrimination using stimulus presentations to the passive finger (Sadato et al., 2002). Activation of medial occipital cortex by Braille reading (relative to rest) occurs in early blind subjects (Cohen et al., 1999; Sadato et al., 2002), whereas the late blind and sighted deactivate these regions (Sadato et al., 2002). However, another study found a stronger temporal correlation in late than early blind subjects' visual cortical areas between the hemodynamic response measured by fMRI and the "boxcar"

function of the block design paradigm alternating between Braille reading and rest (Melzer et al., 2001).

A complementary approach to functional neuroimaging is provided by the technique of TMS. While the former method reveals brain areas that are active during a task, the latter can be used to transiently disrupt the function of a focal cortical zone. If this interferes with performance of the task, it can be inferred that the cortical focus carries out processing that is necessary for the task. TMS over medial occipital cortex impaired the ability of blind subjects to identify Braille or Roman letters and also distorted their subjective percepts of the stimuli (Cohen et al., 1997). These effects (for Roman letters) were absent in sighted subjects, who were more susceptible than their blind counterparts to TMS over the sensorimotor cortex contralateral to the hand used. Thus, visual cortex is actually functionally involved in Braille reading. This conclusion from use of TMS is corroborated by the study of an early blind person who, after an infarct of bilateral occipital cortex, developed alexia for Braille with otherwise normal somatosensory perception (Hamilton et al., 2000). Like the corresponding activation studies cited above, inactivation by TMS of medial occipital cortex disrupted Braille-reading performance in the early blind but not late blind (Cohen et al., 1999), implying that visual cortical involvement in Braille reading depends on cross-modal plasticity that takes place during the critical period of visual development.

Braille reading is, obviously, a complex task that involves not only processing of tactile sensory input but also higher-level cognitive, especially linguistic, operations. In the imaging studies reviewed so far in this section, the control condition comprised a resting state, without any demands for sensory or cognitive processing. Therefore, one cannot distinguish whether sensory or cognitive (including language-related) processes are the ones that account for the differences, in the studies reviewed above, between blind and sighted populations in visual cortical recruitment during Braille-reading tasks compared to rest baselines. Although the use of non-Braille discriminative tasks led to similar results (Sadato et al., 1996), these tasks employed verbal responses and were compared with a rest control, so that a role for linguistic processing in the resultant activations also cannot be excluded. In a PET study of Braille reading that attempted to control for linguistic processes using an auditory word control, with both tasks calling for identification of specific stimulus features, it was found that early as well as late blind subjects activated sensorimotor, superior parietal, superior occipital and fusiform cortex (Büchel et al., 1998a). However, in this study, only the late blind recruited activity in presumptive V1, whereas the early blind did not. The authors suggested that these findings might reflect visual imagery in the late blind. Clearly, these results are at odds with most of the other studies cited, which point to V1 involvement in the early but not late blind. However, a key difference between this study and the previous studies lies in the nature of controls used. As already mentioned, the Büchel et al. (1998a) study used a linguistic control that may have "subtracted" language-related processing out, whereas the other studies cited did not seek to exclude such processing. Could this mean that V1 functions in linguistic rather than perceptual processing when the blind read Braille or perform other tactile tasks? This notion seems even more far-fetched than cross-modal plasticity that is confined to sensory systems, but in fact is supported by a number of recent studies, as elaborated below.

A PET study (Büchel et al., 1998b) compared the activation evoked by words to that evoked by non-words, with the finding that a left occipito-temporal region was active on this contrast during visual presentations to sighted subjects as well as Braille presentations to blind subjects (whether early or late blind). More recently, a pair of fMRI studies examined in detail the visual cortical areas that were recruited in blind subjects during covert verb generation in response to Braille nouns (Burton et al., 2002a) or heard nouns (Burton et al., 2002b). The control condition for the Braille study consisted of feeling the Braille # sign, and that for the auditory study, hearing non-words matched for their auditory characteristics. Interestingly, both studies yielded essentially identical activations in occipital and occipito-temporal visual cortical areas, including V1.

Activation was more extensive in the early than the late blind and also more strongly lateralized to the left hemisphere in the auditory study (Burton et al., 2002b) or to the hemisphere contralateral to the Braille-reading hand in the Braille study (Burton et al., 2002a). These and related findings were reviewed recently (Burton, 2003), and are summarized in Fig. 11.1, which is reprinted from that review. In a follow-up study, it was shown that activity over an extensive region comprising multiple visual cortical areas was stronger during semantic than phonological processing, with again more extensive activity in the early blind (Burton et al., 2003).

Similarly, when congenitally blind subjects listened to sentences to identify incorrect syntactic structures, they activated V1 and other occipital regions, with the magnitude of fMRI activation increasing as a function of both semantic and syntactic complexity (Röder et al., 2002). Another group reported that congenitally blind individuals recruit occipital cortex even during a verbal memory task in the absence of sensory input (Amedi et al., 2003). Further, in this study, the verbal memory task and verb generation in response to heard nouns preferentially activated posterior occipital regions, including V1, whereas Braille reading showed a preference for more anterior regions situated in the lateral occipital complex (LOC). The magnitude of V1 activation correlated with performance on the verbal memory task (Amedi et al., 2003). The overarching conclusion from all these studies is that visual cortex is recruited for language processing in the blind. It remains uncertain whether it is also involved in other non-visual sensory functions.

Apart from the observation cited above that the magnitude of V1 activation correlated with verbal memory ability in the blind (Amedi et al., 2003), it is not known whether any of the neural changes that have been described following blindness (whether in somatosensory or visual cortical areas) are linked to behavioral superiority in non-visual domains. The studies in monkeys cited at the beginning of this section (see above for details) revealed cross-modal neural changes (Hyvärinen et al., 1981) but no improvement in performance was seen (Carlson

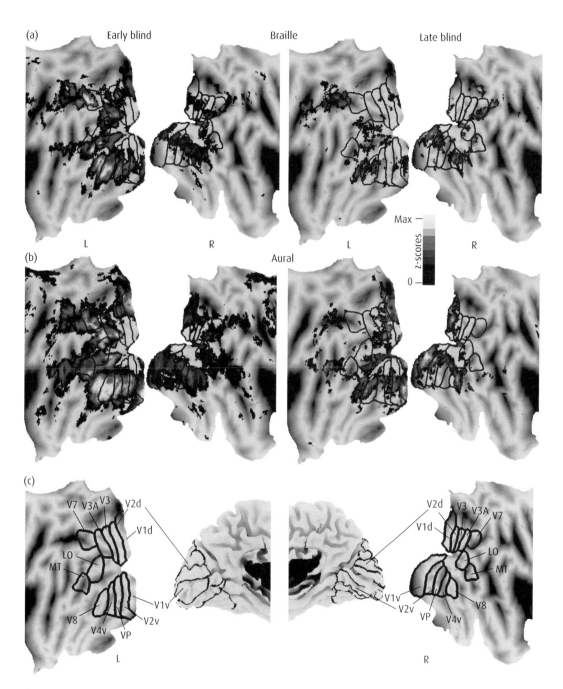

Figure 11.1. Two-dimensional flat maps showing fMRI activations in visual cortical areas in early and late blind subjects, during generation of verbs in response to nouns presented via (a) Braille or (b) aurally. Borders of visual areas are shown in sighted subjects (c). Reprinted, with permission of author and publisher, from Burton (2003); copyright 2003, Society for Neuroscience.

et al., 1989). Whether cross-modal neuroplasticity underlies the generally better high-level non-visual abilities of the blind remains a question to be answered by future research.

11.4 Mental imagery in the blind

It is known that the blind do experience mental imagery, although in the congenitally blind this cannot be visually based, while in acquired blindness the ability to image visually decays over time (Hollins, 1989). A classic mental imagery task, originally introduced for visually presented stimuli (Shepard and Metzler, 1971), involves mental rotation. Blindness, especially when congenital, slows performance of tasks requiring mental rotation of haptic stimuli (Marmor and Zaback, 1976). This suggests that visual imagery can facilitate haptic perception. ERP studies have shown that slow negativities recorded over the parietal scalp during mental rotation of haptic stimuli extend posteriorly over occipital areas in the blind (Rösler et al., 1993; Röder et al., 1997). Similarly, relatively greater occipital negativity was observed in the blind than the sighted during mental imagery of the feel of textures with the fingertips (Uhl et al., 1994). While the precise areas involved could not be localized, these studies indicate that the blind recruit their visual cortices for mental imagery in addition to the language functions discussed earlier. More recent PET studies show that the early blind and sighted activate rather similar areas during mental imagery: superior occipital and superior parietal areas during spatial imagery (Vanlierde et al., 2003) and occipito-temporal areas during form imagery that was visually based in the sighted and haptically based in the blind (De Volder et al., 2001), although there was more extensive activation in the early blind in the latter task.

11.5 Effect of short-term visual deprivation

The effects of blindness on non-visual perceptual abilities and on cerebral cortical function might be attributed to long-term neural plasticity. However, the same cannot apply to similar changes noted, amazingly, after short-term visual deprivation of normally sighted subjects. Simply blindfolding subjects for 90 min resulted in a reversible improvement of performance on discrimination of grating orientation (Facchini and Aglioti, 2003), of similar magnitude to that reported in the blind. Blindfolding for a few days improved the ability to discriminate Braille characters, while (surprisingly) concomitant, intensive Braille training had no effect (Kauffman et al., 2002). After a few days of blindfolding, fMRI studies indicate that occipital cortex, including probable V1, becomes responsive during both tactile discrimination of Braille characters and auditory discrimination of tones (Pascual-Leone and Hamilton, 2001). Moreover, TMS over occipital cortex becomes able to disrupt Braille reading. These findings mimic those reported in the blind, are absent in sighted subjects who are not visually deprived, and revert to normal within 24 h after removing the blindfold (Pascual-Leone and Hamilton, 2001). They suggest that cross-modal activation of visual cortex does not necessarily require the formation of new connections, but could operate on pre-existing connectivity between areas representing individual sensory modalities. The basis of these exciting findings remains unclear, but may be related to the enhanced excitability of visual cortex that has been demonstrated by TMS and fMRI to follow blindfolding (Boroojerdi et al., 2000).

11.6 Cross-modal involvement of visual cortical areas in normal tactile perception

Over the last few years, numerous investigations have revealed that extrastriate visual cortical areas are active during tactile tasks even in sighted people. Although the tasks used in these studies differed from those employed to study the blind, and the precise nature of visual cortical processing in the blind and sighted remains to be elucidated, the findings raise the possibility that visual deprivation simply amplifies the normal range of cross-modal recruitment.

The first report that extrastriate visual cortical areas are active during tactile perception came from our laboratory (Sathian et al., 1997), and was based on a PET study using the grating orientation discrimination task described earlier in this chapter. A contrast between the orientation discrimination task and a control task requiring discrimination of grating groove width yielded activation at a focus in extrastriate visual cortex, close to the parieto-occipital fissure. Others had shown that this focus was active during visual discrimination of grating orientation (Sergent et al., 1992) and tasks requiring spatial mental imagery (Mellet et al., 1996). Its location near the parieto-occipital fissure suggests possible homology to an area in the macaque parieto-occipital fissure (V6/PO), where a high proportion of neurons are orientation-selective (Galletti et al., 1991). To rule out the possibility that parieto-occipital cortical activation in our task was merely an epiphenomenon, we used TMS to test whether blocking processing at this focus disrupts tactile perception. We found that TMS applied directly over the locus of PET activation and at sites close to it (but not at more distant sites) significantly impaired performance in the grating orientation task (Zangaladze et al., 1999). The effect occurred when the TMS pulses were delayed by 180 ms relative to the onset of the tactile stimuli, and was specific for the orientation task, with no effect on discrimination of grating spacing. Thus, we were able to show that the activation found on PET scanning was functionally meaningful.

In another PET study from our laboratory (Prather et al., 2004), we investigated mental rotation of tactile stimuli presented to the immobilized right index fingerpad. The stimuli were upside-down[Js]; subjects reported which of two mirror-image configurations was perceived on each trial. A mental rotation condition, where the stimuli were presented at a 135–180° angle with respect to the long axis of the finger, was contrasted with a pure mirror-image discrimination condition, with the stimuli at 0°. This contrast revealed activity in the left anterior intraparietal sulcus (aIPS). As noted above, posterior parietal cortex was implicated in the mental rotation of tactile stimuli by earlier electrophysiological

studies (Rösler et al., 1993; Röder et al., 1997), but precise localization was not possible. The aIPS focus is also active during mental rotation of visual stimuli (Alivisatos and Petrides, 1997). Other groups have reported that an area involved in perception of visual motion, the MT complex, is also recruited during perception of tactile motion (Hagen et al., 2002; Blake et al., 2004).

The studies reviewed in the preceding paragraphs indicate that regions within the dorsal visual (visuospatial) pathway that are active in particular visual tasks are also engaged when the same tasks are presented tactually. This is also true of the ventral visual pathway, which is specialized for form processing. A ventral visual area known as the LOC is selective for objects compared to lower-level visual stimuli (Malach et al., 1995). We found in a PET study that, relative to a condition requiring discrimination of bar orientation, discrimination of two-dimensional form recruited a focus in the right LOC (Prather et al., 2004). In a related fMRI study from our laboratory (Stoesz et al., 2003), the same form discrimination task evoked greater activity in the LOC bilaterally than a task requiring detection of a gap in bar. The LOC is also recruited during haptic object discrimination (Amedi et al., 2001, 2002; James et al., 2002). However, its lack of activation by object-specific sounds has led to the suggestion that it specifically deals with object geometry (Amedi et al., 2002). Since both visual and haptic object identification engage the LOC, there may be a common neural representation for visual and haptic shape. This idea is supported by psychophysical (Easton et al., 1997a, b; Reales and Ballesteros, 1999) and fMRI (Amedi et al., 2001; James et al., 2002) observations of cross-modal visuo-haptic priming, and by the case report of a patient with visual agnosia resulting from a lesion that presumably damaged the LOC: this patient also had tactile agnosia despite otherwise intact somatosensory function (Feinberg et al., 1986). In a further analysis of bimodal perception of object shape using fMRI (Zhang et al., 2004), we found that both visual and haptic shape perception, relative to texture perception in the respective modality, activated bilateral regions in the superior

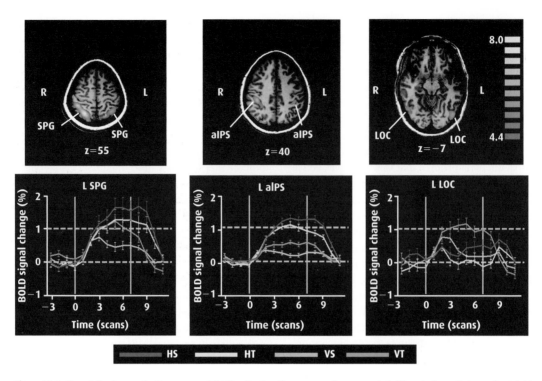

Figure 11.2. Bimodally shape-selective areas and fMRI activation time courses from areas in left hemisphere. Color scale at right represents *t* values. HS: haptic shape; HT: haptic texture; VS: visual shape; VT: visual texture. Modified from Zhang et al. (2004).

parietal gyrus (SPG), the aIPS and the LOC (Fig. 11.2). The time courses illustrated in Fig. 11.2 show the bimodal shape selectivity of these regions, and also show that the LOC preferred visual over haptic stimuli, while the parietal areas preferred haptic over visual stimuli.

11.7 Why are visual cortical areas involved in normal tactile perception?

Taken together, the studies reviewed in the last section establish clearly that tactile perception recruits multiple visual cortical regions in a task-specific manner. However, the mechanisms underlying such recruitment remain uncertain. We have suggested that visual imagery could be responsible. One line of evidence for this stems from comparison of macrospatial tasks (i.e., those requiring discrimination of

relatively large-scale parameters such as global stimulus form and orientation) with microspatial tasks (dealing with smaller-scale parameters, e.g., grating groove width discrimination and gap detection). Macrospatial tasks seem to preferentially involve visual cortical processing, and also show a greater tendency to trigger visual imagery, which is consistent with the idea that visual imagery is responsible for visual cortical involvement in tactile perception (Sathian et al., 1997; Zangaladze et al., 1999; Sathian and Zangaladze, 2001; Stoesz et al., 2003). Thus, visual cortical areas might be recruited through top-down mechanisms, perhaps because they are best adapted to analyzing object geometry. This could exemplify the general principle that information is translated into the format that fits the most adept modality (Freides, 1974). It is relevant that the LOC is active during visual imagery of object shape in sighted subjects (De Volder et al., 2001). However, some have argued against visual imagery as the basis for LOC engagement during haptic shape perception, favoring instead the explanation of a multisensory shape representation (Amedi et al., 2001, 2002; James et al., 2002).

In an attempt to resolve this controversy, we examined correlations across subjects between individual ratings of the vividness of visual imagery and the strength of increase in LOC activation during haptic shape perception compared to haptic texture perception (this indexes the strength of shape-selective activity). Interestingly, we found a dissociation between the left and right LOC: note that the haptic tasks were performed with the right hand. Shape-selective activity in the left LOC was uncorrelated with visual imagery ratings, but in the right LOC was strongly predicted by a multiple regression on two visual imagery scores, one indexing the general vividness of visual imagery in commonplace situations (as measured by the Vividness of Visual Imagery Questionnaire, VVIQ (Marks, 1973)) and the other indexing the vividness of visual imagery utilized during haptic shape perception (Zhang et al., 2004). This study suggests that both visual imagery and other factors could contribute to visual cortical recruitment during non-visual tasks.

Although a number of early neurophysiological studies suggested that non-visual stimuli influence neuronal responses in striate and extrastriate visual cortex (Lömo and Mollica, 1962; Horn, 1965; Murata et al., 1965; Bental et al., 1968; Morrell, 1972; Fishman and Michael, 1973), it is not clear if some of these neurons would still be considered to lie in V1 by today's standards. Moreover, the somatosensory stimuli in these early studies consisted of either shocks or painful stimuli (Lömo and Mollica, 1962; Horn, 1965; Murata et al., 1965), so that non-specific arousal effects cannot be excluded. A modern study in behaving monkeys found that some neurons in area V4 (in the ventral visual pathway) were selective for the orientation of a tactile grating when it served as a cue to be matched to a subsequently presented visual stimulus (Haenny et al., 1988). Such responses were not found in V1. Recent studies have clearly demonstrated multisensory inputs into early sensory

cortical areas that are usually considered as unimodal: these include V1 (Falchier et al., 2002; Rockland and Ojima, 2003) and auditory association cortex (Schroeder et al., 2003). Analysis of these inputs suggests that some are probably top-down (Falchier et al., 2002; Rockland and Ojima, 2003; Schroeder et al., 2003), while there are others that could be bottom-up (Schroeder et al., 2003). Top-down inputs would be a prerequisite for cross-modal imagery. It will be important for future work to delineate the roles of bottom-up and top-down mechanisms in cross-modal cortical recruitment.

11.8 Conclusions

In this chapter, I have reviewed a large body of work that has demonstrated the cross-modal involvement of visual cortical areas in non-visual tasks, both in the sighted and in the blind. Together with the work reviewed in the preceding chapter by Rauschecker, this work attests to the increasing awareness that the senses do not work in isolation from one another, and that neuroplastic mechanisms in response to deprivation of input from one sense modality do not respect the boundaries that are traditionally drawn between modalities. It is reasonable to expect that a fuller understanding of cross-modal processing and plasticity will enhance our ability to design better approaches to neurological rehabilitation, especially for those affected by sensory loss in one or another modality. For instance, the provision of illusory visual input using a mirror can enhance the contralateral referral of touch on the hand to a phantom hand (Ramachandran, 1995) or a hand rendered anesthetic by neurological lesions (Sathian, 2000). Such use of a mirror can also be an aid to post-stroke rehabilitation of hemiparesis (Altschuler et al., 2003) or sensory ataxia (Sathian et al., 2000), and the use of prisms can be helpful to rehabilitate patients with hemineglect (Rossetti et al., 1998). Although the neurological mechanisms underpinning these observations are still largely mysterious, these examples illustrate that creative approaches to neuro-rehabilitation can result from application of cross-modal paradigms. Such approaches merit investigation, and the results will surely be to our patients' benefit. In a broader sense, the extraordinary malleability of sensory pathways represented by these cross-modal paradigms is likely to aid in the development of neural prostheses, which will require that the brain be capable of extracting and interpreting maximum information from greatly reduced sensory inputs (see Volume I, Chapters 32 and 33).

ACKNOWLEDGEMENTS

The author's research has been supported by the NEI and the NINDS. I thank my colleagues for their invaluable contributions.

REFERENCES

Alho, K., Kujala, T., Paavilainen, P., Summala, H. and Näätänen, R. (1993). Auditory processing in visual brain areas of the early blind: evidence from event-related potentials. *EEG Clin Neurophysiol*, **86**, 418–427.

Alivisatos, B. and Petrides, M. (1997). Functional activation of the human brain during mental rotation. *Neuropsychologia*, **36**, 111–118.

Altschuler, E.L., Wisdom, S.B., Stone, L., Foster, C., Galasko, D., Llewellyn, D.M.E. and Ramachandran, V.S. (2003). Rehabilitation of hemiparesis after stroke with a mirror. *Lancet*, **353**, 2035–2036.

Amedi, A., Malach, R., Hendler, T., Peled, S. and Zohary, E. (2001). Visuo-haptic object-related activation in the ventral visual pathway. *Nat Neurosci*, **4**, 324–330.

Amedi, A., Jacobson, G., Hendler, T., Malach, R. and Zohary, E. (2002). Convergence of visual and tactile shape processing in the human lateral occipital complex. *Cereb Cortex*, **12**, 1202–1212.

Amedi, A., Raz, N., Pianka, P., Malach, R. and Zohary, E. (2003). Early "visual" cortex activation correlates with superior verbal memory performance in the blind. *Nat Neurosci*, **6**, 758–766.

Bailes, S.M. and Lambert, R.M. (1986). Cognitive aspects of haptic form recognition by blind and sighted subjects. *Brit J Psychol*, **77**, 451–458.

Bavelier, D. and Neville, H. (2002). Cross-modal plasticity: where and how? *Nat Rev Neurosci*, **3**, 443–452.

Bental, E., Dafny, N. and Feldman, S. (1968). Convergence of auditory and visual stimuli on single cells in the primary visual cortex of unanesthetized unrestrained cats. *Exp Neurol*, **20**, 341–351.

Blake, R., Sobel, K.V. and James, T.W. (2004). Neural synergy between kinetic vision and touch. *Psychol Sci*, **15**, 397–402.

Boroojerdi, B., Bushara, K.O., Corwell, B., Immisch, I., Battaglia, F., Muellbacher, W. and Cohen, L.G. (2000). Enhanced excitability of the human visual cortex induced by short-term light deprivation. *Cereb Cortex*, **10**, 529–534.

Büchel, C., Price, C., Frackowiak, R.S.J. and Friston, K. (1998a). Different activation patterns in the visual cortex of late and congenitally blind subjects. *Brain*, **121**, 409–419.

Büchel, C., Price, C. and Friston, K. (1998b). A multimodal language region in the ventral visual pathway. *Nature*, **394**, 274–277.

Burton, H. (2003). Visual cortex activity in early and late blind people. *J Neurosci*, **23**, 4005–4011.

Burton, H., Snyder, A.Z., Conturo, T.E., Akbudak, E., Ollinger, J.M. and Raichle, M.E. (2002a). Adaptive changes in early and late blind: a fMRI study of Braille reading. *J Neurophysiol*, **87**, 589–607.

Burton, H., Snyder, A.Z., Diamond, J.B. and Raichle, M.E. (2002b). Adaptive changes in early and late blind: a fMRI study of verb generation to heard nouns. *J Neurophysiol*, **88**, 3359–3371.

Burton, H., Diamond, J.B. and McDermott, K.B. (2003). Dissociating cortical regions activated by semantic and phonological tasks: a fMRI study in blind and sighted people. *J Neurophysiol*, **90**, 1965–1982.

Carlson, S., Tanila, H., Linnankoski, I. and Pertovaara, A. (1989). Comparison of tactile discrimination ability of visually deprived and normal monkeys. *Acta Physiol Scand*, **135**, 405–410.

Cohen, L.G., Celnik, P., Pascual-Leone, A., Corwell, B., Faiz, L., Dambrosia, J., Honda, M., Sadato, N., Gerloff, C., Catala, M.D. and Hallett, M. (1997). Functional relevance of cross-modal plasticity in blind humans. *Nature*, **389**, 180–183.

Cohen, L.G., Weeks, R.A., Sadato, N., Celnik, P., Ishii, K. and Hallett, M. (1999). Period of susceptibility for cross-modal plasticity in the blind. *Ann Neurol*, **45**, 451–460.

Craig, J.C. (1988). The role of experience in tactual pattern perception: a preliminary report. *Int J Rehabil Res*, **11**, 167–183.

D'Angiulli, A., Kennedy, J.M. and Heller, M.A. (1998). Blind children recognizing tactile pictures respond like sighted children given guidance in exploration. *Scand J Psychol*, **39**, 187–190.

Davidson, P.W. (1972). Haptic judgments of curvature by blind and sighted humans. *J Exp Psychol*, **93**, 43–55.

De Volder, A.G., Toyama, H., Kimura, Y., Kiyosawa, M., Nakano, H., Vanlierde, A., Wanet-Defalque, M.C., Mishina, M., Oda, K.,

Ishiwata, K. and Senda, M. (2001). Auditory triggered mental imagery of shape involves visual association areas in early blind humans. *Neuroimage*, **14**, 129–139.

Easton, R.D., Greene, A.J. and Srinivas, K. (1997a). Transfer between vision and haptics: memory for 2-D patterns and 3-D objects. *Psychonomic Bull Rev*, **4**, 403–410.

Easton, R.D., Srinivas, K. and Greene, A.J. (1997b). Do vision and haptics share common representations? Implicit and explicit memory within and between modalities. *J Exp Psychol Learn Mem Cogn*, **23**, 153–163.

Facchini, S. and Aglioti, S.M. (2003). Short term light deprivation increases tactile spatial acuity in humans. *Neurology*, **60**, 1998–1999.

Falchier, A., Clavagnier, S., Barone, P. and Kennedy, H. (2002). Anatomical evidence of multimodal integration in primate striate cortex. *J Neurosci*, **22**, 5749–5759.

Feinberg, T.E., Rothi, L.J. and Heilman, K.M. (1986). Multimodal agnosia after unilateral left hemisphere lesion. *Neurology*, **36**, 864–867.

Fishman, M.C. and Michael, C.R. (1973). Integration of auditory information in the cat's visual cortex. *Vision Res*, **13**, 1415–1419.

Foulke, E. and Warm, J.S. (1967). Effects of complexity and redundancy on the tactual recognition of metric figures. *Percept Motor Skills*, **25**, 177–187.

Freides, D. (1974). Human information processing and sensory modality: cross-modal functions, information complexity, memory and deficit. *Psychol Bull*, **81**, 284–310.

Galletti, C., Battaglini, P.P. and Fattori, P. (1991). Functional properties of neurons in the anterior bank of the parieto-occipital sulcus of the macaque monkey. *Eur J Neurosci*, **3**, 452–461.

Goldreich, D. and Kanics, I.M. (2003). Tactile acuity is enhanced in blindness. *J Neurosci*, **23**, 3439–3445.

Grant, A.C., Thiagarajah, M.C. and Sathian, K. (2000). Tactile perception in blind Braille readers: a psychophysical study of acuity and hyperacuity using gratings and dot patterns. *Percept Psychophys*, **62**, 301–312.

Griesbach, H. (1899). Vergleichende Untersuchungen über die Sinnesschärfe Blinder und Sehender. (Comparative studies of perceptual acuity in the blind and sighted.) *Pflügers Arch*, **74**, 577–638.

Haenny, P.E., Maunsell, J.H.R. and Schiller, P.H. (1988). State dependent activity in monkey visual cortex. II. Retinal and extraretinal factors in V4. *Exp Brain Res*, **69**, 245–259.

Hagen, M.C., Franzen, O., McGlone, F., Essick, G., Dancer, C. and Pardo, J.V. (2002). Tactile motion activates the human middle temporal/V5 (MT/V5) complex. *Eur J Neurosci*, **16**, 957–964.

Hamilton, R., Keenan, J.P., Catala, M. and Pascual-Leone, A. (2000). Alexia for Braille following bilateral occipital stroke in an early blind woman. *NeuroReport*, **11**, 237–240.

Heller, M.A. (1989a). Picture and pattern perception in the sighted and the blind: the advantage of the late blind. *Perception*, **18**, 379–389.

Heller, M.A. (1989b). Texture perception in sighted and blind observers. *Percept Psychophys*, **45**, 49–54.

Hollins, M. (1985). Styles of mental imagery in blind adults. *Neuropsychologia*, **23**, 561–566.

Hollins, M. (1989). *Understanding Blindness: An Integrative Approach*, Lawrence Erlbaum Associates, Inc., Hillsdale, New Jersey.

Horn, G. (1965). The effect of somaesthetic and photic stimuli on the activity of units in the striate cortex of unanaesthetized, unrestrained cats. *J Physiol (London)*, **179**, 263–277.

Hyvärinen, J., Carlson, S. and Hyvärinen, L. (1981). Early visual deprivation alters modality of neuronal responses in area 19 of monkey cortex. *Neurosci Lett*, **26**, 239–243.

James, T.W., Humphrey, G.K., Gati, J.S., Servos, P., Menon, R.S. and Goodale, M.A. (2002). Haptic study of three-dimensional objects activates extrastriate visual areas. *Neuropsychologia*, **40**, 1706–1714.

Kauffman, T., Theoret, H. and Pascual-Leone, A. (2002). Braille character discrimination in blindfolded human subjects. *NeuroReport*, **13**, 571–574.

Kujala, T., Alho, K., Paavilainen, P., Summala, H. and Näätänen, R. (1992). Neural plasticity in processing of sound location by the early blind: an event-related potential study. *EEG Clin Neurophysiol*, **84**, 469–472.

Kujala, T., Huotilainen, M., Sinkkonen, J., Ahonen, A.I., Alho, K., Hämäläinen, M.S., Ilmoniemi, R.J., Kajola, M., Knuutila, J.E.T., Lavikainen, J., Salonen, O., Simola, J., Standertskjöld-Nordenstam, C.-G., Tiitinen, H., Tissari, S.O. and Näätänen, R. (1995). Visual cortex activation in blind humans during sound discrimination. *Neurosci Lett*, **183**, 143–146.

Lederman, S.J., Klatzky, R.L., Chataway, C. and Summers, C.D. (1990). Visual mediation and the haptic recognition of two-dimensional pictures of common objects. *Percept Psychophys*, **47**, 54–64.

Lömo, T. and Mollica, A. (1962). Activity of single units in the primary optic cortex in the unanaesthetized rabbit during visual, acoustic, olfactory and painful stimulation. *Arch Ital Biol*, **100**, 86–120.

Malach, R., Reppas, J.B., Benson, R.R., Kwong, K.K., Jiang, H., Kennedy, W.A., Ledden, P.J., Brady, T.J., Rosen, B.R. and Tootell, R.B. (1995). Object-related activity revealed by functional magnetic resonance imaging in human occipital cortex. *Proc Natl Acad Sci USA*, **92**, 8135–8139.

Marks, D.F. (1973). Visual imagery differences in the recall of pictures. *Brit J Psychol*, **64**, 17–24.

Marmor, G.S. and Zaback, L.A. (1976). Mental rotation by the blind: does mental rotation depend on visual imagery? *J Exp Psychol Human Percept Perform*, **2**, 515–521.

Mellet, E., Tzourio, N., Crivello, F., Joliot, M., Denis, M. and Mazoyer, B. (1996). Functional anatomy of spatial mental imagery generated from verbal instructions. *J Neurosci*, **16**, 6504–6512.

Melzer, P., Morgan, V.L., Pickens, D.R., Price, R.R., Wall, R.S. and Ebner, F.F. (2001). Cortical activation during Braille reading is influenced by early visual experience in subjects with severe visual disability: a correlational fMRI study. *Hum Brain Mapp*, **14**, 186–195.

Morrell, F. (1972). Visual system's view of acoustic space. *Nature*, **238**, 44–46.

Morrongiello, B.A., Humphrey, K., Timney, B., Choi, J. and Rocca, P.T. (1994). Tactual object exploration and recognition in blind and sighted children. *Perception*, **23**, 833–848.

Murata, K., Cramer, H. and Bach-y-Rita. P. (1965). Neuronal convergence of noxious, acoustic, and visual stimuli in the visual cortex of the cat. *J Neurophysiol*, **28**, 1223–1240.

Murphy, C. and Cain, W.S. (1986). Odor identification: the blind are better. *Physiol Behav*, **37**, 177–180.

Niemeyer, W. and Starlinger, I. (1981). Do the blind hear better? Investigations on auditory processing in congenital or early acquired blindness. II. Central functions. *Audiology*, **20**, 510–515.

Pascual-Leone, A. and Torres, F. (1993). Plasticity of the sensori-motor cortex representation of the reading finger in Braille readers. *Brain*, **116**, 39–52.

Pascual-Leone, A. and Hamilton, R. (2001). The metamodal organization of the brain. *Prog Brain Res*, **134**, 427–445.

Pascual-Leone, A., Wasserman, E.M., Sadato, N. and Hallett, M. (1995). The role of reading activity on the modulation of motor cortical outputs to the reading hand in Braille readers. *Ann Neurol*, **38**, 910–915.

Prather, S.C., Votaw, J.R. and Sathian, K. (2004). Task-specific recruitment of dorsal and ventral visual areas during tactile perception. *Neuropsychologia*, **42**, 1079–1087.

Ramachandran, V.S. (1995). Touching the phantom limb. *Nature*, **377**, 489–490.

Rauschecker, J.P., Tian, B., Korte, M. and Egert, U. (1992). Crossmodal changes in the somatosensory vibrissa/barrel system of visually deprived animals. *Proc Natl Acad Sci USA*, **89**, 5063–5067.

Reales, J.M. and Ballesteros, S. (1999). Implicit and explicit memory for visual and haptic objects: cross-modal priming depends on structural descriptions. *J Exp Psychol Learn Mem Cogn*, **25**, 644–663.

Reed, C.M., Rubin, S.I., Braida, L.D. and Durlach, N.I. (1978). Analytic study of the Tadoma method: discrimination ability of untrained observers. *J Speech Hearing Res*, **21**, 625–637.

Reed, C.M., Doherty, M.J., Braida, L.D. and Durlach, N.I. (1982). Analytic study of the Tadoma method: further experiments with inexperienced observers. *J Speech Hear Res*, **25**, 216–223.

Rockland, K.S. and Ojima, H. (2003). Multisensory convergence in calcarine visual areas in macaque monkey. *Int J Psychophysiol*, **50**, 19–26.

Röder, B., Rösler, F., Hennighausen, E. and Näcker, F. (1996). Event-related potentials during auditory and somatosensory discrimination in sighted and blind subjects. *Cogn Brain Res*, **4**, 77–93.

Röder, B., Rösler, F. and Hennighausen, E. (1997). Different cortical activation patterns in blind and sighted humans during encoding and transformation of haptic images. *Psychophysiol*, **34**, 292–307.

Röder, B., Teder-Sälejärvi, W., Sterr, A., Rösler, F., Hillyard, S.A. and Neville, H.J. (1999). Improved auditory spatial tuning in blind humans. *Nature*, **400**, 162–166.

Röder, B., Stock, O., Bien, S.N.H. and Rösler, F. (2002). Speech processing activates visual cortex in congenitally blind humans. *Eur J Neurosci*, **16**, 930–936.

Rösler, F., Röder, B., Heil, M. and Hennighausen, E. (1993). Topographic differences of slow event-related brain potentials in blind and sighted adult human subjects during haptic mental rotation. *Cogn Brain Res*, **1**, 145–159.

Rossetti, Y., Rode, G., Pisella, L., Farne, A., Li, L., Boisson, D. and Perenin, M.-T. (1998). Prism adaptation to a rightward optical deviation rehabilitates left hemispatial neglect. *Nature*, **395**, 166–169.

Sadato, N., Pascual-Leone, A., Grafman, J., Ibanez, V., Deiber, M.-P., Dold, G., Hallett, M. (1996). Activation of the primary visual cortex by Braille reading in blind subjects. *Nature*, **380**, 526–528.

Sadato, N., Pascual-Leone, A., Grafman, J., Deiber, M.-P., Ibanez, V. and Hallett, M. (1998). Neural networks for Braille reading by the blind. *Brain*, **121**, 1213–1229.

Sadato, N., Okada, T., Honda, M. and Yonekura, Y. (2002). Critical period for cross-modal plasticity in blind humans: a functional MRI study. *Neuroimage*, **16**, 389–400.

Sathian, K. (2000). Intermanual referral of sensation to anesthetic hands. *Neurology*, **54**, 1866–1868.

Sathian, K. and Zangaladze, A. (2001). Feeling with the mind's eye: the role of visual imagery in tactile perception. *Optometry Vision Sci*, **78**, 276–281.

Sathian, K., Zangaladze, A., Hoffman, J.M. and Grafton, S.T. (1997). Feeling with the mind's eye. *NeuroReport*, **8**, 3877–3881.

Sathian, K., Greenspan, A.I. and Wolf, S.L. (2000). Doing it with mirrors: a case study of a novel approach to neurorehabilitation. *Neurorehabil Neur Rep*, **14**, 73–76.

Schroeder, C.E., Smiley, J., Fu, K.G., McGinnis, T., O'Connell, M.N. and Hackett, T.A. (2003). Anatomical mechanisms and functional implications of multisensory convergence in early cortical processing. *Int J Psychophysiol*, **50**, 5–17.

Sergent, J., Ohta, S. and MacDonald, B. (1992). Functional neuroanatomy of face and object processing. A positron emission tomography study. *Brain*, **115**, 15–36.

Shepard, R.N. and Metzler, J. (1971). Mental rotation of three-dimensional objects. *Science*, **171**, 701–703.

Shimizu, Y., Saida, S. and Shimura, H. (1993). Tactile pattern recognition by graphic display: importance of 3-D information for haptic perception of familiar objects. *Percept Psychophys*, **53**, 43–48.

Starlinger, I. and Niemeyer, W. (1981). Do the blind hear better? Investigations on auditory processing in congenital or early acquired blindness. I. Peripheral functions. *Audiology*, **20**, 503–509.

Sterr, A., Müller, M.M., Elbert, T., Rockstroh, B., Pantev, C. and Taub, E. (1998). Perceptual correlates of changes in cortical representation of fingers in blind multifinger Braille readers. *J Neurosci*, **18**, 4417–4423.

Stevens, J.C., Foulke, E. and Patterson, M.Q. (1996). Tactile acuity, aging and Braille reading in long-term blindness. *J Exp Psychol Appl*, **2**, 91–106.

Stoesz, M., Zhang, M., Weisser, V.D., Prather, S.C., Mao, H. and Sathian, K. (2003). Neural networks active during tactile form perception: common and differential activity during macrospatial and microspatial tasks. *Int J Psychophysiol*, **50**, 41–49.

Toldi, J., Farkas, T. and Völgyi, B. (1994a). Neonatal enucleation induces cross-modal changes in the barrel cortex of rat. A behavioural and electrophysiological study. *Neurosci Lett*, **167**, 1–4.

Toldi, J., Rojik, I. and Feher, O. (1994b). Neonatal monocular enucleation-induced cross-modal effects observed in the cortex of adult rat. *Neuroscience*, **62**, 105–114.

Uhl, F., Kretschmer, T., Lindinger, G., Goldenberg, G., Lang, W., Oder, W. and Deecke, L. (1994). Tactile mental imagery in sighted persons and in patients suffering from peripheral blindness early in life. *EEG Clin Neurophysiol*, **91**, 249–255.

van Boven, R.W. and Johnson, K.O. (1994). The limit of tactile spatial resolution in humans: grating orientation discrimination at the lip, tongue and finger. *Neurology*, **44**, 2361–2366.

van Boven, R.W., Hamilton, R.H., Kauffman, T., Keenan, J.P. and Pascual-Leone, A. (2000). Tactile spatial resolution in blind Braille readers. *Neurology*, **54**, 2230–2236.

Vanlierde, A., De Volder, A.G., Wanet-Defalque, M.-C. and Veraart, C. (2003). Occipito-parietal cortex activation during visuo-spatial imagery in early blind humans. *Neuroimage*, **19**, 698–709.

Veraart, C., De Volder, A.G., Wanet-Defalque, M.-C., Bol, A., Michel, C. and Goffinet, A.M. (1990). Glucose utilization in human visual cortex is abnormally elevated in blindness of early onset but decreased in blindness of late onset. *Brain Res*, **510**, 115–121.

Weeks, R., Horwitz, B., Aziz-Sultan, A., Tian, B., Wessinger, C.M., Cohen, L.G., Hallett, M. and Rauschecker, J.P. (2000). A positron emission tomographic study of auditory localization in the congenitally blind. *J Neurosci*, **20**, 2664–2672.

Zangaladze, A., Epstein, C.M., Grafton, S.T. and Sathian, K. (1999). Involvement of visual cortex in tactile discrimination of orientation. *Nature*, **401**, 587–590.

Zhang, M., Weisser, V.D., Stilla, R., Prather, S.C. and Sathian, K. (2004). Multisensory cortical processing of object shape and its relation to mental imagery. *Cogn Affect Behav Neurosci*, **4**, 251–259.

Zwiers, M.P., Van Opstal, A.J. and Cruysberg, J.R. (2001). A spatial hearing deficit in early-blind humans. *J Neurosci*, **21**, RC142–RC145.

Attentional modulation of cortical plasticity

Bharathi Jagadeesh

Department of Physiology and Biophysics, University of Washington, Seattle, WA, USA

12.1 Introduction

Can willing make it so? (Pollack, 2004). Specifically, in the context of attention and plasticity, can the exercise of conscious selection (attention) make the brain change (cortical plasticity) and is it necessary for the brain to change? If so, a purposeful plan could be a useful tool in changing the brain by inducing cortical plasticity. Knowledge of how plasticity can be induced would, in turn, be invaluable in trying to fix a damaged brain or to optimize learning strategies in a normal brain. In order to understand if this is possible, we need to first understand the definition of attention, its behavioral implications, and its neural and pharmacological basis. We can then turn to whether attention can act as a gating mechanism for plasticity: is it necessary for plasticity to occur? Finally, do these phenomenon act on the same pathways: is attention a prelude to learning? When we begin to understand those questions, we can begin to address whether attention will be a useful tool to manipulate the changes in the brain that underlie learning and recovery from damage.

Attention in this article will refer to selective or focused attention, the conscious exercise of will to chose to select one option, sensory input, or output over others. Attention is most frequently studied in the visual domain, where attention is known to improve the processing of certain visual information at the expense of other information that is presented simultaneously. Attention can be exercised in space (when a certain region of the visual world is selected)

(Moran and Desimone, 1985; Chelazzi et al., 1993; 1998; Corbetta and Shulman, 1998; Corbetta et al., 2000; Muller et al., 2003) or in feature space (when a particular feature, object, or other characteristic is selected) (Chelazzi et al., 1993; 1998; O'Craven et al., 1999; Martinez-Trujillo and Treue, 2004). Analogs exist in the auditory and somatosensory systems, where a particular auditory feature or sounds in a particular location can be selected at the expense of other information or a particular region of the body can be selected for special or extensive processing (Cherry and Taylor, 1954; Hsiao et al., 1993; Johansen-Berg and Lloyd, 2000). Attention can also be compared to a lack of attention, that is the processing of information implicitly, passive stimulation of a sensory pathway, or automatic movements. We will not, here, however, refer to attention for the phenomenon also termed arousal. Arousal means the overall alertness of the learner, as opposed to sleepiness. Instead, by attention we mean volitional interest in a particular activity.

The ultimate proposal to be discussed is whether volitional interest, attention, is necessary for learning or plasticity to occur, or whether learning can occur in the absence of attention. If learning can occur in the absence of attention, is it enhanced when attention is wielded to improve performance? In addition, if attention is necessary for learning, is this requirement limited to the initial acquisition but not performance of a task being learned? Before we can answer these questions, however, a working definition of attention, in its behavioral, neural, and pharmacological manifestations must be developed.

12.2 Attention: behavior, neuron, and pharmacology

Attention: behavior

In 1890, William James wrote "Everyone knows what attention is." (James, 1890). Everyone really does know what attention is, at least in some of its definitions. Try this as an exercise: is it possible to engage in normal conversation for an entire day without using the word attention? James went on to further define some of the aspects of selective attention:

It is the taking possession by the mind, in clear and vivid form, of one out of what seem several simultaneously possible objects or trains of thought. Focalization, concentration of consciousness are of its essence. It implies withdrawal from some things in order to deal effectively with others, and is a condition which has a real opposite in the confused, dazed, scatterbrained state ....

James, 1890

All aspects of this definition have relevance for the relationship between attention and cortical plasticity. Learning, and the plasticity that underlies it could require a focalization of concentration on the activity being learned. In addition, that localization of processing to one activity could imply a withdrawal from other activities, which in turn could mean less learning in those activities. Finally, without active wielding of the attentional process, the learner could be left in a "confused, dazed, scatterbrained state" in which no activity is learned because processing resources are too scattered and disparate.

James' famous quote on attention was built on experiments fleshed out by others that demonstrated both the focalization and withdrawal associated with attention in the processing of visual, auditory, and somatosensory information. Helmholtz demonstrated the action of attention in the visual system (Helmholtz, 1966). Helmholtz presented an array of letters on a screen, and asked people to report letters that appeared at an attended or unattended location. Using short stimulus durations that precluded the movement of the eyes, Helmholtz was able to show, in 1894, that individuals were better able to report the content of information presented at an attended location in space, than in a non-attended location. This relative improvement in performance was independent of the position of the eyes. Parallel experiments in the auditory system involved the "cocktail party" effect, where two different streams of information are sent to the two different ears. When subjects are asked to attend to information from one ear, they are unable to report information that was presented to the other ear. This example emphasizes the loss of information presented at a non-attended location (Cherry and Taylor, 1954). In the somatosensory domain, directing attention to a particular location, or hand, can improve discrimination performance at that location. All of these types of experiments resulted in the initial development of a theory of attention by Broadbent that proposed that sensory information at non-attended information is simply discarded and lost for further processing (Broadbent, 1957; 1962).

This view is overly simplistic, but in the incarnation where un-attended information is discarded, it would be expected that attention would be required for learning, that is, information that is discarded cannot be learned. However, further modifications of the theory followed soon on the footsteps of the original theory. First, highly salient stimuli were found to penetrate through the attentional filter, for example, ones own name in the "cocktail party" task (Broadbent, 1952a,b; Cherry and Taylor, 1954). This lead to a revision of the original theory which suggested that attentional information is merely attenuated (Treisman, 1964; 1966; Treisman and Geffen, 1967; Treisman and Riley, 1969). Attenuated attention would, in turn, also be expected to have an effect on subsequent learning, but learning might occur in spite of the attenuation of non-attended information.

If non-attended information is either discarded or attenuated, sensory representation is modified by attention. Modification of sensory representation is the basis of "early" attention theories. In these theories, the sensory information being used for subsequent processing is modified by attention. By volitional control of attention, individuals change the processing of information in the sensory system.

Other theories of attention propose response selection, rather than sensory modification, as the means through which attention operates in the brain (Deutsch and Deutsch, 1963; Deutsch et al., 1967). In these examples, all information is faithfully maintained until one of the several inputs is chosen among many on which to base a particular behavioral response. These theories, termed "late" attention theories, sensory information is maintained with high fidelity, and thus available for any subsequent learning process, even in the absence of attention.

Attention: neuron

These simple behavioral experiments, demonstrating the profound affects of attention on behavior, were the motivation for neurophysiological experiments that demonstrated the effects of attention on sensory processing. Neurophysiological experiments attacked the proposals of early attention. In early attention, the sensory signal should be modified. Neurophysiological experiments have examined whether attentional interactions modify neural responses in the visual, auditory, and somatosensory systems (Moran and Desimone, 1985; Hsiao et al., 1993; Desimone and Duncan, 1995; Luck et al., 1997; Johansen-Berg and Lloyd, 2000; Martinez-Trujillo and Treue, 2004). In one such experiment, non-human primates were asked to detect, and respond to a visual stimulus that appeared at a particular visual field location, and to ignore that same stimulus if it appeared elsewhere. Other visual stimuli (probes) were presented at attended location while the monkey performed the detection task and neural activity was recorded from extrastriate visual cortex (Moran and Desimone, 1985). The neural response to these probes was enhanced when they were presented at the attended versus unattended location. An example of enhancement of activity, when attention is directed into the receptive field of an individual neuron is shown in Fig. 12.1. In this Figure, the average response of a population of V4 neurons is shown, when attention was either directed within or outside the location of the V4 neurons' receptive field. The gray line shows response when attention was

directed outside the receptive field, the dark line the response when attention is directed within the receptive field. The response, to identical visual stimuli, is enhanced, when attention is directed within the cell's receptive field (Figure modified from Reynolds et al. (2000)). This pattern of activity supported the proposal that attention modifies the sensory signal. Human brain imaging studies have found similar affects on the activity in visual areas following the instruction to attend to particular locations or features of a visual image (Corbetta et al., 1990; 1991a,b; 2000; O'Craven et al., 1997; 1999; Kastner et al., 1998). Attentional modulation of the sensory system depends on both the visual area – it increases in strength as one moves downstream in the visual system, and on the number of elements or objects competing for visual processing (Kastner et al., 1998). In addition, the degree of attentional modulation might depend on overall task demands, stronger modulation with higher loads requiring stronger processing of the image (Rees and Frith, 1998). Parallel experiments in audition and touch have found that responses to auditory signals (Frith and Friston, 1996) and to somatosensory stimulation (Hsiao et al., 1993) are modulated by attention. In each of these cases, the response to the attended stimulus is larger than the same stimulus when it is unattended. Somatosensory cortex and auditory cortex are also upregulated in human functional magnetic resonance imaging (fMRI) experiments by attention (Iguchi et al., 2002). In several experiments (Steinmetz et al., 2000; Fries et al., 2001) attention seems to be accompanied by a greater synchronization among neurons that correspond to an attended stimulus or location.

Both up-modulation of the activity of particular populations of neurons and the increased synchronization of these neurons might be expected to have effects on the likelihood that these attended inputs could undergo plasticity, or experience dependent modification (Hebb, 1949; Magee and Johnston, 1997; Feldman, 2000; Yao and Dan, 2001; Froemke and Dan, 2002).

The neural basis of attention implies the interaction between a bottom-up signal and a top-down signal. The top-down signal is the source of attentional

(a)

(b)

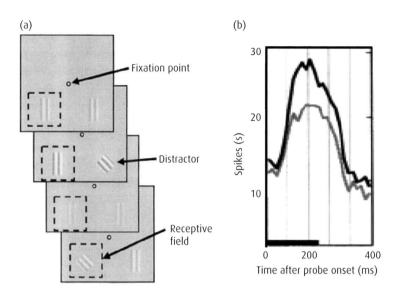

Figure 12.1. Effect of attention on V4 neural responses, modified from Reynolds et al. (2000). (a) Task. Attention is directed to the location of an individual cell's V4 receptive field (by placing a cue around that location on trials before the data is collected). The receptive field indicated with the dashed line. When attention is directed to the location of the receptive field, the monkey performs a task detecting a stimulus at that location, while probe stimuli are also presented at that location. When attention is directed away form the receptive field, the monkey performs a similar task at a location across the vertical meridian from the recorded cell's receptive field. (b) Enhancement of neural response when attention is directed inside a V4 cell's receptive field. Response (in spikes per second) over time from the onset of the stimulus (in milliseconds) to a 10% contrast probe grating, of preferred spatial frequency and orientation (average over 84 neurons). Dark bars at the lower left of each panel indicate stimulus duration (250 ms). Gray lines show average responses to ignored stimuli, when the monkey attended to the location that was across the vertical meridian from the receptive field. Black lines show responses to the identical stimulus when it was attended. The statistical significance of the attention effect within successive 100 ms periods is indicated by asterisks ($P = 0.05$) and double asterisks ($P = 0.001$) along the top of the figure. Responses are binned at 20 ms resolution (figure modified from Fig. 2 and 4, Reynolds et al. (2000)).

modulation of sensory signals, and is consciously wielded by the individual. An individual can choose to attend to one location or object (although attention can also be automatically attracted because of the inherent salience of the stimulus (Broadbent, 1952a; Rees and Frith, 1998; Jagadeesh et al., 2001). When an individual pays attention to a particular region, a top-down signal is produced that modulates the neural response in other areas. Evidence of such a top-down signal has been found in both neurophysiological and imaging studies of the brain. In tasks where an individual is instructed to attend to a particular visual image (by performing a task in a blocked design where the same image is chosen over and over again), neural activity in inferotemporal is biased in favor of those cells that respond well to the visual image (Chelazzi et al., 1993; 1995). This bias shows itself as a change in the baseline-firing rate of cells, a change in the activity of the neurons even when there is no stimulus in their receptive field. Likewise, when monkeys are asked to attend to a particular location in space the activity of cells with receptive fields in that region can be enhanced, even when no stimulus is presented there (Luck et al., 1997, p. 161). Evidence for a bias or top-down signal associated with attention has also been demonstrated in the human brain. When individuals are asked to attend to a particular location in space, the activity of Visual Area 4 (V4) is enhanced in attended locations, and frontal and parietal cortex show enhanced activation during the waiting period between the presentation of stimuli (Kastner et al., 1999; Giesbrecht et al., 2003). These types of top-down signals form a basis for the proposal that attentional modulation can act as a gating signal for neural change in other areas. Are such top-down signals necessary or beneficial to plastic changes in other brain areas?

Attention: pharmacology

Attention is a complex cognitive behavior, with many consequences for how a task is performed, and has close relationships with working memory, and other cognitive processes (Kastner and Ungerleider, 2000). But, attention, as well as related processes appear to have a common pharmacological involvement of cholinergic systems. Cholinergic inputs to frontal and parietal cortices are important for orienting in space (Coull et al., 1999; Bentley et al., 2004) and sustained attention in the presence of distracting stimuli (Gill et al., 2000). One interpretation of the effect of cholinergic inputs is that they are related to the top-down signal produced in frontal cortex; in this explanation, cholinergic inputs are the source of the top-down signal that serve to sharpen or enhance specific bottom-up inputs (Sarter et al., 2001). In this interpretation, cholinergic inputs play a significant role in the attentional modulation of sensory inputs. If cholinergic inputs play that role, it might also be the case that cholinergic inputs act as a gating mechanism for learning dependent plasticity, and that attention gates learning through the effect of cholinergic inputs. This hypothesis raises the possibility that pharmacological interventions might have a significant effect on cortical plasticity.

12.3 Attention and plasticity

With this understanding of attention, we can turn to the question of attention and cortical plasticity. Specifically, is attention necessary for learning to occur, if it is not necessary, is it beneficial, and does it share common substrates with learning and plasticity, that is, is attention necessary during a transient period and unnecessary after learning has occurred?

Evidence that attention or behavioral interaction is required will be addressed first, followed by some examples of plasticity that appears to occur in the absence of behavioral engagement (Godde et al., 1996; 2000; 2003; Erickson et al., 2000). To address the first question, we will first consider studies where attentional modulation or awareness of stimuli was required for learning to occur.

Mere presentation of visual stimuli is thought to be insufficient to cause perceptual learning. Improvement in orientation discrimination, vernier acuity, line orientation discrimination, direction discrimination are all thought to require performance of a discrimination task (Ahissar and Hochstein, 1993; Fahle and Edelman, 1993; Sagi and Tanne, 1994; Ito et al., 1998; Gilbert et al., 2000; Ahissar et al., 2001; Crist et al., 2001). In addition, if subjects perform one task with a set of stimuli (discrimination of overall array orientation) their learning does not transfer to another task performed with identical stimuli (Ahissar and Hochstein, 1993). Thus, when subjects are instructed to base their response on particular characteristics of the stimulus, that is, attend to particular features of the stimulus, improvement in detection other stimulus attributes does not occur, even if they co-vary. In addition, once a particular task is learned, for example, discrimination of array orientation, this learning does not transfer to another set of stimuli (Ahissar and Hochstein, 1993). Cells in primary visual cortex also show an interaction between attention and perceptual learning. In tasks where animals view stimuli, contextual interactions and responses to identical stimuli depend on both task demands (attention) and learning with those stimuli (Ito et al., 1998; Crist et al., 2001). These data suggest that learning only occurs when stimuli are relevant for a particular task, and suggest a possible mechanism, the activation of sensory neurons at the same time that a top-down signal modulates their activity. This pattern would be an attentional gate for learning, and its mechanism would be a modulation of sensory signals by a volitional top-down input that is activated when a task is performed.

In monkey, auditory cortex neuronal evidence also suggests that behavioral relevancy of the task is necessary for plastic changes in the neuronal response (Ahissar et al., 1992; 1998). In these experiments, pairs of neurons were found in auditory cortex and an auditory conditioning stimulus was applied contingent upon firing of one of the neurons in the pair. In some experiments, during this conditioning paradigm, monkeys also performed a behavioral task with the auditory stimuli. The conditioning stimulus weakly enhanced the synaptic connection between the pairs of neurons, expressed as an increase in the cross-correlation of responses between the two neurons through Hebbian-like processes (Stent, 1973). The strength of the increase in correlation was dependent on behavioral task. If the conditioning stimulus was applied while monkeys were performing a task with the stimulus, the increase in correlation was greater than if a similar conditioning paradigm was followed in the absence of a behavioral task (Ahissar et al., 1992; 1998). These results suggest that engagement in the behavioral task produces a signal that allows neuronal response properties in auditory to be altered.

In both auditory and somatosensory system, the tuning properties of cells in primary cortices can change as a function of training in a discrimination task (see Volume I, Chapters 6 and 10). In these experiment, paired stimulation of the auditory system (through the presentation of conditioned sounds) (Bakin and Weinberger, 1990; Bakin et al., 1992; 1996; Weinberger and Bakin, 1998a, b) or the somatosensory system (through the presentation of trained frequencies of vibratory stimuli) can cause changes in the frequency preference of tuning curves as well as the extent of the cortex activated by particular frequencies (Recanzone et al., 1992a, b, c, d; 1993).

In the rodent, a putative mechanism for the top-down signal necessary for synaptic plasticity has been uncovered. Stimulation of the nucleus basalis in rats, paired with stimulation of the auditory system, can induce plasticity similar to that seen with behavioral training of the auditory system (Bakin and Weinberger, 1996; Kilgard and Merzenich, 1998; Kilgard et al., 2002). The nucleus basalis is the source of wide-spread cholinergic input to the cortex, implicating the cholinergic system as a source of the behaviorally controlled gate for plasticity (Hasselmo, 1995; Rasmusson, 2000; Hasselmo and McGaughy, 2004). The cholinergic system has also been implicated in attention, where it appears to play a role in the attentional selection of individual visual stimuli (Voytko et al., 1994; Bentley et al., 2004). Pharmacological inhibition of the cholinergic system, in humans, causes a disruption in tasks involving attention, and a decrease in brain activation in areas thought to be the source of top-down attentional signals (Bentley et al., 2004). Lesions of the nucleus basalis, and thus the disperse cholinergic system, in the primate, impair performance on attentional tasks, but not on short-term working memory tasks, like the delayed match to sample task (Voytko et al., 1994).

These descriptions have concentrated on attentional effects and cortical plasticity in the sensory system, but plasticity that underlies motor learning has also been demonstrated. Motor learning-dependent plasticity appears to require attention and is greatly diminished in the absence of attention (Nissen, 1987; Hazeltine et al., 1997). However, in the case of motor learning, attention, and feedback on correct performance of the motor task being learned might be confounded with more accurate performance of the task itself and the role of good technique in plasticity. In this case, the question is whether cognitive attention to the task is required for learning, or whether performing the motor activity particularly perfectly is sufficient. This question was the basis of an experiment in which Stefan et al. tested whether attention was necessary for motor learning by producing motor learning in the absence of repetitive performance of motor movements (Stefan et al., 2004). In order to induce motor learning under these conditions, they used a pairing protocol where stimulation of cortex was accompanied by a motor movement. They then modulated attention by asking subjects to either attend to the hand being stimulated, or attend away from it by actively engaging in an irrelevant visual task. In these experiments, attention was required for motor learning. When subjects ignored the stimulus being presented to their hand, they showed no improvement in performance after the pairing trials (Stefan et al., 2004).

Although reports that attention, or engagement in a task is required for learning abound, there are examples of learning that seems to occur in the absence of a behavioral task. For example, young infants can learn the statistical probabilities of sounds (distinguishing speech like sounds from non-speech sounds) after repeated exposure to sounds (Saffran et al., 1996). Young infants can also learn statistical relationships within sequences of visual images (Kirkham et al., 2002). Detection can improve as a result of viewing motion stimuli while attention is engaged on other, simultaneously presented stimuli (Watanabe et al., 2002). In this experiment, subjects viewed coherent dot motion stimuli while performing a letter-discrimination task. The coherent dot motion was set at a level at which subjects did not report seeing motion. But, after repeated presentation of this stimulus, while another task was being performed, subjects improved in performance of the motion-discrimination task. This result, with moving stimuli, contrasts with results obtained in previous manipulations of attentional experience where subjects did not show learning about identical stimuli if they were performing a task, and thus attending to other aspects of the stimulus (Ahissar and Hochstein, 1993; Ahissar et al., 2001)

Statistical correlations between inputs seem sufficient to cause learning in the somatosensory system as well (Godde et al., 1996; 2000; 2003). In this study, subjects wore a solenoid on the tip of their index finger that was vibrated at a frequency that caused simultaneous activation of all of the receptive fields at the tip of their finger. After 3 h of this simultaneous activation protocol, subjects' ability to do a two point discrimination with their fingertips was tested. Subjects were pre-trained before the co-activation protocol, and had reached a stable performance of 1.53 mm discrimination. After the activation protocol, all but one subject improved in performance, to reach a median threshold of 1.23 mm. Subjects were instructed to ignore this vibration at their fingertips during the activation period, and permitted to engage in normal activities. However, the stimulation protocol was superthreshold, raising the possibility that subjects were unable to avoid attending to the

activated region. Changing the pattern of activation, so that receptive fields are sequentially activated, rather than simultaneously active destroys the effect on performance (Godde et al., 2003).

Cellular analogs of cortical plasticity in the absence of either a behavioral component of the task, or evidence of learning have also been seen. Pairing paradigms in which activation of a single cell in primary visual cortex is combined with depolarization of the cell with another stimulus can induce a change in that cell's receptive field (Fregnac et al., 1988; 1992; Shulz and Fregnac, 1992). Stimulating V1 cells with stimuli that contain an artificial scotoma, or a hole can cause an expansion of receptive fields in the region (Gilbert and Wiesel, 1992; Gilbert, 1993). Synchronous activation of cells in somatosensory cortex in the rat can cause changes in mapping of cortical receptive fields, in the absence of any task performance (Spengler and Dinse, 1994). In visual cortex, visual stimulation that activates adjacent cortical neurons in sequence causes shifts in receptive fields that depend on the order and interval between the successive stimuli (Fu et al., 2002). This modification occurs in the absence of any behavioral relevance of the stimuli.

In higher-order cortices, two plastic changes in cortical neurons seem to be present in the absence of behavioral interaction with the images. When visual stimuli are presented repeatedly, neurons nearby one another in inferotemporal cortex respond similarly to groups of realistic pictures than when the stimuli are first presented and are novel to the monkey. This increase in the similarity of response in nearby neurons seems to be independent of task: there is no difference in the degree of similar responses for stimuli that are presented repeatedly while the monkeys perform an association task versus a passive fixation task (Erickson et al., 2000). In addition, when monkeys are trained in a paired association task, single neuron can respond similarly to two stimuli that are paired together in individual trials so that one visual stimulus predicts the next. This phenomenon is called pair coding because a single neuron responds similarly to both members of the associated pair. Pair coding can be independent of whether learning about the association is expressed in the monkey's behavior. In experiments where the monkeys show no evidence that they have learned the association (by showing a shorter latency to responding to the second stimulus on paired trials than when an invalid predictor is presented) pair coding is still present. Thus, plasticity occurs independent of behavioral evidence that learning has occurred.

A possible explanation for some of these experiments is that attention has been attracted involuntarily, or through the salience of the stimuli. For example, the brightly colored transiently presented stimuli used in experiments in inferotemporal cortex (Erickson et al., 2000) might attract attention even when the monkey is not required to respond to the stimuli, and is rewarded merely for maintaining fixation on the stimuli. Repeated vibration of the fingertips (Godde et al., 2000; 2003) may attract attention even when subjects are told to ignore the vibration. Moving coherent dots may attract attention because of their salient motion even when resources are devoted to processing other visual stimuli (Watanabe et al., 2002). In addition, the moving dots might be processed in different brain areas, allowing them to operate normally in plasticity in spite of the drawing away of attention from that stimulus to another more relevant stimulus. In early visual cortex, visual stimulation procedures that produced plasticity were done in the presence of stimulation procedures (artificial scotoma with large stimuli) or iontophoresis of inhibitory antagonists that effectively raised overall activity levels in addition to the pairing that produced the specific form of plasticity seen. If the modulatory role of attention operates through an overall enhancement of responsivity in cells undergoing plasticity, these methods of stimulation might bypass the role of attention. In addition, stimulation protocols that effectively control timing might short circuit the role of attention by producing the same conditions attention, such as synchronous firing or increased probability of firing in particular temporal order among groups of neurons (Steinmetz et al., 2000; Fries et al., 2001).

Thus, experiments that show that plasticity can occur in the absence of attention might be relying on the inherent salience of the stimulus used to induce plasticity, attention drawn implicitly by the stimulus, rather than wielded consciously by the individual. And cellular analogs of plasticity that occur in the absence of actively deployed attention might on activating the functional mechanics of attention in the absence of attention in the same way that nucleus basalis stimulation appears to bypass the attentional system by activating its physiological correlate rather than activating the physiological correlate by manipulating behavior (Bakin and Weinberger, 1996; Kilgard and Merzenich, 1998; Kilgard et al., 2001).

The concept of a common pathway for attention and learning is supported by psychophysical studies that show that attentional enhancement of perception and learning enhancement of perception operate on the same substrates. In these experiments (Gilbert et al., 2000) subjects are first trained in a learning task. After their performance has reached asymptotic levels, they are tested to see if deploying attention can further enhance performance. In these experiments it could not. Once perceptual learning had cleaned up the signal available for perception, attention could not improve it further, suggesting a common physiological substrate for the two processes.

Thus, the current body of evidence suggests that attentional modulation plays an important role in inducing cortical plasticity. Experimental evidence suggests that plasticity is most robust under circumstances where attention is wielded, even when it can occur without active deployment of attention. This in turn has implications for both beneficial reorganization of the brain and inhibiting improper reorganization of the brain.

Stimulation protocols that produce cortical plasticity in the somatosensory system (Godde et al., 2000) have been used successfully to ameliorate phantom pain in amputees. Phantom limb pain is thought to be caused by maladaptive cortical plasticity where areas of the cortex that used to be innervated by the missing limb are pathologically encroached by inputs from adjacent brain areas. Pairing protocols that asynchronously activated different areas of the body were able to decrease the perception of phantom limb pain (Huse et al., 2001). These protocols were developed with the idea that attention was not required for the plasticity (and it does not seem to be, in this case) (Godde et al., 2003), but leaves open the possibility that modulating the appropriate pairing protocol with attention might produce even stronger plasticity and thus better performance of the pairing protocol.

In addition, a strong role for attention in plasticity suggests an intriguing role for attention to play in the development of neuroprosthetics (see Volume I, Chapter 32). Early theory about the development of neural prosthetics took as a premise that prosthetic devices would have to be implanted into known input or output areas of the brain. Under this assumption, we need to understand completely the read-out (or read-in) of a particular brain module before we can attach a neural prosthetic to that area. But, more recent experiments in which recordings from monkey motor cortex has been used to control robotic arms suggests that a more successful method will be to give the subject feedback about the correctness of the movement made by the robotic arm and allow the brain to rewire itself (undergo plastic changes) based on this feedback (Nicolelis, 2003). Several assumptions underlie this theory. The first is that the brain can rewire itself in the adult animal (Rouiller and Olivier, 2004). The second is that this rewiring can be under conscious control or the control of a top-down feedback system. The putative candidates for such a system is attention, a top-down signal that can be wielded actively by the subject to attend to particular information while discarding or attenuating other information (Moore and Armstrong, 2003). This top-down signal then acts as a gate allowing plastic changes that rewire the brain so that the brain's neurons can accomplish the task at hand, in particular moving a robot arm (Nicolelis, 2003).

In conclusion we develop a possible model for the role of attention in cortical plasticity. Attention is a means for marking a particular set of inputs for special treatment in the brain. It is normally wielded on a trial by trial or short set of blocks of trials to tune sensory signals for the task at hand, or to improve performance of a particular motor activity. But plasticity is one extreme case of special treatment, and it benefits from this marking for enhanced processing. In this case, the attentional system marks inputs for special treatment, and this special treatment allows the stimulus to gain particular influence on a group of neurons, which undergo plasticity. Attention may operate through increasing overall response levels (Moran and Desimone, 1985; Moore and Armstrong, 2003) by activating cholinergic systems (Bakin and Weinberger, 1996; Kilgard and Merzenich, 1998; Bentley et al., 2004) or by increasing the probabilities of synchronous firing (Steinmetz et al., 2000; Fries et al., 2001). All of these processes have the potential for increasing plasticity in the cortex when particular patterns of stimuli are presented. After learning has been consolidated, however, attention may no longer be required, and have no further benefit (Gilbert et al., 2000; Ahissar et al., 2001).

REFERENCES

Ahissar, M. and Hochstein, S. (1993). Attentional control of early perceptual learning. *Proc Natl Acad Sci USA*, **90**(**12**), 5718–5722.

Ahissar, E., Vaadia, E., et al. (1992). Dependence of cortical plasticity on correlated activity of single neurons and on behavioral context. *Science*, **257**(**5075**), 1412–1415.

Ahissar, E., Abeles, M., et al. (1998). Hebbian-like functional plasticity in the auditory cortex of the behaving monkey. *Neuropharmacology*, **37**(**4–5**), 633–655.

Ahissar, M., Laiwand, R., et al. (2001). Attentional demands following perceptual skill training. *Psychol Sci*, **12**(**1**), 56–62.

Bakin, J.S. and Weinberger, N.M. (1990). Classical conditioning induces CS-specific receptive field plasticity in the auditory cortex of the guinea pig. *Brain Res*, **536**(**1–2**), 271–286.

Bakin, J.S. and Weinberger, N.M. (1996). Induction of a physiological memory in the cerebral cortex by stimulation of the nucleus basalis. *Proc Natl Acad Sci USA*, **93**(**20**), 11219–11224.

Bakin, J.S., Lepan, B., et al. (1992). Sensitization induced receptive field plasticity in the auditory cortex is independent of CS-modality. *Brain Res*, **577**(**2**), 226–235.

Bakin, J.S., South, D.A., et al. (1996). Induction of receptive field plasticity in the auditory cortex of the guinea pig during instrumental avoidance conditioning. *Behav Neurosci*, **110**(**5**), 905–913.

Bentley, P., Husain, M., et al. (2004). Effects of cholinergic enhancement on visual stimulation, spatial attention, and spatial working memory. *Neuron*, **41**(6), 969–982.

Broadbent, D.E. (1952a). Failures of attention in selective listening. *J Exp Psychol*, **44**(6), 428–433.

Broadbent, D.E. (1952b). Listening to one of two synchronous messages. *J Exp Psychol*, **44**(1), 51–55.

Broadbent, D.E. (1957). A mechanical model for human attention and immediate memory. *Psychol Rev*, **64**(3), 205–215.

Broadbent, D.E. (1962). Attention and the perception of speech. *Sci Am*, **206**, 143–151.

Chelazzi, L., Miller, E.K., et al. (1993). A neural basis for visual search in inferior temporal cortex. *Nature*, **363**(6427), 345–347.

Chelazzi, L., Biscaldi, M., et al. (1995). Oculomotor activity and visual spatial attention. *Behav Brain Res*, **71**(1–2), 81–88.

Chelazzi, L., Duncan, J., et al. (1998). Responses of neurons in inferior temporal cortex during memory-guided visual search. *J Neurophysiol*, **80**(6), 2918–2940.

Cherry, E.C. and Taylor, W.K. (1954). Some further experiments on the recognition of speech with one and two ears. *J Acoust Soc Am*, **26**, 554–559.

Corbetta, M. and Shulman, G.L. (1998). Human cortical mechanisms of visual attention during orienting and search. *Philos Trans Roy Soc London B Biol Sci*, **353**(1373), 1353–1362.

Corbetta, M., Miezin, F.M., et al. (1990). Attentional modulation of neural processing of shape, color, and velocity in humans. *Science*, **248**(4962), 1556–1559.

Corbetta, M., Miezin, F.M., et al. (1991a). Selective and divided attention during visual discriminations of shape, color, and speed: functional anatomy by positron emission tomography. *J Neurosci*, **11**(8), 2383–2402.

Corbetta, M., Miezin, F.M., et al. (1991b). Selective attention modulates extrastriate visual regions in humans during visual feature discrimination and recognition. *Ciba Found Symp*, **163**, 165–175; discussion 175–180.

Corbetta, M., Kincade, J.M., et al. (2000). Voluntary orienting is dissociated from target detection in human posterior parietal cortex. *Nat Neurosci*, **3**(3), 292–297.

Coull, J.T., Buchel, C., et al. (1999). Noradrenergically mediated plasticity in a human attentional neuronal network. *Neuroimage*, **10**(6), 705–715.

Crist, R.E., Li, W., et al. (2001). Learning to see: experience and attention in primary visual cortex. *Nat Neurosci*, **4**(5), 519–525.

Desimone, R. and Duncan, J. (1995). Neural mechanisms of selective visual attention. *Annu Rev Neurosci*, **18**, 193–222.

Deutsch, J.A. and Deutsch, D. (1963). Some theoretical considerations. *Psychol Rev*, **70**, 80–90.

Deutsch, J.A., Deutsch, D., et al. (1967). Comments and reply on "Selective attention": perception or response? *Quart J Exp Psychol*, **19**(4), 362–367.

Erickson, C.A., Jagadeesh, B., et al. (2000). Clustering of perirhinal neurons with similar properties following visual experience in adult monkeys. *Nat Neurosci*, **3**(11), 1143–1148.

Fahle, M. and Edelman, S. (1993). Long-term learning in vernier acuity: effects of stimulus orientation, range and of feedback. *Vision Res*, **33**(3), 397–412.

Feldman, D.E. (2000). Timing-based LTP and LTD at vertical inputs to layer II/III pyramidal cells in rat barrel cortex. *Neuron*, **27**(1), 45–56.

Fregnac, Y., Shulz, D., et al. (1988). A cellular analogue of visual cortical plasticity. *Nature*, **333**(6171), 367–370 [published erratum appears in *Nature* 1988, **333**(6175), 786].

Fregnac, Y., Shulz, D., et al. (1992). Cellular analogs of visual cortical epigenesis. I. Plasticity of orientation selectivity. *J Neurosci*, **12**(4), 1280–1300.

Fries, P., Reynolds, J.H., et al. (2001). Modulation of oscillatory neuronal synchronization by selective visual attention. *Science*, **291**(5508), 1560–1563.

Frith, C.D. and Friston, K.J. (1996). The role of the thalamus in "top down" modulation of attention to sound. *Neuroimage*, **4**(3 Pt 1), 210–215.

Froemke, R.C. and Dan, Y. (2002). Spike-timing-dependent synaptic modification induced by natural spike trains. *Nature*, **416**(6879), 433–438.

Fu, Y.X., Djupsund, K., et al. (2002). Temporal specificity in the cortical plasticity of visual space representation. *Science*, **296**(5575), 1999–2003.

Giesbrecht, B., Woldorff, M.G., et al. (2003). Neural mechanisms of top-down control during spatial and feature attention. *Neuroimage*, **19**(3), 496–512.

Gilbert, C., Ito, M., et al. (2000). Interactions between attention, context and learning in primary visual cortex. *Vision Res*, **40**(10–12), 1217–1226.

Gilbert, C.D. (1993). Rapid dynamic changes in adult cerebral cortex. *Curr Opin Neurobiol*, **3**(1), 100–103.

Gilbert, C.D. and Wiesel, T.N. (1992). Receptive field dynamics in adult primary visual cortex. *Nature*, **356**(6365), 150–152.

Gill, T.M., Sarter, M., et al. (2000). Sustained visual attention performance-associated prefrontal neuronal activity: evidence for cholinergic modulation. *J Neurosci*, **20**(12), 4745–4757.

Godde, B., Spengler, F., et al. (1996). Associative pairing of tactile stimulation induces somatosensory cortical reorganization in rats and humans. *NeuroReport*, **8**(1), 281–285.

Godde, B., Stauffenberg, B., et al. (2000). Tactile coactivation-induced changes in spatial discrimination performance. *J Neurosci*, **20**(**4**), 1597–1604.

Godde, B., Ehrhardt, J., et al. (2003). Behavioral significance of input-dependent plasticity of human somatosensory cortex. *NeuroReport*, **14**(**4**), 543–546.

Hasselmo, M.E. (1995). Neuromodulation and cortical function: modeling the physiological basis of behavior. *Behav Brain Res*, **67**(**1**), 1–27.

Hasselmo, M.E. and McGaughy, J. (2004). High acetylcholine levels set circuit dynamics for attention and encoding and low acetylcholine levels set dynamics for consolidation. *Prog Brain Res*, **145**, 207–231.

Hazeltine, E., Grafton, S.T., et al. (1997). Attention and stimulus characteristics determine the locus of motor-sequence encoding. A PET study. *Brain*, **120**(**Pt 1**), 123–140.

Hebb, D.O. (1949). *The Organization of Behavior: A Neuropsychological Theory*, John Wiley & Sons.

Helmholtz, H.V. (1966). *Treatise on Physiological Optics*, Optical Society of America, New York.

Hsiao, S.S., O'Shaughnessy, D.M., et al. (1993). Effects of selective attention on spatial form processing in monkey primary and secondary somatosensory cortex. *J Neurophysiol*, **70**(**1**), 444–447.

Huse, E., Preissl, H., et al. (2001). Phantom limb pain. *Lancet*, **358**(**9286**), 1015.

Iguchi, Y., Hoshi, Y., et al. (2002). Selective attention regulates spatial and intensity information processing in the human primary somatosensory cortex. *NeuroReport*, **13**(**17**), 2335–2339.

Ito, M., Westheimer, G., et al. (1998). Attention and perceptual learning modulate contextual influences on visual perception. *Neuron*, **20**(**6**), 1191–1197.

Jagadeesh, B., Chelazzi, L., et al. (2001). Learning increases stimulus salience in anterior inferior temporal cortex of the macaque. *J Neurophysiol*, **86**(**1**), 290–303.

James, W. (1890). *Principles of Psychology*. Holt, New York.

Johansen-Berg, H. and Lloyd, D.M. (2000). The physiology and psychology of selective attention to touch. *Front Biosci*, **5**, D894–D904.

Kastner, S. and Ungerleider, L.G. (2000). Mechanisms of visual attention in the human cortex. *Annu Rev Neurosci*, **23**, 315–341.

Kastner, S., De Weerd, P., et al. (1998). Mechanisms of directed attention in the human extrastriate cortex as revealed by functional MRI [see comments]. *Science*, **282**(**5386**), 108–111.

Kastner, S., Pinsk, M.A., et al. (1999). Increased activity in human visual cortex during directed attention in the absence of visual stimulation. *Neuron*, **22**(**4**), 751–761.

Kilgard, M.P. and Merzenich, M.M. (1998). Cortical map reorganization enabled by nucleus basalis activity. *Science*, **279**(**5357**), 1714–1718.

Kilgard, M.P., Pandya, P.K., et al. (2001). Sensory input directs spatial and temporal plasticity in primary auditory cortex. *J Neurophysiol*, **86**(**1**), 326–338.

Kilgard, M.P., Pandya, P.K., et al. (2002). Cortical network reorganization guided by sensory input features. *Biol Cybern*, **87**(**5–6**), 333–343.

Kirkham, N.Z., Slemmer, J.A., et al. (2002). Visual statistical learning in infancy: evidence for a domain general learning mechanism. *Cognition*, **83**(**2**), B35–B42.

Luck, S.J., Chelazzi, L., et al. (1997). Neural mechanisms of spatial selective attention in areas V1, V2, and V4 of macaque visual cortex. *J Neurophysiol*, **77**(**1**), 24–42.

Magee, J.C. and Johnston, D. (1997). A synaptically controlled, associative signal for Hebbian plasticity in hippocampal neurons. *Science*, **275**(**5297**), 209–213.

Martinez-Trujillo, J.C. and Treue, S. (2004). Feature-based attention increases the selectivity of population responses in primate visual cortex. *Curr Biol*, **14**(**9**), 744–751.

Moore, T. and Armstrong, K.M. (2003). Selective gating of visual signals by microstimulation of frontal cortex. *Nature*, **421**(**6921**), 370–373.

Moran, J. and Desimone, R. (1985). Selective attention gates visual processing in the extrastriate cortex. *Science*, **229**(**4715**), 782–784.

Muller, N.G., Bartelt, O.A., et al. (2003). A physiological correlate of the "Zoom Lens" of visual attention. *J Neurosci*, **23**(**9**), 3561–3565.

Nicolelis, M.A. (2003). Brain-machine interfaces to restore motor function and probe neural circuits. *Nat Rev Neurosci*, **4**(**5**), 417–422.

Nissen, M.J. (1987). Attentional requirements of learning: evidence from performance measures. *Cognitive Psychol*, **19**, 1–32.

O'Craven, K.M., Rosen, B.R., et al. (1997). Voluntary attention modulates fMRI activity in human MT-MST. *Neuron*, **18**(**4**), 591–598.

O'Craven, K.M., Downing, P.E., et al. (1999). fMRI evidence for objects as the units of attentional selection. *Nature*, **401**(**6753**), 584–587.

Pollack, A. (2004). *With Tiny Brain Implants Thinking May Make It So*, New York Times, New York, p. 5.

Rasmusson, D.D. (2000). The role of acetylcholine in cortical synaptic plasticity. *Behav Brain Res*, **115**(**2**), 205–218.

Recanzone, G.H., Jenkins, W.M., et al. (1992a). Progressive improvement in discriminative abilities in adult owl monkeys performing a tactile frequency discrimination task. *J Neurophysiol*, **67**(**5**), 1015–1030.

Recanzone, G.H., Merzenich, M.M., et al. (1992b). Expansion of the cortical representation of a specific skin field in primary somatosensory cortex by intracortical microstimulation. *Cereb Cortex*, **2**(**3**), 181–196.

Recanzone, G.H., Merzenich, M.M., et al. (1992c). Frequency discrimination training engaging a restricted skin surface results in an emergence of a cutaneous response zone in cortical area 3a. *J Neurophysiol*, **67**(**5**), 1057–1070.

Recanzone, G.H., Merzenich, M.M., et al. (1992d). Topographic reorganization of the hand representation in cortical area 3b owl monkeys trained in a frequency-discrimination task. *J Neurophysiol*, **67**(**5**), 1031–1056.

Recanzone, G.H., Schreiner, C.E., et al. (1993). Plasticity in the frequency representation of primary auditory cortex following discrimination training in adult owl monkeys. *J Neurosci*, **13**(**1**), 87–103.

Rees, G. and Frith, C.D. (1998). How do we select perceptions and actions? Human brain imaging studies. *Philos Trans Roy Soc London B Biol Sci*, **353**(**1373**), 1283–1293.

Reynolds, J.H., Pasternak, T. and Desimone, R. (2000). Attention increases sensitivity of V4 neurons. *Neuron*, **26**, 703–714.

Rouiller, E.M. and Olivier, E. (2004). Functional recovery after lesions of the primary motor cortex. *Prog Brain Res*, **143**, 467–475.

Saffran, J.R., Aslin, R.N., et al. (1996). Statistical learning by 8-month-old infants. *Science*, **274**(**5294**), 1926–1928.

Sagi, D. and Tanne, D. (1994). Perceptual learning: learning to see. *Curr Opin Neurobiol*, **4**(**2**), 195–199.

Sarter, M., Givens, B., et al. (2001). The cognitive neuroscience of sustained attention: where top-down meets bottom-up. *Brain Res Rev*, **35**(**2**), 146–160.

Shulz, D. and Fregnac, Y. (1992). Cellular analogs of visual cortical epigenesis. II. Plasticity of binocular integration. *J Neurosci*, **12**(**4**), 1301–1318.

Spengler, F. and Dinse, H.R. (1994). Reversible relocation of representational boundaries of adult rats by intracortical microstimulation. *NeuroReport*, **5**(**8**), 949–953.

Stefan, K., Wycislo, M., et al. (2004). Modulation of associative human motor cortical plasticity by attention. *J Neurophysiol*, **92**, 66–72.

Steinmetz, P.N., Roy, A., et al. (2000). Attention modulates synchronized neuronal firing in primate somatosensory cortex. *Nature*, **404**(**6774**), 187–190.

Stent, G.S. (1973). A physiological mechanism for Hebb's postulate of learning. *Proc Natl Acad Sci USA*, **70**(**4**), 997–1001.

Treisman, A.M. (1964). Selective attention in man. *Brain Med Bull*, **20**, 12–16.

Treisman, A.M. (1966). Our limited attention. *Adv Sci*, **22**(**104**), 600–611.

Treisman, A. and Geffen, G. (1967). Selective attention: perception or response? *Quart J Exp Psychol*, **19**(**1**), 1–17.

Treisman, A.M. and Riley, J.G. (1969). Is selective attention selective perception or selective response? A further test. *J Exp Psychol*, **79**(**1**), 27–34.

Voytko, M.L., Olton, D.S., et al. (1994). Basal forebrain lesions in monkeys disrupt attention but not learning and memory. *J Neurosci*, **14**(**1**), 167–186.

Watanabe, T., Nanez, Sr., J.E., et al. (2002). Greater plasticity in lower-level than higher-level visual motion processing in a passive perceptual learning task. *Nat Neurosci*, **5**(**10**), 1003–1009.

Weinberger, N.M. and Bakin, J.S. (1998a). Learning-induced physiological memory in adult primary auditory cortex: receptive fields plasticity, model, and mechanisms. *Audiol Neuro-otol*, **3**(**2–3**), 145–167.

Weinberger, N.M. and Bakin, J.S. (1998b). Research on auditory cortex plasticity. *Science*, **280**(**5367**), 1174.

Yao, H. and Dan, Y. (2001). Stimulus timing-dependent plasticity in cortical processing of orientation. *Neuron*, **32**(**2**), 315–323.

Plasticity after injury to the CNS

CONTENTS

Plasticity in the injured spinal cord

Serge Rossignol

Department of Physiology, Centre for Research in Neurological Sciences, Universite de Montreal, Montreal, Quebec, Canada

13.1 Introduction

This chapter is devoted to mechanisms of spinal cord plasticity in animal models as revealed by the recovery of motor functions after a spinal lesion. It will be shown that in cats, rats and mice, motor programs such as locomotion are re-expressed after a complete spinal transection at the low-thoracic level. This suggests that the main neural networks at the basis of these motor programs reside in the spinal cord. Direct evidence for the operation of these circuits as well as cellular properties implicated will be surveyed. On the other hand, modifications of these motor programs by sensory inputs, training and pharmacological stimulation suggest that some of the control mechanisms have some degree of plasticity. Obviously, supraspinal structures normally play a crucial role in the purposeful goal-orienting control of these spinal pattern generators. The deficits observed after complete or partial spinal lesions of ventral/ventrolateral or dorsolateral tracts reveal indeed these important roles. Altogether, these observations lead to the important concept that complex motor functions such as locomotion are largely subserved by intrinsic spinal mechanisms under segmental and suprasegmental controls that are plastic enough to justify the use of rehabilitation approaches to optimize functional locomotor recovery after spinal lesions. Figure 13.1 schematizes the principal structures and mechanisms that will be discussed in this chapter. For related discussions, see Volume I, Chapters 7 and 30, and Volume II, Chapters 3 and 19.

13.2 Locomotor recovery after spinal lesions in cats

Spinal locomotion after complete spinal cord transection in kittens and adults

In most animal species (Delcomyn, 1980) locomotor pattern of the hindlimbs recover after a complete section of the spinal cord at the last thoracic segment (T13). Although such spinal stepping was reported before (Sherrington, 1910; Shurrager and Dykman, 1951), the work of Grillner and associates really started a new era by objectively documenting the kinematics and associated electromyographic (EMG) activity of locomotion after spinalization, especially in kittens (Grillner, 1973; Forssberg et al., 1980a, b). The remarkable observation here, which cannot be stressed enough, is that cats spinalized a few days after birth and before having expressed any spontaneous locomotor pattern, became capable of walking with the hindlimbs at different speeds when held over a treadmill belt. This ability was maintained uninterruptedly for several months. This was the first clear evidence that a full hindlimb locomotor pattern with, plantar foot contact, hindquarter weight support and proper EMG activity could develop as the result of the expression of a genetically determined spinal program that did not require learning, training or pharmacological stimulation. This remains one of the principal concept underlying our understanding of locomotor control as reviewed before (Grillner, 1981; Rossignol, 1996).

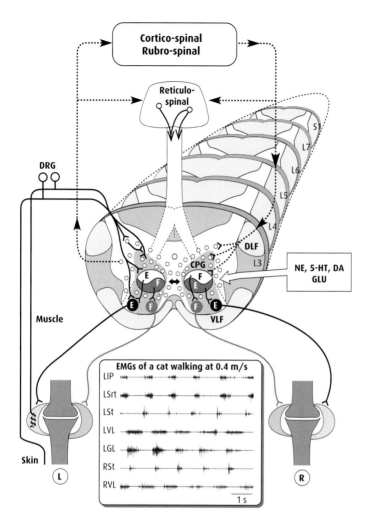

Figure 13.1. *General framework of locomotor control in the cat.* The inset at the bottom center represents the EMG activity for six consecutive steps on a treadmill of a normal cat walking at 0.4 m/s. The EMGs are taken from Iliopsoas (Ip, hip flexor), sartorius (Srt, a hip flexor), semitendinosus (St, a knee flexor/hip extensor), vastus lateralis (VL, a knee extensor), gastrocnemius lateralis (GL, an ankle extensor); L and R refer respectively to left and right sides.Afferents from the skin and muscles with their cell bodies in the dorsal root ganglion (DRG) are graphically fused when they enter the cord. Although this does not represent the reality it allows to illustrate the general principles that the afferent inputs may modulate the locomotor output pattern by acting monosynaptically (proprioceptive Ia afferents) on motoneurons, disynaptically on motoneurons or polysynaptically through the central pattern generator (CPG) or by presynaptic interactions. In the CPG, E and F represent sets of interneurons active during the flexion or extension phase and are connected to extensor (E) or flexor motoneurons (F). Outside the CPG, a shaded area is meant to indicate those interneurons whose excitability changes are governed by the CPG although they are not part of the rhythmogenesis process itself. Other interneurons that may not be rhythmically active are outside this theoretical zone. VLF, ventrolateral funiculus through which course the reticulo spinal pathways; DLF, dorsolateral funiculi through which course the cortico-spinal and rubro-spinal pathways. Again, these descending pathways may make various types of synaptic connections with spinal interneurons. L3-S1 refer to various lumbar and sacral spinal segments that may play specific roles in the elaboration of locomotion; NE, norepinephrine; 5-HT, serotonin, DA, dopamine, Glu, glutamate that are released by descending and/or afferent pathways.

Adult cats can also recover hindlimb locomotion over the treadmill (Barbeau and Rossignol, 1987; Bélanger et al., 1996; Rossignol et al., 2000; 2002). The cat is placed with its forelimb standing on a platform above the treadmill, while the hindlimbs are placed over the moving treadmill belt. Although in the early stage the weight of the hindquarters is taken up mainly by the experimenter, after 2–3 weeks cats can walk with their hindlimbs making plantar foot contacts and supporting the weight of the hindquarters. The experimenter still has to hold the tail mainly to prevent falls on either side since the animal has lost all vestibular balance. Figure 13.2 illustrates the kinematics and EMG discharge of several muscles recorded in the same chronically implanted cat before and after spinalization. Some features merit to be stressed. As far as kinematics is concerned, the step cycles are generally shorter after spinalization, and there is quite often a foot drag at the onset of the swing phase that can last in some cases 20–40% of the swing phase. The EMG pattern in spinal cats is generally very similar to that of the intact cat. The characteristic wave shape of certain muscles is preserved such as the abrupt onset of the ankle extensor (gastrocnemius lateralis, GL) and the gradual onset of the knee extensor (vastus lateralis, VL). The amplitude of extensors may be reduced which corresponds to a decreased ability to support weight. As will be seen later, this might be related to the lesion of reticulo-spinal and vestibulo-spinal pathways since such deficits are also seen with partial spinal lesions including these pathways more specifically (Brustein and Rossignol, 1998). Often, a clonic mode of discharge is seen during the stance phase, as can be observed by the choppy aspect of the EMG discharge in the raw recordings. The flexor muscles can also show some clonic activity. The timing between the flexor muscles acting at different joints is probably the most disturbed feature in spinal cats. Indeed, the usual delay between the initial burst of the knee flexor semitendinosus (St) and the activation of the hip flexor sartorius (Sart) is often lost. This, coupled to an early activation of the ankle flexor tibialis anterior (TA) may explain the foot drag mentioned previously. Indeed, rather than first flexing, the knee to remove the foot from the ground, hip and

ankle flexions are initiated at the same time, which results in a forward movement of the foot on the treadmill belt before it is withdrawn upward. This specific deficit may be related more specifically to damage to the cortico-spinal pathways since selective lesions of the tracts comprising these pathways will result in similar deficits (Jiang and Drew, 1996), as will be seen later.

Effect of locomotor training

Although it is generally considered that younger animals can better express this locomotor pattern after spinalization (Smith et al., 1982; Bregman and Goldberger, 1983; Bradley and Smith, 1988; Howland et al., 1995a, b), it is clear, as shown above, that adult cats can also express this locomotor pattern especially when actively trained on a treadmill. Our work as well as that of others (Edgerton et al., 1991; 1997; de Leon et al., 1998a, b; Roy et al., 1998) has shown that adult spinal cat recover gradually regular, alternate, weight-bearing steps when they are trained several times a week on a treadmill.

We found that the best way to train spinal cats on a treadmill was to hold the hindlimbs over the treadmill while the forelimbs are self-supported on a platform, a few centimeters above the belt. Using perineal stimulation, which can favor the production of rhythmic movements, it is possible to favor the positioning of the feet on the belt and encourage weight-bearing as soon as possible. Although tedious, this method was deemed preferable to devices holding the cat since these devices may often stimulate the groin or the back of the cat, which are very sensitive zones that can completely inhibit locomotion. Although adult cats can recover proper weight-bearing stepping on the treadmill within a few weeks, we have observed that it may take 2–3 months for the locomotor performance to stabilize (Barbeau and Rossignol, 1987), in terms of step cycle duration at a given speed.

The mechanisms of such improvement with locomotor training are still obscure. However, the work of Edgerton has stressed that the main effect of training is not peripheral but central. In other words, the improved performance does not seem to be related to

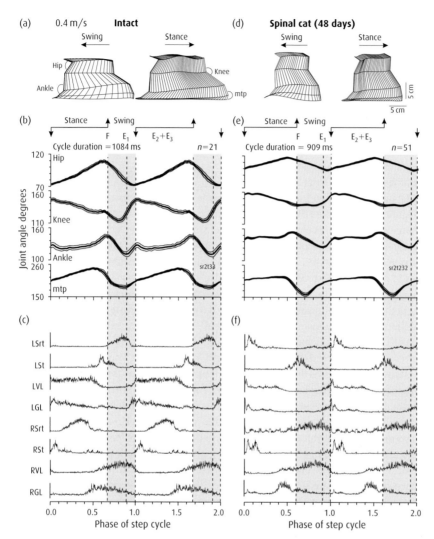

Figure 13.2. *Comparison of hindlimb locomotion at 0.4 m/s in the same cat before and 48 days after spinalization at T13.*
A and D: Stick figures reconstructed from video sequences of one step cycle before and after spinalization. The swing and the stance phases, with arrows pointing in the direction of motion of the leg, are illustrated separately. The orientation of joint angle measurements is given. Note that to prevent overlap of the stick figures, each figure is displaced by an amount equal to the displacement of the foot on the horizontal axis and therefore the horizontal and vertical calibrations are different.
B and E: Angular excursion of the four joints averaged over 21 and 51 cycles, respectively. Flexion always corresponds to a downward deflection of the angular traces. MTP, metatarsophalangeal joint. The vertical dotted lines separate various epochs (F and E1 constitute swing while E2 and E3 constitute stance) of the step cycle (Philippson, 1905). Note that the transition between E2 and E3 is not always obvious and the two sub-phases have been merged together in these examples.
C and F: Average of rectified EMG traces of the corresponding cycles. L, left hindlimb; R, right hindlimb. Muscles are sartorius, anterior head (Srt, a hip flexor and knee extensor), semitendinosus (St, a knee flexor and hip extensor), vastus lateralis (VL, a knee extensor), gastrocnemius lateralis (GL, an ankle extensor). The cycle is normalized to one and the display is repeated twice for clarity of illustration at turning points of the step cycle. The average is synchronized on foot contact (start of E2).

a change in muscle mass or a change in muscle composition of muscle units but rather to central mechanisms. More work is needed to determine which factors are implicated but undoubtedly physiological and neurochemical changes are important. It was suggested for instance that spinal inhibitory mechanisms, documented by measuring enzymes related to the catabolism of gamma amino butyric acid (GABA), were modulated with training (Tillakaratne et al., 2002) such that the decrease of inhibition that may be related to the development of spasticity may be offset by training. Whether or not training induces other changes in the density of receptors of other transmitters remain to be seen (Giroux et al., 1999).

Pharmacological stimulation and evolution of receptors

Neurotransmitter agonists

Pioneering work on L-Dopa in acute spinal cats (Jankowska et al., 1967a, b; Grillner and Zangger, 1979) led to the concept of a central pattern generator for locomotion. Indeed it was shown that intravenous (i.v.) injections of L-Dopa allowed the appearance of long-latency and long-duration discharges in response to nerve stimulation in acutely spinalized and paralyzed cats, sometimes leading to the alternation of long bursts between flexor and extensor nerves. Using nialamide to diminish the degradation of Dopa, Grillner showed that such discharges could be observed for hours, but even more importantly, found that the discharge pattern of characteristic flexor and extensor nerves had a very similar timing to that of the intact cat and even the relative duration of nerve discharge mimicked those found in the intact cat. This description of the detailed locomotor pattern in acute spinal cats that are chemically paralyzed and are therefore motionless was again another important principle for our understanding of locomotion. Indeed, not only is the locomotor pattern generator located in the spinal cord but it can also operate centrally; that is, in the absence of phasic sensory inputs or descending commands. This is the

only type of preparation which allows the use of the expression central pattern generator (CPG). This description also has the merit of linking higher vertebrates to invertebrates where the notion of central pattern generation was already accepted for the flight in locust or in the stomato-gastric ganglion.

Following the work on Dopa, more specific stimulation of adrenergic receptors was utilized. Clonidine was first used in acute spinal cats to initiate locomotion (Forssberg and Grillner, 1973). We have shown further, using adult spinal cats chronically implanted with EMG electrodes, that only the alpha-2 adrenergic agonists could induce locomotion soon after spinalization (Barbeau et al., 1987). Using an intrathecal cannula, we also showed that various alpha-2 adrenergic agonists such as clonidine, tizanidine and oxymetazoline could do the same (Chau et al., 1998). Besides their role in initiating locomotion, alpha-2 agonists also have a profound modulating effect on the spontaneously generated locomotion in spinal cats. Generally, there is an increase in step length and an associated prolongation of EMG bursts, but with little effects on amplitude. The effects are quite specific depending on whether the cat has an intact spinal cord, is completely spinal or partially spinal (Giroux et al., 1998; Rossignol et al., 2001). Whereas clonidine has the striking effect of evoking locomotion in early spinal cats, in the intact state, clonidine has little effect (Giroux et al., 2001). In partial spinal cats, with large bilateral ventral and ventro lateral lesions, clonidine can altogether stop locomotion (Brustein and Rossignol, 1999). This of course raises the important issue that the effect of drugs on the spinal cord will depend on the state of receptivity of receptors.

In our hands, serotonergic agonists such as quipazine, 5-O-DMT or the precursor 5-HTP could not initiate locomotion in acute spinal cats or in the early days after spinalization (Barbeau and Rossignol, 1990). This inability to generate locomotion with these 5-HT agonists raises the issue of the importance of the level of transection. It was indeed suggested that 5-HT receptor subunits important for locomotion may be distributed differentially along spinal segments and that critical segments containing such receptors may be inactivated by a spinalization at T13 (Schmidt and Jordan, 2000). Therefore, not only is the state of responsiveness of receptors important (intact, spinal and partial) but also the level of transection may be important to evaluate the effects of stimulating certain classes of receptors.

Although in T13 spinal cats, 5-HT agonists did not evoke locomotion, they had a profound effect on the output of the spontaneously generated locomotor pattern, such that muscle bursts (especially extensors) were markedly increased in amplitude and other muscles such as periaxial muscles, which are very weakly activated if all in the spinal state become very active (Barbeau and Rossignol, 1990). In partially spinalized cats, 5-HT agonists could increase weight support as well as the time during which cats could walk uninterruptedly (Brustein and Rossignol, 1999). It is interesting to observe here that these pharmacological effects were well integrated in an otherwise voluntarily generated locomotor pattern.

Moreover we were unable to initiate locomotion with N-methyl-D-aspartate (NMDA) in early spinal cats soon after spinalization. Intrathecal injections of NMDA only generated tremor and toe fanning, but no locomotion (Chau et al., 2002; Giroux et al., 2003). This is in contrast to the results obtained in decerebrated cats (Douglas et al., 1993). However, when injected in spinal cats which just started to walk (around 6–7 days), NMDA could potentiate the emerging locomotor pattern and this effect could last several hours, even days (Chau et al., 2002). Interestingly, NMDA had little effects on the locomotor pattern once it was established. The importance of this will be clarified later with the use of NMDA antagonists.

Neurotransmitter antagonists

Antagonists of various neurotransmitter systems have been used either to block the effects of previously injected agonists or to evaluate the role that some receptors may have in spontaneous locomotion.

After intraperitonial (i.p.) injections of clonidine, yohimbine, an alpha-2 adrenergic blocker, largely reverses the effect of clonidine (Barbeau et al., 1987;

Giroux et al., 2001). In a walking chronic spinal cat, the pharmacological block with yohimbine has no effect, suggesting that these receptors are not involved in spinal locomotion as could be expected since they are not longer exposed to the endogenous neurotransmitter after the spinal lesion. However, this work also shows that whether or not these receptors could be activated by other endogenous molecules, they are not important for spinal locomotion. This is in contrast to locomotion in cats with intact spinal cord in which yohimbine induces a marked incoordination of the hindlimbs and a general inability to adequately control the hindquarters, which can walk sideways, uncoordinated with the forelimbs (Giroux et al., 2001).

5-HT blockers were less studied in the cat since 5-HT does not induce locomotion. However, cyproheptadine has a major effect when injected after a 5-HT agonist. The increased output amplitude induced by 5-HT agonists is reduced and locomotion can often be blocked (Barbeau and Rossignol, 1990; 1991).

Blocking NMDA receptors with alkaline phosphatase (AP-5) had some effects in cats with intact spinal cords (reduced weight support resulting in sagging of the hindquarters) but the cats could continue to walk regularly. In the same cats AP-5 completely blocked the spontaneously generated locomotion after spinalization (Giroux et al., 2003), suggesting that NMDA receptors play a critical role in the generation of spinal locomotion.

Evolution of receptors after spinalization

The distribution of α_1 and α_2-noradrenergic receptors, and serotonin$_{1A}$ (5-HT$_{1A}$) receptors was examined in the spinal cord of cats in control conditions as well as from animals spinalized at T13 a few weeks or months previously (Giroux et al., 1999). In control animals, the highest levels of α_1-noradrenergic receptors were found in laminae II, IX and X. The α_2-noradrenergic receptors were found chiefly in laminae II, III and X with moderate densities in lamina IX. Fifteen and thirty days following spinalization binding densities of both receptors significantly increased in lumbar segments. With longer survival times binding densities returned to near control values. The 5-HT_{1A} receptors were found mainly in laminae I–IV and X and, following spinal transection, binding density significantly increased only in laminae II, III and X of lumbar segments at 15 and 30 days. Thereafter, binding returned to control values.

The pronounced up-regulation of various monoaminergic receptors, observed in the lumbar region in the first month after spinal transection, represents a clear neurochemical plastic change and suggests that these receptors might be important during the period when cats normally recover functions such as locomotion of the hindlimbs.

Relative importance of spinal segments for locomotion in the cat

Our pharmacological work with intrathecal cannula suggested that important effects on locomotion could be observed when the intrathecal injections were localized to the rostral spinal segments (Chau et al., 1998; Giroux et al., 2001). Indeed, it was observed that with chronic intrathecal cannula implants that the diffusion of the injected drugs was restricted over the mid-lumbar segments L3–L4. A more direct approach to restricted pharmacological stimulation consisted in making small baths over the cord, to apply drugs, or in microinjecting directly in the cord a noradrenergic agonist or antagonist in various spinal segments of cats during an acute experiment of cats spinalized at T13 1 week before (Marcoux and Rossignol, 2000) as sufficient to induce locomotion of the hindlimbs. Further, locomotion induced in these cats by an i.v. injection of clonidine, which undoubtedly reached all spinal segments, could be blocked by a micro-injection yohimbine restricted to L3–L4. It was further shown that all locomotion could be abolished after lesions at the L4 level. These observations led to the idea that perhaps these midlumbar segments played a key role in locomotion. This was in keeping with the idea that important interneurons are located in these pre-motoneuronal segments and discharge during fictive locomotion (Shefchyk et al., 1990a; Jankowska and Edgley, 1993; Davies and Edgley, 1994; Jankowska et al., 2003). In a series of experiments in chronically implanted cats spinalized at T13, which had recovered spinal locomotion, we performed a second spinalization at more caudal lumbar levels (Langlet and Rossignol, 2005). A second spinalization in rostral L2 or L3 did not interfere with locomotion significantly and did not induce a second spinal shock. However, lesions at caudal L3 and L4 abolished locomotion completely even after several weeks attempting to train the animals. We must conclude that these midlumbar segments, which are largely rostral to the motoneurons of the hindlimbs (Vanderhorst and Holstege, 1997) play a key role in spinal locomotion. Whether the interneurons in these regions play such a role in normal locomotion still has to be characterized. In any event, these segments probably contain key neural elements providing crucial inputs for the operation of the CPG. These might be part of a long chain of propriospinal interneurons activated during locomotion (Shik, 1997; Jordan and Schmidt, 2002). Interneurons recorded during fictive locomotion at L4 level may play such an important role (Edgley et al., 1988; Shefchyk et al., 1990b).

There are a few considerations to make here in relation to the topic of this chapter on plasticity as well on the potential importance for the clinic. It is conceivable that after spinalization, some interneurons that are part of a long chain of propriospinal neurons may evolve to assume a leading role in the expression of spinal locomotion. Such plasticity at the interneuronal level remains to be characterized but other work (Jordan and Schmidt, 2002) suggests that cholinergic propriospinal interneurons appear more numerous using c-fos labeling after intensive locomotion.

Clinically, the notion that certain spinal segments may play a critical role in the control of spinal locomotion may help to somewhat simplify where to target pharmacological stimulation, cell grafts (see later in the rat) or electrical stimulation. Acute experiments in cats have also recently shown that electrical stimulation of the cord may evoke hindlimb locomotion (Barthélemy et al., 2002), and that the locomotion evoked from lower segments is abolished when a spinal lesion, including the ventral quadrants, is performed at L4.

Partial spinal lesions in cats

Medial and medio-lateral pathways

It was suggested that medial and medio-lateral pathways play an irreplaceable role in the control of locomotion (Eidelberg, 1981). Indeed, sparing of a small part of a ventrolateral quadrant was said to be essential for the recovery of locomotion in chronically lesioned cats (Afelt, 1974; Eidelberg et al., 1981a, b; Contamin, 1983). However, other works have indicated that cats (Gorska et al., 1990; 1993a, b; Zmyslowski et al., 1993; Bem et al., 1995; Brustein and Rossignol, 1999; Rossignol et al., 1999) and monkeys (Vilensky et al., 1992) can walk with the hindlimbs even after large lesions of these pathways at the last thoracic segment (T13).

In our experiments (Brustein and Rossignol, 1998; 1999), cats chronically implanted with EMG electrodes were lesioned through a lateral approach of the pedicles and it was observed that the severity of the deficits varied with time after the lesion and on its size. With small lesions, cats recovered voluntary quadrupedal locomotion after 1 to 3 days and could walk quadrupedally on the treadmill at speeds up to 0.7 m/s. However, with large ventral and ventrolateral lesions, sparing only part of the dorsal columns and part of one dorsolateral portion, cats behaved as complete spinal cats and dragged their hindquarters over ground for 3–6 weeks. Eventually, all cats walked voluntarily with all four limbs although animals with the largest lesions could not walk at speeds higher than 0.4 m/s. The intralimb cycle structure was preserved so that coupling between the joints remained normal and there was no paw drag. The interlimb coupling of the hindlimbs remained stable and at around 50% of the cycle. Cats walked with a more crouched position and the hindlimbs – forelimbs coordination was often unstable. They often adopted a pacing gait, that is the forelimb and the hindlimb on one side were coupled so that each would be in swing or in stance at the same time and alternated with the contralateral limbs. The percentage of cycle time spent with three limbs on the ground was higher insuring a strategy of greater locomotor stability. The forelimb and hindlimb could even walk at slightly different mean frequencies leading to

occasional stumbling. Whereas normally cats use their hindlimb to propulse the body, after such lesions the forelimbs became propulsive. Although the voluntary quadrupedal walking was at times unstable on the treadmill, it should be pointed out that they could voluntarily stand up, walk around in the laboratory and overcome natural obstacles on the ground or on the treadmill. When walking up slope, there was an increase in the amplitude of the forelimb elbow extensors to compensate for the increased load. However, there were very little changes in the hindlimb extensors presumably because of a lack of appropriate supraspinal compensation.

At the termination of the experiment, horseradish peroxidase (HRP) was injected below the spinal lesion to evaluate the number and location of surviving cells with spinal projections. In the pontine reticular formation and the medullary reticular formation (MRF), the number of labeled cells amounted to 5–48% of normal values depending on the extent of the lesion. Vestibulo-spinal neurons were eliminated. Rubro-spinal cell counts were found to be either normal or decreased (some of the lesions may have encroached on rubro-spinal axons). It is possible that remaining reticulo-spinal cells and rubro-spinal cells participate in the recovery of locomotion after such lesions. Preliminary evidence suggest that the number of HRP labeled cells was higher in the motor cortex of two lesioned cats compared to two control cats (Rossignol et al., 1999). It is thus possible that a significant compensation from the cortico-spinal pathways contribute to the locomotor recovery. Propriospinal neurons were unfortunately not studied although they could be strategically well-placed neurons to participate in such compensation as suggested (Jordan and Schmidt, 2002).

A number of previous studies may shed light on these results obtained with large ventral-ventrolateral lesions. The important role of the MRF in the initiation and control of locomotion has been well documented (Orlovsky and Shik, 1976; Shik and Orlovsky, 1976; Grillner, 1981; Armstrong, 1986; Rossignol, 1996). The MRF has been shown to play a crucial relay role in the initiation of locomotion by stimulation of the mesencephalic locomotor region. On the other hand, the reduced postural stability during locomotion might be attributed to the role of this region in postural control (Mori, 1987; 1989). Therefore, it could be expected that very large lesions of the MRF should result in a clinical picture of a complete spinalization, at least initially. The return of voluntary quadrupedal locomotion, however, suggests that other pathways coursing through the dorsolateral funiculi (DLF) or propriospinal neurons may participate in the locomotor compensation.

Other work has established the importance of the reticular formation in the step-by-step control of locomotion and this might account for the long-term deficits. Unit recordings of identified reticulospinal (RS) cells in the reticular formation have indicated that RS cells are related to hindlimb extensors and flexors in freely walking cats (Drew and Rossignol, 1986; Drew et al., 1986) as well as during "fictive" locomotion (Orlovsky, 1970; Shimamura et al., 1982; Perreault et al., 1993). Furthermore, microstimulation of the RF gives rise to coupled responses in forelimbs and hindlimbs at rest (Drew and Rossignol, 1990a, b) or during real locomotion in the intact (Drew, 1991) or decerebrate cat (Drew and Rossignol, 1984) as well as during fictive locomotion (Perreault et al., 1994). These results would predict that chronic lesions of the RF should induce an impairment of weight support and interlimb coordination, which is consistent with the main deficits observed in our studies with chronic partial lesions.

Lesions of dorsolateral pathways

After large lesions of the dorsolateral white matter cats can walk overground (Gorska et al., 1993b; Zmyslowski et al., 1993; Bem et al., 1995). Quantitative studies of treadmill locomotion after lesions of the DLF that include the dorsal columns (Jiang and Drew, 1996) showed a brief period of impaired voluntary quadrupedal locomotion, which lasted only 3–10 days. However, cats remained more crouched for 2–3 weeks and the step-cycle duration was increased due to a prolongation at the end of stance contrary to cats with ventrolateral lesions. Also contrary to cats with ventral/ventrolateral lesions, there were changes in the intra cycle characteristics. There was a simultaneous onset of the knee flexor St and the hip flexor Sart (there is normally a delay between the two, St discharging before Srt). This simultaneous coupling was interpreted as a possible mechanism for persistent foot drag. Cats could not modify their gait to voluntarily step over an obstacle on a treadmill (Drew et al., 1996) contrary to cats with ventrolateral lesions. However, cats with dorsolateral lesions could adapt to slopes, with both forelimbs and hindlimbs, imposed on the treadmill.

Importance of sensory inputs: effect of muscle and cutaneous nerve denervation

The previous paragraphs outlined the importance of central spinal mechanisms as well as some of the suprasegmental inputs. Sensory inputs of different modalities are also very important for the control of locomotion and cannot be reviewed here (Rossignol et al., 1988; Pearson, 1995; Rossignol, 1996). Two aspects only will be considered. Firstly, we will consider the consequence of removing specific muscular or cutaneous nerves on the recovery or the expression of spinal locomotion. Second, we will discuss the possibility that plastic changes in spinal reflexes evoked by peripheral afferents may be used to help the recovery of motor functions.

Our first attempt at determining how animals could compensate in the intact and spinal states to a lesion of the periphery consisted in sectioning the major flexor nerves of the ankle on one side (Carrier et al., 1997). With the spinal cord intact, cats could rapidly adapt to such neurectomy by slight modifications in hip and knee flexors so that the kinematics of locomotion were barely altered. Having recovered normal locomotion, cats were then spinalized at T13. Not only did "normal" spinal locomotion never recover but it was characterized by dysfunctional hyperflexions of the denervated hindlimb. This suggested firstly that the exceptional compensation seen when the cord is intact required continuous inputs from supraspinal centers; secondly, that the functional compensation seen in the normal condition was not all transferred to the spinal cord; thirdly, that the spinal cord was nevertheless changed by the chronic adaptation to the neurectomy. Indeed, the abnormal dysfunctional hyperflexions seen after spinalization reveal that the spinal cord was changed. To test whether this was the result of a long-term change in the cord or to the simple effect of ankle flexor denervation in a spinal cat, we performed a similar neurectomy in a cat which already had recovered locomotion. This resulted obviously in a marked decrease of ankle flexion but no dysfunctional hyperflexions as seen in cats spinalized after the neurectomy. In conclusion, changes occurred in the spinal cord itself.

In another experimental series, we lesioned an ankle extensor nerve lateral gastrocnemius-soleus (LGS) on one side in three chronic spinal cats (Bouyer et al., 2001) in a collaborative study with Pearson who had previously studied the effects of such a neurectomy in cats (Pearson et al., 1999). In chronic spinal cats there was a marked yield at the ankle during the first few days post-LGS neurectomy and a large increase in the agonist medial gastrocnemius (MG) EMG activity. This led to a return to almost normal ankle movement within a week and a persistent change in the activity of the MG muscle. Considering that these are spinal cats this finding suggests that the spinal cord is capable of some remarkable adaptation even without the supraspinal systems. This adaptation must result from a complex interplay between the spinal locomotor program and sensory information.

We have developed a model to study locomotor plasticity after cutaneous denervation of the hindpaws. This approach allows us to induce a sensory loss with minimal direct effect on the motor innervation of muscles. This was a confounding issue in the previous models of ankle flexor or extensor muscle denervation. In a first series of experiments, we completely removed the cutaneous inputs from both hind feet without damaging the motor apparatus, except for some intrinsic foot muscles (Bouyer and Rossignol, 2003a, b). After 24–48 h the cats walked almost normally on the treadmill although it took many weeks to be able to walk on an horizontal ladder. This adaptation was accompanied by a consistent increase in knee flexor muscle bursts (amplitude and duration) as well as some increase in extensor muscles during stance with treadmill walking. After complete locomotor adaptation cats were spinalized at T13. Following this, they were no longer capable of plantigrade walking even after several weeks of locomotor training. The cats simply dragged their feet on the dorsum during swing and supported weight on the dorsum during stance. The EMG pattern, especially of the ankle flexor extensor digitorum longus (EDL), was quite perturbed since it now discharged during stance rather than during swing. This is completely different from the "normal" spinal cat with intact somesthetic inputs. This suggests that somesthetic inputs are important for the control of foot placement during locomotion and this is particularly crucial in the spinal cat which, contrary to the intact cat, cannot compensate for the *complete* loss of somesthetic inputs.

In another experiment performed in only one cat we observed that when the cutaneous denervation on one side is progressive the early deficits related to the removal of each successive nerve are compensated within a few days even in the spinal state. Such compensation occurred only until the complete removal of all cutaneous inputs, in which case the cats behaved as other completely denervated cats described before. These findings therefore suggest that the animal, even in the spinal state, is capable of achieving some functional compensation after a *partial* somesthetic denervation.

To initiate studies on reflex compensation as a possible mechanism of adaptation, one cat was subjected to an extensive denervation of the paws leaving only one cutaneous nerve intact (the tibial nerve innervating the plantar surface). For more than 50 days there was a significant and sustained increase in the reflex amplitude in certain flexor muscles such as St and EDL evoked by stimulating the tibial nerve. Such compensatory increases in reflex gain may provide one mechanism by which cats compensate for partial neurectomies. We do not know if such compensation would persist in the spinal state or if such compensation is similar when the neurectomy is performed in the spinal state.

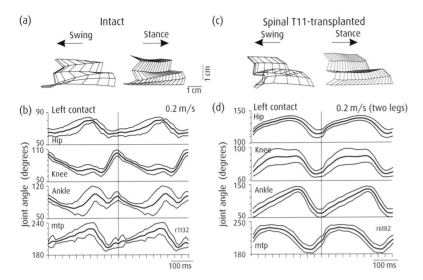

Figure 13.3. *Comparison of rhythmic locomotor activity in an intact rat and a spinal (T8) animal 9 weeks after transplanting 5-HT embryonic cells at T11.*
A and C: reconstruction, as stick diagrams, of treadmill locomotor movements during swing and stance phases at 0.2 m/s.
B and D: Variations of mean angle joints (thick lines) and their standard deviations (thin lines) from six consecutive step cycles. The same normalized step cycle is displayed twice to facilitate viewing the events at around the trigger point (foot contact of the limb facing the camera, downgoing arrow). Modified with permission from (Gimenez y Ribotta et al., 2000).

13.3 The spinal rat

Adult rats spinalized as neonates

Rats spinalized as neonates or weanling rats can recover an extensive spinal locomotor pattern (Stelzner et al., 1975; Weber and Stelzner, 1977). Such rats can also be trained with robotic devices (de Leon et al., 2002) (see also Volume I, Chapter 32). However, adult rats spinalized as adults do not recover any significant locomotion spontaneously. It was found that 5-HT agonists could induce locomotion in adult spinal rats (Feraboli-Lohnherr et al., 1999). Furthermore, it was shown that transplantation of embryonic 5-HT cells below the site of spinal lesion could induce a remarkable recovery of hindlimb locomotion on a treadmill (Feraboli-Lohnherr et al., 1997; Gimenez y Ribotta et al., 1998). Only rats receiving grafts of 5-HT cells re-innervating the rostral L1–L2 levels could display locomotion. Further work has also suggested that chronic exposition of the spinal cord to 5-HT agonists

could improve significantly the spontaneous expression of locomotion (Antri et al., 2002; Orsal et al., 2002) suggesting that the chronic activation of 5-HT receptors may preserve membrane characteristics of motoneurons or interneurons necessary for the operation of the spinal pattern generator. It was indeed shown that a fictive locomotor pattern after paralysis could also be obtained in adult rats that had been transplanted with monoaminergic neurons (Yakovleff et al., 1995) (Fig. 13.3).

Neonatal rat *in vitro* preparations

Bath applications of various neurotransmitters can induce locomotor-like activity in *in vitro* neonatal preparations (Kudo and Yamada, 1987). Serotonergic drugs, alone or with NMDA, have been reported to induce or modulate locomotor activity in the *in vitro* neonatal rat (Cazalets et al., 1992; Sqalli-Houssaini et al., 1993; Cowley and Schmidt, 1994; Kiehn and

Kjaerulff, 1996; Beato et al., 1997; Kiehn et al., 2000). Combined application of 5-HT and NMDA is also more effective in producing a stable and robust locomotor rhythm than in the application of either drug alone (Kiehn and Kjaerulff, 1996). At the cellular level, 5-HT$_{1A}$ agonist (8-OH-DPAT) significantly enhanced the N-methyl-D-aspartate-induced motoneuron depolarizations in the *in vitro* frog spinal cord (Holohean et al., 1992). In these preparations, Noradrenaline (NA) alone does not induce a locomotor pattern but an extremely slow rhythm, which is outside locomotor range, and in which there is a co-activation of flexors and extensors (Sqalli-Houssaini and Cazalets, 2000). On the other hand, NA can decrease the cycle frequency and increase the ventral root burst duration (Kiehn et al., 1999) of the rhythm induced by NMDA/5-HT. It can also reinstate a coordinated rhythm when the NMDA/5-HT-induced locomotor rhythm deteriorates.

The thoraco-lumbar cord was suggested to be of critical importance for the generation of locomotor rhythms (Cazalets and Bertrand, 2000a, b; Bertrand and Cazalets, 2003) although other rhythmogenic capabilities were found in lower lumbar segments (Kudo and Yamada, 1987) and sacral segments (Bonnot and Morin, 1998; Bonnot et al., 1998; Lev-Tov et al., 2000; Cazalets and Bertrand, 2000b). Such regionalization of function was also formulated on the basis of the distribution of receptor subtypes capable of inducing different rhythmic patterns (Jordan and Schmidt, 2002). Other studies in neonatal rats (Ho and O'Donovan, 1993; Bracci et al., 1996; Kjaerulff and Kiehn, 1996) have suggested that the whole spinal cord has rhythmogenic potential but that the upper lumbar segments appear to have a leading role.

With intraspinal injections of an excitotoxin (kainic acid), to destroy the gray matter while sparing the white matter, into the T9 and L2 regions of the spinal cord of rats (Magnuson et al., 1999), it was shown that damage to these segments induced paraplegia in chronically behaving rats. It can thus be concluded that the upper lumbar segments in rats (L1–L2) as well as mid-lumbar segments in cats (L3–L4) play a crucial role in the organization of the spinal locomotor pattern.

13.4 The spinal mouse

With the advent of genetic characterization and the potential for genetic manipulations, the mouse is becoming an increasingly important model for spinal cord injury research (Steward et al., 1999). To complete previous descriptions of mouse locomotion (Fortier et al., 1987; Clarke and Still, 1999; 2001) we have recorded the kinematics and EMGs from normal mice providing a set of basic normal parameters of locomotion (Leblond et al., 2003) as a point of comparison for eventual genetic models (Fig. 13.4). We found that despite the small size of mice we could adapt to some extent the techniques used in cats and rats to characterize locomotion. We found it particularly important to quantify the coupling between limbs, an important feature especially when looking at the effects of treatment after spinal lesions. This should complement the open-field behavioral testing (Basso et al., 1995) often used when studying rodents with spinal lesions (Farooque, 2000; Dergham et al., 2002; Seitz et al., 2002).

Our study (Leblond et al., 2003) has furthermore shown that mice can also recover hindlimb locomotion after a complete spinal section at T8. A second spinal lesion performed at the same level also insured that the recovery was not due to regeneration of descending pathways. This corroborates *in vitro* studies on neonate mouse spinal cord that demonstrate the existence of a central pattern generator (Bonnot et al., 1998). As for the cat (Barbeau and Rossignol, 1987) the locomotor recovery in the mouse took a few weeks. After the normal kinematics of each individual limb was first restored it was followed a few days later by an out-of-phase alternation between the hindlimbs. The ability of the spinal mouse to re-express locomotion was surprising since as mentioned earlier, another rodent, the adult rat, is unable to recover locomotion with their hindlimbs after a complete spinal lesion. This difference between rats and mice has also been suggested in studies with isolated spinal cord of neonates *in vitro*. By recording EMGs in isolated spinal cord with hindlimbs attached *in vitro* (Hernandez et al., 1991) or by recording ventral root discharges in isolated

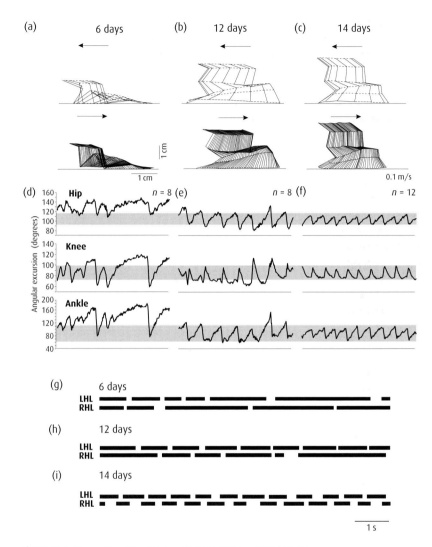

Figure 13.4. *Kinematics of the recovery of locomotion in a spinal mouse.*
A–C: Stick diagram of the left hindlimb of a spinal mouse 6, 12 and 14 days after spinalization.
D–F: Angular excursions of a minimum of eight consecutive step cycles illustrate the timing of locomotor movements. Note that a second spinalization at exactly the same level of the spinal cord was made after day 12 in this mouse. Thus the label 14 days means 14 days after the first spinalization and 2 days after the second one. Modified with permission from (Leblond et al., 2003).

low spinal preparation (Branchereau et al., 2000; Whelan et al., 2000), the lumbar spinal cord of the neonatal mouse has the capacity to generate, without any drugs, a spontaneously rhythmic locomotor pattern, in contrast to rats (Cazalets et al., 1992; 1995; Kiehn and Kjaerulff, 1996).

In another study, complete spinal mice were described as paraplegic for the 12-week period of observation (Farooque, 2000). The animals showed movements of the hindlimbs in the open field but had no coordination or weight support. It should be noted that the spinal mouse, capable of an elaborate pattern of locomotion on the treadmill at 14 days after spinalization, will look "paraplegic" if put in an open-field situation. The hindlimbs will simply drag behind the animal and only some occasional movements will be observed. This should not be interpreted to mean that the spinal cord circuitry cannot generate the locomotor pattern by itself when properly stimulated. This appears particularly important when discussing treatments to promote axonal growth that could act also to stimulate intrinsic spinal circuitry (see Volume I, Chapters 25 and 28). In other words, it is very important in the spinal mouse model to take into account such intrinsic spinal capabilities and be able to differentiate the effects of treatment that can re-establish connections with the sub-lesional spinal cord from other effects that will increase the spinal cord excitability and favor the expression of the intrinsic circuitry capable of generating the locomotor pattern by itself when properly stimulated.

13.5 Concluding remarks

The final characteristics of motor patterns result from an intricate dynamic sensori-motor interaction between the spinal and supraspinal levels. The fact that the CNS can optimize locomotor function after various types of central and/or peripheral lesions suggests a great deal of plasticity at all levels, including the spinal cord (see Volume I, Chapter 7). It is exciting to think that this plasticity can be beneficial for the rehabilitation of movements and can justify the use of different types of stimulation to promote the long-term re-expression of motor patterns even after spinal cord injury in humans (see Volume II, Chapters 3 and 19).

ACKNOWLEDGEMENTS

I wish to thank all the colleagues and students who have participated in one way or the other to the work summarized here. Most of their names appear in the list of references. I would like moreover to thank Janyne Provencher and Daniel Cyr for the iconography of this article. Finally, I would like to thank the Canadian Institute for Health Research for its unfailing support over the past 30 years, as well as the Fonds de la Recherche en Santé du Québec, the Christopher Reeve Paralysis Foundation and the Spinal Cord Research Foundation which all supplemented funding at various stages.

REFERENCES

Afelt, Z. (1974). Functional significance of ventral descending tracts of the spinal cord in the cat. *Acta Neurobiol Exp*, **34**, 393–407.

Antri, M., Orsal, D. and Barthe, J.-Y. (2002). Locomotor recovery in the chronic spinal rat: effects of long-term treatment with a 5-HT2 agonist. *Eur J Neurosci*, **16**, 467–476.

Armstrong, D.M. (1986). Supraspinal contributions to the initiation and control of locomotion in the cat. *Prog Neurobiol*, **26**, 273–361.

Barbeau, H. and Rossignol, S. (1987). Recovery of locomotion after chronic spinalization in the adult cat. *Brain Res*, **412**, 84–95.

Barbeau, H. and Rossignol, S. (1990). The effects of serotonergic drugs on the locomotor pattern and on cutaneous reflexes of the adult chronic spinal cat. *Brain Res*, **514**, 55–67.

Barbeau, H. and Rossignol, S. (1991). Initiation and modulation of the locomotor pattern in the adult chronic spinal cat by noradrenergic, serotonergic and dopaminergic drugs. *Brain Res*, **546**, 250–260.

Barbeau, H., Julien, C. and Rossignol, S. (1987). The effects of clonidine and yohimbine on locomotion and cutaneous reflexes in the adult chronic spinal cat. *Brain Res*, **437**, 83–96.

Barthélemy, D., Leblond, H. and Rossignol, S. (2002). Electrical stimulation of the lumbar spinal cord and the importance of mid lumbar segments in eliciting spinal locomotion. *Soc Neurosci Abst*, **28**[65.19] [Abstract].

Basso, D.M., Beattie, M.S. and Bresnahan, J.C. (1995). A sensitive and reliable locomotor rating scale for open field testing in rats. *J Neurotraum*, **12**, 1–21.

Beato, M., Bracci, E. and Nistri, A. (1997). Contribution of NMDA and non-NMDA glutamate receptors to locomotor pattern generation in the neonatal rat spinal cord. *Proc Roy Soc London B Biol Sci*, **264**, 877–884.

Bélanger, M., Drew, T., Provencher, J. and Rossignol, S. (1996). A comparison of treadmill locomotion in adult cats before and after spinal transection. *J Neurophysiol*, **76**, 471–491.

Bem, T., Gorska, T., Majczynski, H. and Zmyslowski, W. (1995). Different patterns of fore-hindlimb coordination during overground locomotion in cats with ventral and lateral spinal lesions. *Exp Brain Res*, **104**, 70–80.

Bertrand, S. and Cazalets, J.R. (2003). The respective contribution of lumbar segments to the generation of locomotion in the isolated spinal cord of newborn rat. *Eur J Neurosci*, **16**, 1741–1750.

Bonnot, A. and Morin, D. (1998). Hemisegmental localisation of rhythmic networks in the lumbosacral spinal cord of neonate mouse. *Brain Res*, **793**, 136–148.

Bonnot, A., Morin, D. and Viala, D. (1998). Genesis of spontaneous rhythmic motor patterns in the lumbosacral spinal cord of neonate mouse. *Dev Brain Res*, **108**, 89–99.

Bouyer, L.J.G. and Rossignol, S. (2003a). Contribution of cutaneous inputs from the hindpaw to the control of locomotion. I. Intact cats. *J Neurophysiol*, **90**, 3625–3639.

Bouyer, L.J.G. and Rossignol, S. (2003b). Contribution of cutaneous inputs from the hindpaw to the control of locomotion. II. Spinal cats. *J Neurophysiol*, **90**, 3640–3653.

Bouyer, L.J.G., Whelan, P., Pearson, K.G. and Rossignol, S. (2001). Adaptive locomotor plasticity in chronic spinal cats after ankle extensors neurectomy. *J Neurosci*, **21**, 3531–3541.

Bracci, E., Ballerini, L. and Nistri, A. (1996). Localization of rhythmogenic networks responsible for spontaneous bursts induced by strychnine and bicuculline in the rat isolated spinal cord. *J Neurosci*, **16**, 7063–7076.

Bradley, N.S. and Smith, J.L. (1988). Neuromuscular patterns of stereotypic hindlimb behaviors in the first postnatal months. II. Stepping in spinal kittens. *Dev Brain Res*, **38**, 53–67.

Branchereau, P., Morin, D., Bonnot, A., Ballion, B., Chapron, J. and Viala, D. (2000). Development of lumbar rhythmic networks: from embryonic to neonate locomotor-like patterns in the mouse. *Brain Res Bull*, **53**, 711–718.

Bregman, B.S. and Goldberger, M.E. (1983). Infant lesion effect. I. Development of motor behavior following neonatal spinal cord damage in cats. *Develop Brain Res*, **9**, 103–117.

Brustein, E. and Rossignol, S. (1998). Recovery of locomotion after ventral and ventrolateral spinal lesions in the cat. I. Deficits and adaptive mechanisms. *J Neurophysiol*, **80**, 1245–1267.

Brustein, E. and Rossignol, S. (1999). Recovery of locomotion after ventral and ventrolateral spinal lesions in the cat. II. Effects of noradrenergic and serotoninergic drugs. *J Neurophysiol*, **81**, 1513–1530.

Carrier, L., Brustein, L. and Rossignol, S. (1997). Locomotion of the hindlimbs after neurectomy of ankle flexors in intact and spinal cats: model for the study of locomotor plasticity. *J Neurophysiol*, **77**, 1979–1993.

Cazalets, J.R. and Bertrand, S. (2000a). Coupling between lumbar and sacral motor networks in the neonatal rat spinal cord. *Eur J Neurosci*, **12**, 2993–3002.

Cazalets, J.R. and Bertrand, S. (2000b). Ubiquity of motor networks in the spinal cord of vertebrates. *Brain Res Bull*, **53**, 627–634.

Cazalets, J.R., Sqalli-Houssaini, Y. and Clarac, F. (1992). Activation of the central pattern generators for locomotion by serotonin and excitatory amino acids in neonatal rat. *J Physiol*, **455**, 187–204.

Cazalets, J.R., Borde, M. and Clarac, F. (1995). Localization and organization of the central pattern generator for hindlimb locomotion in newborn rat. *J Neurosci*, **15**, 4943–4951.

Chau, C., Barbeau, H. and Rossignol, S. (1998). Effects of intrathecal α_1- and α_2-noradrenergic agonists and norepinephrine on locomotion in chronic spinal cats. *J Neurophysiol*, **79**, 2941–2963.

Chau, C., Giroux, N., Barbeau, H., Jordan, L.M. and Rossignol, S. (2002). Effects of intrathecal glutamatergic drugs on locomotion. I. NMDA in short-term spinal cats. *J Neurophysiol*, **88**, 3032–3045.

Clarke, K.A. and Still, J. (1999). Gait analysis in the mouse. *Physiol Behav*, **66**, 723–729.

Clarke, K.A. and Still, J. (2001). Development and consistency of gait in the mouse. *Physiol Behav*, **73**, 159–164.

Contamin, F. (1983). Sections médullaires incomplètes et locomotion chez le chat. *Bull Acad Nat Med*, **167**, 727–730.

Cowley, K.C. and Schmidt, B.J. (1994). A comparison of motor patterns induced by *N*-methyl-D-aspartate, acetylcholine and serotonin in the *in vitro* neonatal rat spinal cord. *Neurosci Lett*, **171**, 147–150.

Davies, H.E. and Edgley, S.A. (1994). Inputs to group II activated midlumbar interneurones from descending motor pathways in the cat. *J Physiol*, **479**, 463–473.

de Leon, R.D., Hodgson, J.A., Roy, R.R. and Edgerton, V.R. (1998a). Full weight-bearing hindlimb standing following stand training in the adult spinal cat. *J Neurophysiol*, **80**, 83–91.

de Leon, R.D., Hodgson, J.A., Roy, R.R. and Edgerton, V.R. (1998b). Locomotor capacity attributable to step training versus spontaneous recovery after spinalization in adult cats. *J Neurophysiol*, **79**, 1329–1340.

de Leon, R.D., Reinkensmeyer, D.J., Timoszyk, W.K., London, N.J., Roy, R.R. and Edgerton, V.R. (2002). Use of robotics in assessing the adaptive capacity of the rat lumbar spinal cord. *Prog Brain Res*, **137**, 141–150.

Delcomyn, F. (1980). Neural basis of rhythmic behavior in animals. *Science*, **210**, 492–498.

Dergham, P., Ellezam, B., Essagian, C., Avedissian, H., Lubell, W.D. and McKerracher, L. (2002). Rho signaling pathway targeted to promote spinal cord repair. *J Neurosci*, **22**, 6570–6777.

Douglas, J.R., Noga, B.R., Dai, X. and Jordan, L.M. (1993). The effects of intrathecal administration of excitatory amino acid agonists and antagonists on the initiation of locomotion in the adult cat. *J Neurosci*, **13**, 990–1000.

Drew, T. (1991). Functional organization within the medullary reticular formation of the intact unanesthetized cat.III. Microstimulation during locomotion. *J Neurophysiol*, **66**, 919–938.

Drew, T. and Rossignol, S. (1984). Phase-dependent responses evoked in limb muscles by stimulation of medullary reticular formation during locomotion in thalamic cats. *J Neurophysiol*, **52**, 653–675.

Drew, T. and Rossignol, S. (1986). Studies on the medial reticular formation during locomotion in chronic cats using microstimulation and unit recording. In: *Neurobiology of Vertebrate Locomotion, Wenner-Gren International Symposium Series* (eds Grillner, S., Stein, P.S.G., Stuart, D.G., Forssberg, H. and Herman, R.M.), Vol. 45, Macmillan, London, pp. 73–76.

Drew, T. and Rossignol, S. (1990a). Functional organisation within the medullary reticular formation of intact unanaesthetized cat. II. Electromyographic activity evoked by microstimulation. *J Neurophysiol*, **64**, 782–795.

Drew, T. and Rossignol, S. (1990b). Functional organization within the medullary reticular formation of intact unanaesthetized cat. I. Movements evoked by microstimulation. *J Neurophysiol*, **64**, 767–781.

Drew, T., Dubuc, R. and Rossignol, S. (1986). Discharge patterns of reticulospinal and other reticular neurons in chronic, unrestrained cats walking on a treadmill. *J Neurophysiol*, **55**, 375–401.

Drew, T., Jiang, W., Kably, B. and Lavoie, S. (1996). Role of the motor cortex in the control of visually triggered gait modifications. *Can J Physiol Pharmacol*, **74**, 426–442.

Edgerton, V.R., de Guzman, C.P., Gregor, R.J., Roy, R.R., Hodgson, J.A. and Lovely R.G. (1991). Trainability of the spinal cord to generate hindlimb stepping patterns in adult spinalized cats. In: *Neurobiological Basis of Human Locomotion* (eds Shimamura, M., Grillner, S. and Edgerton, V.R.), Japan scientific societies press, Tokyo, pp. 411–423.

Edgerton, V.R., de Leon, R.D., Tillakaratne, N., Recktenwald, M.R., Hodgson, J.A. and Roy, R.R. (1997). Use-dependent plasticity in spinal stepping and standing. *Adv Neurol*, **72**, 233–247.

Edgley, S.A., Jankowska, E. and Shefchyk, S. (1988). Evidence that mid-lumbar neurones in reflex pathways from group II afferents are involved in locomotion in the cat. *J Physiol*, **403**, 57–71.

Eidelberg, E. (1981). Consequences of spinal cord lesions upon motor function, with special reference to locomotor activity. *Prog Neurobiol*, **17**, 185–202.

Eidelberg, E., Story, J.L., Walden, J.G. and Meyer, B.L. (1981a). Anatomical correlates of return of locomotor function after partial spinal cord lesions in cats. *Exp Brain Res*, **42**, 81–88.

Eidelberg, E., Walden, J.G. and Nguyen, L.H. (1981b). Locomotor control in macaque monkeys. *Brain*, **104**, 647–663.

Farooque, M. (2000). Spinal cord compression injury in the mouse: presentation of a model including assessment of motor dysfunction. *Acta Neuropathol*, **100**, 13–22.

Feraboli-Lohnherr, D., Orsal, D., Yakovleff, A., Gimenez y Ribotta, M. and Privat, A. (1997). Recovery of locomotor activity in the adult chronic spinal rat after sublesional transplantation of embryonic nervous cells: specific role of serotonergic neurons. *Exp Brain Res*, **113**, 443–454.

Feraboli-Lohnherr, D., Barthe, J.-Y. and Orsal, D. (1999). Serotonin-induced activation of the network for locomotion in adult spinal rats. *J Neurosci Res*, **55**, 87–98.

Forssberg, H. and Grillner, S. (1973). The locomotion of the acute spinal cat injected with clonidine i.v. *Brain Res*, **50**, 184–186.

Forssberg, H., Grillner, S. and Halbertsma, J. (1980a). The locomotion of the low spinal cat. I. Coordination within a hindlimb. *Acta physiol scand*, **108**, 269–281.

Forssberg, H., Grillner, S., Halbertsma, J. and Rossignol, S. (1980b). The locomotion of the low spinal cat. II. Interlimb coordination. *Acta physiol scand*, **108**, 283–295.

Fortier, P., Smith, A.M. and Rossignol, S. (1987). Locomotor deficits in the mutant mouse, Lurcher. *Exp Brain Res*, **66**, 271–286.

Gimenez y Ribotta, M., Orsal, D., Feraboli-Lohnherr, D., Privat, A., Provencher, J. and Rossignol, S. (1998). Kinematic analysis of recovered locomotor movements of the hindlimbs in paraplegic rats transplanted with monoaminergic embryonic neurons. In: *Neuronal Mechanisms for Generating Locomotor Activity* (eds Kiehn, O., Harris-Warrick, R.M., Jordan, L.M., Hultborn, H. and Kudo, N.), New York, NY, pp. 521–523.

Gimenez y Ribotta, M., Provencher, J., Feraboli-Lohnherr, D., Rossignol, S., Privat, A. and Orsal, D. (2000). Activation of locomotion in adult chronic spinal rats is achieved by transplantation of embryonic raphe cells reinnervating a precise lumbar level. *J Neurosci*, **20**, 5144–5152.

Giroux, N., Brustein, E., Chau, C., Barbeau, H., Reader, T.A. and Rossignol, S. (1998). Differential effects of the noradrenergic agonist clonidine on the locomotion of intact, partially and completely spinalized adult cats. In: *Neuronal Mechanisms for Generating Locomotor Activity* (eds Kiehn, O., Harris-Warrick, R.M., Jordan, L.M., Hulborn, H. and Kudo, N.), New York, pp. 517–520.

Giroux, N., Rossignol, S. and Reader, T.A. (1999). Autoradiographic study of α_1-, α_2-moradrenergic and serotonin $_{1A}$ receptors in the spinal cord of normal and chronically transected cats. *J Comp Neurol*, **406**, 402–414.

Giroux, N., Reader, T.A. and Rossignol, S. (2001). Comparison of the effect of intrathecal administration of clonidine and yohimbine on the locomotion of intact and spinal cats. *J Neurophysiol*, **85**, 2516–2536.

Giroux, N., Chau, C., Barbeau, H., Reader, T.A. and Rossignol, S. (2003). Effects of intrathecal glutamatergic drugs on locomotion. II. NMDA and AP-5 in intact and late spinal cats. *J Neurophysiol*, **90**, 1027–1045.

Gorska, T., Bem, T. and Majczynski, H. (1990). Locomotion in cats with ventral spinal lesions: support patterns and duration of support phases during unrestrained walking. *Acta Neurobiol Exp*, **50**, 191–200.

Gorska, T., Bem, T., Majczynski, H. and Zmyslowski, W. (1993a). Unrestrained walking in cats with partial spinal lesions. *Brain Res Bull*, **32**, 241–249.

Gorska, T., Majczynski, H., Bem, T. and Zmyslowski, W. (1993b). Hindlimb swing, stance and step relationships during unrestrained walking in cats with lateral funicular lesion. *Acta Neurobiol Exp*, **53**, 133–142.

Grillner, S. (1973). Locomotion in the spinal cat. In: *Control of Posture and Locomotion* (eds Stein, R.B., Pearson, K.G., Smith, R.S. and Redford, J.B.), Vol. 7, Plenum Press, NY, pp. 515–535.

Grillner, S. (1981). Control of locomotion in bipeds, tetrapods, and fish. In: *Handbook of Physiology*: The Nervous System II (eds Brookhart, J.M. and Mountcastle, V.B.), SAGE, Bethesda, MD, pp. 1179–1236.

Grillner, S. and Zangger, P. (1979). On the central generation of locomotion in the low spinal cat. *Exp Brain Res*, **34**, 241–261.

Hernandez, P., Elbert, K. and Droge, M.H. (1991). Spontaneous and NMDA evoked motor rhythms in the neonatal mouse spinal cord: an *in vitro* study with comparisons to in situ activity. *Exp Brain Res*, **85**, 66–74.

Ho, S. and O'Donovan, J. (1993). Regionalization and intersegmental coordination of rhythm-generating networks in the spinal cord of the chick embryo. *J Neurosci*, **13**, 1354–1371.

Holohean, A.M., Hackman, J.C., Shope, S.B. and Davidoff, R.A. (1992). Serotonin1A facilitation of frog motoneuron responses to afferent stimuli and to *N*-methyl-D-aspartate. *Neuroscience*, **48**, 469–477.

Howland, D.R., Bregman, B.S. and Goldberger, M.E. (1995a). The development of quadrupedal locomotion in the kitten. *Exp Neurol*, **135**, 93–107.

Howland, D.R., Bregman, B.S., Tessler, A. and Goldberger, M.E. (1995b). Development of locomotor behavior in the spinal kitten. *Exp Neurol*, **135**, 108–122.

Jankowska, E. and Edgley, S. (1993). Interaction between pathways controlling posture and gait at the level of spinal interneurones in the cat. *Prog Brain Res*, **97**, 161–171.

Jankowska, E., Jukes, M.G.M., Lund, S. and Lundberg, A. (1967a). The effect of DOPA on the spinal cord. V. Reciprocal organization of pathways transmitting excitatory action to alpha motoneurones of flexors and extensors. *Acta Physiol Scand*, **70**, 369–388.

Jankowska, E., Jukes, M.G.M., Lund, S. and Lundberg, A. (1967b). The effects of DOPA on the spinal cord. VI. Half centre organization of interneurones transmitting effects from the flexor reflex afferents. *Acta Physiol Scand*, **70**, 389–402.

Jankowska, E., Hammar, I., Slawinska, U., Maleszak, K. and Edgley, S.A. (2003). Neuronal basis of crossed actions from the reticular formation on feline hindlimb motoneurons. *J Neurosci*, **23**, 1867–1878.

Jiang, W. and Drew, T. (1996). Effects of bilateral lesions of the dorsolateral funiculi and dorsal columns at the level of the low thoracic spinal cord on the control of locomotion in the adult cat. I. Treadmill walking. *J Neurophysiol*, **76**, 849–866.

Jordan, L.M. and Schmidt, B.J. (2002). Propriospinal neurons involved in the control of locomotion: potential targets for repair strategies. In: *Spinal Cord Trauma: Neural Repair Recovery* (eds McKerracher, L., Doucet, G. and Rossignol, S.), Elsevier, pp. 125–139.

Kiehn, O. and Kjaerulff, O. (1996). Spatiotemporal characteristics of 5-HT and dopamine-induced rhythmic hindlimb activity in the *in vitro* neonatal rat. *J Neurophysiol*, **75**, 1472–1482.

Kiehn, O., Sillar, K.T., Kjaerulff, O. and McDearmid, J.R. (1999). Effects of noradrenaline on locomotor rhythm-generating networks in the isolated neonatal rat spinal cord. *J Neurophysiol*, **82**, 741–746.

Kiehn, O., Kjaerulff, O., Tresch, M.C. and Harris-Warrick, R.M. (2000). Contributions of intrinsic motor neuron properties to the production of rhythmic motor output in the mammalian spinal cord. *Brain Res Bull*, **53**, 649–659.

Kjaerulff, O. and Kiehn, O. (1996). Distribution of networks generating and coordinating locomotor activity in the neonatal rat spinal cord *in vitro*: a lesion study. *J Neurosci*, **16**, 5777–5794.

Kudo, N. and Yamada, T. (1987). *N*-Methyl-D,L-aspartate-induced locomotor activity in a spinal cord hindlimb muscles preparation of the newborn rat studied *in vitro*. *Neurosci Lett*, **75**, 43–48.

Langlet, C., Leblond, H. and Rossignol, S. (2005). The mid-lumbar segments are needed for the expression of locomotion in chronic spinal cats. *J Neurophysiol*, **93**, 2474–2488.

Leblond, H., L'Espérance, M., Orsal, D. and Rossignol, S. (2003). Treadmill locomotion in the intact and spinal mouse. *J Neurosci*, **23**, 11411–11419.

Lev-Tov, A., Delvolve, I. and Kremer, E. (2000). Sacrocaudal afferents induce rhythmic efferent bursting in isolated spinal cords of neonatal rats. *J Neurophysiol*, **83**, 888–894.

Magnuson, D.S.K., Trinder, T.C., Zhang, Y.P., Burke, D., Morassutti, D.J. and Shields, C.B. (1999). Comparing deficits following excitotoxic and contusion injuries in the thoracic and lumbar spinal cord of the adult rat. *Exp Neurol*, **156**, 191–204.

Marcoux, J. and Rossignol, S. (2000). Initiating or blocking locomotion in spinal cats by applying noradrenergic drugs to restricted lumbar spinal segments. *J Neurosci*, **20**, 8577–8585.

Mori, S. (1987). Integration of posture and locomotion in acute decerebrate cats and in awake, freely moving cats. *Prog Neurobiol*, **28**, 161–195.

Mori, S. (1989). Contribution of postural muscle tone to full expression of posture and locomotor movements: multifaceted analysis of its setting brainstem-spinal cord mechanisms in the cat. *Jpn J Physiol*, **39**, 785–809.

Orlovsky, G.N. (1970). Work of the reticulo-spinal neurones during locomotion. *Biophysics*, **15**, 761–771.

Orlovsky, G.N. and Shik, M.L. (1976). Control of locomotion: a neurophysiological analysis of the cat locomotor system. In: *International Review of Physiology. Neurophysiology II* (ed. Portez, R.), University Park Press, Baltimore, pp. 281–309.

Orsal, D., Barthe, J.Y., Antri, M., Feraboli-Lohnherr, D., Yakovleff, A., Ribotta, M., Privat, A., Provencher, J. and Rossignol, S. (2002). Locomotor recovery in chronic spinal rat: long-term pharmacological treatment or transplantation of embryonic neurons? In: *Spinal Cord Trauma: Regeneration, Neural Repair and Functional Recovery* (eds McKerracher, L., Doucet, G. and Rossignol, S.), Elsevier, NY, pp. 213–230.

Pearson, K.G. (1995). Proprioceptive regulation of locomotion. *Curr Opin Neurobiol*, **5**, 786–791.

Pearson, K.G., Fouad, K. and Misiaszek, J.E. (1999). Adaptive changes in motor activity associated with functional recovery following muscle denervation in walking cats. *J Neurophysiol*, **82**, 370–381.

Perreault, M.-C., Drew, T. and Rossignol, S. (1993). Activity of medullary reticulospinal neurons during fictive locomotion. *J Neurophysiol*, **69**, 2232–2247.

Perreault, M.-C., Rossignol, S. and Drew, T. (1994). Microstimulation of the medullary reticular formation during fictive locomotion. *J Neurophysiol*, **71**, 229–245.

Philippson, M. (1905). L'autonomie et la centralisation dans le système nerveux des animaux. *Trav Lab Physiol Inst Solvay (Bruxelles)*, **7**, 1–208.

Rossignol, S. (1996). Neural control of stereotypic limb movements. In: *Handbook of Physiology, Section 12. Exercise: Regulation and Integration of Multiple Systems* (eds Rowell, L.B. and Sheperd, J.T.), Oxford University Press, NY, pp. 173–216.

Rossignol, S., Lund, J.P. and Drew, T. (1988). The role of sensory inputs in regulating patterns of rhythmical movements in higher vertebrates: a comparison between locomotion, respiration and mastication. In: *Neural Control of Rhythmic Movements in Vertebrates* (eds Cohen, A., Rossignol, S. and Grillner, S.), Wiley and sons Co., NY, pp. 201–283.

Rossignol, S., Drew, T., Brustein, E. and Jiang, W. (1999). Locomotor performance and adaptation after partial or complete spinal cord lesions in the cat. In: *Peripheral and Spinal Mechanisms in the Neural Control of Movement* (ed. Binder, M.D.), Elsevier, Amsterdam, pp. 349–365.

Rossignol, S., Bélanger, M., Chau, C., Giroux, N., Brustein, E., Bouyer, L., Grenier, C.-A., Drew, T., Barbeau, H. and Reader, T. (2000). The spinal cat. In: *Neurobiology of Spinal Cord Injury* (eds Kalb, R.G. and Strittmatter, S.M.), Humana Press, Totowa, pp. 57–87.

Rossignol, S., Giroux, N., Chau, C., Marcoux, J., Brustein, E. and Reader, T. (2001). Pharmacological aids to locomotor training after spinal injury in the cat. *J Physiol*, **533**(1), 65–74.

Rossignol, S., Chau, C., Giroux, N., Brustein, E., Bouyer, L., Marcoux, J., Langlet, C., Barthélemy, D., Provencher, J., Leblond, H., Barbeau, H. and Reader, T.A. (2002). The cat model of spinal injury. In: *Spinal Cord Trauma: Regeneration, Neural Repair and Functional Recovery* (eds McKerracher, L., Doucet, G. and Rossignol, S.), Elsevier, NY, pp. 151–168.

Roy, R.R., Talmadge, R.J., Hodgson, J.A., Zhong, H., Baldwin, K.M. and Edgerton, V.R. (1998). Training effects on soleus of cats spinal cord transected (T12–T13) as adults. *Mus Nerve*, **21**, 63–71.

Schmidt, B.J. and Jordan, L.M. (2000). The role of serotonin in reflex modulation and locomotor rhythm production in the mammalian spinal cord. *Brain Res Bull*, **53**, 689–710.

Seitz, A., Aglow, E. and Heber-Katz, E. (2002). Recovery from spinal cord injury: a new transection model in the C57Bl/6 mouse. *J Neurosci Res*, **67**, 337–345.

Shefchyk, S., McCrea, D.A., Kriellaars, D., Fortier, P. and Jordan, L. (1990a). Activity of interneurons within the L4 spinal segment of the cat during brainstem-evoked fictive locomotion. *Exp Brain Res*, **80**, 290–295.

Shefchyk, S., McCrea, D.A., Kriellaars, D., Fortier, P. and Jordan, L. (1990b). Activity of interneurons within the L4 spinal segment of the cat during brainstem-evoked fictive locomotion. *Exp Brain Res*, **80**, 290–295.

Sherrington, C.S. (1910). Flexion-reflex of the limb, crossed extension-reflex, and reflex stepping and standing. *J Physiol*, **40**, 28–121.

Shik, M.L. (1997). Recognizing propriospinal and reticulospinal systems of initiation of stepping. *Motor Control*, **1**, 310–313.

Shik, M.L. and Orlovsky, G.N. (1976). Neurophysiology of locomotor automatism. *Physiol Rev*, **56**, 465–500.

Shimamura, M., Kogure, I. and Wada, S.I. (1982). Reticular neuron activities associated with locomotion in thalamic cats. *Brain Res*, **231**, 51–62.

Shurrager, P.S. and Dykman, R.A. (1951). Walking spinal carnivores. *J Comp Physiol Psychol*, **44**, 252–262.

Smith, J.L., Smith, L.A., Zernicke, R.F. and Hoy, M. (1982). Locomotion in exercised and non-exercised cats cordotomized at two or twelve weeks of age. *Exp Neurol*, **76**, 393–413.

Sqalli-Houssaini, Y. and Cazalets, J.R. (2000). Noradrenergic control of locomotor networks in the *in vitro* spinal cord of the neonatal rat. *Brain Res*, **852**, 100–109.

Sqalli-Houssaini, Y., Cazalets, J.R. and Clarac, F. (1993). Oscillatory properties of the central pattern generator for locomotion in neonatal rats. *J Neurophysiol*, **70**, 803–813.

Stelzner, D.J., Ershler, W.B. and Weber, E.D. (1975). Effects of spinal transection in neonatal and weanling rats: survival of functions. *Exp Neurol*, **46**, 156–177.

Steward, O., Schauwecker, P.E., Guth, L., Zhang, Z., Fujiki, M., Inman, D., Wrathall, J., Kempermann, G., Gage, F.H., Saatman, K.E., Raghupathi, R. and McIntosh, T. (1999). Genetic approaches to neurotrauma research: opportunities and potential pitfalls of murine models. *Exp Neurol*, **157**, 19–42.

Tillakaratne, N.J., de Leon, R.D., Hoang, T.X., Roy, R.R., Edgerton, V.R. and Tobin, A.J. (2002). Use-dependent modulation of inhibitory capacity in the feline lumbar spinal cord. *J Neurosci*, **22**, 3130–3143.

Vanderhorst, V.G.J.M. and Holstege, G. (1997). Organization of lumbosacral motoneuronal cell groups innervating hindlimb, pelvic floor, and axial muscles in the cat. *J Comp Neurol*, **382**, 46–76.

Vilensky, J.A., Moore, A.M., Eidelberg, E. and Walden, J.G. (1992). Recovery of locomotion in monkeys with spinal cord lesions. *J Motor Behav*, **24**, 288–296.

Weber, E.D. and Stelzner, D.J. (1977). Behavioral effects of spinal cord transection in the developing rat. *Brain Res*, **125**, 241–255.

Whelan, P., Bonnot, A. and O'Donovan, M.J. (2000). Properties of rhythmic activity generated by the isolated spinal cord of the neonatal mouse. *J Neurophysiol*, **84**, 2821–2833.

Yakovleff, A., Cabelguen, J.-M., Orsal, D., Gimenez y Ribotta, M., Rajaofetra, N., Drian, M.-J., Bussel, B. and Privat, A. (1995). Fictive motor activities in adult chronic spinal rats transplanted with embryonic brainstem neurons. *Exp Brain Res*, **106**, 69–78.

Zmyslowski, W., Gorska, T., Majczynski, H. and Bem, T. (1993). Hindlimb muscle activity during unrestrained walking in cats with lesions of the lateral funiculi. *Acta Neurobiol Exp*, **53**, 143–153.

Plasticity after brain lesions

Randolph J. Nudo, Ines Eisner-Janowicz and Ann M. Stowe

Department of Molecular and Integrative Physiology, University of Kansas Medical Center, Kansas City, KS, USA

14.1 Introduction

Throughout this century, neuroscientists have attempted to understand the neurological bases for functional recovery after brain injury (Ogden and Franz, 1917). But until a few years ago neural models were based on poorly understood processes such as diaschisis and substitution (Bach-y-Rita, 1987). At least short-term recovery from cortical injury probably involves the resolution of acute pathophysiologic processes in and around the site of injury. However, since improvement in motor abilities can continue for months, other mechanisms must play a role.

Neurophysiologic studies in animals and neuroimaging and non-invasive stimulation studies in humans over the past 10–15 years have begun to shed light on the neurological bases of motor recovery in greater detail. A common theme in many of these recent studies is that the cerebral cortex undergoes significant alterations in functional organization after peripheral and central nervous system injury, and after specific behavioral experiences (Merzenich et al., 1983; Donoghue and Sanes, 1987; Jenkins and Merzenich, 1987; Kaas et al., 1990; Chollet et al., 1991; Grafton et al., 1992; Nudo et al., 1992; 1996a; Cohen et al., 1993; Recanzone et al., 1993; Pascual-Leone et al., 1995; Seitz et al., 1995; Elbert et al., 1997; Karni et al., 1998; Kleim et al., 1998, and see Volume I, Chapter 8). The high level of interest in these plasticity studies stems from the assumption that the time course and extent of functional recovery is related to the time course and extent of cortical remodeling.

There is growing enthusiasm that new therapeutic approaches for improving function following stroke will be most effective if they are based on the rules underlying neural plasticity (see Volume II, Chapter 36).

14.2 Animal models of plasticity after brain injury

The effects of injury to the cerebral cortex and subcortical structures has been studied in a wide variety of mammalian species to understand the underlying mechanisms involved in recovery of function. Animal models have been especially useful in understanding the role of neuroplasticity in recovery of sensorimotor skills after brain injury. These injury models primarily focus on damage to the sensorimotor cortex and/or basal ganglia, primarily because of the common involvement of these structures in clinical neurological disorders, such as stroke.

The type of injury and the method of induction vary with the specific purposes of the experiment. Typically, injuries are of two types: (1) those designed to mimic traumatic brain injury (TBI) and (2) those designed to mimic cerebral ischemia (or stroke). Of course, other models have been used to damage specific structures or cell types (e.g., 1-methyl-4-phenyl-1,2,3,6 tetrahydropyridine (MPTP) for the destruction of dopaminergic neurons in the substantia nigra), but here, we focus on those most often used in the study of post-injury neuroplasticity.

Models of TBI

The primary methods for inducing TBI are (a) the fluid-percussion model in which saline is rapidly injected into the closed cranium (McIntosh et al., 1989) and (b) the cortical impact model which uses a pneumatic or mechanical impactor to control injury to the exposed brain (Dixon et al., 1991). These studies are performed almost exclusively in rodent species. While TBI models have been used extensively to characterize the histopathological changes in the acute stage post-injury, and have been useful in examining the effects of putative neuroprotective agents, few TBI studies in rats have specifically examined plasticity mechanisms during the later, chronic stages. Thus, the present chapter will focus primarily on ischemia models.

Models of ischemia and stroke

Cerebral ischemia in experimental animal models can be produced using a wide variety of methods (Traystman, 2003). Most commonly used for studies of recovery and plasticity are focal ischemia models, in which cerebral blood flow is reduced in a restricted brain region. Typically, these models employ various techniques for occlusion of the middle cerebral artery (MCAo), either proximally or distally (Fig. 14.1). MCAo is sometimes combined with temporary or permanent occlusion of the internal carotid artery. While MCAo is most commonly employed in rodents, a significant number of primate studies have examined the effects of MCAo, typically for acute experiments (Del Zoppo et al., 1986). The precise location of the MCAo has a significant impact on the extent of the ischemia and the resulting behavioral deficits. Permanent MCAo proximal to the lenticulostriate arteries will create ischemic damage to both cortical structures (especially the somatosensory and motor cortex) and to the basal ganglia. More distal occlusions will spare the basal ganglia, resulting in a pure cortical lesion.

In most studies, the MCA is occluded by tying the artery with suture or wire. An alternative approach is the use of an intraluminal thread gauged to the inside diameter of the proximal MCA. Balloon occlusion has been used, but primarily in non-human primates. Finally, a more recent technique employs the potent vasoconstrictor, endothelin-1 (ET-1). ET-1 can be applied directly to the artery, resulting in a very rapid occlusion. Reperfusion is dependent upon the dose applied (Virley et al., 2004).

In addition to TBI and MCAo to produce brain injury, aspiration lesions (created by vacuum applied through a tapered pipette or stainless steel tube) and electrolytic lesions (created by applying a direct current (DC) for several seconds within the target structure) have been utilized historically, and are still widely applied. It is possible that the presence of necrotic tissue that remains after MCAo, TBI, or

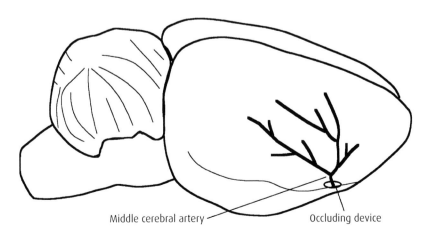

Middle cerebral artery   Occluding device

Figure 14.1. Schematic representation of the distribution of the middle cerebral artery and the location of an occluding device in a typical rodent infarct experiment.

electrolytic lesions, but not after aspiration lesions, will result in an inflammatory response that differs in quality or degree. While the acute pathological events following these differing lesion techniques are clearly different, the long-term consequences of the type of initial insult is still debated (Voorhies and Jones, 2002).

Advantages and disadvantages of common mammalian species in the study of plasticity after brain injury

Animal models of neurological deficits are essential for the assessment of new therapeutic options for stroke. While most studies of stroke and recovery have been conducted in rodents (primarily rats and mice), other models have been developed in larger species (e.g., monkeys, cats, rabbits, etc). The advantages and disadvantages are summarized as below.

Rodent models

The vast majority of studies examining plasticity after brain injury have been conducted in rodent species, primarily in rats, but increasingly in mice. Rodents offer very clear practical advantages:

(a) Genetic homogeneity can be more easily controlled. Due to the ease with which rats can be bred for particular experiments, it is possible to utilize littermate controls, increasing the statistical power of experimental design. Various strains of rats (e.g., spontaneously hypertensive rats) have been employed because of particular anatomical aspects of the MCA distribution (Johansson, 1996).

(b) The relatively low cost of purchasing and maintaining rats is a considerable advantage over non-human primates or other large animal species. This allows a larger number of animals to be used when necessary to power the experiment appropriately. This is particularly important in studies of the effects of interventions after brain injury, as the experimental design may require several parameters to be manipulated.

(c) Reliable sources for rats assure that animals are available whenever needed.

(d) Ages may be specified either by in-house breeding or by purchase of age-specific rats.

(e) Certain euthanasia and fixation procedures are much more feasible in rodent species (e.g., decapitation and quick freezing).

(f) Some histological procedures are easier to perform on small brains.

(g) Finally, the development and proliferation of transgenic and knockout mouse mutants have provided new types of animals to study the genomic and proteomic involvement in mechanisms of cell injury and neuroprotection from ischemia and reperfusion (Traystman, 2003).

Despite these obvious advantages, the use of rodents to model human disease has been controversial on occasion. Due, in part, to the recent failed translation of results from rodents to humans in neuroprotection trials after stroke, it has been suggested that rodents (or, at least, small animal models) are inappropriate for the symptomatic modeling of human disease. It is clear that substantial anatomical differences exist between the brains of rodents and primates, especially in motor systems pathways. Also, the time course of recovery after brain injury may differ considerably.

Nevertheless, a large body of data argues positively for the utility of rodents in brain injury research. Comparative analyses of movements in rats and primates show homology of many motor patterns across species. Rat models of hemiplegia, neglect and tactile extinction are useful in assessing the outcome of ischemic or TBI, and in monitoring the effects of therapeutic interventions. Studies in rodents that emphasize careful behavioral analysis should continue to be developed as effective and inexpensive models that complement studies in primates (Cenci et al., 2002).

Primate models

Although rodent species have been very valuable in the understanding of the cascade of events that follow acute stroke, and have begun to be utilized for studies of recovery mechanisms (Jones, 1999), the need for non-human primate models of stroke has received increasing attention. The primary advantage of non-human primate stroke models is that their vascular and brain structures closely resemble cognate human structures in their anatomy, morphology, cellular physiology, and biochemistry. The species and models are thus uniquely useful in research on the cerebrovascular pathophysiology of focal ischemia resembling human stroke (Fukuda and del Zoppo, 2003). Primate models of stroke are necessary because it is often difficult to extrapolate findings directly from rodents to humans without confirmation in a non-human primate species. Both New World (squirrel monkeys, marmosets) and Old World (baboons, macaques) monkey species have been used in acute and chronic studies of the pathophysiology and behavioral recovery after cerebral ischemia.

While New World monkeys have been used since the late 1960s to examine acute neuropathology after MCAo (Hudgins and Garcia, 1970), more recently these primate species have been used to examine motor and cognitive recovery after focal cortical ischemia. The hand motor area has been the focus of several experiments given that the hand is often affected in human patients with cortical motor infarcts. In some New World monkey species such as the squirrel monkey or marmoset monkey (as well as in prosimian primates), the motor hand area is contained in a relatively flat, unfissured sector of the frontal cortex, allowing direct access for neurophysiological examination and infarct induction. The dexterity of these species is of valuable use as these monkeys can be trained to perform refined movements of the hand for behavioral evaluation. For example, the hand dexterity and prehensile grip of the squirrel monkey allow for discrimination of impairment and functional recovery of skilled hand use. Despite numerous physiological and behavioral dissimilarities between squirrel monkey and man, the primary motor (M1) and premotor cortices of both species appear to be homologous (Nudo and Masterton, 1990). Parallels in the quality and time course of motor recovery after cortical ischemia

supports the use of New World monkey species as reasonable models of the neuronal events contributing to functional recovery after stroke.

Although Old World monkeys (e.g., macaque monkeys) have been used in the past for acute studies after MCAo (Crowell et al., 1981; Mack et al., 2003), few chronic studies have been done until recently (Roitberg et al., 2003). Studies of MCAo in macaques are beginning to employ clinical type assessment measures of motor and cognitive function (Mack et al., 2003). This combination of quantifiable parameters makes this model particularly suitable for studies of the effects of both neuroprotective and regenerative interventions using cell transplantation. In addition to macaque monkeys, baboons have been a popular non-human primate species for acute stroke studies, primarily because of their large size (Fukuda and del Zoppo, 2003). Serial clinical studies can be performed using neurological assessment and neuroimaging after MCAo in this species (Symon et al., 1975; Fukuda and del Zoppo, 2003; Mack et al., 2003), though these studies typically examine events in the acute post-stroke period.

14.3 Plasticity of representational maps after brain lesions

Somatosensory cortex

Studies conducted in cortical sensory areas over the past several years have revealed that representational maps are alterable as a function of the integrity of their sensory inputs, and as a function of experience. While plastic changes in cerebral cortex have long been known to occur developmentally, these studies demonstrating reorganization in adult primates are remarkable in that they suggest that cortical maps are alterable throughout life (Kaas, 2000).

The somatosensory cortex is composed of several regions in the postcentral gyrus, though most plasticity studies have focused on the primary somatosensory cortex, or S1. S1 is somatotopically organized with neurons in the medial portion responding to stimulation of lower extremity skin surfaces, and neurons in the lateral portion responding to stimulation of upper extremity and face skin surfaces. Studies conducted in several different laboratories have revealed that representational maps in somatosensory cortex can be altered by three principal types of manipulation: *peripheral manipulation* (nerve transection, digit amputation, dorsal root section, nerve transection–reconnection, nerve stimulation, island skin transfer, and digital syndactyly), *central manipulation* (spinal cord damage, cortical lesion, chemical manipulation of cortex, microstimulation of cortex), and *experiential manipulation* (behavioral training or other types of environmental distortion). Each type of manipulation results in substantial alterations in functional topography of somatosensory cortex. Reorganization of cortical sensory maps has now been demonstrated in every mammalian species studied.

One of the guiding principles emerging from the plasticity literature in sensory cortex is based on the temporal correlation hypothesis derived from Donald Hebb's conception of synaptic plasticity mechanisms (Hebb, 1949). According to Hebb, cell assemblies are formed because of reinforced coupling of coactive cells. It has been suggested that the normal organization of topographic maps in sensory cortex is an emergent property of temporal coupling in cortical networks (Fig. 14.2). Thus, experimental suturing of two adjacent digits (so-called digital syndactyly) can result in the emergence of atypical double-digit receptive fields in somatosensory cortex (Clark et al., 1988). Increased discriminatory use of the fingertips can lead to an expansion of the stimulated digits (Jenkins et al., 1990; Xerri et al., 1999). Likewise, in visual cortex, differential pairing protocols have demonstrated alteration of ocular dominance, orientation selectivity and other receptive field properties (Fregnac and Shulz, 1999).

It is possible that abnormal coupling within the cerebral cortex may lead to the formation of sensorimotor disabilities. For example, it has been demonstrated that under certain repetitive sensorimotor training conditions in monkeys, especially when vibratory stimuli are delivered to widespread surfaces of the hand, motor performance can deteriorate. The

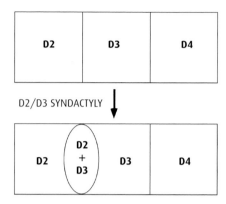

Figure 14.2. Results of a digital syndactyly experiment in which two digits are sutured together to increase temporal contiguity of inputs. Increased probability of simultaneous activation of cutaneous receptors on the two digits results in the emergence of double-digit receptive fields in somatosensory cortex.

monkeys begin to have difficulty in making complete contact with or removing their hand from a handpiece, a condition reminiscent of focal dystonia in typists or musicians. Examination of the somatosensory cortex of these monkeys revealed that the representations of the fingers were substantially altered. The boundaries between individual finger representations were degraded, and individual neurons responded to stimulation of the surface of multiple digits (Byl, 2004). Analogous findings have recently been found in humans with focal hand dystonia (Candia et al., 2003). Thus, it would appear that temporal correlation of inputs in somatosensory cortex may drive both adaptive and maladaptive plasticity.

Focal ischemia in somatosensory finger representations results in a loss of fine sensorimotor skill in the affected digits. However, as skill returns, a concomitant change occurs in the intact somatosensory representations surrounding the infarct, resulting in an eventual return of the lost finger representations (Jenkins and Merzenich, 1987; Xerri et al., 1998). While a cause–effect relationship between the return of cortical reorganization and sensorimotor skill has not yet been adequately established, it is possible that such alterations in functional properties in cerebral

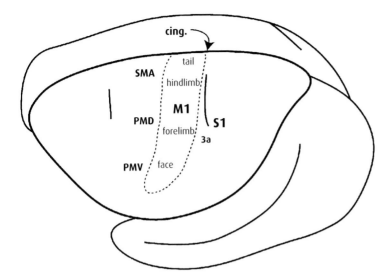

Figure 14.3. Location and somatotopic organization of M1 in a squirrel monkey. Other motor areas include dorsal and ventral premotor cortex (PMD, PMV), the supplementary motor area (SMA), and cingulate motor areas (cing.; along medial wall of cortex). The primary somatosensory area (S1) and area 3a are also indicated. Adapted from (Nudo et al., 1997).

cortex represent the neurophysiological manifestation of vicarious function.

Motor cortex

The primate motor cortex, located in the precentral gyrus, is classically defined as the portion of the cerebral cortex that requires the least amount of electrical stimulation to evoke movement of skeletal musculature. In primate species, including humans, the so-called "motor cortex" is subdivided into several distinct regions based on anatomic, physiologic, and/or functional criteria. These regions include the primary motor cortex (M1) the premotor cortex, the supplementary motor area (SMA), and the cingulated motor area (Fig. 14.3). There is now evidence that at least some of these motor areas can be subdivided into even smaller components.

Primary motor cortex (or M1) is arranged in a medio-lateral strip located rostral to the central sulcus (Fig. 14.3). Representations of the body are organized in a rough topography (or "map") from head-to-toe throughout M1, from the hindlimb and tail in the medial portions and progressing through the trunk (torso), forelimb (arm), and face laterally. The hand representation is located just rostral to the lateral

end of the central sulcus and is composed of representations of the digits, wrist, and forearm, and is also referred to as the distal forelimb representation. The hand area is surrounded on three sides by more proximal representations (elbow, shoulder, face) and caudally by a non-responsive region (at low current levels) that corresponds to somatosensory cortex.

This basic somatotopic arrangement was described in detail by Penfield over 50 years ago based on stimulation of the cortex of neurosurgical patients using surface electrodes and is usually referred to as the motor homunculus, or motor map (Penfield & Rasmussen, 1950; Leyton and Sherrington, 1917). The classic depiction of the homunculus suggests that each part of the body is represented at a single specific location within M1, and that there is a steady progression from one body part to the next across the cortex. Modern cortical mapping studies using intracortical microstimulation (ICMS) in non-human primates, as well as recent neuroimaging studies in human subjects have replicated this basic homuncular somatotopy in M1. Since M1 is frequently involved in clinical stroke, and since the motor deficits following stroke are often severe, it is thought that the integrity of the cortical motor map is essential for the fine control of voluntary movement (Lawrence and Kuypers, 1968).

While a global segregation of body parts is generally evident in functional maps of M1, it is now recognized that the representations of individual movements are widely distributed and overlapping in the motor cortex. The orderly progression implied by the motor homunculus breaks down within each somatotopic subregion. For example, within the cortex devoted to the representation of the upper extremity, there is no clear arrangement of movements of the individual digits, wrist, forearm, elbow, or shoulder; instead, these representations are intermingled in a complex mosaical pattern. Furthermore, individual movements are represented at multiple, spatially discontiguous locations within the forelimb region. In studies where electromyographic (EMG) activity has been recorded in conjunction with ICMS, representations of individual muscles have been found at multiple cortical locations, and individual muscle representations overlap those of other muscles. Further, by examining spike-triggered averaging of EMG activity in awake, behaving monkeys, it has been demonstrated that individual cortical neurons in motor cortex make monosynaptic connections with several motoneuron pools. Finally, local cortical regions containing multiple, overlapping representations communicate via a dense network of intrinsic, horizontal connections.

Several studies in human subjects using contemporary mapping techniques have also demonstrated a distributed organization. Using transcranial magnetic stimulation (TMS), a non-invasive technique in which a focused magnetic field pulse is used to generate an electrical discharge in cortical neurons, multiple and overlapping representations for movements of the arm and hand have been revealed. Functional neuroimaging techniques, such as positron emission tomography (PET) and functional magnetic resonance imaging (fMRI), also suggest that the representations of individual arm, hand, and finger movements are multiple and overlapping. For example, individual finger representations have been shown to overlap each other as well as the representations of the wrist and elbow. It has been suggested that the somatotopic gradients superimposed across a largely distributed representation may account for

observed patterns of separate and overlapping representations. This complex distributed organization may provide the substrate for functional plasticity in motor cortex, at least within each local subregion.

Recent studies have provided substantial evidence that recovery of cortical motor representations can be modified by post-injury behavioral experience, extending hypotheses developed in the early part of this century (Ogden and Franz, 1917). Over the past several years, investigators have begun to examine the effects of focal strokes in the motor cortex of both rats and non-human primates. Primate studies have shown that following injury to a portion of the hand representation in M1, the size of the spared hand representation decreases dramatically (Nudo and Milliken, 1996). However, if the unimpaired hand is restrained and monkeys receive daily rehabilitative training using the impaired hand repetitively in a skilled way, the hand area spared by the lesion is retained (Nudo et al., 1996b; Friel and Nudo, 1998).

These results in non-human primates parallel a recent series of studies in humans. These studies have shown that forced use of the affected limb for 14 days (by constraint of the unaffected limb) results in long-term improvement of motor function of the impaired limb (Taub et al., 1993; see Volume II, Chapter 18). Recent TMS studies in stroke patients confirm that reduced motor cortex representations can be enlarged by constraint- induced movement therapy (Liepert et al., 1998; 2000). It would appear that forced use of the impaired limb has significant functional benefit as well as a modulatory effect on the physiology of the undamaged cortex.

In addition to the M1, non-human and human primate studies have now begun to examine other motor regions of the frontal cortex, such as the premotor cortex and the SMA. For example, the ventral premotor cortex (PMV) is located rostrally and laterally to M1 and contains a smaller but separate and well-defined hand representation.

After a virtually complete ischemic infarct in the M1 hand area, monkeys initially experience a severe deficit in manual skill. While the M1 hand area is virtually completely destroyed, significant spontaneous recovery of hand function still occurs, though residual deficits in fine manual skill remain. Based on the recovery rate and the time to asymptotic performance, these infarcts are functionally equivalent to a moderate stroke in humans (Duncan et al., 2000). Not unexpectedly based on the extent of the injury, spontaneous recovery is not accompanied by a reappearance of M1 hand representations. Also, the adjacent elbow and shoulder representations remain unaltered. This would indicate that, at least under conditions of spontaneous recovery, new hand representations do not emerge within proximal representations. However, it has recently been demonstrated that other motor areas in the injured hemisphere undergo functional alteration. When the M1 hand area damage is extensive, the PMV hand area is enlarged when examined months later (Frost et al., 2003). Small lesions in M1 (<50% of the hand area) do not result in PMV hand area expansion, but when lesions are >50%, the amount of expansion in PMV is proportional to the amount of loss in M1 (Fig. 14.4). This result may indicate that reorganization within the M1 hand area can occur until the extent of damage exceeds some threshold. Once that threshold is reached, then other cortical territories must be recruited to participate in the fine control of movement during recovery.

Further evidence that reorganization of intact, adjacent cortical tissue contributes to functional recovery has come from similar motor mapping studies in rats. In these studies, after bilateral ablation of the forelimb area in rat motor cortex, motor performance was impaired. However, recovery occurred if electrical stimulation of the ventral tegmental nucleus was paired with forelimb responses. The stimulation is thought to have played a motivational role in encouraging forelimb use. When the motor cortex was re-examined following recovery, a novel forelimb representation appeared caudal and lateral to the ablated representation. The size of this representation was directly related to the behavioral performance of the recovered animals. Finally, ablation of the newly emerged forelimb representation resulted in reinstatement of the deficit.

Recent results in monkeys suggest that at least after large lesions of the primary motor cortex, more remote cortical motor areas may participate in recovery. For example, functional alterations have also been reported in the SMA after M1 lesions. Thus, after damage to M1, other motor areas in the injured hemisphere may contribute to recovery of motor skills.

Several non-invasive techniques have been used in humans to examine the effects of cortical injury on the function of intact cortical tissue. Subjects are typically those with cortical lesions (either ischemic or hemorrhagic) or lacunar subcortical lesions involving the internal capsule. These recent studies have

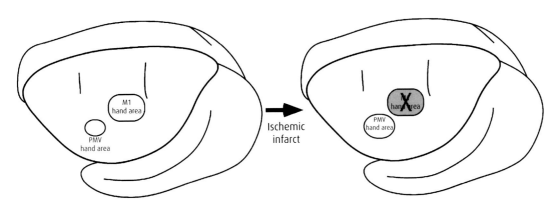

Figure 14.4. Effects of ischemic injury to the M1 hand area on remote motor areas. The PMV hand area expands in proportion to the extent of injury to the M1 hand area.

used non-invasive techniques for mapping the functional organization of the injured cortex, such as PET, fMRI, TMS, and magnetoencephalography (MEG). While the location of the injury is frequently unknown and/or uncontrolled, these studies have consistently shown that functional changes occur in several cortical areas after stroke or other cortical damage, paralleling results from animal experiments. As this review of functional plasticity after cortical injury in humans is not exhaustive, the reader is referred to more complete reviews (Cramer and Bastings, 2000; Cramer, 2004, and see Volume II, Chapter 5).

Using TMS, it has been shown that shortly after stroke, the excitability of the motor cortex is reduced, and the cortical representation of the affected muscles is decreased. It is likely that this effect occurs from a combination of diaschisis-like effects and disuse of the affected limb. Perilesional changes in cortical activity have been shown to occur using a variety of techniques. Further, following 8–10 weeks of rehabilitation treatment, there was an enlargement of the motor map in the injured hemisphere relative to the initial post-injury map. Still further, constraint-induced movement therapy, in which the unimpaired hand is constrained for 2 weeks to induce goal-directed movement with the impaired hand, produces a significant enlargement of the representation of the paretic limb. These results closely parallel the results of rehabilitative training of the impaired hand in primate studies that were described above. For more detailed description of human motor control (see Volume II, Chapter 2).

14.4 Modulation of neurotransmitter systems after cortical injury

Changes in two neurotransmitter systems, gamma-aminobutyric acid (GABA) and glutamate, have been implicated to play a role in functional recovery. Studies of neurotransmitter regulation suggest long-lasting and widespread changes in cortical function after focal injury. In rats, excitability changes have been observed in remote brain areas associated with a downregulation of GABAa, a phenomenon lasting

for weeks (Schiene et al., 1996; Witte and Stoll, 1997; Qu et al., 1998b). This dysfunction in the GABAergic system is associated with facilitation of long-term potentiation, or LTP (Hagemann et al., 1998). (An in-depth review of LTP and long-term depression (LTD) in the motor cortex can be found in Volume I, Chapter 8.) In addition, cortical injury results in enhancement of N-methyl D-aspartate (NMDA) receptors in spared cortical tissue (Mittmann et al., 1998). Regulation of both excitatory and inhibitory neurotransmitters in the cerebral cortex may play a critical role in the reorganizational process that occurs subsequent to focal cortical injury (Hagemann et al., 1998; Qu et al., 1998b).

Behavioral deficits similar to those seen after stroke are found in primates after reversible inactivation of primary motor and premotor cortex by injection of the GABAa agonist muscimol (Kubota, 1996; Schieber and Poliakov, 1998). There is a decrease in the density of inhibitory GABAa receptors and an increase in hyper-excitability in the area adjacent to the lesion following cortical injury in the rat (Schiene et al., 1996). This hyperexcitability has been observed up to 4 months after the lesion. Other studies have shown a bihemi-spheric reduction of GABAa receptors in multiple cortical areas connectionally related to the damaged area in rats (Qu et al., 1998b). Bilateral reductions in inhibitory GABAa receptors and concurrent bilateral increases in excitatory glutamate NMDA receptors occur in spared areas of cortex for up to 4 weeks after MCAo in mice (Qu et al., 1998a). A similar reduction of GABAa receptors and increase in NMDA receptors occurs in the ipsilateral thalamic nucleus projecting to the damaged areas of cortex (Qu et al., 1998a).

A recent study has shown differential downregulation of GABAa receptor subunits in peri-infarct and remote areas after focal cortical infarcts in rats (Redecker et al., 2000). Alterations in subunit composition are associated with changes in electrophysiological and pharmacological properties of GABAa receptors and these changes may be of importance for functional cortical reorganization after injury (Redecker et al., 2000).

Immunohistochemistry of the peri-infarct region in rats has shown that 1 week after injury, parvalbumin-positive interneurons (presumably GABAergic) show signs of degeneration and a reduction in the number of dendrites (Neumann-Haefelin et al., 1998). There is also a reduction in the number of parvalbumin-positive neurons immediately adjacent to the lesion. These results suggest that the downregulation of the GABAergic system, resulting in a decrease in inhibition, also occurs presynaptically.

An upregulation of NMDA receptors in cortex following ischemic lesion appears to be a consistent result in rodents. Other glutamatergic receptors, the alpha-amino-3-hydroxy-5-methyl-4-isoxazolepropionic acid (AMPA) and kainate receptors, have been shown to slightly increase in density in the peri-infarct region, although not significantly (Qu et al., 1998a). Significant changes in the density of AMPA and kainate receptors were not seen in remote areas of cortex away from the lesion (Qu et al., 1998a).

Changes in GABA and glutamate receptor densities may explain increased hyperexcitability following a lesion. Excitability changes in intact tissue following cortical injury have traditionally been thought to be pathological, and thus maladaptive. However, evidence is now accumulating to suggest that excitability changes may be one aspect of post-lesion adaptation in the neuronal network after injury. For example, pharmacological studies have shown that drugs that enhance the effect of GABA result in the potentiation of behavioral deficits following cortical lesion in rats (Schallert et al., 1986). Conversely, drugs that attenuate the effect of GABA speed up the recovery of function following cortical lesion (Hernandez and Schallert, 1988). These results suggest that a downregulation of inhibitory GABA receptors may be an adaptive response to injury, and that a certain degree of hyperexcitability may favor recovery, at least in rodents.

Regulation of specific neurotransmitter systems may play a critical role in the functional reorganizational process that occurs subsequent to cortical injury in primates (see earlier sections above). Perhaps the natural response to injury is a decrease in GABA inhibition that acts to unmask latent horizontal connections (Jacobs and Donoghue, 1991; Rioult-Pedotti et al., 1998). Glutamate is the major neurotransmitter

of the horizontal connections in cortex, and any synaptic modifications that may be necessary for functional reorganization may be mediated by NMDA receptors (Hess et al., 1996).

GABA and glutamate receptor density in primate cortex following injury has yet to be examined. Changes in neurotransmitter systems have not yet been studied in relation to functional reorganization following skilled training in primates. The remote effects of cortical ischemia are believed to be caused by alterations due to electrical or chemical signals emanating from the infarct, alterations along connectivity patterns (diaschisis) and use-dependent adaptations (see Witte and Stoll, 1997 for review). Intact brain areas that are remote from, but contribute information to a damaged motor area may undergo substantial anatomical and neurochemical changes. It is possible that these alterations may contribute to adaptive changes for recovery of lost function, and for learning-dependent plasticity in intact animals.

14.5 Anatomical correlates of functional plasticity after cortical injury

Widespread *structural* changes also occur after injury to motor cortex. In rats, the homotopic cortex opposite sensorimotor cortex lesions undergoes use-dependent dendritic overgrowth, followed by elimination of dendrites in layer V (Jones and Schallert, 1992; Kozlowski et al., 1997; Kozlowski and Schallert, 1998; Schallert and Kozlowski, 1998, and see Volume I, Chapter 8) (See Table 14.1). These changes are dependent upon the increased use of the unimpaired forelimb, since restricting the unimpaired limb prevents dendritic overgrowth (Jones and Schallert, 1994). Post-lesion structural alterations also occur in spared regions of the *damaged* hemisphere, including increased or decreased dendritic branching, decreased dendritic spine density, neural sprouting, and synaptogenesis (Kolb, 1995; Stroemer et al., 1995).

Studies of anatomical changes after unilateral cortical injury have been conducted almost exclusively in rats. After injury to the sensorimotor cortex, rats preferentially use the forelimb ipsilateral to the lesion

Table 14.1. Alterations in intact cortical regions following cortical injury.

Ipsilesional cortex	Contralesional cortex
Decreased dendritic branching	Increased cortical thickness
Decreased spine density	Dendritic growth (up to 18 days)
Increased dendritic branching	Dendritic elimination (after day 18)
Axonal sprouting	Increased spine density (after day 18)
Synaptogenesis	Synaptogenesis (after day 18)
GABAa receptor downregulation	GABAa receptor downregulation
NMDA receptor enhancement	NMDA receptor enhancement
Facilitation of LTP	Neuronal hyperexcitability
Alteration of motor maps	Increased number of synaptic mitochondria per neuron
Angiogenic factors up regulated	
Angiogenesis	
Hypoexcitability (acute)	

for postural support, reaching, and forelimb placing (Castro, 1977; Barth et al., 1990; Whishaw et al., 1991; Jones and Schallert, 1992; Jones et al., 1996; Whishaw and Coles, 1996). This asymmetry is seen within a day or two after the lesion, is maximal during the first 2 weeks post-lesion, and persists for at least 1 month (Jones and Schallert, 1992; Jones et al., 1996). Thus, it is not surprising that compensatory anatomical changes occur in the intact sensorimotor cortex contralateral to the injury.

Dendritic overgrowth, dendritic pruning, and synaptogenesis

As the processes involved in changes on the two sides of the brain differ, especially with respect to the influence of post-injury behavioral experience, these two topics will be discussed separately. Since most of these studies have focused on the contralateral (uninjured) hemisphere, these studies will be discussed first. Then, we review the evidence for similar changes in the injured hemisphere.

Contralateral (uninjured) side

Unilateral damage to the sensorimotor cortex in rats results in a number of time-dependent anatomical alterations in the motor cortex opposite to the side of the lesion. The homotopic cortex opposite to the sensorimotor cortex lesions undergoes a two-phase process of use-dependent dendritic overgrowth, followed by elimination of dendrites in layer V (Jones and Schallert, 1992; 1994; Kozlowski et al., 1997; Kozlowski and Schallert, 1998). Beginning a few days after injury, dendritic branching in layer V neurons begins to increase, reaching its peak at day 18. This increase is primarily in higher order branches (Jones and Schallert, 1992; 1994). At this time point, the volume of dendritic processes in layer V is significantly increased (Jones et al., 1996). At 10 days post-lesion, myelinated axons are reduced in volume fraction (Jones, 1999). At 30 days post-lesion, dendritic branching begins to decrease, suggesting that dendritic pruning has occurred. However, branching is still elevated above normal levels. At this time, the number of synapses and the surface area of dendritic membrane per layer V neuron are increased significantly (Jones et al., 1996). In addition to synaptic density, the proportion of synapses formed by multiple synaptic boutons and perforated post-synaptic densities is significantly elevated at 30 days post-lesion, but not at 10 or 18 days. Single synapse number per neuron did not increase (Jones, 1999). Together, these results suggest that after unilateral sensorimotor cortex lesions, a period of dendritic growth is followed by dendritic pruning, synapse formation, and changes in the specific structure of synaptic connections. The recent findings that the fine structure of synapses changes after injury is particularly interesting since several studies in other systems have suggested that these ultrastructural changes are related to changes in synaptic efficacy (Jones et al., 1997; Neuhoff et al., 1999; Weeks et al., 2000). Other studies suggest that the pruning phase is associated with adaptive changes as well. The administration of the NMDA receptor antagonists MK-801 or ethanol during a critical period after cortical injury can block the pruning process, and disrupt behavioral recovery (Kozlowski et al.,

1994; 1997). Finally, it has recently been shown that the number of synaptic mitochondria per neuron increases in the contralesional cortex after cortical injury (Sakata and Jones, 2003).

There is also evidence that these anatomical changes are dependent upon the increased use of the unimpaired forelimb. After lesions, rats compensate by relying more heavily on the unimpaired limb for postural support (Jones and Schallert, 1992). If the unimpaired forelimb is immobilized during the period of dendritic overgrowth (0–15 days post-lesion), dendritic arborization does not occur in the intact hemisphere and behavioral performance is further degraded (Jones and Schallert, 1994). Dendritic overgrowth is not affected by immobilization of the impaired forelimb. Thus, dendritic overgrowth is closely related to the time of over-reliance on the unimpaired forelimb, while the subsequent dendritic pruning is related to a return of more symmetrical use of the forelimbs. Dendritic overgrowth does not occur after immobilization in sham-operated animals, indicating that the magnitude of morphologic changes results from an interaction of the lesion and post-lesion behavior (Jones and Schallert, 1994). Finally, motor skill training for 28 days after the lesion significantly increased layer V synapses per neuron (Jones et al., 1999). Cortical lesions may therefore trigger the events that lead to use-dependent cortical plasticity in regions interconnected with the damaged cortical area. It is concluded that the changes in the intact cortex are an interactive effect of the lesion and post-lesion behavior.

Other studies appear to contradict these studies of use-dependent growth in the intact hemisphere. After cortical aspiration lesions, increased use of the intact forelimb was not associated with an increase in dendritic arborization of identified corticospinal neurons (Prusky and Whishaw, 1996). Also, after either small electrolytic or more extensive aspiration lesions, no evidence of a use-dependent increase in dendritic aborization was found in the intact hemisphere (Forgie et al., 1996). Both of these negative results were obtained at 18 days post-lesion, the peak of dendritic overgrowth in the previous studies. The authors of the latter two papers propose several possible factors

that might contribute to the discrepancy, including differences in lesion methodology. More recent data confirms that the dendritic growth does not occur after aspiration lesions, or after electrolytic lesions followed by aspiration (T.A. Jones, personal communication and see Voorhies and Jones, 2000). Further, electrolytic lesions may fail to produce dendritic growth if they are too small, a potential factor in some of the negative results with electrolytic lesions (Jones et al., 1996). While the mechanisms controlling this phenomenon are not yet fully understood, it is clear that under certain conditions, use-dependent dendritic overgrowth occurs in the intact hemisphere after motor cortex damage. This effect appears to depend upon the presence of the damaged tissue, and is more likely to occur after large cortical lesions.

Ipsilateral (injured) side

Indirect evidence suggests that anatomical changes occur in the spared cortical tissue surrounding the injury. After focal cortical ischemia in rats, GAP-43 immunoreactivity increased in the surrounding tissue, suggesting axonal sprouting (Stroemer et al., 1993). In addition, synaptophysin immunoreactivity is increased in the surrounding tissue suggesting an increase in the number of synapses in the intact cortex (Stroemer et al., 1992). It is interesting to note that the GAP-43 increase was significantly elevated only at early survival times (3, 7, and 14 days), while the synaptophysin increase was significant at later survival times (14, 30, and 60 days), suggesting that axonal sprouting was followed by synaptogenesis (Stroemer et al., 1995). See Volume I, Chapters 1 and 20 for additional details on sprouting and synaptogenesis, respectively.

After injury to the sensorimotor cortex in rats, extreme use of the affected limb can result in an enlargement of the lesion and further motor impairment (Kozlowski et al., 1996). If the unimpaired limb is placed in a restrictive cast after cortical injury, rats must rely heavily on the impaired limb for posture and locomotion. Forced overuse of the impaired limb during the first week after injury results in expansion of the injury and poorer motor performance (Humm et al., 1998). Forced overuse during the next 7 days does not result in injury expansion, but nonetheless resulted in poorer motor performance. This study strongly suggests that there are specific vulnerable periods for maladaptive effects of use after injury. Timing of these maladaptive effects must be considered along with timing of adaptive effects in any rational therapeutic design for treatment of motor deficits after injury.

In contrast, acrobatic motor training after a similar injury in rats resulted in no detectable increase in the size of the lesion and improved motor performance (Jones et al., 1999). It would appear that the behavioral conditions that follow cortical motor injury are critical in neural processes underlying recovery. The specific conditions that contribute to adaptive plasticity versus those that contribute to maladaptive plasticity are now beginning to come to light.

Subcortical changes

Several lines of evidence suggest that the reorganization seen in motor cortical maps (as well as somatosensory maps) has a substrate at the cortical level. However, at least in the somatosensory system, it is likely that reorganization occurs at several levels of the neuraxis after injury. For example, after massive sensory loss as might occur after amputation, reorganization has been reported at cortical levels, in the thalamus, in the dorsal column nuclei of the brain stem and in the spinal cord (Florence et al., 1998; Jones and Pons, 1998). It has recently been shown that at least after long-term amputation, significant sprouting occurs at the level of the brain stem that might account for massive reorganization in somatosensory cortex. Normally, afferents from the face terminate in the face representation of the trigeminal nucleus. However, 10 years after an amputation, some of these afferents sprout new connections to terminate in the cuneate nucleus, normally the recipient of afferents from the arm (Jain et al., 2000). The growth of face afferents into the deafferented cuneate nucleus in the brain stem appears to contribute substantially to the activation of hand cortex by face afferents.

Despite the growing evidence for subcortical changes in somatosensory structures following amputation, similar data from subcortical motor structures is rare. Mechanisms of cortical reorganization after amputation were recently addressed using TMS techniques and then testing intracortical inhibition and facilitation (Chen et al., 1998). The results suggest that after amputation, motor reorganization occurs predominantly at cortical levels. It is important for future studies to directly assess the contribution of functional and structural plasticity in the motor system (e.g., red nucleus, spinal cord, etc.) after peripheral or central injury.

A few studies have now examined plasticity in subcortical motor structures in adult animal models. After thermocoagulatory lesions, and injection of anterograde tracers into the uninjured hemisphere, labeled fibers were found in the striatum of injured animals contralateral to the injection (i.e., ipsilateral to the injury), suggesting that cortical neurons may undergo axonal sprouting following an injury to the cortex (Napieralski et al., 1996, Cheng et al., 1998). Unusual ultrastructural details have been observed in the newly formed synapses of the deafferented striatum (Cheng et al., 1998). These changes are associated with a variety of changes in gene expression and growth promoting factors (Szele et al., 1995). It is interesting to note that as with studies of morphologic changes in the homotopic, intact cerebral cortex discussed above, if aspiration lesions are made, the sprouting and several growth-related cellular changes are not found (Napieralski et al., 1998).

Axonal sprouting

A large number of studies have reported unusual corticofugal projections after neonatal sensorimotor cortex lesions, including corticorubral, corticopontine, and corticospinal projections (Nah et al., 1980; Castro and Mihailoff, 1983; Rouiller et al., 1991). However, evidence for widespread axonal sprouting or synaptic remodeling in these subcortical pathways is still weak in injury models in adult mammals.

Enhancement of growth factors

Growth factors also have been proposed to enhance neurologic recovery after cortical injury (Finklestein,

1996). In rats, nerve growth factor (NGF), basic fibroblast growth factor (bFGF), and osteogenic protein-1 (OP-1) recently have been found to enhance recovery of sensorimotor function. While efficient delivery of these substances to the central nervous system in humans poses a significant obstacle, it is likely that future recovery strategies will utilize a combination of physical therapeutic and pharmacotherapeutic approaches.

Angiogenesis

One newly emerging and possibly critical field of interest in stroke rehabilitation is angiogenesis following an infarct. In a mouse model of MCAo, a significant increase in the number of new peri-infarct vessels began 48–72 h post-infarct (Marti et al., 2000). A rodent model of distal MCAo, in conjunction with intravital microscopy, confirmed these vessel changes from immediately following stroke to 30 days post-infarct within the same animal (Wei et al., 2001). Clinical evidence of angiogenesis following stroke has also been established as well. Angiogenesis was confirmed in patients with survival times of 5–92 days, with significant increases in vessel numbers in the ipsilateral cortex surrounding

the infarct (Krupinski et al., 1994). Of particular import, however, is the effect of angiogenesis on longevity. In this study, Krupinsky et al. found a significant correlation between the length of patients' survival rates following stroke and the magnitude of peri-infarct angiogenesis.

A great deal of research is needed to determine how angiogenesis and neuronal changes are linked and to what degree the early molecular and excitotoxic events are required for these processes. Neuroanatomical changes may underlie neurophysiological reorganization seen in the remote areas and may require angiogenesis to meet the increase in metabolic demands as growth occurs in a particular area. Therefore, the degree of angiogenesis following stroke may be one of the most important factors in morbidity and functional recovery.

14.6 Assessment of behavioral recovery in animal models

Animal models employ a variety of methods to determine functional outcome in the days to weeks following brain injury (Table 14.2). While the sensitivity of the tests is largely a function of the extent of

Table 14.2. Common behavioral tests of motor function and cognition after cortical injury.

	Sensorimotor	Cognitive
Rodents	Cylinder	Morris water maze
	Forelimb placing	Passive avoidance
	Adhesive removal	
	Rotorod	
	Reach/retrieval	
	Montoya staircase	
	Beam walking/beam balance/grid walking/ladder rung walking	
	Kinematics	
Non-human primates	Reach/retrieval	Six-tube search
	Kinematics	Two-tube choice
	Neurological scales	Neurological scales
	"Staircase" task	
	Adhesive removal (feet)	

the injury and the animal's pre-injury experience with the task, most of these tests will allow a description of a recovery profile, with lasting impairments in some of the measures.

Sensorimotor assessment

Rodents

After a unilateral lesion in sensorimotor cortex in rats, motor impairments with the more affected limb (i.e., the limb contralateral to the injury) can readily be detected during the first several days post-injury. Schallert and colleagues have described several protocols for use in focal ischemia or injury models, and the reader is referred to the original publications for a more detailed description (Schallert et al., 2000). The *cylinder test* depends upon the hyperreliance of the animal to use its less impaired limb for weight shifting and postural control. The animal is placed in a transparent cylinder, and independent use of the left or right forelimb to (a) contact the cylinder wall, or (b) land after a rear, is recorded. Interrater reliability on this task is very high. The *forelimb placing test* examines sensorimotor capacity. Animals are held by their torsos while the experimenter brushes the vibrissae on the edge of a table. This normally results in a quick placement of both forepaws on the table. This task typically requires more skill on the part of the experimenter to obtain reliable results. The *adhesive removal test*, sometimes called the "*sticky tape*" test, tests sensory asymmetry. Small adhesive labels are placed on each forelimb and the experimenter records which label is contacted first and which label is removed first. After unilateral cortical injury, animals will typically remove the label opposite the good hemisphere first. Quantitative assessment of the degree of asymmetry can be achieved by altering the ratio of the size of the labels. The *rotorod test* is widely used to test sensorimotor coordination, but may not be sensitive enough to resolve long-term deficits in chronic studies of recovery after cerebral ischemia (Willing et al., 2002). *Reach training* has begun to be used in several rodent studies of recovery after cortical injury, as these tasks seem to show long-lasting

deficits (Biernaskie and Corbett, 2001). The *Montoya staircase task* has also been used to assess motor function after cerebral ischemia in rats (Bayona et al., 2004). *Beam walking tasks* and *grid walking tasks* are also commonly used to assess accuracy in stepping during locomotion.

Primates

Semiquantitative scales based on human neurological scales have often been used to describe the behavioral deficits resulting from middle occlusion of the cerebral artery either proximally or distally (Fukuda and del Zoppo, 2003). These scales are typically used for acute recovery profiles. More typically, chronic recovery after sensorimotor cortex damage has utilized examination of dexterous use of the impaired hand. For example, the use of the so-called "Klüver board" has been used in a large number of studies for several decades (Nudo et al., 2003). In this task, a familiar food item is placed into one of several wells of various diameter. The dexterity of the hand can be measured either by tallying the number of successful retrievals, the time to retrieve, or the number of total flexions per retrieval (Lawrence and Kuypers, 1968). In some studies, the kinematics of movement patterns has also been examined, similar to studies cited above in rats (Friel and Nudo, 1998).

Cognitive assessment

Rodents

The most common method to assess cognitive performs in rodents remains the Morris Water Maze. Rodents are placed in a pool of opaque liquid and required to swim until they reach a perch. Time to locate the perch reflects spatial abilities of the rats. In variations on the task requirements, both spatial and non-spatial aspects of the cognitive task can be assessed (Harker and Whishaw, 2004). Latency in a passive avoidance task is also frequently used to assess cognitive function in rodents after stroke (Gupta et al., 2002).

Primates

A large number of cognitive studies using various learning paradigms have been developed for use in non-human primate models of brain injury, especially after damage to memory-related structures in macaque monkeys (Alvarado et al., 2002). Recently, cognitive tests have been utilized in New World monkeys to assess deficits after MCAo (Marshall and Ridley, 2003). These tests have included the *Six-tube search task*, which tests spatial neglect, and a *Two-tube choice test*, which tests "extinction".

14.7 Development of treatment strategies based on principles of brain plasticity

The ultimate goal in our understanding of neuro-plasticity mechanisms after brain injury is to provide a theoretical framework from which rational approaches to therapy can be developed. Already, new strategies for promoting recovery that were derived from basic studies in preclinical models are being tested in clinical trials. For example, constraint-induced movement therapy was derived from deaf-ferentation experiments conducted several years ago that resulted in the principle of "learned non-use" (Taub et al., 2002). This therapy is now being tested in clinical populations to determine if intensive physiotherapy can be more effective when the less-impaired limb is restrained (see Volume II, Chapter 18). Neuroplastic changes demonstrated in non-human primates using a similar therapeutic design have provided further impetus to pursue this approach (Nudo et al., 1996b). The supplementation of physical therapy with amphetamine is another approach that was based on studies first conducted in preclinical models (Feeney et al., 1982).

Other potential approaches will likely follow as our understanding of the post-injury plasticity process becomes more clear. Approaches employing neurotrophins, neuromodulators, stem cells, magnetic stimulation, and electrical stimulation are currently under development. Each of the neurophysiological, neurochemical, and neuroanatomical, as well as behavioral changes that have been demonstrated after brain injury are dynamic processes that proceed along predictable time courses. It is imperative to understand the interaction of these processes and the effects of putative therapeutic agents that may modulate neuroplastic events in different ways at different time points. In this way, recovery may be optimized by shaping the inevitable plastic events that take place in the entire brain after focal injury.

REFERENCES

Alvarado, M.C., Wright, A.A. and Bachevalier, J. (2002). Object and spatial relational memory in adult rhesus monkeys is impaired by neonatal lesions of the hippocampal formation but not the amygdaloid complex. *Hippocampus*, **12**, 421–433.

Bach-y-Rita, P. (1987). Processes of recovery from stroke. In: *Stroke Rehabilitation* (eds Brandstater, M.E. and Basmajian, J.V.), Williams and Wilkens, Baltimore, pp. 80–108.

Barth, T.M., Jones, T.A. and Schallert, T. (1990). Functional subdivisions of the rat somatic sensorimotor cortex. *Behav Brain Res*, **39**, 73–95.

Bayona, N.A., Gelb, A.W., Jiang, Z., Wilson, J.X., Urquhart, B.L. and Cechetto, D.F. (2004). Propofol neuroprotection in cerebral ischemia and its effects on low-molecular-weight antioxidants and skilled motor tasks. *Anesthesiology*, **100**, 1151–1159.

Biernaskie, J. and Corbett, D. (2001). Enriched rehabilitative training promotes improved forelimb motor function and enhanced dendritic growth after focal ischemic injury. *J Neurosci*, **21**, 5272–5280.

Byl, N.N. (2004). Focal hand dystonia may result from aberrant neuroplasticity. *Adv Neurol*, **94**, 19–28.

Candia, V., Wienbruch, C., Elbert, T., Rockstroh, B. and Ray, W. (2003). Effective behavioral treatment of focal hand dystonia in musicians alters somatosensory cortical organization. *Proc Natl Acad Sci USA*, **100**, 7942–7946.

Castro, A.J. (1977). Limb preference after lesions of the cerebral hemisphere in adult and neonatal rats. *Physiol Behav*, **18**, 605–608.

Castro, A.J. and Mihailoff, G.A. (1983). Corticopontine remodelling after cortical and/or cerebellar lesions in newborn rat. *J Comp Neurol*, **219**, 112–123.

Cenci, M.A., Whishaw, I.Q. and Schallert, T. (2002). Animal models of neurological deficits: how relevant is the rat? *Nat Rev Neurosci*, **3**, 574–579.

Chen, R., Corwell, B., Yaseen, Z., Hallett, M. and Cohen, L.G. (1998). Mechanisms of cortical reorganization in lower-limb amputees. *J Neurosci*, **18**, 3443–3450.

Cheng, H.W., Tong, J. and McNeill, T.H. (1998). Lesion-induced axon sprouting in the deafferented striatum of adult rat. *Neurosci Lett*, **242**, 69–72.

Chollet, F., DiPiero, V., Wise, R.J., Brooks, D.J., Dolan, R.J. and Frackowiak, R.S. (1991). The functional anatomy of motor recovery after stroke in humans: a study with positron emission tomography. *Ann Neurol*, **29**, 63–71.

Clark, S.A., Allard, T., Jenkins, W.M. and Merzenich, M.M. (1988). Receptive fields in the body-surface map in adult cortex defined by temporally correlated inputs. *Nature*, **332**, 444–445.

Cohen, L.G., Brasil-Neto, J.P., Pascual-Leone, A. and Hallett, M. (1993). Plasticity of cortical motor output organization following deafferentation, cerebral lesions, and skill acquisition. *Adv Neurol*, **63**, 187–200.

Cramer, S.C. (2004). Functional imaging in stroke recovery. *Stroke*, **35**, 2695–2698.

Cramer, S.C. and Bastings, E.P. (2000). Mapping clinically relevant plasticity after stroke. *Neuropharmacology*, **39**, 842–851.

Crowell, R.M., Marcoux, F.W. and DeGirolami, R. (1981). Variability and reversibility of focal cerebral ischemia in unanesthetized monkeys. *Neurology*, **31**, 1295.

Del Zoppo, G.J., Copeland, B.R., Harker, L.A., Waltz, T.A., Zyroff, J., Hanson, S.R. and Battenberg, E. (1986). Experimental acute thrombotic stroke in baboons. *Stroke*, **17**, 1254–1265.

Dixon, C.E., Clifton, G.L., Lighthall, J.W., Yaghmai, A.A. and Hayes, R.L. (1991). A controlled cortical impact model of traumatic brain injury in the rat. *J Neurosci Methods*, **39**, 253–262.

Donoghue, J.P. and Sanes, J.N. (1987). Peripheral nerve injury in developing rats reorganizes representation pattern in motor cortex. *Proc Natl Acad Sci USA*, **84**, 1123–1126.

Duncan, P.W., Lai, S.M. and Keighley, J. (2000). Defining post-stroke recovery: implications for design and interpretation of drug trials. *Neuropharmacology*, **39**, 835–841.

Elbert, T., Sterr, A., Flor, H., Rockstroh, B., Knecht, S., Pantev, C., Wienbruch, C. and Taub, E. (1997). Input-increase and input-decrease types of cortical reorganization after upper extremity amputation in humans. *Exp Brain Res*, **117**, 161–164.

Feeney, D.M., Gonzalez, A. and Law, W.A. (1982). Amphetamine, haloperidol, and experience interact to affect rate of recovery after motor cortex injury. *Science*, **217**, 855–857.

Finklestein, S. (1996). The potential use of neurotrophic growth factors in the treatment of cerebral ischemia. In: *Advances in Neurology, Cellular and Molecular Mechanisms of Ischemic Brain Damage* (eds Siesjö, B. and Wieloch, T.), Vol. 71, Lippincott-Raven, Philadelphia, pp. 413–418.

Florence, S.L., Taub, H.B. and Kaas, J.H. (1998). Large-scale sprouting of cortical connections after peripheral injury in adult macaque monkeys. *Science*, **282**, 1117–1121.

Forgie, M.L., Gibb, R. and Kolb, B. (1996). Unilateral lesions of the forelimb area of rat motor cortex: lack of evidence for use-dependent neural growth in the undamaged hemisphere. *Brain Res*, **710**, 249–259.

Fregnac, Y. and Shulz, D.E. (1999). Activity-dependent regulation of receptive field properties of cat area 17 by supervised Hebbian learning. *J Neurobiol*, **41**, 69–82.

Friel, K.M. and Nudo, R.J. (1998). Recovery of motor function after focal cortical injury in primates: compensatory movement patterns used during rehabilitative training. *Somatosens Mot Res*, **15**, 173–189.

Frost, S.B., Barbay, S., Friel, K.M., Plautz, E.J. and Nudo, R.J. (2003). Reorganization of remote cortical regions after ischemic brain injury: a potential substrate for stroke recovery. *J Neurophysiol*, **89**, 3205–3214.

Fukuda, S. and del Zoppo, G.J. (2003). Models of focal cerebral ischemia in the nonhuman primate. *Ilar J*, **44**, 96–104.

Grafton, S.T., Mazziotta, J.C., Presty, S., Friston, K.J., Frackowiak, R.S. and Phelps, M.E. (1992). Functional anatomy of human procedural learning determined with regional cerebral blood flow and PET. *J Neurosci*, **12**, 2542–2548.

Gupta, Y.K., Sinha, K. and Chaudhary, G. (2002). Transient focal ischemia induces motor deficit but does not impair the cognitive function in middle cerebral artery occlusion model of stroke in rats. *J Neurol Sci*, Nov 15; 203–204, 267–271.

Hagemann, G., Redecker, C., Neumann-Haefelin, T., Freund, H.J. and Witte, O.W. (1998). Increased long-term potentiation in the surround of experimentally induced focal cortical infarction. *Ann Neurol*, **44**, 255–258.

Harker, K.T. and Whishaw, I.Q. (2004). Impaired place navigation in place and matching-to-place swimming pool tasks follows both retrosplenial cortex lesions and cingulum bundle lesions in rats. *Hippocampus*, **14**, 224–231.

Hebb, D.O. (1949). *Organization of Behavior*, John Wiley & Sons, New York.

Hernandez, T.D. and Schallert, T. (1988). Seizures and recovery from experimental brain damage. *Exp Neurol*, **102**, 318–324.

Hess, G., Aizenman, C.D. and Donoghue, J.P. (1996). Conditions for the induction of long-term potentiation in layer II/III horizontal connections of the rat motor cortex. *J Neurophysiol*, **75**, 1765–1778.

Hudgins, W.R. and Garcia, J.H. (1970). Transorbital approach to the middle cerebral artery of the squirrel monkey: a technique for experimental cerebral infarction applicable to ultrastructural studies. *Stroke*, **1**, 107–111.

Humm, J.L., Kozlowski, D.A., James, D.C., Gotts, J.E. and Schallert, T. (1998). Use-dependent exacerbation of brain damage occurs during an early post-lesion vulnerable period. *Brain Res*, **783**, 286–292.

Jacobs, K.M. and Donoghue, J.P. (1991). Reshaping the cortical motor map by unmasking latent intracortical connections. *Science*, **251**, 944–947.

Jain, N., Florence, S.L., Qi, H.X. and Kaas, J.H. (2000). Growth of new brainstem connections in adult monkeys with massive sensory loss. *Proc Natl Acad Sci USA*, **97**, 5546–5550.

Jenkins, W.M. and Merzenich, M.M. (1987). Reorganization of neocortical representations after brain injury: a neurophysiological model of the bases of recovery from stroke. *Prog Brain Res*, **71**, 249–266.

Jenkins, W.M., Merzenich, M.M., Ochs, M.T., Allard, T. and Guic-Robles, E. (1990). Functional reorganization of primary somatosensory cortex in adult owl monkeys after behaviorally controlled tactile stimulation. *J Neurophysiol*, **63**, 82–104.

Johansson, B.B. (1996). Functional outcome in rats transferred to an enriched environment 15 days after focal brain ischemia. *Stroke*, **27**, 324–326.

Jones, E. and Pons, T. (1998). Thalamic and brainstem contributions to large-scale plasticity of primate somatosensory cortex. *Science*, **282**, 1121–1125.

Jones, T.A. (1999). Multiple synapse formation in the motor cortex opposite unilateral sensorimotor cortex lesions in adult rats. *J Comp Neurol*, **414**, 57–66.

Jones, T.A. and Schallert, T. (1992). Overgrowth and pruning of dendrites in adult rats recovering from neocortical damage. *Brain Res*, **581**, 156–160.

Jones, T.A. and Schallert, T. (1994). Use-dependent growth of pyramidal neurons after neocortical damage. *J Neurosci*, **14**, 2140–2152.

Jones, T.A., Kleim, J.A. and Greenough, W.T. (1996). Synaptogenesis and dendritic growth in the cortex opposite unilateral sensorimotor cortex damage in adult rats: a quantitative electron microscopic examination. *Brain Res*, **733**, 142–148.

Jones, T.A., Klintsova, A.Y., Kilman, V.L., Sirevaag, A.M. and Greenough, W.T. (1997). Induction of multiple synapses by experience in the visual cortex of adult rats. *Neurobiol Learn Mem*, **68**, 13–20.

Jones, T.A., Chu, C.J., Grande, L.A. and Gregory, A.D. (1999). Motor skills training enhances lesion-induced structural plasticity in the motor cortex of adult rats. *J Neurosci*, **19**, 10153–10163.

Kaas, J.H. (2000). The reorganization of somatosensory and motor cortex after peripheral nerve or spinal cord injury in primates. *Prog Brain Res*, **128**, 173–179.

Kaas, J.H., Krubitzer, L.A., Chino, Y.M., Langston, A.L., Polley, E.H. and Blair, N. (1990). Reorganization of retinotopic cortical maps in adult mammals after lesions of the retina. *Science*, **248**, 229–231.

Karni, A., Meyer, G., Rey-Hipolito, C., Jezzard, P., Adams, M., Turner, R. and Ungerleider, L. (1998). The acquisition of skilled motor performance: fast and slow experience-driven changes in primary motor cortex. *Proc Natl Acad Sci USA*, **95**, 861–868.

Kleim, J.A., Barbay, S. and Nudo, R.J. (1998). Functional reorganization of the rat motor cortex following motor skill learning. *J Neurophysiol*, **80**, 3321–3325.

Kolb, B. (1995). *Brain Plasticity and Behavior*, Lawrence Erlbaum Associates, Mahwah, NJ.

Kozlowski, D.A. and Schallert, T. (1998). Relationship between dendritic pruning and behavioral recovery following sensorimotor cortex lesions. *Behav Brain Res*, **97**, 89–98.

Kozlowski, D.A., Jones, T.A. and Schallert, T. (1994). Pruning of dendrites and restoration of function after brain damage: role of the NMDA receptor. *Restor Neurol Neurosci*, **7**, 119–126.

Kozlowski, D.A., James, D.C. and Schallert, T. (1996). Use-dependent exaggeration of neuronal injury after unilateral sensorimotor cortex lesions. *J Neurosci*, **16**, 4776–4786.

Kozlowski, D.A., Hilliard, S. and Schallert, T. (1997). Ethanol consumption following recovery from unilateral damage to the forelimb area of the sensorimotor cortex: reinstatement of deficits and prevention of dendritic pruning. *Brain Res*, **763**, 159–166.

Krupinski, J., Kaluza, J., Kumar, P., Kumar, S. and Wang, J.M. (1994). Role of angiogenesis in patients with cerebral ischemic stroke. *Stroke*, **25**, 1794–1798.

Kubota, K. (1996). Motor cortical muscimol injection disrupts forelimb movement in freely moving monkeys. *NeuroReport*, **7**, 2379–2384.

Lawrence, D.G. and Kuypers, H.G.J.M. (1968). The functional organization of the motor system in the monkey. I. The effects of bilateral pyramidal lesions. *Brain*, **91**, 1–14.

Liepert, J., Miltner, W.H., Bauder, H., Sommer, M., Dettmers, C., Taub, E. and Weiller, C. (1998). Motor cortex plasticity during constraint-induced movement therapy in stroke patients. *Neurosci Lett*, **250**, 5–8.

Liepert, J., Bauder, H., Wolfgang, H.R., Miltner, W.H., Taub, E. and Weiller, C. (2000). Treatment-induced cortical reorganization after stroke in humans. *Stroke*, **31**, 1210–1216.

Mack, W.J., King, R.G., Hoh, D.J., Coon, A.L., Ducruet, A.F., Huang, J., Mocco, J., Winfree, C.J., D'Ambrosio, A.L., Nair, M.N., Sciacca, R.R. and Connolly Jr. E.S. (2003). An improved functional neurological examination for use in nonhuman primate studies of focal reperfused cerebral ischemia. *Neurol Res*, **25**, 280–284.

Marshall, J.W. and Ridley, R.M. (2003). Assessment of cognitive and motor deficits in a marmoset model of stroke. *Ilar J*, **44**, 153–160.

Marti, H.J., Bernaudin, M., Bellail, A., Schoch, H., Euler, M., Petit, E. and Risau, W. (2000). Hypoxia-induced vascular endothelial growth factor expression precedes neovascularization after cerebral ischemia. *Am J Pathol*, **156**, 965–976.

McIntosh, T.K., Vink, R., Noble, L., Yamakami, I., Fernyak, S., Soares, H. and Faden, A.L. (1989). Traumatic brain injury in the rat: characterization of a lateral fluid-percussion model. *Neuroscience*, **28**, 233–244.

Merzenich, M.M., Kaas, J.H., Wall, J., Nelson, R.J., Sur, M. and Felleman, D. (1983). Topographic reorganization of somatosensory cortical areas 3b and 1 in adult monkeys following restricted deafferentation. *Neuroscience*, **8**, 33–55.

Mittmann, T., Qu, M., Zilles, K. and Luhmann, H.J. (1998). Long-term cellular dysfunction after focal cerebral ischemia: *in vitro* analyses. *Neuroscience*, **85**, 15–27.

Nah, S.H., Ong, L.S. and Leong, S.K. (1980). Is sprouting the result of a persistent neonatal connection? *Neurosci Lett*, **19**, 39–44.

Napieralski, J.A., Butler, A.K. and Chesselet, M.F. (1996). Anatomical and functional evidence for lesion-specific sprouting of corticostriatal input in the adult rat. *J Comp Neurol*, **373**, 484–497.

Napieralski, J.A., Banks, R.J. and Chesselet, M.F. (1998). Motor and somatosensory deficits following uni- and bilateral lesions of the cortex induced by aspiration or thermocoagulation in the adult rat. *Exp Neurol*, **154**, 80–88.

Neuhoff, H., Roeper, J. and Schweizer, M. (1999). Activity-dependent formation of perforated synapses in cultured hippocampal neurons. *Eur J Neurosci*, **11**, 4241–4250.

Neumann-Haefelin, T., Staiger, J.F., Redecker, C., Zilles, K., Fritschy, J.M., Mohler, H. and Witte, O.W. (1998). Immuno-histochemical evidence for dysregulation of the GABAergic system ipsilateral to photochemically induced cortical infarcts in rats. *Neuroscience*, **87**, 871–879.

Nudo, R.J. and Masterton, R.B. (1990). Descending pathways to the spinal cord, III: sites of origin of the corticospinal tract. *J Comp Neurol*, **296**, 559–583.

Nudo, R.J. and Milliken, G.W. (1996). Reorganization of movement representations in primary motor cortex following focal ischemic infarcts in adult squirrel monkeys. *J Neurophysiol*, **75**, 2144–2149.

Nudo, R.J., Jenkins, W.M., Merzenich, M.M., Prejean, T. and Gedela, R. (1992). Neurophysiological correlates of hand preference in primary motor cortex of adult squirrel monkeys. *J Neurosci*, **12**, 2918–2947.

Nudo, R.J., Milliken, G.W., Jenkins, W.M. and Merzenich, M.M. (1996a). Use-dependent alterations of movement representations in primary motor cortex of adult squirrel monkeys. *J Neurosci*, **16**, 785–807.

Nudo, R.J., Wise, B.M., SiFuentes, F. and Milliken, G.W. (1996b). Neural substrates for the effects of rehabilitative training on motor recovery after ischemic infarct. *Science*, **272**, 1791–1794.

Nudo, R.J., Plautz, E.J. and Milliken, G.W. (1997). Adaptive plasticity of motor cortex as a consequence of behavioral experience and neuronal injury. *Semin Neurosci*, **9**, 13–23.

Nudo, R.J., Larson, D., Plautz, E.J., Friel, K.M., Barbay, S. and Frost, S.B. (2003). A squirrel monkey model of poststroke motor recovery. *Ilar J*, **44**, 161–174.

Ogden, R. and Franz, S.I. (1917). On cerebral motor control: the recovery from experimentally produced hemoplegia. *Psychobiology*, **1**, 33–50.

Pascual-Leone, A., Nguyet, D., Cohen, L.G., Brasil-Neto, J.P., Cammarota, A. and Hallett, M. (1995). Modulation of muscle responses evoked by transcranial magnetic stimulation during the acquisition of new fine motor skills. *J Neurophysiol*, **74**, 1037–1045.

Prusky, G. and Whishaw, I.Q. (1996). Morphology of identified corticospinal cells in the rat following motor cortex injury: absence of use-dependent change. *Brain Res*, **714**, 1–8.

Qu, M., Buchkremer-Ratzmann, I., Schiene, K., Schroeter, M., Witte, O.W. and Zilles, K. (1998a). Bihemispheric reduction of GABAA receptor binding following focal cortical photothrombotic lesions in the rat brain. *Brain Res*, **813**, 374–380.

Qu, M., Mittmann, T., Luhmann, H.J., Schleicher, A. and Zilles, K. (1998b). Long-term changes of ionotropic glutamate and GABA receptors after unilateral permanent focal cerebral ischemia in the mouse brain. *Neuroscience*, **85**, 29–43.

Recanzone, G.H., Schreiner, G.E. and Merzenich, M.M. (1993). Plasticity in the frequency representation of primary auditory cortex following discrimination training in adult owl monkeys. *J Neurophysiol*, **13**, 87–103.

Redecker, C., Fritschy, J.M. and Witte, O.W. (2000). Differential downregulation of GABA(A) receptor subunits after focal cortical infarcts in rats: Regional pattern and time-course. *Soc Neurosci Abstr*, **26**, 2068.

Rioult-Pedotti, M.S., Friedman, D., Hess, G. and Donoghue, J.P. (1998). Strengthening of horizontal cortical connections following skill learning. *Nat Neurosci*, **1**, 230–234.

Roitberg, B., Khan, N., Tuccar, E., Kompoliti, K., Chu, Y., Alperin, N., Kordower, J.H. and Emborg, M.E. (2003). Chronic ischemic stroke model in cynomolgus monkeys: behavioral, neuroimaging and anatomical study. *Neurol Res*, **25**, 68–78.

Rouiller, E.M., Liang, F.Y., Moret, V. and Wiesendanger, M. (1991). Trajectory of redirected corticospinal axons after unilateral lesion of the sensorimotor cortex in neonatal rat; a phaseolus vulgaris-leucoagglutinin (PHA-L) tracing study. *Exp Neurol*, **114**, 53–65.

Sakata, J.T. and Jones, T.A. (2003). Synaptic mitochondrial changes in the motor cortex following unilateral cortical lesions and motor skills training in adult male rats. *Neurosci Lett*, **337**, 159–162.

Schallert, T. and Kozlowski, D.A. (1998). Brain damage and plasticity: use-related enhanced neural growth and overuse-related exaggeration of injury. In: *Cerebrovascular Disease: Pathophysiology, Diagnosis and Management* (eds Ginsberg, M.D. and Bogousslavsky, J.), Blackwell Science, New York, pp. 611–619.

Schallert, T., Hernandez, T.D. and Barth, T.M. (1986). Recovery of function after brain damage: severe and chronic disruption by diazepam. *Brain Res*, **379**, 104–111.

Schallert, T., Fleming, S.M., Leasure, J.L., Tillerson, J.L. and Bland, S.T. (2000). CNS plasticity and assessment of forelimb sensorimotor outcome in unilateral rat models of stroke, cortical ablation, parkinsonism and spinal cord injury. *Neuropharmacology*, **39**, 777–787.

Schieber, M.H. and Poliakov, A.V. (1998). Partial inactivation of the primary motor cortex hand area: effects on individuated finger movements. *J Neurosci*, **18**, 9038–9054.

Schiene, K., Bruehl, C., Zilles, K., Qu, M., Hagemann, G., Kraemer, M. and Witte, O.W. (1996). Neuronal hyperexcitability and reduction of GABAA-receptor expression in the surround of cerebral photothrombosis. *J Cereb Blood Flow Metab*, **16**, 906–914.

Seitz, R.J., Huang, Y., Knorr, U., Tellmann, L., Herzog, H. and Freund, H.J. (1995). Large-scale plasticity of the human motor cortex. *NeuroReport*, **6**, 742–744.

Stroemer, R.P., Kent, T.A. and Hulsebosch, C.E. (1992). Increase in synaptophysin immunoreactivity following cortical infarction. *Neurosci Lett*, **147**, 21–24.

Stroemer, R.P., Kent, T.A. and Hulsebosch, C.E. (1993). Acute increase in expression of growth associated protein GAP-43 following cortical ischemia in rat. *Neurosci Lett*, **162**, 51–54.

Stroemer, R.P., Kent, T.A. and Hulsebosch, C.E. (1995). Neocortical neural sprouting, synaptogenesis, and behavioral recovery after neocortical infarction in rats. *Stroke*, **26**, 2135–2144.

Symon, L., Dorsch, N.W. and Crockard, H.A. (1975). The production and clinical features of a chronic stroke model in experimental primates. *Stroke*, **6**, 476–481.

Szele, F.G., Alexander, C. and Chesselet, M.F. (1995). Expression of molecules associated with neuronal plasticity in the striatum after aspiration and thermocoagulatory lesions of the cerebral cortex in adult rats. *J Neurosci*, **15**, 4429–4448.

Taub, E., Miller, N.E., Novack, T.A., Cook, E.W.I., Fleming, W.C., Nepomuceno, C.S., Connell, J.S. and Crago, J.E. (1993). Technique to improve chronic motor deficit after stroke. *Arch Phys Med Rehabil*, **74**, 347–354.

Taub, E., Uswatte, G. and Elbert, T. (2002). New treatments in neurorehabilitation founded on basic research. *Nat Rev Neurosci*, **3**, 228–236.

Traystman, R.J. (2003). Animal models of focal and global cerebral ischemia. *Ilar J*, **44**, 85–95.

Virley, D., Hadingham, S.J., Roberts, J.C., Farnfield, B., Elliott, H., Whelan, G., Golder, J., David, C., Parsons, A.A. and Hunter, A.J. (2004). A new primate model of focal stroke: endothelin-1-induced middle cerebral artery occlusion and reperfusion in the common marmoset. *J Cereb Blood Flow Metab*, **24**, 24–41.

Voorhies, A.C. and Jones, T.A. (2000). Behavioral and structural effects of aspiration of tissue damaged by cortical injury. *Soc Neurosci Abstr*, **26**, 2294.

Voorhies, A.C. and Jones, T.A. (2002). The behavioral and dendritic growth effects of focal sensorimotor cortical damage depend on the method of lesion induction. *Behav Brain Res*, **133**, 237–246.

Weeks, A.C., Ivanco, T.L., Leboutillier, J.C., Racine, R.J. and Petit, T.L. (2000). Sequential changes in the synaptic structural profile following long-term potentiation in the rat dentate gyrus. II. Induction/early maintenance phase. *Synapse*, **36**, 286–296.

Wei, L., Erinjeri, J.P., Rovainen, C.M. and Woolsey, T.A. (2001). Collateral growth and angiogenesis around cortical stroke. *Stroke*, **32**, 2179–2184.

Whishaw, I.Q. and Coles, B.L.K. (1996). Varieties of paw and digit movement during spontaneous food handling in rats: postures, bimanual coordination, preferences, and the effect of forelimb cortex lesions. *Behav Brain Res*, **77**, 135–148.

Whishaw, I.Q., Pellis, S.M., Gorny, B.P. and Pellis, V.C. (1991). The impairments in reaching and the movements of compensation in rats with motor cortex lesions: an endpoint, videorecording, and movement notation analysis. *Behav Brain Res*, **42**, 77–91.

Willing, A.E., Jiang, L., Nowicki, P., Poulos, S., Milliken, M., Cahill, D.W. and Sanberg, P.R. (2002). Effects of middle cerebral artery occlusion on spontaneous activity and cognitive function in rats. *Int J Neurosci*, **112**, 503–516.

Witte, O.W. and Stoll, G. (1997). Delayed and remote effects of focal cortical infarctions: secondary damage and reactive plasticity. In: *Brain Plasticity, Advances in Neurology* (eds Freund, H.J., Sabel, B.A. and Witte, O.W.), Vol. 73, Lippincott-Raven Publishers, Philadelphia, New York, pp. 179–193.

Xerri, C., Merzenich, M.M., Peterson, B.E. and Jenkins, W. (1998). Plasticity of primary somatosensory cortex paralleling sensorimotor skill recovery from stroke in adult monkeys. *J Neurophysiol*, **79**, 2119–2148.

Xerri, C., Merzenich, M.M., Jenkins, W. and Santucci, S. (1999). Representational plasticity in cortical area 3b paralleling tactual-motor skill acquisition in adult monkeys. *Cereb Cortex*, **9**, 264–276.

From bench to bedside: influence of theories of plasticity on human neurorehabilitation

Agnes Floel and Leonardo G. Cohen

Human Coritical Physiology Section, National Institute of Neurological Disorders and Stroke,
National Institutes of Health, Bethesda, MD, USA

15.1 Introduction

In the last decade, our knowledge about the mechanisms of neurologic injury and recovery has improved. There is now considerable evidence that cortical representations are continuously modulated in response to practice and skill acquisition, a process often referred to as plasticity (Kaas, 1991; Donoghue et al., 1996). Plasticity can also be elicited by lesions in the central and peripheral nervous systems and may take place in cortical as well as subcortical structures (Kaas, 1991; Donoghue et al., 1996; Nudo and Milliken, 1996; Buonomano and Merzenich, 1998; Cohen et al., 1998; Jones and Pons, 1998; see Volume I, Chapters 6, 8 and 14). Cortical plasticity may thus be defined as any enduring change in cortical properties, as, for example, in the strength of internal connections, representation patterns, or neuronal properties, either morphologic or functional (Donoghue et al., 1996). Cortical reorganization can, depending on the settings, contribute to desirable behavioral developments, such as improved performance, or can be linked with unwanted outcomes like phantom pain (Flor et al., 1995; see Volume II, Chapter 15). The primary vehicle for acquiring knowledge on plasticity in the human central nervous system (CNS) has been animal research. Beginning in the 1970s, research from different laboratories (Merzenich et al., 1984; Kaas, 1991) showed that the adult mammalian CNS has the capacity to reorganize after injury. Understanding of mechanisms, development of strategies to purposefully modulate these mechanisms, and translation into rational

strategies to promote recovery of function are the goals of modern neurorehabilitation.

Cortical reorganization may occur rapidly or evolve slowly. One mechanism by which modification of sensory input induces fast changes in cortical representations is called unmasking (Calford and Tweedale, 1991a,b). In animals, blocking inhibition pharmacologically within a small region of the primary motor cortex (M1) immediately unveils new representation patterns (Jacobs and Donoghue, 1991), possibly through unmasking horizontal excitatory connections previously hidden by inhibitory neurons. The strength of these connections, and the balance of excitation and inhibition may shape cortical representations. Corticospinal connections extensively link with other pyramidal tract neurons and with inhibitory interneurons (Landry et al., 1990; McGuire et al., 1991). It is now known that long-term potentiation (LTP), one mechanism of neuroplasticity (see Volume I, Chapter 4), can be induced in these horizontal connections of the adult M1, contributing to lasting associations among neurons within motor cortical areas (Hess and Donoghue, 1994; see Volume I, Chapter 8). Vertical pathways in M1 can express short-term depression, short-term facilitation, long-term depression (LTD), and also LTP (Castro-Alamancos et al., 1995; see Volume I, Chapters 3 and 4). In addition to these relatively rapid processes, slower, progressive plastic changes can be driven by learning (Robertson and Laferriere, 1989; see Volume I, Chapter 2), competition with other inputs (Kaas et al., 1983), and use (Nudo and Milliken, 1996). These mechanisms may underlie practice-dependent improvements in motor learning (Rioult-Pedotti et al., 2000), memory, and activity-dependent plasticity in human health and disease. Furthermore, these mechanisms are likely to operate in multiple areas of human cognition such as learning and memory, and in functional recovery from lesions in the CNS, as in stroke (Buonomano and Merzenich, 1998).

These findings may directly influence how human disease is treated. However, relatively few efforts have been invested in research that translates these advances in the basic science domain to the formulation of new, rational strategies for promoting recovery of function in humans. To accomplish this goal, it would be important to demonstrate that principles similar to those described in animal models apply to the human cerebral cortex in relevant behavioral settings (e.g., peripheral deafferentation, learning, or during stroke recovery).

These needs started in the last few years a process characterized by a tighter connection between basic scientists working in animal models of plasticity and clinicians interested in applying principles of plasticity to the treatment of human disease. The purpose of this chapter is to outline how some of these basic principles moved from the realm of experimentation into clinical settings.

15.2 Influence of training and practice in neurorehabilitation ("practice makes perfect")

Training results in well-documented performance improvements in both animals (Skinner, 1968; Taub et al., 1994; Irvine and Rajan, 1996) and humans (Nissen and Bullemer, 1987; Shadmehr and Holcomb, 1997; Muellbacher et al., 2001; Macaluso and De Vito, 2003). Additionally, training leads to specific changes in brain organization in the motor (Karni et al., 1995; Nudo et al., 1996; Classen et al., 1998), somatosensory (Merzenich et al., 1984; Pons and Kaas, 1986), auditory (Robertson and Laferriere, 1989), and visual (Kaas et al., 1990) domains.

In the motor domain, for example, the size of the primate hand cortical representation correlates with

handedness, probably reflecting the influence of daily use on brain organization (Nudo et al., 1992). Learning to retrieve food pellets from a small well results in reorganization of movement representations in the contralateral motor cortex over the course of hours or days (Nudo et al., 1992). Similar processes appear to operate after brain lesions, since motor training after focal cortical infarcts results in recovery of motor function associated with cortical reorganization in animals (Nudo et al., 1996) and humans (Calautti and Baron, 2003). Brain imaging (functional magnetic resonance imaging (fMRI) and positron emission tomography (PET)), as well as electrophysiologic studies using transcranial magnetic stimulation (TMS) have demonstrated reorganization in primary sensorimotor cortices (Chollet et al., 1991; Calautti et al., 2001) as well as non-primary motor areas in both hemispheres (Chollet et al., 1991; Johansen-Berg et al., 2002; Fridman et al., 2004). After a brain lesion, additional or increased activation in these areas during a specific task may contribute to functional recovery through direct corticomotoneuronal connections and/or corticocortical interactions. Non-pyramidal, cortical efferents could also contribute to the recovery process (Rossini et al., 2003).

Several functional imaging studies in patients with stroke have demonstrated increased activation of motor areas in the intact hemisphere during movement of the affected limb (Chollet et al., 1991; Cramer et al., 1997; Marshall et al., 2000; Carey et al., 2002). One interpretation put forward was that this activity could contribute to functional recovery (Johansen-Berg et al., 2002; Frost et al., 2003). The intact MI may contribute to recovery of function in the paretic hand via interhemispheric, corticoreticular, or direct corticospinal connections. An alternative view proposed that functional recovery relies predominantly on reorganized activity within the injured hemisphere (Traversa et al., 1997; Weiller and Rijntjes, 1999; Frost et al., 2003; Ward et al., 2003; Werhahn et al., 2003; Ward and Cohen, 2004).

Overall, these findings supported the view that motor training could improve performance in patients with stroke, as it does in intact humans, a principle long held in empirical neurorehabilitation for the last century (Shepherd, 2001). Interestingly, only relatively recent studies started to test this formulation in controlled clinical trials. It was demonstrated that a 2-week intervention based on massed training of the affected arm in patients with chronic stroke resulted in improvements in the amount of use that outlasted the intervention period to a larger extent than a control intervention (Taub et al., 1994; Kunkel et al., 1999; Dromerick et al., 2000; Sterr et al., 2002). A randomized National Institute of Neurological Disorders and Stroke (NINDS, USA) sponsored multicenter clinical trial is presently under way to test this hypothesis. Other examples of the role of training in neurorehabilitation include the demonstrations that locomotor functions can improve when patients undergo treadmill-training procedures (Colombo et al., 2001; Hobson and Pace-Schott, 2002; Sullivan et al., 2004). The theoretical background of locomotor therapy is based on experiments in spinalized cats and incompletely lesioned primates, showing an activation of presumed spinal and supraspinal pattern generators by forced locomotor therapy (Lovely et al., 1986). In the language domain, patients with chronic stroke-induced aphasia can also improve after a period of practice (Pulvermuller et al., 2001). In a controlled clinical study, patients underwent a 2-week period of intensive training (extended intensive practice, constraining patients to communicate using speech and shaping speech) that resulted in improved performance on experimental tests of language ability and in the amount of talking done in real life relative to customary care (Pulvermuller et al., 2001).

A different form of motor training has been proposed to improve the disabling consequences of focal dystonia (Candia et al., 2002; Taub et al., 2002), a condition that may be influenced by overuse (Byl et al., 1997; Bara-Jimenez et al., 1998). Dystonia is characterized by involuntary, sustained muscle contractions of agonist and antagonist muscles, causing twisting movements and abnormal postures (Hallett, 1998). Writer's cramp is a focal-action dystonia characterized by dystonic symptoms superimposed on voluntary movement (Cohen and Hallett, 1988). It is usually task-specific, occurring only with writing, typing, playing certain musical instruments (guitar,

piano), engaging in specific sports (golf, darts, or sports that involve throwing), or performing activities that involve repetitive hand movements (Chen and Hallett, 1998).

In a group of musicians with focal hand dystonia, immobilization of the non-dystonic fingers of the hand was used in association with practice of performance of finger motor sequences using the dystonic fingers (Candia et al., 2002). In this study, the guitar and piano players (eight subjects) experienced a significant reduction of dystonic symptoms. Although more information is required to draw firm conclusions, these studies represent examples of strategies that use principles of plasticity to plan interventions geared to improve dystonia.

Training procedures have also been applied to ameliorate the ability of children with specific language impairments to integrate brief and rapidly changing sounds (Tallal et al., 1993; 1996).

In summary, basic science and clinical studies over the last four decades documented the beneficial effects of motor training on performance in the intact and lesioned CNS and its ability to elicit fundamental changes in cortical organization. One challenge has been to develop effective strategies to enhance the beneficial effects of training.

15.3 Mechanisms of human neuroplasticity

Recent work began shedding light on some of the mechanisms underlying the development of human neuroplasticity. Basic science studies demonstrated that neuronal plasticity can be expressed as activity-dependent modifications in the efficacy of existing synapses, including LTP and LTD (Bliss and Gardner, 1973), and generalized changes in post-synaptic excitability (Woody et al., 1991). LTP may contribute to skill acquisition, learning and memory, as well as functional recovery after brain lesions (Lamprecht and LeDoux, 2004). On the molecular level, N-methyl-D-aspartate (NMDA) receptors (Dubnau and Tully, 1998) and GABAergic interneurons (Marty et al., 1997) may play a crucial role in changes of synaptic long-term efficacy such as LTP and LTD.

Acute and chronic alterations in neurotransmitter regulation after injury affect plasticity, and may thus provide a basis for new pharmacologic targets for stroke recovery (Martinsson et al., 2003). Drugs that promote LTP, neural sprouting, and synaptogenesis include enhancers of noradrenergic neurotransmission (Gold et al., 1984) and dopaminergic agents (Jay, 2003). These drugs have also shown beneficial effects for learning and recovery after brain damage (Feeney, 1997). Consistent with this information, drugs that antagonize LTP-like mechanisms lead to delays in rehabilitation (Goldstein, 1998).

The mechanisms of neuroplasticity identified in previous animal studies appear to operate in the human CNS as well. Use-dependent plasticity in intact humans is downregulated by GABAergic agonists such as lorazepam, and NMDA receptor antagonists such as dextrometorphan (Butefisch et al., 2000), consistent with the effect of these drugs on LTP (Hess et al., 1994). Taken together, these results strongly suggest that LTP-like mechanisms operate in the development of use-dependent plasticity in intact humans and can be influenced by drugs acting on central neurotransmitter systems (Butefisch et al., 2000; 2002; Sawaki et al., 2002a). Drugs enhancing noradrenergic transmission may have beneficial effects in rehabilitative settings where re-learning after brain damage is required (Goldstein, 1998; Martinsson et al., 2003), whereas drugs with antinoradrenergic (e.g., some anti-hypertensive medications) or anti-dopaminergic (e.g., anti-psychotic medication like haloperidol) properties should be used with caution (Goldstein, 1998).

15.4 Pharmacologic interventions in stroke rehabilitation

Pharmacologic interventions can influence functional recovery in different ways. Clinical trials of pharmacologic agents have mainly focused on events that need to be modified in the very acute stage, such as restoration of blood flow with thrombolytic therapy or reducing the effects of ischemia with neuroprotective therapy. However, thrombolytic therapy is only effective within the first few hours following the ictal event and so far, no neuroprotective therapy has proven to be definitely efficacious in humans. Thus, there is a great need for new pharmacologic strategies to improve outcome after stroke.

One approach stems from studies in the 1940s suggesting that amphetamines might enhance recovery of motor function following brain injury (Macht, 1950). Several decades later, Feeney and co-workers demonstrated that a single dose of D-amphetamine preceding motor training and administered 24 h following unilateral sensorimotor cortex ablation in the rat results in faster recovery than in a control group (Feeney et al., 1982). The mechanisms underlying this effect are likely to involve alpha adrenergic receptor function since the amphetamine-dependent effect has been mimicked by infusions of noradrenaline in the brain 24 h following injury (Boyeson and Feeney, 1990). Several animal studies have now demonstrated a beneficial effect on recovery for increased concentration of norepinephrine at the synapse (Stroemer et al., 1998). Pairing drug administration with appropriate rehabilitative treatment showed the most prominent effect.

Experimental studies in healthy humans demonstrated that pre-medication with D-amphetamine enhanced the effects of motor training on use-dependent plasticity (Butefisch et al., 2002). Motor training resulted in increased magnitude, faster development, and longer lasting duration of use-dependent plasticity relative to placebo, a possible mechanism mediating the beneficial effect of this drug on functional recovery after cortical lesions. A follow-up study demonstrated that D-amphetamine combined with motor training could elicit use-dependent plasticity in individuals poorly responsive to training alone (Sawaki et al., 2002b). Administration of a single dose of 10 mg of D-amphetamine preceding training led to use-dependent plasticity in a subgroup of these subjects.

In patients with stroke, Crisostomo et al. (1988) reported eight patients with stable motor deficits randomized within 10 days of an ischemic stroke to a placebo or D-amphetamine group. Within 3 h of drug/placebo administration patients underwent intensive physical therapy. The following day, the patients' abilities to use their affected limbs were reassessed. Overall, the amphetamine-treated group had a significant improvement in motor performance whereas there was little change in the placebo-treated group. From a clinical standpoint, the study involved only a small group of highly selected patients and only two of the four receiving D-amphetamine experienced substantial motor improvement. Walker-Batson et al. (1995) later performed a double-blind, placebo-controlled trial. This study included five patients in the D-amphetamine group and another five in the placebo group. A single oral dose of 10 mg D-amphetamine was administered every 4 days for 10 sessions beginning from 15 to 30 days after stroke. Each dose was given in conjunction with a session of intensive physical therapy. One week after the end of the intervention, patients in the D-amphetamine group experienced more significant motor recovery than those in the placebo group. The difference was maintained a year later. The authors raised the hypothesis of the existence of a window of opportunity for D-amphetamine intervention, thought to operate in the initial few weeks following the stroke (Walker-Batson, 2000).

Beneficial effects of amphetamines have also been reported in speech and language function therapy after stroke. Aphasic patients between 16 and 40 days after stroke received single oral doses of 10 mg D-amphetamine or placebo 30 min before language therapy. Patients in the treated group experienced better recovery than those in the placebo group, a benefit that was maintained a year later independent of the amount of tissue loss (Walker-Batson, 2000). An interesting concept raised during these investigations was that, since D-amphetamine intake results in substantial release of neurotransmitters, daily administration could deplete CNS storage and result in paradoxical effects. For this reason, most protocols utilize single oral doses of this drug every 4 days, a period considered appropriate to allow restoration of neurotransmitter pools.

Although the few clinical studies conducted so far have not reported clinically important adverse events (Crisostomo et al., 1988; Walker-Batson et al.,

1995) potentially dangerous cardiovascular side-effects by systemic administration of amphetamine remain a potential risk, especially in the mostly elderly and often multimorbid stroke population. Furthermore, physical and psychologic dependence cannot be excluded which restricts the use of these drugs (Weiner, 1980). Overall, tentative conclusions raised by these studies included: (a) the identified documented therapeutic window for these effects is up to 30 days after stroke (it remains to be determined if D-amphetamine can influence recovery if applied closer to the ictal event or in the chronic stage), (b) multiple sessions of drug and physical therapy administration appear to provide greater therapeutic benefit than single sessions, and (c) beneficial effects in the treated versus the placebo group lasted for at least 12 months, suggesting that, once the maximal recovery is accomplished, prolonged drug administration may be unnecessary. At this point, this approach does not represent "customary treatment" partly because trials so far have been inconclusive and partly because many patients shortly after stroke cannot receive this type of drug. A multicenter NINDS-funded study is under way to clarify some of these aspects.

Another potentially useful drug in neurorehabilitation, which affects the central dopaminergic neurotransmitter system, has recently emerged: levodopa. It is well known that endogenous dopamine modulates corticostriatal activity by enhancing transmission at active synapses while suppressing it at inactive ones (Wickens et al., 1995). The effect of dopamine release in the vicinity of highly active corticostriatal terminations could be to increase the signal-to-noise ratio by strengthening that synapse while suppressing neighboring ones. Furthermore, dopamine modulates working memory and LTP, a putative cellular mechanism underlying long-term memory consolidation (Schultz, 2000; Centonze et al., 2001). Dopamine appears to be a key regulator in specific synaptic changes observed at certain stages of learning and memory processes (Jay, 2003). Interestingly, dopamine agonists can reduce the severity of experimentally induced neglect (Corwin et al., 1986) while dopamine receptor antagonists reinstate

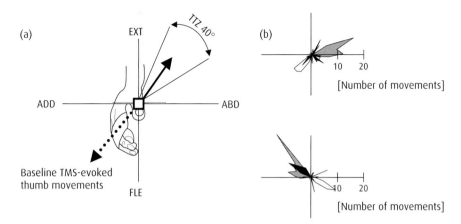

Figure 15.1. Use-dependent plasticity after training + placebo and training + levodopa. (a) Diagram showing measurement of thumb movements with an accelerometer positioned on the distal interphalangeal joint (rectangle on the thumb). Baseline TMS-evoked thumb movements in this example fell in a flexion–adduction direction (dotted arrow). Training voluntary thumb motions were performed in the opposite direction (extension–abduction, solid arrow). At the end of the training period, we measured the percentage of TMS-evoked thumb movements falling in the training target zone (TTZ), the endpoint measure of the study (modified from Floel et al. (in press a)). (b) TMS-evoked movement directions displayed as circular histograms in a representative elderly subject in the placebo (upper histogram) and levodopa (lower histogram) sessions. TMS-evoked movement directions at baseline are displayed in white, voluntary training movements in gray, and TMS-evoked movement directions after training in black. Only levodopa + training (lower) but not placebo + training (upper) induced a substantial increase of movements falling in the TTZ. Please note that baseline direction of TMS-evoked thumb movements was not always in flexion/adduction.

neglect in recovered animals (Vargo et al., 1989). Furthermore, Grondin and colleagues (Grondin et al., 2000) found that dopaminergic therapy can improve upper limb motor function in aged non-human primates. Experimental studies in healthy humans, using a model of motor training that leads to use-dependent plasticity (Classen et al., 1998), showed that pre-medication with levodopa immediately preceding motor training enhances use-dependent plasticity in healthy elderly volunteers and chronic stroke patients (Floel et al., in press a) (see Fig. 15.1). Similarly, a recent study demonstrated that oral administration of the dopamine precursor levodopa improved language learning (speed, overall success and long-term retention of an artificial vocabulary) in healthy volunteers (Knecht et al., 2004; Scheidtmann et al., 2001). A prospective, randomized, placebo-controlled, double-blind study of levodopa after stroke showed that motor function was significantly better for patients on levodopa than those on placebo after 3 and 6 weeks. A randomized,

double-blind, multicenter study testing the effectiveness of ropinirole, a dopamine receptor agonist, in enhancing motor rehabilitation in chronic stroke patients, is currently under way (Cramer and Dobkin, 2004). Levodopa appears to exert a beneficial effect on the rehabilitation of hemineglect following stroke (Pahlke and Scheidtmann, 2003).

One of the advantages of using dopaminergic agents relative to D-amphetamine is that it exhibits less side-effects. In summary, dopaminergic agents show promise to enhance recovery after brain lesions due to stroke. Larger clinical trials are now needed to further clarify its effectiveness in the chronic stage after stroke.

15.5 Influence of somatosensory input on functional recovery

Somatosensory input is required for proper motor performance and for skill acquisition in both animals and humans (Bastian, 1887; Sakamoto et al., 1989; Pavlides et al., 1993; Pearson, 2000). Reduction of somatosensory input in non-human primates, for example by surgical abolition of sensation from a forelimb, results in clumsy movements, and disuse (Mott and Sherrington, 1895). In humans, reduction of somatic input by local anesthesia impairs motor control in the anesthesized body part (Edin and Johansson, 1995; Aschersleben et al., 2001). Consistent with this information, patients with large-fiber sensory neuropathy and substantially decreased proprioception display abnormal motor behavior (Rothwell et al., 1982; Gordon et al., 1995). In patients with stroke, somatosensory deficits are associated with slower recovery of motor function (Reding and Potes, 1988). Thus, it is possible that modulation of somatosensory input could influence motor behavior in stroke patients.

Somatosensory stimulation

Peripheral nerve stimulation leads to changes in the cortical representations of the stimulated body part (Recanzone et al., 1990; Kaas, 1991; 2000). In the motor cortex, peripheral nerve stimulation results in increased motor cortical excitability that outlast the stimulation period (Luft et al., 2002). Similar results have been reported in humans, in whom a period of peripheral nerve stimulation leads to a lasting increase in corticomotoneuronal excitability to the stimulated body parts (Hamdy et al., 1998b; Stefan et al., 2000; Ridding and Taylor, 2001; Kaelin-Lang et al., 2002) (see Fig. 15.2(a)). For example, Stefan et al. showed that peripheral nerve stimulation applied in synchrony with TMS to the contralateral motor cortex induced an increment in motor cortical excitability, as demonstrated by larger motor-evoked potential (MEP) amplitudes. This effect developed rapidly, persisted for approximately 30–60 min, and had topographic specificity (Stefan et al., 2000). Similarly, prolonged ulnar nerve stimulation led to enlarged MEPs of the first dorsal interosseus and abductor digiti minimi muscles, but not of the median nerve-innervated muscles (Ridding and Taylor, 2001; Kaelin-Lang et al., 2002). Different studies are presently under way to determine if

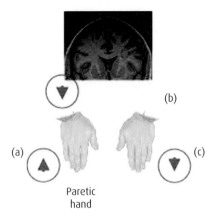

Figure 15.2. Interventional strategies in chronic stroke patients. Motor performance of the paretic hand can be influenced by different operational strategies, including increased somatosensory input from the paretic hand; (a); anesthesia of the upper arm proximal to the paretic hand, (b); reduction of somatosensory input from the intact hand, and (c) (Ward and Cohen, 2004).

longer periods of peripheral nerve stimulation applied on different days could elicit longer lasting changes in motor cortical function.

This approach was initially used in clinical settings with the expectation of eliciting beneficial effects on motor behavior in stroke patients (Johansson et al., 1993; Powell et al., 1999; Wong et al., 1999; Conforto et al., 2002; Dobkin and Havton, 2004). For example, Conforto et al. provided preliminary evidence that peripheral nerve stimulation leads to an improvement in functional measures of motor performance, such as pinch muscle strength. Eight chronic stroke patients were exposed in a randomized cross-over experiment to either median nerve electrical stimulation or placebo stimulation to determine changes in pinch strength. After 2 h of nerve stimulation, pinch strength increased in a manner proportional to the intensity of the stimulation. Two patients reported that they could write better and hold objects and play cards more accurately, a perception that lasted for approximately 24 h. This proposal is consistent with other studies (Struppler et al., 2003a, b). For swallowing functions after stroke, it was found that the return of swallowing after dysphagic stroke is associated with increased

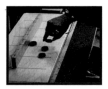

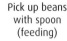

Pick up beans
with spoon
(feeding)

Stacking
checkers

Moving cans
(light and
heavy)

Figure 15.3. JTT of Hand Function. The JTT of hand function is widely used to assess a broad range of hand functions required for activities of daily living (Jebsen et al., 1969). Subtests of the JTT include picking up beans with a teaspoon placing them in a can (mimicking a feeding function), stacking checkers, moving large light cans, and heavy cans.

pharyngeal representation in the unaffected hemisphere (Hamdy et al., 1998a), and that the magnitude of cortical reorganization induced by pharyngeal stimulation in stroke patients correlates with functional recovery (Fraser et al., 2002). Somatosensory stimulation may also enhance use-dependent plasticity in patients after chronic stroke (Sawaki et al., 2004). Moreover, a recent randomized, double-blind study in stroke patients with chronic weakness of one hand demonstrated that 2-h somatosensory stimulation of the median, ulnar, and radial nerves, compared to stimulation of three leg nerves, leads to performance improvements in activity of daily living involving the hand (Jebsen–Taylor test (JTT), see Fig. 15.3) (Wu et al., 2004). While not conclusive, these studies are consistent with the view that somatosensory stimulation can be purposefully used to influence motor function after stroke and they provide preliminary evidence to design more definite clinical trials.

Somatosensory input is also relevant in the setting of dystonia. Animal studies suggested that focal hand dystonia may be associated with abnormal processing of somatosensory input. Electrophysiologic mapping performed in non-human primates with a form of focal dystonia demonstrated a breakdown of normally separated finger representations in the somatosensory cortex accompanied by an enlargement of receptive fields (Byl et al., 1996; Merzenich et al., 1996). Human patients with focal hand dystonia have shown similar abnormalities of the homuncular representation in the somatosensory cortex (Byl et al., 1996; Bara-Jimenez et al., 1998) as

well as abnormalities in graphesthesia, stereagnosia (Byl et al., 1996; Merzenich et al., 1996), and perception of tonic vibration reflex (Grunewald et al., 1997), the ability to interpret sensory information immediately preceding and during voluntary movement (Murase et al., 2000), decreased tactile spatial acuity and tactile spatial localization, and abnormal temporal discrimination of somatosensory stimuli (Bara-Jimenez et al., 2000a, b). Together, these findings are consistent with the view that abnormal sensorimotor integration is a prominent feature in this condition (Odergren et al., 1996). Indeed, Zeuner et al. trained patients with focal hand dystonia and normal matched volunteers to perform a difficult tactile discrimination task (read Braille) as a strategy to decrease the overlap in finger cortical representations (Sterr et al., 1998; 1999). A training period of 8 weeks resulted in improvements in spatial tactile acuity that correlated with improvement in dystonic symptoms (Zeuner et al., 2002).

Disruption of somatosensory input

Anesthesia, nerve lesions or amputations involving one body part result in reorganization in the contralateral somatosensory cortex, by which nearby body part representations often expand over the deafferented one (see Volume I, Chapter 6). For example, after epidural nerve block, neurons in the cat primary somatosensory cortex (S1) that originally respond to stimulation of the anesthetized area become responsive to stimulation of adjacent, unanesthetized regions (Metzler and Marks, 1979).

Similar findings have been documented after peripheral nerve lesions or amputations (Kaas et al., 1983; Kolarik et al., 1994; Tinazzi et al., 1997). In the motor domain, nerve lesions also induce changes in the contralateral motor cortex characterized by a rapid expansion of motor cortical representations near the deafferented one (Sanes et al., 1988; Donoghue et al., 1990).

In humans, changes in brain organization by modulation of somatosensory input have likewise been demonstrated. Transient deafferentation induced by regional anesthesia or ischemic nerve block has profound implications in motor cortical function (Brasil-Neto et al., 1992; Brasil-Neto et al., 1993; Sadato et al., 1995; Ziemann et al., 2001; Werhahn et al., 2002a). Motor cortical excitability targeting arm muscles immediately proximal to the level of ischemic nerve block (elbow) and measured as MEP to TMS increased several fold within minutes after nerve block and returned to control values within 20 min after termination of ischemia (Ziemann et al., 1998). PET studies showed that during forearm ischemia, resting regional cerebral blood flow (rCBF) was increased in the sensorimotor cortex (SM1) bilaterally, suggesting that increased excitability of the motor cortex was associated with increased synaptic activity (Sadato et al., 1995). Another experiment demonstrated that this form of plasticity may have important behavioral implications. Ziemann et al. showed that training-induced improvements in the ability to perform a ballistic elbow flexion are more prominent during hand deafferentation (Ziemann et al., 2001). The hypothesis raised by this study is that motor performance and possibly learning by one body part (in this case, upper arm) could be favored by deafferentation of a nearby body part (in this case, the hand).

A preliminary study tested this hypothesis in human stroke patients in whom the purpose is to ameliorate hand motor function (i.e., "competition among adjacent body parts for territory in the brain", see Fig. 15.2(b)) (Muellbacher et al., 2002). In this trial, patients with motor deficits subsequent to chronic stroke trained in the presence of brachial plexus anesthesia selectively anesthetizing the upper arm,

but not the hand. This intervention resulted in transient improvements in paretic hand motor function and increases in corticomotor excitability targeting hand muscles, as measured by TMS.

Interestingly, reduction of somatosensory input from one limb results in the emergence of new receptive fields of individual neurons in the hemisphere contralateral to the deafferented one as well (Calford and Tweedale, 1990). These findings suggest that manipulation of somatosensory input originated in one limb results in well-defined measurable changes in cortical organization in both cerebral hemispheres. One study showed that ischemic anesthesia of one hand in healthy volunteers resulted in increases in corticomotor excitability targeting the homonymous non-deafferented hand (Werhahn et al., 2002b). More importantly, transient anesthesia of one hand led to surprising improvements in tactile discriminative skills in the non-deafferented hand (Werhahn et al., 2002b). These behavioral gains were accompanied by enhanced processing of somatosensory information as reflected by somatosensory-evoked potentials. These findings suggest that success of lateralized behavior, movements or processing of somatosensory or visual information, rely on a proper balance of interhemispheric interactions (Werhahn et al., 2002a; Murase et al., 2004). If so, it is conceivable that transient reduction of somatosensory input from the intact hand of patients with stroke could influence motor function in the paretic hand. A recent small open-label trial in patients with chronic motor stroke started to address this hypothesis. It was shown that performance of a dynamic finger motor task, but not an arm motor task, improved significantly with anesthesia of the intact hand but not of the intact foot (see Fig. 15.2(c)) (Floel et al., 2004).

15.6 Brain–computer interfaces

One of the strategies proposed to enhance functional recovery and sensory substitution is to use mechanical devices interfaced with human sensory afferents or interacting with the CNS. Modern pursuits of this goal have been driven by concrete technologic and clinical goals (see Volume I, Chapter 32). Overall, the idea has been to utilize these technologic advances to replace lost senses (i.e., audition in the case of cochlear implants) or to translate "thoughts into action" (i.e., use of electroencephalogram (EEG) activity to express language in patients with advanced amyotrophic lateral sclerosis).

Vision-substitution systems

Somatosensory input may be used to convey spatial information to blind individuals. In this case, a camera transduces visual information into electrical stimulation that is applied to the tongue (Bach-y-Rita et al., 1998). Different patterns of stimulation provide information on spatial features of the environment to the blind. Future developments in these areas could lead to higher independence in blind individuals.

Cochlear implants

Another fruitful approach for sensory prosthesis is the development of cochlear implants for the deaf. Here, understanding of cochlear function (Simmons, 1966) has led to cochlear implants that transduce sound waves into electrical stimuli to the cochlea. With training, these stimuli are interpreted as hearing sensations. The development of digital intracochlear multichannel systems allows now close-to-normal auditory functioning (Clark et al., 1979).

"Thought translation devices" in paralyzed individuals

Brain–computer interface (BCI) technology has the potential to enable severely disabled people to express volition through the use of computers (see Volume I, Chapter 33. This work stems from research that studied the effects of brain stimulation on behavior (Cooper, 1981) and also the influence of behavior on brain activity. The first use of invasive CNS recordings as control signals did not occur until advances in microelectrode, electronics, and computer technologies made the approach technically feasible (Mussa-Ivaldi and Miller, 2003). In a

first experiment, rats were trained to retrieve drops of water by pressing a lever controlling the rotation of a robotic arm (Wessberg et al., 2000). Subsequently, other groups demonstrated real-time control of robotic arms (Serruya et al., 2002; Taylor et al., 2002).

Work in humans has focused so far on the use of non-invasive physiologic recordings (EEG) as a vehicle of volition (Birbaumer et al., 1999; Curran and Stokes, 2003; Mussa-Ivaldi and Miller, 2003). For example, paralyzed individuals have been trained to control EEG activity in order to drive a cursor on a computer screen (Wolpaw and McFarland, 1994; McFarland et al., 1997). This approach has been used by Birbaumer et al. to train locked-in patients with amyotrophic lateral sclerosis to operate a spelling device by regulating slow cortical potentials (SCP) (Birbaumer et al., 1999). Visual feedback of SCP was provided on a screen for each trial, in the form of a ball that moved toward or away from a box, depending on the direction in which the SCP deviated from baseline. At the end of the training period, subjects were able to identify letters and form words on a computer screen by voluntary modulation of SCPs. Advances in this field may carry important implications for neurorehabilitation of patients with brain lesions (Donoghue, 2002; Mussa-Ivaldi and Miller, 2003) allowing them, for example, to make more involved decisions about their lives. This has obvious ethical and legal implications. Other possibilities include controlling wheelchairs and various environmental control systems (Curran and Stokes, 2003).

Cortical stimulation and functional recovery

It has been reported that electrical stimulation applied to a body part representation in the rodent motor cortex results in an increase in motor maps corresponding to the body part (Nudo et al., 1990). Consistent with this finding, human studies demonstrated that non-invasive stimulation using TMS can increase or decrease motor cortical excitability (Pascual-Leone et al., 1994). More recent work showed that brain stimulation can not only influence cortical excitability, but also cortical plasticity. Ziemann et al. showed that cortical stimulation in the form of TMS applied to a reorganized motor cortex increased the magnitude of deafferentation-induced plasticity, possibly through strengthening (e.g., LTP) of pre-existent synaptic connections (Ziemann et al., 1998). This effect is topographically specific, since it is shown with TMS of the same body part representation (i.e., the arm), but does not occur with stimulation of nearby representations (i.e., the face, hand, or leg) (Ziemann et al., 2002). Similar principles seem to influence cortical plasticity elicited by motor training. In a recent study, Butefisch et al. demonstrated that TMS synchronously applied to a motor cortex engaged in a motor training task enhances UDP (Buetefisch et al., 2004). The longevity of UDP was significantly enhanced by TMS applied in synchrony to the cortex contralateral to the training hand. In this protocol, the results demonstrated that use-dependent encoding of a motor memory can be enhanced by synchronous Hebbian stimulation of the motor cortex that drives the training task (Hebb, 1949). Overall, these results raise the exciting hypothesis that cortical stimulation could be used as an adjuvant to motor training in neurorehabilitation (Plautz et al., 2003; Hummel et al., 2005; Hummel and Cohen, 2005; Mansur et al., 2005; Martin et al., 2004).

15.7 Stem cells

Stem cells are pluripotential undifferentiated precursor cells that have the capacity to differentiate into mature cell types, for example, brain cell, under the appropriate conditions (see Volume I, Chapter 18). The quintessential source of stem cells is the embryo, but such cells may also exist in bone marrow and peripheral blood (especially in the umbilical cord blood). Chopp and colleagues reported that intraparenchymal implant of marrow stromal cells (MSC) in a rat model of stroke results in better recovery (Chen et al., 2001). When MSC are administered within the first few days after stroke onset, the functional effects appear to be rapid, with functional improvement occurring within a day or two. When MSC are administered intravenously, they

seem to cross the damaged blood–brain barrier and to cluster at the borders of infarcted tissue. Immunohistochemical studies show that most administered MSC do not differentiate into mature brain neurons or glia but seem to remain in a relatively undifferentiated state. This observation, coupled with the rapidity of functional effects, suggests MSC may have a trophic effect. That is, these cells seem to act as miniature "factories" for trophic substances rather than behaving in a cellular manner by structurally reconstituting the damaged brain. Similar results have been obtained in rodent stroke models using human umbilical cored blood cells (HUCB). Intravenous HUCB infusion (Chen et al., 2001) may have a beneficial effect on recovery processes (Borlongan et al., 1997; Schallert et al., 1997). Human trials are presently under way to test the safety and feasibility of this approach (Kondziolka et al., 2000).

15.8 Growth factors

Growth factors are involved in differentiation, maintenance, and proliferation of brain cells (see Volume I, Chapter 23). Neurotrophin basic fibroblast growth factor (bFGF), transforming growth factors a and b, insulin-like growth factor, and platelet-derived growth factor families appear to influence CNS function. Factors with effects on neurons are termed neurotrophic, whereas those with effects on glia or blood vessels can be termed gliotrophic or angiogenic, respectively. Growth factors seem to exert their effects by local processes including autocrine, paracrine, and juxtacrine stimulation. The expression of many growth factors is increased after stroke, and may have different spatial and temporal profiles, suggesting different roles for these substances. Several studies in animal models of stroke have demonstrated the neuroprotective effects of bFGF. This substance was first shown to reduce infarct size by 25% in rats given a continuous intraventricular infusion for 3 days before permanent middle cerebral artery (MCA) infarction (Koketsu et al., 1994). Subsequent studies showed that bFGF, given intravenously to rats for 3 h, beginning 30 min after MCA occlusion, decreases infarct size and neurologic deficit (Fisher et al., 1995; Sugimori et al., 2001). The neuroprotective effects are most likely exerted in the ischemic penumbra (Ay et al., 2001). The bFGF has also been shown in several animal studies to promote recovery (for review see Cairns and Finklestein, 2003). However, results from human studies are not encouraging. Clinical trials in North America of intravenous bFGF as a neuroprotective agent in acute stroke were stopped because of unanticipated side-effects of bFGF (Lutsep and Clark, 2000). In European and Australian trials, however, these same dosages given over a longer time period (24 h) appeared to be safe (Bogousslavsky et al., 2000).

15.9 Conclusion

Basic science findings over the last few years led to improved understanding the mechanisms underlying plasticity in the human CNS. Understanding of these principles is stimulating the involvement of new investigators and the development of more rational strategies to promote recovery of function and will likely result in improvements in patient care.

REFERENCES

Aschersleben, G., Gehrke, J., et al. (2001). Tapping with peripheral nerve block: a role for tactile feedback in the timing of movements. *Exp Brain Res*, **136**(3), 331–339.

Ay, I., Sugimori, H., et al. (2001). Intravenous basic fibroblast growth factor (bFGF) decreases DNA fragmentation and prevents downregulation of Bcl-2 expression in the ischemic brain following middle cerebral artery occlusion in rats. *Brain Res Mol Brain Res*, **87**(1), 71–80.

Bach-y-Rita, P., Kaczmarek, K.A., et al. (1998). Form perception with a 49-point electrotactile stimulus array on the tongue: a technical note. *J Rehabil Res Dev*, **35**(4), 427–430.

Bara-Jimenez, W., Catalan, M.J., et al. (1998). Abnormal somatosensory homunculus in dystonia of the hand. *Ann Neurol*, **44**(5), 828–831.

Bara-Jimenez, W., Shelton, P., et al. (2000a). Spatial discrimination is abnormal in focal hand dystonia. *Neurology*, **55**(12), 1869–1873.

Bara-Jimenez, W., Shelton, P., et al. (2000b). Sensory discrimination capabilities in patients with focal hand dystonia. *Ann Neurol*, **47**(3), 377–380.

Bastian, H.C. (1887). The "muscular sense"; its nature and cortical localization. *Brain*, **10**, 1–137.

Birbaumer, N., Ghanayim, N., et al. (1999). A spelling device for the paralysed. *Nature*, **398**(6725), 297–298.

Bliss, T.V. and Gardner, M.A. (1973). Long-lasting potentiation of synaptic transmission in the dentate area of the unanaesthetized rabbit following stimulation of the perforant path. *J Physiol London*, **232**, 357–374.

Bogousslavsky, J., Victor, S.J., et al. (2000). Fiblast (trafermin) in acute stroke: results of the European–Australian phase II/III safety and efficacy trial. *Cerebrovasc Dis*, **10**(**Suppl. 2**), 1–16 (abstract).

Borlongan, C.V., Koutouzis, T.K., et al. (1997). Neural transplantation as an experimental treatment modality for cerebral ischemia. *Neurosci Biobehav Rev*, **21**(1), 79–90.

Boyeson, M.G. and Feeney, D.M. (1990). Intraventricular norepinephrine facilitates motor recovery following sensorimotor cortex injury. *Pharmacol Biochem Behav*, **35**(3), 497–501.

Brasil-Neto, J.P., Cohen, L.G., et al. (1992). Rapid reversible modulation of human motor outputs after transient deafferentation of the forearm: a study with transcranial magnetic stimulation. *Neurology*, **42**(7), 1302–1306.

Brasil-Neto, J.P., Valls-Sole, J. et al. (1993). Rapid modulation of human cortical motor outputs following ischaemic nerve block. *Brain*, **116**(Pt 3), 511–525.

Buetefisch, C.M., Khurana, V., et al. (2004). Enhancing encoding of a motor memory in the primary motor cortex by cortical stimulation. *J Neurophysiol*, **91**(5), 2110–2116.

Buonomano, D.V. and Merzenich, M.M. (1998). Cortical plasticity: from synapses to maps. *Annu Rev Neurosci*, **21**, 149–186.

Butefisch, C.M., Davis, B.C., et al. (2000). Mechanisms of use-dependent plasticity in the human motor cortex. *Proc Natl Acad Sci USA*, **97**(7), 3661–3665.

Butefisch, C.M., Davis, B.C., et al. (2002). Modulation of use-dependent plasticity by D-amphetamine. *Ann Neurol*, **51**(1), 59–68.

Byl, N.N., Merzenich, M.M., et al. (1996). A primate genesis model of focal dystonia and repetitive strain injury. I. Learning-induced dedifferentiation of the representation of the hand in the primary somatosensory cortex in adult monkeys. *Neurology*, **47**(2), 508–520.

Byl, N.N., Merzenich, M.M., et al. (1997). A primate model for studying focal dystonia and repetitive strain injury: effects on the primary somatosensory cortex. *Phys Ther*, **77**(3), 269–284.

Cairns, K. and Finklestein, S.P. (2003). Growth factors and stem cells as treatments for stroke recovery. *Phys Med Rehabil Clin N Am*, **14**(**Suppl. 1**), S135–S142.

Calautti, C. and Baron, J.C. (2003). Functional neuroimaging studies of motor recovery after stroke in adults: a review. *Stroke*, **34**(6), 1553–1566.

Calautti, C., Leroy, F., et al. (2001). Dynamics of motor network overactivation after striatocapsular stroke: a longitudinal PET study using a fixed-performance paradigm. *Stroke*, **32**(11), 2534–2542.

Calford, M.B. and Tweedale, R. (1990). Interhemispheric transfer of plasticity in the cerebral cortex. *Science*, **249**(4970), 805–807.

Calford, M.B. and Tweedale, R. (1991a). Acute changes in cutaneous receptive fields in primary somatosensory cortex after digit denervation in adult flying fox. *J Neurophysiol*, **65**(2), 178–187.

Calford, M.B. and Tweedale, R. (1991b). Immediate expansion of receptive fields of neurons in area 3b of macaque monkeys after digit denervation. *Somatosens Mot Res*, **8**(3), 249–260.

Candia, V., Schafer, T., et al. (2002). Sensory motor retuning: a behavioral treatment for focal hand dystonia of pianists and guitarists. *Arch Phys Med Rehabil*, **83**(10), 1342–1348.

Carey, J.R., Kimberley, T.J., et al. (2002). Analysis of fMRI and finger tracking training in subjects with chronic stroke. *Brain*, **125**(Pt 4), 773–788.

Castro-Alamancos, M.A., Donoghue, J.P., et al. (1995). Different forms of synaptic plasticity in somatosensory and motor areas of the neocortex. *J Neurosci*, **15**(7 Pt 2), 5324–5333.

Centonze, D., Picconi, B., et al. (2001). Dopaminergic control of synaptic plasticity in the dorsal striatum. *Eur J Neurosci*, **13**(6), 1071–1077.

Chen, J., Sanberg, P.R., et al. (2001). Intravenous administration of human umbilical cord blood reduces behavioral deficits after stroke in rats. *Stroke*, **32**(11), 2682–2688.

Chen, R. and Hallett, M. (1998). Focal dystonia and repetitive motion disorders. *Clin Orthop*, **351**, 102–106.

Chollet, F., DiPiero, V., et al. (1991). The functional anatomy of motor recovery after stroke in humans: a study with positron emission tomography. *Ann Neurol*, **29**(1), 63–71.

Clark, G.M., Pyman, B.C., et al. (1979). The surgery for multiple-electrode cochlear implantation. *J Laryngol Otol*, **93**, 215–223.

Classen, J., Liepert, J., et al. (1998). Rapid plasticity of human cortical movement representation induced by practice. *J Neurophysiol*, **79**(2), 1117–1123.

Cohen, L.G. and Hallett, M. (1988). Hand cramps: clinical features and electromyographic patterns in a focal dystonia. *Neurology*, **38**(7), 1005–1012.

Cohen, L.G., Ziemann, U., et al. (1998). Studies of neuroplasticity with transcranial magnetic stimulation. *J Clin Neurophysiol*, **15**(4), 305–324.

Colombo, G., Wirz, M., et al. (2001). Driven gait orthosis for improvement of locomotor training in paraplegic patients. *Spinal Cord*, **39**(5), 252–255.

Conforto, A.B., Kaelin-Lang, A., et al. (2002). Increase in hand muscle strength of stroke patients after somatosensory stimulation. *Ann Neurol*, **51**(1), 122–125.

Cooper, I.S. (1981). Twenty-five years of experience with physiological neurosurgery. *Neurosurgery*, **9**, 190–200.

Corwin, J.V., Kanter, S., et al. (1986). Apomorphine has a therapeutic effect on neglect produced by unilateral dorsomedial prefrontal cortex lesions in rats. *Exp Neurol*, **94**(3), 683–698.

Cramer, S.C. and Dobkin, B.H. (2004). Ropinirole in the treatment of motor deficits after stroke: a randomized, placebo-controlled, double-blind pilot trial. *Proceedings of the International Stroke Conference*, Vancouver, BC (confererence abstract).

Cramer, S.C., Nelles, G., et al. (1997). A functional MRI study of subjects recovered from hemiparetic stroke. *Stroke*, **28**(12), 2518–2527.

Crisostomo, E.A., Duncan, P.W., et al. (1988). Evidence that amphetamine with physical therapy promotes recovery of motor function in stroke patients. *Ann Neurol*, **23**(1), 94–97.

Curran, E.A. and Stokes, M.J. (2003). Learning to control brain activity: a review of the production and control of EEG components for driving brain–computer interface (BCI) systems. *Brain Cogn*, **51**(3), 326–336.

Dobkin, B.H. and Havton, L.A. (2004). Basic advances and new avenues in therapy of spinal cord injury. *Annu Rev Med*, **55**, 255–282.

Donoghue, J., Hess, G., et al. (1996). Substrates and mechanisms for learning in motor cortex. In: *Acquisition of Motor Behavior in Vertebrates* (eds Bloedel, J., Ebner, T. and Wise, S.), MIT Press, Cambridge, MA.

Donoghue, J.P. (2002). Connecting cortex to machines: recent advances in brain interfaces. *Nat Neurosci*, **5**(**Suppl.**), 1085–1088.

Donoghue, J.P., Suner, S., et al. (1990). Dynamic organization of primary motor cortex output to target muscles in adult rats. II. Rapid reorganization following motor nerve lesions. *Exp Brain Res*, **79**(3), 492–503.

Donoghue, J.P., Hess, G., et al. (1996). Substrates and mechanisms for learning in motor cortex. In: *Acquisition of Motor Behavior in Vertebrates* (ed. Wise, S.P.), pp. 363–386. MIT Press, Cambridge, MA.

Dromerick, A.W., Edwards, D.F., et al. (2000). Does the application of constraint-induced movement therapy during acute rehabilitation reduce arm impairment after ischemic stroke? *Stroke*, **31**(12), 2984–2988.

Dubnau, J. and Tully, T. (1998). Gene discovery in *Drosophila*: new insights for learning and memory. *Annu Rev Neurosci*, **21**, 407–444.

Edin, B.B. and Johansson, N. (1995). Skin strain patterns provide kinaesthetic information to the human central nervous system. *J Physiol*, **487**(Pt 1), 243–251.

Feeney, D.M. (1997). From laboratory to clinic: noradrenergic enhancement of physical therapy for stroke or trauma patients. *Adv Neurol*, **73**, 383–394.

Feeney, D.M., Gonzalez, A., et al. (1982). Amphetamine, haloperidol, and experience interact to affect rate of recovery after motor cortex injury. *Science*, **217**(4562), 855–857.

Fisher, M., Meadows, M.M., et al. (1995). Delayed treatment with intravenous basic fibroblast growth factor reduces infarct size following permanent focal cerebral ischemia in rats. *J Cereb Blood Flow Metab*, **15**(6), 953–959.

Floel, A., Nagorsen, U., Werhahn, K.J., Ravindran, S., Birbaumer, N., Knecht, S. and Cohen, L.G. (2004). Influence of somatosensory input on motor function in patients with chronic stroke. *Ann Neurol*, **56**, 206–212.

Floel, A., Breitenstein, C., et al. (2005). Dopaminergic influences on formation of a motor memory. *Ann Neurol*, in press.

Floel, A., Hummel, F., et al. (in press). Dopaminergic effects on encoding of a motor memory in chronic stroke. *Neurology*.

Flor, H., Elbert, T., et al. (1995). Phantom-limb pain as a perceptual correlate of cortical reorganization following arm amputation. *Nature*, **375**(6531), 482–484.

Fraser, C., Power, M., et al. (2002). Driving plasticity in human adult motor cortex is associated with improved motor function after brain injury. *Neuron*, **34**(5), 831–840.

Fridman, E.A., Hanakawa, T., et al. (2004). Reorganization of the human ipsilesional premotor cortex after stroke. *Brain*, **127**(4), 747–758.

Frost, S.B., Barbay, S., et al. (2003). Reorganization of remote cortical regions after ischemic brain injury: a potential substrate for stroke recovery. *J Neurophysiol*, **89**(6), 3205–3214.

Gold, P.E., Delanoy, R.L., et al. (1984). Modulation of long-term potentiation by peripherally administered amphetamine and epinephrine. *Brain Res*, **305**(1), 103–107.

Goldstein, L.B. (1998). Potential effects of common drugs on stroke recovery. *Arch Neurol*, **55**(4), 454–456.

Gordon, J., Ghilardi, M.F., et al. (1995). Impairments of reaching movements in patients without proprioception. I. Spatial errors. *J Neurophysiol*, **73**(1), 347–360.

Grondin, R., Zhang, Z., et al. (2000). Dopaminergic therapy improves upper limb motor performance in aged rhesus monkeys. *Ann Neurol*, **48**(2), 250–253.

Grunewald, R.A., Yoneda, Y., et al. (1997). Idiopathic focal dystonia: a disorder of muscle spindle afferent processing? *Brain*, **120**(Pt 12), 2179–2185.

Hallett, M. (1998). Physiology of dystonia. *Adv Neurol*, **78**, 11–18.

Hamdy, S., Aziz, Q., et al. (1998a). Recovery of swallowing after dysphagic stroke relates to functional reorganization in the intact motor cortex. *Gastroenterology*, **115**(5), 1104–1112.

Hamdy, S., Enck, P., et al. (1998b). Spinal and pudendal nerve modulation of human corticoanal motor pathways. *Am J Physiol*, **274**(2 Pt 1), G419–G423.

Hebb, D.O. (1949). *The Organization of Behavior*, Wiley, New York.

Hess, G. and Donoghue, J.P. (1994). Long-term potentiation of horizontal connections provides a mechanism to reorganize cortical motor maps. *J Neurophysiol*, **71**(6), 2543–2547.

Hess, G., Jacobs, K.M., et al. (1994). *N*-methyl-D-aspartate receptor mediated component of field potentials evoked in horizontal pathways of rat motor cortex. *Neuroscience*, **61**(2), 225–235.

Hobson, J.A. and Pace-Schott, E.F. (2002). The cognitive neuroscience of sleep: neuronal systems, consciousness and learning. *Nat Rev Neurosci*, **3**(9), 679–693.

Hummel, F. and Cohen, L.G. (2005). Improvement of motor function with noninvasive cortical stimulation in a patient with chronic stroke. *Neurorehabil Neural Repair*, **19**, 14–19.

Hummel, F., Celnik, P., Giraux, P., Floel, A., Wu, W.H., Gerloff, C. and Cohen, L.G. (2005). Effects of non-invasive cortical stimulation on skilled motor function in chronic stroke. *Brain*, **128**, 490–499.

Irvine, D.R. and Rajan, R. (1996). Injury- and use-related plasticity in the primary sensory cortex of adult mammals: possible relationship to perceptual learning. *Clin Exp Pharmacol Physiol*, **23**(10–11), 939–947.

Jacobs, K.M. and Donoghue, J.P. (1991). Reshaping the cortical motor map by unmasking latent intracortical connections. *Science*, **251**(4996), 944–947.

Jay, T.M. (2003). Dopamine: a potential substrate for synaptic plasticity and memory mechanisms. *Prog Neurobiol*, **69**(6), 375–390.

Jebsen, R.H., Taylor, N., et al. (1969). An objective and standardized test of hand function. *Arch Phys Med Rehabil*, **50**(6), 311–309.

Johansen-Berg, H., Rushworth, M.F., et al. (2002). The role of ipsilateral premotor cortex in hand movement after stroke. *Proc Natl Acad Sci USA*, **99**(22), 14518–14523.

Johansson, K., Lindgren, I., et al. (1993). Can sensory stimulation improve the functional outcome in stroke patients? *Neurology*, **43**(11), 2189–2192.

Jones, E.G. and Pons, T.P. (1998). Thalamic and brainstem contributions to large-scale plasticity of primate somatosensory cortex. *Science*, **282**(5391), 1121–1125.

Kaas, J.H. (1991). Plasticity of sensory and motor maps in adult mammals. *Annu Rev Neurosci*, **14**, 137–167.

Kaas, J.H. (2000). The reorganization of somatosensory and motor cortex after peripheral nerve or spinal cord injury in primates. *Prog Brain Res*, **128**, 173–179.

Kaas, J.H., Merzenich, M.M., et al. (1983). The reorganization of somatosensory cortex following peripheral nerve damage in adult and developing mammals. *Annu Rev Neurosci*, **6**, 325–356.

Kaas, J.H., Krubitzer, L.A., et al. (1990). Reorganization of retinotopic cortical maps in adult mammals after lesions of the retina. *Science*, **248**(**4952**), 229–231.

Kaelin-Lang, A., Luft, A.R., et al. (2002). Modulation of human corticomotor excitability by somatosensory input. *J Physiol*, **540**(**Pt 2**), 623–633.

Karni, A., Meyer, G., et al. (1995). Functional MRI evidence for adult motor cortex plasticity during motor skill learning. *Nature*, **377**(**6545**), 155–158.

Knecht, S., Breitenstein, C., et al. (2004). Levodopa: faster and better word learning in normal humans. *Ann Neurol*, **56**, 20–26.

Koketsu, N., Berlove, D.J., et al. (1994). Pretreatment with intraventricular basic fibroblast growth factor decreases infarct size following focal cerebral ischemia in rats. *Ann Neurol*, **35**(**4**), 451–457.

Kolarik, R.C., Rasey, S.K., et al. (1994). The consistency, extent, and locations of early-onset changes in cortical nerve dominance aggregates following injury of nerves to primate hands. *J Neurosci*, **14**(**7**), 4269–4288.

Kondziolka, D., Wechsler, L., et al. (2000). Transplantation of cultured human neuronal cells for patients with stroke. *Neurology*, **55**(**4**), 565–569.

Kunkel, A., Kopp, B., et al. (1999). Constraint-induced movement therapy for motor recovery in chronic stroke patients. *Arch Phys Med Rehabil*, **80**(**6**), 624–628.

Lamprecht, R. and LeDoux, J. (2004). Structural plasticity and memory. *Nat Rev Neurosci*, **5**(**1**), 45–54.

Landry, C.F., Ivy, G.O., et al. (1990). Developmental expression of glial fibrillary acidic protein mRNA in the rat brain analyzed by in situ hybridization. *J Neurosci Res*, **25**(**2**), 194–203.

Lovely, R.G., Gregor, R.J., et al. (1986). Effects of training on the recovery of full-weight-bearing stepping in the adult spinal cat. *Exp Neurol*, **92**(**2**), 421–435.

Luft, A.R., Kaelin-Lang, A., et al. (2002). Modulation of rodent cortical motor excitability by somatosensory input. *Exp Brain Res*, **142**(**4**), 562–569.

Lutsep, H.L. and Clark, W.M. (2000). Association of intracranial stenosis with cortical symptoms or signs. *Neurology*, **55**(**5**), 716–718.

Macaluso, A. and De Vito, G. (2004). Muscle strength, power and adaptations to resistance training in older people. *Eur J Appl Physiol*, **91**(**4**), 450–472.

Macht, M.B. (1950). Effects of D-amphetamine on hemidecorticate, decorticate, and decerebrate cats. *Am J Physiol*, **163**, 731–732.

Mansur, C.G., Fregni, F., Boggio, P.S., Riberto, M., Gallucci-Neto, J., Santos, C.M., Wagner, T., Rigonatti, S.P., Marcolin, M.A. and Pascual-Leone, A. (2005). A sham stimulation-controlled trial of rTMS of the unaffected hemisphere in stroke patients. *Neurology*, **64**, 1802–1804.

Marshall, R.S., Perera, G.M., et al. (2000). Evolution of cortical activation during recovery from corticospinal tract infarction. *Stroke*, **31**(**3**), 656–661.

Martin, P.I., Naeser, M.A., Theoret, H., Tormos, JM., Nicholas, M., Kurland, J., Fregni, F., Seekins, H., Doron, K. and Pascual-Leone, A. (2004). Transcranial magnetic stimulation as a complementary treatment for aphasia. *Semin Speech Lang*, **25**, 181–191.

Martinsson, L., Wahlgren, N.G., et al. (2003). Amphetamines for improving recovery after stroke. *Cochrane Database Syst Rev*, **3**, CD002090.

Marty, S., Berzaghi Mda, P., et al. (1997). Neurotrophins and activity-dependent plasticity of cortical interneurons. *Trend Neurosci*, **20**(**5**), 198–202.

McFarland, D.J., McCane, L.M., et al. (1997). Spatial filter selection for EEG-based communication. *Electroencephalogr Clin Neurophysiol*, **103**(**3**), 386–394.

McGuire, B.A., Gilbert, C.D., et al. (1991). Targets of horizontal connections in macaque primary visual cortex. *J Comp Neurol*, **305**(**3**), 370–392.

Merzenich, M., Wright, B., et al. (1996). Cortical plasticity underlying perceptual, motor, and cognitive skill development: implications for neurorehabilitation. *Cold Spring Harb Symp Quant Biol*, **61**, 1–8.

Merzenich, M.M., Nelson, R.J., et al. (1984). Somatosensory cortical map changes following digit amputation in adult monkeys. *J Comp Neurol*, **224**(**4**), 591–605.

Metzler, J. and Marks, P.S. (1979). Functional changes in cat somatic sensory-motor cortex during short-term reversible epidural blocks. *Brain Res*, **177**(**2**), 379–383.

Mott, F.W. and Sherrington, C.S. (1895). Experiments upon the influence of sensory nerves upon movement and nutrition of the limbs. *Proc Natl Acad Sci USA*, **57**, 481–488.

Muellbacher, W., Ziemann, U., et al. (2001). Role of the human motor cortex in rapid motor learning. *Exp Brain Res*, **136**(**4**), 431–438.

Muellbacher, W., Richards, C., et al. (2002). Improving hand function in chronic stroke. *Arch Neurol*, **59**(**8**), 1278–1282.

Murase, N., Kaji, R., et al. (2000). Abnormal premovement gating of somatosensory input in writer's cramp. *Brain*, **123**(**Pt 9**), 1813–1829.

Murase, N., Duque, J., et al. (2004). Influence of interhemispheric interactions on motor function in chronic stroke. *Ann Neurol*, **55**(**3**), 400–409.

Mussa-Ivaldi, F.A. and Miller, L.E. (2003). Brain-machine interfaces: computational demands and clinical needs meet basic neuroscience. *Trend Neurosci*, **26**(**6**), 329–334.

Nissen, M.J. and Bullemer, P. (1987). Attentional requirements of learning: evidence from performance measures. *Cogn Psychol*, **19**, 1–32.

Nudo, R.J. and Milliken, G.W. (1996). Reorganization of movement representations in primary motor cortex following focal ischemic infarcts in adult squirrel monkeys. *J Neurophysiol*, **75**(**5**), 2144–2149.

Nudo, R.J., Jenkins, W.M., et al. (1990). Repetitive microstimulation alters the cortical representation of movements in adult rats. *Somatosens Mot Res*, **7**(**4**), 463–483.

Nudo, R.J., Jenkins, W.M., et al. (1992). Neurophysiological correlates of hand preference in primary motor cortex of adult squirrel monkeys. *J Neurosci*, **12**(**8**), 2918–2947.

Nudo, R.J., Wise, B.M., et al. (1996). Neural substrates for the effects of rehabilitative training on motor recovery after ischemic infarct. *Science*, **272**(**5269**), 1791–1794.

Odergren, T., Iwasaki, N., et al. (1996). Impaired sensory-motor integration during grasping in writer's cramp. *Brain*, **119**(**Pt 2**), 569–583.

Pahlke, K. and Scheidtmann, K. (2003). Levodopa steigert die Effektivität des Explorationstrainings bei linksseitigem Neglect [Levodopa boosts efficacy of exploration training after left-sided neglect]. *Aktuel Neurol*, **30**(**S1**), S131.

Pascual-Leone, A., Valls-Sole, J., et al. (1994). Responses to rapid-rate transcranial magnetic stimulation of the human motor cortex. *Brain*, **117**(**Pt 4**), 847–858.

Pavlides, C., Miyashita, E., et al. (1993). Projection from the sensory to the motor cortex is important in learning motor skills in the monkey. *J Neurophysiol*, **70**(**2**), 733–741.

Pearson, K. (2000). Motor systems. *Curr Opin Neurobiol*, **10**(**5**), 649–654.

Plautz, E.J., Barbay, S., et al. (2003). Post-infarct cortical plasticity and behavioral recovery using concurrent cortical stimulation and rehabilitative training: a feasibility study in primates. *Neurol Res*, **25**(**8**), 801–810.

Pons, T.P. and Kaas, J.H. (1986). Corticocortical connections of area 2 of somatosensory cortex in macaque monkeys: a correlative anatomical and electrophysiological study. *J Comp Neurol*, **248**(**3**), 313–335.

Powell, J., Pandyan, A.D., et al. (1999). Electrical stimulation of wrist extensors in poststroke hemiplegia. *Stroke*, **30**(**7**), 1384–1389.

Pulvermuller, F., Neininger, B., et al. (2001). Constraint-induced therapy of chronic aphasia after stroke. *Stroke*, **32**, 1621–1626.

Recanzone, G.H., Allard, T.T., et al. (1990). Receptive-field changes induced by peripheral nerve stimulation in SI of adult cats. *J Neurophysiol*, **63**(**5**), 1213–1225.

Reding, M.J. and Potes, E. (1988). Rehabilitation outcome following initial unilateral hemispheric stroke. Life table analysis approach. *Stroke*, **19**(**11**), 1354–1358.

Ridding, M.C. and Taylor, J.L. (2001). Mechanisms of motor-evoked potential facilitation following prolonged dual peripheral and central stimulation in humans. *J Physiol*, **537**(**Pt 2**), 623–631.

Rioult-Pedotti, M.S., Friedman, D., et al. (2000). Learning-induced LTP in neocortex. *Science*, **290**(**5491**), 533–536.

Robertson, A. and Laferriere, A. (1989). Disruption of the connections between the mediodorsal and sulcal prefrontal cortices alters the associability of rewarding medial cortical stimulation to place and taste stimuli in rats. *Behav Neurosci*, **103**(**4**), 770–778.

Rossini, P.M., Calautti, C., et al. (2003). Post-stroke plastic reorganisation in the adult brain. *Lancet Neurol*, **2**(**8**), 493–502.

Rothwell, J.C., Traub, M.M., et al. (1982). Manual motor performance in a deafferented man. *Brain*, **105**(**Pt 3**), 515–542.

Sadato, N., Zeffiro, T.A., et al. (1995). Regional cerebral blood flow changes in motor cortical areas after transient anesthesia of the forearm. *Ann Neurol*, **37**(**1**), 74–81.

Sakamoto, T., Arissian, K., et al. (1989). Functional role of the sensory cortex in learning motor skills in cats. *Brain Res*, **503**(**2**), 258–264.

Sanes, J.N., Suner, S., et al. (1988). Rapid reorganization of adult rat motor cortex somatic representation patterns after motor nerve injury. *Proc Natl Acad Sci USA*, **85**(**6**), 2003–2007.

Sawaki, L., Boroojerdi, B., et al. (2002a). Cholinergic influences on use-dependent plasticity. *J Neurophysiol*, **87**(**1**), 166–171.

Sawaki, L., Cohen, L.G., et al. (2002b). Enhancement of use-dependent plasticity by D-amphetamine. *Neurology*, **59**(**8**), 1262–1264.

Sawaki, L., Wu, C.W.H., et al. (2004). Enhancement of use-dependent plasticity by peripheral nerve stimulation in patients with chronic stroke. *Proceedings of the Conference of the 5th World Stroke Congress*, Vancouver, BC, Canada (conference abstract).

Schallert, T., Kozlowski, D.A., et al. (1997). Use-dependent structural events in recovery of function. *Adv Neurol*, **73**, 229–238.

Scheidtmann, K., Fries, W., et al. (2001). Effect of levodopa in combination with physiotherapy on functional motor recovery after stroke: a prospective, randomised, double-blind study. *Lancet*, **358**(**9284**), 787–790.

Schultz, W. (2000). Multiple reward signals in the brain. *Nat Rev Neurosci*, **1**(**3**), 199–207.

Serruya, M.D., Hatsopoulos, N.G., et al. (2002). Instant neural control of a movement signal. *Nature*, **416**(**6877**), 141–142.

Shadmehr, R. and Holcomb, H.H. (1997). Neural correlates of motor memory consolidation. *Science*, **277**(**5327**), 821–825.

Shepherd, E.B. (2001). Exercise and training to optimize functional motor performance in stroke: driving neural reorganization? *Neural Plast*, **8**, 121–129.

Simmons, F.B. (1966). Electrical stimulation of the auditory nerve in man. *Arch Otolaryngol*, **84**, 2–54.

Skinner, B.F. (1968). *The Technology of Teaching*, Appleton-Century-Crofts, New York.

Stefan, K., Kunesch, E., et al. (2000). Induction of plasticity in the human motor cortex by paired associative stimulation. *Brain*, **123**(**Pt 3**), 572–584.

Sterr, A., Muller, M.M., et al. (1998). Perceptual correlates of changes in cortical representation of fingers in blind multi-finger Braille readers. *J Neurosci*, **18**(**11**), 4417–4423.

Sterr, A., Muller, M., et al. (1999). Development of cortical reorganization in the somatosensory cortex of adult Braille students. *Electroencephalogr Clin Neurophysiol Suppl*, **49**, 292–298.

Sterr, A., Elbert, T., et al. (2002). Longer versus shorter daily constraint-induced movement therapy of chronic hemiparesis: an exploratory study. *Arch Phys Med Rehabil*, **83**(**10**), 1374–1377.

Stroemer, R.P., Kent, T.A., et al. (1998). Enhanced neocortical neural sprouting, synaptogenesis, and behavioral recovery with D-amphetamine therapy after neocortical infarction in rats. *Stroke*, **29**(**11**), 2381–2393; discussion 2393–2395.

Struppler, A., Angerer, B., et al. (2003a). Modulation of sensorimotor performances and cognition abilities induced by RPMS: clinical and experimental investigations. *Suppl Clin Neurophysiol*, **56**, 358–367.

Struppler, A., Havel, P., et al. (2003b). Facilitation of skilled finger movements by repetitive peripheral magnetic stimulation (RPMS) – a new approach in central paresis. *Neurorehabilitation*, **18**(**1**), 69–82.

Sugimori, H., Speller, H., et al. (2001). Intravenous basic fibroblast growth factor produces a persistent reduction in infarct volume following permanent focal ischemia in rats. *Neurosci Lett*, **300**(**1**), 13–16.

Sullivan, K.J., Knowlton, B.J. and Dobkin, B.H. (2002). Step training with body weight support: effect of treadmill speed and practice paradigms on poststroke locomotor recovery. *Arch Phys Med Rehabil*, **83**, 683–691.

Tallal, P., Miller, S., et al. (1993). Neurobiological basis of speech: a case for the preeminence of temporal processing. *Ann NY Acad Sci*, **682**, 27–47.

Tallal, P., Miller, S.L., et al. (1996). Language comprehension in language-learning impaired children improved with acoustically modified speech. *Science*, **271**(**5245**), 81–84.

Taub, E., Crago, J.E., et al. (1994). An operant approach to rehabilitation medicine: overcoming learned nonuse by shaping. *J Expo Anal Behav*, **61**(**2**), 281–293.

Taub, E., Uswatte, G., et al. (2002). New treatments in neurorehabilitation founded on basic research. *Nat Rev Neurosci*, **3**(**3**), 228–236.

Taylor, D.M., Tillery, S.I., et al. (2002). Direct cortical control of 3D neuroprosthetic devices. *Science*, **296**(**5574**), 1829–1832.

Tinazzi, M., Zanette, G., et al. (1997). Selective gating of lower limb cortical somatosensory evoked potentials (SEPs) during passive and active foot movements. *Electroencephalogr Clin Neurophysiol*, **104**(**4**), 312–321.

Traversa, R., Cicinelli, P., et al. (1997). Mapping of motor cortical reorganization after stroke. A brain stimulation study with focal magnetic pulses. *Stroke*, **28**(**1**), 110–117.

Vargo, J.M., Richard-Smith, M., et al. (1989). Spiroperidol reinstates asymmetries in neglect in rats recovered from left or right dorsomedial prefrontal cortex lesions. *Behav Neurosci*, **103**(**5**), 1017–1027.

Walker-Batson, D. (2000). Use of pharmacotherapy in the treatment of aphasia. *Brain Lang*, **71**(**1**), 252–254.

Walker-Batson, D., Smith, P., et al. (1995). Amphetamine paired with physical therapy accelerates motor recovery after stroke. Further evidence. *Stroke*, **26**(**12**), 2254–2259.

Ward, N.S. and Cohen, L.G. Mechanisms underlying recovery of motor function in stroke. *Arch Neurol*, **61**(**12**), 1844–1848 (in press).

Ward, N.S., Brown, M.M., et al. (2003). Neural correlates of outcome after stroke: a cross-sectional fMRI study. *Brain*, **126**(**Pt 6**), 1430–1448.

Weiller, C. and Rijntjes, M. (1999). Learning, plasticity, and recovery in the central nervous system. *Exp Brain Res*, **128**(**1–2**), 134–138.

Weiner, N. (1980). Norepinephrine, epinephrine, and the sympathomimetic amines. In: *The Pharmacological Basis of Therapeutics* (eds Gilman, A.G., Doodman, L.S. and Filman, A.), Macmillan Publishing, New York, pp. 138–175.

Werhahn, K.J., Mortensen, J., et al. (2002a). Cortical excitability changes induced by deafferentation of the contralateral hemisphere. *Brain*, **125**(**Pt 6**), 1402–1413.

Werhahn, K.J., Mortensen, J., et al. (2002b). Enhanced tactile spatial acuity and cortical processing during acute hand deafferentation. *Nat Neurosci*, **5**(**10**), 936–938.

Werhahn, K.J., Conforto, A.B., et al. (2003). Contribution of the ipsilateral motor cortex to recovery after chronic stroke. *Ann Neurol*, **54**(**4**), 464–472.

Wessberg, J., Stambaugh, C.R., et al. (2000). Real-time prediction of hand trajectory by ensembles of cortical neurons in primates. *Nature*, **16**, 361–365.

Wickens, J.R., Kotter, R., et al. (1995). Effects of local connectivity on striatal function: stimulation and analysis of a model. *Synapse*, **20**(**4**), 281–298.

Wolpaw, J.R. and McFarland, D.J. (1994). Multichannel EEG-based brain–computer communication. *Electroencephalogr Clin Neurophysiol*, **90**(**6**), 444–449.

Wong, A.M., Su, T.Y., et al. (1999). Clinical trial of electrical acupuncture on hemiplegic stroke patients. *Am J Phys Med Rehabil*, **78**(**2**), 117–122.

Woody, C.D., Gruen, E., et al. (1991). Changes in membrane currents during Pavlovian conditioning of single cortical neurons. *Brain Res*, **539**(**1**), 76–84.

Wu, W.H., Seo, H.J., et al. (2004). Improvement of paretic hand function by somatosensory stimulation in chronic stroke. *Proceedings of the Conference of the 5th World Stroke Congress*. Vancouver, BC (conference abstract).

Zeuner, K.E., Bara-Jimenez, W., et al. (2002). Sensory training for patients with focal hand dystonia. *Ann Neurol*, **51**(**5**), 593–598.

Ziemann, U., Corwell, B., et al. (1998). Modulation of plasticity in human motor cortex after forearm ischemic nerve block. *J Neurosci*, **18**(**3**), 1115–1123.

Ziemann, U., Muellbacher, W., et al. (2001). Modulation of practice-dependent plasticity in human motor cortex. *Brain*, **124**(**Pt 6**), 1171–1181.

Ziemann, U., Wittenberg, G.F., et al. (2002). Stimulation-induced within-representation and across-representation plasticity in human motor cortex. *J Neurosci*, **22**(**13**), 5563–5571.

Neural repair

Contents

Basic cellular and molecular processes

CONTENTS

Neuronal death and rescue: neurotrophic factors and anti-apoptotic mechanisms

Thomas W. Gould and Ronald W. Oppenheim

Department of Neurobiology and Anatomy, and the Neuroscience Program, Wake Forest University School of Medicine, NC, USA

16.1 Introduction

Developmental cell death

One of the most counter-intuitive events during the normal development of the nervous system is the massive loss of neurons that characterizes virtually all populations in the central and peripheral nervous system (CNS and PNS) (Oppenheim, 1991; Pettmann and Henderson, 1998; Oppenheim and Johnson, 2003); counter-intuitive, because as a general rule, development is a progressive process whereby new cells, tissues and organs are gradually built-up over time, whereas cell death is a prototypical regressive process. Although precise numbers are not available, as adults we are in the seemingly unenviable position of having many fewer nerve cells (several millions less!) than were present during fetal and early postnatal development. Since most of this loss occurs prior to birth,[1] it cannot be attributed to aging, pathology or other life history events such as puberty, although, as we discuss below, pathologic neuronal loss by contrast can occur at virtually any stage in the life cycle. Rather, the developmental cell death we refer to is an entirely normal event in most

tissues (Raff, 1992). In fact, the perturbation of this normal developmental cell death (i.e., too little or too much cell loss) may be a major factor in the generation of many developmental defects (Ikonomidou et al., 2001; Oppenheim and Johnson, 2003). Accordingly, it is now generally accepted that developmental cell death is a fundamental and integral part of the many adaptive strategies employed during ontogeny for generating the mature nervous system.

As the major focus of this book is neural repair and rehabilitation, it is reasonable to ask why the topic of normal **developmental** neuronal death is included here. **First**, as described below, there is increasing evidence that some of the mechanisms that regulate the death and survival of developing neurons, on the one hand, and that of mature neurons following injury or in neurologic disease, on the other hand, are similar (e.g., Vila and Przedborski, 2003). Importantly, much of the basic biology of these mechanisms has been established in the developing nervous system (Yuan and Yankner, 2000; Oppenheim and Johnson, 2003). **Second**, developmental models are commonly used as *in vitro* and *in vivo* bioassays for testing suspected therapeutic agents that may be potentially applicable to rescuing adult neurons from death following injury or disease (Elliott and Snider, 1999; Hilt et al., 1999).

Although it is beyond the scope of this chapter to provide a comprehensive review of the field of neuronal death during development, it is nonetheless important to briefly describe some of the key

---

[1] An important exception to the restriction of the normal loss of neurons during early development is the equally massive loss of newly generated neurons in a few specific regions of the brain where adult neurogenesis persists. For example, more than one-half of adult generated neurons in the mammalian hippocampus normally undergo cell death (Cameron and McKay, 2001; Sun et al., 2004).

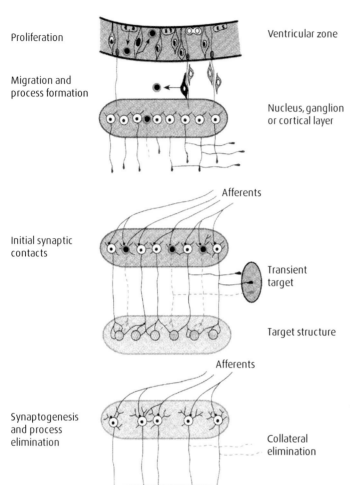

Proliferation

Ventricular zone

Migration and
process formation

Nucleus, ganglion
or cortical layer

Afferents

Initial synaptic
contacts

Transient
target

Target structure

Afferents

Synaptogenesis
and process
elimination

Collateral
elimination

Synapse
elimination

Figure 16.1. Stages of neuronal development when PCD occurs. PCD can occur at all stages between proliferation and synaptogenesis. Once synaptic connections are stabilized, normal PCD ceases. Following the period of PCD, axonal pathways and synaptic connections are defined by collateral and synapse elimination. Round red cells with a dark center represent cells undergoing PCD (from Oppenheim and Johnson, 2003).

features of this process in order to place what follows in an appropriate framework for comparison with the mechanisms involved in injury- and disease-related cell death.

Beginning with multi-potent proliferative progenitor cells in the ventricular and sub-ventricular zones of the developing brain and spinal cord and continuing up to the initiation of synaptogenesis between neurons or between neurons and their non-neuronal targets (e.g., muscle), a large proportion of developing cells in the CNS and PNS will undergo programmed cell death (PCD, Fig. 16.1). As

shown in Fig. 16.1, a major phase of neuronal PCD occurs as neurons form connections with efferents and afferent targets. Because the loss of neurons following injury or disease also typically involves mature post-mitotic neurons with well-established connectivity, it seems reasonable that the mechanisms involved in this type of developmental PCD are likely to be relevant to the later pathologic loss of neurons. As a general rule, the number of neurons present prior to this phase of PCD exceeds the number that persist in the adult nervous system by 15–70% (average of 50%). As synaptogenesis

Table 16.1. Some possible functions of PCD in the nervous system.

Category	Example
1 Removal of cells that appear to have no function	Death of neurons in either males or females for creating sexually dimorphic structures
2 Removal of cells of an inappropriate phenotype	Death of neuronal precursors located in regions of the spinal cord, such as the roof or floor plate, that lack neurons in the adult
3 Pattern formation and morphogenesis	Death of neural crest cells in specific segments of the hindbrain
4 Systems matching	Creation of optimal levels of innervation between interconnected groups of neurons and between neurons and their non-neuronal targets
5 Error corrections	Death of neurons with inappropriate synaptic connections or aberrant pathway projections
6 Guidance	Loss of neurons or glia that guide neuronal migration or axonal growth at specific stages of development
7 Transient function	Death of sensory, motor and CNS neurons that serve a transient physiologic/behavioral function during development (e.g., Rohon-Beard SNs in tadpoles)
8 Removal of harmful cells	Death of cells with defective DNA or infected by viruses
9 A means of evolutionary change	Adaptive changes in the ontogenetic death and survival of cells in response to genetic mutation (e.g., the production of excess neurons could be used for innervation of new targets made available by the evolution of limbs)

proceeds, neurons compete for limiting amounts of survival signals derived from targets, afferents and non-neuronal (e.g., glial) sources resulting in the survival of only those cells that win the competition. These then go on to complete their differentiation and comprise the mature nervous system. By contrast, the losers in the competition undergo an active, gene-regulated degeneration and are ultimately removed by being engulfed and further degraded by phagocytic cells (Savill et al., 2003). The over-production and subsequent loss of developing neurons by PCD serves a variety of adaptive functions (Table 16.1). Since the different modes by which developing neurons undergo PCD, and the different genetic and biochemical pathways involved have been reasonably well characterized, these are now a major focus of studies of pathologic cell death.

Different types of cell death

Characterizing the specific morphologic and histologic changes exhibited by degenerating cells is of considerable interest because differences in the mode of degeneration may provide insights into the cellular and molecular pathways by which cells are destroyed. This may, in turn, provide clues for protecting cells from death. More than a century ago two major modes of cell death were recognized **necrosis** and **spontaneous cell death** (Clarke and Clarke, 1996). Necrosis referred to pathologic cell death, whereas spontaneous cell death was used to describe the normal death of cells during tissue turnover in adult animals (e.g., the periodic regression of ovarian follicles or mammary gland cells). Beginning in the 1970s and continuing up to the present, a similar dichotomy has been used to distinguish between pathologic cell death ("necrosis") and normal occurring ("spontaneous") cell death whether it occurs during development or in adult animals. The Greek term **apoptosis** was coined to describe this normal cell death process (Kerr et al., 1972). Initially, morphologic criteria were used to define each type of death and only later were biochemical, molecular and genetic criteria utilized. For example, apoptosis was characterized by cytoplasmic condensation, nuclear pyknosis, chromatin condensation, DNA fragmentation, cytoskeletal degradation, cell fragmentation into membrane-bound apoptotic bodies and finally, phagocytosis. By contrast, necrosis was characterized by an initial swelling of the cell, modest condensation of chromatin, cytoplasmic vacuolization, degradation of organelles, rupture of the cell membrane, externalization of cytoplasmic contents and localized inflammation (see Fig. 16.6). In general, necrosis reflects malfunctioning biochemical pathways that mediate normal functions in unstressed/uninjured cells. Although the necrosis–apoptosis dichotomy has been of considerable heuristic value, it has outlived its usefulness. It is now recognized that this dichotomy is an oversimplification (Clarke, 1990). Regardless of whether one uses morphologic, biochemical or genetic criteria, there are several modes of cell death which may or may not meet all

of the criteria for either necrosis or apoptosis (Fig. 16.2). Accordingly, there is a growing consensus that the death of cells should not be defined as being either necrotic or apoptotic, but rather that cell death should be defined operationally, by using the specific morphologic, biochemical, molecular and genetic features displayed by a specific cell type in a specific situation (Clarke, 1990; Leist and Jäättelä, 2001; Oppenheim and Johnson, 2003). Only in this way will it be possible to develop neuroprotective treatment strategies that target the appropriate pathways for each pathologic condition. As described below, because of the remarkable progress that has occurred in the last 10–15 years in characterizing pathways of cell death and survival (Pettmann and Henderson, 1998; Hengartner, 2000; Yuan and Yankner, 2000; Syntichaki and Tavernarakis, 2003),

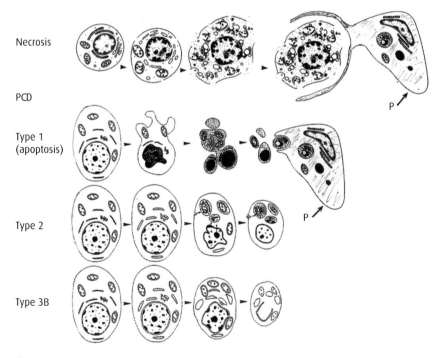

Necrosis

PCD

Type 1
(apoptosis)

Type 2

Type 3B

Figure 16.2. Schematic representation of necrotic cell death and three of the commonest types of PCD observed at the ultrastructural level (see Clarke, 1990). Only type 1 PCD meets most of the criteria for defining apoptosis. The cells on the right marked P represent phagocytic cells engulfing necrotic cell corpses and apoptotic bodies. Phagocytosis also occurs in the other types of PCD but is not shown (from Oppenheim and Johnson, 2003).

future prospects appear promising for developing clinically relevant strategies for reducing or preventing pathologic cell death in the nervous system.

Molecular regulation of cell death and survival

As most normal cell death in the developing nervous system of vertebrates appears to be attributable to a failure of individual neurons to compete successfully for trophic support, it is appropriate to begin this section with a brief description of how the availability of neurotrophic factors (NTFs) regulates the

decision to live or die. In the past it was generally believed that NTFs were required to prevent the passive degeneration of developing neurons. In the absence of sufficient NTF, neurons were thought to die by a process analogous to starvation. As summarized below, it is now clear that death following NTF deprivation is not passive at all but rather is a metabolically active process requiring new gene transcription and protein expression. The binding of NTFs to cell surface receptors on nerve processes for example initiates a complex signaling cascade that is transmitted retrogradely to the cell body and nucleus (Fig. 16.3). One consequence of this

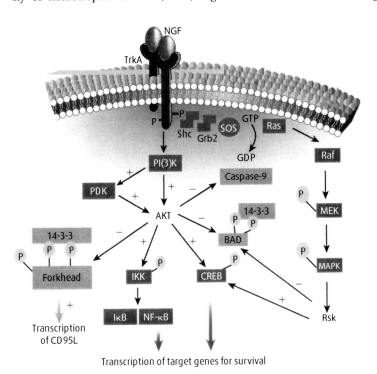

Figure 16.3. Neuronal survival pathways induced by the binding of NGF to its tropomyosin-related kinase A (TrkA) receptor. NGF induces the autophosphorylation of TrkA which provides docking sites for signal transduction molecules such as phospholipase C, PI(3)K and the adaptor protein Shc. Activated PI(3)K induces the activation of Akt through 3′-phosphorylated phosphatidylinositol as well as phosphoinositide-dependent kinase (PDK), which in turn phosphorylates and activates Akt. The phosphorylation of CREB and IKK stimulates the transcription of pro-survival factors; whereas the phosphorylation of Bad, Forkhead and caspase-9 inhibits the pro-apoptotic pathway. In a parallel pathway, the interaction of Shc-Grb2 and SOS activates the Ras-Raf-MEK-ERK pathway, resulting in the activation of Rsk. Bad and CREB are also the targets of Rsk that might act synergistically with Akt to activate the survival pathway (from Yuan and Yankner, 2000).

signaling cascade is the activation of survival promoting second messenger pathways such as the mitogen-activated protein kinase (MAPK) and phosphoinositide-3-kinase (P1(3)K)pathways, which in turn regulate the expression of pro- and anti-apoptotic proteins such as the Bcl-2 family members. A central integrator of the life-death decision for a developing neuron is the mitochondrion. By monitoring the expression of relative amounts of pro- and anti-apoptotic Bcl-2 family members, the mitochondrion modulates cell survival by the regulated release of mitochondrial molecules such as cytochrome-c that then activates downstream proteases (caspases) that either directly or indirectly degrade cytoplasmic and nuclear substrates (Fig. 16.4). Once activated this execution phase represents an irreversible step leading inexorably to death. A commonly used assay for detecting this apoptotic-like cell death visualizes individual cells in tissue sections in which the DNA has been degraded during the execution phase (Fig. 16.5). This technique known as terminal-deoxyneucleotidyl-transferase-mediated dUTP nick-end labeling (TUNEL) utilizes deoxynucleotidyl transferase (TdT)-mediated dUPT-biotin nick end labeling and relies on the specific binding of terminal TdT to expose 3'-OH ends of damaged DNA (Ben-Sasson et al., 1995). However, the gold standard for demonstrating whether cell death is apoptotic remains the morphologic approach using ultrastructural criteria (e.g., Fig. 16.6).

Although the most common and best understood mechanisms of normal neuronal cell death is the evolutionarily conserved apoptotic pathway, it is becoming increasingly recognized that there are alternative pathways that resemble autophagy or necrosis and which may also be caspase or NTF-independent, as well as others that by-pass the mitochondrion, some of which involve death receptors and others that exhibit changes in intracellular calcium levels mediated by extracellular glutamate and *N*-methyl-D-aspartate (NMDA) receptors. Depending on the specific pathologic condition, each of these death pathways represent potential targets for therapeutic intervention (Olney and Ishimaru, 1999; Raoul et al., 2000; Leist and Jäättelä, 2001).

16.2 Neuronal death and rescue after disease and injury

Amyotrophic lateral sclerosis

Amyotrophic lateral sclerosis (ALS) is an adult-onset neurodegenerative disease resulting in the death of cranial and spinal motoneurons (lower MNs) as well as neurons in the motor cortex (upper MNs). MN death leads to paralysis and, within 3–5 years, death due to impaired respiration caused by denervation of the diaphragm. Pathologically, the predominant findings include vacuolization of mitochondria within the cell bodies and axons of MNs as well as neurofilament-containing inclusions in the proximal ventral root. While the preponderance of ALS is sporadic, about 5% of ALS is familial (FALS), and a subset of these patients inherit dominant mutations in the gene encoding copper/zinc superoxide dismutase (Brown, 1995). Transgenic mice overexpressing various mutated forms of human SOD1 in all tissues recapitulate the cell specific, delayed-onset MN degeneration observed in ALS and form the major genetic model of this disease.

MN death occurs in sporadic and FALS by a process that in several respects is similar to apoptosis. Similarly, transgenic mice expressing the G93A mutation of human SOD1, which develop motor symptoms at postnatal day (P)90 and succumb by P140, show increases in MN expression and activation of pro-apoptotic Bcl-2 family proteins and caspases, respectively (Guégan et al., 2001). Interestingly, increases in caspase-1 activity occur at about P45, when MN axons exhibit the first signs of terminal denervation (Frey et al., 2000). These temporal correlates indicate an intimate link between early neuronal dysfunction and activation of the cell death pathway. What is less clear is the subcellular compartment which initiates this process: **the cell body**, implying nuclear-controlled cell-autonomous dysfunction or insults deriving from afferent input or adjacent glia; **the axon**, suggesting transport dysfunction, aggregate formation or Schwann cell-derived apoptotic signals; **the target**, indicating a potential role of decreased NTF stimulation and/or

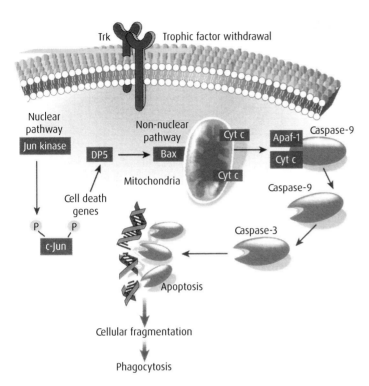

Nuclear pathway

Non-nuclear pathway

Trophic factor withdrawal

Trk

Jun kinase

DP5 → Bax

Cell death genes

Mitochondria

Cyt c

Cyt c

Apaf-1

Cyt c

Caspase-9

Caspase-9

P   P

c-Jun

Caspase-3

Apoptosis

Cellular fragmentation

Phagocytosis

Figure 16.4. Activation of apoptosis in sympathetic neurons by trophic factor withdrawal. Trophic factor withdrawal induces JNK activation and the phosphorylation of c-Jun, which in turn induces the expression of DP5/Bim, "BH3-domain only" members of the Bcl-2 family. DP5 and Bim might activate Bax, causing mitochondrial damage, which results in the release of cytochrome c. Formation of the cytochrome c/Apaf-1/caspase-9 complex induces the activation of caspase-9. Activated caspase-9 in turn activates caspase-3, resulting in apoptosis. A lack of trophic factor signaling also induces a non-nuclear competence-to-die pathway that facilitates the formation of the cytochrome c/Apaf-1/caspase-9 complex, resulting in caspase-9 activation (modified from Yuan and Yankner, 2000).

loss of innervation; or **organelle disruption** within the MN, offering a direct pathway to cell death. Several prominent hypotheses of the etiology of ALS are presented and discussed with respect to this spatial framework.

Excitotoxicity and/or other forms of oxidative stress

Deficits in high-affinity glutamate transport, the primary mechanism by which extracellular glutamate is removed from the synapse, are observed in synaptic preparations derived from cortex and spinal cord but not other CNS regions of patients with ALS, providing a mechanism for MN selectivity (Bar-Peled and Rothstein, 1999). These reductions in transport result from RNA editing errors and therefore reduced protein levels of excitatory amino acid transporter 2 (EAAT2), a glial-derived glutamate transporter. Conversely, experimentally induced decreases in the level of EAAT2 are sufficient to cause MN degeneration and paralysis (Bar-Peled and Rothstein, 1999). These results implicate glia as potential regulators of MN survival, a hypothesis supported by the finding that certain SOD1 mutations produce glial-containing aggregates and diminished EAAT2 expression preceding MN dysfunction (Cleveland, 1999). Astrocyte-restricted overexpression of mutant SOD1, however,

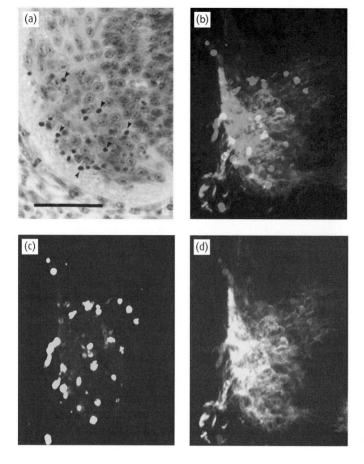

Figure 16.5. Photomicrographs of transverse sections through the cervical spinal cord of a 4-day-old chick embryo showing the distribution of dying neurons in the ventral horn. (a) Hematoxylin and eosin staining. (b–d) Labeling with the TUNEL method and spinal cord-1 (SC-1) (a marker for ventral horn neurons) immunohistochemistry. (b) TUNEL + SC-1. (c) TUNEL (d) SC-1. Scale bars. 50 μm *Arrows* in (a) indicate pyknotic profiles of degenerating neurons (from Yaginuma et al., 1996).

is insufficient to cause MN neurodegeneration. Nevertheless, a recent study which constructed chimeric mice expressing high levels of mutant SOD1 only in MNs showed that these mice develop ALS much later than mice with mutant SODI in all cells, indicating that signals originating from sources other than MNs are sufficient to induce MN death (Clement et al., 2003).

Increases in glutamate may trigger pathologic elevations of intracellular calcium through classic excitotoxic mechanisms (Olney and Ishimaru, 1999). Alternatively, excessive intracellular calcium levels may result from diminished expression of intracellular calcium-buffering proteins or calcium-impermeable glutamate receptor subunits in MNs (such

as GluR2). This finding is strengthened by the recent report that RNA editing errors which reduce GluR2 function are found selectively in the spinal cord of a subset of patients with sporadic ALS (Kawahara et al., 2004). Therefore, deleterious effects of chronically elevated intracellular calcium on neuronal survival may be responsible for the mitochondrial dysfunction and vacuolization observed in ALS. Alternatively, oxidative stress within the mitochondria itself, derived from the overexpression of mutant SOD1, may increase the production of reactive oxygen species (ROS) through altered metal oxidation (Valentine, 2002). Intriguingly, whereas reductions in mitochondrial oxidative phosphorylation and release of cytochrome c into the cytosol

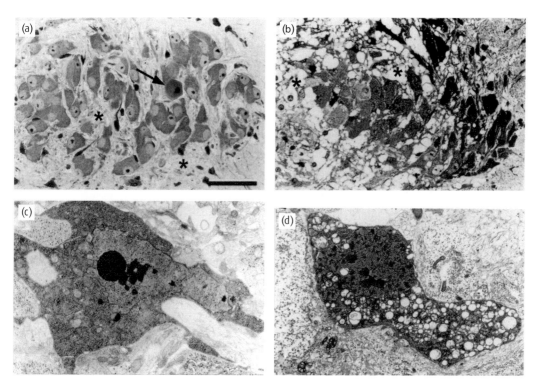

Figure 16.6. Degenerating spinal MNs in the chick embryo. (a) Ventral horn from a control embryo. Note that only one cell (arrow) is undergoing apoptotic PCD and the neuropil (*) is intact. (b) Ventral horn from an embryo following an excitotoxic (glutamate) lesion. Most neurons are undergoing a necrotic cell death (dark cells) and the neuropil is disintegrating (*). Apoptotic (c) and necrotic MNs (d) in the chick embryo spinal cord as seen with an electron microscope (from Oppenheim and Johnson, 2003).

occur near the onset of symptoms in the mutant SOD1 mice, morphologic swellings are observed far earlier. Probing the mechanism as well as consequence of this early abnormality may help lead to effective therapies.

Interference with axonal transport and/or protein aggregation

Neurofilament (NF) accumulations are a pathologic hallmark of ALS (Julien, 1999). Transgenic mice over-expressing various NF subunits exhibit NF accumulation and MN degeneration; conversely, inhibiting the expression or transport of NFs in SOD1 mutant mice dramatically extends survival (Cleveland, 1999).

Additionally, axonal transport is diminished in the axons of mutant SOD1 transgenic mice long before the onset of behavioral symptoms (Cleveland, 1999). Furthermore, a significant number of mutations have been identified in a region of the large NF subunit NF-H in patients with familial and sporadic ALS (Al-Chalabi et al., 1999). Together, these findings suggest that alterations in the delivery of intra-axonal cargo arise early from a novel property of mutant SOD1. Indeed, experimental disruption of transport itself is sufficient to cause a late-onset MN-specific neurodegenerative disorder, and mutations in the transport machinery have recently been documented in FALS (Hafezparast et al., 2003). One potential consequence of impaired axonal transport and denervation may be a reduction in target-derived NTF signaling, as it has recently been shown that mutations in one NTF are sufficient to cause selective MN degeneration (Oosthuyse et al., 2001).

Therapeutic strategies for ALS

Riluzole, a drug which blocks sodium channel function and reduces glutamate release, is the only drug approved for treatment of ALS. Although clinical trials for a number of NTFs failed to ameliorate disease progression, genetic delivery to MNs of retrogradely transported viral vectors expressing insulin-like-growth factor type 1 (IGF-1) extend the lifespan of mutant SOD1 mice (Kaspar et al., 2003). Transgenic or genetic delivery of hepatocyte growth factor (HGF) or glial cell line-derived neurotrophic factor (GDNF), respectively, also attenuates disease progression (Sun et al., 2002; Wang et al., 2002). Conversely, interference with cell death pathways by inhibiting caspase-1 activity or overexpressing Bcl-2 results in only a modest delay in symptom onset and survival (but see Kang et al., 2003). Other strategies targeting excitotoxic pathways have demonstrated a potent rescue effect in transgenic mice with "cocktails" of three drugs, including riluzole, minocycline, which stabilizes mitochondrial function, and nimodipine, which inhibits voltage-sensitive calcium channels (Kriz et al., 2003). Finally, preserving mitochondrial homeostasis by administering creatine or minocycline alone, or together, increases lifespan (Zhang et al., 2003).

Huntington's disease

Huntington's disease (HD) is an autosomal-dominant, adult-onset neurodegenerative disorder characterized by abnormal cognitive and motor function, including its hallmark, choreiform movement. HD results in the selective loss of spiny GABAergic interneurons in the caudate and putamen, while sparing proximal neostriatal cholinergic interneurons. Degeneration of cortical layer V and layer VI projection neurons is also observed in HD. The mutation

causing HD is an expanded tract of glutamine residues (>40) in the first exon of the huntingtin gene product (Htt), a 350-kDa protein of unknown function (HD Collaborative Research Group, 1993). It is one member in the family of so-called CAG triplet repeat or polyglutamine (polyQ) repeat diseases, which also includes spinobulbar muscular atrophy (SBMA), dentatorubral-pallidoluysian atrophy and the spinocerebellar ataxias (SCA) 1, 2, 3, 6 and 7. A distinctive neuropathologic finding in HD is the presence of intracellular inclusions containing mutant Htt in cortex and striatum, although it is unclear whether they contribute to disease pathogenesis. Four different types of models exist to study the pathophysiology and therapeutic intervention of HD: excitotoxic lesions, transgenic mice, transgenic flies and *in vitro* transformation of primary or clonal cells.

Abnormal proteolytic processing

Neuronal cell death observed in the brains of HD patients, mutant Htt-expressing transgenic mice or neurotoxin-treated rats occurs through apoptosis (Portera-Cailliau et al., 1995). One mechanism by which mutant Htt may initiate a pathologic cellular response is caspase cleavage, which generates truncated N-terminal regions of mutant Htt (Wellington et al., 2002). Indeed, transgenic overexpression of only a small N-terminal fragment of mutant Htt (containing the polyQ tract) is more neurotoxic than expression of the entire mutant protein, supporting a role for caspase cleavage in disease pathogenesis (Martindale et al., 1998). Inhibition of caspase cleavage, which occurs in the cytoplasm before other signs of neurodegeneration in striatal cells *in vitro* and *in vivo*, reduces mutant Htt toxicity. Wild-type Htt is also cleaved by caspases, suggesting that production of mutant Htt fragments, rather than proteolytic cleavage of mutant full-length Htt *per se*, contributes to neuronal toxicity (Wellington et al., 2002). These findings led to the "toxic peptide hypothesis", which, similar to the role of caspase-3 cleavage of amyloid precursor protein (APP) in Alzheimer's disease (AD), proposes a feedback mechanism progressing from early cleavage of cytotoxic mutant proteins to activation of cell death molecules such as caspases, which in turn increase cytotoxicity by generating more mutant fragments as well as by activating the caspase cascade (Gervais et al., 1999). Wild-type and mutant Htt proteins are also processed by calcium-dependent cysteine proteases μ- and m-calpain (Kim et al., 2001). Cleavage by calpain yields smaller N-terminal mutant Htt fragments than by caspases, and elimination of consensus recognition sites within mutant Htt reduces its cleavage by calpain and decreases its neurotoxicity (Gafni et al., 2004).

Altered energy metabolism caused by excitotoxicity and/or oxidative stress

Cerebral glucose metabolism, which requires intact mitochondrial function, is decreased in patients with HD selectively in the neostriatum and cortex. Additionally, biochemical studies reveal decreased mitochondrial respiratory chain complex activities I, II and III in the neostriatum but not cortex of human HD brain and transgenic mice expressing mutant Htt (Grünewald and Beal, 1999). Similarly, mitochondrial adenosine triphosphate (ATP) synthesis is diminished in mutant Htt mice. Together with the discovery that both GluR2 agonists and mitochondrial complex II inhibitors reproduce HD pathogenesis, these findings suggest a link between excitotoxicity, mitochondrial dysfunction and mutant Htt. Striatal mitochondrial deficits in calcium handling are detected in mutant Htt transgenic mice months before other signs of neurodegeneration occur (Panov et al., 2002). Additionally, internal calcium concentration is regulated by the ER-derived type 1 inositol (1,4,5)-triphosphate receptor, which acts as an intracellular calcium release channel and is modulated directly by mutant Htt (Tang et al., 2003). Therefore, mutant Htt may disrupt calcium homeostasis at multiple checkpoints, leading to cell death of striatal neurons. Subsequent decreases in mitochondrial oxidative phosphorylation are also accompanied by increases in cytotoxic ROS and protein oxidation, both of which are observed in striatal and cortical neurons in human HD brain.

Inhibition of NTF signaling: disruption of transcription

Wild-type but not mutant Htt inhibits an endogenous repressor of brain-derived neurotrophic factor (BDNF) transcription, suggesting that HD may reflect in part a loss of Htt function (Zuccato et al., 2003). Indeed, BDNF rescues mutant Htt-expressing striatal neurons *in vitro* (Humbert et al., 2002). Furthermore, cortical expression of BDNF is dramatically reduced in patients with HD as well as in mutant Htt transgenic mice, suggesting that one source of afferent trophic support for striatal neurons may be reduced in HD (Zuccato et al., 2003). Additionally, mutant Htt sequesters the transcription cofactor cAMP-response element binding (*CREB*) *P*rotein (CBP), which participates in the co-activation of the cell survival-regulating transcription factor CREB (Steffan et al., 2001). Indeed, disruption of CREB function is sufficient to induce striatal neurodegeneration (Mantamadiotis et al., 2002). Mutant Htt may also affect transcription indirectly through its ability to disrupt the proteosome and thus inhibit degradation of pro-apoptotic transcription factors such as p53 (Jana et al., 2001).

Interference with axonal transport

Recent studies demonstrate that mutant Htt forms small fibrillar protease-dependent aggregates in the cytoplasm (Feany and La Spada, 2003). These studies, as well as others which fail to find such aggregates, show impaired axonal transport in neurons overexpressing mutant Htt (Feany and La Spada, 2003). Interestingly, decreases in wild-type Htt also result in an impairment of axonal transport, but not apoptosis. Together with findings that mutant Htt traps proteins required for transport into cytoplasmic aggregates, these results suggest simultaneous loss and gain of function phenotypes may operate in the axon, while mutant Htt-induced neuronal death may represent an additional toxic gain of function in the nucleus. Similar mechanisms may underlie the pathogeneses of other neurodegenerative disorders, as mutations in axonal motor proteins are sufficient to induce neurodegeneration (see section on ALS).

Therapeutic intervention of HD

Mice deficient in caspase-1 activity delay disease onset when bred into lines of mice overexpressing mutant Htt, demonstrating that the inhibition of pathologic proteolysis may provide one target (Ona et al., 1999). Two recent reports indicate that dietary restriction or environmental enrichment upregulates BDNF levels in the cortex of mutant Htt-expressing transgenic mice and increases their survival (Duan et al., 2003; Spires et al., 2004). Finally, histone deacetylase inhibitors impede polyQ-induced neurotoxicity in *Drosophila*, suggesting that aberrant transcription can be targeted as well (Steffan et al., 2001).

Parkinson's disease

The second most common neurodegenerative disorder, Parkinson's disease (PD), affects 1% of all people above the age of 65 and results in distinctive motor impairments including akinesia, bradykinesia, resting tremor, postural impairment and rigidity (see Volume II, Chapter 35). PD results in the degeneration of dopaminergic (DAergic) neurons in the substantia nigra pars compacta (sensory neuron, SN), a midbrain structure which innervates the striatum in the so-called nigrostriatal pathway. Hallmark neuropathologic inclusions within these cells, known as Lewy bodies, are finely ordered spherical aggregates containing a number of proteins whose function is thought to contribute to the pathogenesis of this disease. Indeed, a dominant mutation in one of these proteins, α-synuclein, has been linked to a familial form of PD (Maries et al., 2003). A recessive mutation causing another inherited form of PD has identified parkin as a potential regulator of the formation of Lewy bodies (Maries et al., 2003). In contrast, the cause of most sporadic PD is unknown but may utilize similar pathogenetic mechanisms. Two factors resulting in non-genetic forms of PD include exposure to pesticide and intoxication with the drug 1-methyl-4-phenyl-1,2,3,6-tetrahydropyridine (MPTP), both of which have been reproduced in animals to investigate the pathogenesis of PD. Additional animal models include mice, flies and monkeys that express α-synuclein and parkin mutations; each of these five models exhibit deficits which partly or completely reproduce PD neuropathology and behavior (Maries et al., 2003).

Dopamine-mediated oxidative stress

Ample evidence suggests that DAergic SN neurons undergo apoptosis in PD, including ultrastructural analysis of morphology, TUNEL labeling and activation of pro-apoptotic proteins (Burke and Kholodilov, 1998). Recent studies reveal a striking continuity in the molecular mechanisms by which apoptosis occurs in the various animal models of PD. Systemic treatment of rats with rotenone, a plant-derived pesticide which inhibits mitochondrial respiratory chain complex I, results in Lewy body formation, progressive degeneration of the SN and motor dysfunction such as bradykinesia and unsteady gait, leading to the suggestion that DAergic cells are uniquely sensitive to agents which cause oxidative stress. Indeed, multiple studies of PD postmortem brain tissue demonstrate oxidative damage to lipids, proteins and DNA within the SN (Jenner, 1998). Similarly, administration of MPTP, another mitochondrial complex I inhibitor, results in PD-type degeneration and dysfunction. The metabolite of MPTP is MPP$^+$, which binds to the dopamine (DA) transporter with high affinity and thus gains selective entrance into DAergic neurons. In addition to interfering with DAergic oxidative phosphorylation, MPP$^+$ increases the production of ROS; overexpressing or knocking out various anti-oxidants reduces or enhances, respectively, MPTP neurotoxicity (Beal, 2001). Furthermore, MPP$^+$ binds the vesicular DA transporter, suggesting that this agent may redistribute DA to the cytoplasm and subject it to a myriad of enzymatic activities which render it cytotoxic (Lotharius and Brundin, 2003). Such oxidative damage compromises the integrity of membranes, proteins and nucleic acids, increases intracellular calcium concentration, and initiates proteolytic processing and pro-apoptotic gene transcription.

Interestingly, overexpression of wild-type α-synuclein in DAergic but not non-DAergic neurons causes apoptosis, suggesting that excess amounts of this protein may also selectively promote DA-mediated toxicity (Xu et al., 2002). Indeed, *Drosophila* overexpressing either wild-type or mutant α-synuclein develop neuronal inclusions, DAergic cell loss and motor dysfunction (Feany and Bender, 2000). Furthermore, a recent study discovered genomic triplication of the region containing α-synuclein as the sole genetic defect underlying a familial form of PD (Singleton et al., 2003). The deleterious effects of α-synuclein overexpression may be mediated by the formation of oxidative and highly toxic forms of DA; these DA species increase and stabilize the formation of α-synuclein aggregates, which themselves are thought to be toxic and ROS-producing (Conway et al., 2001). Additionally, familial mutations in α-synuclein result in aggregates which rupture vesicles and thus contribute to cytoplasmic DA redistribution and oxidative stress (Volles et al., 2001). Finally, mice deficient in α-synuclein are resistant to MPTP-induced neurotoxicity, indicating that this protein is required for DAergic oxidative stress-induced neurodegeneration (Dauer et al., 2002). These studies indicate that slight perturbations in DA storage (neurotoxin) or α-synuclein function (familial mutation) or expression level (genomic triplication or transgenic study) may initiate a self-perpetuating cycle of neurotoxicity and thus contribute to PD pathogenesis.

Disruption of protein degradation

In addition to its role in initiating cell death through DA-containing ROS, α-synuclein may stimulate other cell death pathways indirectly through its accumulation into aggregates and eventually, Lewy bodies. These pathologic inclusions contain ubiquitin and thus may reflect evidence of aborted protein degradation by the ubiquitin proteasomal pathway (UPP). This hypothesis has been strengthened by recent findings which demonstrate an inhibition of the UPP in the SN of PD brain as well as direct inhibition of the UPP by α-synuclein or Lewy body aggregates (Eriksen et al., 2003). A tantalizing link between mutations underlying two different forms of PD was established by the report that parkin can mitigate the toxicity of mutant α-synuclein (Cookson, 2003). While the mechanisms by which this interaction occurs are unclear, it appears that in the absence of parkin, α-synuclein may form ubiquitinated aggregates which perturb either proteasomal activity or the degradation of other key proteins such as p53, either of which may contribute directly to cell death.

Treatment strategies for PD

Treatment strategies targeting PD can be divided into three categories: inhibitors of α-synuclein aggregation, anti-oxidants and inhibitors of cell death pathways. As development of α-synuclein into fibrils initiates Lewy bodies, agents that prevent this pathogenic oligomerization, such as chaperone proteins or β or γ-synuclein, may be therapeutic. Secondly, inhibiting oxidative stress with agents such as minocycline prevents neurodegeneration in MPTP-lesioned mice (Wu et al., 2002). Thirdly, inhibiting intrinsic cell death pathway genes such as Apaf-1 or Bax provides neuroprotection in MPTP models of PD (Vila and Przedborski, 2003); conversely, treatment with NTFs, especially GDNF, stimulates not only DAergic survival but also striatal innervation and function (Kirik et al., 2004; see Volume I, Chapters 29 and 34). Finally, grafts of embryonic DA neurons or stem cells offer another potential therapeutic strategy in PD (see Volume I, Chapter 34 and Volume II, Chapter 6).

AD

AD is the most prevalent neurodegenerative disorder, affecting 15 million people worldwide and occurring mainly in the seventh decade of life. AD patients suffer from memory impairment, dementia and global cognitive decline, neurologic deficits which are associated with decreased function of the hippocampus, limbic system and cortex (see

Volume II, Chapter 31). Hallmark histopathologic signs of AD, including intracellular tangles consisting of hyperphosphorylated tau protein and extracellular β-amyloid (Aβ) plaques, occur predominantly in these regions. Decreases in brain acetylcholine levels are observed early in AD and coincide with the dysfunction of cholinergic projection neurons innervating the hippocampus and cortex. Genetic forms of early onset AD are caused by dominant mutations in one of three genes, APP, presenilin-1 and -2; all three of these gene defects result in pathologically enhanced cleavage and secretion of a toxic peptide fragment of APP known as Aβ42 (Younkin, 1998). The ratio of this peptide, compared to normal Aβ40, is increased in AD versus control patients, leading to the formation of toxic Aβ-containing oligomers and fibrils that are rudiments of the extracellular plaques observed in affected regions of AD brain. Patients with Down's Syndrome (DS) also develop Aβ plaques, and a variety of other neurodegenerative disorders exhibit tau-containing fibrillary tangles (so-called tauopathies). Further evidence that levels of APP and/or Aβ processing contribute to the etiology of AD is based on the finding that APP is located on chromosome 21, which is triplicated in patients with DS. The fact that Aβ plaques are observed in DS and familial and sporadic AD led to the generation of numerous transgenic models based on these inherited mutations. These models reproduce some but not all elements of the pathologic and behavioral dysfunction observed in AD, however, and illustrate the potential involvement of other pathophysiologic mechanisms of the disease, including toxicity mediated by altered metal metabolism and oxidative stress. Indeed, multiple studies establish a role for Aβ both in the induction of and inhibition of oxidative stress, depending on cellular and extracellular context (Smith et al., 2002).

Aβ-mediated oxidative stress

Several studies report that neuronal death in AD is apoptotic, findings consistent with elevated levels of pro-apoptotic Bcl-2 family members and of activated caspases-3, -8 and -9 in human AD brain (Behl, 2000).

Additionally, exogenous administration of Aβ peptides (multiple peptide-length species of Aβ referred to simply as Aβ) kills neurons *in vitro* through apoptosis (Loo et al., 1993). This effect proceeds through mitochondrial and ER-specific pathways, as overexpression of Bcl-2 or deletion of caspase-12 inhibits Aβ-induced death (Bruce-Keller et al., 1998; Nakagawa et al., 2000). Furthermore, exogenous Aβ directly inhibits mitochondrial oxidative phosphorylation and induces the liberation of ROS (Parks et al., 2001). One intriguing mechanism by which Aβ may induce oxidative damage is through complexing with zinc, which is present in exceedingly high concentration at extracellular, synaptic regions in the cortex. Indeed, both zinc and copper induce the precipitation of Aβ and contribute to the induction of ROS, which increases Aβ aggregation and leads to toxic, extracellular Aβ-containing plaques; elimination of the zinc transporter ZnT3 dramatically reduces the levels of these plaques in a mouse model of AD. Similarly, treatment of AD transgenic mice with clioquinol, a copper/zinc chelator, markedly reduces Aβ plaques and improves behavior (Bush and Tanzi, 2002).

In contrast to these studies, systematic *in vitro* expression of physiologically appropriate amounts of mutant APP, which generates both intracellular and secreted forms of Aβ, *fails* to induce apoptosis but renders neurons more sensitive to oxidative stress-induced insults (Eckert et al., 2003). Higher-level overexpression of either mutant or wild-type APP, however, induces apoptosis *in vitro*, suggesting that Aβ dosage may indeed contribute to toxicity (Niikura et al., 2002). Together, these findings are consistent with two prevailing, but opposing, hypotheses regarding the role of deregulated Aβ: that Aβ is completely sufficient to cause neuronal dysfunction and subsequent apoptosis; or that it is insufficient on its own to cause neuronal death but contributes to oxidative-stress-induced neurodegeneration (Selkoe, 2002; Smith et al., 2002).

Therapies for AD: anti-amyloid

The predominance of therapeutic approaches toward AD rest on the assumption that interference with Aβ aggregation is sufficient to prevent disease pathogenesis, largely because early stage aggregates of Aβ are sufficient to inhibit neuronal dysfunction (Selkoe, 2002). In order to discuss these therapies, it is necessary to briefly describe the molecular mechanisms of Aβ production. The 40–43 peptide-length species of Aβ are generated from APP by the activity of two protease complexes, namely β- and γ-secretases. Presenilin was identified as a critical member of the γ-secretase complex, indicating that mutations in APP near these cleavage sites or in other members of the secretase complex largely determine the expression level, species size and hence toxicity of Aβ (Younkin, 1998). Strategies aimed at reducing such Aβ toxicity therefore include the prevention of these proteolytic activities. An early target was the activity of the γ-secretase itself, but targeted deletion of one known component, presenilin, led to embryonic lethality, suggesting the existence of other γ-secretase substrates critical for early development. In contrast to γ-secretase, the protein BACE-1 appears to completely mediate β-secretase activity, and its genetic inactivation completely eliminates the formation of Aβ and rescues the neuropathologic and neurologic deficits observed in animal models of AD (Ohno et al., 2004). Additional therapeutic strategies aimed at reducing the levels of Aβ include enhancing the activity of a third intracellular protease, known as α-secretase, which produces the secretion of a non-Aβ fragment, and stimulating extracellular proteases that degrade secreted Aβ. Alternatively, agents that alter cholesterol homeostasis and biogenesis have emerged as good candidates to lower extracellular Aβ levels, consistent with reports that identify a genetic variant of apolipoprotein E (ApoE), which is the major cholesterol transporter in the brain, as a major genetic risk factor for AD (Puglielli et al., 2003). Clinical trials using antibodies directed against Aβ, which yielded extraordinary results in animals, have been discontinued in human clinical trials due to the stimulation of toxic levels of inflammation (Nicoll et al., 2003). Finally, because of perturbation of cortical cholinergic systems in AD, nerve growth factor (NGF), which regulates the survival and

maintenance of cortical cholinergic cells, may be an effective therapeutic agent in the disease (Tuszynski and Blesch, 2004). For additional details on the pathogenesis and potential therapeutic approaches to AD, see Volume I, Chapter 31.

Spinal cord injury

Traumatic injury to the spinal cord (SCI) results in the paralysis of at least 15,000 people per year. In addition to the acute loss of neurons and glia observed at the primary site of trauma, a second wave of neuronal and glial apoptosis occurs distal to this site and over the course of several weeks (Keane et al., 2001). This secondary degeneration, occurring predominantly within oligodendrocytes and microglia, results in significant demyelination and Wallerian degeneration of white matter axons whose cell bodies are not affected by the primary mechanical insult, and thus magnifies the injury. Additional complications resulting from SCI include the inhibition of remyelination, re-growth and re-innervation of damaged axons in the CNS, which perpetuates the death process by depriving neurons of trophic support. Whereas acute cell death proceeds through both apoptotic and necrotic pathways, secondary cell death is predominantly apoptotic, based on histologic and molecular analyses. The following sections describe the cellular and molecular events of SCI and suggest potential strategies for therapeutic rescue. Additional clinical discussion can be found in Volume II, Chapter 37.

Pathophysiology of SCI

Animal models developed to mimic the most common forms of SCI include the weight drop method for a blunt impact trauma and spinal cord hemisection or transection. Acute SCI-induced inflammation includes pathologic processes such as invasion by non-resident immune cells (including neutrophils and leukocytes), endothelial activation and damage, edema, release of pro-inflammatory cytokines and prostaglandins, and toxic accumulation of glutamate. Expression within neurons of the glucocorticoid receptor (GR) protein occurs as early as 15 min after injury and is downregulated by 24 h. Similarly, tumor necrosis factor-α (TNF-α), an inflammatory cytokine, is upregulated acutely after injury and maintained for 2 weeks after injury. Additionally, increased levels of fas ligand (fasL) and its receptor (fas) are also detected in neurons and glia 1–3 days after injury (Demjen et al., 2004). Vascular permeability is often compromised after SCI, leading to alterations of the blood-spinal cord barrier and to edema and immunologic invasion. A hallmark cellular reaction to the disruption of vascular permeability is the migration of activated glia around the primary lesion site: the so-called glial scar. Though initiated as a protective mechanism against inflammation, the glial scar prevents the passage through the lesion of damaged axons due to the deposition of a dense matrix of growth-inhibiting proteoglycans (see Volume I, Chapter 22). Damaged axons and glia exhibit degraded structural proteins and myelin within the first hour after SCI (Ray et al., 2003). In addition to the formidable barriers presented by glial scars, the death of oligodendrocytes causes demyelination in a population of CNS axons after SCI, impairing axonal conductance and initiating the process of Wallerian degeneration. Indeed, it was recently demonstrated that a spinal transection results in the apoptosis of corticospinal neurons in the motor cortex (Hains et al., 2003). Finally, the myelin of surviving oligodendrocytes is highly enriched in proteins which inhibit axonal regrowth, such as Nogo, myelin-associated glycoprotein (MAG) and oligodendrocyte myelin glycoprotein (OMG; see Volume I, Chapter 21). Together, these phenomena lead to the devastating destruction of spinal circuits and long-lasting motor dysfunction.

Cell death in SCI

Secondary apoptosis in response to SCI can be divided into an initial 24 h acute phase and a later phase lasting several weeks. Neurons appear to die mostly within the first 24 h, whereas glial apoptosis peaks at 24 h and then again at 7 days (Liu et al., 1997). Glutamate-induced excitotoxicity has emerged as a likely candidate to underlie SCI-induced apoptosis, as large increases of this neurotransmitter are observed very early after SCI, leading to a marked increase in intracellular free calcium. Administration of the α-amino-3-hydroxy-5-methylisoxazole-4-propionic acid (AMPA) receptor antagonist NBQX immediately after injury rescues both oligodendrocyte and neurons and reduces motor deficits (Wrathall et al., 1994). The second peak of oligodendrocyte apoptosis is also regulated by signaling through the TNF-α receptor superfamily member p75, whose expression in the spinal cord is initiated 5 days after SCI; genetic elimination of this receptor greatly reduces oligodendrocyte apoptosis. The pro-apoptotic ligand for p75, proNGF, appears within meningeal tissue and activated astrocytes of the glial scar (Beattie et al., 2002).

Excess glutamate may induce acute secondary apoptosis through excess intracellular calcium, disrupted mitochondrial function and ROS production. Alternatively, macrophage-derived nitric oxide may initiate cell death through similar mechanisms after SCI. Indeed, intraspinally administered peroxynitrite, an ROS induced by elevated nitric oxide signaling, is sufficient to induce neuronal caspase-3 activation and death (Bao and Liu, 2003). Other calcium-activated degenerative events after SCI include the cleavage of cytoskeletal proteins and myelin by the calpain proteases (Ray et al., 2003). Additionally, activity of the calcium-dependent phosphatase calcineurin is required for the translocation of pro-apoptotic Bcl-2 family members to the mitochondrion (Springer et al., 2000). Finally, expression of fasL and activation of caspase-8 suggest a potential contribution to apoptosis from this extrinsic cell death pathway (Demjen et al., 2004). Together, these upstream events initiate the activation of the executor caspases-3 and -9, which bring about the demise of the cell through the inactivation of the inhibitors of apoptosis (IAPs) (Keane et al., 2001).

Therapy of SCI

High doses of the steroid methylprednisolone, delivered within 8 h post-injury and lasting for 24–48 h, is currently the only approved pharmacologic therapy for human SCI. Early treatment with glucocorticoids reduces TNF-α secretion, NF-κb activation and secondary apoptosis. Antibody treatment targeting fasL but not TNF-α dramatically reduces secondary apoptosis and preserves motor function in spinal cord-injured mice (Demjen et al., 2004). Agents inhibiting the vascular pathway also attenuate SCI-induced apoptosis and damage (Akiyama et al., 2003). Administration of drugs which reduce calpain activity prevent the proteolysis of myelin and NFs, reduce apoptosis and ameliorate motor dysfunction (Ray et al., 2003). Trophic stimulation with gene-based therapies promotes regeneration and reduces apoptosis (see Volume I, Chapter 29). Inhibition of the pro-apoptotic Bcl-2 protein bax reduces the retraction and Wallerian degeneration of axons after the injury and thereby reduces oligondendrocyte apoptosis (Dong et al., 2003). Finally, pharmacologic inhibition of caspases fails to attenuate SCI-induced degeneration (Ozawa et al., 2002). Strategies aimed not at preventing apoptosis but rather at preventing demyelination and growth inhibition have shown that proteoglycan protease treatment permits axons to enter and cross the lesion and re-establish functional circuits (see Volume I, Chapter 22). Similarly, an ionic treatment aimed at inhibiting the efflux of potassium from demyelinated axons has proven therapeutic (Hayes et al., 2003). Finally, the intrinsically non-permissive environment of post-injury glia and myelin can be surmounted by experimental elevation of an intracellular signaling molecule, cAMP (see Volume I, Chapters 21 and 24). If initiated promptly, combinations of these different approaches to inhibit apoptosis, demyelination and growth inhibition may be sufficient to restore function after SCI.

16.3 Conclusion

In the 30 years since the term apoptosis was coined by Kerr et al. (1972), numerous advances have been made into the molecular pathways underlying this process during neuronal development. Many, if not all, of these pathways appear to serve the same purpose during the course of disease and injury, thus begging the obvious question: are anti-apoptotic therapeutic measures, including NTFs, sufficient to ameliorate these pathologies? At least for the neurodegenerative diseases, it appears that the simple answer is no; inhibition of bax translocation or caspase activation, although it does delay disease progression, is generally insufficient to stave off the inexorable onslaught of auxiliary molecular death processes which eventually compensate for the inhibition of these pathways and kill the cell. Similarly, the addition of generic anti-oxidants at best delays but does not prevent disease, despite clear evidence for the presence of oxidative stress. This then leads to the viewpoint that the most suitable effective strategy to combat neurodegeneration is through manipulation of the most upstream molecular events (Selkoe, 2002). While this is undoubtedly the most sound approach from a logical perspective, should the "most upstream event" reach consensus, it need not be the only technique to guide neuro-restorative strategies aimed at preserving function. For example, although no link exists between pathologically reduced GDNF signaling or GDNF receptor expression and the onset of PD pathogenesis, treatment with this NTF improves motor function in patients with PD (Kirik et al., 2004). Whether this enhancement occurs through the ability of GDNF to prevent apoptosis or induce new growth and innervation is unclear; nevertheless, it represents a therapeutic strategy completely separable from those aimed directly at disaggregating α-synuclein or reducing oxidative stress. In contrast to apoptosis occurring during disease, cell death after traumatic injury such as SCI may greatly benefit from the inhibition of canonical apoptotic pathways, which are activated after a fairly well-defined sequence of events. However, the additional problem of restoring neuronal connectivity must also be solved in conjunction with the inhibition of apoptosis. In conclusion, therefore, it seems that anti-apoptotic agents, including NTFs, will be necessary but not exclusive components of any effective therapy for neurodegenerative disease and neuronal injury.

ACKNOWLEDGEMENTS

We would like to acknowledge the many primary research contributions which we were not able to cite in this chapter. Where possible, we cited reviews from the same laboratories from which the original reports were made.

REFERENCES

Akiyama, C., Yuguchi, T., Nishio, M., Fujinaka, T., Taniguchi, M., Nakajima, Y. and Yoshimine, T. (2003). Src family kinase inhibitor PP1 improves motor function by reducing edema after spinal cord contusion in rats. *Acta Neurochir Suppl*, **86**, 421–423.

Al-Chalabi, A., Andersen, P.M., Nilsson, P., Chioza, B., Andersson, J.L., Russ, C., Shaw, C.E., Powell, J.F. and Leigh, P.N. (1999). Deletions of the heavy neurofilament subunit tail in amyotrophic lateral sclerosis. *Hum Mol Genet*, **8**, 157–164.

Bao, F. and Liu, D. (2003). Peroxynitrite generated in the rat spinal cord induces apoptotic cell death and activates caspase-3. *Neuroscience*, **116**, 59–70.

Bar-Peled, O. and Rothstein, J.D. (1999). Antiglutamate therapies for neurodegenerative disease: the case of amyotrophic lateral sclerosis. In: *Cell Death and Diseases of the Nervous System* (eds Koliatsos, V. and Ratan, R.), Humana Press, Totowa, NJ, pp. 633–647.

Beal, M.F. (2001). Experimental models of Parkinson's disease. *Nat Rev Neurosci*, **2**, 325–334.

Beattie, M.S., Harrington, A.W., Lee, R., Kim, J.Y., Boyce, S.L., Longo, F.M., Bresnahan, J.C., Hempstead, B.L. and Yoon, S.O. (2002). ProNGF induces p75-mediated death of oligodendrocytes following spinal cord injury. *Neuron*, **36**, 375–386.

Behl, C. (2000). Apoptosis and Alzheimer's disease. *J Neural Transm*, **107**, 1325–1344.

Ben-Sasson, S.A., Sherman, Y. and Gavrieli, Y. (1995). Identification of dying cells – in situ staining. *Methods Cell Biol*, **46**, 29–39.

Brown Jr., R.H. (1995). Amyotrophic lateral sclerosis: recent insights from genetics and transgenic mice. *Cell*, **80**, 687–692.

Bruce-Keller, A.J., Begley, J.G., Fu, W., Butterfield, D.A., Bredesen, D.E., Hutchins, J.B., Hensley, K. and Mattson, M.P. (1998). Bcl-2 protects isolated plasma and mitochondrial membranes against lipid peroxidation induced by hydrogen peroxide and amyloid beta-peptide. *J Neurochem*, **70**, 31–39.

Burke, R.E. and Kholodilov, N.G. (1998). Programmed cell death: does it play a role in Parkinson's disease? *Ann Neurol*, **44**, S126–S133.

Bush, A.I. and Tanzi, R.E. (2002). The galvanization of beta-amyloid in Alzheimer's disease. *Proc Natl Acad Sci USA*, **99**, 7317–7319.

Cameron, H.A. and McKay, R.D. (2001). Adult neurogenesis produces a large pool of new granule cells in the dentate gyrus. *J Comp Neurol*, **435**, 406–417.

Clarke, P.G. (1990). Developmental cell death: morphological diversity and multiple mechanisms. *Anat Embryol (Berlin)*, **181**, 195–213.

Clarke, P.G. and Clarke, S. (1996). Nineteenth century research on naturally occurring cell death and related phenomena. *Anat Embryol (Berlin)*, **193**, 81–99.

Clement, A.M., Nguyen, M.D., Roberts, E.A., Garcia, M.L., Boillee, S., Rule, M., McMahon, A.P., Doucette, W., Siwek, D., Ferrante, R.J., Brown Jr., R.H., Julien, J.P., Goldstein, L.S. and Cleveland, D.W. (2003). Wild-type nonneuronal cells extend survival of SOD1 mutant motor neurons in ALS mice. *Science*, **302**, 113–117.

Cleveland, D.W. (1999). From Charcot to SOD1: mechanisms of selective motor neuron death in ALS. *Neuron*, **24**, 515–520.

Conway, K.A., Rochet, J.C., Bieganski, R.M. and Lansbury Jr., P.T. (2001). Kinetic stabilization of the alpha-synuclein protofibril by a dopamine-alpha-synuclein adduct. *Science*, **294**, 1346–1349.

Cookson, M. (2003). Neurodegeneration: how does parkin prevent Parkinson's disease? *Curr Biol*, **13**, R522–R524.

Dauer, W., Kholodilov, N., Vila, M., Trillat, A.C., Goodchild, R., Larsen, K.E., Staal, R., Tieu, K., Schmitz, Y., Yuan, C.A., Rocha, M., Jackson-Lewis, V., Hersch, S., Sulzer, D., Przedborski, S., Burke, R. and Hen, R. (2002). Resistance of alpha-synuclein null mice to the parkinsonian neurotoxin MPTP. *Proc Natl Acad Sci USA*, **99**, 14524–14529.

Demjen, D., Klussmann, S., Kleber, S., Zuliani, C., Stieltjes, B., Metzger, C., Hirt, U.A., Walczak, H., Falk, W., Essig, M., Edler, L., Krammer, P.H. and Martin-Villalba, A. (2004). Neutralization of CD95 ligand promotes regeneration and functional recovery after spinal cord injury. *Nat Med*, epub, March 7.

Dong, H., Fazzaro, A., Xiang, C., Korsmeyer, S.J., Jacquin, M.F. and McDonald, J.W. (2003). Enhanced oligodendrocyte survival after spinal cord injury in Bax-deficient mice and mice with delayed Wallerian degeneration. *J Neurosci*, **23**, 8682–8691.

Duan, W., Guo, Z., Jiang, H., Ware, M., Li, X.J. and Mattson, M.P. (2003). Dietary restriction normalizes glucose metabolism and BDNF levels, slows disease progression, and increases survival in huntingtin mutant mice. *Proc Natl Acad Sci USA*, **100**, 2911–2916.

Eckert, A., Keil, U., Marques, C.A., Bonert, A., Frey, C., Schussel, K. and Muller, W.E. (2003). Mitochondrial dysfunction, apoptotic cell death, and Alzheimer's disease. *Biochem Pharmacol*, **66**, 1627–1634.

Elliott, J.L. and Snider, W.D. (1999). Axotomy-induced motor neuron death. In: *Cell Death and Diseases of the Nervous System* (eds Koliatsos, V. and Ratan, R.), Humana Press, Totowa, NJ, pp. 181–195.

Eriksen, J.L., Dawson, T.M., Dickson, D.W. and Petrucelli, L. (2003). Caught in the act: alpha-synuclein is the culprit in Parkinson's disease. *Neuron*, **40**, 453–456.

Feany, M.B. and Bender, W.W. (2000). A *Drosophila* model of Parkinson's disease. *Nature*, **404**, 394–398.

Feany, M.B. and La Spada, A.R. (2003). Polyglutamines stop traffic: axonal transport as a common target in neurodegenerative diseases. *Neuron*, **40**, 1–2.

Frey, D., Schneider, C., Xu, L., Borg, J., Spooren, W. and Caroni, P. (2000). Early and selective loss of neuromuscular synapse subtypes with low sprouting competence in motoneuron diseases. *J Neurosci*, **20**, 2534–2542.

Gafni, J., Hermel, E., Young, J.E., Wellington, C.L., Hayden, M.R. and Ellerby, L.M. (2004). Inhibition of calpain cleavage of huntingtin reduces toxicity: accumulation of calpain/caspase fragments in the nucleus. *J Biol Chem*, epub, February 23.

Gervais, F.G., Xu, D., Robertson, G.S., Vaillancourt, J.P., Zhu, Y., Huang, J., LeBlanc, A., Smith, D., Rigby, M., Shearman, M.S., Clarke, E.E., Zheng, H., Van Der Ploeg, L.H., Ruffolo, S.C., Thornberry, N.A., Xanthoudakis, S., Zamboni, R.J., Roy, S. and Nicholson, D.W. (1999). Involvement of caspases in proteolytic cleavage of Alzheimer's amyloid-beta precursor protein and amyloidogenic A beta peptide formation. *Cell*, **97**, 395–406.

Grünewald, T. and Beal, M.F. (1999). Bioenergetics in Huntington's disease. *Ann NY Acad Sci*, **893**, 203–213.

Guégan, C., Vila, M., Rosoklija, G., Hays, A.P. and Przedborski, S. (2001). Recruitment of the mitochondrial-dependent apoptotic pathway in amyotrophic lateral sclerosis. *J Neurosci*, **21**, 6569–6576.

Hafezparast, M., Ahmad-Annuar, A., Hummerich, H., Shah, P., Ford, M., Baker, C., Bowen, S., Martin, J.E. and Fisher, E.M. (2003). Paradigms for the identification of new genes in motor neuron degeneration. *Amyotroph Lateral Scler Other Motor Neuron Disord*, **4**, 249–257.

Hains, B.C., Black, J.A. and Waxman, S.G. (2003). Primary cortical motor neurons undergo apoptosis after axotomizing spinal cord injury. *J Comp Neurol*, **462**, 328–341.

Hayes, K.C., Katz, M.A., Devane, J.G., Hsieh, J.T., Wolfe, D.L., Potter, P.J. and Blight, A.R. (2003). Pharmacokinetics of an immediate-release oral formulation of fampridine (4-aminopyridine) in normal subjects and patients with spinal cord injury. *J Clin Pharmacol*, **43**, 379–385.

Hengartner, M.O. (2000). The biochemistry of apoptosis. *Nature*, **407**, 770–776.

Hilt, D.C., Miller, J.A. and Malta, E. (1999). Early experiences with trophic factors as drugs for neurological disease: brain-derived neurotrophic factor and ciliary neurotrophic factor for ALS. In: *Cell Death and Diseases of the Nervous System* (eds Koliatsos, V. and Ratan, R.), Humana Press, Totowa, NJ, pp. 593–607.

Humbert, S., Bryson, E.A., Cordelieres, F.P., Connors, N.C., Datta, S.R., Finkbeiner, S., Greenberg, M.E. and Saudou, F. (2002). The IGF-1/Akt pathway is neuroprotective in Huntington's disease and involves huntingtin phosphorylation by Akt. *Dev Cell*, **2**, 831–837.

The Huntington's Disease Collaborative Research Group (1993). A novel gene containing a trinucleotide repeat that is expanded and unstable on Huntington's disease chromosomes. *Cell*, **72**, 971–983.

Ikonomidou, C., Bittigau, P., Koch, C., Genz, K., Hoerster, F., Felderhoff-Mueser, U., Tenkova, T., Dikranian, K. and Olney, J.W. (2001). Neurotransmitters and apoptosis in the developing brain. *Biochem Pharmacol*, **4**, 401–405.

Jana, N.R., Zemskov, E.A., Wang, G.H. and Nukina, N. (2001). Altered proteasomal function due to the expression of polyglutamine-expanded truncated N-terminal huntingtin induces apoptosis by caspase activation through mitochondrial cytochrome c release. *Hum Mol Genet*, **10**, 1049–1059.

Jenner, P. (1998). Oxidative mechanisms in nigral cell death in Parkinson's disease. *Mov Disord*, **13**(1), 24–34.

Julien, J.P. (1999). Neurofilament functions in health and disease. *Curr Opin Neurobiol*, **9**, 554–560.

Kang, S.J., Sanchez, I., Jing, N. and Yuan, J. (2003). Dissociation between neurodegeneration and caspase-11-mediated activation of caspase-1 and caspase-3 in a mouse model of amyotrophic lateral sclerosis. *J Neurosci*, **23**, 5455–5460.

Kaspar, B.K., Llado, J., Sherkat, N., Rothstein, J.D. and Gage, F.H. (2003). Retrograde viral delivery of IGF-1 prolongs survival in a mouse ALS model. *Science*, **301**, 839–842.

Kawahara, Y., Ito, K., Sun, H., Aizawa, H., Kanazawa, I. and Kwak, S. (2004). Glutamate receptors: RNA editing and death of motor neurons. *Nature*, **427**, 801.

Keane, R.W., Kraydieh, S., Lotocki, G., Bethea, J.R., Krajewski, S., Reed, J.C. and Dietrich, W.D. (2001). Apoptotic and anti-apoptotic mechanisms following spinal cord injury. *J Neuropathol Exp Neurol*, **60**, 422–429.

Kerr, J.F., Wyllie, A.H. and Currie, A.R. (1972). Apoptosis: a basic biological phenomenon with wide-ranging implications in tissue kinetics. *Brit J Cancer*, **26**, 239–257.

Kim, Y.J., Yi, Y., Sapp, E., Wang, Y., Cuiffo, B., Kegel, K.B., Qin, Z.H., Aronin, N. and DiFiglia, M. (2001). Caspase 3-cleaved N-terminal fragments of wild-type and mutant huntingtin are present in normal and Huntington's disease brains, associate with membranes, and undergo calpain-dependent proteolysis. *Proc Natl Acad Sci USA*, **98**, 12784–12789.

Kirik, D., Georgievska, B. and Björklund, A. (2004). Localized striatal delivery of GDNF as a treatment for Parkinson's disease. *Nat Neurosci*, **7**, 105–110.

Kriz, J., Gowing, G. and Julien, J.P. (2003). Efficient three-drug cocktail for disease induced by mutant superoxide dismutase. *Ann Neurol*, **53**, 429–436.

Leist, M. and Jäättelä, M. (2001). Four deaths and a funeral: from caspases to alternative mechanisms. *Nat Rev Mol Cell Biol*, **2**, 589–598.

Liu, X.Z., Xu, X.M., Hu, R., Du, C., Zhang, S.X., McDonald, J.W., Dong, H.X., Wu, Y.J., Fan, G.S., Jacquin, M.F., Hsu, C.Y. and Choi, D.W. (1997). Neuronal and glial apoptosis after traumatic spinal cord injury. *J Neurosci*, **17**, 5395–5406.

Loo, D.T., Copani, A., Pike, C.J., Whittemore, E.R., Walencewicz, A.J. and Cotman, C.W. (1993). Apoptosis is induced by beta-amyloid in cultured central nervous system neurons. *Proc Natl Acad Sci USA*, **90**, 7951–7955.

Lotharius, J. and Brundin P. (2003). Pathogenesis of Parkinson's disease: dopamine, vesicles and alpha-synuclein. *Nat Rev Neurosci*, **3**, 932–942.

Mantamadiotis, T., Lemberger, T., Bleckmann, S.C., Kern, H., Kretz, O., Martin Villalba, A., Tronche, F., Kellendonk, C., Gau, D., Kapfhammer, J., Otto, C., Schmid, W. and Schutz, G. (2002). Disruption of CREB function in brain leads to neurodegeneration. *Nat Genet*, **31**, 47–54.

Maries, E., Dass, B., Collier, T.J., Kordower, J.H. and Steece-Collier, K. (2003). The role of alpha-synuclein in Parkinson's disease: insights from animal models. *Nat Rev Neurosci*, **4**, 727–738.

Martindale, D., Hackam, A., Wieczorek, A., Ellerby, L., Wellington, C., McCutcheon, K., Singaraja, R., Kazemi-Esfarjani, P., Devon, R., Kim, S.U., Bredesen, D.E., Tufaro, F. and Hayden, M.R. (1998). Length of huntingtin and its polyglutamine tract influences localization and frequency of intracellular aggregates. *Nat Genet*, **18**, 150–154.

Nakagawa, T., Zhu, H., Morishima, N., Li, E., Xu, J., Yankner, B.A. and Yuan, J. (2000). Caspase-12 mediates endoplasmic-reticulum-specific apoptosis and cytotoxicity by amyloid-beta. *Nature*, **403**, 98–103.

Nicoll, J.A., Wilkinson, D., Holmes, C., Steart, P., Markham, H. and Weller, R.O. (2003). Neuropathology of human Alzheimer disease after immunization with amyloid-beta peptide: a case report. *Nat Med*, **9**, 448–452.

Niikura, T., Hashimoto, Y., Tajima, H. and Nishimoto, I. (2002). Death and survival of neuronal cells exposed to Alzheimer's insults. *J Neurosci Res*, **70**, 380–391.

Ohno, M., Sametsky, E.A., Younkin, L.H., Oakley, H., Younkin, S.G., Citron, M., Vassar, R. and Disterhoft, J.F. (2004). BACE1 deficiency rescues memory deficits and cholinergic dysfunction in a mouse model of Alzheimer's disease. *Neuron*, **41**, 27–33.

Olney, J.W. and Ishimaru, M.J. (1999). Excitotoxic cell death. In: *Cell Death and Diseases of the Nervous System* (eds Koliatsos, V. and Ratan, R.), Humana Press, Totowa, NJ, pp. 197–219.

Oosthuyse, B., Moons, L., Storkebaum, E., Beck, H., Nuyens, D., Brusselmans, K., Van Dorpe, J., Hellings, P., Gorselink, M., Heymans, S., Theilmeier, G., Dewerchin, M., Laudenbach, V., Vermylen, P., Raat, H., Acker, T., Vleminckx, V., Van Den Bosch, L., Cashman, N., Fujisawa, H., Drost, M.R., Sciot, R., Bruyninckx, F., Hicklin, D.J., Ince, C., Gressens, P., Lupu, F., Plate, K.H., Robberecht, W., Herbert, J.M., Collen, D. and Carmeliet, P. (2001). Deletion of the hypoxia-response element in the vascular endothelial growth factor promoter causes motor neuron degeneration. *Nat Genet*, **28**, 131–138.

Ona, V.O., Li, M., Vonsattel, J.P., Andrews, L.J., Khan, S.Q., Chung, W.M., Frey, A.S., Menon, A.S., Li, X.J., Stieg, P.E., Yuan, J., Penney, J.B., Young, A.B., Cha, J.H. and Friedlander, R.M. (1999). Inhibition of caspase-1 slows disease progression in a mouse model of Huntington's disease. *Nature*, **399**, 263–267.

Oppenheim, R.W. (1991). Cell death during development of the nervous system. *Annu Rev Neurosci*, **14**, 453–501.

Oppenheim, R.W. and Johnson, J.E. (2003). Programmed cell death and neurotrophic factors. In: *Fundamental Neuroscience* (eds Zigmond, M.J., Bloom, F.E., Landis, S.C., Roberts, J.L. and Squire, L.R.), 2nd edn., Academic Press, San Diego, CA, pp. 499–531.

Ozawa, H., Keane, R.W., Marcillo, A.E., Diaz, P.H. and Dietrich, W.D. (2002). Therapeutic strategies targeting caspase inhibition following spinal cord injury in rats. *Exp Neurol*, **177**, 306–313.

Panov, A.V., Gutekunst, C.A., Leavitt, B.R., Hayden, M.R., Burke, J.R., Strittmatter, W.J. and Greenamyre, J.T. (2002). Early mitochondrial calcium defects in Huntington's disease are a direct effect of polyglutamines. *Nat Neurosci*, **5**, 731–736.

Parks, J.K., Smith, T.S., Trimmer, P.A., Bennett Jr., J.P. and Parker Jr., W.D. (2001). Neurotoxic A3 peptides increase oxidative stress *in vivo* through NMDA-receptor and nitric-oxide-synthase mechanisms, and inhibit complex IV activity and induce a mitochondrial permeability transition *in vitro*. *J Neurochem*, **76**, 1050–1056.

Pettmann, B. and Henderson, C.E. (1998). Neuronal cell death. *Neuron*, **20**, 633–647.

Portera-Cailliau, C., Hedreen, J.C., Price, D.L. and Koliatsos, V.E. (1995). Evidence for apoptotic cell death in Huntington disease and excitotoxic animal models. *J Neurosci*, **15**, 3775–3787.

Puglielli, L., Tanzi, R.E. and Kovacs, D.M. (2003). Alzheimer's disease: the cholesterol connection. *Nat Neurosci*, **6**, 345–351.

Raff, M.C. (1992). Social controls on cell survival and cell death. *Nature*, **356**, 397–400.

Raoul, C., Pettmann, B. and Henderson, C.E. (2000). Active killing of neurons during development and following stress: a role for p75 (NTR) and Fas? *Curr Opin Neurobiol*, **10**, 111–117.

Ray, S.K., Hogan, E.L. and Banik, N.L. (2003). Calpain in the pathophysiology of spinal cord injury: neuroprotection with calpain inhibitors. *Brain Res Brain Res Rev*, **42**, 169–185.

Savill, J., Gregory, C. and Haslett, C. (2003). Cell biology. Eat me or die. *Science*, **302**, 1516–1517.

Selkoe, D.J. (2002). Alzheimer's disease is a synaptic failure. *Science*, **298**, 789–791.

Singleton, A.B., Farrer, M., Johnson, J., Singleton, A., Hague, S., Kachergus, J., Hulihan, M., Peuralinna, T., Dutra, A., Nussbaum, R., Lincoln, S., Crawley, A., Hanson, M., Maraganore, D., Adler, C., Cookson, M.R., Muenter, M., Baptista, M., Miller, D., Blancato, J., Hardy, J. and Gwinn-Hardy, K. (2003). Alpha-synuclein locus triplication causes Parkinson's disease. *Science*, **302**, 841.

Smith, M.A., Drew, K.L., Nunomura, A., Takeda, A., Hirai, K., Zhu, X., Atwood, C.S., Raina, A.K., Rottkamp, C.A., Sayre, L.M., Friedland, R.P. and Perry, G. (2002). Amyloid-beta, tau alterations and mitochondrial dysfunction in Alzheimer disease: the chickens or the eggs? *Neurochem Int*, **40**, 527–531.

Spires, T.L., Grote, H.E., Varshney, N.K., Cordery, P.M., van Dellen, A., Blakemore, C. and Hannan, A.J. (2004). Environmental enrichment rescues protein deficits in a mouse model of Huntington's disease, indicating a possible disease mechanism. *J Neurosci*, **24**, 2270–2276.

Springer, J.E., Azbill, R.D., Nottingham, S.A. and Kennedy, S.E. (2000). Calcineurin-mediated BAD dephosphorylation activates the caspase-3 apoptotic cascade in traumatic spinal cord injury. *J Neurosci*, **20**, 7246–7251.

Steffan, J.S., Bodai, L., Pallos, J., Poelman, M., McCampbell, A., Apostol, B.L., Kazantsev, A., Schmidt, E., Zhu, Y.Z., Greenwald, M., Kurokawa, R., Housman, D.E., Jackson, G.R., Marsh, J.L. and Thompson, L.M. (2001). Histone deacetylase inhibitors arrest polyglutamine-dependent neurodegeneration in *Drosophila*. *Nature*, **413**, 739–743.

Sun, W., Funakoshi, H. and Nakamura, T. (2002). Overexpression of HGF retards disease progression and prolongs life span in a transgenic mouse model of ALS. *J Neurosci*, **22**, 6537–6548.

Sun, W., Winseck, A., Vinsant, S., Park, O., Kim, H. and Oppenheim, R.W. (2004). Programmed cell death of adult-generated hippocampus neurons is medated by the pro-apoptotic gene bod. *J Neurosci*, **24**, 11205–11213.

Syntichaki, P. and Tavernarakis, N. (2003). The biochemistry of neuronal necrosis: rogue biology? *Nat Rev Neurosci*, **4**, 672–684.

Tang, T.S., Tu, H., Chan, E.Y., Maximov, A., Wang, Z., Wellington, C.L., Hayden, M.R. and Bezprozvanny, I. (2003). Huntingtin and Huntingtin-associated protein 1 influence neuronal calcium signaling mediated by inositol-(1,4,5) triphosphate receptor type 1. *Neuron*, **39**, 227–239.

Tuszynski, M.H. and Blesch, A. (2004). Nerve growth factor: from animal models of cholinergic neuronal degeneration to gene therapy in Alzheimer's disease. *Prog Brain Res*, **146**, 441–449.

Valentine, J.S. (2002). Do oxidatively modified proteins cause ALS? *Free Radic Biol Med*, **33**, 1314–1320.

Vila, M. and Przedborski, S. (2003). Targeting programmed cell death in neuro-degenerative diseases. *Nat Rev Neurosci*, **4**, 365–375.

Volles, M.J., Lee, S.J., Rochet, J.C., Shtilerman, M.D., Ding, T.T., Kessler, J.C. and Lansbury Jr., P.T. (2001). Vesicle permeabilization by protofibrillar alpha-synuclein: implications for the pathogenesis and treatment of Parkinson's disease. *Biochemistry*, **40**, 7812–7819.

Wang, L.J., Lu, Y.Y., Muramatsu, S., Ikeguchi, K., Fujimoto, K., Okada, T., Mizukami, H., Matsushita, T., Hanazono, Y., Kume, A., Nagatsu, T., Ozawa, K. and Nakano, I. (2002). Neuroprotective effects of glial cell line-derived neurotrophic factor mediated by an adeno-associated virus vector in a transgenic animal model of amyotrophic lateral sclerosis. *J Neurosci*, **22**, 6920–6928.

Wellington, C.L., Ellerby, L.M., Gutekunst, C.A., Rogers, D., Warby, S., Graham, R.K., Loubser, O., van Raamsdonk, J., Singaraja, R., Yang, Y.Z., Gafni, J., Bredesen, D., Hersch, S.M., Leavitt, B.R., Roy, S., Nicholson, D.W. and Hayden, M.R. (2002). Caspase cleavage of mutant huntingtin precedes neurodegeneration in Huntington's disease. *J Neurosci*, **22**, 7862–7872.

Wrathall, J.R., Choiniere, D. and Teng, Y.D. (1994). Dose-dependent reduction of tissue loss and functional impairment after spinal cord trauma with the AMPA/kainate antagonist NBQX. *J Neurosci*, **14**, 6598–6607.

Wu, D.C., Jackson-Lewis, V., Vila, M., Tieu, K., Teismann, P., Vadseth, C., Choi, D.K., Ischiropoulos, H. and Przedborski, S. (2002). Blockade of microglial activation is neuroprotective in the 1-methyl-4-phenyl-1,2,3,6-tetrahydropyridine mouse model of Parkinson disease. *J Neurosci*, **22**, 1763–1771.

Xu, J., Kao, S.Y., Lee, F.J., Song, W., Jin, L.W. and Yankner, B.A. (2002). Dopamine-dependent neurotoxicity of alpha-synuclein: a mechanism for selective neurodegeneration in Parkinson disease. *Nat Med*, **8**, 600–606.

Yaginuma, H., Tomita, M., Takashita, N., McKay, S.E., Cardwell, C., Yin, Q.W. and Oppenheim, R.W. (1996). A novel type of programmed neuronal death in the cervical spinal cord of the chick embryo. *J Neurosci*, **16**, 3685–3703.

Younkin, S.G. (1998). The role of Aβ42 in Alzheimer's disease. *J Physiol Paris*, **92**, 289–292.

Yuan, J. and Yankner, B.A. (2000). Apoptosis in the nervous system. *Nature*, **407**, 802–809.

Zhang, W., Narayanan, M. and Friedlander, R.M. (2003). Additive neuroprotective effects of minocycline with creatine in a mouse model of ALS. *Ann Neurol*, **53**, 267–270.

Zuccato, C., Tartari, M., Crotti, A., Goffredo, D., Valenza, M., Conti, L., Cataudella, T., Leavitt, B.R., Hayden, M.R., Timmusk, T., Rigamonti, D. and Cattaneo, E. (2003). Huntingtin interacts with REST/NRSF to modulate the transcription of NRSE-controlled neuronal genes. *Nat Genet*, **35**, 76–83.

Axon degeneration and rescue

John W. Griffin, Ahmet Höke and Thien T. Nguyen

Departments of Neurology and Neuroscience, Johns Hopkins University, School of Medicine, Baltimore, MD, USA

17.1 Introduction

In the mid-19th century Augustus Waller found that the distal stump of a severed axon underwent degeneration, while the axon proximal to the site of injury survived (Waller, 1850). Waller's seminal contribution was made in England only 2 years after Schleiden and Schwann articulated the cell theory in 1848. It had previously been recognized that following transection of a nerve, the muscles were paralyzed. Waller brought to such experiments the advent of microscopy. In the frog hypoglossal nerve he observed that distal to the site of section the fibers survived for only a few days, then degenerated so that the "axis cylinders" – the axons – disappeared (Waller, 1850). Proximal to the site of section they survived.

Implicit in the findings of Waller the idea that the nerve cell body is a nutritive source for the axon, without which the axon can only survive for short periods. This observation identified the nerve cell body as the "nourishing mother" of a dependent axon, and suggested that the separation of the severed axon from the cell body resulted in passive starvation of the axon. Waller's inferences have proved largely correct: most macromolecular synthesis occurs largely in the nerve cell body, so that the axon is largely a metabolically dependent structure. Yet the inescapable lesson of the last two decades of research is that Wallerian degeneration is not passive, but an energy-requiring, temperature-sensitive active process of self-destruction, conceptually analogous to apoptotic mechanisms of cell death (see Volume I, Chapter 16). The destruction of the axon sets in motion a cascade of alterations in cell–cell interactions that are integral to the later stages of Wallerian degeneration, and that set the stage for the possibility of regeneration.

Subtler insults than axotomy can ultimately engage the axon death cascade. Early pathologists studying peripheral nerve diseases observed that the distal regions of long fibers often degenerate first and "die back" over time. They ascribed this pattern to the distance of the ends of long fibers from the cell body. Today an open question is whether all axonal degeneration follows the same cascade of changes seen in Wallerian degeneration after axonal transection. That is, are chronic axonal degenerations such as dying back, axonal degeneration after ischemic/anoxic injury, axonal degeneration in demyelination, and axonal degeneration in disorders of axonal transport all fundamentally the same? We will review the sequence of changes in Wallerian degeneration after transection, and suggest that the late stages are similar in all of these disorders.

17.2 Wallerian degeneration

Immediately distal to the site of transection the pathology represents the consequence of the focal interruption of retrograde axonal transport (Zelena et al., 1968; Ranish and Ochs, 1972; Griffin et al., 1977). The axons develop swellings containing densely packed accumulations of mitochondria, dense bodies and multivesicular bodies. In settings where interrupted axons survive for long periods, such as the *Wlds* (*W*allerian-*l*ike *d*egeneration *s*low) mouse that is discussed below, there is also an accumulation of neurofilaments (Glass and Griffin, 1991). Neurofilament proteins were initially recognized to move in the slow anterograde phase of axonal transport (Hoffman and Lasek, 1975; Hirokawa, 1984). The morphologic observation of slow neurofilament accumulation at the proximal end of the distal stump is consistent with data indicating that neurofilament proteins can undergo slow retrograde transport (Glass and Griffin, 1991).

From the time of axonal transection until onset of axonal breakdown is a period termed the latent phase. During this time the axonal structure is nearly normal (Ballin and Thomas, 1969), axonal transport continues at normal rates and roughly normal abundance (Ranish and Ochs, 1972; Lubinska and Niemierko, 1977), and nerve conduction velocities and the amplitudes remain nearly normal. The duration of the latent phase varies with the species, the length of distal stump (longer with a longer stump (Miledi and Slater, 1970; Lubinska, 1982)), the temperature (longer in cooler distal stump (Cancalon, 1985; Tsao et al., 1999)), and possibly the location (peripheral versus central nervous system.

After the initial latent period axonal breakdown generally begins in the axonal terminal and also near the site of transection. From this latter site it moves distally down the nerve with time (Lubinska, 1977; Lubinska, 1982; Cancalon, 1983). After lumbar dorsal rhizotomy degeneration of the central process of dorsal root ganglion sensory neurons begins close to the transection and spreads rostrally up the dorsal columns (away from the cell body) at a rate of about 3–7 mm/h (George and Griffin, 1994).

The axon terminals may precede breakdown of the preterminal axon (George and Griffin, 1994). For example, in motor nerve terminals nonquantal and quantal release of acetylcholine persists during a latent period that ranges from less than 24 h in short nerves of the rodent (Miledi and Slater, 1970) to several days in man (Chaudhry et al., 1992). The latent period ends with the abrupt loss of the ability to elicit end plate potentials (epps) by nerve stimulation physiologically and swelling of the terminal

with loss of cytoskeletal elements and particulate organelles morphologically, followed shortly by disappearance of the terminal itself (Miledi and Slater, 1970).

The pivotal morphologic change in axonal breakdown is *granular degeneration of the cytoskeleton*. It consists of conversion of the normal cytoskeleton to granular and amorphous debris. It is the first morphologic change that appears to be irreversible. The development of granular disintegration is abrupt and explosive. Evidence that it is an abrupt "all or none" phenomenon comes from the observation that at any cross sectional level partially degenerated axoplasm is rarely seen. The axolemma and some particulate organelles may remain as morphologic features for short periods after granular degeneration ensues (Franson and Ronnevi, 1984; George and Griffin, 1994). Granular degeneration reflects a rise in intraaxonal calcium and activation of calcium-sensitive proteases, as discussed below.

Calcium and granular degeneration: The onset of granular disintegration of the cytoskeleton is triggered by an increase in intraaxonal calcium concentration, and a consequent activation of the calcium-sensitive proteases, the calpains. The process is delayed by lowering temperature (Cancalon, 1985; Tsao et al., 1999), by maintaining nerves in low concentrations of calcium (Schlaepfer and Bunge, 1973), and by membrane-permeant inhibitors of calpains (Schlaepfer and Micko, 1979; Glass et al., 1994; George et al., 1995). The rise in intraaxonal calcium is due, at least in part, to entry of extracellular calcium (Schlaepfer and Bunge, 1973). This influx of calcium was necessary to activate calpains (calcium-dependent cysteine proteases) and result in granular degradation of the axoplasm (Schlaepfer, 1974; George et al., 1995). Blockage of entry of calcium or of activation of calpains is sufficient to delay the axonal cytoskeletal degradation (Schlaepfer and Hasler, 1979; George et al., 1995).

Reversal of the sodium-calcium exchanger has been shown to underlie calcium entry in ischemic optic nerve (Stys et al., 1990; Stys et al., 1991). The exchanger normally moves one molecule of calcium out of the cell for every three molecules of sodium that enter. In energy deprivation the exchange reverses, so that calcium enters the axon. Some data also suggests that calcium entry may occur via calcium channels, but the status of calcium channels along the axon remains unresolved (Agullo and Garcia, 1992). There is also evidence for a release of calcium from intracellular stores. Ouardouz and colleagues (Ouardouz et al., 2003) showed that in the rat spinal cord dorsal column, ischemia results an increase in intraaxonal calcium levels even in the absence of extracellular calcium. This release of calcium from intracellular stores is blocked by ryanodine. At the initial stages of axonal degeneration, local increases in intraaxonal calcium around endoplasmic reticulum profiles lead to dissolution of neurofilaments. Although this process was initiated by ischemia rather than axonal transection, and therefore might be different than classical Wallerian degeneration, rise in intraaxonal calcium and degradation of neurofilaments is very similar to what happens during granular disintegration of the axon.

Wallerian degeneration is an active process: The concept that the axon depends day-to-day on materials received via axonal transport was implicitly challenged by the increasing data that some proteins can be synthesized within the axon and by observations that axons survive at least for many days in the face of apparently complete blockade of axonal transport. The most dramatic basis for reconsideration was the identification of profoundly retarded Wallerian degeneration in a substrain of mice (C57Bl/Ola, now called *Wlds*) (Lunn et al., 1989; Perry et al., 1990a; Perry et al., 1990b; Glass et al., 1993). In this spontaneously occurring substrain degeneration of the transected axons is significantly slower. In a wild-type animal, transection of the sciatic nerve results in loss of electrical conductivity in the distal portion within a day or two, followed by dissolution of the axoplasm. In contrast, a transected axon in a *Wlds* mouse continues to conduct electricity for up to 2 weeks (Lunn et al., 1989). A dramatic example of the effect of the *Wlds* mutation is in cultured nerve growth factor (NGF)-dependent neurons from which NGF is withdrawn. In wild-type neurons the axon and the neuronal perikaryon

degenerate over the next day. *Wlds* cell bodies degeneratre on a similar time scale, but their axons survive for a few days longer, producing the singular picture of axons living without cell bodies (Deckwerth and Johnson, Jr. 1993).

The *Wlds* mutation in the mouse is an 85-kb tandem triplication on the distal arm of the mouse chromosome 4 that contains a translocation. This encodes a fusion protein that includes 70 amino acids of the ubiquitin fusion degradation protein 2 (*Ufd2*) and a protein identical to human nicotinamide mononucleotide acetyltransferase, *NMNAT*. Overexpression of the latter enzyme appears to be responsible for prolonged axonal survival. This NAD synthetic enzyme is involved in the NAD salvage pathway. NAD in turn is involved in activation of protein deacetylases within the nucleus. Araki and colleagues (2004) have demonstrated that the NAD-dependent acetylase SIRT1 appears to be the target of the increased NAD. The site of action is in the neuronal nucleus. An antibody generated against the N-terminal of the fusion protein gave only a punctate nuclear staining in both the transgenic mouse and the original *Wlds* mouse. There was no accumulation of the fusion protein at the swollen endbulbs of transected axons suggesting that there was no axonal transport of the *Ube4b/NMNAT* fusion protein. Thus the *Wlds* protein, through increased NAD levels, appears to produce deacetylation of transcription factors involved in synthesis of as yet unknown proteins that promote axonal survival. Importantly, this effect could be achieved by increased NAD levels by exogenous administration in neuronal cultures (Araki et al., 2004).

17.3 Distal axonal degeneration (dying back)

Length-dependent axonal neuropathies are prevalent neurologic problems. Causes include diabetic (see Volume II, Chapter 40) polyneuropathy (Dyck et al., 1987), including the painful neuropathy seen with impaired glucose tolerance (IGT), before frank diabetes (Singleton et al., 2001a; Singleton et al.,

2001b; Sumner et al., 2003); the sensory neuropathy of AIDS (So et al., 1990; Blum et al., 1996; Cornblath and McArthur, 1995), neuropathies caused by some neurotoxic drugs including antiretroviral (Cornblath and McArthur, 1995) and some cancer chemotherapeutic agents (Chaudhry et al., 1994), nutitional neuropathies, and many others (Holland et al., 1998; Periquet et al., 1999). All of these disorders are characterized by distally predominant axonal degeneration (here termed "distal axonal degeneration" or DAD). The degeneration of the ends of axons in a long-before-short sequence was termed "dying back" by the father of the field, John Cavanagh at Queens Square in London. It has gone under a series of other names including "central–peripheral distal axonopathy" by Spencer and Schaumburg (Spencer and Schaumburg, 1976), and is clinically recognized as "length-dependent axonal degeneration". In all these terms the implication is that long axons degenerate before short ones, that degeneration begins in the distal-most region of the axon and proceeds proximally with time, and that in dorsal root ganglion (DRG) neurons with processes ascending the dorsal columns, in general, the ends of the peripheral and central processes degenerate roughly synchronously. A fourth element used to be taught – that large-caliber axons degenerate before small-caliber ones (Spencer and Schaumburg, 1976; Spencer and Schaumburg, 1977). Recent studies have proved that concept is often incorrect, because small fibers are involved synchronously or before large fibers in many neuropathies (v.i.).

The pathology of "dying back" was recognized in human nerve and cord diseases in the 19th century. The pathology suggested that the end of the axon was at greatest risk because it was farthest from the cell body. In this view the distal axon might be viewed as the "last field of irrigation". A corollary was that the basis for DAD might be sought in defects in the cell body. A lesson from the past 10 years is that in most of these models the responsible defects appear to be in axonal transport, especially retrograde transport, or related functions. In the mature nervous system most of the growth factors derive from the target of innervation. This finding inverts the "last field of irrigation" concept, suggesting that the *target* is in fact the "alma mater", that the cell body receives this trophic support from the periphery via retrograde transport and translates it into the materials that the axon terminals will receive via anterograde transport.

The importance of defects in axonal transport have become especially clear in genetic disorders where molecules involved in axonal transport have been responsible for human length-dependent neuropathies. Abnormalities in the retrograde motor system, based on dynein, have been identified, including predominantly motor neuropathies associated with abnormalities in dynamitin and dynamin. In hereditary spastic paraparesis (HSP) one of the identified mutatuions is in spastin, an ATPase associated with microtubule severing. One of the most frequent causes of axonal Charcot–Marie-tooth disease, a dominantly inherited DAD, is a mutation in mitofusin-2, a gene involved in mitochondrial fusion. Fusion is likely to be important in renewal of transported mitochondria in axons.

Deficiency in growth factors leads to a reprogramming of perikaryal synthesis and axonal transport. In the PNS separation from that target initiates a series of changes that move the axon away from a high radial growth, high stability, low plasticity state to one in which longitudinal growth and plasticity are favored and radial caliber is reduced. The biochemical changes fit with this reprogramming: (1) neurofilaments (NFs), major determinants of axonal caliber, are reduced in both message and protein (Hoffman et al., 1987; Greenberg and Lasek, 1988), and (2) the amount of pulse-labeled NF protein undergoing axonal transport is also reduced (Hoffman et al., 1984; Hoffman et al., 1985; Hoffman, 1988; Hoffman et al., 1988). A consequence is centrifugally spreading atrophy of the axon, moving from the perikaryon down the axon. Tubulins and actin, required for longitudinal growth, are increased (Hoffman and Cleveland, 1988), as is the growth-associated protein-43 (GAP-43) and other growth cone molecules.

The axotomized PNS axon can find growth factors "packaged" and presented in the plasmalemma of denervated Schwann cell bands – the Bungner bands. This arrangement provides an ever-changing growth factor gradient that drives the growing axon down individual bands. No comparable longitudinal structural scaffolding or presentation is found in the CNS. Ironically, to get regenerating axons pass the pia-glial junction of the cord and regenerate intraparenchymally has required higher levels of growth factors to be supplied (Ramer et al., 2000) or perikaryal cAMP to be raised (Qiu et al., 2002; Lu et al., 2004).

17.4 Demyelination and Wallerian-like degeneration

Progressive and extensive axonal loss occurs in multiple sclerosis (MS) and other demyelinating diseases, and contributes to the neurologic deficits (Trapp et al., 1998) (see Volume II, Chapter 38). In MS and other human and experimental settings with inflammatory demyelination, axonal degeneration and loss can result from focal axonal interruption consequent to the presence of nearby inflammatory cells and inflammatory mediators. Acute intralesional axonal damage correlates with the degree of inflammation (Bjartmar et al., 2003). In experimental allergic encephalomyelitis (EAE) axonal loss increases with number of relapses (Wujek et al., 2002). Changes in axonal cytoskeletal elements, including hyperphosphorylation and aggregation of tau, have been observed in EAE but not noninflammatory models of demyelination (Schneider et al., 2004).

A large body of evidence indicates that long-standing or recurrent demyelination *in itself* predictably produces changes in the axonal phenotype and can lead to axonal degeneration and loss (reviewed in Griffin and Sheikh, 1999). In this setting, even perfect suppression of inflammation may not prevent late axonal loss. This type of axonal loss is likely to be due to faulty glial/axonal signaling. An attractive hypothesis is that in intact axons the same ligand/receptor systems that inhibit neurite outgrowth after injury, thereby discouraging longitudinal axonal growth and plasticity, may promote radial growth, axonal stability, and long-term survival.

Demyelination leads to axonal loss: One of the characteristic features of peripheral neuropathies with predominantly "demyelinating" phenotype has been that the degree of clinical severity is associated with the progressive axonal loss rather than the degree of "demyelination". In recent years, as the genes underlying many of the inherited human demyelinating neuropathies have been identified, animal models of these diseases have been developed. In all of these animal models, the genetic abnormality is in proteins expressed primarily by the myelinating cells, oligodendrocytes and Schwann cells, and results in disturbances of proper myelination. However, although there are minor differences, a common theme among all of these genetic disturbances has been the age-related progressive distal axonal loss. Heritable mutations in obligate intrinsic myelin proteins, such as the demyelinating forms of Charcot–Marie-tooth disease (CMT-1A, -1B, and X), as well as PLP/DM20 HSP (Garbern et al., 2002; Shy et al., 1992), CNPase deficiency, and other CNS disorders, develop DAD. All produce recurrent demyelination and slowed nerve conduction, but the clinical manifestations are partly (or in the case of in CMT almost entirely) explained by the late progressive axonal loss (Berciano et al., 1986; Krajewski et al., 2000), which begins in the distal regions of the axon (farthest from the nerve cell body), and progresses more proximally with time ("dying back"). In CMT this leads to weakness of intrinsic foot muscles, foot deformities, and atrophic distal calf muscles ("stork legs") and in HSP to greater involvement of the legs and spastic paraparesis. DAD occurs in many mouse models of human demyelinating diseases, including P_o and connexin 32 mutations, PMP22 duplication, and PLP/DM20 and CNPase null animals (Martini and Toyka, 2004).

Demyelination promptly alters the phenotype of the axon in that segment: Myelination changes the phenotype of the axon directly beneath the myelinated segment. For example, myelin substantially increases the caliber of the underlying axon. Axonal caliber in the internodes of large fibers correlates with neurofilament content (Hoffman et al., 1985; Hoffman et al., 1987) and spacing (Hsieh et al., 1994). The greater spacing of neighboring neurofilaments that is seen in myelinated internodes reflects greater phosphorylation of the carboxyterminal tail domains of NF-H and NF-M than in nonmyelinated or demyelinated segments of the same fiber (Aguayo et al., 1977; Yeung et al., 1991; deWaegh et al., 1992; Hsieh et al., 1994; Sternberger and Sternberger, 1983). Demyelination produces a reduction in axonal diameter to approximately 30–50% of its previous cross-sectional area (Gombault, 1873; Raine et al., 1969; Aguayo et al., 1977), so that the axon resembles the initial segments and nodes. This reduction in caliber correlates with, and is largely caused by, a decrease in neurofilament phosphorylation and neurofilament spacing (Aguayo et al., 1977; Garcia et al., 2003; Rao et al., 2002a, b, 2003; Yin et al., 1998).

Demyelination also affects fast bidirectional axonal transport (Aguayo et al., 1977). The PLP/DM20 null animals have disrupted transport, with retrogradely transported organelles accumulating distal to nodes (Edgar et al., 2004). Cell transplantation studies unequivocally show that both the axonal pathology and the defects in axonal transport are the consequence of the abnormal overlying oligodendrocytes (Edgar et al., 2004).

Myelin-associated glycoprotein is involved in maintenance of the myelinated axonal phenotype and in axonal survival: Myelin-associated glycoprotein (MAG) is involved normally in signaling from the oligodendrocyte to the axon. MAG is normally located in the adaxonal oligodendrocyte plasmalemma (as well as the paranodal loops, Schmidt–Lanterman incisures, and mesaxons) (Trapp and Quarles, 1982). MAG is present in all myelinated internodes. It is located in noncompacted membranes including the adaxonal plasmalemma, the paranodal loops in the paranode, the inner and outer mesaxons, and the Schmidt–Lanterman incisures (Trapp, 1988; Trapp et al., 1989). Demyelination results in prompt loss of MAG from these membranes (Trapp et al., 1984; Gendelman et al., 1985; Trapp, 1988). MAG is not necessary for myelination (Owens and Bunge,

1991), and myelin sheaths from MAG−/− mice are largely normal (Yin et al., 1998). Importantly, exposure of cortical neurons to MAG in *vitro* results in prompt phosphorylation of the NF proteins, tau, MAP1b, and other axonal proteins (Dashiell et al., 2002), and MAG−/− mice have an axonal phenotype identical to that of nonmyelinated and demyelinated axons in terms of NF phosphorylation, NF spacing, and axonal caliber (Yin et al., 1998). Progressive DAD is seen in the CNS and PNS in MAG−/−mice.

MAG may signal through multiple mechanisms: MAG is known to be lost from the adaxonal plasmalemma with demyelination (Gendelman et al., 1985; Trapp, 1988), and this correlates with prompt phenotypic changes in the underlying axon. Mice genetically engineered to lack MAG have phenotypic changes in their axons comparable to those produced by demyelination, and that their axons undergo slowly progressive distal degeneration and loss (Yin et al., 1998). This suggests that the late axonal loss may be consequent to altered signaling from myelin-forming cells to the axons, and that MAG can be at least one participant in this normal signaling mechanism.

Demyelination and axonal transport: One potential mechanism by which demyelination can lead to axonal degeneration is disruption of axonal transport through demyelinated segments (Rao et al., 1981; Guy et al., 1989; Munoz-Martinez et al., 1994; Kirkpatrick et al., 2001). This is more apparent in the optic nerve system where local injections of very small quantities of anti-Gal-C antibody can lead to focal demyelination and abnormal axonal cytoskeleton and axonal transport through the demyelinated segment (Zhu et al., 1999). Similarly, in animal models of experimental allergic neuritis, there are axonal transport deficits in the optic nerve (Rao et al., 1981; Guy et al., 1989). The issue is less clear in the PNS; demyelination in the sciatic nerve induced by focal injection of a neurotoxin from K. humboldtiana causes slowed fast axonal transport (Munoz-Martinez et al., 1994), but demyelination induced by intraneural injection of anti-galactocerebroside does not have any effect on fast axonal transport (Armstrong et al., 1987).

REFERENCES

Aguayo, A.J., Attiwell, M., Trecarten, J., Perkins, S. and Bray, G.M. (1977). Abnormal myelination in transplanted trembler mouse Schwann cells. *Nature*, **265**, 73–75.

Agullo, L. and Garcia, A. (1992). Different receptors mediate stimulation of nitric oxide-dependent cyclic GMP formation in neurons and astrocytes in culture. *Biochem Biophys Res Commun*, **182**, 1362–1368.

Araki, T., Sasaki, Y. and Milbrandt, J. (2004). Increased nuclear NAD biosynthesis and SIRT1 activation prevent axonal degeneration. *Science*, **305**(**5686**), 1010–1013.

Armstrong, R., Toews, A.D. and Morell, P. (1987). Rapid axonal transport in focally demyelinated sciatic nerve. *J Neurosci*, **7**(**12**), 4044–4053.

Ballin, R.H.M. and Thomas, P.K. (1969). Changes at the node of Ranvier during Wallerian degeneration: an electron microscopic study. *Acta Neuropathol*, **14**, 237–249.

Berciano, J., Combarros, O., Figols, J., Calleja, J., Cabello, A., Silos, I. and Coria, F. (1986). Hereditory motor and sensory neuropathy type II. Clinicopathological study of a family. *Brain*, **109**, 897–914.

Bjartmar, C., Wujek, J.R. and Trapp, B.D. (2003). Axonal loss in the pathology of MS: consequences for understanding the progressive phase of the disease. *J Neurol Sci*, **206**(**2**), 165–171.

Blum, A.S., Dal Pan, G.J., Feinberg, J., Raines, C., Mayjo, K., Cornblath, D.R. and McArthur, J.C. (1996). Low-dose zalcitabine (ddC)-related toxic neuropathy: frequency, natural history, and risk factors. *Neurology*, **46**, 999–1003.

Cancalon, P. (1983). Proximodistal degeneration of C-fibers detached from their perikarya. *J Cell Biol*, **97**, 6–14.

Cancalon, P. (1985). Influence of temperature on various mechanisms associated with neuronal growth and nerve regeneration. *Prog Neurobiol*, **25**, 27–92.

Chaudhry, V., Glass, J.D. and Griffin, J.W. (1992). Wallerian degeneration in peripheral nerve disease. In:*Peripheral Neuropathy: New Concepts and Treatments* (*Neurologic Clinics*) (ed. Dyck, P. J.), Vol. 10, W.B. Saunders, Philadelphia, pp. 613–627.

Chaudhry, V., Rowinsky, E.K., Sartorius, S.E., Donehower, R.C. and Cornblath, D.R. (1994). Peripheral neuropathy from taxol and cisplatin combination chemotherapy: clinical and electrophysiological studies. *Ann Neurol*, **35**, 304–311.

Cornblath, D.R. and McArthur, J.C. (1995). Peripheral neuropathies in human immunodeficiency virus type 1 infection. In: *Peripheral Nerve Disorders* (eds Asbury, A.K. and Thomas, P.K.), 2nd edn., Butterworth Heinemann, Oxford, pp. 223–237.

Dashiell, S.M., Tanner, S.L., Pant, H.C. and Quarles, R.H. (2002). Myelin-associated glycoprotein modulates expression and phosphorylation of neuronal cytoskeletal elements and their associated kinases. *J Neurochem*, **81**(**6**), 1263–1272.

Deckwerth, T.L. and Johnson, Jr., E.M. (1993). Neurites can remain viable after destruction of the neuronal soma by programmed cell death (apoptosis) (1993). *Dev Biol*, **165**, 63–72.

deWaegh, S.M., Lee, V.M.Y. and Brady, S.T. (1992). Local modulation of neurofilament phosphorylation, axonal caliber, and slow axonal transport by myelinating Schwann cells. *Cell*, **68**, 451–463.

Dyck, P.J., Thomas, P.K., Asbury, A.K., Winegrad, A.J. and Porte, D. (1987). *Diabetic Neuropathy*, W.B. Saunders, Philadelphia.

Edgar, J.M., McLaughlin, M., Yool, D., Zhang, S.C., Fowler, J.H., Montague, P., Barrie, J.A., McCulloch, M.C., Duncan, I.D., Garbern, J., Nave, K.A. and Griffiths, I.R. (2004). Oligodendroglial modulation of fast axonal transport in a mouse model of hereditary spastic paraplegia. *J Cell Biol*, **166**(**1**), pp. 121–131.

Franson, P. and Ronnevi, L.-O. (1984). Myelin breakdown and elimination in the posterior funiculus of the adult cat after dorsal rhizotomy: a light and electron microscopic qualitative and quantitative study. *J Comp Neurol*, **223**, 138–151.

Garbern, J.Y., Yool, D.A., Moore, G.J., Wilds, I.B., Faulk, M.W., Klugmann, M., Nave, K.A., Sistermans, E.A., Van Der Knaap, M.S., Bird, T.D., Shy, M.E., Kamholz, J.A. and Griffiths, I.R. (2002). Patients lacking the major CNS myelin protein, proteolipid protein 1, develop length-dependent axonal degeneration in the absence of demyelination and inflammation. *Brain*, **125**(**Pt 3**), 551–561.

Gendelman, H.E., Pereshkpour, G.H., Pressman, N.J., Wolinksy, J.S., Quarles, R.H., Dobersen, M.J., Trapp, B.D., Kitt, C.A., Aksamit, A. and Johnson, R.T. (1985). A quantitation of myelin-associated glycoprotein and myelin basic protein in different demyelinating diseases. *Ann Neurol*, **18**, 324–328.

George, R. and Griffin, J.W. (1994). The proximo-distal spread of axonal regeneration in the dorsal columns of the rat. *J Neurocytol*, **23**, 657–667.

George, E.B., Glass, J. and Griffin, J.W. (1995). Axotomy-induced axonal degeneration is mediated by calcium influx through ion-specific channels. *J Neurosci*, **15**, 6445–6452.

Glass, J.D. and Griffin, J.W. (1991). Neurofilament redistribution in transected nerves: evidence for bidirectional transport of neurofilaments. *J Neurosci*, **11**, 3146–3154.

Glass, J.D., Brushart, T.M., George, E.B. and Griffin, J.W. (1993). Prolonged survival of transected nerve fibres in C57BL/Ola mice is an intrinsic characteristic of the axon. *J Neurocytol*, **22**, 311–321.

Glass, J.D., Schryer, B.L. and Griffin, J.W. (1994). Calcium-mediated degeneration of the axonal cytoskeleton in the Ola mouse. *J Neurochem*, **62**, 2472–2475.

Gombault, F.A.A. (1873). Contribution a l'histoire anatomique de l'atrophie musculaire saturnine. *Arch de Physiologie*, **5**, 592.

Greenberg, S.G. and Lasek, R.J. (1988). Neurofilament protein synthesis in DRG neurons decreases more after peripheral axotomy than after central axotomy. *J Neurosci*, **8**, 1739–1746.

Griffin, J.W. and Sheikh, K.A. (1999). Schwann cell-axon interactions in Charcot–Marie-tooth disease. *Ann NY Acad Sci*, **883**, 77–90.

Griffin, J.W., Price, D.L., Engel, W.K. and Drachman, D.B. (1977). The pathogenesis of reactive axonal swellings: role of axonal transport. *J Neuropathol Exp Neurol*, **36**, 214–227.

Guy, J., Ellis, E.A., Tark, III, E.F., Hope, G.M. and Rao, N.A. (1989). Axonal transport reductions in acute experimental allergic encephalomyelitis: qualitative analysis of the optic nerve. *Curr Eye Res*, **8**(3), 261–269.

Hoffman, P.N. (1988). Distinct roles of neurofilament and tubulin gene expression in axonal growth. In: *Ciba Found Symp: Plast Neuromusc Sys*, **138**, 192–204.

Hoffman, P.N. and Cleveland, D.W. (1988). Neurofilament and tubulin expression recapitulates the developmental program during axonal regeneration: induction of a specific beta tubulin isotype. *Proc Natl Acad Sci USA*, **85**, 4530–4533.

Hoffman, P.N., Griffin, J.W. and Price, D.L. (1984). Control of axonal caliber by neurofilament transport. *J Cell Biol*, **99**, 705–714.

Hoffman, P.N., Thompson, G.W., Griffin, J.W. and Price, D.L. (1985). Changes in neurofilament transport coincide temporally with alterations in the caliber of axons in regenerating motor fibers. *J Cell Biol*, **101**, 1332–1340.

Hoffman, P.N., Cleveland, D.W., Griffin, J.W., Landes, P.W., Cowan, N.J. and Price, D.L. (1987). Neurofilament gene expression: a major determinant of axonal caliber. *Proc Natl Acad Sci USA*, **84**, 3472–3476.

Hoffman, P.N., Koo, E.H., Muma, N.A., Griffin, J.W. and Price, D.L. (1988). Role of neurofilaments in the control of axonal caliber in myelinated nerve fibers. In: *Intrinsic Determinants of Neuronal Form and Function* (eds Lasek, R.J. and Black, M.M.), Alan R. Liss, New York, pp. 389–402.

Holland, N.R., Crawford, T.O., Hauer, P., Cornblath, D.R., Griffin, J.W. and McArthur, J.C. (1998). Small-fiber sensory neuropathies: clinical course and neuropathology of idiopathic cases. *Ann Neurol*, **44**(1), 47.

Hsieh, S.-T., Kidd, G.J., Crawford, T.O., Xu, Z., Lin, W.-M., Trapp, B.D., Cleveland, D.W. and Griffin, J.W. (1994). Regional modulation of neurofilament organization by myelination in normal axons. *J Neurosci*, **14**, 6392–6401.

Kirkpatrick, L.L., Witt, A.S., Payne, H.R., Shine, H.D. and Brady, S.T. (2001). Changes in microtubule stability and density in myelin-deficient shiverer mouse CNS axons. *J Neurosci*, **21**(7), 2288–2297.

Krajewski, K.M., Lewis, R.A., Fuerst, D.R., Turansky, C., Hinderer, S.R., Garbern, J., Kamholz, J. and Shy, M.E. (2000). Neurological dysfunction and axonal degeneration in Charcot–Marie-tooth disease type 1A. *Brain*, **123**(Pt 7), 1516–1527.

Lu, P., Yang, H., Jones, L.L., Filbin, M.T. and Tuszynski, M.H. (2004). Combinatorial therapy with neurotrophins and cAMP promotes axonal regeneration beyond sites of spinal cord injury. *J Neurosci*, **24**(28), 6402–6409.

Lubinska, L. (1977). Early course of Wallerian degeneration in myelinated fibers of the rat phrenic nerve. *Brain Res*, **130**, 47–63.

Lubinska, L. (1982). Patterns of Wallerian degeneration of myelinated fibres in short and long peripheral stumps and in isolated segments of rat phrenic nerve. Interpretation of the role of axoplasmic flow of the trophic factor. *Brain Res*, **233**, 227–240.

Lubinska, L. and Niemierko, S. (1977). Velocity and intensity of bidirectional migration of acetylcholinesterase in transected nerves. *Brain Res*, **27**, 329–342.

Lunn, E.R., Perry, V.H., Brown, M.C., Rosen, H. and Gordon, S. (1989). Absence of Wallerian degeneration does not hinder regeneration in peripheral nerve. *Eur J Neurosci*, **1**, 27–33.

Miledi, R. and Slater, C.K. (1970). On the degeneration of rat neuromuscular junctions after nerve section. *J Physiol*, **207**, 507–528.

Munoz-Martinez, E.J., Cuellar-Pedroza, L.H., Rubio-Franchini, C., Jauregui-Rincon, J. and Joseph-Nathan, P. (1994). Depression of fast axonal transport in axons demyelinated by intraneural injection of a neurotoxin from *K. humboldtiana*. *Neurochem Res*, **19**(11), 1341–1348.

Ouardouz, M., Nikolaeva, M.A., Coderre, E., Zamponi, G.W., McRory, J.E., Trapp, B.D., Yin, X., Wang, W., Woulfe, J. and Stys, P.K. (2003). Depolarization-induced Ca^{2+} release in ischemic spinal cord white matter involves L-type Ca^{2+} channel activation of ryanodine receptors. *Neuron*, **40**(1), 53–63.

Owens, G.C. and Bunge, R.P. (1991). Schwann cells infected with a recombinant retrovirus expressing myelin-associated glycoprotein antisense RNA do not form myelin. *Neuron*, **7**, 565–575.

Periquet, M.I., Novak, V., Collins, M.P., Nagaraja, H.N., Erdem, S., Nash, S.M., Freimer, M.L., Sahenk, Z., Kissel, J.T. and Mendell, J.R. (1999). Painful sensory neuropathy: prospective evaluation using skin biopsy. *Neurology*, **53**(8), 1641–1647.

Perry, V.H., Brown, M.C., Lunn, E.R., Tree, P. and Gordon, S. (1990a). Evidence that very slow Wallerian degeneration in C57BL/Ola mice is an intrinsic property of the peripheral nerve. *Eur J Neurosci*, **2**, 802–808.

Perry, V.H., Lunn, E.R., Brown, M.C., Cahusac, S. and Gordon, S. (1990b). Evidence that the rate of Wallerian degeneration is controlled by a single autosomal dominant gene. *Eur J Neurosci*, **2**, 408–413.

Qiu, J., Cai, D., Dai, H., McAtee, M., Hoffman, P.N., Bregman, B.S. and Filbin, M.T. (2002). Spinal axon regeneration induced by elevation of cyclic AMP. *Neuron*, **34**(6), 895–903.

Raine, C.S., Wisniewski, H. and Prineas, J. (1969). An ultrastructural study of experimental demyelination and remyelination. *Lab Invest*, **21**, 316–327.

Ramer, M.S., Priestley, J.V. and McMahon, S.B. (2000). Functional regeneration of sensory axons into the adult spinal cord. *Nature*, **403**, 312–316.

Ranish, N. and Ochs, S. (1972). Fast axoplasmic transport of acetylcholinesterase in mammalian nerve fibers. *J Neurochem*, **19**, 2641–2649.

Rao, N.A., Guy, J. and Sheffield, P.S. (1981). Effects of chronic demyelination on axonal transport in experimental allergic optic neuritis. *Invest Ophthalmol Vis Sci*, **21**(4), 606–611.

Schlaepfer, W.W. (1974). Calcium-induced degeneration of axoplasm in isolated segments of rat phrenic nerve. *Brain Res*, **69**, 203–215.

Schlaepfer, W.W. and Bunge, R.P. (1973). Effects of calcium ion concentration on the degradation of amputated axons in tissue culture. *J Cell Biol*, **59**, 456–470.

Schlaepfer, W.W. and Hasler, M.B. (1979). Characterization of the calcium-induced disruption of neurofilaments in rat peripheral nerves. *Brain Res*, **168**, 299–309.

Schlaepfer, W.W. and Micko, S. (1979). Calcium-dependent alterations of neurofilament proteins of rat peripheral nerve. *J Neurochem*, **32**, 211–219.

Schneider, A., Araujo, G.W., Trajkovic, K., Herrmann, M.M., Merkler, D., Mandelkow, E.M., Weissert, R. and Simons, M. (2004). Hyperphosphorylation and aggregation of tau in experimental autoimmune encephalomyelitis. *J Biol Chem*, **279**(53), 55833–55839.

Singleton, J.R., Smith, A.G. and Bromberg, M.B. (2001a). Increased prevalence of impaired glucose tolerance in patients with painful sensory neuropathy. *Diabetes Care*, **24**(8), 1448–1453.

Singleton, J.R., Smith, A.G. and Bromberg, M.B. (2001b). Painful sensory polyneuropathy associated with impaired glucose tolerance. *Muscle Nerve*, **24**(9), 1225–1228.

So, Y.T., Engstrom, J.W. and Olney, R.K. (1990). The spectrum of electrodiagnostic abnormalities in patients with human immunodeficiency virus infection. *Muscle Nerve* **13**, 855. (abstract).

Spencer, P.S. and Schaumburg, H.H. (1976). Central–peripheral distal axonopathy – the pathogenesis of dying-back polyneuropathies. In: *Progress in Neuropathology* (ed. Zimmerman, H.), Vol. 3, Grune and Stratton, New York, pp. 253–295.

Spencer, P.S. and Schaumburg, H.H. (1977). Ultrastructural studies of the dying back process. III. The evolution of experimental peripheral giant axonal degeneration. *J Neuropathol Exp Neurol*, **36**, 276–299.

Stys, P.K., Ransom, B.R. and Waxman, S.G. (1990). Effects of polyvalent cations and dihydropyridine calcium channel blockers on recovery of CNS white matter from anoxia. *Neurosci Lett*, **115**, 293–299.

Stys, P.K., Waxman, S.G. and Ransom, B.R. (1991). Na^+–Ca^{2+} exchanger mediates Ca^{2+} influx during anoxia in mammalian central nervous system white matter. *Ann Neurol*, **30**, 375–380.

Sumner, C.J., Sheth, S., Griffin, J.W., Cornblath, D.R. and Polydefkis, M. (2003). The spectrum of neuropathy in diabetes and impaired glucose tolerance. *Neurology*, **60**(1), 108–111.

Trapp, B.D. (1988). Distribution of the myelin-associated glycoprotein and P_0 protein during myelin compaction in quaking mouse peripheral nerve. *J Cell Biol*, **107**, 675–685.

Trapp, B.D. and Quarles, R.H. (1982). Presence of the myelin-associated glycoprotein correlates with alterations in the periodicity of peripheral myelin. *J Cell Biol*, **92**, 877–882.

Trapp, B.D., Quarles, R.H. and Suzuki, K. (1984). Immunocytochemical studies of quaking mice support a role for the myelin-associated glycoprotein in forming and maintaining the periaxonal space and periaxonal cytoplasmic collar of myelinating Schwann cells. *J Cell Biol*, **99**, 594–606.

Trapp, B.D., Andrews, S.B., Wong, A., O'Connell, M. and Griffin, J.W. (1989). Co-localization of the myelin-associated glycoprotein and the microfilament components f-actin and spectrin in Schwann cells of myelinated fibers. *J Neurocytol*, **18**, 47–60.

Trapp, B.D., Peterson, J., Ransohoff, R.M., Rudick, R., Mork, S. and Bo, L. (1998). Axonal transection in the lesions of multiple sclerosis. *New Engl J Med*, **338**(5), 278–285.

Tsao, J.W., George, E.B. and Griffin, J.W. (1999). Temperature modulation reveals three distinct stages of Wallerian degeneration. *J Neurosci*, **19**(**12**), 4718–4726.

Waller, A. (1850). Experiments on the section of glossopharyngeal and hypoglossal nerves of the frog and observations of the alternatives produced thereby in the structure of their primitive fibers. *Philos Trans Roy Soc London*, **140**, 423.

Wujek, J.R., Bjartmar, C., Richer, E., Ransohoff, R.M., Yu, M., Tuohy, V.K. and Trapp, B.D. (2002). Axon loss in the spinal cord determines permanent neurological disability in an animal model of multiple sclerosis. *J Neuropathol Exp Neurol*, **61**(**1**), 23–32.

Yeung, K.B., Thomas, P.K., King, R.H.M., Waddy, H., Will, R.G., Hughes, R.A.C., Gregson, N.A. and Leibowitz, S. (1991). The clinical spectrum of peripheral neuropathies associated with benign monoclonal IgM, IgG and IgA paraproteinemia: comparative clinical, immunological and nerve biopsy findings. *J Neurol*, **238**, 383–391.

Yin, X., Crawford, T.O., Griffin, J.W., Tu, P., Lee, V.M.Y., Li, C., Roder, J. and Trapp, B.D. (1998). Myelin-associated glycoprotein is a myelin signal that modulates the caliber of myelinated axons. *J Neurosci*, **18**(**6**), 1953–1962.

Zelena, J., Lubinska, L. and Gutmann, E. (1968). Accumulation of organelles at the ends of interrupted axons. *Z Zellforsch Mikrosk Anat*, **91**, 200–219.

Zhu, B., Moore, G.R., Zwimpfer, T.J., Kastrukoff, L.F., Dyer, J.K., Steeves, J.D., Paty, D.W. and Cynader, M.S. (1999). Axonal cytoskeleton changes in experimental optic neuritis. *Brain Res*, **824**(**2**), 204–217.

18

Adult neurogenesis and neural precursors, progenitors, and stem cells in the adult CNS

Jeffrey D. Macklis and Gerd Kempermann

*Department of Neurology, MGH–HMS Center for Nervous System Repair, Harvard Medical School, Boston, MA, USA
and Max Delbrück Center for Molecular Medicine (MDC), Berlin-Buch, Germany*

> Take note: the precursor of the oboe goes back to antiquity.
>
> *From a program booklet of the Boston
> Symphony Orchestra, 2003*

18.1 Introduction

Over most of the past century of modern neuroscience, it was thought that the adult brain was completely incapable of generating new neurons or having neurons added to its complex circuitry. However, in the last decade, the development of new techniques has resulted in an explosion of new research showing that neurogenesis, the birth of new neurons, normally occurs in only two regions of the adult mammalian brain, and that there are significant numbers of multipotent neural precursors, or "stem cells", in many parts of the adult mammalian brain (Reynolds et al., 1992; Lois and Alvarez-Buylla, 1993; Palmer et al., 1995).

The idea of "making new neurons" is appealing for neurodegenerative disease or selective neuronal loss – whenever neurons are lost causing chronic neurological or psychiatric disorders. As is so often the case in science, however, the path from the intuitive idea and first reports of general feasibility to clinical realization has turned out to be a long one. However, contrary to previously widely held beliefs, we now know that the brain itself demonstrates how new neurons can be generated from neural precursors ("neurogenesis") (Altman and Das, 1965; Altman, 1969; Cameron et al., 1993; Eriksson et al., 1998). One goal of neural precursor biology is to learn from this regionally limited, constitutive neurogenesis how to manipulate neural precursors toward therapeutic neuronal repopulation. Elucidation of the relevant molecular controls might allow both control over transplanted precursor cells and the development of neuronal replacement therapies based on the recruitment of endogenous cells.

This chapter deals with "adult neurogenesis" and what is known about the behavior and function of precursor cells in the adult brain. In the context of nervous system repair and regeneration, this is important for two main reasons:

1 Adult neurogenesis and precursor cell function might play an important role for the function of the healthy and diseased brain – it might be a particular aspect of neuronal plasticity, that is the adaptation of the structure in response to functional demands.
2 Study of precursor cell biology in the adult brain teaches us about the molecular, cellular, and other requirements for neuronal development in the adult brain – information that lies at the core of all attempts to guide neuronal development from neural precursors in the adult brain for therapeutic purposes.

A number of definitions are important. Rigorously defined, adult central nervous system (CNS) "stem cells" are cells with three cardinal features:

1 They are "self-renewing", with the theoretically unlimited ability to produce progeny indistinguishable from themselves.

2 They are proliferative, continuing to undergo mitosis (though perhaps with quite long cell cycle times).

3 They are multipotent for the different neuroectodermal lineages of the CNS, including the multitude of different neuronal and glial sub-types.

Multipotent progenitors of the adult brain are proliferative cells with only limited self-renewal that can differentiate into at least two different cell lineages (multipotency) (Gage et al., 1995b; Weiss et al., 1996b; McKay, 1997). Lineage-specific precursors or progenitors are cells with restriction to one lineage (e.g. neuronal, astroglial, glial, oligodendroglial). Together, CNS stem cells and all precursor/progenitor types are "precursors", broadly defined. We favor reserving the term "stem cell" as rigorously defined above, and using "precursor" or "progenitor" for most forms of multipotent or lineage-restricted mitotic cells. We use "precursor cell" as a generic term encompassing both stem and progenitor cells.

In the classical model, rarely dividing stem cells generate transit amplifying progenitor or precursor cells, which generate the bulk of newborn cells (Seaberg and van der Kooy, 2003). To some degree, this model is academic and based on traditional concepts in the field. Still, at present, there is considerable evidence that such a hierarchy of stem and precursor/progenitor cells exists, arguing against abandoning this model (Alvarez-Buylla et al., 2001; Seaberg and van der Kooy, 2003).

In practice, however, the use of the terms "stem cell", "progenitor", or "precursor" is largely operational. It is very likely that only molecular criteria will one day allow a clear definition. In the following chapter, we largely refer to "precursor" cells, indicating that the degree of "stemness" of particular cells is not usually known, but often can be inferred by the available data.

Adult neurogenesis, the birth of new neurons, comprises the entire set of events of neuronal development, beginning with the division of a precursor cell and ending with the presence and survival of a mature, integrated, functioning new neuron. Neurogenesis is sometimes incorrectly used only in the sense of "precursor cell proliferation", but this definition clearly falls short. Precursor cell proliferation is not predictive of net neurogenesis. True neuronal integration depends on many complex variables and progressive events.

The most pivotal caveat, however, is that precursor cells in the adult mammalian brain are heterogeneous. While all of these criteria might apply in many cases, it is not clear how many of the sometimes amazing observations in neural precursor biology can be broadly generalized and how many reflect particulars of a certain brain region or a certain condition.

While the identity of "true" CNS stem cells is as yet unknown, limiting some conclusions, the heterogeneity and seeming variety of neural precursor cells is also an important aspect of the promise of such cells. Their variable specialization and differentiation competence provide great promise for application in medicine. The idea that "one cell fits all" might turn out to be as unrealistic as it is unnecessary. Adult neural precursors with partial fate restriction may, in some cases, allow for more efficient production of desired cell types. The brain itself may provide the environmental determinants for the different forms of adult neurogenesis and gliogenesis, and may powerfully enable and direct specific lineage development.

Neurogenesis in the adult brain shares many characteristics with, but also differs considerably from, neurogenesis during embryogenesis, because adult neurogenesis occurs under spatial and tissue conditions that are generally difficult for neuronal development and circuit integration. This lack of neurogenic permissiveness is considered one key to the conspicuous lack of neuroregeneration in neurological disorders.

Recent work has partially elucidated the normal behavior of endogenous adult precursors, including their ability to migrate to select brain regions, differentiate into neurons, integrate into normal neural circuitry, and, finally, functionally integrate into the adult brain. Research is also beginning to identify and describe molecular and activity-related controls over constitutively occurring neurogenesis. The location, identity, and differentiation potential of endogenous adult precursors are beginning to be understood. In this chapter, we will outline the few examples of normally occurring neurogenesis in the mammalian CNS, describe adult neural precursors, and mention a few lines of recent research demonstrating that endogenous neural precursors can be induced to differentiate into neurons in regions of the adult brain that do not normally undergo neurogenesis.

18.2 Functional adult neurogenesis occurs in non-mammalian vertebrates

Functional adult neurogenesis also occurs in many non-mammalian vertebrates. The medial cerebral cortex of lizards, which resembles the dentate gyrus (DG) of mammals, undergoes postnatal neurogenesis and can regenerate in response to injury (Lopez-Garcia et al., 1992). Newts can regenerate their tails, limbs, jaws, and ocular tissues, and the neurons that occupy these regions (Brockes, 1997). Goldfish continue retinal neurogenesis through adulthood (Johns and Easter, 1977; Hitchcock et al., 1992). Although some non-mammalian animals can undergo quite dramatic regeneration of neural tissue, it is unclear how relevant this is to mammals. It is thought that selective evolutionary pressures have led mammals to lose such abilities during normal life (Rakic, 2002).

Birds, complex vertebrates whose brains are much closer to mammals in complexity, also exhibit postnatal neurogenesis. Lesioned postnatal avian retina undergoes some neurogenesis, with the new neurons most likely arising from Müller glia (Fischer and Reh, 2001). In songbirds, new neurons are constantly added to the high vocal center (Goldman and Nottebohm, 1983; Nottebohm, 1985; Alvarez-Buylla et al., 1998), a portion of the brain necessary for the production of learned song (Nottebohm and Arnold, 1976; Simpson and Vicario, 1990), as well as to specific regions elsewhere in the brain (but not all neuronal populations). It is possible to experimentally manipulate the extent to which new neurons are produced in at least one songbird, the zebrafinch, which does not normally, seasonally replace high vocal center

robust nucleus of the archistriatum (HVC–RA) projection neurons in the song production network, for example as canaries do (Scharff et al., 2000). Inducing cell death of HVC–RA neurons in zebrafinches leads to deterioration in song. Neurogenesis increases following induced cell death, and birds variably recover their ability to produce song coincident with the formation of new projections from area HVC to area RA, suggesting that induced neuronal replacement can restore a learned behavior.

18.3 The discovery of constitutively occurring adult mammalian neurogenesis

Joseph Altman was the first to use techniques sensitive enough to detect the ongoing cell genesis that occurs in adult brain. Using tritiated thymidine as a mitotic label, he published evidence that neurogenesis constitutively occurs in the hippocampus (Altman and Das, 1965) and olfactory bulb (Altman, 1969) of the adult mammalian brain. These results were later replicated using tritiated thymidine labeling followed by electron microcopy (Kaplan and Hinds, 1977). However, the absence of neuron-specific immunocytochemical markers at the time resulted in identification of putatively newborn neurons being made on purely morphological criteria. These limitations led to a widespread lack of acceptance of these results, and made research in the field difficult.

The field of adult neurogenesis was rekindled in 1992, when it was shown that precursor cells isolated from the forebrain can differentiate into neurons *in vitro* (Reynolds and Weiss, 1992; Richards et al., 1992). These results and technical advances, including the development of immunocytochemical reagents that could more easily and accurately identify the phenotype of various neural cells, led to an explosion of research in the field.

18.4 Neurogenic versus non-neurogenic regions in the adult brain

In the adult mammalian brain, neurogenesis normally occurs only in the olfactory bulb and the DG of the hippocampus. In the olfactory system, precursor cells reside in the sub-ventricular zone (SVZ; sometimes also called the sub-ependymal zone) in the walls of the lateral ventricles, migrate via "chain migration" through a structure surrounding the obliterated olfactory ventricle (the rostral migratory stream (RMS)) into the olfactory bulb, and differentiate into two types of interneurons in the granule cell layer and peri-glomerular regions of the bulb (Lois and Alvarez-Buylla, 1993; Luskin, 1993; Goldman, 1995; Doetsch et al., 1999). In the DG of the hippocampus, the precursor cell population is found in the sub-granular zone of the DG. Here, new granule cell neurons are produced. These two brain regions are referred to as the "neurogenic regions". Additionally, there have been controversial isolated reports of adult neurogenesis in the amygdala (Bernier et al., 2002), area CA1 of the hippocampus (Rietze et al., 2000), and the substantia nigra (Zhao et al., 2003), though this last result, for example, has been disputed (Lie et al., 2002; Frielingsdorf, 2004). Similarly, reports of extremely low level constitutive neurogenesis in the normal neocortex have been disputed (Gould et al., 1999c; 2001), primarily for methodological reasons. In addition, this same group later modified their interpretation by stating that the existence of these neurons was only transient (Gould et al., 2001).

No constitutive cortical neurogenesis has been found by many groups in a variety of species from mouse to primate (Magavi et al., 2000; Kornack and Rakic, 2001; Ehninger and Kempermann, 2003; Koketsu et al., 2003). If neurogenesis does indeed occur in what are typically considered non-neurogenic regions, it is an exceptionally rare event.

Transplantation studies support the concept of neurogenic and non-neurogenic regions, and provide evidence about the role of the microenvironment in realizing the potential of neuronal stem or progenitor cells. If precursor cells are transplanted into neurogenic regions, they can differentiate into neurons in a region-specific way (Gage et al., 1995a; Suhonen et al., 1996; Takahashi et al., 1998a; Shihabuddin et al., 2000). When implanted outside the neurogenic regions, precursor cells generate

only glia. These data further support the interpretation that neurogenesis is a function of a permissive microenvironment, and not so much of regionally different properties of stem or progenitor cells.

Neurogenic regions are defined by the neurogenic permissiveness of the local microenvironment, rather than by the presence of neural precursor cells. Precursor cells have been found in a large number of brain regions, including white matter tracts (Palmer et al., 1999). It is possible that the entire brain contains precursor cells, albeit at very low density. These widely distributed precursor cells do not seem to differ fundamentally, although they are far from homogenous, with dramatically different growth kinetics and differentiation potential. Their function outside the classical neurogenic regions is neither not known, nor is their relation to the precursor cells of the neurogenic regions. For example, precursor cells from the spinal cord behave *in vitro* much like their counterparts from the sub-granular zone (SGZ) and SVZ (Shihabuddin et al., 1997), and are multipotent after implantation into the hippocampus, producing granule cell neurons, but generate only glial cells and no neurons in situ or when transplanted back to their original site in the spinal cord (Shihabuddin et al., 2000). *In vivo*, no neurogenesis can be found in the adult rodent spinal cord (Horner et al., 2000).

Thus, there is an important conceptual distinction between neurogenic and non-neurogenic regions, but it might turn out that this distinction reflects complex molecular and functional states rather than a fixed cellular environment. Can non-neurogenic regions be molecularly modified to promote neurogenesis? Could this occur under certain pathological conditions? There are strong natural precedents in other vertebrate systems, for example the avian telencephalon and the olfactory epithelium, for the concept that selective neuronal death can alter the differentiation of precursors, thereby increasing or inducing neurogenesis (Herzog and Otto, 1999; Scharff et al., 2000).

In recent work, several groups have demonstrated the induction of modest levels of neurogenesis in normally non-neurogenic regions in response to selective neuronal death or degeneration. Magavi et al. found that endogenous multipotent precursors normally located in the adult brain can be induced to differentiate into neurons in the normally non-neurogenic adult mammalian neocortex, without transplantation (Magavi et al., 2000). More recently, other groups have reported similar and complementary results in a normally non-neurogenic region of the hippocampus (Nakatomi et al., 2002) and in the striatum (Arvidsson et al., 2002; Parent et al., 2002). These reports of seemingly regenerative neurogenesis in the vicinity of targeted cortical neuron degeneration and cerebral ischemia suggest that the lack of normal neurogenic permissiveness in these regions is not unalterable (Magavi et al., 2000; Arvidsson et al., 2002; Nakatomi et al., 2002; Parent et al., 2002). The as-yet controversial examples of reportedly extremely low-level constitutive neurogenesis outside the classical neurogenic regions might also support this possibility, potentially as "leakage" from normally tightly inhibited systems.

The situation in the literature is far from clear, but it is important to remain critical and cautious in interpretation, maintaining "reserved optimism". After all, the brain does regenerate poorly. There is as-yet little evidence that neurogenesis outside normally neurogenic regions could by itself significantly contribute to brain repair. Attempts toward endogenous repair might require exogenous support. Restorative neurobiology focusing on this approach aims at awakening the potential that lies in precursor cells in the neurogenic and non-neurogenic regions of the adult brain.

18.5 Neurogenesis in the olfactory bulb

Adult olfactory bulb neurogenesis has been most extensively studied in the rodent, with some studies conducted in non-human primates (Lois and Alvarez-Buylla, 1993; Kornack and Rakic, 1999; Pencea et al., 2001). *In vitro* (Kirschenbaum et al., 1994; Pincus et al., 1998) and *in vivo* (Sanai et al., 2004) evidence suggest that such neuronal precursors also exist in humans. Several experiments show that the

precursors that contribute to olfactory bulb neurogenesis reside in the anterior portion of the SVZ. When retroviruses (Lois and Alvarez-Buylla, 1994), tritiated thymidine (Lois and Alvarez-Buylla, 1994), vital dyes (Lois and Alvarez-Buylla, 1994; Doetsch and Alvarez-Buylla, 1996), or virally labeled SVZ cells (Luskin and Boone, 1994; Doetsch and Alvarez-Buylla, 1996) are microinjected into the anterior portion of the SVZ, labeled cells are eventually found in the olfactory bulb. To reach the olfactory bulb, the neuroblasts undergo a unique process of tangential chain migration though the RMS into the olfactory bulb (Lois and Alvarez-Buylla, 1994; Rousselot et al., 1994), may occur differently in humans (Sanai et al., 2004). Once in the olfactory bulb, the neurons migrate away from the RMS and differentiate into interneurons.

The ratio of granular neuron to peri-glomerular neuron neurogenesis is about 200 : 1 (Winner et al., 2002). Most of the cells that are born in the SVZ die before they have matured into neurons (Winner et al., 2002). Thus, a principle of embryonic development is repeated here: new neurons are generated in surplus and only a subset of them survives to maturation and functional integration, whereas the remainder die (Oppenheim, 1991). Consistent with this, high levels of cell death can be detected in the neurogenic regions of the adult brain (Biebl et al., 2000). Adult neurogenesis in the olfactory bulb appears to be both replacing old neurons and adding new ones. In contrast to the hippocampus, there is evidence of both neuronal turnover and a net increase in neurons (Winner et al., 2002). While the function of the new neurons is not known, one theory has been that high turnover of receptor neurons in the olfactory epithelium requires a similar degree of plasticity at the level of the synaptic targets in the olfactory bulb (Petreanu and Alvarez-Buylla, 2002). Recent evidence has identified an entirely novel function of adult-born olfactory bulb granule neurons – they are especially responsive to novel odorants and undergo experience-dependent modification in response to familiarization with novel odorants presented as the neurons are integrating into functional circuitry (Magavi, 2005). Although neural precursors residing in the SVZ in rodents and in non-human primates have been found to undergo chain migration through RMS and into the olfactory bulb, recent evidence in humans has raised the possibility that despite the presence of progenitors in the SVZ, these cells may not undergo chain migration through the RMS in humans (Sanai et al., 2004). The complexity of the human brain is considerably greater than that of rodents, and the introduction of new neurons into such a complex pre-existing system may be a far more challenging feat in humans than in rodents or non-human primates. Understanding the factors that contribute to normal SVZ precursor migration could be important in developing approaches to induce such precursors to migrate to injured or degenerating regions of the brain.

The effort to identify the neural precursors that contribute to olfactory bulb neurogenesis has generated a great deal of controversy. The predominant precursor cell population of the adult SVZ appears to be astrocyte-like cells, termed "B-cells", which reside in the sub-ependymal layer and send out one ciliated process touching the ventricular surface (Doetsch et al., 1999). These multipotent neural precursors have astrocytic morphology and express glial fibrillary acidic protein (GFAP) (Doetsch et al., 1999; Alvarez-Buylla et al., 2001; Seri et al., 2001). Additional independent reports provide support for the concept that multipotent neural precursors with similarities to astrocytes contribute to adult neurogenesis (Laywell et al., 2000). Other investigators suggested that a subset of ependymal cells themselves act as the precursors of this region (Johansson et al., 1999), though this interpretation has been challenged (Chiasson et al., 1999). As it is potentially difficult to distinguish a true ependymal cell from a sub-ependymal cell with a process in the ependymal layer, both sets of observations might actually correspond to the identical cell type. B-cells give rise to neuroblasts, still able to divide, which migrate in the ventricular wall and later in RMS.

It is important to distinguish between true astroglia and a distinct class of precursor cells that may also express GFAP. GFAP, while generally a reliable marker for activated astrocytes, has been used as a sole phenotypic marker in reports suggesting that astrocytes are multipotent neural precursors or "stem cells". It is quite possible that at least some multipotent neural precursors may also express GFAP, while remaining distinct from astroglia. However, these findings are additionally compelling when combined with recent data from embryogenesis that glia-like cells could serve as neural precursors. Radial glia not only guide migrating neurons to their proper position in the cortex, but a subset possesses multipotent neural precursor properties and generate neurons during development of the neocortex (Malatesta et al., 2000; Heins et al., 2002; Noctor et al., 2002).

In vitro, SVZ precursors have been exposed to a number of factors to determine their responses. Generally, precursor cells have been isolated from the brain, dissociated, and cultured in endothelial growth factor (EGF) or basic fibroblast growth factor (Bfgf). The growth factor is then removed, and the cells are exposed to differentiation conditions. The details of this process, including the particular regions from which the cells are derived, the media in which they are grown, and the substrates on which they are plated, can have significant effects on the fate of the precursors. EGF and bFGF (Gritti et al., 1995; 1996; 1999) both induce the proliferation of SVZ precursors, and can influence their differentiation. EGF tends to direct cells to a glial fate, and bFGF more toward a neuronal fate (Whittemore et al., 1999). Bone morphogenetic proteins (BMPs) promote differentiation of SVZ precursors into astroglial fates (Gross et al., 1996), while platelet derived growth factor (PDGF) (Williams et al., 1997; Whittemore et al., 1999) and insulin like growth factor (IGF-1) (Arsenijevic and Weiss, 1998) promote SVZ precursors to differentiate into neurons. There are ambiguous results regarding whether brain-derived neurotrophic factor (BDNF) promotes the survival (Kirschenbaum and Goldman, 1995) or differentiation of SVZ precursors *in vitro* (Ahmed et al., 1995).

The effects of several growth factors have also been tested *in vivo*. Intracerebroventricularly (ICV) infused EGF or TGF-α induced a dramatic increase in SVZ precursor proliferation, and bFGF induced a smaller increase in proliferation (Craig et al., 1996; Kuhn et al., 1997). Even subcutaneously delivered bFGF can induce the proliferation of SVZ precursors (Tao et al., 1996). But despite the fact that mitogen-induced newborn cells disperse into regions of the brain surrounding the ventricles, these newborn cells generally do not differentiate into neurons (Kuhn et al., 1997). Other factors have also emerged as potentially important regulators of neurogenesis, most notably vascular EGF (VEGF) (Jin et al., 2002) and BDNF (Zigova et al., 1998; Pencea et al., 2001). Intraventricularly infused BDNF increased the number of newly born neurons found in the olfactory bulbs of adult animals (Zigova et al., 1998). Further studies have shown that intraventricularly administered BDNF is not only capable of increasing the proliferation of SVZ precursors, but is additionally able to promote neuronal migration into areas such as the neostriatum, septum, thalamus, and hypothalamus (Benraiss et al., 2001; Pencea et al., 2001). Some skepticism regarding the feasibility of such approaches is also justified, however; intracerebroventricular EGF infusions have also been reported to cause massive hyperplasia of the ventricular walls (Kuhn et al., 1997).

Several studies have attempted to establish the differentiation potential of SVZ multipotent precursors, but have yielded conflicting results. Postnatal mouse SVZ precursors can differentiate into neurons in a number of regions in the developing neuraxis (Lim et al., 1997), while their fate is more limited to astroglia when they are transplanted into adult brain (Herrera et al., 1999). Adult mouse SVZ precursors injected intravenously into sub-lethally irradiated mice have been reported to differentiate into hematopoietic cells, interpreted as demonstrating the broad potential of neural precursors for differentiation and interlineage "trans-differentiation". However, it is possible that either cell fusion or a chance transformation of cultured SVZ cells led to a single transformant precursor accounting for this finding (Alvarez-Dolado et al., 2003). Labeled multipotent neural precursors, derived from adult mouse and transplanted into stage 4 chick embryos or developing mouse morulae or blastocysts, have

been reported to integrate into the heart, liver, and intestine, and express proteins specific for each of these sites (Clarke et al., 2000), though the same alternate interpretations of fusion and transformation might apply here. Adult multipotent neural precursors may not be pluripotent, but they appear to be capable of differentiating into a variety of cell types under appropriate conditions. Providing the cellular and molecular signals for appropriate differentiation and integration of new neurons will be critical for neuronal replacement therapies in which endogenous neural precursors are either transplanted or manipulated in situ.

18.6 Neurogenesis in the adult hippocampus

Neurogenesis in the DG of the adult hippocampus has been extensively studied, due at least partially to the tantalizing connection between the hippocampus and the formation of memory. Does hippocampal neurogenesis play a part in memory formation? This question has only begun to be answered, but our understanding of hippocampal neurogenesis is already quite significant (Kempermann et al., 2004b). Of particular interest is the fact that hippocampal neurogenesis can be modulated by physiological and behavioral events such as aging, stress, seizures, learning, and exercise.

Hippocampal neurogenesis has been described *in vivo* in adult rodents (Altman and Das, 1965), monkeys (Gould et al., 1998; 1999b; Kornack and Rakic, 1999) and adult humans (Eriksson et al., 1998). Newborn cells destined to become neurons are generated along the innermost aspect of the granule cell layer, the SGZ, of the DG of the adult hippocampus. The cells migrate a short distance into the granule cell layer, send dendrites into the molecular layer of the hippocampus, and send their axons into the CA3 region of the hippocampus (Stanfield and Trice, 1988; Hastings and Gould, 1999; Markakis and Gage, 1999).

The SGZ is highly vascularized, and a close proximity between blood vessels and the dividing precursor

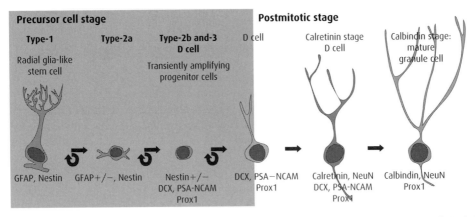

Figure 18.1. Neuronal development in the adult hippocampus proceeds through stages from precursor cells, including radial glia-like precursors, to new post-mitotic intermediate and mature DG granule neurons. Combinations of progressive differentiation markers allow the identification of distinct stages and have helped to elucidate that neuronal development in the adult brain is regulated at several stages of development.

cells has been noted (Palmer et al., 2000). Based on morphological criteria and antigenic properties, three different types of proliferative cells have been distinguished by multiple groups (Fig. 18.1) (Kempermann et al., 2004a):

1. Radial glia-like precursors termed "B cells" or "type-1 cells".
2. Nestin-expressing "type-2 cells", which lack glial features.
3. Doublecortin-positive, nestin-negative "type-3 cells".

The rarely dividing cells with radial glia-like appearance have been identified as the predominant precursors of this region (Seri et al., 2001), although the degree of "stemness" of these hippocampal cells is still controversial (Seaberg and van der Kooy, 2002). These cells, termed B-cells or "type-1 cells" by different groups, have astrocytic properties, among them characteristic electrophysiological properties and vascular end-feet, but do not express S100 beta, a marker of mature astrocytes (Seri et al., 2001; Filippov et al., 2003; Fukuda et al., 2003). These cells are thought to give rise to progenitor cells via asymmetric divisions. Type-2 cells can be sub-divided into doublecortin-positive "type-2a" and negative cells "type-2b" cells (Kronenberg et al., 2003).

Proliferation of precursor cells is an important part of neurogenic regulation. Under resting conditions, type-2a cells are most actively dividing, and physiologic mitogenic stimuli (such as physical activity) seem to affect primarily these early types of precursors. Type-1 cells are rarely dividing, and their proliferation is not induced by the experimental manipulations studied so far. Behavioral stimuli such as in environmental enrichment, which are thought to be more specific for the DG in the sense that they are closer to presumed hippocampal functions, have a limited effect on dividing progenitors, and affect later, nestin-negative stages. A subset of type-3 cells becomes post-mitotic and begins to express postmitotic neuronal markers such as NeuN. The maturing granule cells also transiently express calretinin, and it is believed that this phase is the one during which the new neurons extend their axons along the mossy fiber tract to CA3 (Brandt et al., 2003). The cells also send out dendrites into the molecular layer of the DG. In mice, adult-born granule neurons mature functionally and become electrophysiologically similar or identical to older granule neurons over 1 or 2 months (van Praag et al., 2002). The newly generated granule neurons later exchange their calcium-binding protein calretinin for calbindin (Brandt et al., 2003).

During this early postmitotic stage the new neurons apparently are recruited into function or otherwise die (Kempermann et al., 2004a).

Hippocampal precursors are studied *in vitro* much like SVZ precursors: they are removed from the brain, dissociated, and typically cultured in EGF or bFGF; the mitogen is then removed; and the cells are exposed to differentiation conditions such as retinoic acid. Hippocampal precursors proliferate in response to FGF-2 and can differentiate into astroglia, oligodendroglia, and neurons *in vitro* (Gage, 1998). Further demonstrating the existence of precursors in the adult human, multipotent precursors derived from the adult human hippocampus can be cultured *in vitro* (Kukekov et al., 1999; Roy et al., 2000).

Hippocampal neurogenesis occurs throughout adulthood, but declines with age (Kuhn et al., 1996). Understanding what causes this age-related decrease in neurogenesis may be important in assessing the possible utility of potential future neuronal replacement therapies based on manipulation of endogenous precursors. Although aged rats have dramatically lower levels of neurogenesis than young rats, adrenalectomized aged rats have levels of neurogenesis very similar to those of young adrenalectomized rats (Cameron and McKay, 1999; Montaron et al., 1999). These results suggest that it is at least partially increased corticosteroids, which are produced by the adrenal glands, and not a decrease in the number of multipotent precursors, that leads to age-related decreases in neurogenesis.

Seizures can also increase hippocampal neurogenesis. However, it appears that seizure-induced neurogenesis may contribute to inappropriate plasticity, highlighting the fact that newly introduced neurons need to be appropriately integrated into the brain in order to have beneficial effects. Chemically or electrically induced seizures induce the proliferation of sub-granular zone precursors, the majority of which differentiate into neurons in the granule cell layer (Bengzon et al., 1997; Parent et al., 1997). However, some newborn cells differentiate into granule cell neurons in ectopic locations in the hilus or molecular layers of the hippocampus and form aberrant connections to the inner molecular layer of the DG,

in addition to the CA3 pyramidal cell region (Parent et al., 1997; Huang et al., 1999). It is hypothesized that these ectopic cells and aberrant connections may contribute to hippocampal kindling (Represa et al., 1995; Parent et al., 1997; 1999; Parent and Lowenstein, 2002).

Hippocampal cell death or activity-related signals resulting from seizures may modify signals that lead to increased neurogenesis. Granule cells might either physiologically suppress neurogenesis, or surrounding cells produce signals that induce neurogenesis as they die. However, since neurogenesis is also increased by less pathological levels of electrophysiological activity (Derrick et al., 2000), it is possible that signals induced by electrophysiological activity play a role in seizure-induced hippocampal neurogenesis.

Events occurring in the hippocampus dramatically demonstrate that behavior and environment can have a direct influence on the brain's microcircuitry. Animals living in an enriched environment containing toys and social stimulation contain more newborn cells in their hippocampus than control mice living in standard cages (Kempermann et al., 1997). Experiments to further assess which aspects of the enriched environment contribute to increased neurogenesis revealed that part of the increase can be attributed to simply exercise via running (van Praag et al., 1999). Associative learning tasks that involve the hippocampus also appear to increase neurogenesis (Gould et al., 1999a). Stress, on the other hand, can reduce neurogenesis in both rodents (Tanapat et al., 1998) and primates (Gould et al., 1998). While still quite speculative, it is possible that the processes mediating these effects on neurogenesis may underlie some of the benefits that physical and social therapies provide for patients with stroke and brain injury.

There is some evidence that essentially all DG neurons that have survived the initial 2 weeks will mature and persist (Kempermann et al., 2003). Regulation of adult hippocampal neurogenesis occurs at the level of differentiation and survival of precursor cells. Most of the newly generated cells in the SGZ die, presumably by apoptotic mechanisms

(Kempermann et al., 2003). This is not unlike the process found during development, where a surplus of neurons is generated and only a proportion of these are recruited into function.

Some of the molecular mechanisms that mediate behavioral influences on hippocampal neurogenesis have begun to be elucidated. For instance, IGF-I, which increases adult hippocampal neurogenesis (Aberg et al., 2000), is preferentially transported into the brain in animals that are allowed to exercise. Blocking IGF-I activity in exercising animals reduces hippocampal neurogenesis (Carro et al., 2000), suggesting that IGF-I at least partially mediates the effects of exercise on neurogenesis (Trejo et al., 2001). Stress increases systemic adrenal steroid levels and reduces hippocampal neurogenesis (Tanapat et al., 1998). Adrenalectomy, which reduces adrenal steroids, including corticosteroids, increases hippocampal neurogenesis (Gould et al., 1992; Cameron and Gould, 1994), suggesting that adrenal hormones might mediate the effects of stress on hippocampal neurogenesis. Serotonin is a strong positive regulator of adult hippocampal neurogenesis (Brezun and Daszuta, 1999; 2000). Drugs that increase serotonin action, such as antidepressants, increase neurogenesis (Malberg et al., 2000). Modifying such systemic signals, and not only local ones, may be useful in developing potential future neuronal replacement therapies involving manipulation of endogenous precursors.

After transplantation, adult hippocampal multipotent precursors can adopt a variety of fates *in vivo*, suggesting that they may be able to appropriately integrate into neuronal microcircuitry outside of the DG of the hippocampus. Hippocampal precursors transplanted into neurogenic regions of the brain can differentiate into neurons, whereas precursors transplanted into non-neurogenic regions do not. Adult rat hippocampal precursors transplanted into RMS migrate to the olfactory bulb and differentiate into a neuronal sub-type not found in the hippocampus, tyrosine-hydroxylase-positive neurons (Suhonen et al., 1996). However, although adult hippocampal precursors transplanted into the retina can adopt neuronal fates and extend neurites, they do not

differentiate into photoreceptors, demonstrating at least conditional limitation of their differentiation fate potential (Takahashi et al., 1998b; Young et al., 2000). These results highlight that, although adult hippocampal precursors can adopt a variety of neuronal fates, they may not be able to adopt every neuronal fate.

Some recent correlative evidence suggests that newly generated neurons in the adult hippocampus may participate in some way in hippocampal-dependent memory. Non-specifically inhibiting hippocampal neurogenesis using a systemic mitotic toxin impairs trace conditioning in a manner not seen in relevant controls, suggesting a role for newly born neurons in the formation of memories (Shors et al., 2001). These correlative results, along with direct analysis of electrophysiologic integration by newborn granule neurons (van Praag et al., 2002) and an increasing responsiveness of new neurons to external stimuli (Jessberger and Kempermann, 2003), suggest that adult-born hippocampal neurons integrate functionally into the adult mammalian brain.

18.7 Cortical neurogenesis – a controversy in the field

The vast majority of studies report the absence of normally occurring adult cortical neurogenesis. Rigorous studies employing serial-section analysis and three-dimensional confocal reconstruction demonstrated a complete absence of constitutively occurring neurogenesis in the murine neocortex (Magavi et al., 2000). These experiments simultaneously demonstrated satellite glial cells closely apposed to neurons in normal neocortex that could be mistakenly interpreted as adult-born neurons when, in fact, a newborn glial cell overlies a pre-existent neuronal nucleus. However, a few studies reported low level, constitutively occurring neurogenesis in specific regions of the neocortex of adult primates (Gould et al., 1999c; 2001). In Gould et al. (1999c), neurogenesis of 2–3 new neurons/mm^3 was reported in prefrontal, inferior temporal, and posterior parietal cortex of the adult macaque, but not in striate cortex, interpreted by the authors as being because this is a simpler primary sensory area. These authors later reported that these cells are transient and do not survive (Gould et al., 2001). Other more recent reports have been unable to reproduce these findings, and report a complete absence of constitutive cortical neurogenesis in both rodents and primates (Kornack and Rakic, 2001; Ehninger and Kempermann, 2003; Koketsu et al., 2003). There exists a single report of neurogenesis in the visual cortex of the adult rat (Kaplan, 1981), but this study used tritiated thymidine and purely morphological cell type identification, and has not been confirmed by any other group.

Isolated neural precursor cells *in vitro*

Cells with precursor cell properties have successfully been isolated from the adult brain. These cells were first found in the hippocampus and the SVZ (Reynolds and Weiss, 1992; Palmer et al., 1995). Following these first reports, cells with similar properties have been isolated from many other adult mammalian brain regions as well, including neocortex, striatum proper, corpus callosum, optic nerve, spinal cord, retina, and hypothalamus (Shihabuddin et al., 1997; Palmer et al., 1999; Tropepe et al., 2000; Lie et al., 2002). *In vitro*, these cells are self-renewing and produce differentiated cells of the three neural lineages: astroglia, oligodendroglia, and neurons.

Neural precursor cells can be propagated in two main forms: in adherent cultures (Palmer et al., 1995 1999) and under floating conditions, in which they aggregate to form heterogeneous ball-like structures, termed "neurospheres" (Reynolds and Weiss, 1992). While it has become standard for some groups to use this so-called "sphere-forming" assay as the key criterion for "neural stem cells", the ability to form a "sphere", alone, is not a sufficiently reliable hallmark of stem cells and does not fully differentiate between various mitotic and precursor cell populations (Seaberg and van der Kooy, 2003). Clonal analysis provides important additional information. By sub-cloning individual cells, it can be tested whether an individual cell from these spheres can again give rise to secondary spheres, which upon transfer into differentiation conditions can produce all lineages.

Although this all contributes useful information, cell culture systems are highly artificial in many respects. *In vivo*, precursor cells are never alone. Their relationship to a neurogenic microenvironment might be inseparable from their inherent properties. Adherent cultures might acknowledge this requirement somewhat better, but the central problem remains. Not surprisingly, the importance of tissue conditions for precursor cell function, for example factors contributed by astroglia, has become more and more apparent (Song et al., 2002a).

The effectiveness of individual factors such as EGF, FGF2, BDNF, or VEGF *in vitro* does not prove that they play that role in neurogenic permissiveness *in vivo*. Conversely, regional differences *in vivo* can be equalized by treating all precursor cells with the same regimen of culture conditions to standardize comparative analysis.

18.8 The location of adult mammalian multipotent precursors

The precursors derived from all brain regions investigated so far can self-renew and differentiate into neurons, astroglia, and oligodendroglia *in vitro*. It is thought that they normally differentiate only into glia or die *in vivo*. Cells from each region have different requirements for their proliferation and differentiation. Precursors derived from septum, striatum, cortex, and optic nerve are reported to require bFGF to proliferate and differentiate into neurons *in vitro*. There are conflicting reports on whether bFGF is sufficient to culture spinal cord precursors (Weiss et al., 1996a; Shihabuddin et al., 1997). Retinal precursors do not require any mitogens in order to divide *in vitro*, although they do respond to both EGF and bFGF. As with all primary cultures, the particular details of the protocols used can strongly influence the proliferation, differentiation, and viability of the cultured cells, so it is difficult to compare results from different labs. In addition to the undifferentiated multipotent precursors that are found in various portions of the brain, there are controversial reports that mature neurons themselves can be induced to divide (Brewer, 1999; Gu et al., 2000). While it seems unlikely that a neuron could maintain the elaborate neurochemical and morphologic differentiation state of a mature neuron while replicating its DNA and remodeling its nucleus and soma, it is still theoretically possible. Though it is generally accepted that other neural cells, such as astroglia, can divide, most reports suggest that any attempt by differentiated neurons to re-enter the cell cycle results in aborted cycling and ultimately, death (Yang et al., 2001). Significant evidence would need to be presented to convincingly demonstrate that mature neurons in the adult brain are capable of mitosis.

18.9 Methodological considerations for studying neural precursor cells *in vivo*

Other aspects of neural precursor cell biology require a closer look at the putative precursor cells in their natural microenvironments *in vivo*. Unfortunately, no marker proteins are yet known that allow a prospective identification of precursor cells in the adult brain. The intermediate filament nestin is a very useful marker (Lendahl et al., 1990; Yamaguchi et al., 2000), but its sensitivity and specificity are only partial, and the limits of each are not fully known. Other markers are of great interest, for example sox-2 (D'Amour and Gage, 2003) and brain lipid binding protein (BLPB) (Rousselot et al., 1997).

In essentially all of this research, the "stemness" of certain cells *in vivo* has been inferred from:

1 The fact that after having been labeled as dividing cells, the cells give rise to neurons and glia.
2 Ex *vivo* evidence regarding precursor cells in this same brain region.

Thymidine analogs are typically used as proliferation markers, to label dividing cells permanently and pass labeling on to the progeny. In most recent studies, tritiated thymidine has been replaced by bromodeoxyuridine (BrdU), because BrdU can be detected immunocytochemically and thus allows double- and triple-labeling with cell type-specific markers and confocal microscopic analysis (Kuhn et al., 1996). The use of BrdU and multilabel confocal microscopy has allowed the study of adult neurogenesis in much greater detail, but has raised some technical issues. One question is whether BrdU labeling might identify cells undergoing DNA repair rather than proliferation. This has been discussed in detail elsewhere (Cooper-Kuhn and Kuhn, 2002). There is no evidence that adult neurogenesis as detected with standard BrdU assessment would confuse cells with ongoing DNA repair (Palmer et al., 2000). However, another issue is the use of BrdU under pathological conditions. There is some evidence that dying neurons can enter into an abortive cell cycle (Yang et al., 2003), which includes an S-phase and thus potentially BrdU-incorporation. However, such terminally sick neurons do not survive for long periods, so experiments with long survivals do not risk confusion. An additionally important approach is to study development of labeled cells from at least two different times of investigation. If, for example, early after the pathological event, only immature cells or precursors contain BrdU, and only at long survival times are mature neurons labeled, this eliminates confusion by ruling out BrdU incorporation by dying cells.

Retroviral labeling can also identify mitotic cells and allow more complete cellular morphologic and/or electrophysiologic analysis by expression of green fluorescent protein family members or other reporter genes. Retroviruses carrying a reporter gene require full cell division for integration, rather than only S-phase. Unfortunately, labeling efficiency is considerably lower than with BrdU, making quantitative analysis or analysis of rare cell divisions difficult. Neurogenesis has been confirmed and further investigated electrophysiologically and functionally in the hippocampus (van Praag et al., 2002) and also in the olfactory bulb (Carleton et al., 2003; Magavi SSP, Mitchell BD,

Szentirmai O, Carter BS, Macklis JD, 2005) by labeling dividing cells with retroviruses.

A second methodological issue concerns criteria for identification of cellular phenotype. Currently, NeuN has become the standard immunocytochemical marker to identify neurons. GFAP and S100beta are used as astroglial markers. In mice, nestin (the best known precursor cell marker *in vivo*) is notoriously difficult to detect within neurogenic regions, except under pathological conditions, when it appears to be up-regulated. Transgenic mice expressing green fluorescent protein under a neurally specific element of the nestin promoter has been very helpful in identifying precursor cells *in vivo* (Yamaguchi et al., 2000; Filippov et al., 2003), but conclusions can only be drawn regarding those cells that are labeled; no conclusions can be drawn about cells in which the nestin promoter is not active.

The most problematic point in this context, however, is the potential pitfall in identifying the phenotype of any newborn cell by a single marker, for example a BrdU-labeled "neuron" solely by its expression of NeuN (Magavi and Macklis, 2002a, b). For the classical neurogenic regions, neurogenesis has been confirmed by other markers, for example with Prox-1 and calbindin in the hippocampus, and with the neurotransmitter gamma-amino butyric acid (GABA) and the dopaminergic-associated enzyme tyrosine hydroxylase in the olfactory bulb. Cellular morphology provides one of the most reliable markers in the nervous system, and sub-cellular distribution of antigens can be additionally helpful. Electrophysiological studies (Song et al., 2002b; van Praag et al., 2002) and retrograde labeling of axons (Stanfield and Trice, 1988; Hastings and Gould, 1999; Markakis and Gage, 1999; Magavi et al., 2000; Catapano et al., 2002) can powerfully assess and further confirm the neuronal identity of newly generated cells. Additional important evidence can be obtained by analysis of progressive differentiation in the sense of progression through different markers of increasing neuronal (or other cell type) differentiation over time after the cell division (Arvidsson et al., 2002; Magavi and Macklis, 2002b; Kronenberg et al., 2003).

18.10 Induction of neurogenesis in non-neurogenic regions of the adult brain

Induced neurogenesis in non-neurogenic regions can be envisioned in at least two basic forms:

1 either local precursor cells might be activated to generate new neurons upon a stimulus attached either to the pathological event or to a therapeutic intervention; or
2 precursor cells from normally neurogenic regions, for example the SVZ, might migrate into the damaged region.

The first evidence that regenerative neurogenesis is generally possible was reported by Magavi et al. (2000); this work served as a "proof-of-concept" for the induction of adult mammalian neurogenesis by other groups in the hippocampus and striatum. Known properties of endogenous multipotent precursors led Magavi et al. to investigate the fate of these precursors in an adult cortical environment manipulated in a manner previously demonstrated to support neurogenesis (Wang et al., 1998; Scharff et al., 2000). Although they are rare, precursors throughout the adult brain have broad potential; they can differentiate into astroglia, oligodendroglia, and neurons, receive afferents, and extend axons to their targets, given an appropriate *in vitro* or *in vivo* environment. Population-specificity of neuronal death was found to be essential, allowing maintenance of local circuitry and survival of surrounding cells that alter gene expression to direct precursors (Wang et al., 1998; Fricker-Gates et al., 2002).

In agreement with the prior data, it was found that endogenous multipotent precursors could be induced to differentiate into neurons in the adult mouse neocortex, without transplantation (Fig. 18.2) (Magavi et al., 2000). They induced synchronous apoptotic degeneration of corticothalamic projection neurons and examined the fates of newborn cells within cortex, using markers of progressive neuronal differentiation. These experiments demonstrated that endogenous neural precursors (from the SVZ and possibly from the parenchyma of the cortex itself) could be induced in situ to differentiate into

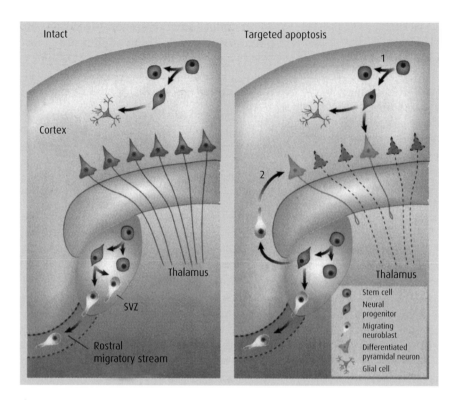

Figure 18.2. Induction of neurogenesis in the neocortex of adult mice. Cartoon showing targeted apoptosis of corticothalamic projection neurons and subsequent recruitment of new neurons from endogenous neural precursors, without transplantation, in adult mouse neocortex. (a) In intact adult mouse neocortex, endogenous precursors exist in the cortex itself, and in the underlying SVZ. Normally, these precursors produce only glia in cortex. Neurons produced in the anterior SVZ migrate along RMS to the olfactory bulb (not shown). (b) When corticothalamic projection neurons are induced to undergo synchronous targeted apoptosis, new migratory neuroblasts are born from endogenous precursors. These migrate into cortex, differentiate progressively into mature neurons, and a subset send long-distance projections to the thalamus, the appropriate original target of the neurons being replaced. The new neurons appeared to be recruited from SVZ precursors and potentially also from precursors resident in cortex itself. Adapted from Bjorklund and Lindvall, *Nature* (News and Views, Re: Magavi et al., *Nature*, 2000), **405**, 892–894, 2000. Reprinted by permission from *Nature*; copyright 2000 Macmillan Magazines Ltd.

cortical neurons, survive for many months, and form appropriate long-distance connections in the adult mammalian brain. These results indicated that the normal absence of constitutive cortical neurogenesis does not reflect an intrinsic limitation of the endogenous neural precursors' potential, but more likely results from a lack of appropriate microenvironmental signals necessary for neuronal differentiation or survival. Elucidation of these signals could enable CNS repair.

Other groups have reported similar and complementary results in hippocampus (Nakatomi et al., 2002) and striatum (Arvidsson et al., 2002; Parent et al., 2002) confirming and further supporting this direction of research. Nakatomi and colleagues (2002) used an *in vivo* ischemia model by which it was found that repopulation of neurons in the CA1 region of the hippocampus is possible following the elimination of these neurons in the CA1 region. It was found that the overwhelming majority of adult-born neurons repopulating the damaged CA1 region originated from a proliferative response in the posterior periventricle, and this proliferative response could be augmented by infusion of high levels of FGF-2 and EGF, dramatically increasing the number of neurons able to migrate into and repopulate the damaged CA1 region. While the levels of FGF-2 and EGF substantially exceeded those reasonable for human application, these experiments serve as a proof-of-principle for enhancement of an endogenous neurogenic response.

Taken together, these results demonstrate that endogenous neural precursors can be induced to differentiate into CNS neurons in a region-specific manner and at least partially replace neuronal populations that do not normally undergo neurogenesis. It appears that these results are generalizable to at least some other classes of projection neurons, including corticospinal motor neurons (Chen et al., 2004). Microenvironmental factors can support and instruct the neuronal differentiation and axon extension of endogenous precursors.

18.11 Consequences of disturbed adult neurogenesis

As so little has been known about the physiological function of adult neurogenesis, it has been difficult to evaluate the possible consequences of disturbed neurogenesis. Nonetheless, altered adult hippocampal neurogenesis has been suggested as playing a role in a number of medical conditions. The soundest data exist for temporal lobe epilepsy (Bengzon et al., 1997; Parent et al., 1997). Ectopic neurons can form in seizure-induced neurogenesis, and that their activity might contribute to ictogenesis (Scharfman et al., 2000).

Other studies suggested a possible role of disturbed neurogenesis in the pathogenesis of dementias. For example, presenilin mutations alter both amyloid processing and processing of the developmentally important molecule "Notch". It has been reported that such dysregulation leads to premature neuronal differentiation from precursors and depletion

of the adult precursor population (Handler et al., 2000). Although there may be a connection, it is difficult to merge this idea with the overt lack of normal mammalian forebrain neurogenesis, and very few studies specifically deal with this quite speculative hypothesis (Feng, 2002).

More experimental data have been gathered to support the speculative hypothesis that failure of adult hippocampal neurogenesis might underlie major depression (Jacobs et al., 2000; D'Sa and Duman, 2002; Kempermann and Kronenberg, 2003). Patients with long-lasting depression have global hippocampal atrophy (however, it should be stressed that this is not limited to the neurogenic DG) (Sheline et al., 1996), and essentially all modes of antidepressant therapy also appear to increase at least some aspect of adult DG neurogenesis (Malberg et al., 2000). Consistent with this hypothesis, stress-related glucocorticoids are associated with a decrease in neurogenesis, and increased serotonin levels are associated with an increase in neurogenesis (Brezun and Daszuta, 1999; Jacobs et al., 2000). Santarelli et al. (2003) eliminated cell proliferation in the SGZ by selective irradiation and showed that this manipulation attenuated the effects of antidepressants on performance on an anxiety task. However, the interpretation of these experiments is somewhat controversial, because this behavioral test is not widely accepted as a model for depression, and because irradiation causes damage to the microvasculature of the SGZ (and potentially other structures) and thus alters this brain region beyond affecting neurogenesis (Monje et al., 2002). Further, in general, depression is not thought to be primarily a hippocampal disorder, and the presumed link to adult neurogenesis would need to strongly depend on the functional contribution of new DG neurons to hippocampal function (Kempermann and Kronenberg, 2003). The fact that neurogenesis occurs only in the DG, while hippocampal atrophy in depression and positive effects of therapies are widespread throughout the hippocampus, argue that these are not directly linked. The most important aspect of the "neurogenesis theory" of depression might be that it brings neurons and hippocampal circuitry into a context that has been largely dominated by biochemical considerations and transmitter dysbalances. In any case, this theory should still be considered speculative and in need of considerable rigorous analysis and investigation.

18.12 Conclusions and medical implications

Neurogenesis and precursor cells in the adult brain are interesting for medicine in two regards. First, from the point of view of bio-engineering, adult brain precursor/"stem cell" biology is highly relevant, because the generation, insertion, and functional integration of new neurons is possible in the adult brain, and we may be able to "engineer" the process toward therapies using cellular and molecular tools (see Volume I, Chapter 29). Second, from a more fundamental point of view, it is important to learn about the normal role of precursor cells and the normal function of neurogenesis in the neurogenic regions of the adult brain. Circuit plasticity at the level of individual cells, neuronal or glial, adds a new layer of complexity to our understanding of how brain structure and function interact. Better understanding of these issues may enable the prevention of disease and dysfunction. Protection of normal brain function may offer chances for rehabilitation beyond currently realistic chances for repair.

A better understanding of the cellular and molecular controls over differentiation of neural precursor cells during development and in the adult CNS will be critical to potential cellular therapeutic approaches to repopulating damaged or diseased areas of the nervous system (Arlotta, Molyneaux et al., 2005; Molyneaux, Arlotta et al., 2005). The future prospect of directing the development and integration of precursors in the adult mammalian brain, toward the replacement of lost neurons or glia, is exciting indeed, and several recent lines of work provide remarkable progress toward this aim. Specifically, recent findings regarding the presence of neural precursors in a number of areas in the adult mammalian brain, ongoing adult mammalian neurogenesis, and the possibility of activating even limited neurogenesis in normally non-neurogenic regions of the adult brain are advancing the field toward the goal of cellular repopulation and repair.

Although constitutive neurogenesis normally occurs in only two areas of the adult mammalian brain (SVZ and DG), recent research suggests that it may be possible to manipulate endogenous neural precursors in situ to undergo neurogenesis in other regions of the adult brain, toward future neuronal (or oligodendroglial) replacement therapy for neurodegenerative disease and other CNS injury. Multipotent precursors in many regions of the adult brain have considerable plasticity, and, although they may have limitations in their integration into some areas of the CNS, appear capable of differentiation into neurons appropriate to a wide variety of regions, when either heterotopically transplanted, or, more recently, recruited in situ. Taken together, these results indicate that there exists a sequence and combination of molecular signals by which neurogenesis can be induced in regions of the adult mammalian brain where it does not normally occur.

Neuronal replacement therapies based on manipulation of endogenous precursors may be possible in the future. However, many questions must be answered before neuronal replacement therapies using endogenous precursors become a reality. The multiple signals that are responsible for endogenous precursor division, migration, differentiation, axon extension, and survival will need to be elucidated in order for such therapies to be developed efficiently. These challenges also exist for neuronal replacement strategies based on transplantation of precursors, since donor cells, whatever their source, must interact with an extremely complex and intricate mature CNS environment in order to integrate into the brain.

Looking forward, it may be possible to induce the cellular repopulation of the diseased brain via specific activation and differentiation of endogenous neural precursors along desired neuronal or glial lineages. However, this field is just at the beginning of understanding the complex interplay between neural precursors' potential and signals in their local microenvironment; much can be learned about precursor heterogeneity and how to take advantage of what may be partial cell-type restriction, permissive and instructive developmental signals, and modulation of specific aspects of neuronal differentiation and survival. Progress over the past decade has been great, and the coming decades promise to offer significant insight into these and other critical issues for the field.

REFERENCES

Aberg, M.A., Aberg, N.D., Hedbacker, H., Oscarsson, J. and Eriksson, P.S. (2000). Peripheral infusion of IGF-I selectively induces neurogenesis in the adult rat hippocampus. *J Neurosci*, **20**, 2896–2903.

Ahmed, S., Reynolds, B.A. and Weiss, S. (1995). BDNF enhances the differentiation but not the survival of CNS stem cell-derived neuronal precursors. *J Neurosci*, **15**, 5765–5778.

Altman, J. (1969). Autoradiographic and histological studies of postnatal neurogenesis. IV. Cell proliferation and migration in the anterior forebrain, with special reference to persisting neurogenesis in the olfactory bulb. *J Comp Neurol*, **137**, 433–457.

Altman, J. and Das, G.D. (1965). Autoradiographic and histologic evidence of postnatal neurogenesis in rats. *J Comp Neurol*, **124**, 319–335.

Alvarez-Buylla, A., Garcia-Verdugo, J.M., Mateo, A.S. and Merchant-Larios, H. (1998). Primary neural precursors and intermitotic nuclear migration in the ventricular zone of adult canraries. *J Neurosci*, **18**, 1020–1037.

Alvarez-Buylla, A., Garcia-Verdugo, J.M. and Tramontin, A.D. (2001). A unified hypothesis on the lineage of neural stem cells. *Nat Rev Neurosci*, **2**, 287–293.

Alvarez-Dolado, M., Pardal, R., Garcia-Verdugo, J.M., Fike, J.R., Lee, H.O., Pfeffer, K., Lois, C., Morrison, S.J. and Alvarez-Buylla, A. (2003). Fusion of bone-marrow-derived cells with Purkinje neurons, cardiomyocytes and hepatocytes. *Nature*, **425**, 968–973.

Arlotta, P., Molyneaux, B.J., Chen, J., Inoue, J., Kominami, R. and Macklis, J.D. (2005). Neuronal subtype specific genes that control corticospinal motor neuron development *in vivo*. *Neuron*, **45**, 207–221.

Arsenijevic, Y. and Weiss, S. (1998). Insulin-like growth factor-I is a differentiation factor for postmitotic stem cell-derived neuronal precursors: distinct actions form those of brain-derived neurotrophic factor. *J Neurosci*, **18**, 2118–2128.

Arvidsson, A., Collin, T., Kirik, D., Kokaia, Z. and Lindvall, O. (2002). Neuronal replacement from endogenous precursors in the adult brain after stroke. *Nat Med*, **8**, 963–970.

Bengzon, J., Kokaia, Z., Elmér, E., Nanobashvili, A., Kokaia, M. and Lindvall, O. (1997). Apoptosis and proliferation of dentate gyrus neurons after single and intermittent limbic seizures. *Proc Natl Acad Sci USA*, **94**, 10432–10437.

Benraiss, A., Chmielnicki, E., Lerner, K., Roh, D. and Goldman, S.A. (2001). Adenoviral brain-derived neurotrophic factor induces both neostriatal and olfactory neuronal recruitment from endogenous progenitor cells in the adult forebrain. *J Neurosci*, **21**, 6718–6731.

Bernier, P.J., Bedard, A., Vinet, J., Levesque, M. and Parent, A. (2002). Newly generated neurons in the amygdala and adjoining cortex of adult primates. *Proc Natl Acad Sci USA*, **99**, 11464–11469.

Biebl, M., Cooper, C.M., Winkler, J. and Kuhn, H.G. (2000). Analysis of neurogenesis and programmed cell death reveals a self-renewing capacity in the adult rat brain. *Neurosci Lett*, **291**, 17–20.

Brandt, M.D., Jessberger, S., Steiner, B., Kronenberg, G., Reuter, K., Bick-Sander, A., Von der Behrens, W. and Kempermann, G. (2003). Transient calretinin-expression defines early postmitotic step of neuronal differentiation in adult hippocampal neurogenesis of mice. *Mol Cell Neurosci*, **24**, 603–613.

Brewer, G.J. (1999). Regeneration and proliferation of embryonic and adult rat hippocampal neurons in culture. *Exp Neurol*, **159**, 237–247.

Brezun, J.M. and Daszuta, A. (1999). Depletion in serotonin decreases neurogenesis in the dentate gyrus and the subventricular zone of adult rats. *Neuroscience*, **89**, 999–1002.

Brezun, J.M. and Daszuta, A. (2000). Serotonin may stimulate granule cell proliferation in the adult hippocampus, as observed in rats grafted with foetal raphe neurons. *Eur J Neurosci*, **12**, 391–396.

Brockes, J.P. (1997). Amphibian limb regeneration: rebuilding a complex structure. *Science*, **276**, 81–87.

Cameron, H.A. and Gould, E. (1994). Adult neurogenesis is regulated by adrenal steroids in the dentate gyrus. *Neuroscience*, **61**, 203–209.

Cameron, H.A. and McKay, R.D. (1999). Restoring production of hippocampal neurons in old age. *Nat Neurosci*, **2**, 894–897.

Cameron, H.A., Woolley, C.S., McEwen, B.S. and Gould, E. (1993). Differentiation of newly born neurons and glia in the dentate gyrus of the adult rat. *Neuroscience*, **56**, 337–344.

Carleton, A., Petreanu, L.T., Lansford, R., Alvarez-Buylla, A. and Lledo, P.M. (2003). Becoming a new neuron in the adult olfactory bulb. *Nat Neurosci*, **6**, 507–518.

Carro, E., Nunez, A., Busiguina, S. and Torres-Aleman, I. (2000). Circulating insulin-like growth factor I mediates effects of exercise on the brain. *J Neurosci*, **20**, 2926–2933.

Catapano, L.A., Magavi, S.S. and Macklis, J.D. (2002). Neuroanatomical tracing of neuronal projections with Fluoro-Gold. *Methods Mol Biol*, **198**, 299–304.

Chen, J., Magavi, S.S. and Macklis, J.D. (2004). Neurogenesis of corticospinal motor neurons extending spinal projections in adult mice. *Proc Natl Acad Sci USA*, **101**, 16357–16362.

Chiasson, B.J., Tropepe, V., Morshead, C.M. and van der Kooy, D. (1999). Adult mammalian forebrain ependymal and subependymal cells demonstrate proliferative potential, but only subependymal cells have neural stem cell characteristics. *J Neurosci*, **19**, 4462–4471.

Clarke, D.L., Johansson, C.B., Wilbertz, J., Veress, B., Nilsson, E., Karlstrom, H., Lendahl, U. and Frisen, J. (2000). Generalized potential of adult neural stem cells. *Science*, **288**, 1660–1663.

Cooper-Kuhn, C.M. and Kuhn, H.G. (2002). Is it all DNA repair? Methodological considerations for detecting neurogenesis in the adult brain. *Brain Res Dev Brain Res*, **134**, 13–21.

Craig, C.G., Tropepe, V., Morshead, C.M., Reynolds, B.A., Weiss, S. and van der Kooy, D. (1996). *In vivo* growth factor expansion of endogenous subependymal neural precursor cell populations in the adult mouse brain. *J Neurosci*, **16**, 2649–2658.

D'Amour, K.A. and Gage, F.H. (2003). Genetic and functional differences between multipotent neural and pluripotent embryonic stem cells. *Proc Natl Acad Sci USA*, **100**(**Suppl. 1**), 11866–11872.

D'Sa, C. and Duman, R.S. (2002). Antidepressants and neuroplasticity. *Bipolar Disord*, **4**, 183–194.

Derrick, B.E., York, A.D. and Martinez Jr., J.L. (2000). Increased granule cell neurogenesis in the adult dentate gyrus following mossy fiber stimulation sufficient to induce long-term potentiation. *Brain Res*, **857**, 300–307.

Doetsch, F. and Alvarez-Buylla, A. (1996). Network of tangential pathways for neuronal migration in adult mammalian brain. *Proc Natl Acad Sci USA*, **93**, 14895–14900.

Doetsch, F., Caille, I., Lim, D.A., Garcia-Verdugo, J.M. and Alvarez-Buylla, A. (1999). Subventricular zone astrocytes are neural stem cells in the adult mammalian brain. *Cell*, **97**, 703–716.

Ehninger, D. and Kempermann, G. (2003). Regional effects of wheel running and environmental enrichment on cell genesis and microglia proliferation in the adult murine neocortex. *Cereb Cortex*, **13**, 845–851.

Eriksson, P.S., Perfilieva, E., Björk-Eriksson, T., Alborn, A.M., Nordborg, C., Peterson, D.A. and Gage, F.H. (1998). Neurogenesis in the adult human hippocampus. *Nat Med*, **4**, 1313–1317.

Feng, R., Rampon, C., Tang, Y.P., Shrom, D., Jin, J., Kyin, M., Sopher, B., Miller, M.W., Ware, C.B., Martin, G.M., Kim, S.H., Langdon, R.B., Sisodia, S.S. and Tsien, J.Z. (2002). Deficient neurogenesis in forebrain-specific presenilin-1 knockout mice is associated with reduced clearance of hippocampal memory traces. *Neuron*, **32**, 911–926. Erratum in *Neuron* (2002), **33**, 313.

Filippov, V., Kronenberg, G., Pivneva, T., Reuter, K., Steiner, B., Wang, L.P., Yamaguchi, M., Kettenmann, H. and Kempermann, G. (2003). Subpopulation of nestin-expressing progenitor cells in the adult murine hippocampus shows electrophysiological and morphological characteristics of astrocytes. *Mol Cell Neurosci*, **23**, 373–382.

Fischer, A.J. and Reh, T.A. (2001). Muller glia are a potential source of neural regeneration in the postnatal chicken retina. *Nat Neurosci*, **4**, 247–252.

Fricker-Gates, R.A., Shin, J.J., Tai, C.C., Catapano, L.A. and Macklis, J.D. (2002). Late-stage immature neocortical neurons reconstruct interhemispheric connections and form synaptic contacts with increased efficiency in adult mouse cortex undergoing targeted neurodegeneration. *J Neurosci*, **22**, 4045–4056.

Frielingsdorf, H., Schwarz, K., Brundin, P. and Mohapel, P. (2004). No evidence for new dopaminergic neurons in the adult mammalian substantia. *Proc Natl Acad Sci USA*, **101**, 10177–10182.

Fukuda, S., Kato, F., Tozuka, Y., Yamaguchi, M., Miyamoto, Y. and Hisatsune, T. (2003). Two distinct subpopulations of nestin-positive cells in adult mouse dentate gyrus. *J Neurosci*, **23**, 9357–9366.

Gage, F.H. (1998). Stem cells of the central nervous system. *Curr Opin Neurobiol*, 671–676.

Gage, F.H., Coates, P.W., Palmer, T.D., Kuhn, H.G., Fisher, L.J., Suhonen, J.O., Peterson, D.A., Suhr, S.T. and Ray, J. (1995a). Survival and differentiation of adult neuronal progenitor cells transplanted to the adult brain. *Proc Natl Acad Sci USA*, **92**, 11879–11883.

Gage, F.H., Ray, J. and Fisher, L.J. (1995b). Isolation, characterization, and use of stem cells from the CNS. *Annu Rev Neurosci*, **18**, 159–192.

Goldman, S.A. (1995). Neuronal precursor cells and neurogenesis in the adult forebrain. *Neuroscientist*, **1**, 338–350.

Goldman, S.A. and Nottebohm, F. (1983). Neuronal production, migration and differentiation in a vocal control nucleus of the adult female canary brain. *Proc Acad Sci USA*, **80**, 2390–2394.

Gould, E., Cameron, H.A., Daniels, D.C., Woolley, C.S. and McEwen, B.S. (1992). Adrenal hormones suppress cell division in the adult rat dentate gyrus. *J Neurosci*, **12**, 3642–3650.

Gould, E., Tanapat, P., McEwen, B.S., Flügge, G. and Fuchs, E. (1998). Proliferation of granule cell precursors in the dentate gyrus of adult monkeys is diminished by stress. *Proc Natl Acad Sci USA*, **95**, 3168–3171.

Gould, E., Beylin, A., Tanapat, P., Reeves, A. and Shors, T.J. (1999a). Learning enhances adult neurogenesis in the hippoampal formation. *Nat Neurosci*, **2**, 260–265.

Gould, E., Reeves, A.J., Fallah, M., Tanapat, P., Gross, C.G. and Fuchs, E. (1999b). Hippocampal neurogenesis in adult old world primates. *Proc Natl Acad Sci USA*, **96**, 5263–5267.

Gould, E., Reeves, A.J., Graziano, M.S. and Gross, C.G. (1999c). Neurogenesis in the neocortex of adult primates. *Science*, **286**, 548–552.

Gould, E., Vail, N., Wagers, M. and Gross, C.G. (2001). Adult-generated hippocampal and neocortical neurons in macaques have a transient existence. *Proc Natl Acad Sci USA*, **98**, 10910–10917.

Gritti, A., Cova, L., Parati, E.A., Galli, R. and Vescovi, A.L. (1995). Basic fibroblast growth factor supports the proliferation of epidermal growth factor-generated neuronal precursor cells of the adult mouse CNS. *Neurosci Lett*, **185**, 151–154.

Gritti, A., Parati, E.A., Cova, L., Frolichsthal, P., Galli, R., Wanke, E., Faravelli, L., Morassutti, D.J., Roisen, F., Nickel, D.D. and Vescovi, A.L. (1996). Multipotential stem cells from the adult mouse brain proliferate and self-renew in response to basic fibroblast growth factor. *J Neurosci*, **16**, 1091–1100.

Gritti, A., Frolichsthal-Schoeller, P., Galli, R., Parati, E.A., Cova, L., Pagano, S.F., Bjornson, C.R. and Vescovi, A.L. (1999). Epidermal and fibroblast growth factors behave as mitogenic regulators for a single multipotent stem cell-like population from the subventricular region of the adult mouse forebrain. *J Neurosci*, **19**, 3287–3297.

Gross, R.E., Mehler, M.F., Mabie, P.C., Zang, Z., Santschi, L. and Kessler, J.A. (1996). Bone morphogenetic proteins promote astroglial lineage commitment by mammalian subventricular zone progenitor cells. *Neuron*, **17**, 595–606.

Gu, W., Brannstrom, T. and Wester, P. (2000). Cortical neurogenesis in adult rats after reversible photothrombotic stroke. *J Cereb Blood Flow Metab*, **20**, 1166–1173.

Handler, M., Yang, X. and Shen, J. (2000). Presenilin-1 regulates neuronal differentiation during neurogenesis. *Development*, **127**, 2593–2606.

Hastings, N.B. and Gould, E. (1999). Rapid extension of axons into the CA3 region by adult-generated granule cells. *J Comp Neurol*, **413**, 146–154.

Heins, N., Malatesta, P., Cecconi, F., Nakafuku, M., Tucker, K.L., Hack, M.A., Chapouton, P., Barde, Y.A. and Gotz, M. (2002). Glial cells generate neurons: the role of the transcription factor Pax6. *Nat Neurosci*, **5**, 308–315.

Herrera, D.G., Garcia-Verdugo, J.M. and Alvarez-Buylla, A. (1999). Adult-derived neural precursors transplanted into multiple regions in the adult brain. *Ann Neurol*, **46**, 867–877.

Herzog, C. and Otto, T. (1999). Regeneration of olfactory receptor neurons following chemical lesion: time course and enhancement with growth factor administration. *Brain Res*, **849**, 155–161.

Hitchcock, P.F., Lindsey Myhr, K.J., Easter Jr., S.S., Mangione-Smith, R. and Jones, D.D. (1992). Local regeneration in the retina of the goldfish. *J Neurobiol*, **23**, 187–203.

Horner, P.J., Power, A.E., Kempermann, G., Kuhn, H.G., Palmer, T.D., Winkler, J., Thal, L.J. and Gage, F.H. (2000). Proliferation and differentiation of progenitor cells throughout the intact adult rat spinal cord. *J Neurosci*, **20**, 2218–2228.

Huang, L., Cilio, M.R., Silveira, D.C., McCabe, B.K., Sogawa, Y., Stafstrom, C.E. and Holmes, G.L. (1999). Long-term effects of neonatal seizures: a behavioral, electrophysiological, and histological study. *Brain Res Dev Brain Res*, **118**, 99–107.

Jacobs, B.L., Praag, H. and Gage, F.H. (2000). Adult brain neurogenesis and psychiatry: a novel theory of depression. *Mol Psychiatry*, **5**, 262–269.

Jessberger, S. and Kempermann, G. (2003). Adult-born hippocampal neurons mature into activity-dependent responsiveness. *Eur J Neurosci*, **18**, 2707–2712.

Jin, K., Zhu, Y., Sun, Y., Mao, X.O., Xie, L. and Greenberg, D.A. (2002). Vascular endothelial growth factor (VEGF) stimulates neurogenesis *in vitro* and *in vivo*. *Proc Natl Acad Sci USA*, **99**, 11946–11950.

Johansson, C.B., Momma, S., Clarke, D.L., Risling, M., Lendahl, U. and Frisen, J. (1999). Identification of a neural stem cell in the adult mammalian central nervous system. *Cell*, **96**, 25–34.

Johns, P.R. and Easter Jr., S.S. (1977). Growth of the adult goldfish eye. II. Increase in retinal cell number. *J Comp Neurol*, **176**, 331–341.

Kaplan, M.S. (1981). Neurogenesis in the 3-month-old rat visual cortex. *J Comp Neurol*, **195**, 323–338.

Kaplan, M.S. and Hinds, J.W. (1977). Neurogenesis in the adult rat: electron microscopic analysis of light radioautographs. *Science*, **197**, 1092–1094.

Kempermann, G. and Kronenberg, G. (2003). Depressed new neurons? Adult hippocampal neurogenesis and a cellular plasticity hypothesis of major depression. *Biol Psychiatr* **54**, 499–503.

Kempermann, G., Kuhn, H.G. and Gage, F.H. (1997). More hippocampal neurons in adult mice living in an enriched environment. *Nature*, **386**, 493–495.

Kempermann, G., Gast, D., Kronenberg, G., Yamaguchi, M. and Gage, F.H. (2003). Early determination and long-term persistence of adult-generated new neurons in the hippocampus of mice. *Development*, **130**, 391–399.

Kempermann, G., Jessberger, S., Steiner, B. and Kronenberg, G. (2004a). Milestones of neuronal development in the adult hippocampus. *Trend Neurosci* (in press).

Kempermann, G., Wiskott, L. and Gage, F.H. (2004b). Functional significance of adult neurogenesis. *Curr Opin Neurobiol*, **14**, 186–191.

Kirschenbaum, B. and Goldman, S.A. (1995). Brain-derived neurotrophic factor promotes the survival of neurons arising from the adult rat forebrain subependymal zone. *Proc Natl Acad Sci USA*, **92**, 210–214.

Kirschenbaum, B., Nedergaard, M., Preuss, A., Barami, K., Fraser, R.A. and Goldman, S.A. (1994). *In vitro* neuronal production and differentiation by precursor cells derived from the adult human forebrain. *Cerebral Cortex*, **6**, 576–589.

Koketsu, D., Mikami, A., Miyamoto, Y. and Hisatsune, T. (2003). Nonrenewal of neurons in the cerebral neocortex of adult macaque monkeys. *J Neurosci*, **23**, 937–942.

Kornack, D.R. and Rakic, P. (1999). Continuation of neurogenesis in the hippocampus of the macaque monkey. *Proc Natl Acad Sci USA*, **96**, 5768–5773.

Kornack, D.R. and Rakic, P. (2001). Cell proliferation without neurogenesis in adult primate neocortex. *Science*, **294**, 2127–2130.

Kronenberg, G., Reuter, K., Steiner, B., Brandt, M.D., Jessberger, S., Yamaguchi, M. and Kempermann, G. (2003). Subpopulations of proliferating cells of the adult hippocampus respond differently to physiologic neurogenic stimuli. *J Comp Neurol*, **467**, 455–463.

Kuhn, H.G., Dickinson-Anson, H. and Gage, F.H. (1996). Neurogenesis in the dentate gyrus of the adult rat: age-related decrease of neuronal progenitor proliferation. *J Neurosci*, **16**, 2027–2033.

Kuhn, H.G., Winkler, J., Kempermann, G., Thal, L.J. and Gage, F.H. (1997). Epidermal growth factor and fibroblast growth factor-2 have different effects on neural progenitors in the adult rat brain. *J Neurosci*, **17**, 5820–5829.

Kukekov, V.G., Laywell, E.D., Suslov, O., Davies, K., Scheffler, B., Thomas, L.B., O'Brien, T.F., Kusakabe, M. and Steindler, D.A. (1999). Multipotent stem/progenitor cells with similar properties arise from two neurogenic regions of adult human brain. *Exp Neurol*, **156**, 333–344.

Laywell, E.D., Rakic, P., Kukekov, V.G., Holland, E.C. and Steindler, D.A. (2000). Identification of a multipotent astrocytic stem cell in the immature and adult mouse brain. *Proc Natl Acad Sci USA*, **97**, 13883–13888.

Lendahl, U., Zimmerman, L.B. and McKay, R.D.G. (1990). CNS Stem cells express a new class of intermediate filament protein. *Cell*, **60**, 585–595.

Lie, D.C., Dziewczapolski, G., Willhoite, A.R., Kaspar, B.K., Shults, C.W. and Gage, F.H. (2002). The adult substantia nigra contains progenitor cells with neurogenic potential. *J Neurosci*, **22**, 6639–6649.

Lim, D.A., Fishell, G.J. and Alvarez-Buylla, A. (1997). Postnatal mouse subventricular zone neuronal precursors can migrate and differentiate within multiple levels of the developing neuraxis. *Proc Natl Acad Sci USA*, **94**, 14832–14836.

Lois, C. and Alvarez-Buylla, A. (1993). Proliferating subventricular zone cells in the adult mammalian forebrain can differentiate into neurons and glia. *Proc Natl Acad Sci USA*, **90**, 2074–2077.

Lois, C. and Alvarez-Buylla, A. (1994). Long-distance neuronal migration in the adult mammalian brain. *Science*, **264**, 1145–1148.

Lopez-Garcia, C., Molowny, A., Martinez-Guijarro, F.J., Blasco-Ibanez, J.M., Luis de la Iglesia, J.A., Bernabeu, A. and Garcia-Verdugo, J.M. (1992). Lesion and regeneration in the medial cerebral cortex of lizards. *Histol Histopathol*, **7**, 725–746.

Luskin, M.B. (1993). Restricted proliferation and migration of postnatally generated neurons derived from the forebrain subventricular zone. *Neuron*, **11**, 173–189.

Luskin, M.B. and Boone, M.S. (1994). Rate and pattern of migration of lineally-related olfactory bulb interneurons generated postnatally in the subventricular zone of the rat. *Chem Senses*, **19**, 695–714.

Magavi, S., Leavitt, B. and Macklis, J. (2000). Induction of neurogenesis in the neocortex of adult mice. *Nature*, **405**, 951–955.

Magavi, S.S. and Macklis, J.D. (2002a). Identification of newborn cells by BrdU labeling and immunocytochemistry *in vivo*. *Method Mol Biol*, **198**, 283–290.

Magavi, S.S. and Macklis, J.D. (2002b). Immunocytochemical analysis of neuronal differentiation. *Method Mol Biol*, **198**, 291–297.

Magavi, S.S.P., Mitchell, B.D., Szentirmai, O., Carter, B.S. and Macklis, J.D. (2005). Adult-born and pre-existing olfactory granule neurons undergo distinct experience-dependent modifications of their olfactory responses *in vivo*. *J Neurosci* (in press).

Malatesta, P., Hartfuss, E. and Gotz, M. (2000). Isolation of radial glial cells by fluorescent-activated cell sorting reveals a neuronal lineage. *Development*, **127**, 5253–5263.

Malberg, J.E., Eisch, A.J., Nestler, E.J. and Duman, R.S. (2000). Chronic antidepressant treatment increases neurogenesis in adult rat hippocampus. *J Neurosci*, **20**, 9104–9110.

Markakis, E. and Gage, F.H. (1999). Adult-generated neurons in the dentate gyrus send axonal projections to the field CA3 and are surrounded by synaptic vesicles. *J Comp Neurol*, **406**, 449–460.

McKay, R. (1997). Stem cells in the central nervous system. *Science*, **276**, 66–71.

Molyneaux, B.J., Arlotta, P., Hirata, T., Hibi, M. and Macklis, J.D. (2005). Fezl is required for the birth and specification of corticospinal motor neurons. *Neuron* (in press).

Monje, M.L., Mizumatsu, S., Fike, J.R. and Palmer, T.D. (2002). Irradiation induces neural precursor-cell dysfunction. *Nat Med*, **8**, 955–962.

Montaron, M.F., Petry, K.G., Rodriguez, J.J., Marinelli, M., Aurousseau, C., Rougon, G., Le Moal, M. and Abrous, D.N. (1999). Adrenalectomy increases neurogenesis but not PSA-NCAM expression in aged dentate gyrus. *Eur J Neurosci*, **11**, 1479–1485.

Nakatomi, H., Kuriu, T., Okabe, S., Yamamoto, S., Hatano, O., Kawahara, N., Tamura, A., Kirino, T. and Nakafuku, M. (2002). Regeneration of hippocampal pyramidal neurons after ischemic brain injury by recruitment of endogenous neural progenitors. *Cell*, **110**, 429–441.

Noctor, S.C., Flint, A.C., Weissman, T.A., Wong, W.S., Clinton, B.K. and Kriegstein, A.R. (2002). Dividing precursor cells of the embryonic cortical ventricular zone have morphological and molecular characteristics of radial glia. *J Neurosci*, **22**, 3161–3173.

Nottebohm, F. (1985). Neuronal replacement in adulthood. *Ann NY Acad Sci*, **457**, 143–161.

Nottebohm, F. and Arnold, A.P. (1976). Sexual dimorphism in vocal control areas of the songbird brain. *Science*, **194**, 211–213.

Oppenheim, R.W. (1991). Cell death during development of the nervous system. *Annu Rev Neurosci*, **14**, 453–501.

Palmer, T.D., Ray, J. and Gage, F.H. (1995). FGF-2-responsive neuronal progenitors reside in proliferative and quiescent regions of the adult rodent brain. *Mol Cell Neurosci*, **6**, 474–486.

Palmer, T.D., Markakis, E.A., Willhoite, A.R., Safar, F. and Gage, F.H. (1999). Fibroblast Growth Factor-2 activates a latent neurogenic program in neural stem cells from divers regions of the adult CNS. *J Neurosci*, **19**, 8487–8497.

Palmer, T.D., Willhoite, A.R. and Gage, F.H. (2000). Vascular niche for adult hippocampal neurogenesis. *J Comp Neurol*, **425**, 479–494.

Parent, J.M. and Lowenstein, D.H. (2002). Seizure-induced neurogenesis: are more new neurons good for an adult brain? *Prog Brain Res*, **135**, 121–131.

Parent, J.M., Yu, T.W., Leibowitz, R.T., Geschwind, D.H., Sloviter, R.S. and Lowenstein, D.H. (1997). Dentate granule cell neurogenesis is increased by seizures and contributes to aberrant network reorganization in the adult rat hippocampus. *J Neurosci*, **17**, 3727–3738.

Parent, J.M., Tada, E., Fike, J.R. and Lowenstein, D.H. (1999). Inhibition of dentate granule cell neurogenesis with brain irradiation does not prevent seizure-induced mossy fiber synaptic reorganization in the rat. *J Neurosci*, **19**, 4508–4519.

Parent, J.M., Vexler, Z.S., Gong, C., Derugin, N. and Ferriero, D.M. (2002). Rat forebrain neurogenesis and striatal neuron replacement after focal stroke. *Ann Neurol*, **52**, 802–813.

Pencea, V., Bingaman, K.D., Wiegand, S.J. and Luskin, M.B. (2001). Infusion of brain-derived neurotrophic factor into the lateral ventricle of the adult rat leads to new neurons in the parenchyma of the striatum, septum, thalamus, and hypothalamus. *J Neurosci*, **21**, 6706–6717.

Petreanu, L. and Alvarez-Buylla, A. (2002). Maturation and death of adult-born olfactory bulb granule neurons: role of olfaction. *J Neurosci*, **22**, 6106–6113.

Pincus, D.W., Keyoung, H.M., Harrison-Restelli, C., Goodman, R.R., Fraser, R.A., Edgar, M., Sakakibara, S., Okano, H., Nedergaard, M. and Goldman, S.A. (1998). Fibroblast growth factor-2/brain-derived neurotrophic factor-associated maturation of new neurons generated from adult human subependymal cells. *Ann Neurol*, **43**, 576–585.

Rakic, P. (2002). Neurogenesis in adult primate neocortex: an evaluation of the evidence. *Nat Rev Neurosci*, **3**, 65–71.

Represa, A., Niquet, J., Pollard, H. and Ben-Ari, Y. (1995). Cell death, gliosis, and synaptic remodeling in the hippocampus of epileptic rats. *J Neurobiol*, **26**, 413–425.

Reynolds, B.A. and Weiss, S. (1992). Generation of neurons and astrocytes from isolated cells of the adult mammalian central nervous system. *Science*, **255**, 1707–1710.

Reynolds, B.A., Tetzlaff, W. and Weiss, S. (1992). A multipotent EGF-responsive striatal embryonic progenitor cell produces neurons and astrocytes. *J Neurosci*, **12**, 4565–4574.

Richards, L.J., Kilpatrick, T.J. and Bartlett, P.F. (1992). De novo generation of neuronal cells from the adult mouse brain. *Proc Natl Acad Sci USA*, **89**, 8591–8595.

Rietze, R., Poulin, P. and Weiss, S. (2000). Mitotically active cells that generate neurons and astrocytes are present in multiple regions of the adult mouse hippocampus. *J Comp Neurol*, **424**, 397–408.

Rousselot, P., Lois, C. and Alvarez-Buylla, A. (1994). Embryonic (PSA) N-CAM reveals chains of migrating neuroblasts between the lateral ventricle and the olfactory bulb of adult mice. *J Comp Neurol*, **351**, 51–61.

Rousselot, P., Heintz, N. and Nottebohm, F. (1997). Expression of brain lipid binding protein in the brain of the adult canary and its implications for adult neurogenesis. *J Comp Neurol*, **385**, 415–426.

Roy, N.S., Wang, S., Jiang, L., Kang, J., Benraiss, A., Harrison-Restelli, C., Fraser, R.A., Couldwell, W.T., Kawaguchi, A.,

Okano, H., Nedergaard, M. and Goldman, S.A. (2000). *In vitro* neurogenesis by progenitor cells isolated from the adult human hippocampus. *Nat Med*, **6**, 271–277.

Sanai, N., Tramontin, A.D., Quinones-Hinojosa, A., Barbaro, N.M., Gupta, N., Kunwar, S., Lawton, M.T., McDermott, M.W., Parsa, A.T., Manuel-Garcia Verdugo, J., Berger, M.S. and Alvarez-Buylla, A. (2004). Unique astrocyte ribbon in adult human brain contains neural stem cells but lacks chain migration. *Nature*, **427**, 740–744.

Santarelli, L., Saxe, M., Gross, C., Surget, A., Battaglia, F., Dulawa, S., Weisstaub, N., Lee, J., Duman, R., Arancio, O., Belzung, C. and Hen, R. (2003). Requirement of hippocampal neurogenesis for the behavioral effects of antidepressants. *Science*, **301**, 805–809.

Scharff, C., Kirn, J.R., Grossman, M., Macklis, J.D. and Nottebohm, F. (2000). Targeted neuronal death affects neuronal replacement and vocal behavior in adult songbirds. *Neuron*, **25**, 481–492.

Scharfman, H.E., Goodman, J.H. and Sollas, A.L. (2000). Granule-like neurons at the hilar/CA3 border after status epilepticus and their synchrony with area CA3 pyramidal cells: functional implications of seizure-induced neurogenesis. *J Neurosci*, **20**, 6144–6158.

Seaberg, R.M. and van der Kooy, D. (2002). Adult rodent neurogenic regions: the ventricular subependyma contains neural stem cells, but the dentate gyrus contains restricted progenitors. *J Neurosci*, **22**, 1784–1793.

Seaberg, R.M. and van der Kooy, D. (2003). Stem and progenitor cells: the premature desertion of rigorous definitions. *Trend Neurosci*, **26**, 125–131.

Seri, B., Garcia-Verdugo, J.M., McEwen, B.S. and Alvarez-Buylla, A. (2001). Astrocytes give rise to new neurons in the adult mammalian hippocampus. *J Neurosci*, **21**, 7153–7160.

Sheline, Y.I., Wang, P.W., Gado, M.H., Csernansky, J.G. and Vannier, M.W. (1996). Hippocampal atrophy in recurrent major depression. *Proc Natl Acad Sci USA*, **93**, 3908–3913.

Shihabuddin, L.S., Ray, J. and Gage, F.H. (1997). FGF-2 is sufficient to isolate progenitors found in the adult mammalian spinal cord. *Exp Neurol*, **148**, 577–586.

Shihabuddin, L.S., Horner, P.J., Ray, J. and Gage, F.H. (2000). Adult spinal cord stem cells generate neurons after transplantation in the adult dentate gyrus. *J Neurosci*, **20**, 8727–8735.

Shors, T.J., Miesegaes, G., Beylin, A., Zhao, M., Rydel, T. and Gould, E. (2001). Neurogenesis in the adult is involved in the formation of trace memories. *Nature*, **410**, 372–376.

Simpson, H.B. and Vicario, D.S. (1990). Brain pathways for learned and unlearned vocalizations differ in zebra finches. *J Neurosci*, **10**, 1541–1556.

Song, H., Stevens, C.F. and Gage, F.H. (2002a). Astroglia induce neurogenesis from adult neural stem cells. *Nature*, **417**, 39–44.

Song, H.J., Stevens, C.F. and Gage, F.H. (2002b). Neural stem cells from adult hippocampus develop essential properties of functional CNS neurons. *Nat Neurosci*, **5**, 438–445.

Stanfield, B.B. and Trice, J.E. (1988). Evidence that granule cells generated in the dentate gyrus of adult rats extend axonal projections. *Exp Brain Res*, **72**, 399–406.

Suhonen, J.O., Peterson, D.A., Ray, J. and Gage, F.H. (1996). Differentiation of adult hippocampus-derived progenitors into olfactory neurons *in vivo*. *Nature*, **383**, 624–627.

Takahashi, M., Palmer, T.D., Takahashi, J. and Gage, F.H. (1998a). Widespread integration and survival of adult-derived neural progenitor cells in the developing optic retina. *Mol Cell Neurosci*, **12**, 340–348.

Takahashi, M., Palmer, T.D., Takahashi, J. and Gage, F.H. (1998b). Widespread integration and survival of adult-derived neural progenitor cells in the developing optic retina. *Mol Cell Neurosci*, **12**, 340–348.

Tanapat, P., Galea, L.A. and Gould, E. (1998). Stress inhibits the proliferation of granule cell precursors in the developing dentate gyrus. *Int J Dev Neurosci*, **16**, 235–239.

Tao, Y., Black, I.B. and DiCicco-Bloom, E. (1996). Neurogenesis in neonatal rat brain is regulated by peripheral injection of basic fibroblast growth factor (bFGF). *J Comp Neurol*, **376**, 653–663.

Trejo, J.L., Carro, E. and Torres-Aleman, I. (2001). Circulating insulin-like growth factor I mediates exercise-induced increases in the number of new neurons in the adult hippocampus. *J Neurosci*, **21**, 1628–1634.

Tropepe, V., Coles, B.L., Chiasson, B.J., Horsford, D.J., Elia, A.J., McInnes, R.R. and van der Kooy, D. (2000). Retinal stem cells in the adult mammalian eye. *Science*, **287**, 2032–2036.

van Praag, H., Kempermann, G. and Gage, F.H. (1999). Running increases cell proliferation and neurogenesis in the adult mouse dentate gyrus. *Nat Neurosci*, **2**, 266–270.

van Praag, H., Schinder, A.F., Christie, B.R., Toni, N., Palmer, T.D. and Gage, F.H. (2002). Functional neurogenesis in the adult hippocampus. *Nature*, **415**, 1030–1034.

Wang, Y., Sheen, V.L. and Macklis, J.D. (1998). Cortical interneurons upregulate neurotrophins *in vivo* in response to targeted apoptotic degeneration of neighboring pyramidal neurons. *Exp Neurol*, **154**, 389–402.

Weiss, S., Dunne, C., Hewson, J., Wohl, C., Wheatley, M., Peterson, A.C. and Reynolds, B.A. (1996a). Multipotent CNS stem cells are present in the adult mammalian spinal cord and ventricular neuroaxis. *J Neurosci*, **16**, 7599–7609.

Weiss, S., Reynolds, B.A., Vescovi, A.L., Morshead, C., Craig, C.G. and van der Kooy, D. (1996b). Is there a neural stem cell in the mammalian forebrain? *Trend Neurosci*, **19**, 387–393.

Whittemore, S.R., Morassutti, D.J., Walters, W.M., Liu, R.H. and Magnuson, D.S. (1999). Mitogen and substrate differentially affect the lineage restriction of adult rat subventricular zone neural precursor cell populations. *Exp Cell Res*, **252**, 75–95.

Williams, B.P., Park, J.K., Alberta, J.A., Muhlebach, S.G., Hwang, G.Y., Roberts, T.M. and Stiles, C.D. (1997). A PDGF-regulated immediate early gene response initiates neuronal differentiation in ventricular zone progenitor cells. *Neuron*, **18**, 553–562.

Winner, B., Cooper-Kuhn, C.M., Aigner, R., Winkler, J. and Kuhn, H.G. (2002). Long-term survival and cell death of newly generated neurons in the adult rat olfactory bulb. *Eur J Neurosci*, **16**, 1681–1689.

Yamaguchi, M., Saito, H., Suzuki, M. and Mori, K. (2000). Visualization of neurogenesis in the central nervous system using nestin promoter-GFP transgenic mice. *NeuroReport*, **11**, 1991–1996.

Yang, Y., Geldmacher, D.S. and Herrup, K. (2001). DNA replication precedes neuronal cell death in Alzheimer's disease. *J Neurosci*, **21**, 2661–2668.

Yang, Y., Mufson, E.J. and Herrup, K. (2003). Neuronal cell death is preceded by cell cycle events at all stages of Alzheimer's disease. *J Neurosci*, **23**, 2557–2563.

Young, M.J., Ray, J., Whiteley, S.J., Klassen, H. and Gage, F.H. (2000). Neuronal differentiation and morphological integration of hippocampal progenitor cells transplanted to the retina of immature and mature dystrophic rats. *Mol Cell Neurosci*, **16**, 197–205.

Zhao, M., Momma, S., Delfani, K., Carlen, M., Cassidy, R.M., Johansson, C.B., Brismar, H., Shupliakov, O., Frisen, J. and Janson, A.M. (2003). Evidence for neurogenesis in the adult mammalian substantia nigra. *Proc Natl Acad Sci USA*, **100**, 7925–7930.

Zigova, T., Pencea, V., Wiegand, S.J. and Luskin, M.B. (1998). Intraventricular administration of BDNF increases the number of newly generated neurons in the adult olactory bulb. *Mol Cell Neurosci*, **11**, 234–245.

19

Axon guidance during development and regeneration

Simon W. Moore and Timothy E. Kennedy

Department of Neurology and Neurosurgery, Center for Neuronal Survival, Montreal Neurological Institute, McGill University, Montreal, Quebec, Canada

During neural development, many neurons must extend an axon across a relatively large distance in order to reach their targets and make appropriate synaptic connections. Several models were contemplated during the 20th century to explain axon guidance. Late in the 19th century, Santiago Ramón y Cajal proposed a chemotropic model (Ramón y Cajal, 1892), speculating that axons reach their targets by sensing molecular cues. Later, based on observations of live neurons in cell culture, Ross Granville Harrison and Paul Weiss put forth a stereotropic model, proposing a form of mechanical guidance whereby axons respond to relatively nonspecific physical constraints. This was inspired by finding that axons tend to follow mechanical discontinuities on a substrate, such as scratches on the bottom of a glass cell culture dish (Harrison, 1914; Weiss, 1934). Paul Weiss elaborated on this model by proposing the resonance principle, which argues that a rough layout of neuronal connections established by stereotropism is subsequently refined by matching an axon's electrical activity with that of its target (Weiss, 1941). It was not until the early 1940s that Roger Sperry, a student of Paul Weiss, revived the hypothesis that chemical cues direct axon growth by demonstrating that axons regenerating along the frog optic nerve reconnect with their original targets in the tectum (reviewed in Sperry, 1963). Many subsequent studies, utilizing a variety of organisms and systems have established that, although activity may refine neuronal connections once they have been established, molecular cues are the major influence directing axons to their targets during development.

This chapter provides an overview of molecular mechanisms that guide axon extension during neural development. It begins by introducing the growth cone, a specialized motile structure at the tip of the axon responsible for sensing and responding to guidance cues. This is followed by a description of the trajectory of embryonic spinal commissural axons, which serves to illustrate fundamental characteristics of axon guidance. A brief overview of key axonal guidance cues is then presented, followed by a description of our growing understanding of the cellular and molecular mechanisms that transduce extracellular guidance cues into directed axon growth. The chapter concludes with a brief discussion of the possibility that cues now known to regulate axon guidance during development may subsequently influence axon regeneration in the adult central nervous system (CNS).

19.1 The growth cone

The growth cone at the tip of an axon is a motile structure that is exquisitely sensitive to guidance cues in its environment. Santiago Ramón y Cajal, who gave the growth cone its name, described it as "a concentration of protoplasm of conical form, endowed with amoeboid movements" (Ramón y Cajal, 1890). While Ramón y Cajal hypothesized that the growth cone was a motile structure from his

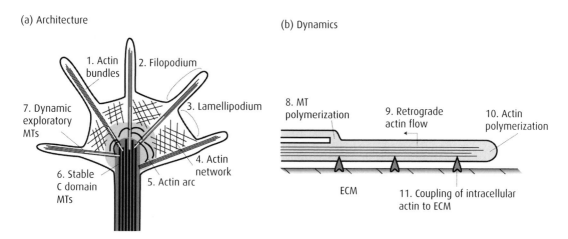

Figure 19.1. *Architecture and dynamics of the growth cone cytoskeleton.* The growth cone is composed of three domains: a central domain (dark shading), a peripheral domain (no shading), and transition zone (light shading). F-actin bundles (1) are located in filopodia (2), F-actin networks (4) in the peripheral domain and F-actin arcs (5) in the transition zone. F-actin polymerization (10) occurs at the leading edge of filopodia (2) and lamellipodia (3). F-actin networks and bundles move by retrograde flow towards the central domain of the growth cone (9). Dynamic unbundled MTs (7) polymerize into the peripheral domain (8) along filopodial F-actin bundles and are simultaneously cleared by depolymerization and coupling to retrograde F-actin flow (9). Protrusions are stabilized by bridging intracellular F-actin to the ECM (11).

studies of fixed tissue, direct evidence of this was provided by Ross Granville Harrison in 1907 based on his examination of neurons extending axons into a three-dimensional matrix in cell culture (Harrison, 1907). Notably, this first report provided an indication of just how motile growth cones can be, with Harrison commenting that, "close observation reveals a continual change in form, especially as regards the origin and branching of the filaments. In fact the changes are so rapid that it is difficult to draw the details accurately." The first description of growth cones imaged within a living organism, a frog tadpole, was provided by Carl Caskey Speidel in 1933 (Speidel, 1933).

The peripheral domain of neuronal growth cones is made up of filopodia and lamellipodia, highly dynamic membrane protrusions at the motile leading edge of many cells (reviewed in Bentley and O'Connor, 1994). Filopodia are thin finger-like extensions that can reach out dozens of microns to probe the surrounding environment. Lamellipodia are flattened veils of ruffling membrane between the

filopodia (Fig. 19.1(a)). Disruption of these structures causes errors in axon guidance (Keshishian and Bentley, 1983; Bentley and Toroian-Raymond, 1986; Chien et al., 1993; Zheng et al., 1996). Conversely, contact of the tip of a single filopodium with an appropriate extracellular target is sufficient to cause a growth cone to turn (O'Connor et al., 1990; Chien et al., 1993), indicating that receptors for guidance cues are present, and perhaps enriched, at the tips of growth cone filopodia.

Growth cone morphology is a direct consequence of the organization of the two main components of its cytoskeleton, microtubules, and filamentous actin (F-actin, Fig. 19.1(a)). Both F-actin and microtubules are polarized polymers, both are tightly regulated, and both are required to be stable at some times and dynamic at others (reviewed in Schaefer et al., 2002; Dent and Gertler, 2003). Microtubules form a dense parallel array in the axon shaft and splay apart as they enter the growth cone (Letourneau, 1983; Forscher and Smith, 1988; Dailey and Bridgman, 1991; Tanaka and Kirschner, 1991). Although microtubules are the major cytoskeletal element of the axon shaft and the central domain of the growth cone (Fig. 19.1(a)), they continuously probe into the growth cone periphery and will even extend into filopodia (Schaefer et al., 2002). In contrast, F-actin is concentrated in the peripheral domain of growth cones where it is arranged in two types of arrays: extended parallel bundles form the core of filopodia, while a meshwork underlies lamellipodia (Fig. 19.1(a)). Like microtubules, actin filaments are also polarized, and grow through polymerization of their barbed end located near the membrane. A retrograde flow of F-actin travels back from the leading edge of growth cone filopodia and lamellipodia (Fig. 19.1(b)) (Forscher and Smith, 1988; Welnhofer et al., 1997; Mallavarapu and Mitchison, 1999). This retrograde flow can be slowed or stopped if a receptor that is linked intracellularly to F-actin becomes bound to an immobilized extracellular ligand, such as a component of the extracellular matrix (ECM). Reducing retrograde flow in this way will promote local extension due to the polymerization of F-actin that builds out the cytoskeleton and supports a leading edge of membrane (reviewed by Suter and Forscher, 2000). As growth cones probe their environment through fits of polymerization and depolymerization that extend and retract filopodia and lamellipodia, guidance in one direction or another is thought to occur through selective stabilization of these F-actin-based membrane protrusions on one side, coupled with the withdrawal and collapse of the trailing edge on the opposite side.

19.2 Axon guidance during development

An axon seeking its target faces enormous challenges in the embryo. Not only must it correctly interpret a multitude of cues present in a very rich environment, but the distance separating it from its final destination can be relatively large. Axons appear to use three main strategies to reach their goal: they extend early during development when distances are smaller, they utilize intermediate targets that break up long complex trajectories into smaller more

manageable steps, and axons that extend later in development often fasciculate with and follow earlier pioneer axons. Factors that influence axon extension can be broadly divided into permissive and instructive cues. Permissive and non-permissive cues either promote or inhibit axon extension, respectively, but without necessarily exerting a directional influence on axon growth. In contrast, an instructive cue directs axon extension, either attracting or repelling the growth cone. It has also been useful to describe axon guidance cues as having either short-range or long-range functions (Tessier-Lavigne and Goodman, 1996). Short-range refers to cues that remain close to or attached to the surface of the cell that synthesized them. These include membrane-associated secreted proteins and transmembrane guidance cues. In contrast, a secreted long-range cue may be presented to a growth cone which may be many cell diameters from the cell that produced it. In some cases, a gradient of an axon guidance cue may be established by graded expression of a short-range cue across a field of cells. Alternatively gradients may be generated by secretion of a long-range cue that polarizes the embryonic neural epithelium.

To illustrate the mechanisms employed by extending axons, we describe the trajectory followed by embryonic spinal sensory interneurons that pioneer the ventral commissure. This axonal projection can be broken into at least five distinct steps as illustrated in Fig. 19.2(a):

1 Initially, commissural axons are repelled ventrally along the lateral edge of the embryonic spinal cord by BMP7 and GDF7, members of the bone morphogeneic family of proteins secreted by the roof plate at the dorsal midline, an example of long-range chemorepulsion (Augsburger et al., 1999; Butler and Dodd, 2003).

2 Complementary to this, netrin-1 and sonic hedgehog (Shh) secreted by the floor plate attract commissural axons to the ventral midline, illustrating long-range chemoattraction (Kennedy et al., 1994; Serafini et al., 1994; Charron et al., 2003).

3 As the axons cross the floor plate, a contact mediated interaction between the cell adhesion

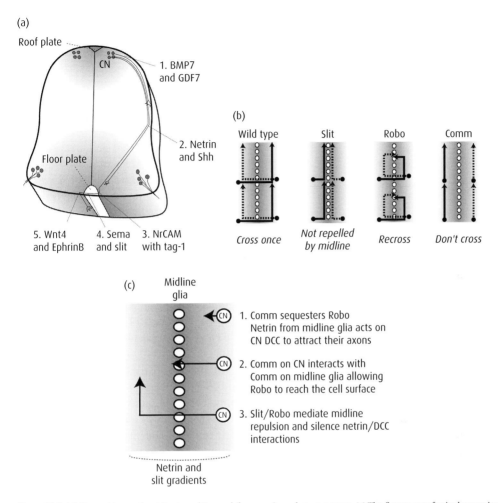

Figure 19.2. *Midline guidance of vertebrate and* Drosophila *commissural neuron axons.* (a) The five stages of spinal commissural neuron (CN) axon guidance in vertebrates. (b) Schematic of the behavior of CN axons in *Comm, Slit,* and *Robo* genetic mutants (adapted from Kidd et al., 1999). (c) Summary of the mechanisms regulating the response to guidance cues in *Drosophila* CN axon extension.

molecules tag-1 (called axonin-1 in chick) on the growth cone and Nr-CAM on floor plate cells is required for commissural axons to traverse the midline (Stoeckli et al., 1997), a short-range permissive action of these cues.

4 Once the axons have crossed to the contralateral side of the developing spinal cord, most extend longitudinally towards the head. Although the mechanisms regulating this turn are not well understood, expression of B-class

ephrins and Wnt4 by the floor plate are implicated (Imondi and Kaprielian, 2001; Lyuksyutova et al., 2003).

5 As they extend longitudinally, commissural axons are directed by semaphorin and Slit family members, secreted repellents that prevent them from re-crossing the midline and direct them out of the gray matter where they fasiculate into different longitudinal tracks (Zou et al., 2000; Long et al., 2004).

These cues are described in more detail below, but the point to be made here is that commissural axons make their way along a complex trajectory by sequentially responding to guidance cues that are precisely positioned in the developing neural epithelium, first being directed circumferentially, then across the ventral midline, and finally longitudinally toward their ultimate synaptic targets.

19.3 Axon guidance cues and their receptors

Although multiple families of axon guidance cues have been identified and their number continues to increase, the diversity of known cues still seems small in light of the immense complexity of the nervous system. The following provides an overview of several well-described families of axon guidance proteins, illustrating the range of molecules now known to direct axons to their targets.

Laminins

Multiple ECM components influence axon extension during neural development (reviewed in Reichardt and Tomaselli, 1991). Among these, the laminin family is notable for several reasons. Many types of neurons, derived from either the CNS or peripheral nervous system (PNS), readily extend axons on laminin, and laminin-1 is very commonly used as a permissive substrate that promotes axon outgrowth in cell culture. Laminins are a major component of basement membranes, a layer of ECM at the base of epithelia (Colognato and Yurchenco, 2000). Notably, the basal lamina secreted by Schwann cells in peripheral nerves promotes axon regeneration following injury (Ide et al., 1983). Depletion of laminin from preparations of peripheral nerve myelin substantially reduces its capacity to promote axon growth, indicating that laminin is a key component of peripheral nerve basal lamina responsible for promoting regeneration. Interestingly, preparations of CNS myelin that are potent inhibitors of axon

growth, actually promote axon growth following the addition of exogenous laminin-1, indicating that laminin-1 is a powerful stimulant of axon extension that can mask some of the growth inhibitory properties of CNS myelin (David et al., 1995).

Laminins are secreted as large cruciform heterotrimers made up of one α, one β, and one γ subunit (Fig. 19.3) (reviewed in Beck et al., 1990; Engvall and Wewer, 1996). Ten different laminin chains and at least 12 different heterotrimers have been documented *in vivo* (reviewed in Erickson and Couchman, 2000). Multiple laminins are expressed early during embryonic development (Lentz et al., 1997). Among many important functions, they influence neural crest cell migration, Schwann cell migration, axon extension, and nerve-muscle synapse formation. Mutations of genes encoding specific laminins indicate that they make numerous essential contributions to the development of both the CNS and PNS (reviewed by Colognato and Yurchenco, 2000). Although laminins are secreted, proteins and axons will migrate up a gradient of a peptide fragment of laminin-1 (Adams et al., 2005), evidence for laminin gradients directing axon extension *in vivo* has not been obtained (McKenna and Raper, 1988; Matsuzawa et al., 1998; Dertinger et al., 2002).

Multiple proteins interact with laminins. Of particular importance as laminin receptors are the integrins, a large family of receptors for ECM proteins (Fig. 19.3). Integrins are transmembrane heterodimers composed of combinations drawn from at least 16α and 8β subunits. They are linked intracellularly to F-actin and by acting as a transmembrane bridge between the ECM and the cytoskeleton, integrins function as key regulators of cell-ECM adhesion and of cell motility, including growth cone motility (Belkin and Stepp, 2000).

Netrins

Netrins, named for the Sanskrit word meaning "one who guides", are a small family of axon proteins that direct axon outgrowth during embryogenesis. They are bifunctional, attracting some axons and

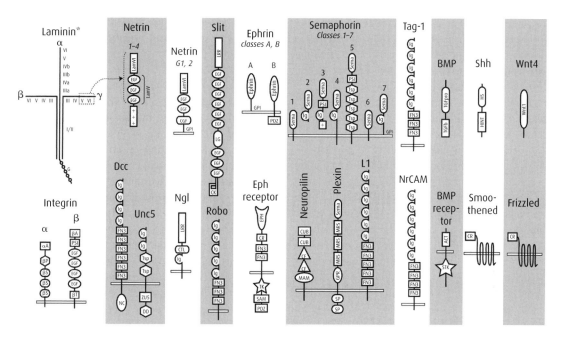

Figure 19.3. *Axon guidance cues and their receptors.* For membrane proteins, domains above the plasma membrane are extracellular, while those below it are intracellular. *Due to its size, the domains of laminin are omitted. Domain abbreviations: ACT: activin types I and II receptor; LG: lamin G (also known as an ALPS spacer, agrin, laminin, perlecan, and Slit); βP: β propeller; βS: β sandwich; βT: β tail; CF: coagulation faction V, VIII homology; CGF: cripto growth factor; CK: cysteine knot; CR: cysteine rich; CTL: carboxy terminal leucine rich repeat; CUB: complement binding; DD: death domain; EPH: ephrin binding; Ephrin: Eph receptor binding; FN3: fibronectin type III; Hint: Hedgehog/intein; HS: Hedgehog signaling; GPR: glycine–proline-rich region; LamVI: laminin N-terminal domain VI; LamV: laminin N-terminal domain V; MAM: meprin, A5, Mu domain; MRS: met related sequence; NC: neogenin C-terminus; PSI: plexins, semaphorins and integrins; SAM: sterile alpha motif; SP: sex-plexin, STK: serine/threonine kinase; TGFb: transforming growth factor beta like; TGFpro: TGF-beta propeptide; TK: tyrosine kinase; Tsp: thrombospondin type I; +: basic/positively charged. Domains were drawn based on NCBI conserved domain database.

repelling others. Six netrins have been identified in vertebrates: netrins 1–4 and netrins G1 and G2 (reviewed in Manitt and Kennedy, 2002). All are ~75 kDa glycoproteins, with sequence homology to the amino-terminus of laminins (Fig. 19.3). Netrins 1–4 are secreted proteins, while netrins G1 and G2 contain a GPI (glycosylphosphatidylinositol) that attaches them to the plasma membrane. Although netrins 1–4 are secreted, their carboxyl terminal domain, a domain unrelated to laminins, contains many charged amino acids and netrin-1 binds heparin with high affinity (Kappler et al., 2000). Consistent with this, the majority of netrin-1 in the CNS is bound to cell surfaces and ECM

(Serafini et al., 1994; Manitt et al., 2001; Manitt and Kennedy, 2002).

The functional assays used to identify netrins were based on the proposal, and subsequent demonstration, that the axons of embryonic spinal commissural neurons are attracted to the ventral midline of the neural tube by a cue secreted by the floor plate (Ramón y Cajal, 1899; Weber, 1934; Tessier-Lavigne et al., 1988; Placzek et al., 1990). Consistent with this, a source of netrin-1 attracts commissural axons, and netrin-1 is strongly expressed by floor plate cells at the ventral midline of the embryonic neural tube (Kennedy et al., 1994). Furthermore, netrin-1 is required for formation of the corpus callosum, hippocampal commissure, and ventral spinal commissure, indicating that it is essential for the normal development of multiple axonal projections to the ventral midline of the developing CNS (Serafini et al., 1996).

Candidate netrin receptors were first identified genetically in *C. elegans*. *Unc-5* mutation caused defects in axon trajectories directed away from netrin expressing cells, while mutation of *unc-40* caused defects in axon extension toward these cells. Mutation of the *C. elegans* netrin homolog *unc-6* produced defects in both trajectories (Hedgecock et al., 1990; Ishii et al., 1992; Wadsworth et al., 1996). Both *unc-40* and *unc-5* encode transmembrane immunoglobulin (Ig) superfamily members (Leung-Hagesteijn et al., 1992; Chan et al., 1996). Deleted in colorectal cancer (DCC), the mammalian homolog of unc-40 (Keino-Masu et al., 1996), binds netrin-1, is expressed by spinal commissural neurons and is required for chemoattractant responses to netrin-1 (Fazeli et al., 1997). Members of the Unc-5 homolog family also bind netrin-1 and mediate the repellent response to netrin-1. Four have been identified in mammals, Unc5h1 to 4 (Ackerman et al., 1997; Leonardo et al., 1997; Engelkamp, 2002). Many neurons express both an Unc5 homolog and DCC. The two classes of receptors interact, forming a netrin receptor complex, and neurons that express both can respond to netrin-1 as an attractant or a repellent (Hong et al., 1999). Interestingly, integrins have recently been shown to bind to the extreme carboxyl-terminus of netrin-1 (Yebra et al., 2003), however a role for this interaction in axon guidance has not been demonstrated.

Slits

A key challenge for axons that cross the midline during development is that once they have crossed to the contralateral side of the CNS, they must remain crossed and ignore the cues that directed them to the midline. An interesting group of mutations in *Drosophila melanogaster* led to the initial molecular insights into this process. The *Drosophila Slit* mutant phenotype was first identified over 20 years ago

(Nusslein-Volhard et al., 1984) and then cloned in 1988, but its role in axon guidance was not appreciated until 10 years later (Rothberg et al., 1988; Brose et al., 1999; Kidd et al., 1999; Li et al., 1999). The ventral nerve cord of a fly embryo is composed of symmetrical longitudinal projections connected by a series of commissures, making a ladder-like structure (Fig. 19.2(b)). In *Slit* loss of function mutants, the commissures disappear, and the longitudinal projections merge (Kidd et al., 1999). *Slit* is expressed by specialized midline glia at the ventral midline of the *Drosophila* CNS and encodes a large secreted protein composed of leucine rich repeats (LRR), epidermal growth factor repeats (EGF), and a laminin G domain (Rothberg et al., 1990). Slit is an essential midline repellent that inhibits ipsilaterally projecting neurons from approaching the midline and prevents contralaterally projecting neurons from recrossing (Kidd et al., 1999; Rajagopalan et al., 2000; Simpson et al., 2000).

A complementary mutation, *Roundabout* (*Robo*), identified the Slit receptor (Seeger et al., 1993). In *Robo* mutant fly embryos, axons that would normally project ipsilaterally and contralaterally instead cross and recross the midline repeatedly (Fig. 19.2(b)). Named after the circular roundabouts found at British intersections, loss of Robo function generates a phenotype where the CNS collapses into a series of circles that are essentially repeated commissural crossings that go nowhere.

Robo is a single pass transmembrane protein that binds Slit. In mammals, three Robo homologs, Robo1, Robo2, and Rig-1, and three Slits, Slit1–3, have been identified (Taguchi et al., 1996; Holmes et al., 1998; Itoh et al., 1998; Brose et al., 1999; Yuan et al., 1999). Analogous to their role in *Drosophila*, Slits are expressed in the ventral embryonic spinal cord where they repel ipsilaterally projecting axons and prevent recrossing by contralaterally projecting axons (Long et al., 2004). Slits also regulate axon branching (Wang et al., 1999) and are important guidance cues for axons in the dentate gyrus of the hippocampus, olfactory bulb, and retina (Li et al., 1999; Nguyen Ba-Charvet et al., 1999; Erskine et al., 2000; Long et al., 2004).

Semaphorins

Semaphorins, named after semaphore, a flag-based method of signaling once used between ships and along railroads, constitute a large family of secreted and membrane-associated proteins. The first evidence that semaphorins might function as axonal chemorepellents was provided by the demonstration that collapsin-1, subsequently named semaphorin 3A, could collapse sensory ganglion growth cones *in vitro* (Luo et al., 1993). The semaphorin family is divided into eight subclasses. Five of these (classes 3–7) are found in vertebrates and play major roles as axon guidance cues during neural development (reviewed in Raper, 2000). Classes 1 and 2 are expressed in invertebrates. Interestingly, class "V" is viral. All semaphorins share a characteristic 500 amino acid "sema" extracellular domain, and may be secreted, transmembrane, or GPI linked (Fig. 19.3). Secreted class 3 semaphorins are well characterized for their role organizing the central projections of dorsal root ganglion sensory neurons into different laminae of the embryonic spinal cord (Messersmith et al., 1995). Although they are best understood for their role as repellents that affect axon steering, fasciculation, and branching (reviewed in Kolodkin and Ginty, 1997; de Wit and Verhaagen, 2003), like many axon guidance cues, they are bifunctional and also promote the growth of some axons (Wong et al., 1997; Song et al., 1998; Wong et al., 1999). These semaphorins signal via a receptor complex composed of a neuropilin family member, the ligand-binding component, and a plexin family member, which activates intracellular signaling (reviewed in Tamagnone and Comoglio, 2000). In addition, L1, a transmembrane Ig superfamily cell adhesion molecule, interacts with neuropilin-1 and is required for repellent responses to Sema3A (Castellani et al., 2000).

Ephrins

In the early 1940s, Roger Sperry's findings generated the chemospecificity hypothesis of axon guidance (reviewed in Sperry, 1963). Sperry's experiments took advantage of the capability of some lower vertebrates, such as frogs, to regenerate the precise array of axonal connections made between the retina and visual tectum. He demonstrated that if, following transection of the optic nerve, the eye was rotated 180° and reimplanted, the misaligned axons were able to find and reconnect with their original targets in the tectum. The rotated eye then generated a grossly misaligned visual signal that produced equivalently inappropriate motor responses, such as a frog jumping upward when aiming for a fly placed on the ground. The conclusion of such behavioral findings, confirmed by subsequent anatomic and physiologic analyses, was that the regenerating axons found their targets by responding to precise distributions of chemical cues in the cellular environment, and not by responding to mechanical constraints, or based on activity directing the formation of appropriate connections.

It is now clear that graded expression of ephrins across the tectum, and complementary gradients of their receptors, the Eph tyrosine kinases, in the retina, play key roles directing the spatiotopic projection of the retina to the tectum. Eph receptors make up the largest family of receptor tyrosine kinases in the mammalian genome. Ephrins are either transmembrane (ephrinB1–B3) and bind EphB receptors (EphB1–B6), or GPI linked (ephrinA1–A5) and bind EphA receptors (EphA1–A9) (reviewed in Himanen and Nikolov, 2003). Graded expression of EphA receptors by retinal ganglion cells and ephrinAs in the tectum direct the topographic projection of retinal ganglion cell axons along the tectal anterior/posterior axis. Complementing this, graded expression of EphB receptors by retinal ganglion cells and ephrinBs in the tectum directs the formation of lateral to medial projections into the tectum (reviewed in McLaughlin et al., 2003). Ephrins influence multiple CNS axonal projections including those of the vomeronasal axons, anterior commissure, corpus callosum, and corticospinal tract (Drescher et al., 1995; Orioli et al., 1996; Coonan et al., 2001; Kullander et al., 2001; Yokoyama et al., 2001). Both classes of ephrins are membrane attached, and the interaction between ephrins and Eph receptors generates bi-directional signaling into both the "ligand" and the "receptor" expressing cells (reviewed in Kullander and Klein, 2002). Although ephrins have been intensively studied for their role as repellent axon guidance cues, it is now clear that they also influence adhesive interactions between cells, synaptic plasticity, cell migration, and vascular development (reviewed in Holmberg and Frisen, 2002; Knoll and Drescher, 2002). Reflecting this diversity of function, "Eph" is derived from their expression by an *e*rythropoietin-*p*roducing human *h*epatocellular carcinoma cell line (Eph Nomenclature Committee, 1997), and "ephrin" from the contraction of "*Eph* family *r*eceptor *in*teracting protein", and ephoros, the ancient Greek word for overseer or controller.

Morphogens as guidance cues: Wnts, BMPs, and Hedgehogs

The Wingless (Wg)/Wnt, BMP (bone morphogenic protein), and Hedgehog families are all well-characterized morphogens: secreted proteins that direct target cells to adopt a particular fate. Surprisingly, members of each of these protein families have now been implicated as axon guidance cues during embryogenesis. In the embryonic spinal cord, the BMP family members BMP7 and GDF7, are secreted by roof plate cells and act as repellents that direct the initial outgrowth of commissural axons ventrally (Augsburger et al., 1999; Butler and Dodd, 2003). In contrast, Shh secreted by the floor plate attracts commissural neurons to the ventral midline, and this chemoattractant response requires the Shh receptor, Smoothened (Charron et al., 2003). Wnt4 and its receptor Frizzled3 have been implicated in reorienting commissural axon growth longitudinally, once the axons have crossed the ventral midline (Lyuksyutova et al., 2003). Although known receptors for these proteins have been implicated as influencing axon guidance in some cases, the signal transduction mechanisms

underlying their effect on growth cone motility are not well understood.

19.4 Regulation of the growth cone cytoskeleton

Growth cones integrate inputs from many guidance cues to produce directed motility. Although our understanding of the intracellular signaling mechanisms used by the receptors for guidance cues is currently incomplete, a point of convergence for guidance cue signal transduction is their influence on the organization of the growth cone cytoskeleton (Fig. 19.4(a)). The Rho family of small GTPases are key regulators of the organization of F-actin in both neuronal and non-neuronal cells (reviewed in Hall, 1998; Dickson, 2001). They function as molecular switches that are inactive when bound to GDP and active when bound to GTP (Fig. 19.4(b)). Cycling between GDP and GTP bound states is tightly regulated by multiple mechanisms. Guanine nucleotide exchange factors (GEFs) activate Rho GTPases by promoting the exchange of GDP for GTP. GTPase activating proteins (GAPs) inhibit Rho GTPases by promoting the hydrolysis of GTP to GDP. Guanine nucleotide dissociation inhibitors (GDIs) remove the GTPase from the membrane and prevent dissociation of GDP, thereby maintaining the GTPase in an inactive state. Downstream of the Rho GTPases, over 30 target effector proteins have been identified (reviewed in Bishop and Hall, 2000).

In many cell types, the Rho family members Cdc42 and Rac1 regulate the formation of filopodia and lamellipodia, respectively. RhoA activation directs the formation of F-actin stress fibers and activates myosin contractility, potentially leading to increased retrograde flow of F-actin and process retraction. A current model suggests that attractant guidance cues will activate Cdc42 and Rac in growth cones, while repellents trigger growth cone collapse by activating RhoA (Fig. 19.4(c)). Substantial experimental support for this model has now been obtained: netrins, ephrins, slits, and the semaphorins

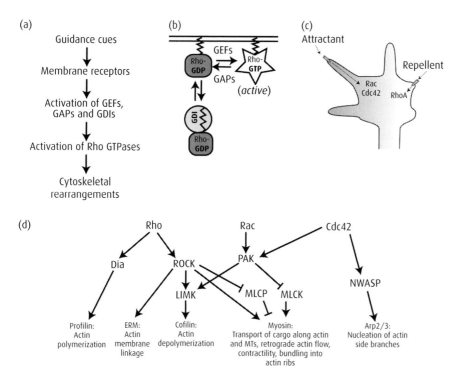

Figure 19.4. *Intracellular signaling mechanisms that regulates F-actin architecture.* (a) Flowchart of how guidance cues affect the growth cone's cytoskeleton. (b) The cycling of Rho GTPases between inactive and active GTP-bound states is under the control of GEFs, GAPs, and GDIs. (c) Activation of Rac and Cdc42 is correlated with a response to attractants, while activation of RhoA is correlated with a response to repellents. (d) Examples of how RhoA, Rac, and Cdc42 activation can lead to remodeling of the actin cytoskeleton.

all influence axon extension by signaling via the Rho GTPases and the mechanisms by which these cues regulate Rho GTPase activity in neurons are currently under intense scrutiny (reviewed in Govek et al., 2005).

19.5 Modulating the response of growth cones to guidance cues

As an axon extends along its trajectory, its growth cone has the capacity to rapidly change its response to local guidance cues. This is well illustrated by an interesting twist in the Robo/Slit story that first presented itself as the following paradox. If Slit prevents commissural axons from recrossing the midline, why are the axons not prevented from crossing as

they approach the midline the first time? At least two mechanisms have now been identified that contribute to overcoming this challenge. In *Drosophila*, a protein named Commissureless (Comm), describing its loss of function phenotype (Fig. 19.2(b)), regulates the vesicular traffic that carries newly synthesized Robo to the plasma membrane (Keleman et al., 2002). Before crossing the midline, commissural neurons express Comm, which targets newly synthesized Robo for degradation, and therefore the growth cone remains insensitive to Slit. In ipsilaterally projecting neurons and in commissural neurons after they have crossed the midline, Comm is not expressed. This allows newly synthesized Robo to travel unimpeded to the plasma membrane and the axons are repelled by midline-derived Slit. Interestingly, a mammalian homolog of Comm has not been identified thus far. In contrast, a divergent member of the Robo family, Rig1, inhibits the ability of precrossing embryonic commissural axons to respond to Slits, although it does not appear to do this by regulating sorting analogous to Comm function in *Drosophila* (Marillat et al., 2004; Sabatier et al., 2004). In addition to turning on the response to Slit as they cross the midline, Robo binds to DCC inhibiting it, thereby silencing the response to the midline attractant netrin-1 (Stein and Tessier-Lavigne, 2001). These findings indicate that their encounter with the midline changes the commissural neurons, silencing their response to midline attractants, while activating their sensitivity to midline repellents, thereby allowing them to cross once and then preventing recrossing (Fig. 19.2(c)).

Growth cones must rapidly respond to local guidance cues and this ability exhibits substantial autonomy from the neuronal cell body. Growth cones will even continue to migrate and respond to guidance cues hours after severing the axon, completely independent of any connection to the cell body (Shaw and Bray, 1977; Harris et al., 1987; Campbell and Holt, 2001; Brittis et al., 2002). Mechanisms that modify the response of growth cones to guidance cues include regulated presentation of receptors on the cell surface, receptor inactivation, degradation of receptors by proteolysis, and local protein synthesis in the growth cone (reviewed in Yu and Bargmann, 2001; Piper and Holt, 2004). In addition, the intracellular concentrations of the cyclic nucleotide cAMP and cGMP are key regulators of growth cone responsiveness (reviewed in Song and Poo, 1999). Decreasing the concentration of cAMP, or in some cases cGMP, in the neuron can convert attraction to repulsion (Ming et al., 1997; Hopker et al., 1999). Conversely, increasing the concentration of cAMP or cGMP can convert a repellent response to attraction. These findings suggest that extracellular cues that regulate the concentration of cAMP or cGMP in the growth cone may exert a profound influence on the response to guidance cues presented in parallel. An example of this is provided by Hopker et al. (1999) who demonstrated that regulation of the concentration of cAMP in the growth

cone by Laminin-1, changes the response of retinal ganglion cell axons to netrin-1 from attraction to repulsion as they exit the eye and enter the optic nerve.

A decrease in the intracellular concentration of cAMP also contributes importantly to the reduced capacity of neurons to regenerate during maturation (Cai et al., 2001). Increasing the intraneuronal concentration of cAMP, thereby activating protein kinase A (PKA), a major downstream effector of cAMP, enhances axon growth in the presence of myelin-associated inhibitors of axon extension (Cai et al., 2001), including promoting axon regeneration in the mature mammalian CNS following injury (Neumann et al., 2002; Qiu et al., 2002). PKA induces increased expression of intracellular polyamines, which contribute to enhanced axon regeneration (Cai et al., 2002). Consistent with a requirement for changes in gene expression, the ability of PKA to promote regeneration also requires the activation of the transcription factor, such as cAMP response element binding protein (CREB) (Gao et al., 2004). PKA also recruits the netrin receptor DCC to the cell surface enhancing axon outgrowth in response to netrin-1 (Bouchard et al., 2004). This suggests that PKA-dependent regulation of the complement of receptors on the growth cone may influence the capacity of an axon to regenerate (Volume I, Chapter 21). PKA can also regulate the activity of the Rho GTPases, in particular, directly phosphorylating and inhibiting RhoA (Lang et al., 1996; Ellerbroek et al., 2003). As described below, inhibiting RhoA has a dramatic influence on the capacity of axons to regenerate in the CNS.

19.6 Axon guidance during regeneration

Inhibitors of axon regeneration

Although many neurons in the adult CNS have the capacity to regenerate a severed axon (David and Aguayo, 1981), maturation, and in particular myelination, in the mammalian CNS coincides with a dramatic decrease in the ability of injured axons to regenerate (Volume I, Chapter 24). CNS white matter contains multiple myelin-associated inhibitors of axon outgrowth and regeneration (Volume I, Chapter 21). Identified inhibitors include myelin-associated glycoprotein (MAG), oligodendrocyte-myelin glycoprotein (OMgp), and Nogo (McKerracher et al., 1994; Mukhopadhyay et al., 1994; Chen et al., 2000; GrandPre et al., 2000; Prinjha et al., 2000; Kottis et al., 2002; Wang et al., 2002). MAG is a transmembrane Ig superfamily member expressed by myelinating glia in the PNS and CNS. OMgp is a GPI-linked membrane protein component of CNS myelin. Nogo is expressed by oligodendrocytes, but not Schwann cells, and is the protein recognized by IN-1, a monoclonal antibody that enhances axon outgrowth on substrates of myelin *in vitro* and promotes axon regeneration in the mammalian CNS (reviewed in Schwab and Bartholdi, 1996). Remarkably, these three structurally unrelated proteins all interact with the same cell surface receptor, NgR, a GPI-linked membrane protein widely expressed by neurons that was first identified as a receptor for Nogo (Fig. 19.5) (Fournier et al., 2001; Domeniconi et al., 2002; Liu et al., 2002; Wang et al., 2002). Although MAG, OMgp, and Nogo all influence axon extension, their functional role during development and in the intact adult CNS are not known. In addition to these three identified myelin-associated inhibitors, components of the glial scar that forms following injury, such as chondroitin sulfate proteoglycans, are also potent inhibitors of axon regeneration (reviewed in Morgenstern et al., 2002).

RhoA activity inhibits regeneration

Similar to their role downstream of axon guidance cues during neural development, the small Rho GTPases, and in particular RhoA, are thought to be a point of convergence for neuronal signal transduction mechanisms that inhibit axon regeneration in the adult (Volume I, Chapter 24). Inhibiting RhoA blocks growth cone collapse and promotes axon extension, both on myelin substrates *in vitro* and in the adult CNS following lesion (Jalink et al., 1994; Jin and Strittmatter, 1997; Lehmann et al., 1999; Dergham et al., 2002; Winton et al., 2002; Dubreuil et al., 2003;

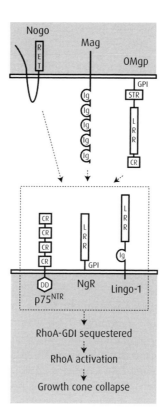

Figure 19.5. *Common signaling pathway of Nogo, MAG and OMgp.* Nogo, MAG, and OMgp all lead to RhoA activation by acting through a receptor complex containing the GPI-linked Nogo receptor (NgR), P75NTR, and Lingo-1 (Mi et al., 2004). Intracellular space is shaded.

Fournier et al., 2003). Importantly, NgR, the receptor for MAG, Omgp and Nogo, forms a functional complex with the p75 neurotrophin receptor (p75NTR) (Wang et al., 2002; Wong et al., 2002), a key upstream regulator of RhoA in neurons (Yamashita et al., 1999). Myelin-associated inhibitors cause the intracellular domain of p75NTR to sequester a Rho-GDI (Yamashita and Tohyama, 2003) leading to the activation of RhoA. These findings support a model whereby the GDI membrane-linked NgR acts as the ligand-binding component of a myelin-associated-inhibitor receptor complex, leading to RhoA activation by p75NTR, growth cone collapse, and termination of axon regeneration (Fig. 19.5).

Roles for developmental cues during regeneration

Interestingly, several of the cues that guide axons during development are also expressed in the adult CNS, raising the possibility that they may also influence axon regeneration following injury. The semaphorins currently present the strongest case for an embryonic axon guidance cue subsequently influencing axon regeneration in the adult nervous system. Sema3A expression increases following lesion in the adult CNS, and this increased expression appears to contribute to restricting or blocking axon regeneration (Tanelian et al., 1997; Pasterkamp et al., 1998a, b, 1999b; Williams-Hogarth et al., 2000). Notably, sema3A is strongly expressed by fibroblast-like cells at the core of the scar that forms following lesion (Pasterkamp et al., 1999a). Additionally, sema4D, a transmembrane semaphorin shown to inhibit axon extension, is expressed by mature myelinating oligodendrocytes and strongly upregulated by oligodendrocytes at the edge of an adult spinal cord injury (Moreau-Fauvarque et al., 2003).

Netrin-1 is also expressed by mature oligodendrocytes in the adult CNS, making it a candidate myelin-associated inhibitor of axon regeneration. If this is the case, neurons attempting to regenerate following injury should express Unc-5 homologs, receptors required for the repellent response to netrin-1. Both DCC and Unc5h2 expression persists in retinal ganglion cells following axotomy as their axons attempt to regenerate along the optic nerve or into a growth permissive peripheral nerve graft (Petrausch et al., 2000; Ellezam et al., 2001). Interestingly, studies carried out in lamprey, a primitive vertebrate with the ability to recover significant function following spinal cord transection (Cohen et al., 1988), have revealed a correlation between Unc-5 expression and poor axonal regeneration following lesion (Shifman and Selzer, 2000).

Although these axon guidance cues are expressed in the adult mammalian CNS, the functional significance of this expression remains unknown. An intriguing hypothesis is that proteins such as semaphorins and netrins function in the intact adult CNS as barriers that restrain axonal sprouting. During maturation of the spinal cord, neuronal expression of Unc5 homologs increases, while expression of DCC decreases, suggesting that Unc5 homolog repellent signaling may be the dominant response to netrin in the adult spinal cord (Manitt et al., 2004). Notably, injection of antibodies that mask Nogo into the intact adult cerebellum causes axonal sprouting of uninjured Purkinje cells (Buffo et al., 2000). These findings suggest that such cues may play an important role maintaining appropriate connections in the intact CNS by restraining inappropriate axonal sprouting. However, the price paid for this is that they subsequently inhibit the re-establishment of connections following injury.

19.7 Concluding remarks

Overcoming the inhibition of axon growth characteristic of the adult CNS following injury is a major goal of contemporary neuroscience. Ultimately, functional recovery will require connecting regenerated axons to their appropriate targets. Although it is now clear that multiple guidance cues for axons in the embryo continue to be expressed in the adult intact CNS, the extent to which these cues will assist, block or misdirect regenerative growth, or might be manipulated to promote the regeneration of appropriate connections, remains to be determined (for additional discussion, see Volume I, Chapter 24).

REFERENCES

Ackerman, S.L., Kozak, L.P., Przyborski, S.A., Rund, L.A., Boyer, B.B. and Knowles, B.B. (1997). The mouse rostral cerebellar malformation gene encodes an UNC-5-like protein. *Nature*, **386**, 838–842.

Adams, D.N., Kao, E.Y., Hypolite, C.L., Distefano, M.D., Hu, W.S. and Letourneau, P.C. (2005). Growth cones turn and migrate up an immobilized gradient of the laminin IKVAV peptide. *J Neurobiol*, **62**, 134–147.

Augsburger, A., Schuchardt, A., Hoskins, S., Dodd, J. and Butler, S. (1999). BMPs as mediators of roof plate repulsion of commissural neurons. *Neuron*, **24**, 127–141.

Beck, K., Hunter, I. and Engel, J. (1990). Structure and function of laminin: anatomy of a multidomain glycoprotein. *FASEB J*, **4**, 148–160.

Belkin, A.M. and Stepp, M.A. (2000). Integrins as receptors for laminins. *Microsc Res Tech*, **51**, 280–301.

Bentley, D. and O'Connor, T.P. (1994). Cytoskeletal events in growth cone steering. *Curr Opin Neurobiol*, **4**, 43–48.

Bentley, D. and Toroian-Raymond, A. (1986). Disoriented pathfinding by pioneer neurone growth cones deprived of filopodia by cytochalasin treatment. *Nature*, **323**, 712–715.

Bishop, A.L. and Hall, A. (2000). Rho GTPases and their effector proteins. *Biochem J*, **348**(Pt 2), 241–255.

Bouchard, J.F., Moore, S.W., Tritsch, N.X., Roux, P.P., Shekarabi, M., Barker, P.A. and Kennedy, T.E. (2004). Protein kinase A activation promotes plasma membrane insertion of DCC from an intracellular pool: a novel mechanism regulating commissural axon extension. *J Neurosci*, **24**, 3040–3050.

Brittis, P.A., Lu, Q. and Flanagan, J.G. (2002). Axonal protein synthesis provides a mechanism for localized regulation at an intermediate target. *Cell*, **110**, 223–235.

Brose, K., Bland, K.S., Wang, K.H., Arnott, D., Henzel, W., Goodman, C.S., Tessier-Lavigne, M. and Kidd, T. (1999). Slit proteins bind Robo receptors and have an evolutionarily conserved role in repulsive axon guidance. *Cell*, **96**, 795–806.

Buffo, A., Zagrebelsky, M., Huber, A.B., Skerra, A., Schwab, M.E., Strata, P. and Rossi, F. (2000). Application of neutralizing antibodies against NI-35/250 myelin-associated neurite growth inhibitory proteins to the adult rat cerebellum induces sprouting of uninjured purkinje cell axons. *J Neurosci*, **20**, 2275–2286.

Butler, S.J. and Dodd, J. (2003). A role for BMP heterodimers in roof plate-mediated repulsion of commissural axons. *Neuron*, **38**, 389–401.

Cai, D., Qiu, J., Cao, Z., McAtee, M., Bregman, B.S. and Filbin, M.T. (2001). Neuronal cyclic AMP controls the developmental loss in ability of axons to regenerate. *J Neurosci*, **21**, 4731–4739.

Cai, D., Deng, K., Mellado, W., Lee, J., Ratan, R.R. and Filbin, M.T. (2002). Arginase I and polyamines act downstream from cyclic AMP in overcoming inhibition of axonal growth MAG and myelin *in vitro*. *Neuron*, **35**, 711–719.

Campbell, D.S. and Holt, C.E. (2001). Chemotropic responses of retinal growth cones mediated by rapid local protein synthesis and degradation. *Neuron*, **32**, 1013–1026.

Castellani, V., Chedotal, A., Schachner, M., Faivre-Sarrailh, C. and Rougon, G. (2000). Analysis of the L1-deficient mouse phenotype reveals cross-talk between Sema3A and L1 signaling pathways in axonal guidance. *Neuron*, **27**, 237–249.

Chan, S.S., Zheng, H., Su, M.W., Wilk, R., Killeen, M.T., Hedgecock, E.M. and Culotti, J.G. (1996). UNC-40, a *C. elegans* homolog of DCC (deleted in colorectal cancer), is required in motile cells responding to UNC-6 netrin cues. *Cell*, **87**, 187–195.

Charron, F., Stein, E., Jeong, J., McMahon, A.P. and Tessier-Lavigne, M. (2003). The morphogen sonic hedgehog is an axonal chemoattractant that collaborates with netrin-1 in midline axon guidance. *Cell*, **113**, 11–23.

Chen, M.S., Huber, A.B., van der Haar, M.E., Frank, M., Schnell, L., Spillmann, A.A., Christ, F. and Schwab, M.E. (2000). Nogo-A is a myelin-associated neurite outgrowth inhibitor and an antigen for monoclonal antibody IN-1. *Nature*, **403**, 434–439.

Chien, C.B., Rosenthal, D.E., Harris, W.A. and Holt, C.E. (1993). Navigational errors made by growth cones without filopodia in the embryonic Xenopus brain. *Neuron*, **11**, 237–251.

Cohen, A.H., Mackler, S.A. and Selzer, M.E. (1988). Behavioral recovery following spinal transection: functional regeneration in the lamprey CNS. *Trend Neurosci*, **11**, 227–231.

Colognato, H. and Yurchenco, P.D. (2000). Form and function: the laminin family of heterotrimers. *Dev Dyn*, **218**, 213–234.

Coonan, J.R., Greferath, U., Messenger, J., Hartley, L., Murphy, M., Boyd, A.W., Dottori, M., Galea, M.P. and Bartlett, P.F. (2001). Development and reorganization of corticospinal projections in EphA4 deficient mice. *J Comp Neurol*, **436**, 248–262.

Dailey, M.E. and Bridgman, P.C. (1991). Structure and organization of membrane organelles along distal microtubule segments in growth cones. *J Neurosci Res*, **30**, 242–258.

David, S. and Aguayo, A.J. (1981). Axonal elongation into peripheral nervous system "bridges" after central nervous system injury in adult rats. *Science*, **214**, 931–933.

David, S., Braun, P.E., Jackson, D.L., Kottis, V. and McKerracher, L. (1995). Laminin overrides the inhibitory effects of peripheral nervous system and central nervous system myelin-derived inhibitors of neurite growth. *J Neurosci Res*, **42**, 594–602.

de Wit, J. and Verhaagen, J. (2003). Role of semaphorins in the adult nervous system. *Prog Neurobiol*, **71**, 249–267.

Dent, E.W. and Gertler, F.B. (2003). Cytoskeletal dynamics and transport in growth cone motility and axon guidance. *Neuron*, **40**, 209–227.

Dergham, P., Ellezam, B., Essagian, C., Avedissian, H., Lubell, W.D. and McKerracher, L. (2002). Rho signaling pathway targeted to promote spinal cord repair. *J Neurosci*, **22**, 6570–6577.

Dertinger, S.K., Jiang, X., Li, Z., Murthy, V.N. and Whitesides, G.M. (2002). Gradients of substrate-bound laminin orient axonal specification of neurons. *Proc Natl Acad Sci USA*, **99**, 12542–12547.

Dickson, B.J. (2001). Rho GTPases in growth cone guidance. *Curr Opin Neurobiol*, **11**, 103–110.

Domeniconi, M., Cao, Z., Spencer, T., Sivasankaran, R., Wang, K., Nikulina, E., Kimura, N., Cai, H., Deng, K., Gao, Y., He, Z. and Filbin, M. (2002). Myelin-associated glycoprotein interacts with the Nogo66 receptor to inhibit neurite outgrowth. *Neuron*, **35**, 283–290.

Drescher, U., Kremoser, C., Handwerker, C., Loschinger, J., Noda, M. and Bonhoeffer, F. (1995). *In vitro* guidance of retinal ganglion cell axons by RAGS, a 25 kDa tectal protein related to ligands for Eph receptor tyrosine kinases. *Cell*, **82**, 359–370.

Dubreuil, C.I., Winton, M.J. and McKerracher, L. (2003). Rho activation patterns after spinal cord injury and the role of activated Rho in apoptosis in the central nervous system. *J Cell Biol*, **162**, 233–243.

Ellerbroek, S.M., Wennerberg, K. and Burridge, K. (2003). Serine phosphorylation negatively regulates RhoA *in vivo*. *J Biol Chem*, **278**, 19023–19031.

Ellezam, B., Selles-Navarro, I., Manitt, C., Kennedy, T.E. and McKerracher, L. (2001). Expression of netrin-1 and its receptors DCC and UNC-5H2 after axotomy and during regeneration of adult rat retinal ganglion cells. *Exp Neurol*, **168**, 105–115.

Engelkamp, D. (2002). Cloning of three mouse Unc5 genes and their expression patterns at mid-gestation. *Mech Dev*, **118**, 191–197.

Engvall, E. and Wewer, U.M. (1996). Domains of laminin. *J Cell Biochem*, **61**, 493–501.

Eph Nomenclature Committee (1997). Unified nomenclature for Eph family receptors and their ligands, the ephrins. *Cell*, **90**, 403–404.

Erickson, A.C. and Couchman, J.R. (2000). Still more complexity in mammalian basement membranes. *J Histochem Cytochem*, **48**, 1291–1306.

Erskine, L., Williams, S.E., Brose, K., Kidd, T., Rachel, R.A., Goodman, C.S., Tessier-Lavigne, M. and Mason, C.A. (2000). Retinal ganglion cell axon guidance in the mouse optic chiasm: expression and function of robos and slits. *J Neurosci*, **20**, 4975–4982.

Fazeli, A., Dickinson, S.L., Hermiston, M.L., Tighe, R.V., Steen, R.G., Small, C.G., Stoeckli, E.T., Keino-Masu, K., Masu, M., Rayburn, H., Simons, J., Bronson, R.T., Gordon, J.I.,

Tessier-Lavigne, M. and Weinberg, R.A. (1997). Phenotype of mice lacking functional deleted in colorectal cancer (Dcc) gene. *Nature*, **386**, 796–804.

Forscher, P. and Smith, S.J. (1988). Actions of cytochalasins on the organization of actin filaments and microtubules in a neuronal growth cone. *J Cell Biol*, **107**, 1505–1516.

Fournier, A.E., GrandPre, T. and Strittmatter, S.M. (2001). Identification of a receptor mediating Nogo-66 inhibition of axonal regeneration. *Nature*, **409**, 341–346.

Fournier, A.E., Takizawa, B.T. and Strittmatter, S.M. (2003). Rho kinase inhibition enhances axonal regeneration in the injured CNS. *J Neurosci*, **23**, 1416–1423.

Gao, Y., Deng, K., Hou, J., Bryson, J.B., Barco, A., Nikulina, E., Spencer, T., Mellado, W., Kandel, E.R. and Filbin, M.T. (2004). Activated CREB is sufficient to overcome inhibitors in myelin and promote spinal axon regeneration *in vivo*. *Neuron*, **44**, 609–621.

Govek, E.E., Newey, S.E. and Van Aelst, L. (2005). The role of the Rho GTPases in neuronal development. *Gene Dev*, **19**, 1–49.

GrandPre, T., Nakamura, F., Vartanian, T. and Strittmatter, S.M. (2000). Identification of the Nogo inhibitor of axon regeneration as a reticulon protein. *Nature*, **403**, 439–444.

Hall, A. (1998). Rho GTPases and the actin cytoskeleton. *Science*, **279**, 509–514.

Harris, W.A., Holt, C.E. and Bonhoeffer, F. (1987). Retinal axons with and without their somata, growing to and arborizing in the tectum of Xenopus embryos: a time-lapse video study of single fibres *in vivo*. *Development*, **101**, 123–133.

Harrison, C.J. (1914). The reaction of embryonic cells to solid structures. *J Exp Zool*, **17**, 521–544.

Harrison, R.G. (1907). Observations on the living developing nerve fiber. *Proc Soc Exp Biol Med*, **4**, 140–143.

Hedgecock, E.M., Culotti, J.G. and Hall, D.H. (1990). The unc-5, unc-6, and unc-40 genes guide circumferential migrations of pioneer axons and mesodermal cells on the epidermis in *C. elegans*. *Neuron*, **4**, 61–85.

Himanen, J.P. and Nikolov, D.B. (2003). Eph signaling: a structural view. *Trend Neurosci*, **26**, 46–51.

Holmberg, J. and Frisen, J. (2002). Ephrins are not only unattractive. *Trend Neurosci*, **25**, 239–243.

Holmes, G.P., Negus, K., Burridge, L., Raman, S., Algar, E., Yamada, T. and Little, M.H. (1998). Distinct but overlapping expression patterns of two vertebrate slit homologs implies functional roles in CNS development and organogenesis. *Mech Dev*, **79**, 57–72.

Hong, K., Hinck, L., Nishiyama, M., Poo, M.M., Tessier-Lavigne, M. and Stein, E. (1999). A ligand-gated association between cytoplasmic domains of UNC5 and DCC family receptors converts netrin-induced growth cone attraction to repulsion. *Cell*, **97**, 927–941.

Hopker, V.H., Shewan, D., Tessier-Lavigne, M., Poo, M. and Holt, C. (1999). Growth-cone attraction to netrin-1 is converted to repulsion by laminin-1. *Nature*, **401**, 69–73.

Ide, C., Tohyama, K., Yokota, R., Nitatori, T. and Onodera, S. (1983). Schwann cell basal lamina and nerve regeneration. *Brain Res*, **288**, 61–75.

Imondi, R. and Kaprielian, Z. (2001). Commissural axon pathfinding on the contralateral side of the floor plate: a role for B-class ephrins in specifying the dorsoventral position of longitudinally projecting commissural axons. *Development*, **128**, 4859–4871.

Ishii, N., Wadsworth, W.G., Stern, B.D., Culotti, J.G. and Hedgecock, E.M. (1992). UNC-6, a laminin-related protein, guides cell and pioneer axon migrations in *C. elegans*. *Neuron*, **9**, 873–881.

Itoh, A., Miyabayashi, T., Ohno, M. and Sakano, S. (1998). Cloning and expressions of three mammalian homologues of *Drosophila* slit suggest possible roles for Slit in the formation and maintenance of the nervous system. *Brain Res Mol Brain Res*, **62**, 175–186.

Jalink, K., van Corven, E.J., Hengeveld, T., Morii, N., Narumiya, S. and Moolenaar, W.H. (1994). Inhibition of lysophosphatidate- and thrombin-induced neurite retraction and neuronal cell rounding by ADP ribosylation of the small GTP-binding protein Rho. *J Cell Biol*, **126**, 801–810.

Jin, Z. and Strittmatter, S.M. (1997). Rac1 mediates collapsin-1-induced growth cone collapse. *J Neurosci*, **17**, 6256–6263.

Kappler, J., Franken, S., Junghans, U., Hoffmann, R., Linke, T., Muller, H.W. and Koch, K.W. (2000). Glycosaminoglycan-binding properties and secondary structure of the C-terminus of netrin-1. *Biochem Biophys Res Commun*, **271**, 287–291.

Keino-Masu, K., Masu, M., Hinck, L., Leonardo, E.D., Chan, S.S., Culotti, J.G. and Tessier-Lavigne, M. (1996). Deleted in colorectal cancer (DCC) encodes a netrin receptor. *Cell*, **87**, 175–185.

Keleman, K., Rajagopalan, S., Cleppien, D., Teis, D., Paiha, K., Huber, L.A., Technau, G.M. and Dickson, B.J. (2002). Comm sorts robo to control axon guidance at the *Drosophila* midline. *Cell*, **110**, 415–427.

Kennedy, T.E., Serafini Jr., de la Torre, J.R. and Tessier-Lavigne, M. (1994). Netrins are diffusible chemotropic factors for commissural axons in the embryonic spinal cord. *Cell*, **78**, 425–435.

Keshishian, H. and Bentley, D. (1983). Embryogenesis of peripheral nerve pathways in grasshopper legs. I. The initial nerve pathway to the CNS. *Dev Biol*, **96**, 89–102.

Kidd, T., Bland, K.S. and Goodman, C.S. (1999). Slit is the midline repellent for the robo receptor in *Drosophila*. *Cell*, **96**, 785–794.

Knoll, B. and Drescher, U. (2002). Ephrin-As as receptors in topographic projections. *Trend Neurosci*, **25**, 145–149.

Kolodkin, A.L. and Ginty, D.D. (1997). Steering clear of semaphorins: neuropilins sound the retreat. *Neuron*, **19**, 1159–1162.

Kottis, V., Thibault, P., Mikol, D., Xiao, Z.C., Zhang, R., Dergham, P. and Braun, P.E. (2002). Oligodendrocyte-myelin glycoprotein (OMgp) is an inhibitor of neurite outgrowth. *J Neurochem*, **82**, 1566–1569.

Kullander, K. and Klein, R. (2002). Mechanisms and functions of Eph and ephrin signalling. *Nat Rev Mol Cell Biol*, **3**, 475–486.

Kullander, K., Croll, S.D., Zimmer, M., Pan, L., McClain, J., Hughes, V., Zabski, S., DeChiara, T.M., Klein, R., Yancopoulos, G.D. and Gale, N.W. (2001). Ephrin-B3 is the midline barrier that prevents corticospinal tract axons from recrossing, allowing for unilateral motor control. *Gene Dev*, **15**, 877–888.

Lang, P., Gesbert, F., Delespine-Carmagnat, M., Stancou, R., Pouchelet, M. and Bertoglio, J. (1996). Protein kinase A phosphorylation of RhoA mediates the morphological and functional effects of cyclic AMP in cytotoxic lymphocytes. *EMBO J*, **15**, 510–519.

Lehmann, M., Fournier, A., Selles-Navarro, I., Dergham, P., Sebok, A., Leclerc, N., Tigyi, G. and McKerracher, L. (1999). Inactivation of Rho signaling pathway promotes CNS axon regeneration. *J Neurosci*, **19**, 7537–7547.

Lentz, S.I., Miner, J.H., Sanes, J.R. and Snider, W.D. (1997). Distribution of the ten known laminin chains in the pathways and targets of developing sensory axons. *J Comp Neurol*, **378**, 547–561.

Leonardo, E.D., Hinck, L., Masu, M., Keino-Masu, K., Ackerman, S.L. and Tessier-Lavigne, M. (1997). Vertebrate homologues of *C. elegans* UNC-5 are candidate netrin receptors. *Nature*, **386**, 833–838.

Letourneau, P.C. (1983). Differences in the organization of actin in the growth cones compared with the neurites of cultured neurons from chick embryos. *J Cell Biol*, **97**, 963–973.

Leung-Hagesteijn, C., Spence, A.M., Stern, B.D., Zhou, Y., Su, M.W., Hedgecock, E.M. and Culotti, J.G. (1992). UNC-5, a transmembrane protein with immunoglobulin and thrombospondin type 1 domains, guides cell and pioneer axon migrations in *C. elegans*. *Cell*, **71**, 289–299.

Li, H.S., Chen, J.H., Wu, W., Fagaly, T., Zhou, L., Yuan, W., Dupuis, S., Jiang, Z.H., Nash, W., Gick, C., Ornitz, D.M., Wu, J.Y. and Rao, Y. (1999). Vertebrate slit, a secreted ligand for the transmembrane protein roundabout, is a repellent for olfactory bulb axons. *Cell*, **96**, 807–818.

Liu, B.P., Fournier, A., GrandPre, T. and Strittmatter, S.M. (2002). Myelin-associated glycoprotein as a functional ligand for the Nogo-66 receptor. *Science*, **297**, 1190–1193.

Long, H., Sabatier, C., Ma, L., Plump, A., Yuan, W., Ornitz, D.M., Tamada, A., Murakami, F., Goodman, C.S. and Tessier-Lavigne, M. (2004). Conserved roles for Slit and Robo proteins in midline commissural axon guidance. *Neuron*, **42**, 213–223.

Luo, Y., Raible, D. and Raper, J.A. (1993). Collapsin: a protein in brain that induces the collapse and paralysis of neuronal growth cones. *Cell*, **75**, 217–227.

Lyuksyutova, A.I., Lu, C.C., Milanesio, N., King, L.A., Guo, N., Wang, Y., Nathans, J., Tessier-Lavigne, M. and Zou, Y. (2003). Anterior-posterior guidance of commissural axons by Wnt-frizzled signaling. *Science*, **302**, 1984–1988.

Mallavarapu, A. and Mitchison, T. (1999). Regulated actin cytoskeleton assembly at filopodium tips controls their extension and retraction. *J Cell Biol*, **146**, 1097–1106.

Manitt, C. and Kennedy, T.E. (2002). Where the rubber meets the road: netrin expression and function in developing and adult nervous systems. *Prog Brain Res*, **137**, 425–442.

Manitt, C., Colicos, M.A., Thompson, K.M., Rousselle, E., Peterson, A.C. and Kennedy, T.E. (2001). Widespread expression of netrin-1 by neurons and oligodendrocytes in the adult mammalian spinal cord. *J Neurosci*, **21**, 3911–3922.

Manitt, C., Thompson, K.M. and Kennedy, T.E. (2004). Developmental shift in expression of netrin receptors in the rat spinal cord: predominance of UNC-5 homologues in adulthood. *J Neurosci Res*, **77**, 690–700.

Marillat, V., Sabatier, C., Failli, V., Matsunaga, E., Sotelo, C., Tessier-Lavigne, M. and Chedotal, A. (2004). The slit receptor Rig-1/Robo3 controls midline crossing by hindbrain precerebellar neurons and axons. *Neuron*, **43**, 69–79.

Matsuzawa, M., Tokumitsu, S., Knoll, W. and Liesi, P. (1998). Molecular gradient along the axon pathway is not required for directional axon growth. *J Neurosci Res*, **53**, 114–124.

McKenna, M.P. and Raper, J.A. (1988). Growth cone behavior on gradients of substratum bound laminin. *Dev Biol*, **130**, 232–236.

McKerracher, L., David, S., Jackson, D.L., Kottis, V., Dunn, R.J. and Braun, P.E. (1994). Identification of myelin-associated glycoprotein as a major myelin-derived inhibitor of neurite growth. *Neuron*, **13**, 805–811.

McLaughlin, T., Hindges, R. and O'Leary, D.D. (2003). Regulation of axial patterning of the retina and its topographic mapping in the brain. *Curr Opin Neurobiol*, **13**, 57–69.

Messersmith, E.K., Leonardo, E.D., Shatz, C.J., Tessier-Lavigne, M., Goodman, C.S. and Kolodkin, A.L. (1995). Semaphorin III can function as a selective chemorepellent to pattern sensory projections in the spinal cord. *Neuron*, **14**, 949–959.

Mi, S., Lee, X., Shao, Z., Thill, G., Ji, B., Relton, J., Levesque, M., Allaire, N., Perrin, S., Sands, B., Crowell, T., Cate, R.L., McCoy, J.M. and Pepinsky, R.B. (2004). LINGO-1 is a component of the Nogo-66 receptor/p75 signaling complex. *Nat Neurosci*, **7**, 221–228.

Ming, G.L., Song, H.J., Berninger, B., Holt, C.E., Tessier-Lavigne, M. and Poo, M.M. (1997). cAMP-dependent growth cone guidance by netrin-1. *Neuron*, **19**, 1225–1235.

Moreau-Fauvarque, C., Kumanogoh, A., Camand, E., Jaillard, C., Barbin, G., Boquet, I., Love, C., Jones, E.Y., Kikutani, H., Lubetzki, C., Dusart, I. and Chedotal, A. (2003). The transmembrane semaphorin Sema4D/CD100, an inhibitor of axonal growth, is expressed on oligodendrocytes and upregulated after CNS lesion. *J Neurosci*, **23**, 9229–9239.

Morgenstern, D.A., Asher, R.A. and Fawcett, J.W. (2002). Chondroitin sulphate proteoglycans in the CNS injury response. *Prog Brain Res*, **137**, 313–332.

Mukhopadhyay, G., Doherty, P., Walsh, F.S., Crocker, P.R. and Filbin, M.T. (1994). A novel role for myelin-associated glycoprotein as an inhibitor of axonal regeneration. *Neuron*, **13**, 757–767.

Neumann, S., Bradke, F., Tessier-Lavigne, M. and Basbaum, A.I. (2002). Regeneration of sensory axons within the injured spinal cord induced by intraganglionic cAMP elevation. *Neuron*, **34**, 885–893.

Nguyen Ba-Charvet, K.T., Brose, K., Marillat, V., Kidd, T., Goodman, C.S., Tessier-Lavigne, M., Sotelo, C. and Chedotal, A. (1999). Slit2-mediated chemorepulsion and collapse of developing forebrain axons. *Neuron*, **22**, 463–473.

Nusslein-Volhard, C., Wiechaus, E. and Kluding, H. (1984). Mutations affecting the pattern of the larval cuticle in *Drosophila melanogaster*. I. Zygotic loci on the second chromosome. *Wilhelm Roux's Archiv Develop Biol*, **193**, 267–283.

O'Connor, T.P., Duerr, J.S. and Bentley, D. (1990). Pioneer growth cone steering decisions mediated by single filopodial contacts in situ. *J Neurosci*, **10**, 3935–3946.

Orioli, D., Henkemeyer, M., Lemke, G., Klein, R. and Pawson, T. (1996). Sek4 and Nuk receptors cooperate in guidance of commissural axons and in palate formation. *EMBO J*, **15**, 6035–6049.

Pasterkamp, R.J., De Winter, F., Holtmaat, A.J. and Verhaagen, J. (1998a). Evidence for a role of the chemorepellent semaphorin III and its receptor neuropilin-1 in the regeneration of primary olfactory axons. *J Neurosci*, **18**, 9962–9976.

Pasterkamp, R.J., Giger, R.J. and Verhaagen, J. (1998b). Regulation of semaphorin III/collapsin-1 gene expression during peripheral nerve regeneration. *Exp Neurol*, **153**, 313–327.

Pasterkamp, R.J., Giger, R.J., Ruitenberg, M.J., Holtmaat, A.J., de Wit, J., De Winter, F. and Verhaagen, J. (1999a). Expression of the gene encoding the chemorepellent semaphorin III is induced in the fibroblast component of neural scar tissue formed following injuries of adult but not neonatal CNS. *Mol Cell Neurosci*, **13**, 143–166.

Pasterkamp, R.J., Ruitenberg, M.J. and Verhaagen, J. (1999b). Semaphorins and their receptors in olfactory axon guidance. *Cell Mol Biol (Noisy. -le-grand)* **45**, 763–779.

Petrausch, B., Jung, M., Leppert, C.A. and Stuermer, C.A. (2000). Lesion-induced regulation of netrin receptors and modification of netrin-1 expression in the retina of fish and grafted rats. *Mol Cell Neurosci*, **16**, 350–364.

Piper, M. and Holt, C. (2004). RNA translation in axons. *Annu Rev Cell Dev Biol*, **20**, 505–523.

Placzek, M., Tessier-Lavigne, M., Jessell, T. and Dodd, J. (1990). Orientation of commissural axons *in vitro* in response to a floor plate-derived chemoattractant. *Development*, **110**, 19–30.

Prinjha, R., Moore, S.E., Vinson, M., Blake, S., Morrow, R., Christie, G., Michalovich, D., Simmons, D.L. and Walsh, F.S. (2000). Inhibitor of neurite outgrowth in humans. *Nature*, **403**, 383–384.

Qiu, J., Cai, D., Dai, H., McAtee, M., Hoffman, P.N., Bregman, B.S. and Filbin, M.T. (2002). Spinal axon regeneration induced by elevation of cyclic AMP. *Neuron*, **34**, 895–903.

Rajagopalan, S., Vivancos, V., Nicolas, E. and Dickson, B.J. (2000). Selecting a longitudinal pathway: Robo receptors specify the lateral position of axons in the *Drosophila* CNS. *Cell*, **103**, 1033–1045.

Ramón y Cajal, S. (1890). À quelle époque apparaissent les expansions des cellules nerveuses de la moëlle épinière du poulet? *Anat Anzeiger*, **21–22**, 609–639.

Ramón y Cajal, S. (1892). La rétine des vertèbres. *Cellule*, **9**, 119–258.

Ramón y Cajal, S. (1899). Textura del sistema nervioso del hombre y de los vertebrados estudios sobre el plan estructural y composición histológica de los centros nerviosos adicionados de consideraciones fisiológicas fundadas en los nuevos descubrimientos. N. Moya, Madrid.

Raper, J.A. (2000). Semaphorins and their receptors in vertebrates and invertebrates. *Curr Opin Neurobiol*, **10**, 88–94.

Reichardt, L.F. and Tomaselli, K.J. (1991). Extracellular matrix molecules and their receptors: functions in neural development. *Annu Rev Neurosci*, **14**, 531–570.

Rothberg, J.M., Hartley, D.A., Walther, Z. and Artavanis-Tsakonas, S. (1988). Slit: an EGF-homologous locus of *D. melanogaster* involved in the development of the embryonic central nervous system. *Cell*, **55**, 1047–1059.

Rothberg, J.M., Jacobs, J.R., Goodman, C.S. and Artavanis-Tsakonas, S. (1990). Slit: an extracellular protein necessary for development of midline glia and commissural axon pathways contains both EGF and LRR domains. *Gene Dev*, **4**, 2169–2187.

Sabatier, C., Plump, A.S., Le, M., Brose, K., Tamada, A., Murakami, F., Lee, E.Y. and Tessier-Lavigne, M. (2004). The divergent Robo family protein rig-1/Robo3 is a negative regulator of slit responsiveness required for midline crossing by commissural axons. *Cell*, **117**, 157–169.

Schaefer, A.W., Kabir, N. and Forscher, P. (2002). Filopodia and actin arcs guide the assembly and transport of two populations of microtubules with unique dynamic parameters in neuronal growth cones. *J Cell Biol*, **158**, 139–152.

Schwab, M.E. and Bartholdi, D. (1996). Degeneration and regeneration of axons in the lesioned spinal cord. *Physiol Rev*, **76**, 319–370.

Seeger, M., Tear, G., Ferres-Marco, D. and Goodman, C.S. (1993). Mutations affecting growth cone guidance in *Drosophila*: genes necessary for guidance toward or away from the midline. *Neuron*, **10**, 409–426.

Serafini, T., Kennedy, T.E., Galko, M.J., Mirzayan, C., Jessell, T.M. and Tessier-Lavigne, M. (1994). The netrins define a family of axon outgrowth-promoting proteins homologous to *C. elegans* UNC-6. *Cell*, **78**, 409–424.

Serafini, T., Colamarino, S.A., Leonardo, E.D., Wang, H., Beddington, R., Skarnes, W.C. and Tessier-Lavigne, M. (1996). Netrin-1 is required for commissural axon guidance in the developing vertebrate nervous system. *Cell*, **87**, 1001–1014.

Shaw, G. and Bray, D. (1977). Movement and extension of isolated growth cones. *Exp Cell Res*, **104**, 55–62.

Shifman, M.I. and Selzer, M.E. (2000). Expression of the netrin receptor UNC-5 in lamprey brain: modulation by spinal cord transection. *Neurorehabil Neural Repair*, **14**, 49–58.

Simpson, J.H., Bland, K.S., Fetter, R.D. and Goodman, C.S. (2000). Short-range and long-range guidance by Slit and its Robo receptors: a combinatorial code of Robo receptors controls lateral position. *Cell*, **103**, 1019–1032.

Song, H., Ming, G., He, Z., Lehmann, M., McKerracher, L., Tessier-Lavigne, M. and Poo, M. (1998). Conversion of neuronal growth cone responses from repulsion to attraction by cyclic nucleotides. *Science*, **281**, 1515–1518.

Song, H.J. and Poo, M.M. (1999). Signal transduction underlying growth cone guidance by diffusible factors. *Curr Opin Neurobiol*, **9**, 355–363.

Speidel, C.C. (1933). Studies of living nerves. II. Activities of amoeboid growth cones, sheath cells and myelin segments, as revealed by prolonged observation of individual fibers in frog tadpoles. *Am J Anat*, **52**, 1–79.

Sperry, R.W. (1963). Chemoaffinity in the orderly growth of nerve fiber patterns and connections. *Proc Natl Acad Sci USA*, **50**, 703–710.

Stein, E. and Tessier-Lavigne, M. (2001). Hierarchical organization of guidance receptors: silencing of netrin attraction by slit through a Robo/DCC receptor complex. *Science*, **291**, 1928–1938.

Stoeckli, E.T., Sonderegger, P., Pollerberg, G.E. and Landmesser, L.T. (1997). Interference with axonin-1 and NrCAM interactions unmasks a floor-plate activity inhibitory for commissural axons. *Neuron*, **18**, 209–221.

Suter, D.M. and Forscher, P. (2000). Substrate-cytoskeletal coupling as a mechanism for the regulation of growth cone motility and guidance. *J Neurobiol*, **44**, 97–113.

Taguchi, A., Wanaka, A., Mori, T., Matsumoto, K., Imai, Y., Tagaki, T. and Tohyama, M. (1996). Molecular cloning of novel leucine-rich repeat proteins and their expression in the developing mouse nervous system. *Brain Res Mol Brain Res*, **35**, 31–40.

Tamagnone, L. and Comoglio, P.M. (2000). Signalling by semaphorin receptors: cell guidance and beyond. *Trend Cell Biol*, **10**, 377–383.

Tanaka, E.M. and Kirschner, M.W. (1991). Microtubule behavior in the growth cones of living neurons during axon elongation. *J Cell Biol*, **115**, 345–363.

Tanelian, D.L., Barry, M.A., Johnston, S.A., Le, T. and Smith, G.M. (1997). Semaphorin III can repulse and inhibit adult sensory afferents *in vivo*. *Nat Med*, **3**, 1398–1401.

Tessier-Lavigne, M. and Goodman, C.S. (1996). The molecular biology of axon guidance. *Science*, **274**, 1123–1133.

Tessier-Lavigne, M., Placzek, M., Lumsden, A.G., Dodd, J. and Jessell, T.M. (1988). Chemotropic guidance of developing axons in the mammalian central nervous system. *Nature*, **336**, 775–778.

Wadsworth, W.G., Bhatt, H. and Hedgecock, E.M. (1996). Neuroglia and pioneer neurons express UNC-6 to provide global and local netrin cues for guiding migrations in *C. elegans*. *Neuron*, **16**, 35–46.

Wang, K.H., Brose, K., Arnott, D., Kidd, T., Goodman, C.S., Henzel, W. and Tessier-Lavigne, M. (1999). Biochemical purification of a mammalian slit protein as a positive regulator of sensory axon elongation and branching. *Cell*, **96**, 771–784.

Wang, K.C., Kim, J.A., Sivasankaran, R., Segal, R. and He, Z. (2002). P75 interacts with the Nogo receptor as a co-receptor for Nogo, MAG and OMgp. *Nature*, **420**, 74–78.

Weber, A. (1934). Croissance des fibres nerveuses commissurales lors de lésions de la moelle épinière chez de jeunes embryons de poulet. *Biomorphosis*, **1**, 30–35.

Weiss, P.A. (1934). *In vitro* experiments on the factors determining the course of the outgrowing nerve fiber. *J Exp Zool*, **68**, 393–448.

Weiss, P.A. (1941). Self-differentiation of the basic patterns of coordination. *Comparat Psychol Monogr*, **17**, 1–96.

Welnhofer, E.A., Zhao, L. and Cohan, C.S. (1997). Actin dynamics and organization during growth cone morphogenesis in Helisoma neurons. *Cell Motil Cytoskel*, **37**, 54–71.

Williams-Hogarth, L.C., Puche, A.C., Torrey, C., Cai, X., Song, I., Kolodkin, A.L., Shipley, M.T. and Ronnett, G.V. (2000). Expression of semaphorins in developing and regenerating olfactory epithelium. *J Comp Neurol*, **423**, 565–578.

Winton, M.J., Dubreuil, C.I., Lasko, D., Leclerc, N. and McKerracher, L. (2002). Characterization of new cell permeable C3-like proteins that inactivate Rho and stimulate neurite outgrowth on inhibitory substrates. *J Biol Chem*, **277**, 32820–32829.

Wong, J.T., Yu, W.T. and O'Connor, T.P. (1997). Transmembrane grasshopper semaphorin I promotes axon outgrowth *in vivo*. *Development*, **124**, 3597–3607.

Wong, J.T., Wong, S.T. and O'Connor, T.P. (1999). Ectopic semaphorin-1a functions as an attractive guidance cue for developing peripheral neurons. *Nat Neurosci*, **2**, 798–803.

Wong, S.T., Henley, J.R., Kanning, K.C., Huang, K.H., Bothwell, M. and Poo, M.M. (2002). A p75(NTR) and Nogo receptor complex mediates repulsive signaling by myelin-associated glycoprotein. *Nat Neurosci*, **5**, 1302–1308.

Yamashita, T. and Tohyama, M. (2003). The p75 receptor acts as a displacement factor that releases Rho from Rho-GDI. *Nat Neurosci*, **6**, 461–467.

Yamashita, T., Tucker, K.L. and Barde, Y.A. (1999). Neurotrophin binding to the p75 receptor modulates Rho activity and axonal outgrowth. *Neuron*, **24**, 585–593.

Yebra, M., Montgomery, A.M., Diaferia, G.R., Kaido, T., Silletti, S., Perez, B., Just, M.L., Hildbrand, S., Hurford, R., Florkiewicz, E., Tessier-Lavigne, M. and Cirulli, V. (2003). Recognition of the neural chemoattractant netrin-1 by integrins alpha6beta4 and alpha3beta1 regulates epithelial cell adhesion and migration. *Dev Cell*, **5**, 695–707.

Yokoyama, N., Romero, M.I., Cowan, C.A., Galvan, P., Helmbacher, F., Charnay, P., Parada, L.F. and Henkemeyer, M.

(2001). Forward signaling mediated by ephrin-B3 prevents contralateral corticospinal axons from recrossing the spinal cord midline. *Neuron*, **29**, 85–97.

Yu, T.W. and Bargmann, C.I. (2001). Dynamic regulation of axon guidance. *Nat Neurosci*, **4(Suppl. 4)**, 1169–1176.

Yuan, S.S., Cox, L.A., Dasika, G.K. and Lee, E.Y. (1999). Cloning and functional studies of a novel gene aberrantly expressed in RB-deficient embryos. *Dev Biol*, **207**, 62–75.

Zheng, J.Q., Wan, J.J. and Poo, M.M. (1996). Essential role of filopodia in chemotropic turning of nerve growth cone induced by a glutamate gradient. *J Neurosci*, **16**, 1140–1149.

Zou, Y., Stoeckli, E., Chen, H. and Tessier-Lavigne, M. (2000). Squeezing axons out of the gray matter: a role for slit and semaphorin proteins from midline and ventral spinal cord. *Cell*, **102**, 363–375.

20

Synaptogenesis

Matthew S. Kayser and Matthew B. Dalva

Department of Neuroscience, University of Pennsylvania School of Medicine, Philadelphia, PA, USA

Synaptic connections are highly specialized sites of cell–cell contact that allow information to pass between neurons. Each central nervous system (CNS) neuron must form thousands of these connections for proper brain function. The establishment of neuronal contacts during development is a precise and specific phenomenon, in which axons are guided to the vicinity of their targets and appropriate pre- and postsynaptic partners are able to connect. The signaling cascades and molecular interactions regulating synaptogenesis must provide for synapse formation to occur between the correct cells, on the correct portion of a cell, and with the correct alignment of essential components within a synapse. Following contact, some nascent synapses stabilize and mature while others are lost, resulting in a dynamic neuronal circuitry thought to underlie information processing and storage.

In this chapter, we detail the process of synapse development, focusing on the signaling and molecular cues involved in the formation of mammalian central excitatory synapses. We provide an overview of synapse structure and describe the initial contact between axon and dendrite. We then discuss the differentiation of those pre- and postsynaptic compartments, and the large number of molecules implicated in the regulation of synaptogenesis. Finally, we address how activity might be involved in the formation and/or maturation of synaptic contacts, and how control of this intricate process might differ in young animals compared to adults or following neural injury.

20.1 The neuromuscular synapse

At both central excitatory chemical synapses and the peripheral neuromuscular junction (NMJ), a synapse is characterized by tightly opposed, asymmetric pre- and postsynaptic terminals, each containing specialized proteins present in far higher concentrations than anywhere else in the cell (Sanes and Lichtman, 1999). Much is know regarding NMJ synapse development, organization, and modulation, due largely to its accessibility, size, and homogeneity; the molecular signals controlling NMJ formation have served as a foundation for study of the more complex CNS (Sanes and Lichtman, 1999).

The NMJ forms through a relatively well-defined series of events. The first step in NMJ formation is prepatterning of the muscle fiber, which requires the muscle-specific tyrosine kinase (MuSK) but can occur in the absence of presynaptic input (Lin et al., 2001; Yang et al., 2001). The arriving presynaptic motor neuron secretes the proteoglycan agrin, inducing clusters of postsynaptic acetylcholine receptors (AChRs) via MuSK activation (DeChiara et al., 1996; Glass et al., 1996). MuSK promotes AChR clustering through the effector protein rapsyn, and also increases AChR synthesis by enhancing the concentration of the neuregulin-binding ErbB receptors (Sanes and Lichtman, 1999). While many characteristics of NMJ and CNS synapse development may be shared, obvious distinctions are apparent, due largely to the different structure and function of the central synapse. A mature muscle fiber is innervated by a single axon, and the synapse is specialized to reliably produce an action potential in the muscle fiber given presynaptic input (Sanes and Lichtman, 1999). In contrast, CNS neurons are innervated by hundreds or thousands of axons, and most synapses are specialized to allow integration of numerous inputs that can sum to cause a neuronal action potential.

20.2 CNS synapse structure

Mature pre- and postsynaptic terminals have characteristic morphologic and molecular components that allow for transmission of neuronal activity between cells. Presynaptic compartments are filled with thousands of neurotransmitter-containing synaptic vesicles and a specialized set of proteins that control vesicle fusion in a calcium-dependent fashion, including SNAP receptor (SNARE) proteins and Munc-18 (Hata et al., 1993; Rizo and Sudhof, 2002). The postsynaptic region is defined by an electron dense area known as the postsynaptic density (PSD), which contains clustered neurotransmitter receptors and associated proteins that mediate and modulate synaptic transmission. Mass-spectrometry has enabled the postsynaptic complex of proteins to be purified from adult brain (Peng et al., 2004). Remarkably, this work suggests that hundreds of different proteins may reside at the postsynaptic density. In addition to those that are directly involved in transmission, such as N-methyl-D-aspartate (NMDA) and di-alpha-amino-3-hydroxy-5-methyl-4-isoxazone-propionate (AMPA) type glutamate receptors, a host of other molecules are involved in synapse formation and stability, or play a role in modulating synaptic strength and shape (Fig. 20.1).

Not only are specific sets of proteins found at synapses, but the majority of mature excitatory synapses in the CNS occur on small, bulbous morphologic specializations known as dendritic spines (Harris, 1999); the brain contains more than 10^{13} spines (Nimchinsky et al., 2002). Dendritic spines may behave as electrical compartments (Koch and Poggio, 1983; Nimchinsky et al., 2002) or as chemical

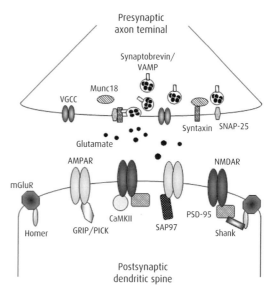

Figure 20.1. *Diagram of a glutamatergic excitatory synapse.* The postsynaptic dendritic compartment contains hundreds of proteins, a subset of which are depicted here. AMPA- and NMDA-type glutamate receptors are the primary mediators of excitatory synaptic transmission, and are located in the PSD; metabotropic glutamate receptors (mGluRs) are located more peripherally. Each of these receptors binds to scaffolding and signaling molecules (PSD-95, GRIP/PICK, Homer, CaMKII) via specific intracellular domain binding motifs. The presynaptic terminal contains synaptic vesicles and exocytic machinery. Calcium flux through voltage-gated calcium channels (VGCC) causes formation of the SNARE complex (synaptobrevin, syntaxin, SNAP-25) and fusion of synaptic vesicles with the presynaptic membrane to release neurotransmitter into the synaptic cleft.

compartments, particularly for calcium (Sabatini et al., 2001). Regardless, their vast number and relatively stereotyped shape suggests that spines have functional importance. Mushroom-shaped spines, with large heads and short constricted necks, are thought to be the most mature morphology (Hering and Sheng, 2001; Nimchinsky et al., 2002). Dendritic protrusions can also be classified into other shapes, including thin and stubby spines, and filopodia (Fig. 20.2; Hering and Sheng, 2001; Pak et al., 2001). The long, thin, motile filopodia-like protrusions on

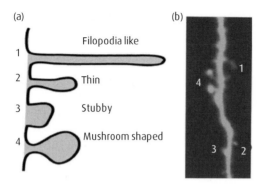

Figure 20.2. *Morphology of dendritic spines.* (a) Dendritic protrusions are found with relatively stereotyped shapes, ranging from filopodia like (thought to be the most immature) to mushroom shaped (thought to be the most stable and mature). (b) A small portion of dendrite from a cortical neuron in brain slice culture labeled with GFP reveals each of these protrusion shapes in a living cell.

dendrites are widely thought to be precursors of spines; they are abundant early on and replaced by the predominant mushroom-shaped spines in the adult brain (Fiala et al., 1998). Interestingly, spine morphology is abnormal in a number of human disorders with cognitive deficits, such as Fragile X syndrome, Rett syndrome, and Downs' syndrome, in which filopodia rather than mature spines predominate (O'Donnell and Warren, 2002). In sum, examination of the mature synapse suggests that synaptogenesis likely consists of two types of events: recruitment of the correct sets of proteins and formation of the proper morphological structures.

20.3 Synaptic contact

Contact between an axon and dendrite is the integral step in CNS synapse initiation. How do these pre- and postsynaptic elements come together? Two main models exist for how contact is initiated: regulation by the dendrite and regulation by the axon. With use of time-lapse imaging of neurons in culture, it has been observed that dendritic filopodia can initiate contact with axons (Ziv and Smith,

1996); these filopodia-axon contacts appear to be synapses, as there is synaptic vesicle recycling (Ziv and Smith, 1996) and a stepwise assembly of pre- and postsynaptic components at the sites (Marrs et al., 2001; Okabe et al., 2001). Furthermore, stimuli thought to induce the formation of new synapses increase the density of dendritic filopodia (Engert and Bonhoeffer, 1999; Maletic-Savatic et al., 1999).

Not all spines form from filopodia, as early on many synapses occur directly on the dendritic shaft where from stable spines can emerge (Fiala et al., 1998; Parnass et al., 2000), suggesting a role for axons in this process of contact formation. Over twenty years ago it was shown that growth cones begin to release neurotransmitter before reaching their targets (Hume et al., 1983; Young and Poo, 1983). Moreover, growth cone filopodia, which extend from the core of the growth cone and are often first to the contact a cell, also contain cycling synaptic vesicles (Sabo and McAllister, 2003). This presynaptic neurotransmitter release prior to target contact could contribute to synaptogenesis during development. In hippocampal mossy fibers, glutamate release initially increases motility of axonal filopodia, possibly to assist in finding a synaptic target, and then inhibits filopodia motility once contact has been made, potentially stabilizing the connection (Tashiro et al., 2000; Chang and De Camilli, 2001). Although synaptic transmission is not required for synapses to form correctly (Verhage et al., 2000), synaptogenesis might be facilitated on axonal filopodia with high levels of activity (Tashiro et al., 2000). Contact between axon and dendrite occurs both *en passent* along the shaft of the axon and at its growing tip (Ahmari et al., 2000), just as synapses form both on dendritic protrusions and the dendritic shaft (Fiala et al., 1998). Clearly, much remains to be explored with regard to how synaptic contact proceeds under these different circumstances and in different areas of the brain. As will be discussed below, whether the axon, dendrite, or both initiate contact, trans-synaptic adhesion molecules are thought to play a major role in not only holding the synaptic terminals tightly aligned but also the maturation of those terminals.

20.4 Synaptic differentiation

Once a contact between axon and dendrite has formed, how do the requisite components reach the nascent synapse? Incredibly, in Xenopus nerve-muscle cultures, synaptic transmission begins within seconds of muscle-neurite contact, suggesting that pre- and postsynaptic machinery is in place even before opposing terminals reach one another (Chow and Poo, 1985). In the CNS, immunostaining of synaptic protein markers combined with time-lapse imaging indicates that synapse assembly occurs within 1–2 hours after axon-dendrite contact (Friedman et al., 2000). Functional synaptic transmission may well occur much more rapidly, however, as these techniques require that a relatively large cluster of protein form to be detectable. Even so, this time scale is faster than previously expected from static images (Friedman et al., 2000). How might this process occur so rapidly? One model suggests that the presynaptic apparatus forms from pre-assembled cytoplasmic transport packets containing synaptic vesicle and/or active zone proteins (Ahmari et al., 2000; Zhai et al., 2001). These pre-assembled packets can arrive within 30 min of synaptic contact (Friedman et al., 2000). In hippocampal neuronal cultures, GFP-tagged presynaptic vesicle protein VAMP is transported along axons in discrete packets along with active zone molecules such as calcium channels and endocytic proteins (Fig. 20.3; Ahmari et al., 2000). Other studies have described a different mobile complex of active zone components that includes the scaffolding molecules Piccolo and Bassoon, vesicle exocytosis machinery, and the cell adhesion molecule Neuronal (N)-cadherin, though no markers for synaptic vesicles (Zhai et al., 2001). It is not known whether these two types of presynaptic packets function independently or are part of the same process. Regardless, both types of packets are highly dynamic and mobile, traveling anterogradely and retrogradely along axons before becoming immobilized at sites of dendrite contact – presumably the initiation of a functional synaptic connection (Ahmari et al., 2000; Zhai et al., 2001).

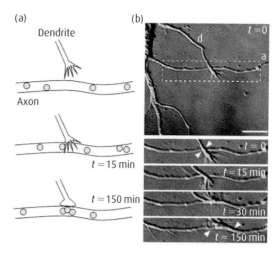

Figure 20.3. *Rapid recruitment of presynaptic transport packets following axon-dendrite contact.* (a) Schematic of dendrite-initiated contact with an axon depicts the rapid accumulation of fluorescently labeled pre-assembled transport packets at the site of contact. These packets have been shown to contain a host of presynaptic active zone proteins. (b) DIC and fluorescence image overlay of a hippocampal neuron transfected with VAMP-GFP (d = dendrite, a = axon; scale bar, 10 μm). Time-lapse imaging demonstrates formation of a stable contact and recruitment of VAMP-GFP to that site. White arrowheads at *t* = 0 and *t* = 150 min indicate the contact area, and reveal continued accumulation of VAMP-GFP to this area throughout the experiment (adapted from Ahmari et al., 2000).

The details of how the postsynaptic complex of proteins is rapidly assembled during synaptogenesis remain less clear. One of the earliest events is arrival of the scaffolding molecule PSD-95 and NMDA receptors (Friedman et al., 2000). There is little consensus, however, as to exactly when these molecules arrive. Evidence for PSD-95 reaching postsynaptic sites first comes from Garner, Ziv, and colleagues, who have demonstrated that PSD-95 can colocalize with presynaptic marker proteins 30–45 min after synaptic vesicle recycling has commenced (Friedman et al., 2000; Bresler et al., 2001; Shapira et al., 2003). Yet, is the presence of PSD-95 the critical event in postsynaptic organization? Reports in the late 1990s demonstrated that PSD-95 clusters are at synaptic sites prior to NMDA receptors

(NMDARs) (Rao et al., 1998; Friedman et al., 2000), consistent with the hypothesized role of PSD-95 in initiating postsynaptic differentiation and NMDAR clustering (Kim and Huganir, 1999). However, recent work has challenged these findings by demonstrating that NMDARs can be recruited to sites of axo-dendritic contact within minutes, often in the absence of PSD-95 (Washbourne et al., 2002).

Are postsynaptic molecules delivered rapidly in transport packets, analogous to trafficking during presynaptic differentiation? PSD-95 clusters are often transient, and constantly increasing or decreasing in size (Okabe et al., 1999). Further, the clusters have not been observed to travel over long distances like presynaptic packets, and an overwhelming percentage of PSD-95 clusters are colocalized to presynaptic markers (Marrs et al., 2001). Taken together, it would seem that the arrival of PSD-95 to synaptic sites occurs from a diffuse cytoplasmic pool rather than discrete vesicular units traveling along the dendrite (but see Prange and Murphy, 2001). The dynamics of glutamate receptor trafficking during postsynaptic development is more controversial. Washbourne and colleagues (Washbourne et al., 2002) found that both NMDA and AMPA receptors may move along dendrites in modular transport packets, and that NMDAR clusters are highly mobile before settling at sites of contact. Thus, glutamatergic synapses could form rapidly via delivery of discrete packets of glutamate receptors, allowing for differentiation of the postsynaptic terminal on a time scale similar to presynaptic formation. Consensus has not yet been reached, however, as other investigators have not been able to identify postsynaptic packets (Bresler et al., 2004). It remains unclear how we can account for these differences, but various ages and types of cells are often used in otherwise similar studies of synaptogenesis, and trafficking of proteins could change as cells mature. Furthermore, CNS synapses and neurons are heterogeneous and could be guided by a diverse array of synaptogenic mechanisms even within a given cell population. These concerns point to the need for continued studies to define the sequence of events that occur as synapses mature.

20.5 Molecular regulators of synaptogenesis

In discerning how the development of synaptic compartments is regulated, two major types of signals have been implicated: those that are membrane bound and thus activated by cell–cell contact, and those that are factors secreted by neurons or glia. Additionally, some molecules may be particularly important for recruiting synaptic components rather than inductive in the process of synapse formation. Below, we discuss various candidate molecules that appear to play a role in the formation or maturation of excitatory synapses.

Trans-synaptic molecules

A number of trans-synaptic signaling complexes have been identified that may function in cell–cell contact and adhesion, yet also be able to trigger the assembly of synaptic specializations on one or both sides of the cleft (Fig. 20.4). These trans-synaptic complexes may be matching pairs of proteins on axon and dendrite (homophilic) or receptor/ligand interactions pre- and postsynaptically (heterophilic). It has been postulated that homophilic proteins dictate appropriate and specific connectivity, while heterophilic interactions offer co-ordinated but distinct cues for the pre- and postsynaptic terminals (Scheiffele, 2003).

Cadherins

Cadherins are calcium-dependent junctional complex homophilic adhesion molecules found in many different cell types throughout the body. The N-cadherin is localized to both pre- and postsynaptic membranes in the CNS, and via the cadherin-binding proteins αN- and β-catenin, can modify the actin cytoskeleton of dendritic spines. Loss of N-cadherin activity with use of dominant negative N-cadherin results in a decrease in spine and increase in filopodia density, along with decreased clustering of the synaptic vesicle protein synapsin and postsynaptic scaffolding molecule PSD-95 (Togashi et al., 2002).

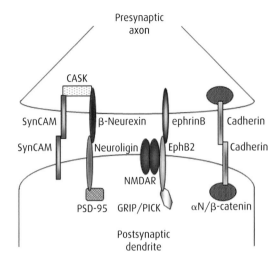

Figure 20.4. *Trans-synaptic signaling complexes are involved in synaptic differentiation during development.* SynCAM and β-Neurexin both bind CASK (protein containing calcium/calmodulin-dependent kinase) through their cytoplasmic tails and are able to direct presynaptic differentiation *in vitro*. Neuroligin interacts with PSD-95 and thus may have a role in postsynaptic development as well. EphB2 interacts directly with the NMDAR through its extracellular domain and also binds AMPAR-interacting proteins PICK and GRIP through its cytoplasmic tail. N-cadherin binds αN- and β-catenin to modify the actin cytoskeleton of dendritic spines (adapted from Li and Sheng (2003)).

Presynaptic vesicular recycling is also impaired, as shown with FM dye labeling. Knock-out mice lacking αN-catenin do not demonstrate alterations in the localization of pre- and postsynaptic marker proteins (Togashi et al., 2002) but dendritic spines are longer and more motile, indicating possible defects in synaptic stability (Togashi et al., 2002; Abe et al., 2004); overexpression of αN-catenin results in an increase in spine density (Abe et al., 2004). Studies in mice lacking β-catenin show that it controls the clustering and localization of synaptic vesicles, though without affecting PSD-95 localization (Bamji et al., 2003). An inclusive picture for how these catenins function together has not emerged, just as whether cadherins have a primary role in

adhesion, formation, or maintenance of synapses has yet to be elucidated.

SynCAM

Through a search for proteins with extracellular immunoglobulin domains and intracellular PDZ-binding motifs, characteristics that might yield cell adhesion and synaptogenic properties for a given molecule, the protein SynCAM was recently identified (Biederer et al., 2002). SynCAM can mediate homophilic cell–cell adhesion in a calcium-independent manner and interact via its cytoplasmic domain with synaptic scaffolding molecules (Biederer et al., 2002). When expressed in nonneuronal cells, SynCAM is sufficient to induce cocultured neurons to form presynaptic specializations at sites of contact; overexpression of SynCAM in neurons results in an increase in spontaneous presynaptic activity. Though its significance *in vivo* has not been demonstrated, this homophilic interaction does provide a viable means by which opposing synaptic membranes might be held together and the presynaptic compartment instructed to differentiate at the earliest stages, even prior to calcium flux in synaptic terminals.

Neurexins and Neuroligins

The heterophilic interaction between the postsynaptic neuroligin and presynaptic β-neurexin is also sufficient to organize a functional presynaptic terminal in neuronal granule cell culture, as neuroligin expressed in nonneuronal cells triggers presynaptic development in contacting axons (Scheiffele et al., 2000). Identified as calcium-dependent heterophilic synaptic adhesion molecules (Song et al., 1999), neuroligins bind PSD-95 (Irie et al., 1997) and neurexins bind presynaptic scaffolding molecules CASK and Mint, leading to recruitment of Munc18, a protein essential for synaptic vesicle exocytosis (Biederer and Sudhof, 2000). Overexpression of neuroligins in dissociated hippocampal cell culture results in increased postsynaptic differentiation and increased density of dendritic spines (Chih et al., 2005).

Neuroligin/neurexin interactions may therefore act to cooperatively assemble pre- and postsynaptic terminals (Dean et al., 2003). Interestingly, mice lacking α-neurexin, transcribed from the same genes but different promoter than β-neurexin, exhibit abnormalities in presynaptic calcium channel activity, and consequently neurotransmitter release (Missler et al., 2003). Thus, α-neurexin likely has a role in differentiation of the presynaptic terminal *in vivo*, while the *in vivo* significance of β-neurexin remains unknown.

Recently, a role for neurexin/neuroligin signaling *in* excitation/inhibition (E/I) balance has emerged. Neurexins expressed in nonneuronal cells induce differentiation of not only glutamatergic but also GABAergic neuroligins-1, -3, and -4, paly a role in glutamatergic synapse differentiation, whereas neuroligin-2 contributes to both glutamatergic and GABAergic synaptogenesis (Graf et al., 2004; Chih et al., 2005). The neuroligin/PSD-95 intracellular interaction is important for determining the distribution of neuroligins to excitatory vs. inhibitory synapses, and in turn, the balance of excitatory to inhibitory synaptic input in hippocampal neurons (Prange et al., 2004; Graf et al., 2004; Chih et al., 2005), loss of neuroligins *in vitro* results in a particular deficit of inhibitory synapse function, and disruption of E/I balance (Chih et al., 2005). Interestingly, genetic mutations in neuroligin family members have been associated with autism (Jamain et al., 2003; Laumonnier et al., 2004), suggesting a role for neurexin/neuroligin signaling and E/I balance in this human spectrum of disease.

Ephs and ephrins

The Eph receptor family consists of transmembrane signaling molecules that are largest known family of receptor tyrosine kinases in the human genome, and are another set of heterophilic synaptic signaling molecules. Interestingly, Eph receptors are activated only when the membrane-bound ephrin ligands are clustered (Davis et al., 1994). Upon ligand binding, multimerized receptors autophosphorylate the intracellular tyrosine residues (Kullander and Klein, 2002).

Ephs are highly expressed in the developing and mature nervous system, with well-known functions mediating repulsive axon guidance cues and target recognition (Flanagan and Vanderhaeghen, 1998; see Volume I, Chapter 19). EphB receptors have recently been localized to postsynaptic sites (Torres et al., 1998; Buchert et al., 1999) and found to cause an increase in pre- and postsynaptic specializations when activated by ephrin-B in neuronal culture (Dalva et al., 2000). Activated EphB2 also interacts directly with the NMDA receptor via their extracellular domains, and causes an increase in NMDAR-mediated calcium influx and gene expression (Takasu et al., 2002). Mice lacking EphB2 show reduced synaptic NMDAR-mediated currents and ~40% decrease in NR1 associated with the postsynaptic density, indicating that EphB2 is crucial for appropriate targeting of NMDARs to synaptic sites (Henderson et al., 2001). Additionally, certain forms of NMDAR-mediated synaptic plasticity are impaired in these mice (Grunwald et al., 2001; Henderson et al., 2001). Knowing that the NMDAR has a critical role in activity-dependent organization and modulation of CNS synapses (Katz and Shatz, 1996), it has been suggested that EphB activity might bridge early steps in synaptogenesis to subsequent activity-mediated modulatory events (Takasu et al., 2002; Goda and Davis, 2003). Cultured neurons from knock-out mice lacking all three EphB subtypes expressed in the brain, EphB1-3, show severe synaptic abnormalities with few dendritic spines and synapses, a predominance of filopodia, and a drastic reduction in NMDA and AMPA receptor clustering (Henkemeyer et al., 2003). Furthermore, EphB is coupled to the dendritic spine cytoskeleton through syndecans (Ethell et al., 2001) and small GTPases (Penzes et al., 2003); activation of EphB results in a rapid increase in the density of spines (Penzes et al., 2001; Henkemeyer et al., 2003). Despite extensive evidence for its role in proper synapse development, whether EphB acts primarily as an organizer or stabilizer of synaptic structure is not yet clear.

Secreted factors

In addition to trans-synaptic molecules, a number of secreted factors appear to have important roles in synaptogenesis. Wnts, which are known best

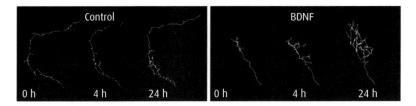

Figure 20.5. *BDNF increases retinal ganglion cell (RGC) axon arborization and GFP-synaptobrevin puncta in vivo.* Tracings of three-dimensional arbors illustrate the effects of BDNF on axon arbor complexity and synapse number. Individual RGC axons double-labeled with GFP-synaptobrevin and DsRed were visualized by confocal microscopy in the live, developing tadpole after direct tectal injection of vehicle solution (control) or BDNF. BDNF not only increases axon arbor complexity but also increases the number and density of GFP-synaptobrevin clusters per axon terminal. Note the high proportion of branch points with synaptic clusters in these arbors (from Alsina et al. (2001)).

for their roles during embryonic development (see Volume I, Chapter 19), are synthesized and secreted by postsynaptic cerebellar granule cells, and act as retrograde signals to regulate the structure of presynaptic mossy fiber axons and growth cones (Burden, 2000; Hall et al., 2000). WNT-7a also induces synapsin clustering at the remodeled fibers, and synaptogenesis is delayed in Wnt-7a mutant mice *in vivo* (Hall et al., 2000). Wnts are expressed throughout the brain and could play a role in synapse formation in areas outside of cerebellum.

The growth factor BDNF (see Volume I, Chapter 23), important in neuronal survival, promotes growth and arborization of dendrites and axons, a process which is dynamic during development (Alsina et al., 2001; Vicario-Abejon et al., 2002). Via double labeling of retinal ganglion cells (RGCs) in *Xenopus* with a red fluorescent probe to visualize axonal arbors and GFP-tagged synaptobrevin (a synaptic vesicle marker) to visualize synapses, a direct correlation was found between arbor growth and synapse formation (Fig. 20.5; Alsina et al., 2001). BDNF has also been demonstrated to increase the number and synaptic localization of NMDARs in neuronal culture (Elmariah et al., 2004). BDNF could cause this increase in the density of excitatory synapses by permissive or instructive cues: more synapses might be formed because of increased surface area due to arborization, or the neurotrophin might directly promote the recruitment of synaptic components (Vicario-Abejon et al., 2002).

Recently, two unexpected and intriguing signals were demonstrated to have critical roles in synapse formation: glial-derived factors and fibroblast growth factor. First, although it has long been thought that glial cells comprise only a support system upon which neurons perform the hard labor of brain development and function, Frank Pfrieger and Ben Barres produced a number of studies showing that retinal ganglion cells form few synaptic connections in the absence of astrocytes; coculturing neurons with these glial cells causes a sevenfold increase in synapse number on each neuron (Pfrieger and Barres, 1997; Nagler et al., 2001; Ullian et al., 2001). Two groups have purified an active factor secreted by astrocytes, one identifying thrombospondins, which are extacellular matrix proteins that mediate cell–cell interactions, and the other cholesterol (Mauch et al., 2001; Christopherson et al., 2005). The group that found thrombospondins, however, reported cholesterol to enhance synaptic efficacy but not number (Christopherson et al., 2005). Though the identity of the active factor remains controversial, these studies of glial-derived substances clearly demonstrate that synapse formation is not only determined by intrinsic neuronal cues, but can be modulated by external signals (Ullian et al., 2004).

In vertebrate systems, most factors found to be involved in synapse formation have been identified by a candidate approach where proteins are tested in culture for their synaptogenic potential. As noted, few have definitive roles *in vivo*. FGF-22 and closely related family members not only cause presynaptic differentiation in neuronal cell culture, but injection of a soluble FGF receptor (FGFR) fusion protein *in vivo*, which neutralizes FGF activity, results in decreased number and size of synaptic vesicle clusters (Umemori et al., 2004). Further, conditional deletion of the FGFR2 impairs presynaptic differentiation of cerebellar mossy fibers *in vivo*, with no effect on granule cell migration, neurite growth, or granule cell density (Umemori et al., 2004). FGFs are target-derived factors, appearing to serve as retrograde signals for presynaptic differentiation, and are only expressed by specific neuronal populations during the period that they receive synapses (Umemori et al., 2004). FGFs have classically been studied in regards to cell proliferation, migration, tissue repair, and response to injury (Dono, 2003; Reuss et al., 2003). How the current findings fit in with these other roles will be of great interest, particularly whether the function of FGFs in synaptogenesis and injury response can be co-ordinated.

Organizing the postsynaptic terminal

A number of proteins that play a specific role in the function of the postsynaptic terminal may also be important in differentiation of the postsynaptic structure. Overexpression studies point to the significance of these postsynaptic proteins. The scaffold molecule PSD-95 has been shown to drive maturation of glutamatergic synapses, as well as increase the number and size of dendritic spines, when overexpressed in hippocampal neurons (El-Husseini et al., 2000). Overexpression of the N-terminal domain alone of the GluR2 subunit of AMPA receptors increases spine size and density in hippocampal neurons, and even induces spine formation in normally aspiney gamma amino butyric acid (aspiney GABA) releasing interneurons (Passafaro et al., 2003). Additionally, overexpression of the postsynaptic scaffold protein Shank promotes spine maturation and enhancement of presynaptic function without impacting spine number (Sala et al., 2001). These results suggest that a number of molecules are able to orchestrate synapse maturation, though whether

they are actually necessary for the process to occur is less clear.

Some factors identified as candidate synaptogenic molecules may also function to specifically promote postsynaptic development. EphB, with its ability to bind directly to and cluster NMDARs, certainly appears to have a particular role in the rapid differentiation of the postsynaptic terminal during synapse formation (Dalva et al., 2000); at later time points, BDNF can mediate changes in NMDAR accumulation at synapses, possibly part of the neuron's homeostatic mechanism to balance excitatory and inhibitory synaptic transmission (Elmariah et al., 2004). The secreted factor Narp triggers accumulation of AMPA receptors (AMPARs) and an increase in the number of excitatory synapses when overexpressed in spinal neuronal culture, though with no effect on presynaptic proteins (O'Donnell and Warren, 2002). Lastly, TNFα secreted by glia also increases the surface expression of AMPARs, and its presence is required for maintenance of synaptic strength at excitatory synapses (O'Donnell and Warren, 2002). These factors may work together during the first few weeks of development to properly organize and stabilize postsynaptic compartments.

20.6 Specificity of synaptic connections

For the brain to function normally, synapses must occur between the correct pre- and postsynaptic partners. Once guided to the vicinity of their final destination, how is an axon able to choose (or be led to) its appropriate target? Interestingly, a number of the molecules already discussed may help in this process as well as the formation of a functional synapse. In *Drosophila*, selective removal of N-cadherin from photoreceptors causes those neurons to synapse on the wrong cells (Lee et al., 2001). Interestingly, cadherins are one of many families capable of diverse expression, with generation of multiple mRNAs via differential promoter utilization or splicing (Suzuki et al., 1997; Serafini, 1999; Wu and Maniatis, 1999). Dscam, an immunoglobulin superfamily protein required for the formation of neuronal connections in *Drosophila*, gives rise to over 38,000 isoforms, each with different binding specificities (Wojtowicz et al., 2004). It has been proposed the preferential homophilic binding with such a large number of isoforms on either side of a synapse could regulate specificity of connections (Wojtowicz et al., 2004). Another possibility is that non-neuronal cells determine where and between what neurons connections are made. In *Caenorhabditis elegans*, the transmembrane immunoglobulin protein SYG-2 is expressed on epithelial guidepost cells and directs SYG-1 expressing presynaptic cells to differentiate and recruit the appropriate postsynaptic partner (Shen et al., 2004). In the mammalian system, an intriguing feature of the neurexin family is the vast number of alternatively spliced variants (over 1000 neurexin isoforms) expressed differentially throughout the CNS (Scheiffele, 2003), giving rise to the suggestion that this family also might play a role in axon and target specification (Li and Sheng, 2003; Scheiffele, 2003). Likewise, EphB/ephrin-B signaling is essential for proper mapping of retinal axons in the mammalian midbrain during development (Hindges et al., 2002), and through its interaction with NMDARs could play a role in activity-dependent refinement and specification of those connections. While the nature of specificity in synaptic contacts still exceeds the variety of isoforms of identified molecules, it is conceivable that within given brain regions, this kind of molecular recognition might bring appropriate synaptic partners together.

20.7 Role of activity in synapse formation and elimination

While neuronal activity has a significant function in the refinement and modulation of synaptic connections (Katz and Shatz, 1996; Malenka and Nicoll, 1999), its role in synapse formation is not as well understood. One particularly striking study demonstrates that mice lacking Munc18, resulting in complete and permanent loss of synaptic transmission due to an inability to release synaptic vesicles, have grossly normal brains (Verhage et al., 2000). Synapses in mutant animals are indistinguishable from wild-type, with normal morphology and expression levels of synaptic proteins. Spontaneous action potentials are present in these null animals and may be necessary for axon guidance and establishment of functional circuits, but synaptic transmission appears not to be (Verhage et al., 2000). As might be expected given the importance of neural activity as a trophic factor, extensive cell death occurs in the null animals as development proceeds. Other studies have demonstrated, however, that activity may be required during synapse formation in circumstances once thought to be activity-independent (Tessier-Lavigne and Goodman, 1996). For example, activity is necessary for proper thalamo-cortical axon guidance (Catalano and Shatz, 1998) and activity can alter the response of a growth cone to a guidance molecule from attractive to repulsive (Ming et al., 2001).

As discussed previously, activity does play at least a modulatory role as synapses are forming and beyond. Glutamate release from presynaptic terminals may control axonal filopodia motility and selection of postsynaptic targets (Tashiro et al., 2000). Sensory deprivation in rat barrel cortex *in vivo* also reduces the motility of what are otherwise highly dynamic dendritic protrusions (Lendvai et al., 2000). Further, studies on dendritic arbors in developing tectum demonstrate that NMDAR activity promotes arborization and, in turn, increased numbers of synapses; this same affect has been observed *in vivo* with enhanced visual activity driving arbor growth (Cline, 2001; Sin et al., 2002; see Volume I, Chapter 9). Synaptic activity is also well-known to recruit synaptic glutamate receptors during development, possibly converting newly formed glutamatergic transmission mediated by NMDARs ("silent" synapses) to synapses that contain AMPARs as well (Wu et al., 1996; Isaac et al., 1997; Zhang and Poo, 2001).

During synaptogenesis, more synapses are formed than will ultimately be retained in the mature brain. Activity has a role in this pruning of synaptic contacts, which is a vital step in development of neuronal circuits. At the neuromuscular junction, multiple motor axons initially innervate each muscle fiber but this number is reduced to one in adulthood (Sanes and Lichtman, 1999), a process that relies on activity-dependent competition between inputs (Thompson et al., 1979; Balice-Gordon and Lichtman, 1994; Goda and Davis, 2003). In the CNS, the stabilization or elimination of synapses has also long been thought to be activity dependent (Hebb, 1949). Relative competition of inputs again dictates synapse survival: in the visual system, if one eye is deprived of input during early life, most visual cortical neurons will become responsive to stimuli only from the eye that remained open (Shatz and Stryker, 1978). Anatomic studies indicate that axonal arbors of afferents from the occluded eye rapidly withdraw from their postsynaptic targets and shrink in size (Antonini and Stryker, 1993; Goda and Davis, 2003), and disassembly of synapses occurs before branch elimination, as most branches that are eliminated do not express presynaptic marker proteins before retraction (Alsina et al., 2001; Cohen-Cory, 2002). Little is known regarding the molecular underpinnings of synapse elimination, though experiments have implicated neurotrophin signaling, NMDAR activation, and CaMKII as necessary for this process during synaptic development (Goda and Davis, 2003). It does appear that synapse elimination is reversible, and might be considered as one part in a continual course of synapse refinement. Both at the NMJ (Walsh and Lichtman, 2003) and in the CNS (Antonini et al., 1998) synapse assembly and disassembly is a dynamic process modulated by experience, still without well-defined cellular mechanisms.

20.8 Synapse formation in the adult brain

Adult synaptogenesis is less well defined than that in the developing brain, as the vast majority of new synapses are made during development. In adult female rats, however, it has been demonstrated that the density of synapses in hippocampus is sensitive to estradiol levels during the estrous cycle: low levels of estradiol correlate with lower synaptic density and high levels with high synaptic density (Woolley and McEwen, 1992). Recent results indicate that new synapses may also form in adulthood to support experience-dependent plasticity. With extended *in vivo* imaging of adult mouse barrel cortex using two-photon microscopy, Trachtenberg and colleagues (2002) found that spines remain surprisingly transient into adulthood; 50% of the spine population was observed to persist for at least a month with the remainder only present for a few days or less. Sensory deprivation by whisker trimming caused a specific decrease in the stability of those spines in the corresponding receptive field, indicating that spines are directly affected by experience. As spines are the site of most excitatory synapses (Harris, 1999), development of new spines might indicate new synapses. Here, the formation and retraction of spines was demonstrated to be associated with synapse formation and elimination, respectively (Trachtenberg et al., 2002). Notably, all of the observed synaptic changes were local, with no alterations in axonal and dendritic branching. The authors postulate that while synapse formation and elimination continues into adulthood, the absence of alterations in branching would ensure that plasticity is reversible, as presynaptic partners and dendritic branches remain in place (Trachtenberg et al., 2002).

In contrast to the plastic state of local dendritic morphology in the Trachtenberg study, Grutzendler and colleagues (2002) reported in a direct comparison of young to adult mice that filopodia, abundant in young animals, are nearly absent in adults; furthermore, ~73% of spines are stable over 1 month in young animals, whereas ~96% of spines remain stable in adults over that time period, with a half-life of over 1 year. The results provide an attractive structural basis for long-term memory, but indicate much less dynamism of dendritic spines, and possibly synapse formation, in adult brain.

Studies of neuronal plasticity also suggest that although synapse formation is present in the adult brain, it has different properties than that during development. There exists far more plasticity of neural circuits in younger animals, particularly during the critical period, when compared to adults (Kirkwood et al., 1995). Long-term potentiation (LTP) inducing paradigms have been found to cause rapid growth of new dendritic protrusions in young animals (Maletic-Savatic et al., 1999), but does the same occur even with the less robust LTP induced in adults? And will synapse formation onto new dendritic protrusions in an adult brain be mechanistically similar to that during development? Furthermore, many insults to the CNS, such as epilepsy and stroke, result in increased axonal sprouting and often lowered thresholds for induction of synaptic plasticity (Coulter and DeLorenzo, 1999; Carmichael, 2003). Do these changes result in increased levels of synaptogenesis, and are the same molecular regulators of synapse formation active? While few questions have been answered regarding how synapses are created in adults and after injury or disease, there have been great strides in understanding regulation of synapse formation during normal development, bringing the field closer towards addressing synaptogenesis under pathologic conditions.

REFERENCES

Abe, K., Chisaka, O., Van Roy, F. and Takeichi, M. (2004). Stability of dendritic spines and synaptic contacts is controlled by alpha N-catenin. *Nat Neurosci*, **7**, 357–363.

Ahmari, S.E., Buchanan, J. and Smith, S.J. (2000). Assembly of presynaptic active zones from cytoplasmic transport packets. *Nat Neurosci*, **3**, 445–451.

Alsina, B., Vu, T. and Cohen-Cory, S. (2001). Visualizing synapse formation in arborizing optic axons *in vivo*: dynamics and modulation by BDNF. *Nat Neurosci*, **4**, 1093–1101.

Antonini, A. and Stryker, M.P. (1993). Rapid remodeling of axonal arbors in the visual cortex. *Science*, **260**, 1819–1821.

Antonini, A., Gillespie, D.C., Crair, M.C. and Stryker, M.P. (1998). Morphology of single geniculocortical afferents and functional recovery of the visual cortex after reverse monocular deprivation in the kitten. *J Neurosci*, **18**, 9896–9909.

Balice-Gordon, R.J. and Lichtman, J.W. (1994). Long-term synapse loss induced by focal blockade of postsynaptic receptors. *Nature*, **372**, 519–524.

Bamji, S.X., Shimazu, K., Kimes, N., Huelsken, J., Birchmeier, W., Lu, B. and Reichardt, L.F. (2003). Role of beta-catenin in synaptic vesicle localization and presynaptic assembly. *Neuron*, **40**, 719–731.

Barres, B.A. and Smith, S.J. (2001). Neurobiology. Cholesterol – making or breaking the synapse. *Science*, **294**, 1296–1297.

Biederer, T. and Sudhof, T.C. (2000). Mints as adaptors. Direct binding to neurexins and recruitment of munc18. *J Biol Chem*, **275**, 39803–39806.

Biederer, T., Sara, Y., Mozhayeva, M., Atasoy, D., Liu, X., Kavalali, E.T. and Sudhof, T.C. (2002). SynCAM, a synaptic adhesion molecule that drives synapse assembly. *Science*, **297**, 1525–1531.

Bresler, T., Ramati, Y., Zamorano, P.L., Zhai, R., Garner, C.C. and Ziv, N.E. (2001). The dynamics of SAP90/PSD-95 recruitment to new synaptic junctions. *Mol Cell Neurosci*, **18**, 149–167.

Bresler, T., Shapira, M., Boeckers, T., Dresbach, T., Futter, M., Garner, C.C., Rosenblum, K., Gundelfinger, E.D. and Ziv, N.E. (2004). Postsynaptic density assembly is fundamentally different from presynaptic active zone assembly. *J Neurosci*, **24**, 1507–1520.

Buchert, M., Schneider, S., Meskenaite, V., Adams, M.T., Canaani, E., Baechi, T., Moelling, K. and Hovens, C.M. (1999). The junction-associated protein AF-6 interacts and clusters with specific Eph receptor tyrosine kinases at specialized sites of cell–cell contact in the brain. *J Cell Biol*, **144**, 361–371.

Burden, S.J. (2000). Wnts as retrograde signals for axon and growth cone differentiation. *Cell*, **100**, 495–497.

Carmichael, S.T. (2003). Plasticity of cortical projections after stroke. *Neuroscientist*, **9**, 64–75.

Catalano, S.M. and Shatz, C.J. (1998). Activity-dependent cortical target selection by thalamic axons. *Science*, **281**, 559–562.

Chang, S. and De Camilli, P. (2001). Glutamate regulates actin-based motility in axonal filopodia. *Nat Neurosci*, **4**, 787–793.

Chih, B. and Engelman, H. (2005). Control of excitatory and inhibitory synapse formation by neuroligins. *Science*, **307**, 1324–1328.

Chow, I. and Poo, M.M. (1985). Release of acetylcholine from embryonic neurons upon contact with muscle cell. *J Neurosci*, **5**, 1076–1082.

Christopherson, K.S., Ullian, E.M., Stokes, C.C., Mullowney, C.E., Hell, J.W., Agah, A., Lawler, J., Mosher, D.F., Bornstein, P., Barres, B.A. (2005). Thrombospondins are astrocyte-secreted proteins that promote CNS synaptogenesis. *Cell*, **120**, 421–433.

Cline, H.T. (2001). Dendritic arbor development and synaptogenesis. *Curr Opin Neurobiol*, **11**, 118–126.

Cohen-Cory, S. (2002). The developing synapse: construction and modulation of synaptic structures and circuits. *Science*, **298**, 770–776.

Coulter, D.A. and DeLorenzo, R.J. (1999). Basic mechanisms of status epilepticus. *Adv Neurol*, **79**, 725–733.

Dalva, M.B., Takasu, M.A., Lin, M.Z., Shamah, S.M., Hu, L., Gale, N.W. and Greenberg, M.E. (2000). EphB receptors interact with NMDA receptors and regulate excitatory synapse formation. *Cell*, **103**, 945–956.

Davis, S., Gale, N.W., Aldrich, T.H., Maisonpierre, P.C., Lhotak, V., Pawson, T., Goldfarb, M. and Yancopoulos, G.D. (1994). Ligands for EPH-related receptor tyrosine kinases that require membrane attachment or clustering for activity. *Science*, **266**, 816–819.

Dean, C., Scholl, F.G., Choih, J., DeMaria, S., Berger, J., Isacoff, E. and Scheiffele, P. (2003). Neurexin mediates the assembly of presynaptic terminals. *Nat Neurosci*, **6**, 708–716.

DeChiara, T.M., Bowen, D.C., Valenzuela, D.M., Simmons, M.V., Poueymirou, W.T., Thomas, S., Kinetz, E., Compton, D.L., Rojas, E., Park, J.S., Smith, C., DiStefano, P.S., Glass, D.J., Burden, S.J. and Yancopoulos, G.D. (1996). The receptor tyrosine kinase MuSK is required for neuromuscular junction formation *in vivo*. *Cell*, **85**, 501–512.

Dono, R. (2003). Fibroblast growth factors as regulators of central nervous system development and function. *Am J Physiol Regul Integr Comp Physiol*, **284**, R867–R881.

El-Husseini, A.E., Schnell, E., Chetkovich, D.M., Nicoll, R.A. and Bredt, D.S. (2000). PSD-95 involvement in maturation of excitatory synapses. *Science*, **290**, 1364–1368.

Elmariah, S.B., Crumling, M.A., Parsons, T.D. and Balice-Gordon, R.J. (2004). Postsynaptic TrkB-mediated signaling modulates excitatory and inhibitory neurotransmitter receptor clustering at hippocampal synapses. *J Neurosci*, **24**, 2380–2393.

Engert, F. and Bonhoeffer, T. (1999). Dendritic spine changes associated with hippocampal long-term synaptic plasticity. *Nature*, **399**, 66–70.

Ethell, I.M., Irie, F., Kalo, M.S., Couchman, J.R., Pasquale, E.B. and Yamaguchi, Y. (2001). EphB/syndecan-2 signaling in dendritic spine morphogenesis. *Neuron*, **31**, 1001–1013.

Fiala, J.C., Feinberg, M., Popov, V. and Harris, K.M. (1998). Synaptogenesis via dendritic filopodia in developing hippocampal area CA1. *J Neurosci*, **18**, 8900–8911.

Flanagan, J.G. and Vanderhaeghen, P. (1998). The ephrins and Eph receptors in neural development. *Annu Rev Neurosci*, **21**, 309–345.

Friedman, H.V., Bresler, T., Garner, C.C. and Ziv, N.E. (2000). Assembly of new individual excitatory synapses: time course and temporal order of synaptic molecule recruitment. *Neuron*, **27**, 57–69.

Glass, D.J., DeChiara, T.M., Stitt, T.N., DiStefano, P.S., Valenzuela, D.M. and Yancopoulos, G.D. (1996). The receptor tyrosine kinase MuSK is required for neuromuscular junction formation and is a functional receptor for agrin. *Cold Spring Harb Symp Quant Biol*, **61**, 435–444.

Goda, Y. and Davis, G.W. (2003). Mechanisms of synapse assembly and disassembly. *Neuron*, **40**, 243–264.

Graf, E.R., Zhang, X., Jin, S.X., Linhoff, M.W. and Craig, A.M. (2004). Neurexins induce differentiation of GABA and glutamate postsynaptic specializations via neuroligins. *Cell*, **119**, 1013–1026.

Grunwald, I.C., Korte, M., Wolfer, D., Wilkinson, G.A., Unsicker, K., Lipp, H.P., Bonhoeffer, T. and Klein, R. (2001). Kinase-independent requirement of EphB2 receptors in hippocampal synaptic plasticity. *Neuron*, **32**, 1027–1040.

Grutzendler, J., Kasthuri, N. and Gan, W.B. (2002). Long-term dendritic spine stability in the adult cortex. *Nature*, **420**, 812–816.

Hall, A.C., Lucas, F.R. and Salinas, P.C. (2000). Axonal remodeling and synaptic differentiation in the cerebellum is regulated by WNT-7a signaling. *Cell*, **100**, 525–535.

Harris, K.M. (1999). Structure, development, and plasticity of dendritic spines. *Curr Opin Neurobiol*, **9**, 343–348.

Hata, Y., Slaughter, C.A. and Sudhof, T.C. (1993). Synaptic vesicle fusion complex contains unc-18 homologue bound to syntaxin. *Nature*, **366**, 347–351.

Hebb, D.O. (1949). *The Organization of Behavior*, John Wiley Inc., NY.

Henderson, J.T., Georgiou, J., Jia, Z., Robertson, J., Elowe, S., Roder, J.C. and Pawson, T. (2001). The receptor tyrosine kinase EphB2 regulates NMDA-dependent synaptic function. *Neuron*, **32**, 1041–1056.

Henkemeyer, M., Itkis, O.S., Ngo, M., Hickmott, P.W. and Ethell, I.M. (2003). Multiple EphB receptor tyrosine kinases shape dendritic spines in the hippocampus. *J Cell Biol*, **163**, 1313–1326.

Hering, H. and Sheng, M. (2001). Dendritic spines: structure, dynamics and regulation. *Nat Rev Neurosci*, **2**, 880–888.

Hindges, R., McLaughlin, T., Genoud, N., Henkemeyer, M. and O'Leary, D.D. (2002). EphB forward signaling controls directional branch extension and arborization required for dorsal–ventral retinotopic mapping. *Neuron*, **35**, 475–487.

Hume, R.I., Role, L.W. and Fischbach, G.D. (1983). Acetylcholine release from growth cones detected with patches of acetylcholine receptor-rich membranes. *Nature*, **305**, 632–634.

Irie, M., Hata, Y., Takeuchi, M., Ichtchenko, K., Toyoda, A., Hirao, K., Takai, Y., Rosahl, T.W. and Sudhof, T.C. (1997). Binding of neuroligins to PSD-95. *Science*, **277**, 1511–1515.

Isaac, J.T., Crair, M.C., Nicoll, R.A. and Malenka, R.C. (1997). Silent synapses during development of thalamocortical inputs. *Neuron*, **18**, 269–280.

Jamain, S., Quach, H., Betancur, C., Rastam, M., Colineaux, C., Gillberg, I.C., Soderstrom, H., Giros, B., Leboyer, M., Gillberg, C., Bourgeron, T. and Paris Autism Research International Sibpair Study (2003). Mutations of the

X-linked genes encoding neuroligins NLGN3 and NLGN4 are associated with autism. *Nat Genet*, **34**, 27–29.

Katz, L.C. and Shatz, C.J. (1996). Synaptic activity and the construction of cortical circuits. *Science*, **274**, 1133–1138.

Kim, J.H. and Huganir, R.L. (1999). Organization and regulation of proteins at synapses. *Curr Opin Cell Biol*, **11**, 248–254.

Kirkwood, A., Lee, H.K. and Bear, M.F. (1995). Co-regulation of long-term potentiation and experience-dependent synaptic plasticity in visual cortex by age and experience. *Nature*, **375**, 328–331.

Koch, C. and Poggio, T. (1983). A theoretical analysis of electrical properties of spines. *Proc Roy Soc London B Biol Sci*, **218**, 455–477.

Kullander, K. and Klein, R. (2002). Mechanisms and functions of Eph and ephrin signalling. *Nat Rev Mol Cell Biol*, **3**, 475–486.

Laumonnier, F., Bonnet-Brilhault, F., Gomot, M., Blanc, R., David, A., Moizard, M.P., Raynaud, M., Ronce, N., Lemonnier, E., Calvas, P., Laudier, B., Chelly, J., Fryns, J.P., Ropers, H.H., Hamel, B.C., Andres, C., Barthelemy, C., Moraine, C. and Briault, S. (2004). X-linked mental retardation and autism are associated with a mutation in the NLGN4 gene, a member of the neuroligin family. *Am J Hum Genet*, **74**, 552–557.

Lee, C.H., Herman, T., Clandinin, T.R., Lee, R. and Zipursky, S.L. (2001). N-cadherin regulates target specificity in the Drosophila visual system. *Neuron*, **30**, 437–450.

Lendvai, B., Stern, E.A., Chen, B. and Svoboda, K. (2000). Experience-dependent plasticity of dendritic spines in the developing rat barrel cortex *in vivo*. *Nature*, **404**, 876–881.

Li, Z. and Sheng, M. (2003). Some assembly required: the development of neuronal synapses. *Nat Rev Mol Cell Biol*, **4**, 833–841.

Lin, W., Burgess, R.W., Dominguez, B., Pfaff, S.L., Sanes, J.R. and Lee, K.F. (2001). Distinct roles of nerve and muscle in postsynaptic differentiation of the neuromuscular synapse. *Nature*, **410**, 1057–1064.

Malenka, R.C. and Nicoll, R.A. (1999). Long-term potentiation – a decade of progress? *Science*, **285**, 1870–1874.

Maletic-Savatic, M., Malinow, R. and Svoboda, K. (1999). Rapid dendritic morphogenesis in CA1 hippocampal dendrites induced by synaptic activity. *Science*, **283**, 1923–1927.

Marrs, G.S., Green, S.H. and Dailey, M.E. (2001). Rapid formation and remodeling of postsynaptic densities in developing dendrites. *Nat Neurosci*, **4**, 1006–1013.

Mauch, D.H., Nagler, K., Schumacher, S., Goritz, C., Muller, E.C., Otto, A. and Pfrieger, F.W. (2001). CNS synaptogenesis promoted by glia-derived cholesterol. *Science*, **294**, 1354–1357.

Ming, G., Henley, J., Tessier-Lavigne, M., Song, H. and Poo, M. (2001). Electrical activity modulates growth cone guidance by diffusible factors. *Neuron*, **29**, 441–452.

Missler, M., Zhang, W., Rohlmann, A., Kattenstroth, G., Hammer, R.E., Gottmann, K. and Sudhof, T.C. (2003). Alpha-neurexins couple Ca^{2+} channels to synaptic vesicle exocytosis. *Nature*, **423**, 939–948.

Nagler, K., Mauch, D.H. and Pfrieger, F.W. (2001). Glia-derived signals induce synapse formation in neurones of the rat central nervous system. *J Physiol*, **533**, 665–679.

Nimchinsky, E.A., Sabatini, B.L. and Svoboda, K. (2002). Structure and function of dendritic spines. *Annu Rev Physiol*, **64**, 313–353.

O'Donnell, W.T. and Warren, S.T. (2002). A decade of molecular studies of fragile X syndrome. *Annu Rev Neurosci*, **25**, 315–338.

Okabe, S., Kim, H.D., Miwa, A., Kuriu, T. and Okado, H. (1999). Continual remodeling of postsynaptic density and its regulation by synaptic activity. *Nat Neurosci*, **2**, 804–811.

Okabe, S., Miwa, A. and Okado, H. (2001). Spine formation and correlated assembly of presynaptic and postsynaptic molecules. *J Neurosci*, **21**, 6105–6114.

Pak, D.T., Yang, S., Rudolph-Correia, S., Kim, E. and Sheng, M. (2001). Regulation of dendritic spine morphology by SPAR, a PSD-95-associated RapGAP. *Neuron*, **31**, 289–303.

Parnass, Z., Tashiro, A. and Yuste, R. (2000). Analysis of spine morphological plasticity in developing hippocampal pyramidal neurons. *Hippocampus*, **10**, 561–568.

Passafaro, M., Nakagawa, T., Sala, C. and Sheng, M. (2003). Induction of dendritic spines by an extracellular domain of AMPA receptor subunit GluR2. *Nature*, **424**, 677–681.

Peng, J., Kim, M.J., Cheng, D., Duong, D.M., Gygi, S.P. and Sheng, M. (2004). Semiquantitative proteomic analysis of rat forebrain postsynaptic density fractions by mass spectrometry. *J Biol Chem*, **279**, 21003–21011.

Penzes, P., Johnson, R.C., Sattler, R., Zhang, X., Huganir, R.L., Kambampati, V., Mains, R.E. and Eipper, B.A. (2001). The neuronal Rho-GEF Kalirin-7 interacts with PDZ domain-containing proteins and regulates dendritic morphogenesis. *Neuron*, **29**, 229–242.

Penzes, P., Beeser, A., Chernoff, J., Schiller, M.R., Eipper, B.A., Mains, R.E. and Huganir, R.L. (2003). Rapid induction of dendritic spine morphogenesis by trans-synaptic ephrinB-EphB receptor activation of the Rho-GEF kalirin. *Neuron*, **37**, 263–274.

Pfrieger, F.W. and Barres, B.A. (1997). Synaptic efficacy enhanced by glial cells *in vitro*. *Science*, **277**, 1684–1687.

Prange, O. and Murphy, T.H. (2001). Modular transport of postsynaptic density-95 clusters and association with stable spine precursors during early development of cortical neurons. *J Neurosci*, **21**, 9325–9333.

Prange, O., Wong, T.P., Gerrow, K., Wang, Y.T. and El-Husseini, A. (2004). A balance between excitatory and inhibitory synapses is controlled by PSD-95 and neuroligin. *Proc Natl Acad Sci*, **101**, 13915–13920.

Rao, A., Kim, E., Sheng, M. and Craig, A.M. (1998). Heterogeneity in the molecular composition of excitatory postsynaptic sites during development of hippocampal neurons in culture. *J Neurosci*, **18**, 1217–1229.

Reuss, B., von Bohlen and Halbach, O. (2003). Fibroblast growth factors and their receptors in the central nervous system. *Cell Tissue Res*, **313**, 139–157.

Rizo, J. and Sudhof, T.C. (2002). Snares and Munc18 in synaptic vesicle fusion. *Nat Rev Neurosci*, **3**, 641–653.

Sabatini, B.L., Maravall, M. and Svoboda, K. (2001). Ca(2+) signaling in dendritic spines. *Curr Opin Neurobiol*, **11**, 349–356.

Sabo, S.L. and McAllister, A.K. (2003). Mobility and cycling of synaptic protein-containing vesicles in axonal growth cone filopodia. *Nat Neurosci*, **6**, 1264–1269.

Sala, C., Piech, V., Wilson, N.R., Passafaro, M., Liu, G. and Sheng, M. (2001). Regulation of dendritic spine morphology and synaptic function by Shank and Homer. *Neuron*, **31**, 115–130.

Sanes, J.R. and Lichtman, J.W. (1999). Development of the vertebrate neuromuscular junction. *Annu Rev Neurosci*, **22**, 389–442.

Scheiffele, P. (2003). Cell–cell signaling during synapse formation in the CNS. *Annu Rev Neurosci*, **26**, 485–508.

Scheiffele, P., Fan, J., Choih, J., Fetter, R. and Serafini, T. (2000). Neuroligin expressed in nonneuronal cells triggers presynaptic development in contacting axons. *Cell*, **101**, 657–669.

Serafini, T. (1999). Finding a partner in a crowd: neuronal diversity and synaptogenesis. *Cell*, **98**, 133–136.

Shapira, M., Zhai, R.G., Dresbach, T., Bresler, T., Torres, V.I., Gundelfinger, E.D., Ziv, N.E. and Garner, C.C. (2003). Unitary assembly of presynaptic active zones from Piccolo-Bassoon transport vesicles. *Neuron*, **38**, 237–252.

Shatz, C.J. and Stryker, M.P. (1978). Ocular dominance in layer IV of the cat's visual cortex and the effects of monocular deprivation. *J Physiol*, **281**, 267–283.

Shen, K., Fetter, R.D. and Bargmann, C.I. (2004). Synaptic specificity is generated by the synaptic guidepost protein SYG-2 and its receptor, SYG-1. *Cell*, **116**, 869–881.

Sin, W.C., Haas, K., Ruthazer, E.S. and Cline, H.T. (2002). Dendrite growth increased by visual activity requires NMDA receptor and Rho GTPases. *Nature*, **419**, 475–480.

Song, J.Y., Ichtchenko, K., Sudhof, T.C. and Brose, N. (1999). Neuroligin 1 is a postsynaptic cell-adhesion molecule of excitatory synapses. *Proc Natl Acad Sci USA*, **96**, 1100–1105.

Suzuki, S.C., Inoue, T., Kimura, Y., Tanaka, T. and Takeichi, M. (1997). Neuronal circuits are subdivided by differential expression of type-II classic cadherins in postnatal mouse brains. *Mol Cell Neurosci*, **9**, 433–447.

Takasu, M.A., Dalva, M.B., Zigmond, R.E. and Greenberg, M.E. (2002). Modulation of NMDA receptor-dependent calcium influx and gene expression through EphB receptors. *Science*, **295**, 491–495.

Tashiro, A., Minden, A. and Yuste, R. (2000). Regulation of dendritic spine morphology by the rho family of small GTPases: antagonistic roles of Rac and Rho. *Cereb Cortex*, **10**, 927–938.

Tessier-Lavigne, M. and Goodman, C.S. (1996). The molecular biology of axon guidance. *Science*, **274**, 1123–1133.

Thompson, W., Kuffler, D.P. and Jansen, J.K. (1979). The effect of prolonged, reversible block of nerve impulses on the elimination of polyneuronal innervation of new-born rat skeletal muscle fibers. *Neuroscience*, **4**, 271–281.

Togashi, H., Abe, K., Mizoguchi, A., Takaoka, K., Chisaka, O. and Takeichi, M. (2002). Cadherin regulates dendritic spine morphogenesis. *Neuron*, **35**, 77–89.

Torres, R., Firestein, B.L., Dong, H., Staudinger, J., Olson, E.N., Huganir, R.L., Bredt, D.S., Gale, N.W. and Yancopoulos, G.D. (1998). PDZ proteins bind, cluster, and synaptically colocalize with Eph receptors and their ephrin ligands. *Neuron*, **21**, 1453–1463.

Trachtenberg, J.T., Chen, B.E., Knott, G.W., Feng, G., Sanes, J.R., Welker, E. and Svoboda, K. (2002). Long-term *in vivo* imaging of experience-dependent synaptic plasticity in adult cortex. *Nature*, **420**, 788–794.

Ullian, E.M., Sapperstein, S.K., Christopherson, K.S. and Barres, B.A. (2001). Control of synapse number by glia. *Science*, **291**, 657–661.

Ullian, E.M., Christopherson, K.S. and Barres, B.A. (2004). Role for glia in synaptogenesis. *Glia*, **47**, 209–216.

Umemori, H., Linhoff, M.W., Ornitz, D.M. and Sanes, J.R. (2004). FGF22 and its close relatives are presynaptic organizing molecules in the mammalian brain. *Cell*, **118**, 257–270.

Verhage, M., Maia, A.S., Plomp, J.J., Brussaard, A.B., Heeroma, J.H., Vermeer, H., Toonen, R.F., Hammer, R.E., van den Berg, T.K., Missler, M., Geuze, H.J. and Sudhof, T.C. (2000). Synaptic assembly of the brain in the absence of neurotransmitter secretion. *Science*, **287**, 864–869.

Vicario-Abejon, C., Owens, D., McKay, R. and Segal, M. (2002). Role of neurotrophins in central synapse formation and stabilization. *Nat Rev Neurosci*, **3**, 965–974.

Walsh, M.K. and Lichtman, J.W. (2003). *In vivo* time-lapse imaging of synaptic takeover associated with naturally occurring synapse elimination. *Neuron*, **37**, 67–73.

Washbourne, P., Bennett, J.E. and McAllister, A.K. (2002). Rapid recruitment of NMDA receptor transport packets to nascent synapses. *Nat Neurosci*, **5**, 751–759.

Wojtowicz, W.M., Flanagan, J.J., Millard, S.S., Zipursky, S.L. and Clemens, J.C. (2004). Alternative splicing of Drosophila Dscam generates axon guidance receptors that exhibit isoform-specific homophilic binding. *Cell*, **118**, 619–633.

Woolley, C.S. and McEwen, B.S. (1992). Estradiol mediates fluctuation in hippocampal synapse density during the estrous cycle in the adult rat. *J Neurosci*, **12**, 2549–2554.

Wu, G., Malinow, R. and Cline, H.T. (1996). Maturation of a central glutamatergic synapse. *Science*, **274**, 972–976.

Wu, Q. and Maniatis, T. (1999). A striking organization of a large family of human neural cadherin-like cell adhesion genes. *Cell*, **97**, 779–790.

Yang, X., Arber, S., William, C., Li, L., Tanabe, Y., Jessell, T.M., Birchmeier, C. and Burden, S.J. (2001). Patterning of muscle acetylcholine receptor gene expression in the absence of motor innervation. *Neuron*, **30**, 399–410.

Young, S.H. and Poo, M.M. (1983). Spontaneous release of transmitter from growth cones of embryonic neurones. *Nature*, **305**, 634–637.

Zhai, R.G., Vardinon-Friedman, H., Cases-Langhoff, C., Becker, B., Gundelfinger, E.D., Ziv, N.E. and Garner, C.C. (2001). Assembling the presynaptic active zone: a characterization of an active one precursor vesicle. *Neuron*, **29**, 131–143.

Zhang, L.I. and Poo, M.M. (2001). Electrical activity and development of neural circuits. *Nat Neurosci* **4**(**Suppl.**), 1207–1214.

Ziv, N.E. and Smith, S.J. (1996). Evidence for a role of dendritic filopodia in synaptogenesis and spine formation. *Neuron*, **17**, 91–102.

Determinants or regeneration in the injured nervous system

CONTENTS

Inhibitors of axonal regeneration

Tim Spencer, Marco Domeniconi and Marie T. Filbin

Department of Biological Sciences, Hunter College of the City, University of New York, New York, NY, USA

21.1 Introduction

The adult mammalian central nervous system (CNS) is one of the most sophisticated and intricate structures found in nature. It is also, however, one of the most delicate. Injuries to the mammalian brain or spinal cord often result in a loss of sensory and/or motor function which is invariably considered to be "untreatable". The ancient Egyptians were the first to recognize this fact and, since then, doctors and scientists have sought to understand why, following injury, neurons of the mammalian CNS fail to regrow cut or damaged axons whereas their peripheral nervous system (PNS) counterparts often do. Research conducted in many laboratories over the past 25 years, have resulted in the elucidation of some of the causes and mechanisms of this regenerative failure and, indeed, have also suggested potential targets for therapeutic intervention thus indicating that these ailments may, in fact, not be "untreatable."

Why *do* injured CNS neurons fail to regenerate? Do these neurons lose their intrinsic capacity to grow with development, or are there extrinsic factors which prevent repair? The answers to these questions appear to lie in the study of the local CNS environment. In 1981, Sam David and Albert Aguayo were the first to suggest that perhaps this lack of regeneration may not be entirely cell autonomous. Axons from damaged CNS neurons will, in fact, exhibit some regeneration if provided a permissive environment such as a peripheral nerve graft (David and Aguayo, 1981). The following year, Martin Berry also found that products of the breakdown of the myelin sheath, which are released after CNS injury, can inhibit the regrowth of damaged axons (Berry, 1982). In addition, several years later, work by Martin Schwab's group identified specific myelin membrane-associated protein fractions that displayed axonal growth inhibitory properties (Caroni and Schwab, 1988a). Since these seminal findings, several molecules, associated with myelin, have been found which may be primary factors in the lack of CNS regeneration.

In order for a molecule to be considered to be an inhibitor of CNS regeneration *in vivo*, it must, of course, be present in the adult mammalian CNS and be in a position to encounter an extending axon following neuronal injury and the associated damage. To date, three major inhibitors of axonal regeneration associated with myelin have been identified: myelin-associated glycoprotein (MAG), Nogo and oligodendrocyte-myelin glycoprotein (OMgp) (Fig. 21.1). Recent evidence from several labs has shown, interestingly, that all three of these molecules enact their effects via binding to the same receptors, the NgR-LINGO-p75^{NTR} complex (Domeniconi et al., 2002; Fournier et al., 2001; Liu et al., 2002; Wang et al., 2002a; Wong et al., 2002a, b; Mi et al., 2004). All three of these inhibitory molecules appear to be present in the adult mammalian CNS and *in vitro* data suggests that they may each be sufficient to block regeneration after CNS injury (McKerracher et al., 1994; Mukhopadhyay et al., 1994; Chen et al., 2000; GrandPre et al., 2000; Prinjha et al., 2000; Wang et al., 2002b). While their respective distribution and abundance in CNS myelin varies, all are present and able to bind receptor(s) on the neuronal surface

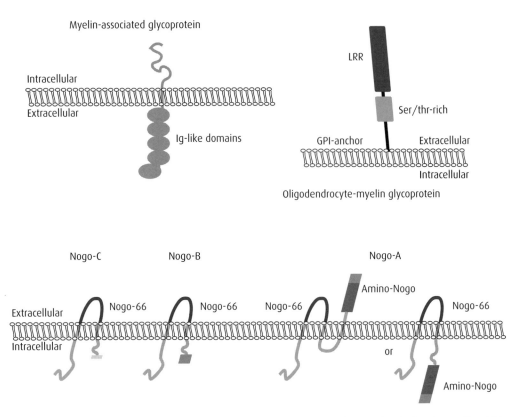

Figure 21.1. *The myelin-associated inhibitors of regeneration*: The three known inhibitory molecules found in myelin exhibit very different physical structures but all are able to potently inhibit axonal regeneration.

following injury and myelin fragmentation. Interestingly, these molecules are also thought to be present in the PNS as well. Why, then, do PNS axons readily regenerate after injury while CNS axons do not? One hypothesis suggests that the process of rapid Wallerian degeneration – which includes an influx of immune responsive elements such as macro-phages, which occurs after injury to the PNS, resulting in the clearing of myelin debris – results in the rapid removal of the myelin-associated inhibitors, thereby allowing regeneration. Evidence for this hypothesis can be seen in the C57BL/6WLD/ OLA (Wld^S) mice. These Wallerian degeneration-slowed mice exhibit retarded regeneration following PNS injury (Brown et al., 1991; 1992; Perry et al., 1991; Bisby et al., 1995). Conversely, in the immune-privileged CNS, myelin clearing proceeds much more slowly and, therefore,

the inhibitors are still present and, indeed, more accessible, following injury.

In addition to the myelin-associated inhibitors, axonal regeneration can be blocked by the formation of a structure called the glial scar. This structure, indicated by the increase in reactive gliosis which occurs after injury to the CNS, forms both a chemical and physical barrier to regenerating axons. Furthermore, there also exist several molecules which act as repulsive or inhibitory guidance cues during development. While these molecules are able to induce growth cone collapse or turning in embryonic and adult neurons, it is not clear if these molecules are in fact active in the mature nervous system and so their physiological role as inhibitors of axonal regeneration remain questionable (see Volume I, Chapter 24). These molecules and structures will be discussed in more detail later in this chapter.

21.2 Inhibitors of axonal regeneration in myelin

The myelin sheath is, simply put, a membranous extension which encircles an axon in a multilayered, concentric fashion. This structure serves as an "electrical insulator" which increases the velocity of conducted action potentials via a process called saltatory conduction. In the PNS, myelin is produced by cytoplasmic extensions from Schwann cells with a single Schwann cell myelinating a single axonal segment. In the CNS, however, myelination is performed by oligodendrocytes. Here, oligodendrocytes send out projections which, upon encountering an axon, begin the process of membrane extension and axonal envelopment. In the CNS, a single oligodendrocyte can myelinate many axons. In either system, however, myelin is essential for proper neuronal signal propagation. Myelination failure or disorders which result in demyelination, such as multiple sclerosis, invariably result in loss of effective sensory and motor function or death.

During the processes of myelination in both the CNS and PNS, changes occur in the expression and localization of myelin membrane proteins. The completion of myelination also correlates with a precipitous drop in axonal sprouting and growth (Savio and Schwab, 1990; Kapfhammer and Schwab, 1994a, b; Keirstead et al., 1995; Schwegler et al., 1995). This loss of growth potential may be attributed to the expression of the myelin-associated inhibitors of regeneration. Since these myelinated axons have already reached their targets prior to the final stages of myelination, it is believed that the aforementioned inhibitors may act to prevent inadvertent sprouting and improper synapse formation. While this blockage of axonal growth by the myelin-associated inhibitors is essential following the termination of development, it also has the unfortunate effect of blocking any attempts by damaged adult axons to regenerate after injury.

Despite the differences in cellular origin, however, both PNS and CNS myelin express the proteins associated with inhibition of axonal regeneration. The myelin-associated inhibitors all appear to be present in undamaged myelin and may have roles other than the block of regeneration or inadvertent sprouting. For example, MAG is found in the periaxonal surface of CNS myelin and is thought to be responsible for maintaining the 12–14 nm space between myelin and the axonal membrane (Trapp and Quarles, 1982; Trapp, 1988; 1990). In the CNS, MAG and Nogo have been shown to be present in the periaxonal internode and OMgp is believed to be enriched in the paranodal loops. However, following injury, all of these proteins may become exposed to any potentially regenerating axons as a result of fragmentation of the myelin.

21.3 The myelin-associated inhibitors

Nogo

In the late 1980s several investigators reported that both CNS and PNS neurons could extend neurites through a sciatic nerve explant but failed to enter an explant from the optic nerve. Since the two explants differed only in their myelin producing cells, Schwann cells in the sciatic nerve and oligodendrocytes in the optic nerve, it was proposed that the oligodendrocytes were the deciding factor in the lack of neurite outgrowth seen within the CNS tracts and, subsequently, myelin was proposed as an inhibitor of regeneration (Berry, 1982). In a seminal study on this CNS-specific inhibition, Martin Schwab and colleagues at the University of Zurich examined CNS myelin's inhibitory properties and found that the main inhibitory components were membrane-bound and associated with the protein fraction of CNS myelin (Caroni and Schwab, 1988b). The inhibitory components of myelin could be recovered after separation in sodium dodecyl sulfate polyacrylamide gel electrophoresis (SDS-PAGE) as two minor myelin-associated proteins with relative molecular masses of 35 and 250 kDa (then called neurite growth inhibitors NI-35 and NI-250, respectively) (Caroni and Schwab, 1988b).

When the same group generated a monoclonal antibody, IN-1, against the two proteins, they showed that the addition of IN-1 to cultures reduced the inhibitory activity of myelin (Caroni and Schwab, 1988a). Notably, IN-1 injected into the injured spinal cord resulted in regeneration of 5% of the damaged axons and improvements in functional recovery in injured adult rats (Schnell and Schwab, 1990; Bregman et al., 1995).

Using peptide sequences derived from the bovine homolog of NI-250 (Spillmann et al., 1998), three groups independently identified the IN-1 antigen(s) as products of the *Nogo* gene (Chen et al., 2000; GrandPre et al., 2000; Prinjha et al., 2000).

Three Nogo isoforms, Nogo-A, -B and -C, are encoded from a single gene by alternative splicing and/or promoter usage. In human and rat fetal tissue, Nogo-A mRNA is strongly expressed in the ventral spinal cord, dorsal root and autonomic ganglia. The same expression pattern is observed in the adult spinal cord and ganglia. High levels of Nogo-A message are present in oligodendrocytes, motor neurons and sensory ganglia neurons, but not in astrocytes or Schwann cells. Minor expression is also observed in developing muscle tissue (Josephson et al., 2001). Western blot analysis of adult tissue reveals that Nogo-A protein is present in brain and spinal cord, and at low levels in the testis and heart (Huber et al., 2002). After spinal cord injury, Nogo-A is up regulated to a moderate degree (Wang, X., et al., 2002), whereas traumatic lesions to the cortex do not change Nogo-A expression (Huber et al., 2002). Nogo-B and -C have a much wider expression profile in neurons, skeletal muscle and various peripheral tissues.

The *Nogo* products show a high degree of homology with the reticulon protein family (van de Velde et al., 1994) and contain a dilysine endoplasmic reticulum (ER) retention sequence. Interestingly, Nogo proteins are mostly localized to the ER with a small percentage present at the plasma membrane (GrandPre et al., 2000). Throughout the adult CNS, Nogo-A has been detected by confocal and electron-immuno-microscopy on oligodendrocyte processes in the periaxonal and outermost myelin membranes

(Huber et al., 2002; Wang, X., et al., 2002). Furthermore, it has been suggested that Nogo-A may have two different membrane topologies, one in which both the N- and C-terminus are oriented cytoplasmically, and a second in which both termini are oriented extracellularly (Oertle et al., 2002).

All three Nogo isoforms contain a 66-amino acid extracellular region (Nogo-66) which displays neuron-specific growth inhibitory activity *in vitro* (GrandPre et al., 2000). An additional domain which is specific to Nogo-A, termed Amino-Nogo, has been localized to a 195-amino acid stretch near the N-terminus which was shown to inhibit neurite outgrowth as well as abrogate 3T3 fibroblast spreading (Fournier et al., 2001; Prinjha et al., 2002) (Fig. 21.1). Schwab's team generated a transgenic mouse expressing Nogo-A under the control of the Schwann cell-specific P0 promoter which is strongly induced 7 days post-peripheral nerve injury at the onset of remyelination (Gupta et al., 1988). These transgenic mice displayed an impaired recovery from sciatic nerve crush injury suggesting that Nogo-A was capable of inhibiting axonal growth *in vivo* (Pot et al., 2002).

Several groups using different strategies have created Nogo knockout mice but, at the present time, there is a lack of consensus on the effects of the Nogo deletion. Strittmatter and colleagues utilized a retroviral gene trap insertion technique in order to disrupt exon 3 (specific to Nogo-A) of the Nogo gene. The resultant mice, however, were found to lack both Nogo-A and -B with Nogo-C levels remaining unaffected (Kim et al., 2003). In this study, Strittmatter's group reports limited regeneration in several young animals, but these improvements appear to be lost as the animals age (Kim et al., 2003). Conversely, Tessier-Lavigne's group generated two different mouse models. In the first, they induced a deletion in the exon 1 region of the Nogo gene, thereby disrupting Nogo-A and -B expression but without affecting Nogo-C expression. The second model featured a selected deletion of the C-terminal region which is common to all three isoforms, thereby eliminating all Nogo expression. In both of these mouse models, Tessier-Lavigne and colleagues failed to observe any improvements in axonal regeneration following injury (Zheng et al., 2003). Finally, Schwab and colleagues report another Nogo-deficient mouse model where selected disruption of the Nogo-A-specific exon (exon 3) resulted in a complete loss of Nogo-A expression. Surprisingly, however, this group also reported a robust, compensatory increase in Nogo-B expression. In regeneration studies performed on these mice, only limited axonal regeneration, and no improvements in functional recovery, was observed *in vivo* (Simonen et al., 2003). It appears likely that the limited/failed regeneration observed in these mice may be attributable to the other, still-present inhibitory proteins found in myelin. This idea is supported by the finding that inhibition of neurite outgrowth *in vitro* by Nogo-A −/− myelin is primarily reduced and these remaining, residual effects are completely abolished by application of anti-MAG antibodies (Kim et al., 2003).

MAG

MAG is a member of the sialic acid binding immune globulin (Ig)-like lectin (siglec) family of adhesion molecules (Siglec 4) (Crocker et al., 1998). MAG contains a short cytoplasmic domain and a single transmembrane region while its extracellular domain consists of five Ig-like domains (Lai et al., 1987; Salzer et al., 1987; 1990) (Fig. 21.1). MAG expression is limited to the myelin forming cells, oligodendrocytes in the CNS and Schwann cells in the PNS, although with varying expression patterns within uncompacted myelin areas (Trapp et al., 1989; Trapp, 1990). In the CNS, MAG comprises 1% of the total myelin protein and it is localized solely to the periaxonal membrane in the internodal segments of the myelin sheath (Trapp, 1990). In the PNS, MAG is expressed in the paranodal regions, Schmidt-Lanterman incisures, and outer mesaxon segments, though it only represents 0.1% of the total PNS myelin protein (Trapp, 1990). Due to its molecular structure, which is closely related to that of N-CAM, and due to its localization, MAG is hypothesized to play a role in the stabilization of the axon-glia interface (Quarles, 1983; Salzer et al.,

1990; Trapp, 1990; Filbin, 1995). This idea is supported by studies indicating that in older MAG-deficient (MAG −/−) mice, generated via homologous recombination-induced deletion of the MAG gene (Li et al., 1994; Montag et al., 1994), these mice exhibit normal products of the first myelination events however, they eventually acquire altered periaxonal architecture and an increase in axonal loss (Fruttiger et al., 1995).

In 1994, two investigators independently identified MAG as a major inhibitor of axonal growth *in vitro* (McKerracher et al., 1994; Mukhopadhyay et al., 1994). Primary CNS neurons cultured on monolayers of MAG-expressing cells display a drastic reduction in axonal growth as compared to neurons plated on control cells. NG108 cells (a neuronal cell line) also fail to extend neurites when plated on slides coated with myelin or MAG. Furthermore, a soluble, proteolytic fragment of MAG, consisting of the entire extracellular domain and found *in vivo*, was shown to inhibit neurite outgrowth *in vitro* and *in vivo* (Tang et al., 1997b; 2001). In an effort to further elucidate the role of MAG in the inhibition of axonal regeneration, several groups sought to compare neurite outgrowth on myelin purified from the MAG −/− mice. In these studies, two separate groups found that the MAG −/− myelin exhibited an impaired ability to inhibit axonal growth from primary neurons *in vitro* (Li et al., 1996; Shen et al., 1998) while a third group found that while neurite length from NG108 cells was improved, there was no effect on the growth of primary neurons (Bartsch et al., 1995). It is likely that this discrepancy in inhibitory ability may be due in part to the existence of the other now-identified myelin-associated inhibitors as well as due to the methods used for myelin preparation (Filbin, 1996).

However, further evidence supporting MAG activity *in vivo* was gathered using the mutant Wld[S] mice. As mentioned earlier, the Wld[S] mice exhibit very slow Wallerian degeneration following peripheral nerve injury with impaired axonal regeneration (Brown et al., 1991). The dramatic differences in the clearance of myelin debris could account, at least in part, for the difference in regenerating ability seen between CNS and PNS neurons. Furthermore, Martini and colleagues crossbred

Wld^S mice with MAG $-/-$ mice and studied axonal regrowth *in vivo* (Schafer et al., 1996). Following peripheral nerve injury, analysis of MAG-deficient/ Wld^S mice revealed that the number of myelin sheets associated with regrowing axons doubled as compared to Wld^S mice (Schafer et al., 1996). These results further support the notion that MAG-deficient myelin is less inhibitory than the wild type myelin.

OMgp

The latest addition to the group of myelin-based inhibitors is OMgp (Kottis et al., 2002; Wang et al., 2002b), a minor component of CNS myelin whose expression in development coincides closely with the caudal to rostral progression of CNS myelination (Habib et al., 1998; Vourc'h and Andres, 2004). OMgp is detectable by western blot analysis in the brains of post-natal rats and its concentration peaks at the late stages of myelination (Habib et al., 1998; Vourc'h et al., 2003a). The majority of the protein is found in diverse groups of neurons, particularly in large projection neurons such as the pyramidal cells of the hippocampus, the Purkinje cells of the cerebellum, motor neurons in the brainstem, and anterior horn cells of the spinal cord (Habib et al., 1998). However, OMgp is not confined to these cells and it is expressed in oligodendrocytes as well (Habib et al., 1998). Although its "normal" function is still unknown, recent observations suggest that OMgp could be involved in the regulation of oligodendrocytes growth as well as in the arrest of myelination or compaction of myelin. Regardless of this proposed function, it was also demonstrated to inhibit axonal growth *in vitro* (Kottis et al., 2002; Wang et al., 2002b). Originally identified in the late 1980s (Mikol and Stefansson, 1988), OMgp is an extracellular membrane protein anchored to the cell surface through a glycosylphosphatidylinositol (GPI) lipid intermediate and it contains a highly conserved leucine-rich repeat (LRR) domain which is necessary for proper receptor binding (Fig. 21.1). The deletion of this LRR domain is responsible for a total loss of inhibitory function in an *in vitro* neurite outgrowth assay (Wang et al., 2002b; Vourc'h et al., 2003b).

21.4 Receptors for the myelin inhibitors

Nogo-66 receptor

The receptor for Nogo-66 (NgR) was identified using an alkaline phosphatase (AP) fusion protein to screen a mouse brain cDNA library transfected into COS-7 cells (Fournier et al., 2001). NgR is a 473 amino acid GPI-anchored protein. Its globular structure consists of a translocation signal sequence, eight LRR motifs, which are capped by N-terminal and C-terminal cysteine-rich modules (termed LRR-NT and LRR-CT segments, respectively), and a unique C-terminal region proximal to the anchoring site (Fournier et al., 2001). The functional specificity of NgR was demonstrated by a gain-of-function experiment in chick early embryonic retinal ganglion cells (RGC), which are insensitive to Nogo-66-induced growth cone collapse. Viral-mediated NgR expression in embryonic day 7 (E7) RGCs renders these neurons sensitive to the Nogo-66 activity (Fournier et al., 2001). Also, a truncated, soluble NgR antagonizes Nogo-66-dependent inhibition of neurite extension by E13 DRGs (Fournier et al., 2002). The expression pattern of NgR is consistent with a role in the inhibition of axonal regeneration. Transcripts are present predominantly in the adult and maturing brain where the NgR protein is found in a wide variety of neurons but not in oligodendrocytes (Hunt et al., 2002b). Expression is minimal prior to myelination and there are no detectable changes after trauma (Hunt et al., 2002b).

NgR functions as a common receptor mediating the inhibition of axonal growth by at least the three myelin-based inhibitors discussed so far, Nogo-66, MAG and OMgp (Fournier et al., 2001; Domeniconi et al., 2002; Liu et al., 2002; Wang et al., 2002b). The additional Nogo-A domain Amino-Nogo does not seem to interact with NgR (Hunt et al., 2002a). Notably, the structurally unrelated ligands all bind to NgR with high affinities (Fournier et al., 2001;

Domeniconi et al., 2002; Liu et al., 2002; Wang et al., 2002b). Mutation analysis demonstrated that the receptor-ligand interaction is localized to the LRR motifs. The structural basis for the ligand recognition has been partially clarified by the resolution of NgR crystal structure (Barton et al., 2003; He et al., 2003). The multiple LRR motifs result in a concave groove which contains a putative degenerate binding site, hence accounting for the similar interactions with such different ligands. The structure also suggests a possible co-receptor binding site within the unique C-terminal region and the deletion studies support this idea.

Some groups have also reported that sialylated glycans are mediators of MAG inhibition of neurite outgrowth and that MAG inhibition is a result of carbohydrate recognition (Vinson et al., 2001; Vyas et al., 2002). MAG specifically binds gangliosides GT1b and GD1a, which are both expressed on the surface of MAG-responsive neurons. It is also known that multivalent immunoglobulin M (IgM) antibody cross-linking of cell surface GT1b mimics the effect of MAG (Vinson et al., 2001). However, other studies indicate that removal of sialic acid residues by sialidase treatment does not affect MAG's inhibitory activity (Tang et al., 1997a). Since the addition to outgrowth assays of IgM Fab fragments generated from either anti-GT1b or anti-GD1a antibodies mimics MAG inhibitory activity, it is likely that this interaction is not specific to an MAG pathway. Current data supports a model in which the recognition of sialylated glycans, while not essential for inhibition of neurite outgrowth by MAG, may result in a weak, transient activation of the inhibitory pathway, independent of the NgR-dependent effects. Furthermore, *in vivo*, the effects of ganglioside-mediated binding of MAG may serve to potentiate the inhibitory effects of the NgR-mediated pathway. One possible interpretation of these events is that MAG has two discrete functions: first, to hinder aberrant sprouting and generate structural axon-glia stability via interaction with gangliosides, and, second, to strongly inhibit outgrowth via interaction with a functional high-affinity receptor.

21.4.2 The p75 neurotrophin receptor

Due to the GPI-linked nature of NgR, the ability of this receptor to initiate a signaling pathway requires the presence of at least one co-receptor. Indeed, it was recently found that the inhibition of axonal elongation induced by all three of the myelin-associated inhibitors, Nogo-66, MAG and OMgp, depends on the association of NgR with the p75 neurotrophin receptor (p75[NTR]) (Wong et al., 2002; Wang et al., 2002a). This is evidenced by the fact that cultured primary neurons from p75[NTR] null mice are insensitive to the activity of the myelin-associated inhibitors (Wang et al., 2002a). The extracellular domain of p75[NTR] contains four cysteine-rich motifs, which are necessary for nerve growth factor (NGF) binding (Dostaler et al., 1996). Thus far, it is unclear if these motifs are also responsible for NgR binding, although it should be noted that simultaneous treatment with NGF does not abrogate nor does it reduce myelin-mediated inhibition of growth from Trk-A negative neurons (Cai et al., 1999). The p75[NTR] intracellular domain does not have an intrinsic enzymatic activity and the signal transduction takes place through interaction with several adaptor proteins (Bandtlow and Dechant, 2004; Barker, 2004). The cytoplasmic segment of p75[NTR] contains a palmitoylation site, two TNFR-associated factor (TRAF) binding sites, a type II death domain, a small G-protein activating domain, and a PSD-95, Discs-large, ZD-1 (PDZ) domain-binding motif.

During early development p75[NTR] is expressed in a wide variety of cells within the CNS and PNS, as well as many non-neuronal tissues such as kidney, testis, lung and muscle (Ryffel and Mihatsch, 1993). Post-natally, p75[NTR] levels are reduced in most tissues and restricted to a narrower range of cells (Ryffel and Mihatsch, 1993). Trauma to the nervous system induces p75[NTR] expression in many cell types (Ebadi et al., 1997). After injury, increased mRNA and protein levels have been documented in motor, corticospinal and hippocampal neurons, as well as oligodendrocytes, Schwann and Purkinje cells, microglia and macrophages (Ebadi et al., 1997).

21.4.3 Lingo

A third molecule has been associated with the NgR/p75[NTR] complex. Lingo-1 is a human homolog of SLIT – a Drosophila axonal guidance molecule which binds the neuronal receptor Robo – which is highly expressed in CNS tissue and is undetectable in non-neuronal tissue (Mi et al., 2004). Like p75[NTR], its expression is upregulated following trauma. The protein consists of 12 LRR motifs, one Ig-like domain, a transmembrane domain and a short cytoplasmic tail (Mi et al., 2004). The cytoplasmic tail contains a canonical epidermal growth factor receptor-like tyrosine phosphorylation site. Lingo-1 interacts with both NgR and p75[NTR] and its absence reduces the inhibitory activity of myelin proteins. It has been demonstrated that concurrent expression of NgR, p75[NTR] and Lingo-1 into the non-neuronal cell line COS-7 confers sensitivity to OMgp (Mi et al., 2004).

21.5 Signaling by inhibitors

Following the binding of each of the myelin-associated inhibitors to the NgR-p75[NTR]-LINGO receptor complex, there is an induction of a signaling pathway which eventually leads to the blockage of neurite extension from damaged or naïve adult neurons. While the entire pathway and all of its constituent members have yet to be elucidated, some of the prime movers in this pathway have begun to reveal themselves.

It has been known for several years that the MAG-mediated block of axonal regeneration is dependent on the activity of the small GTPase, RhoA (Lehmann et al., 1999). Work from the lab of Lisa McKerracher has shown that blocking RhoA activity can promote axonal regeneration both in the presence of MAG or purified myelin *in vitro* or following the application of a CNS injury *in vivo* (Lehmann et al., 1999; Dergham et al., 2002; Winton et al., 2002). Furthermore, recent findings have also suggested that the activation of p75[NTR] upon binding of the receptor complex by MAG results in activation of RhoA (Yamashita et al., 2002; Wang et al., 2002a) in a protein kinase C

(PKC)-dependent manner (Sivasankaran et al., 2004) and that this RhoA activation may work via the sequestration of the Rho-GDP dissociation inhibitor, Rho-GDI, by p75[NTR] following activation of the signaling complex (Yamashita and Tohyama, 2003). A further elucidation of the role of Rho in the inhibition of axonal regeneration can be found in Chapter 24 of this volume.

Beside its role in transducing the inhibitory signal from myelin-based inhibitors, p75[NTR] is involved a wide array of biological activities, requiring it to interact with multiple ligands, surface receptors and adaptor proteins (Dechant and Barde, 2002; Bandtlow and Dechant, 2004; Barker, 2004). Evidence indicates that p75[NTR] can bind all known neurotrophins with similar affinities as well as pro-neurotrophins (Lee et al., 2001). In addition, several non-neurotrophin ligands have been shown to associate with the receptor. Among these are the neurotoxic prion protein fragment PrP (26–106) (Della-Bianca et al., 2001) and the Aβ-peptide of the amyloid precursor protein (APP) (Perini et al., 2002). At the cell surface, p75[NTR] also associates with a growing number of membrane proteins. It can interact with itself to form homodimers, with gangliosides such as GT1b (Yamashita et al., 2002), the three Trk receptors and the ankyrin repeat–rich membrane spanning protein (ARMS) (Kong et al., 2001).

A member of the tumor necrosis factor (TNF) superfamily, p75[NTR] can regulate cell death and survival (Chao et al., 1998; Lee et al., 2001). Among the ligands that activate p75[NTR] cell death pathways, pro-neurotrophins seem to be the most effective (Lee et al., 2001). This function is carried out by novel interaction with Sortilin (Nykjaer et al., 2004). Regulation of life and death pathways in different contexts requires that p75[NTR] interacts with a plethora of cytoplasmic adaptors like the neurotrophin receptor interacting factors 1 and 2 (NRIF1 and NRIF2) (Casademunt et al., 1999), the IAP-binding protein neurotrophin receptor – interacting microarray and gene expression (MAGE) homolog (NRAGE or MAGED1) (Salehi et al., 2000), FAS-associated phosphatase-1 (FAP-1) (Irie et al., 1999), the p75[NTR]-associated cell death executor (NADE)

(Mukai et al., 2000), and several of the TNF receptor associated factors (TRAFs) (Ye et al., 1999). Furthermore, p75^{NTR} interacts with caveolin (Bilderback et al., 1997) and with protein kinases such as the interleukin-1 receptor associated kinase (IRAK) (Mamidipudi et al., 2002) and the mitogen-activated protein kinases (MAPK) extracellular-regulated kinase (ERK1 and ERK2) (Volonte et al., 1993) and P38β2 (Wang et al., 2000).

Some of the adaptor proteins that interact with p75^{NTR} block cell-cycle progression when expressed in cultured cells. These adaptors include: the zinc finger proteins SC-1 (Chittka et al., 2004), NRIF1 and NRIF2, as well as NRAGE. Interestingly, a recent study indicates that p75^{NTR} can affect synaptic transmission between sympathetic neurons and cardiac myocytes (Yang et al., 2002). In this system, single neurons can release two different and "contrasting" neurotransmitters: norepinephrine, which increases the twitching frequency of myocytes, and acetylcholine, which has the opposite effect (Furshpan et al., 1976). While the addition of NGF to co-cultures increases the release of norepinephrine in a TrkA-dependent manner (Lockhart et al., 1997), the addition of brain-derived neurotrophic factor (BDNF) increases inhibitory transmission by promoting acetylcholine release (Yang et al., 2002).

Overcoming the myelin-induced block of regeneration

One of the most intriguing and encouraging aspects of the axonal regeneration paradigm is the afore-mentioned finding that all three of the myelin-associated inhibitors bind and exert their effects via the same receptor complex. This fact suggests a redundancy in the activity of these various inhibitory proteins and also provides a host of potential targets for therapeutic intervention to encourage axonal regeneration. If the binding or signaling of a single receptor complex can be compromised, it may be possible to permit sufficient regeneration in the adult mammalian CNS after injury, particularly prior to formation of the glial scar.

Blocking inhibition with antibodies and peptides

The concept of inhibitor and receptor-specific targeting in regeneration-encouraging paradigms was born with the discovery of the NI-35 and NI-250-blocking antibody, IN-1 (Caroni and Schwab, 1988a). *In vivo* application of this inhibition-blocking antibody following CNS injury was shown to mediate moderate regeneration of injured fibers and this improved regeneration could be correlated with an increase in recovery of function (Bregman et al., 1995; Schnell and Schwab, 1990). Since this time, many studies have followed which sought to examine the effects on regeneration of blocking the myelin-associated inhibitors. One particularly interesting study found that if adult mice are immunized against myelin-associated protein components – including the myelin-associated inhibitors of regeneration – some regeneration is observed following dorsal column lesioning *in vivo*, and that this improved regeneration occurs in the absence of a cellular inflammatory response (Huang et al., 1999).

Another method for blocking the inhibitory effects of the myelin-associated inhibitors is the use of function-blocking antibodies to the receptor complex. Indeed, it has been shown that if the binding of the myelin inhibitors to NgR is blocked via addition of an anti-NgR antibody *in vitro*, axotomized neurons will extend long processes even on purified myelin (Domeniconi et al., 2002). Furthermore, recent work by several groups have shown that expression of small antagonistic peptides may also provide a potential avenue for intervention. Application of a small peptide which consists of the first 40 amino acids of the Nogo-66 domain (NEP 1–40) will effectively bind to NgR and block the inhibitory signaling of the Nogo-66 inhibitor (GrandPre et al., 2002). Conversely, introduction of non-signaling peptide fragments of the receptor complex such as p75-Fc (Wang et al., 2002a), a truncated fragment of NgR (NgR-Ecto) (Liu et al., 2002) or LINGO-Fc (Mi et al., 2004) are all able to effectively compromise the binding and/or signaling of the inhibitor–receptor interaction, thereby promoting axonal regeneration *in vitro*. Further work may soon elucidate the efficiency of these therapies *in vivo* following injury.

The convergence of the inhibitory effects of all three inhibitors is consistent with findings that modulations of the activity or expression of certain intracellular signaling molecules can simultaneously abrogate the inhibitory effects of all the inhibitors. To this end, it may be possible to target some of the downstream effectors of the NgR-LINGO-p75^{NTR} signaling cascade and thereby block the functional effects of these inhibitors. One such method is via blockage of the small GTPase, RhoA. Evidence suggests that blocking Rho signaling can promote axonal regeneration both in the presence of all of the myelin-associated inhibitors *in vitro* and following injury to the adult CNS *in vivo*. Work from the McKerracher lab has shown that inactivation of Rho, via application of the exoenzyme C3 transferase, or blocking the signaling cascade via inhibition of the downstream effector, Rho-associated kinase (ROCK) can effectively block the axonal growth inhibitory effects of the myelin-associated inhibitors both *in vitro* and *in vivo* (Lehmann et al., 1999; Dergham et al., 2002; Winton et al., 2002). For further discussion on this topic, see Chapter 24 of this volume.

In addition to the blockage of the inhibitors or the signaling receptor complex, it is also possible to encourage axonal regeneration via induction of changes in the intrinsic growth state of the neuron such that it no longer responds to the myelin-associated inhibitors. It has been well characterized for many years that the axons of embryonic (or, in a few cases, neonatal) neurons are not inhibited in their growth potential by myelin and its inhibitors. It has been surmised that this is a result in a difference in the intrinsic growth state of the neuron rather than a difference in the inhibitory components in the environment. Thus, the question becomes, what are the modulatory signals that differentiate the growth state of embryonic versus adult CNS neurons?

Cyclic-adenosine monophosphate

An answer to this question can be found in the levels of one of the usual cellular "suspects": the ubiquitous

signaling messenger, cyclic-adenosine monophosphate (cAMP). In the nervous system, cAMP signaling has been implicated in a variety of neuronal processes including memory and learning (Alberini et al., 1995; Frey et al., 1993; Wong et al., 1999; Wu et al., 1995), neurotransmitter modulation (Byrne and Kandel, 1996; Castellucci et al., 1980; 1982; Milner et al., 1998) and axonal growth cone turning and developmental guidance. Indeed, significant evidence exists to suggest that the levels of intracellular cAMP can modulate the turning and growth induction effects of guidance cues on an extending growth cone (Song et al., 1997; 1998). This phenomenon will be examined in more detail later in this chapter.

The role of cAMP levels and signaling during development, however, are not limited to the modulation of responses to guidance cues. As stated earlier, it is commonly accepted that embryonic neurons are able to extend long axons both during normal development or following axotomy at the embryonic stages. Therefore, not surprisingly, examinations into the role of cAMP perinatally have revealed that the cAMP levels of embryonic neurons are significantly higher than that of their adult counterparts and that this elevation can account for the ability of these neurons to extend axons in the inhibitory CNS environment (Cai et al., 2001). Furthermore, the loss of regenerative ability which occurs post-natally directly correlates with a precipitous decrease in endogenous cAMP levels. Even in neuronal types which retain their regenerative abilities in the neonatal stages, cAMP levels appear to remain high until the developmental switch occurs.

Thus, it is reasonable to assume that if the elevated cAMP levels observed in regeneration-competent embryonic neurons could be replicated in the adult animal, perhaps axonal regeneration and repair post-injury could indeed be possible. Recent evidence suggests that this may, in fact, be the case. Elevation of intracellular cAMP levels via addition of chemical analogs can indeed improve the regenerative capacity of post-natal neurons on an inhibitory substrate *in vitro*. Interestingly, it was also noted that pre-treatment of neurons with neurotrophins like BDNF, called "priming", can also mediate improved regeneration on myelin-associated inhibitor-containing substrates. Not surprisingly though, it was found that even this mechanism is mediated by the induction of elevated cAMP levels and the associated signaling (Cai et al., 1999). Furthermore, the pro-regenerative effects of cAMP elevation are not limited to abrogation of myelin-associated inhibitor signaling. The growth inhibitory properties of several glial scar-associated proteoglycans as well as certain repulsive guidance cues can be overcome by induction of cAMP elevation (Shearer et al., 2003).

Evidence for the regeneration-promoting effects of cAMP elevation exists in a variety of animal model systems as well. One commonly employed tool utilizes the easily observable RGCs as a model for improving CNS regeneration. Indeed, evidence exists which suggests that application of chemical cAMP analogs (Monsul et al., 2004) or adenylyl-cyclase activators along with neurotrophic factors (Watanabe et al., 2003) can mediate improved regeneration of adult mammalian RGCs *in vivo*.

cAMP elevation has also been implicated in another regeneration paradigm, the conditioning-lesion effect. Dorsal root ganglion neurons (DRG) are unique in that they possess two branches, one which extends into the spinal cord (the CNS branch) and another which extends into the periphery. It has been well established that if a "pre-conditioning" lesion is applied to the peripheral branch of a DRG neuron and, 1 day or 1 week later, a second lesion is introduced into the dorsal column (the CNS branch), CNS regeneration is observed. Regenerating axons will extend processes into a peripheral nerve graft at the lesion site (Richardson and Issa, 1984; Richardson and Verge, 1986) and even in the absence of such a graft, into and beyond the site of injury (Neumann and Woolf, 1999). This effect, as well, has been shown to be cAMP-dependent (Neumann et al., 2002; Qiu et al., 2002). In fact, a single injection of dibutyryl-cAMP (db-cAMP), a non-hydrolyzable analog of cAMP, can mimic the conditioning lesion effect, even in the absence of the peripheral lesion (Qiu et al., 2002) (Fig. 21.2). Furthermore, a more recent study by the Tuszynski laboratory has demonstrated that the injection of db-cAMP into DRG neurons may be combined with other therapeutic techniques, such as injection of the neurotrophin NT-3 and bone marrow stromal cells directly into the lesion site to improve overall regeneration after a cervical spinal cord injury (Lu et al., 2004).

These findings have helped to elucidate an essential portion of the regeneration-invoking signaling pathway but neither application of a pre-conditioning lesion nor direct injection of db-cAMP are viable avenues for therapeutic intervention in human spinal cord injury patients. Therefore, more recent work has focused on less intrusive and post-injury applied methods for elevation neuronal cAMP levels. One such method for achieving this is to elevate cAMP levels by blocking its degradation. Recent evidence from several labs has indicated that application of the phosphodiesterase 4 inhibitor, rolipram, can effectively induce an increase in cAMP levels *in vitro* and post-injury *in vivo* and can improve regeneration and functional recovery, particularly when combined with other therapeutic methods (Nikulina et al., 2004; Pearse et al., 2004). The reason that rolipram is so attractive as a potential spinal cord injury therapeutic is due to the fact that it is blood–brain barrier permeable and, therefore, can be injected subcutaneously, thereby alleviating the need for intrusive surgery.

However, since cAMP has many roles in a multitude of signaling pathways in neuronal cells, the artificial elevation of cAMP alone may not be a valid therapeutic approach. Therefore, it is essential to comprehend the entire complexity of the cAMP signaling pathway, particularly the downstream effectors that mediate this improved regenerative capacity. Understanding this signaling pathway may present yet another potential target for therapeutic intervention in the hopes of encouraging regeneration in the adult.

Downstream effectors

It is well known that elevated cAMP levels result in an activation of the cAMP-dependent protein kinase, or protein kinase A (PKA) – and, indeed, both the

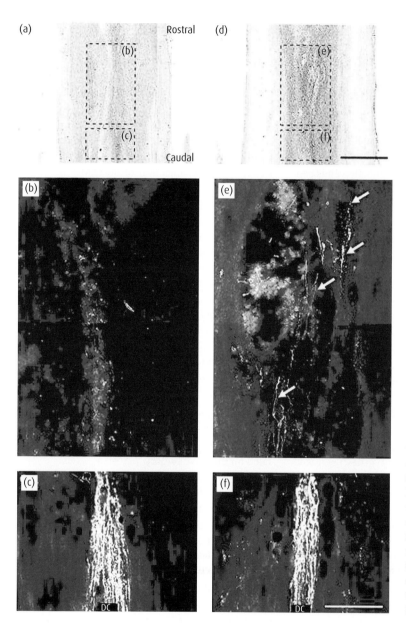

Figure 21.2. *Injection of db-cAMP induces regeneration of dorsal column axons in vivo*: Either saline (a–c) or 50 mM db-cAMP (d–f) was injected into L5 dorsal root ganglia and 1 week later dorsal column axons were lesioned. Axonal regeneration was assessed at 2 weeks post-injury. Darkfield images caudal to the lesion show that in both the control (c) and db-cAMP-injected (f) animals, regenerating axons approach the lesion site. However, the db-cAMP-treated (e) animals exhibit robust regeneration into and beyond the lesion site (arrows) as compared to the saline-injected controls (b). Scale bars: (a and d), 500 μm; (b, c, e and f), 150 μm (reprinted from Qui et al. (2002) *Neuron*, **34**, 895–903).

improved regenerative growth observed following priming *in vitro* (Cai et al., 1999) and following a conditioning lesion *in vivo* are dependent on PKA activation (Neumann et al., 2002; Qiu et al., 2002) – but recent evidence suggests that another well-known signaling component may also be involved in the regeneration-promoting signal. Induction of the neurotrophin-induced elevation of cAMP also appears to be mediated by an ERK-dependent process. Activation of ERK by neurotrophin binding results in a transient inhibition of the neuronal-enriched phosphodiesterase, PDE4. As mentioned above, inhibition of PDE4, results in an accumulation of cAMP, thereby increasing intracellular levels and inducing subsequent signaling modules. Blocking the activation of this MAPK abrogates the improved regeneration observed after cAMP elevation *in vitro* and therefore, it is an essential member of this regeneration-promoting signal (Gao et al., 2003).

In neurons, PKA and MAPK have many cellular targets, including activation of the cAMP-response element binding protein (CREB) and the subsequent induction of gene transcription. And, indeed, recently published evidence suggests that the phosphorylation and activation of CREB is an integral part of the cAMP-mediated axonal growth (Gao et al., in press). This coincides with evidence which suggests that in the regenerative paradigms illustrated above, the cAMP-induced promotion of axonal growth is, initially, PKA dependent but later becomes independent of PKA activation (Qiu et al., 2002) and sensitive to pharmacological inhibitors of transcription (Cai et al., 2002). These facts, coupled with the latency of response observed in the conditioning lesion effect, suggest that cAMP-mediated genetic transcription is essential for axonal regeneration. Therefore, the question then becomes which genes are upregulated in response to elevated cAMP levels and what are their roles in the axonal regeneration paradigm?

The induction of cAMP-mediated gene transcription often results in an upregulation of many immediate early gene products. However, only some of these products play a role in regeneration. Recently, evidence has emerged which suggests a role for a family of known cytoskeletal regulators, the polyamines. Activation or overexpression of the protein Arginase I, a key enzyme in the polyamine synthesis pathway, or application of the polyamine family member, putrescene, can induce improved growth on inhibitory substrates. Conversely, blocking the synthesis of these molecules can abrogate the cAMP-mediated regenerative increase (Cai et al., 2002). Furthermore, an upregulation of Arginase I temporally coincides with either conditioning-lesion (unpublished data) or artificially induced elevated cAMP levels. The polyamines are known modulators of cytoskeletal rearrangement, a step which is ultimately necessary for the induction of axonal growth and regeneration, and it is this

activity which makes the polyamines encouraging targets for therapeutic intervention following spinal cord injury.

Further elucidation of the signaling cascade and cytoskeletal targets which mediate the cAMP-induced axonal regeneration (Fig. 21.3) may soon follow, thereby providing new and, potentially, more specific targets for therapeutic intervention and induction of regeneration after injury *in vivo*.

Guidance cues of development

In the developing mammalian CNS, the neurons which will comprise the sensory and motor systems must extend their axons from the location of the cell body – often in the brain or spinal cord – to their eventual targets (which can be as far as hundreds of centimeters in humans) and form synaptic connections. As noted earlier, the embryonic CNS environment is not inhibitory toward these growing axons and, indeed, at this juncture, myelination has not begun in earnest and therefore, many of the myelin-associated inhibitors may not be present in abundance. However, these pioneering axonal processes do not find their proper targets on their own. How, then, do these developing axons determine the proper pathways and target locations? Once again, the local environment of the CNS provides the answer. While the aforementioned myelin-associated inhibitors are either not yet present or unable to affect axonal growth, there are many "cues" which act on each of these developing axons to "nudge" or "draw" them in the proper direction. These molecules are called developmental axonal guidance cues (for more details see Volume I, Chapter 19).

There are primarily four types of guidance "forces" found in the developing CNS: chemoattraction, chemorepulsion, contact attraction and contact repulsion.

The "contact" type of forces often work over short distances and are mediated by membrane or extracellular matrix (ECM) bound molecules. This mode of guidance acts much like the large highway: the attractive cues often provide the "roadway" on which the axons grow and subsequently follow and

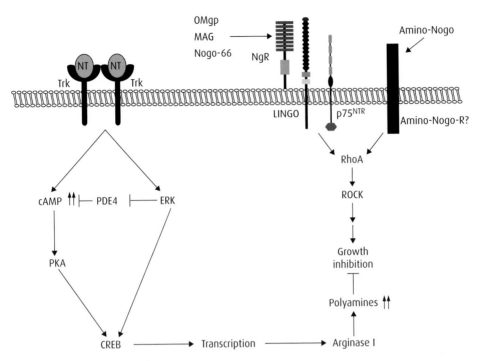

Figure 21.3. *The signaling pathways of regeneration and inhibition*: The signaling induced by all the myelin-associated inhibitors of regeneration is believed to work in a Rho-A-dependent manner. However, elevation of intracellular cAMP levels by a variety of methods (treatment with neurotrophins, blocking phosphodiesterases or application of analogs) can block the inhibitory signaling and improve regeneration by inducing gene transcription and induction of polyamine synthesis.

the repulsive cues are the "guardrails", preventing any wayward axons from wandering off the "road".

The chemo forces are usually more "long-range" in their effects and are mediated by diffusible factors which bind receptors on the surface of the developing growth cone. Often, subtle gradients of these diffusible factors determine the growth mode and direction of these axonal processes: gradients of attractive cues will "pull" the growth cone toward the proper pathway while repulsive cues prevent growth into inappropriate regions or away from incorrect targets.

The guidance-associated molecules

To date, several molecules have been identified as potential developmental guidance cues. These molecules include, but are not limited to, the slits,

ephrins, netrins and semaphorins. Each of these factors, while normally associated with one type of chemotactic modulation, has shown bifunctional properties under a variety of conditions. Each of these molecules is expressed during the initial stages of development of the nervous system and aid extending axons in assuming the correct pathfinding mode and direction. To this end, these molecules may attract, repel or even inhibit the growth of these developing axons. With this in mind, one may ask whether or not these factors may play the same roles in the adult organism, specifically after CNS injury. In other words, can these guidance cues be another set of axonal regeneration inhibitors?

While the presence and effects of these molecules are undeniable in the developing nervous system, the question that remains unanswered is whether or not they are in fact present in the mature CNS and, if so, whether they can still induce growth modulation in a regenerating axon. To answer this question, we must first examine some of the more prominent guidance molecules.

Netrin

Netrins are bifunctional molecules, generally diffusible in nature, which can act to either attract or repel developing axons. Netrin binds to axonal processes via two receptor complexes: the deleted in colorectal cancer (DCC) receptor or the UNC-5 receptors. The attractive or repellant nature of netrin binding is dependent on several factors, including receptor choice and intracellular levels of key signaling molecules. It has been shown that binding of netrin to the DCC receptor mediates the chemoattractive signal while UNC-5 receptor-binding results in a repulsive response. This receptor-mediated activation is coupled to downstream signaling components which subsequently generate the growth response. The attractive response of the growth cone to netrin signaling may be broken down into two components: the attractive turning response and the axonal growth response. The attractive component of this response appears to be mediated by the induction of a multifaceted signaling cascade involving the activation of phospholipase C (PLC) (Ming et al., 1999), MAP kinase (Forcet et al., 2002; Ming et al., 2002), phosphatidylinositol 3-kinase (PI3K) (Ming et al., 1999) and the small GTPases Rac and Cdc42 (Li et al., 2002; Shekarabi and Kennedy, 2002). Conversely, axonal extension involves a calcium-dependent activation of the cellular phosphatase calcineurin, activation of the nuclear transcription factor NFAT (nuclear factor of activated T cells) and subsequent gene transcription (Graef et al., 2003). The UNC5-mediated signaling which results in growth cone repulsion, however, is less well understood. Following ligand binding the UNC-5 receptor becomes phosphorylated via a mechanism which may involve the src family of kinases (Tong et al., 2001). What other downstream components are induced following this induction of signaling have yet to be elucidated.

The activity of netrin on an extending growth cone involves induction of highly regulated signaling molecules and therefore, not unexpectedly, intracellular levels of ubiquitous signaling molecules such as cAMP and calcium appear to be involved in determining this axonal response. High levels of either of these two molecules results in a chemoattractive response to netrin, whereas constitutively low-levels results in axonal repulsion (Hong et al., 2000; Ming et al., 1997; Nishiyama et al., 2003; Song et al., 1997; 1998). In vitro, modulation of these factors does, in fact, mediate axonal growth and turning as well as repulsion/inhibition. And while netrin and its receptors are constitutively expressed in the adult CNS, what role, if any, netrin plays in regeneration – or lack thereof – after injury is still unclear.

Semaphorins

The semaphorins are a family of either secreted or membrane-bound chemotactic molecules which have been shown to exhibit both repulsive and, under certain conditions, attractive properties for developing axons. Semaphorins have been classified into eight distinct subclasses. Class 1 and 2 are exclusive to the invertebrates. Among the vertebrate semaphorins, class 3 is a secreted protein while the semaphorin classes 4–7 are all linked to the membrane via GPI-anchors. In addition, there is a viral class of semaphorin which is also secreted.

The soluble (secreted) semaphorin molecules have been shown to bind to the neuropilin class of receptors, of which there are two, neuropilin-1 and -2. Conversely, the membrane-bound semaphorin family members bind via the plexin receptors. The intracellular domain of the neuropilins, however, are very short and do not appear to be able to initiate signaling and therefore, they are unable to mediate the semaphorin-induced effects alone. Thus induction of the signaling cascade is dependent on the formation of a receptor complex which consists of a heterodimer of the neuropilin and plexin receptors. Indeed, the precise types of complexes formed upon binding may determine the binding specificity of these interactions. While differential dimerization patterns and ligand binding activates differing downstream effectors, the subsequent induction of Rho-dependent cytoskeletal rearrangement results in the repulsion of the axonal growth cone. However, one class of semaphorin, Sema7A, has been shown to bind the $\beta 1$ integrin molecule, a cell adhesion-associated receptor. Upon binding to this receptor, an ERK-dependent pathway is initiated which leads to attraction and axonal outgrowth instead of repulsion.

While the role of these molecules in the guidance of developing axons is undeniable, recent evidence has also suggested that they may play a role in the inhibition of axonal regeneration after injury. The semaphorin family member, Sema3A, in particular, may be active in regulating regeneration after CNS injury. Secreted by both fibroblasts and neurons, Sema3A binds neuropilin-1 on the neuronal cell surface and the complete receptor complex forms upon subsequent binding by the signaling co-receptor, plexinA1. Binding and formation of this ligand-receptor complex appears to be sufficient to induce growth cone collapse via a signaling cascade which involves activation of the collapsin response mediator protein (CRMP) and, not surprisingly, RhoA. Sema3A and the components of its receptor complex have all been shown to be expressed in the adult mammalian CNS after injury (Pasterkamp et al., 1998a; 1999; 2001; Pasterkamp and Verhaagen, 2001). In addition, it has been demonstrated that these molecules can inhibit axonal sprouting after injury and even induce cell death via a pro-apoptotic pathway. Interestingly, it has also been shown that Sema3A is downregulated in the PNS (an environment where axonal regeneration is readily observed) after injury and that levels remain low until regeneration is complete (Pasterkamp et al., 1998b). Thus, the semaphorins may indeed have a post-developmental role and may also participate in cell death and inhibition of axonal regeneration in the CNS after injury.

Slits

The slits are a secreted family of proteins which were initially characterized as modulators of embryonic patterning. In 1999, however, several investigators identified the slit proteins as repellant cues for developing commissural axons (Brose et al., 1999; Kidd et al., 1999; Li et al., 1999). The slit-induced axonal repulsion is mediated via binding to the Roundabout (robo) receptor family and have been shown to induce axonal repulsion in a several neuronal types (including commissural and retinal). Following ligand binding, the robo receptors initiate a signaling cascade which includes activation of the mammalian enabled (Mena) and, interestingly, modulation of a Rho GTPase family member. The proline-rich CC3 region of the robo receptor has been shown to bind a subfamily of Rho GTPase activating proteins (GAPs) called srGAPs (Wong et al., 2001). Slit-induced growth cone repulsion appears to be mediated by the inhibition of the Rho GTPase, Cdc42, which results in modulation of actin dynamics and subsequent repulsive turning in the extending axon. In the adult CNS, both the slit ligands and their robo receptors have been observed and, indeed, may exhibit elevated levels as compared to embryonic expression (Marillat et al., 2002). Furthermore, recent studies suggest that slit2 is expressed in reactive astrocytes after injury (Hagino et al., 2003), thus indicating that these slit ligands may, in fact, be available at the right place and time to act as a regeneration inhibitor, but there is no evidence, as yet, to indicate that they do so.

Ephrins

The ephrins are yet another family of axon guidance molecules. The ephrins exist as membrane-bound proteins which bind the surface receptors, Eph-A and -B. The ephrin ligands and the Eph receptors are expressed on both the neuronal and astocyte cell membranes. The ephrin-A molecules are anchored to the cell membrane via a GPI linkage while the ephrin-B moieties include both transmembrane and intracellular domains which may be involved in "reverse" signaling. These molecules generally act to mediate a contact repulsive guidance cue, serving to direct developing axons away from inappropriate areas and toward their targets. However, evidence exists which indicates that in some circumstances, the ephrins may also induce growth cone adhesion and attraction (Hassen et al., 2004; Knoll and Drescher, 2002).

The Ephs are tyrosine kinase receptors which, following ligand binding, autophosphorylate tyrosine residues in the intracellular domain which then become docking sites for the SH2-containing proteins. Like virtually all other growth cone inhibitory molecules, ephrin signaling appears to be mediated via activation of the small GTPase, RhoA. Ligand binding and induction of the signaling cascade results in the activation of a Rho guanine exchange factor (GEF) termed ephexin. This ephexin-mediated Rho activation, coupled with a simultaneous inactivation of both Rac and Cdc42, results in the modulation of the actin cytoskeleton and the subsequent repulsion or collapse of the extending growth cone (Wahl et al., 2000).

While their expression in the adult CNS has been confirmed (Janis et al., 1999; Miranda et al., 1999; Winslow et al., 1995; Willson et al., 2002; Bundesen et al., 2003), no evidence yet exists to indicate that they may in fact play a role in the inhibition of axonal regeneration after injury. Instead, it has been suggested that since the developmental expression patterns of the ephrins have been demonstrated to persist in the adult superior colliculus (McLaughlin and O'Leary, 1999; Knoll et al., 2001), the role of ephrins post-injury may be the same as during development: the precise guidance of growing axons toward their proper targets.

The glial scar

Injury to the adult mammalian nervous system often causes extensive damage to the spinal cord and surrounding tissue. As elucidated above, this can induce the release of many molecules from injured cells of the CNS, including the myelin-associated inhibitors of regeneration with the end result being a block of spontaneous regeneration by injured axons. However, the myelin-associated inhibitors are not the only factors which prevent regeneration. Following injury and the associated ancillary damage, one may observe the formation of

a structure called the glial scar which forms both a physical and chemical barrier to regeneration *in vivo*. In the following section, we will briefly describe the role of the glial scar following injury. However, the structure and function of the glial scar in the adult mammalian CNS is addressed in more detail by Jared H. Miller and Jerry Silver in Chapter 22 of this volume.

During glial scar formation, astrocytes in the area of the lesion undergo a process which is referred to as "reactive gliosis". Hypertrophic reactive astrocytes will exhibit changes in both cellular morphology and in protein expression patterns (Barrett et al., 1981; Yang et al., 1994). One effect of these morphological changes is the formation of a sturdy, intransigent membrane which effectively forms a "wall" through which regenerating axons cannot pass the glial scar. This regeneration-inhibiting wall, however, can often take several weeks to fully form following injury.

In addition to the formation of this physical barrier, reactive astrocytes express a class of molecules called proteoglycans (Gallo et al., 1987). These extracellular-matrix molecules consist of a protein core connected to a sulfated glycosaminoglycan (GAG) chain containing repeating disaccharides. One group of these proteoglycans, called the chondroitin sulfate proteoglycans (CSPGs) have been shown to be upregulated in the glial scar following injury to the CNS of adult animals (McKeon et al., 1999; Jones et al., 2003; Tang et al., 2003) and have also been implicated in axonal regenerative failure after injury both *in vitro* (McKeon et al., 1991; Smith-Thomas et al., 1994; Niederost et al., 1999) and *in vivo* (Davies et al., 1999). These reports are further supported by recent findings which have indicated that removal of the chondroitin sulfate GAG chains using the enzyme chondroitinase ABC improves regeneration and functional recovery after CNS injury (Bradbury et al., 2002). Interestingly, evidence from several groups suggest that the growth inhibitory effects of CSPGs in the glial scar appear to mediated via a signaling pathway which, like the NgR-LINGO-p75[NTR]-induced pathway, utilizes the small GTPase, Rho and its downstream effector, ROCK (Dergham et al.,

2002; Borisoff et al., 2003; Monnier et al., 2003). This finding has important implications for the development of potential therapeutics since it suggests a viable target for pharmacological or genetic intervention which may effectively block the regenerative inhibition induced by both the myelin-associated inhibitors as well as the glial scar proteoglycans.

21.6 Conclusions

In this chapter, we have outlined some of the various components which may contribute to the observed lack of regeneration which occurs after injury to the adult mammalian CNS. With the recent elucidation of these molecular players and some of the neuronal signaling pathways which they modulate, a host of new targets have emerged which may prove to be therapeutically relevant with regards to encouraging regeneration and functional recovery in human patients with brain and spinal cord injuries. Further work in this field may now take many directions. Firstly, a more complete understanding of the downstream signaling pathways which mediate both axonal growth inhibition as well as the cAMP-mediated block of this inhibition must be undertaken so that aforementioned therapeutic approaches may be more specifically targeted, thereby minimizing the disruption of "standard" cellular metabolic signaling. Secondly, the viability of the multitude of potential therapeutic methods and/or delivery systems must be assessed. And finally, while these new therapeutics may indeed result in improved recovery after spinal cord injury *in vivo*, the true efficacy of these treatments may only be seen in the acute injury. The true "holy grail" of CNS regenerative therapy is treatment and recovery of the chronically injured patient and these recent advances are but the first step in achieving this eventual goal.

Thus, it appears that while the obstacles that need to be overcome after CNS injury are indeed formidable, this relatively recent explosion in our understanding of the molecules and mechanisms involved lead one to believe that the days of classifying spinal cord injuries as "untreatable" may, in fact, be numbered.

REFERENCES

Alberini, C.M., Ghirardi, M., Huang, Y.Y., Nguyen, P.V. and Kandel, E.R. (1995). A molecular switch for the consolidation of long-term memory: cAMP-inducible gene expression. *Ann NY Acad Sci*, **758**, 261–286.

Bandtlow, C. and Dechant, G. (2004). From cell death to neuronal regeneration, effects of the p75 neurotrophin receptor depend on interactions with partner subunits. *Sci STKE*, pe24.

Barker, P.A. (2004). p75NTR is positively promiscuous: novel partners and new insights. *Neuron*, **42**, 529–533.

Barrett, C.P., Guth, L., Donati, E.J. and Krikorian, J.G. (1981). Astroglial reaction in the gray matter lumbar segments after midthoracic transection of the adult rat spinal cord. *Exp Neurol*, **73**, 365–377.

Barton, W.A., Liu, B.P., Tzvetkova, D., Jeffrey, P.D., Fournier, A.E., Sah, D., Cate, R., Strittmatter, S.M. and Nikolov, D.B. (2003). Structure and axon outgrowth inhibitor binding of the Nogo-66 receptor and related proteins. *Embo J*, **22**, 3291–3302.

Bartsch, U., Bandtlow, C.E., Schnell, L., Bartsch, S., Spillmann, A.A., Rubin, B.P., Hillenbrand, R., Montag, D., Schwab, M.E. and Schachner, M. (1995). Lack of evidence that myelin-associated glycoprotein is a major inhibitor of axonal regeneration in the CNS. *Neuron*, **15**, 1375–1381.

Berry, M. (1982). Post-injury myelin-breakdown products inhibit axonal growth: an hypothesis to explain the failure of axonal regeneration in the mammalian central nervous system. *Bibl Anat*, **23**, 1–11.

Bilderback, T.R., Grigsby, R.J. and Dobrowsky, R.T. (1997). Association of p75(NTR) with caveolin and localization of neurotrophin-induced sphingomyelin hydrolysis to caveolae. *J Biol Chem*, **272**, 10922–10927.

Bisby, M.A., Tetzlaff, W. and Brown, M.C. (1995). Cell body response to injury in motoneurons and primary sensory neurons of a mutant mouse, Ola (Wld), in which Wallerian degeneration is delayed. *J Comp Neurol*, **359**, 653–662.

Borisoff, J.F., Chan, C.C., Hiebert, G.W., Oschipok, L., Robertson, G.S., Zamboni, R., Steeves, J.D. and Tetzlaff, W. (2003). Suppression of Rho-kinase activity promotes axonal growth on inhibitory CNS substrates. *Mol Cell Neurosci*, **22**, 405–416.

Bradbury, E.J., Moon, L.D., Popat, R.J., King, V.R., Bennett, G.S., Patel, P.N., Fawcett, J.W. and McMahon, S.B. (2002).

Chondroitinase ABC promotes functional recovery after spinal cord injury. *Nature*, **416**, 636–640.

Bregman, B.S., Kunkel-Bagden, E., Schnell, L., Dai, H.N., Gao, D. and Schwab, M.E. (1995). Recovery from spinal cord injury mediated by antibodies to neurite growth inhibitors. *Nature*, **378**, 498–501.

Brose, K., Bland, K.S., Wang, K.H., Arnott, D., Henzel, W., Goodman, C.S., Tessier-Lavigne, M. and Kidd, T. (1999). Slit proteins bind robo receptors and have an evolutionarily conserved role in repulsive axon guidance. *Cell*, **96**, 795–806.

Brown, M.C., Booth, C.M., Lunn, E.R. and Perry, V.H. (1991). Delayed response to denervation in muscles of C57BL/Ola mice. *Neuroscience*, **43**, 279–283.

Brown, M.C., Lunn, E.R. and Perry, V.H. (1992). Consequences of slow Wallerian degeneration for regenerating motor and sensory axons. *J Neurobiol*, **23**, 521–536.

Bundesen, L.Q., Scheel, T.A., Bregman, B.S. and Kromer, L.F. (2003). Ephrin-B2 and EphB2 regulation of astrocyte-meningeal fibroblast interactions in response to spinal cord lesions in adult rats. *J Neurosci*, **23**, 7789–7800.

Byrne, J.H. and Kandel, E.R. (1996). Presynaptic facilitation revisited: state and time dependence. *J Neurosci*, **16**, 425–435.

Cai, D., Shen, Y., De Bellard, M., Tang, S. and Filbin, M.T. (1999). Prior exposure to neurotrophins blocks inhibition of axonal regeneration by MAG and myelin via a cAMP-dependent mechanism. *Neuron*, **22**, 89–101.

Cai, D., Qiu, J., Cao, Z., McAtee, M., Bregman, B.S. and Filbin, M.T. (2001). Neuronal cyclic AMP controls the developmental loss in ability of axons to regenerate. *J Neurosci*, **21**, 4731–4739.

Cai, D., Deng, K., Mellado, W., Lee, J., Ratan, R.R. and Filbin, M.T. (2002). Arginase I and polyamines act downstream from cyclic AMP in overcoming inhibition of axonal growth MAG and myelin *in vitro*. *Neuron*, **35**, 711–719.

Caroni, P. and Schwab, M.E. (1988a). Antibody against myelin-associated inhibitor of neurite growth neutralizes nonpermissive substrate properties of CNS white matter. *Neuron*, **1**, 85–96.

Caroni, P. and Schwab, M.E. (1988b). Two membrane protein fractions from rat central myelin with inhibitory properties for neurite growth and fibroblast spreading. *J Cell Biol*, **106**, 1281–1288.

Casademunt, E., Carter, B.D., Benzel, I., Frade, J.M., Dechant, G. and Barde, Y.A. (1999). The zinc finger protein NRIF interacts with the neurotrophin receptor p75(NTR) and participates in programmed cell death. *Embo J*, **18**, 6050–6061.

Castellucci, V.F., Kandel, E.R., Schwartz, J.H., Wilson, F.D., Nairn, A.C. and Greengard, P. (1980). Intracellular injection of the catalytic subunit of cyclic AMP-dependent protein kinase simulates facilitation of transmitter release underlying behavioral sensitization in Aplysia. *Proc Natl Acad Sci USA*, **77**, 7492–7496.

Castellucci, V.F., Nairn, A., Greengard, P., Schwartz, J.H. and Kandel, E.R. (1982). Inhibitor of adenosine 3′,5′-monophosphate-dependent protein kinase blocks presynaptic facilitation in Aplysia. *J Neurosci*, **2**, 1673–1681.

Chao, M., Casaccia-Bonnefil, P., Carter, B., Chittka, A., Kong, H. and Yoon, S.O. (1998). Neurotrophin receptors: mediators of life and death. *Brain Res Brain Res Rev*, **26**, 295–301.

Chen, M.S., Huber, A.B., van der Haar, M.E., Frank, M., Schnell, L., Spillmann, A.A., Christ, F. and Schwab, M.E. (2000). Nogo-A is a myelin-associated neurite outgrowth inhibitor and an antigen for monoclonal antibody IN-1. *Nature*, **403**, 434–439.

Chittka, A., Arevalo, J.C., Rodriguez-Guzman, M., Perez, P., Chao, M.V. and Sendtner, M. (2004). The p75NTR-interacting protein SC1 inhibits cell cycle progression by transcriptional repression of cyclin E. *J Cell Biol*, **164**, 985–996.

Crocker, P.R., Clark, E.A., Filbin, M., Gordon, S., Jones, Y., Kehrl, J.H., Kelm, S., Le Douarin, N., Powell, L., Roder, J., et al. (1998). Siglecs: a family of sialic-acid binding lectins. *Glycobiology*, **8**, v.

David, S.J. and Aguayo, A.J. (1981). Axonal elongation into peripheral nervous system "bridges" after central nervous system injury in adult rats. *Science*, **214**, 931–933.

Davies, S.J., Goucher, D.R., Doller, C. and Silver, J. (1999). Robust regeneration of adult sensory axons in degenerating white matter of the adult rat spinal cord. *J Neurosci*, **19**, 5810–5822.

Dechant, G. and Barde, Y.A. (2002). The neurotrophin receptor p75(NTR): novel functions and implications for diseases of the nervous system. *Nat Neurosci*, **5**, 1131–1136.

Della-Bianca, V., Rossi, F., Armato, U., Dal-Pra, I., Costantini, C., Perini, G., Politi, V. and Della Valle, G. (2001). Neurotrophin p75 receptor is involved in neuronal damage by prion peptide. *J Biol Chem*, **276**(**106–126**), 38929–38933.

Dergham, P., Ellezam, B., Essagian, C., Avedissian, H., Lubell, W.D. and McKerracher, L. (2002). Rho signaling pathway targeted to promote spinal cord repair. *J Neurosci*, **22**, 6570–6577.

Domeniconi, M., Cao, Z., Spencer, T., Sivasankaran, R., Wang, K., Nikulina, E., Kimura, N., Cai, H., Deng, K., Gao, Y., et al. (2002). Myelin-associated glycoprotein interacts with the Nogo66 receptor to inhibit neurite outgrowth. *Neuron*, **35**, 283–290.

Dostaler, S.M., Ross, G.M., Myers, S.M., Weaver, D.F., Ananthanarayanan, V. and Riopelle, R.J. (1996). Characterization of a distinctive motif of the low molecular weight neurotrophin receptor that modulates NGF-mediated neurite growth. *Eur J Neurosci*, **8**, 870–879.

Ebadi, M., Bashir, R.M., Heidrick, M.L., Hamada, F.M., Refaey, H.E., Hamed, A., Helal, G., Baxi, M.D., Cerutis, D.R. and Lassi, N.K. (1997). Neurotrophins and their receptors in nerve injury and repair. *Neurochem Int*, **30**, 347–374.

Filbin, M.T. (1995). Myelin-associated glycoprotein: a role in myelination and in the inhibition of axonal regeneration? *Curr Opin Neurobiol*, **5**, 588–595.

Filbin, M.T. (1996). The Muddle with MAG. *Mol Cell Neurosci*, **8**, 84–92.

Forcet, C., Stein, E., Pays, L., Corset, V., Llambi, F., Tessier-Lavigne, M. and Mehlen, P. (2002). Netrin-1-mediated axon outgrowth requires deleted in colorectal cancer-dependent MAPK activation. *Nature*, **417**, 443–447.

Fournier, A.E., GrandPre, T. and Strittmatter, S.M. (2001). Identification of a receptor mediating Nogo-66 inhibition of axonal regeneration. *Nature*, **409**, 341–346.

Fournier, A.E., Gould, G.C., Liu, B.P. and Strittmatter, S.M. (2002). Truncated soluble Nogo receptor binds Nogo-66 and blocks inhibition of axon growth by myelin. *J Neurosci*, **22**, 8876–8883.

Frey, U., Huang, Y.Y. and Kandel, E.R. (1993). Effects of cAMP simulate a late stage of LTP in hippocampal CA1 neurons. *Science*, **260**, 1661–1664.

Fruttiger, M., Montag, D., Schachner, M. and Martini, R. (1995). Crucial role for the myelin-associated glycoprotein in the maintenance of axon-myelin integrity. *Eur J Neurosci*, **7**, 511–515.

Furshpan, E.J., MacLeish, P.R., O'Lague, P.H. and Potter, D.D. (1976). Chemical transmission between rat sympathetic neurons and cardiac myocytes developing in microcultures: evidence for cholinergic, adrenergic, and dual-function neurons. *Proc Natl Acad Sci USA*, **73**, 4225–4229.

Gallo, V., Bertolotto, A. and Levi, G. (1987). The proteoglycan chondroitin sulfate is present in a subpopulation of cultured astrocytes and in their precursors. *Dev Biol*, **123**, 282–285.

Gao, Y., Nikulina, E., Mellado, W. and Filbin, M.T. (2003). Neurotrophins elevate cAMP to reach a threshold required to overcome inhibition by MAG through extracellular signal-regulated kinase-dependent inhibition of phosphodiesterase. *J Neurosci*, **23**, 11770–11777.

Gao, Y., Deng, K., Hou, J., Bryson, J.B., Barco, A., Nikulina, E., Spencer, T., Mellado, W., Kandel, E.R. and Filbin, M.T. (2004). Activated CREB is sufficient to overcome inhibitors in myelin and promote spinal axon regeneration *in vivo*. *Neuron*, **44**, 609–621.

Graef, I.A., Wang, F., Charron, F., Chen, L., Neilson, J., Tessier-Lavigne, M. and Crabtree, G.R. (2003). Neurotrophins and

netrins require calcineurin/NFAT signaling to stimulate outgrowth of embryonic axons. *Cell*, **113**, 657–670.

GrandPre, T., Nakamura, F., Vartanian, T. and Strittmatter, S.M. (2000). Identification of the Nogo inhibitor of axon regeneration as a Reticulon protein. *Nature*, **403**, 439–444.

GrandPre, T., Li, S. and Strittmatter, S.M. (2002). Nogo-66 receptor antagonist peptide promotes axonal regeneration. *Nature*, **417**, 547–551.

Gupta, S.K., Poduslo, J.F. and Mezei, C. (1988). Temporal changes in P0 and MBP gene expression after crush-injury of the adult peripheral nerve. *Brain Res*, **464**, 133–141.

Habib, A.A., Marton, L.S., Allwardt, B., Gulcher, J.R., Mikol, D.D., Hognason, T., Chattopadhyay, N. and Stefansson, K. (1998). Expression of the oligodendrocyte-myelin glycoprotein by neurons in the mouse central nervous system. *J Neurochem*, **70**, 1704–1711.

Hagino, S., Iseki, K., Mori, T., Zhang, Y., Hikake, T., Yokoya, S., Takeuchi, M., Hasimoto, H., Kikuchi, S. and Wanaka, A. (2003). Slit and glypican-1 mRNAs are coexpressed in the reactive astrocytes of the injured adult brain. *Glia*, **42**, 130–138.

Hansen, M.J., Dallal, G.E. and Flanagan, J.G. (2004). Retinal axon response to ephrin-as shows a graded, concentration-dependent transition from growth promotion to inhibition. *Neuron*, **42**, 717–730.

He, X.L., Bazan, J.F., McDermott, G., Park, J.B., Wang, K., Tessier-Lavigne, M., He, Z. and Garcia, K.C. (2003). Structure of the Nogo receptor ectodomain: a recognition module implicated in myelin inhibition. *Neuron*, **38**, 177–185.

Hong, K., Nishiyama, M., Henley, J., Tessier-Lavigne, M. and Poo, M. (2000). Calcium signalling in the guidance of nerve growth by netrin-1. *Nature*, **403**, 93–98.

Huang, D.W., McKerracher, L., Braun, P.E. and David, S. (1999). A therapeutic vaccine approach to stimulate axon regeneration in the adult mammalian spinal cord. *Neuron*, **24**, 639–647.

Huber, A.B., Weinmann, O., Brosamle, C., Oertle, T. and Schwab, M.E. (2002). Patterns of Nogo mRNA and protein expression in the developing and adult rat and after CNS lesions. *J Neurosci*, **22**, 3553–3567.

Hunt, D., Coffin, R.S. and Anderson, P.N. (2002a). The Nogo receptor, its ligands and axonal regeneration in the spinal cord; a review. *J Neurocytol*, **31**, 93–120.

Hunt, D., Mason, M., Campbell, G., Coffin, R. and Anderson, P. (2002b). Nogo receptor mRNA expression in intact and regenerating CNS neurons. *Mol Cell Neurosci*, **20**, 537.

Irie, S., Hachiya, T., Rabizadeh, S., Maruyama, W., Mukai, J., Li, Y., Reed, J.C., Bredesen, D.E. and Sato, T.A. (1999). Functional interaction of Fas-associated phosphatase-1 (FAP-1) with p75(NTR) and their effect on NF-kappaB activation. *FEBS Lett*, **460**, 191–198.

Janis, L.S., Cassidy, R.M. and Kromer, L.F. (1999). Ephrin-A binding and EphA receptor expression delineate the matrix compartment of the striatum. *J Neurosci*, **19**, 4962–4971.

Jones, L.L., Margolis, R.U. and Tuszynski, M.H. (2003). The chondroitin sulfate proteoglycans neurocan, brevican, phosphacan, and versican are differentially regulated following spinal cord injury. *Exp Neurol*, **182**, 399–411.

Josephson, A., Widenfalk, J., Widmer, H.W., Olson, L. and Spenger, C. (2001). NOGO mRNA expression in adult and fetal human and rat nervous tissue and in weight drop injury. *Exp Neurol*, **169**, 319–328.

Kapfhammer, J.P. and Schwab, M.E. (1994a). Increased expression of the growth-associated protein GAP-43 in the myelin-free rat spinal cord. *Eur J Neurosci*, **6**, 403–411.

Kapfhammer, J.P. and Schwab, M.E. (1994b). Inverse patterns of myelination and GAP-43 expression in the adult CNS: neurite growth inhibitors as regulators of neuronal plasticity? *J Comp Neurol*, **340**, 194–206.

Keirstead, H.S., Dyer, J.K., Sholomenko, G.N., McGraw, J., Delaney, K.R. and Steeves, J.D. (1995). Axonal regeneration and physiological activity following transection and immunological disruption of myelin within the hatchling chick spinal cord. *J Neurosci*, **15**, 6963–6974.

Kidd, T., Bland, K.S. and Goodman, C.S. (1999). Slit is the midline repellent for the robo receptor in drosophila. *Cell*, **96**, 785–794.

Kim, J.E., Li, S., GrandPre, T., Qiu, D. and Strittmatter, S.M. (2003). Axon regeneration in young adult mice lacking Nogo-A/B. *Neuron*, **38**, 187–199.

Knoll, B. and Drescher, U. (2002). Ephrin-As as receptors in topographic projections. *Trend Neurosci*, **25**, 145–149.

Knoll, B., Isenmann, S., Kilic, E., Walkenhorst, J., Engel, S., Wehinger, J., Bahr, M. and Drescher, U. (2001). Graded expression patterns of ephrin-as in the superior colliculus after lesion of the adult mouse optic nerve. *Mech Dev*, **106**, 119–127.

Kong, H., Boulter, J., Weber, J.L., Lai, C. and Chao, M.V. (2001). An evolutionarily conserved transmembrane protein that is a novel downstream target of neurotrophin and ephrin receptors. *J Neurosci*, **21**, 176–185.

Kottis, V., Thibault, P., Mikol, D., Xiao, Z.C., Zhang, R., Dergham, P. and Braun, P.E. (2002). Oligodendrocyte-myelin glycoprotein (OMgp) is an inhibitor of neurite outgrowth. *J Neurochem*, **82**, 1566–1569.

Lai, C., Brow, M.A., Nave, K.A., Noronha, A.B., Quarles, R.H., Bloom, F.E., Milner, R.J. and Sutcliffe, J.G. (1987). Two forms of 1B236/myelin-associated glycoprotein, a cell adhesion molecule for postnatal neural development, are produced by alternative splicing. *Proc Natl Acad Sci USA*, **84**, 4337–4341.

Lee, R., Kermani, P., Teng, K.K. and Hempstead, B.L. (2001). Regulation of cell survival by secreted proneurotrophins. *Science*, **294**, 1945–1948.

Lehmann, M., Fournier, A., Selles-Navarro, I., Dergham, P., Sebok, A., Leclerc, N., Tigyi, G. and McKerracher, L. (1999). Inactivation of Rho signaling pathway promotes CNS axon regeneration. *J Neurosci*, **19**, 7537–7547.

Li, C., Tropak, M.B., Gerlai, R., Clapoff, S., Abramow-Newerly, W., Trapp, B., Peterson, A. and Roder, J. (1994). Myelination in the absence of myelin-associated glycoprotein. *Nature*, **369**, 747–750.

Li, H.S., Chen, J.H., Wu, W., Fagaly, T., Zhou, L., Yuan, W., Dupuis, S., Jiang, Z.H., Nash, W., Gick, C., et al. (1999). Vertebrate slit, a secreted ligand for the transmembrane protein roundabout, is a repellent for olfactory bulb axons. *Cell*, **96**, 807–818.

Li, M., Shibata, A., Li, C., Braun, P.E., McKerracher, L., Roder, J., Kater, S.B. and David, S. (1996). Myelin-associated glycoprotein inhibits neurite/axon growth and causes growth cone collapse. *J Neurosci Res*, **46**, 404–414.

Li, X., Saint-Cyr-Proulx, E., Aktories, K. and Lamarche-Vane, N. (2002). Rac1 and Cdc42 but not RhoA or Rho kinase activities are required for neurite outgrowth induced by the Netrin-1 receptor DCC (deleted in colorectal cancer) in N1E-115 neuroblastoma cells. *J Biol Chem*, **277**, 15207–15214.

Liu, B.P., Fournier, A., GrandPre, T. and Strittmatter, S.M. (2002). Myelin-associated glycoprotein as a functional ligand for the Nogo-66 receptor. *Science*, **297**, 1190–1193.

Lockhart, S.T., Turrigiano, G.G. and Birren, S.J. (1997). Nerve growth factor modulates synaptic transmission between sympathetic neurons and cardiac myocytes. *J Neurosci*, **17**, 9573–9582.

Lu, P., Yang, H., Jones, L.L., Filbin, M.T. and Tuszynski, M.H. (2004). Combinatorial therapy with neurotrophins and cAMP promotes axonal regeneration beyond sites of spinal cord injury. *J Neurosci*, **24**, 6402–6409.

Mamidipudi, V., Li, X. and Wooten, M.W. (2002). Identification of interleukin 1 receptor-associated kinase as a conserved component in the p75-neurotrophin receptor activation of nuclear factor-kappa B. *J Biol Chem*, **277**, 28010–28018.

Marillat, V., Cases, O., Nguyen-Ba-Charvet, K.T., Tessier-Lavigne, M., Sotelo, C. and Chedotal, A. (2002). Spatiotemporal expression patterns of slit and robo genes in the rat brain. *J Comp Neurol*, **442**, 130–155.

McKeon, R.J., Schreiber, R.C., Rudge, J.S. and Silver, J. (1991). Reduction of neurite outgrowth in a model of glial scarring following CNS injury is correlated with the expression of inhibitory molecules on reactive astrocytes. *J Neurosci*, **11**, 3398–3411.

McKeon, R.J., Jurynec, M.J. and Buck, C.R. (1999). The chondroitin sulfate proteoglycans neurocan and phosphacan are expressed by reactive astrocytes in the chronic CNS glial scar. *J Neurosci*, **19**, 10778–10788.

McKerracher, L., David, S., Jackson, D.L., Kottis, V., Dunn, R.J. and Braun, P.E. (1994). Identification of myelin-associated glycoprotein as a major myelin-derived inhibitor of neurite growth. *Neuron*, **13**, 805–811.

McLaughlin, T. and O'Leary, D.D. (1999). Functional consequences of coincident expression of EphA receptors and ephrin-A ligands. *Neuron*, **22**, 636–639.

Mi, S., Lee, X., Shao, Z., Thill, G., Ji, B., Relton, J., Levesque, M., Allaire, N., Perrin, S., Sands, B., et al. (2004). LINGO-1 is a component of the Nogo-66 receptor/p75 signaling complex. *Nat Neurosci*, **7**, 221–228.

Mikol, D.D. and Stefansson, K. (1988). A phosphatidylinositol-linked peanut agglutinin-binding glycoprotein in central nervous system myelin and on oligodendrocytes. *J Cell Biol*, **106**, 1273–1279.

Milner, B., Squire, L.R. and Kandel, E.R. (1998). Cognitive neuroscience and the study of memory. *Neuron*, **20**, 445–468.

Ming, G., Song, H., Berninger, B., Inagaki, N., Tessier-Lavigne, M. and Poo, M. (1999). Phospholipase C-gamma and phosphoinositide 3-kinase mediate cytoplasmic signaling in nerve growth cone guidance. *Neuron*, **23**, 139–148.

Ming, G.L., Song, H.J., Berninger, B., Holt, C.E., Tessier-Lavigne, M. and Poo, M.M. (1997). cAMP-dependent growth cone guidance by netrin-1. *Neuron*, **19**, 1225–1235.

Ming, G.L., Wong, S.T., Henley, J., Yuan, X.B., Song, H.J., Spitzer, N.C. and Poo, M.M. (2002). Adaptation in the chemotactic guidance of nerve growth cones. *Nature*, **417**, 411–418.

Miranda, J.D., White, L.A., Marcillo, A.E., Willson, C.A., Jagid, J. and Whittemore, S.R. (1999). Induction of Eph B3 after spinal cord injury. *Exp Neurol*, **156**, 218–222.

Monnier, P.P., Sierra, A., Schwab, J.M., Henke-Fahle, S. and Mueller, B.K. (2003). The Rho/ROCK pathway mediates neurite growth-inhibitory activity associated with the chondroitin sulfate proteoglycans of the CNS glial scar. *Mol Cell Neurosci*, **22**, 319–330.

Monsul, N.T., Geisendorfer, A.R., Han, P.J., Banik, R., Pease, M.E., Skolasky Jr., R.L. and Hoffman, P.N. (2004). Intraocular injection of dibutyryl cyclic AMP promotes axon regeneration in rat optic nerve. *Exp Neurol*, **186**, 124–133.

Montag, D., Giese, K.P., Bartsch, U., Martini, R., Lang, Y., Bluthmann, H., Karthigasan, J., Kirschner, D.A., Wintergerst, E.S. and Nave, K.A. (1994). Mice deficient for the myelin-associated glycoprotein show subtle abnormalities in myelin. *Neuron*, **13**, 229–246.

Mukai, J., Hachiya, T., Shoji-Hoshino, S., Kimura, M.T., Nadano, D., Suvanto, P., Hanaoka, T., Li, Y., Irie, S., Greene, L.A. and Sato, T.A. (2000). NADE, a p75NTR-associated cell death executor, is involved in signal transduction mediated by the common neurotrophin receptor p75NTR. *J Biol Chem*, **275**, 17566–17570.

Mukhopadhyay, G., Doherty, P., Walsh, F.S., Crocker, P.R. and Filbin, M.T. (1994). A novel role for myelin-associated glycoprotein as an inhibitor of axonal regeneration. *Neuron*, **13**, 757–767.

Neumann, S. and Woolf, C.J. (1999). Regeneration of dorsal column fibers into and beyond the lesion site following adult spinal cord injury. *Neuron*, **23**, 83–91.

Neumann, S., Bradke, F., Tessier-Lavigne, M. and Basbaum, A.I. (2002). Regeneration of sensory axons within the injured spinal cord induced by intraganglionic cAMP elevation. *Neuron*, **34**, 885–893.

Niederost, B.P., Zimmermann, D.R., Schwab, M.E. and Bandtlow, C.E. (1999). Bovine CNS myelin contains neurite growth-inhibitory activity associated with chondroitin sulfate proteoglycans. *J Neurosci*, **19**, 8979–8989.

Nikulina, E., Tidwell, J.L., Dai, H.N., Bregman, B.S. and Filbin, M.T. (2004). The phosphodiesterase inhibitor rolipram delivered after a spinal cord lesion promotes axonal regeneration and functional recovery. *Proc Natl Acad Sci USA*, **101**, 8786–8790.

Nishiyama, M., Hoshino, A., Tsai, L., Henley, J.R., Goshima, Y., Tessier-Lavigne, M., Poo, M.M. and Hong, K. (2003). Cyclic AMP/GMP-dependent modulation of Ca^{2+} channels sets the polarity of nerve growth-cone turning. *Nature*, **424**, 990–995.

Nykjaer, A., Lee, R., Teng, K.K., Jansen, P., Madsen, P., Nielsen, M.S., Jacobsen, C., Kliemannel, M., Schwarz, E., Willnow, T.E., et al. (2004). Sortilin is essential for proNGF-induced neuronal cell death. *Nature*, **427**, 843–848.

Oertle, T., Buss, A., Dodd, D., van der Haar, M.E., Robeva, A., Burfeind, P., Vallon, R. and Schwab, M.E. (2002). Membrane topologies and receptors of the oligodendrocyte protein Nogo-A. Program No. 333.10. Paper presented at: Society for Neuroscience, Washington, DC.

Pasterkamp, R.J. and Verhaagen, J. (2001). Emerging roles for semaphorins in neural regeneration. *Brain Res Brain Res Rev*, **35**, 36–54.

Pasterkamp, R.J., De Winter, F., Holtmaat, A.J. and Verhaagen, J. (1998a). Evidence for a role of the chemorepellent semaphorin III and its receptor neuropilin-1 in the regeneration of primary olfactory axons. *J Neurosci*, **18**, 9962–9976.

Pasterkamp, R.J., Giger, R.J. and Verhaagen, J. (1998b). Regulation of semaphorin III/collapsin-1 gene expression during peripheral nerve regeneration. *Exp Neurol*, **153**, 313–327.

Pasterkamp, R.J., Giger, R.J., Ruitenberg, M.J., Holtmaat, A.J., De Wit, J., De Winter, F. and Verhaagen, J. (1999). Expression of the gene encoding the chemorepellent semaphorin III is induced in the fibroblast component of neural scar tissue formed following injuries of adult but not neonatal CNS. *Mol Cell Neurosci*, **13**, 143–166.

Pasterkamp, R.J., Anderson, P.N. and Verhaagen, J. (2001). Peripheral nerve injury fails to induce growth of lesioned ascending dorsal column axons into spinal cord scar tissue expressing the axon repellent Semaphorin3A. *Eur J Neurosci*, **13**, 457–471.

Pearse, D.D., Pereira, F.C., Marcillo, A.E., Bates, M.L., Berrocal, Y.A., Filbin, M.T. and Bunge, M.B. (2004). cAMP and Schwann cells promote axonal growth and functional recovery after spinal cord injury. *Nat Med*, **10**, 610–616.

Perini, G., Della-Bianca, V., Politi, V., Della Valle, G., Dal-Pra, I., Rossi, F. and Armato, U. (2002). Role of p75 neurotrophin receptor in the neurotoxicity by beta-amyloid peptides and synergistic effect of inflammatory cytokines. *J Exp Med*, **195**, 907–918.

Perry, V.H., Brown, M.C. and Lunn, E.R. (1991). Very slow retrograde and Wallerian degeneration in the CNS of C57BL/Ola Mice. *Eur J Neurosci*, **3**, 102–105.

Pot, C., Simonen, M., Weinmann, O., Schnell, L., Christ, F., Stoeckle, S., Berger, P., Rulicke, T., Suter, U. and Schwab, M.E. (2002). Nogo-A expressed in Schwann cells impairs axonal regeneration after peripheral nerve injury. *J Cell Biol*, **159**, 29–35.

Prinjha, R., Moore, S.E., Vinson, M., Blake, S., Morrow, R., Christie, G., Michalovich, D., Simmons, D.L. and Walsh, F.S. (2000). Inhibitor of neurite outgrowth in humans. *Nature*, **403**, 383–384.

Prinjha, R.K., Hill, C., Irving, E., Roberts, J., Campbell, C., Parsons, A., Davis, R., Morrow, R., Woodhams, P.L., Philpott, K.L., et al. (2002). Mapping the functional inhibitory sites of Nogo-A. Discovery of regulated expression following neuronal injury. Program No. 333.12. Paper presented at: Society for Neuroscience, Washington, DC.

Qiu, J., Cai, D., Dai, H., McAtee, M., Hoffman, P.N., Bregman, B.S. and Filbin, M.T. (2002). Spinal axon regeneration induced by elevation of cyclic AMP. *Neuron*, **34**, 895–903.

Quarles, R.H. (1983). Myelin-associated glycoprotein in development and disease. *Dev Neurosci*, **6**, 285–303.

Richardson, P.M. and Issa, V.M. (1984). Peripheral injury enhances central regeneration of primary sensory neurones. *Nature*, **309**, 791–793.

Richardson, P.M. and Verge, V.M. (1986). The induction of a regenerative propensity in sensory neurons following peripheral axonal injury. *J Neurocytol*, **15**, 585–594.

Ryffel, B. and Mihatsch, M.J. (1993). TNF receptor distribution in human tissues. *Int Rev Exp Pathol*, **34**(**Pt B**), 149–156.

Salehi, A.H., Roux, P.P., Kubu, C.J., Zeindler, C., Bhakar, A., Tannis, L.L., Verdi, J.M. and Barker, P.A. (2000). NRAGE, a novel MAGE protein, interacts with the p75 neurotrophin receptor and facilitates nerve growth factor-dependent apoptosis. *Neuron*, **27**, 279–288.

Salzer, J.L., Holmes, W.P. and Colman, D.R. (1987). The amino acid sequences of the myelin-associated glycoproteins: homology to the immunoglobulin gene superfamily. *J Cell Biol*, **104**, 957–965.

Salzer, J.L., Pedraza, L., Brown, M., Struyk, A., Afar, D. and Bell, J. (1990). Structure and function of the myelin-associated glycoproteins. *Ann NY Acad Sci*, **605**, 302–312.

Savio, T. and Schwab, M.E. (1990). Lesioned corticospinal tract axons regenerate in myelin-free rat spinal cord. *Proc Natl Acad Sci USA*, **87**, 4130–4133.

Schafer, M., Fruttiger, M., Montag, D., Schachner, M. and Martini, R. (1996). Disruption of the gene for the myelin-associated glycoprotein improves axonal regrowth along myelin in C57BL/Wlds mice. *Neuron*, **16**, 1107–1113.

Schnell, L. and Schwab, M.E. (1990). Axonal regeneration in the rat spinal cord produced by an antibody against myelin-associated neurite growth inhibitors. *Nature*, **343**, 269–272.

Schwegler, G., Schwab, M.E. and Kapfhammer, J.P. (1995). Increased collateral sprouting of primary afferents in the myelin-free spinal cord. *J Neurosci*, **15**, 2756–2767.

Shearer, M.C., Niclou, S.P., Brown, D., Asher, R.A., Holtmaat, A.J., Levine, J.M., Verhaagen, J. and Fawcett, J.W. (2003). The astrocyte/meningeal cell interface is a barrier to neurite outgrowth which can be overcome by manipulation of inhibitory molecules or axonal signalling pathways. *Mol Cell Neurosci*, **24**, 913–925.

Shekarabi, M. and Kennedy, T.E. (2002). The netrin-1 receptor DCC promotes filopodia formation and cell spreading by activating Cdc42 and Rac1. *Mol Cell Neurosci*, **19**, 1–17.

Shen, Y.J., DeBellard, M.E., Salzer, J.L., Roder, J. and Filbin, M.T. (1998). Myelin-associated glycoprotein in myelin and expressed by Schwann cells inhibits axonal regeneration and branching. *Mol Cell Neurosci*, **12**, 79–91.

Simonen, M., Pedersen, V., Weinmann, O., Schnell, L., Buss, A., Ledermann, B., Christ, F., Sansig, G., van der Putten, H. and Schwab, M.E. (2003). Systemic deletion of the myelin-associated outgrowth inhibitor Nogo-A improves regenerative and plastic responses after spinal cord injury. *Neuron*, **38**, 201–211.

Sivasankaran, R., Pei, J., Wang, K.C., Zhang, Y.P., Shields, C.B., Xu, X.M. and He, Z. (2004). PKC mediates inhibitory effects of myelin and chondroitin sulfate proteoglycans on axonal regeneration. *Nat Neurosci*, **7**, 261–268.

Smith-Thomas, L.C., Fok-Seang, J., Stevens, J., Du, J.S., Muir, E., Faissner, A., Geller, H.M., Rogers, J.H. and Fawcett, J.W. (1994). An inhibitor of neurite outgrowth produced by astrocytes. *J Cell Sci*, **107**(Pt 6), 1687–1695.

Song, H., Ming, G., He, Z., Lehmann, M., McKerracher, L., Tessier-Lavigne, M. and Poo, M. (1998). Conversion of neuronal growth cone responses from repulsion to attraction by cyclic nucleotides. *Science*, **281**, 1515–1518.

Song, H.J., Ming, G.L. and Poo, M.M. (1997). cAMP-induced switching in turning direction of nerve growth cones. *Nature*, **388**, 275–279.

Spillmann, A.A., Bandtlow, C.E., Lottspeich, F., Keller, F. and Schwab, M.E. (1998). Identification and characterization of a bovine neurite growth inhibitor (bNI-220). *J Biol Chem*, **273**, 19283–19293.

Tang, S., Shen, Y.J., DeBellard, M.E., Mukhopadhyay, G., Salzer, J.L., Crocker, P.R. and Filbin, M.T. (1997a). Myelin-associated glycoprotein interacts with neurons via a sialic acid binding site at ARG118 and a distinct neurite inhibition site. *J Cell Biol*, **138**, 1355–1366.

Tang, S., Woodhall, R.W., Shen, Y.J., deBellard, M.E., Saffell, J.L., Doherty, P., Walsh, F.S. and Filbin, M.T. (1997b). Soluble myelin-associated glycoprotein (MAG) found *in vivo* inhibits axonal regeneration. *Mol Cell Neurosci*, **9**, 333–346.

Tang, S., Qiu, J., Nikulina, E. and Filbin, M.T. (2001). Soluble myelin-associated glycoprotein released from damaged white matter inhibits axonal regeneration. *Mol Cell Neurosci*, **18**, 259–269.

Tang, X., Davies, J.E. and Davies, S.J. (2003). Changes in distribution, cell associations, and protein expression levels of NG2, neurocan, phosphacan, brevican, versican V2, and tenascin-C during acute to chronic maturation of spinal cord scar tissue. *J Neurosci Res*, **71**, 427–444.

Tong, J., Killeen, M., Steven, R., Binns, K.L., Culotti, J. and Pawson, T. (2001). Netrin stimulates tyrosine phosphorylation of the UNC-5 family of netrin receptors and induces Shp2 binding to the RCM cytodomain. *J Biol Chem*, **276**, 40917–40925.

Trapp, B.D. (1988). Distribution of the myelin-associated glycoprotein and P0 protein during myelin compaction in quaking mouse peripheral nerve. *J Cell Biol*, **107**, 675–685.

Trapp, B.D. (1990). Myelin-associated glycoprotein. Location and potential functions. *Ann NY Acad Sci*, **605**, 29–43.

Trapp, B.D. and Quarles, R.H. (1982). Presence of the myelin-associated glycoprotein correlates with alterations in the periodicity of peripheral myelin. *J Cell Biol*, **92**, 877–882.

Trapp, B.D., Andrews, S.B., Cootauco, C. and Quarles, R. (1989). The myelin-associated glycoprotein is enriched in multivesicular bodies and periaxonal membranes of actively myelinating oligodendrocytes. *J Cell Biol*, **109**, 2417–2426.

van de Velde, H.J., Roebroek, A.J., Senden, N.H., Ramaekers, F.C. and Van de Ven, W.J. (1994). NSP-encoded reticulons, neuroendocrine proteins of a novel gene family associated with membranes of the endoplasmic reticulum. *J Cell Sci*, **107**, 2403–2416.

Vinson, M., Strijbos, P.J., Rowles, A., Facci, L., Moore, S.E., Simmons, D.L. and Walsh, F.S. (2001). Myelin-associated glycoprotein interacts with ganglioside GT1b. A mechanism for neurite outgrowth inhibition. *J Biol Chem*, **276**, 20280–20285.

Volonte, C., Ross, A.H. and Greene, L.A. (1993). Association of a purine-analogue-sensitive protein kinase activity with p75 nerve growth factor receptors. *Mol Biol Cell*, **4**, 71–78.

Vourc'h, P. and Andres, C. (2004). Oligodendrocyte myelin glycoprotein (OMgp): evolution, structure and function. *Brain Res Brain Res Rev*, **45**, 115–124.

Vourc'h, P., Dessay, S., Mbarek, O., Marouillat Vedrine, S., Muh, J.P. and Andres, C. (2003a). The oligodendrocyte-myelin glycoprotein gene is highly expressed during the late stages of myelination in the rat central nervous system. *Brain Res Dev Brain Res*, **144**, 159–168.

Vourc'h, P., Moreau, T., Arbion, F., Marouillat-Vedrine, S., Muh, J.P. and Andres, C. (2003b). Oligodendrocyte myelin glycoprotein growth inhibition function requires its conserved leucine-rich repeat domain, not its glycosylphosphatidyl–inositol anchor. *J Neurochem*, **85**, 889–897.

Vyas, A.A., Patel, H.V., Fromholt, S.E., Heffer-Lauc, M., Vyas, K.A., Dang, J., Schachner, M. and Schnaar, R.L. (2002). Gangliosides are functional nerve cell ligands for myelin-associated glycoprotein (MAG), an inhibitor of nerve regeneration. *Proc Natl Acad Sci USA*, **99**, 8412–8417.

Wahl, S., Barth, H., Ciossek, T., Aktories, K. and Mueller, B.K. (2000). Ephrin-A5 induces collapse of growth cones by activating Rho and Rho kinase. *J Cell Biol*, **149**, 263–270.

Wang, J.J., Tasinato, A., Ethell, D.W., Testa, M.P. and Bredesen, D.E. (2000). Phosphorylation of the common neurotrophin receptor p75 by p38beta2 kinase affects NF-kappaB and AP-1 activities. *J Mol Neurosci*, **15**, 19–29.

Wang, K.C., Kim, J.A., Sivasankaran, R., Segal, R. and He, Z. (2002a). p75 interacts with the Nogo receptor as a co-receptor for Nogo, MAG and OMgp. *Nature*, **420**, 74–78.

Wang, K.C., Koprivica, V., Kim, J.A., Sivasankaran, R., Guo, Y., Neve, R.L. and He, Z. (2002b). Oligodendrocyte-myelin glycoprotein is a Nogo receptor ligand that inhibits neurite outgrowth. *Nature*, **417**, 941–944.

Wang, X., Chun, S.J., Treloar, H., Vartanian, T., Greer, C.A. and Strittmatter, S.M. (2002). Localization of Nogo-A and Nogo-66 receptor proteins at sites of axon–myelin and synaptic contact. *J Neurosci*, **22**, 5505–5515.

Watanabe, M., Tokita, Y., Kato, M. and Fukuda, Y. (2003). Intravitreal injections of neurotrophic factors and forskolin enhance survival and axonal regeneration of axotomized beta ganglion cells in cat retina. *Neuroscience*, **116**, 733–742.

Willson, C.A., Irizarry-Ramirez, M., Gaskins, H.E., Cruz-Orengo, L., Figueroa, J.D., Whittemore, S.R. and Miranda, J.D. (2002). Upregulation of EphA receptor expression in the injured adult rat spinal cord. *Cell Transplant*, **11**, 229–239.

Winslow, J.W., Moran, P., Valverde, J., Shih, A., Yuan, J.Q., Wong, S.C., Tsai, S.P., Goddard, A., Henzel, W.J., Hefti, F., et al. (1995). Cloning of AL-1, a ligand for an Eph-related tyrosine kinase receptor involved in axon bundle formation. *Neuron*, **14**, 973–981.

Winton, M.J., Dubreuil, C.I., Lasko, D., Leclerc, N. and McKerracher, L. (2002). Characterization of new cell permeable C3-like proteins that inactivate Rho and stimulate neurite outgrowth on inhibitory substrates. *J Biol Chem*, **277**, 32820–32829.

Wong, K., Ren, X.R., Huang, Y.Z., Xie, Y., Liu, G., Saito, H., Tang, H., Wen, L., Brady-Kalnay, S.M., Mei, L., et al. (2001). Signal transduction in neuronal migration: roles of GTPase activating proteins and the small GTPase Cdc42 in the slit-robo pathway. *Cell*, **107**, 209–221.

Wong, S.T., Athos, J., Figueroa, X.A., Pineda, V.V., Schaefer, M.L., Chavkin, C.C., Muglia, L.J. and Storm, D.R. (1999). Calcium-stimulated adenylyl cyclase activity is critical for hippocampus-dependent long-term memory and late phase LTP. *Neuron*, **23**, 787–798.

Wong, S.T., Henley, J.R., Kanning, K.C., Huang, K.H., Bothwell, M. and Poo, M.M. (2002a). A p75(NTR) and Nogo receptor complex mediates repulsive signaling by myelin-associated glycoprotein. *Nat Neurosci*, **5**, 1302–1308.

Wu, Z.L., Thomas, S.A., Villacres, E.C., Xia, Z., Simmons, M.L., Chavkin, C., Palmiter, R.D. and Storm, D.R. (1995). Altered behavior and long-term potentiation in type I adenylyl cyclase mutant mice. *Proc Natl Acad Sci USA*, **92**, 220–224.

Yamashita, T. and Tohyama, M. (2003). The p75 receptor acts as a displacement factor that releases Rho from Rho-GDI. *Nat Neurosci*, **6**, 461–467.

Yamashita, T., Higuchi, H. and Tohyama, M. (2002). The p75 receptor transduces the signal from myelin-associated glycoprotein to Rho. *J Cell Biol*, **157**, 565–570.

Yang, B., Slonimsky, J.D. and Birren, S.J. (2002). A rapid switch in sympathetic neurotransmitter release properties mediated by the p75 receptor. *Nat Neurosci*, **5**, 539–545.

Yang, H.Y., Lieska, N., Shao, D., Kriho, V. and Pappas, G.D. (1994). Proteins of the intermediate filament cytoskeleton as markers for astrocytes and human astrocytomas. *Mol Chem Neuropathol*, **21**, 155–176.

Ye, X., Mehlen, P., Rabizadeh, S., VanArsdale, T., Zhang, H., Shin, H., Wang, J.J., Leo, E., Zapata, J., Hauser, C.A., et al. (1999). TRAF family proteins interact with the common neurotrophin receptor and modulate apoptosis induction. *J Biol Chem*, **274**, 30202–30208.

Zheng, B., Ho, C., Li, S., Keirstead, H., Steward, O. and Tessier-Lavigne, M. (2003). Lack of enhanced spinal regeneration in Nogo-deficient mice. *Neuron*, **38**, 213–224.

22

Effects of the glial scar and extracellular matrix molecules on axon regeneration

Jared H. Miller and Jerry Silver

Department of Neurosciences, School of Medicine, Case Western Reserve University, Cleveland, OH, USA

Following injury to the adult central nervous system (CNS), injured axons are unable to regenerate past the lesion. Within the site of injury, referred to as the glial scar, reactive astrocytes produce chondroitin and keratan sulfate proteoglycans (CSPG/KSPG). These molecules are among the major inhibitory extracellular matrix (ECM) molecules believed to play a role in regeneration failure. The environment of the glial scar will be discussed in this chapter, with particular focus placed on the role of CSPGs in regeneration failure. The balance between CSPGs and growth promoting molecules produced by reactive astrocytes in the glial scar will be considered, as well as the behavior of regenerating neurons in the environment of CNS injury.

22.1 Introduction

The glial scar

With the exception of a small pathway in the hypothalamus (Chauvet et al., 1998) and the olfactory sensory projections within the olfactory bulb (Monti Graziadei et al., 1980; Morrison and Costanzo, 1995), severed axons within long myelinated tracks of the central nervous system (CNS) are capable only of abortive sprouting that provides little functional recovery (Ramón y Cajal, 1928; Li and Raisman, 1995). One of the major barriers to regeneration is the glial scar, in addition to myelin inhibitors (see Volume I, Chapter 21). In lesions that spare the dura mater the scar is composed primarily of astrocytes but in more severe lesions that open the meninges, astroglia become mixed with invading connective tissue elements (Fig. 22.1; Windle and Chambers, 1950; Windle et al., 1952; Clemente and Windle, 1954; Windle, 1956; Clemente, 1958). Astrocytes in the area of injury undergo reactive gliosis (i.e. more glia). However, in most types of injury the actual amount of glial cell division is relatively small and confined to the immediate penumbra surrounding the lesion core (Faulkner et al., 2003). Astrocyte hypertrophy occurs to a much greater extent than proliferation, identified by increased production of intermediate filaments (Bignami and Dahl, 1976; Fitch and Silver, 1999). One can identify hypertrophic reactive astrocytes by immunocytochemical methods that reveal increases in the astrocyte specific intermediate filament glial fibrillary acidic protein (GFAP) (Bignami and Dahl, 1974; Barret et al., 1981; Eng, 1985) as well as other intermediate filament proteins, such as vimentin (reviewed by Yang et al., 1994). Identification of enlarged and entangled reactive astrocytes surrounding dystrophic endballs at the tips of non-regenerating fibers indicates that reactive glia are responsible for failed regeneration through the formation of a physical barrier.

The physical barrier of the glial scar evolves over considerable time into a rubbery, tenacious membrane (Fig. 22.2). Recent evidence suggests that the walling off phenomenon begins early and may provide several important beneficial functions for stabilizing CNS tissue that is especially fragile

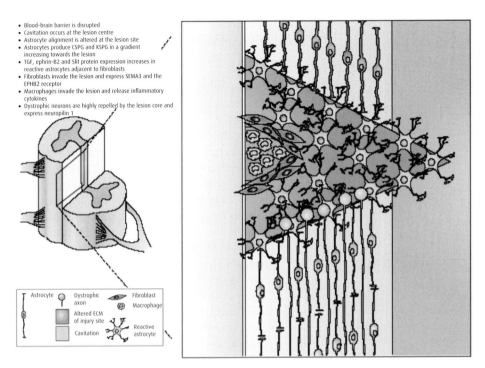

- Blood–brain barrier is disrupted
- Cavitation occurs at the lesion centre
- Astrocyte alignment is altered at the lesion site
- Astrocytes produce CSPG and KSPG in a gradient increasing towards the lesion
- TGF, ephrin-B2 and Slit protein expression increases in reactive astrocytes adjacent to fibroblasts
- Fibroblasts invade the lesion and express SEMA3 and the EPHB2 receptor
- Macrophages invade the lesion and release inflammatory cytokines
- Dystrophic neurons are highly repelled by the lesion core and express neuropilin 1

Astrocyte	Dystrophic axon	Fibroblast	
	Altered ECM of injury site	Macrophage	
	Cavitation	Reactive astrocyte	

Figure 22.1. *Schematic representation of a stereotypical CNS lesion*: Representative stab lesion that penetrates the meninges and allows for fibroblast and macrophage invasion. Axons are highly repulsed by the increasing gradient of CSPGs and KSPGs, but a number of other inhibitory molecules are also made in this type of injury and are especially prevalent in the core of the lesion (figure excerpted from Silver and Miller, 2004).

following injury. Experiments from the Sofroniew lab (Bush et al., 1999; Faulkner et al., 2004) have utilized an ingenious combinatorial technique employing avian herpes simplex viral infection of mammalian astrocytes and gancyclovir delivery to produce targeted depletion of the subpopulation of reactive astrocytes that undergo mitosis immediately surrounding the core of the lesion. It appears that following injury, these cells serve to repair the blood–brain barrier, prevent an overwhelming inflammatory response, and limit cellular degeneration. Thus, it is now clear that one role of the glial scar is to seclude the injury site from healthy tissue, preventing a cascading wave of uncontrolled tissue damage. Unfortunately, the protective effects of glial scarring come at the cost of failed long distance

functional regeneration in warm-blooded animals (Faulkner et al., 2003).

Immature reactive astrocytes do not prevent regeneration

Injury to mature animals results in a glial scar that prevents regeneration. However, regeneration failure does not occur in very young animals. The differences in ability of axons to regenerate in very young versus old mammals appear to be due, in part, to changes in the astroglial reaction to injury. When nitrocellulose is impaled into the brain of both young and old animals, it is possible to then remove the tightly adherent reactive astrocytes, and other cells, that respond to and become embedded in the

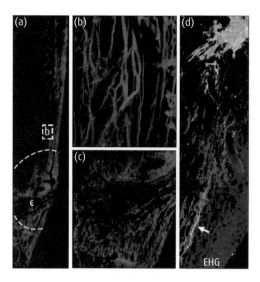

Figure 22.2. *The glial scar 9 months after a spinal cord stab lesion:* (a) Sagittal section of the spinal cord illustrating astrocyte hypertrophy (gray) and chondroitin sulfate proteoglycan (CSPG) upregulation (denoted by dashed lines). Note the longitudinal, thickened bands of reactive astrocytes forming an extremely dense wall of cells. (b) High magnification of the banded, reactive astrocytes, further demonstrating the extreme hypertrophy of astroglia at this late time point after the lesion. (c) High magnification of the injury region clearly illustrates the presence of CSPG still remaining, along with the fibrous banding of reactive astrocytes. (d) Regenerating axons from a microtransplanted DRG (arrow) can grow almost everywhere within the zone of Wallerian degeneration and reactive gliosis (gray) rostral to the lesion even at 9 months following injury. However, the regrowing axons are excluded from a zone of extremely dense fibrous reactive astrocytes (right of arrow). Note the lack of proteoglycans in this region of the scar. This form of axon repulsion seems to be caused by the mechanical constraints of the reactive tissue (EHG: extremely hypertrophic glia) (figure taken from Silver and Miller, 2004).

implant. The wound tissues harvested from animals at different ages can then be used to examine the outgrowth of identified populations of neurons *in vitro* (Rudge and Silver, 1990). Hippocampal neurons cultured on "scar-in-a-dish" explants from neonatal animals extended neurites with much greater vigor than those cultured on explants taken

from mature animals. The results suggested that scar tissues from younger animals were growth supportive, whereas scar tissue from older animals was inhibitory, at least *in vitro*. Similar results were obtained when retinal ganglion cells were cultured on newborn reactive optic nerve astrocytes and extended processes over greater distances and with greater velocity than retinal ganglion cells cultured on adult reactive astrocytes. Adult reactive astrocytes completely inhibited growth of both embryonic and adult neurons *in vitro*, whereas young astrocytes promoted outgrowth from both embryonic and adult neurons (Bahr et al., 1995). Interestingly, adult reactive astrocytes do allow for the growth of dendrites, but not axons *in vitro* perhaps via a different complement of adhesion molecules (Le Roux and Reh, 1996).

In vivo studies further illustrate the differences between immature and mature astrocytes in the context of injury. Untreated Millipore implants placed in the brains of adult acallosal mice normally produce glial scarring and tissue degeneration (Smith et al., 1986). However, when the implant was placed into young acallosal mice, highly reactive astrocytes integrated into the implant. Even in the reactive state, young astrocytes supported regeneration of callosal axons across the implant at least until postnatal day 8 when the critical period for regeneration closes. Furthermore, immature, but not mature, reactive astrocytes transplanted into adult brains on nitrocellulose (Smith and Silver, 1988) or directly as cell suspensions (Smith and Miller, 1991) suppressed glial scar formation by integrating with host tissue and modifying the scar environment.

22.2 Formation of the glial scar

The role of inflammation

Many injuries of the CNS occur with an accompanying opening of the blood–brain barrier. Non-CNS molecules entering the brain parenchyma through the disrupted blood–brain barrier have significant effects on the immune system and subsequent development of the glial scar (Preston et al., 2001).

The blood–brain barrier remains porous to blood and serum components for up to 14 days after brain or spinal cord injury. It is in these areas of greatest blood–brain barrier breakdown that the greatest amount of macrophage activation occurs along with the greatest level of glial scarring and proteoglycan deposition. The yeast cell wall extract, Zymosan, can be used to aggressively stimulate macrophages in a sterile environment (Fitch et al., 1999). This treatment produced rapid astrocyte migration away from the inflammatory focus, CNS cavitation, glial scarring, and upregulation of inhibitory proteoglycans around the cavity. Furthermore, *in vitro*, the observed astrocyte migration resulted in secondary stretching and axotomy in the region of inflammation. These studies indicate that blood, or a serum component, along with activated macrophages play a critical role in the upregulation of inhibitory extracellular matrix (ECM) component and other phenomena related to formation of the glial scar.

The search for the initial molecular trigger of inhibitory gliosis continues. One of the most interesting potential inducers is TGFβ. TGFβ1 expression increases immediately after injury in the injured brain and spinal cord. TGFβ2 expression increases more slowly near the wound in astrocytes and endothelial cells (Lagord et al., 2002). TGFβ2 has been shown to significantly increase the production of proteoglycans by astroglia (Asher et al., 2000). Attenuating TGFβ1 and TGFβ2 activity with antibody application (Moon and Fawcett, 2001), reduces glial scarring. However, this occurs without a reduction in macrophage invasion and was not sufficient to allow for long distance regeneration. Another candidate family of scar inducers is the interleukins. Injection of interleukin-1, a protein produced by mononuclear phagocytes, helps initiate the inflammatory response in a variety of cells, including astrocytes, which take on the reactive state (Giulian et al., 1988). TGFβ1, 2, and interleukin-1 are thus implicated as mediators of macrophage induced glial scarring but there may be others.

Interferon-γ (IFNγ) and basic fibroblast growth factor (FGF2) are two inflammatory cytokines whose interactions play a role in the induction of the glial scar. In culture, limiting IFNγ activity reduces the mitogenic effects of activated T-lymphocytes and the addition of recombinant IFNγ induces astrocyte proliferation and increases the extent of glial scarring *in vivo* (Yong et al., 1991). After injury, the levels of FGF2 increase in both the brain and spinal cord (Logan et al., 1992; Mocchetti et al., 1996), and FGF2 has also been shown to increase astrocyte proliferation in culture (DiProspero et al., 1997). It has been proposed that IFNγ and FGF2 modulate the effects of one another following injury. Interestingly, IFNγ antagonizes the pro-mitogenic effects of FGF2 (DiProspero et al., 1997). However, it should be reiterated that following injury in the vicinity of blood–brain barrier extravasation, much of the glial scar forms without astrocyte proliferation; but rather with a switch to the reactive state followed by inhibitory ECM production and then hypertrophy (Miyake et al., 1988). This rather complex discussion further illustrates our own ignorance of the complex, yet important, role that inflammation plays in the induction of the glial scar. Perhaps, with a greater understanding of the inflammatory signals that lead to glial scarring, steps can be taken to effectively reduce scarring and enhance regeneration.

Cellular components of the glial scar

Injuries to the CNS occur with varying degrees of severity which alters the cellular make-up of the glial scar. In extremely small lesions of the CNS, a microlesion, minimal alteration in astrocyte morphology occurs (Davies et al., 1996). There is an increase in GFAP immunoreactivity in astrocytes adjacent to the lesion, but alignment is largely unaltered. Only macrophages migrate into the site of these micro-lesions.

In more severe lesions of the CNS, the number of different cell types that are contained within in the glial scar increases (Fig. 22.1; reviewed by Fawcett and Asher, 1999). The majority of the cells are reactive astrocytes that form a tightly interconnected lacework of cellular processes. Many of the oligodendrocytes contained with in the injury site survive the insult and are contained within the glial scar along with myelin debris. Macrophages and microglia also invade the lesion site, and may play a role in the development of the glial scar. Lastly, oligodendrocyte precursor cells and multipotential progenitor cells invade the lesion, possibly in an attempt to remake the lesion, but their role is not well defined.

22.3 Glial production of growth inhibitory molecules

Chondroitin sulfate proteoglycans

Very tiny lesions of the mature CNS do not result in an obviously obstructive terrain. Do such minute lesions allow for regeneration? In fact, even the most minimal of CNS lesions, which do not alter astrocytic alignment (Pindzola et al., 1993; Davies et al., 1996; 1997), causes completely aborted regeneration. Observations such as these, as well as those demonstrating failed regeneration after a critical period discussed above, suggested that there must be a molecular basis for scar mediated inhibition that changes during maturation. This hypothesis has lead to a search for what these molecules might be (McKeon et al., 1991; Bovolenta et al., 1993; Pindzola et al., 1993; Geisert et al., 1996; Huber and Schwab, 2000; Jones et al., 2003; Tang et al., 2003).

In addition to growth promoting molecules, which will be discussed later (Wyss-Coray et al., 1995; Canning et al., 1996), astrocytes produce a class of molecules referred to as proteoglycans (Gallo et al., 1987; Gallo and Bertolotto, 1990). These ECM molecules consist of a protein core linked by four sugar moieties to a sulfated glycosaminoglycan (GAG) chain that contains repeating disaccharide units. Astrocytes produce four classes of proteoglycans: heparan sulfate (HS), dermatan sulfate (DS), keratan sulfate (KS) and chondroitin sulfate (CSPG) (Johnson-Green et al., 1991). Chondroitin sulfate proteoglycans (CSPGs) include a number of molecules that comprise their own relatively large family, including among others aggrecan, brevican, neurocan, NG2, phosphacan (sometimes appearing as a KSPG), and versican, all of which share chondroitin sulfate side chains. They differ in the protein core, as well as the number, length, and pattern of sulfation of the side chains (Margolis and Margolis, 1993; Grimpe and Silver, 2002; Morgenstern et al., 2002). The expression of these CSPGs increases in the glial scar following brain and spinal cord injury (McKeon et al., 1999; Jones et al., 2003; Tang et al., 2003).

Developmental evidence has implicated proteoglycans as barriers to axon outgrowth in the roof plate of the spinal cord (Snow et al., 1990b; Katoh-Semba et al., 1995), in the midline rhombencephalon and mesencephalon (Cole and McCabe, 1991; Wu et al., 1998), at the dorsal root entry zone (DREZ) (Pindzola et al., 1993), in retinal pattern development (Brittis et al., 1992; Jhaveri, 1993), and at the optic chiasm and distal optic tract (Chung et al., 2000; Becker and Becker, 2002). Furthermore, extensive work has demonstrated that CSPGs are extremely inhibitory to axon outgrowth in culture. Neurites growing on alternating stripes of laminin and laminin/CSPG (aggrecan) had robust outgrowth on laminin but turned away at the sharp interface between the two surfaces. The turning behavior is not usually mediated via collapse of the entire growth cone, but rather by selective retraction of filopodia in contact with CSPG and enhanced motility of those on laminin (Snow et al., 1990a; Hynds and Snow, 1999). These effects of CSPGs are not limited to laminin, in fact, CSPGs inhibit other growth promoting molecules, including fibronectin and L1 (Dou and Levine, 1994; Snow et al., 1996).

In the early 1990s the first evidence emerged that these CSPGs important in developmental boundaries might be playing a role in the failure of regeneration in the CNS following injury. CSPGs are produced in excess by astrocytes when induced to become reactive *in vivo* following small lesions of the DREZ (Pindzola et al., 1993). The upregulated CSPGs were present at the right time and place to potentially inhibit sensory axons from regenerating in the dorsal columns or through the DREZ. CSPGs are upregulated and excreted extracellularly following a wide variety of CNS injuries (Asher et al., 2000; Jones et al., 2002; Moon et al., 2002). Importantly, precritical period embryonic reactive astroglia do not upregulate CSPGs following injury (McKeon et al., 1991) and there is minimal upregulation of CSPGs on reactive glia in cold blooded species (Becker and Becker, 2002).

In mature mammals, CSPGs are secreted rapidly after injury and can persist for many months (Fig. 22.2; McKeon et al., 1999; Jones et al., 2003; Tang et al., 2003). Most importantly, it was shown in a number of *in vitro* assays of highly reactive mature astrocytes that upregulated proteoglycans within the complex ECM made by reactive astroglia does, indeed, inhibit axonal outgrowth (McKeon et al., 1991; Canning et al., 1993; Dou and Levine, 1994; Smith-Thomas et al., 1994). To further demonstrate that the GAG portion of CSPGs are inhibitory to neurite outgrowth in models of the glial scar in culture, the *Proteus vulgaris* extract chondroitinase (Ch'ase), a class of enzymes that selectively removes a major portion of the CSPG GAG side chain and renders CSPGs less inhibitory (see below), was applied to mature glial scar explants using the nitrocellulose harvesting model. Retinal ganglion cells cultured on the scar explants were only able to extend long neurites following enzyme treatment, indicating that digestion of CSPGs was essential to enhance regeneration and that CSPGs may be potent inhibitors *in vivo* (McKeon et al., 1995). Furthermore, when laminin (which is also produced by astroglia in these scar explants) was blocked with antibodies, the growth enhancing effects of Ch'ase treatment was reduced. These findings indicated that neurite extension may depend on a balance of growth promoting and growth inhibiting molecules at the site of injury or that CSPGs might be blocking outgrowth indirectly by interfering with the growth promoting effects of laminin.

Differential effects of CSPGs on axon regeneration

CSPGs retard growth of different populations of neurons to varying degrees *in vitro* (Snow and Letourneau, 1992). To demonstrate this, embryonic dorsal root ganglion (DRG) neurons, retinal ganglion neurons, or forebrain neurons were cultured on a gradient of laminin and CSPG, in which the concentration of CSPG increased in a stepwise fashion while the concentration of laminin was

unchanged. Neurons were placed on laminin alone and the ability of each neuronal population to extend neurites from the laminin onto and up the step gradient was analyzed. Interestingly, all neurons were able to extend some distance up the gradient, but the retinal ganglion cells were able to extend furthest. Not only does this work demonstrate that different populations of neurons respond to CSPGs differently, but that neurons are capable of outgrowth on CSPGs when there is a balance of growth promotion and inhibition. Once a critical threshold of inhibition is reached, the balance is altered such that growth ceases. Furthermore, time-lapse microscopy of fully adult DRG neuron growth cones on a more smoothly constructed spot gradient of CSPG indicates that growth cones can extend along a gradient of proteoglycan until a highly inhibitory region is reached resulting in cessation of forward extension along with the formation of an unusual type of dystrophic ending (Tom et al., 2002).

The differential abilities of different neuronal populations to regenerate into a proteoglycan enriched lesion has also been demonstrated in the spinal cord (Inman and Steward, 2003). After injury, regenerating motor axons were unable to enter the lesion directly, but were capable of sprouting in the region adjacent to the lesion. Seritonergic neurons were also only capable of regenerating to the edge of the lesion; however, sensory axons were capable of deeper penetration, albeit not all the way through the lesion. This study reiterates that some neurons have a higher intrinsic threshold for dealing with a terrain laden with proteoglycans, especially when they are presented in a gradient. At some point, however, usually near the lesion epicenter, all regenerating fibers become dystrophic and finally succumb to their increasingly inhibitory environment.

Removal of CSPGs enhances regeneration

Further evidence that CSPGs inhibit regeneration arises from experiments in which digestion of CSPGs enhances regeneration. One strategy to accomplish this is to enzymatically degrade them *in vivo* following injury to axonal pathways using Ch'ase which removes the sugar chain from CSPGs leaving the protein core behind. Ch'ase is very effective at digesting CSPGs. In fact, a single injection of Ch'ase into the brain results in decreased levels of intact CSPG that persists for up to 4 weeks (Brückner et al., 1998). Experiments to be discussed demonstrate that Ch'ase is an effective method to reduce inhibition and shift the balance towards regeneration.

Treatment with Ch'ase following nigrostriatal tract lesioning enhanced regeneration of dopaminergic neurons back to their desired targets (Moon et al., 2001). Ch'ase applied intrathecally to animals with bilateral dorsal column lesions digested CSPGs at the lesion site and allowed for both ascending sensory and descending motor axon regeneration through and past the lesion (Bradbury et al., 2002). Furthermore, treatment resulted in limited recovery of locomotor and proprioceptive function. Additional, yet preliminary, studies have shown that CSPG digestion can improve regeneration following spinal cord hemisection in the cat (Tester et al., 2003) and in contusive injuries to the rat (Caggiano et al., 2003) which is a more relevant model of the typical human spinal cord injury. In another strategy, treatment with Ch'ase enhances the ability of regenerating axons to enter as well as exit peripheral nerve grafts transplanted into CNS lesions in order to provide a Schwann cell laden highway and possible bypass of the injury site (Xu et al., 1995; Mayes and Houle, 2003). Lastly, results in our laboratory indicate that preventing the synthesis of CSPGs after injury by inhibiting the synthetic enzymes for GAG chain assembly also enhances regeneration (Grimpe and Silver, 2004). Thus, removal of CSPGs has now been demonstrated to reduce the inhibitory environment of the glial scar *in vivo* enhancing regeneration and providing some measure of functional recovery.

Additional inhibitory molecules in the glial scar

CSPGs are not the only inhibitory molecules upregulated following injury. Several other molecules are now known to be upregulated, especially in the core of the lesion, and contribute to the growth retarding effects of the glial scar. One such molecule is the secreted protein Sema 3, a member of the semaphorin gene family (see Volume I, Chapter 19). Sema 3 acts through its high-affinity receptor, neuropilin-1 as a chemorepellent. Following lesions of the lateral olfactory tract (Pasterkamp et al., 1999), cortex (Pasterkamp et al., 1999), or spinal cord (Pasterkamp et al., 1999, 2001; De Winter et al., 2002), Sema 3 expression increases in fibroblasts deeply penetrating the lesion and neuropilin-1 expression increases in neurons that project to the lesion site. Regenerating axons were excluded from central areas of the lesion containing Sema 3, essentially creating an exclusion zone at the heart of the lesion.

Recent work by Bundeson and colleagues (2003) has implicated ephrin-B2 and its receptor EphB2 in inhibition of regeneration following spinal cord transection. In normal development, this ligand-receptor pairing plays diverse roles in cell migration, axonal guidance, and tissue patterning (see Volume I, Chapter 19). The interactions of these partners becomes important again after injury, when ephrin-B2 expression increases in astrocytes and EphB2 expression increases in fibroblasts. At first, astrocytes and fibroblasts co-mingle, but then as ephrin-B2 and EphB2 expression increases, they signal cell type segregation, creating bands of fibroblasts and astrocytes, and more importantly, the cellular structure of the so-called glial/mesenchymal scar.

One last protein to consider is the slit family of proteins (see Volume I, Chapter 19). These proteins play important roles as regulators of axon guidance and cell migration by inhibiting axon growth (reviewed by Brose and Tessier-Lavigne, 2000) and signal via the glypican-1 heparan sulfate proteoglycan in the CNS (Ronca et al., 2001). Slit proteins expression increases in reactive astrocytes, along with glypican-1 receptors, following cortical injury (Hagino et al., 2003). This correlative evidence implicates the slit proteins in regeneration failure as well. Together, Sema 3, ephrin-B2, and slit proteins add additional levels of complexity to the inhibition of regeneration in the adult CNS following injury.

22.4 Growth promoting molecules in the glial scar

Not only are growth inhibitory molecules upregulated in the glial scar following CNS injury, but many molecules implicated in promoting axon growth are also present (Eddleston and Mucke, 1993; Fitch and Silver, 1999). The growth inhibitory and growth promoting molecules exist in a balance that favors stalled regeneration of axons (see below), but it is important to reiterate that non-regenerating axons still bay need to be supported if they are to remain indefinitely in the vicinity of the lesion. Reactive astrocytes secrete laminin following injury (Liesi et al., 1984) and adult neurons sprout into areas of the glial scar where laminin persists (Frisén et al., 1995). Additionally, reactive astrocytes secrete normal basal lamina, which includes laminin, collagen IV, and heparin sulfate (Bernstein et al., 1985). The basal lamina may appear normal, but it is produced in excessive levels in ectopic locations, contributing to the glial scar. Bands of basal lamina coalesce and can support limited adult neurite sprouting (Risling et al., 1993) and even more extensive outgrowth when trophic factors are added to the milieu (Kawaja and Gage, 1991).

Many examples of reactive gliosis in which laminin expression is increased also result in increased production of the growth promoting molecule fibronectin. Examples include production of laminin and fibronectin by immature and mature astrocytes in the previously described "scar-in-a-dish" (McKeon et al., 1991) and by immature and mature reactive optic nerve astrocytes (Hirsch and Bähr, 1999). Fibronectin expression also increases in reactive astrocytes associated with neuritic plaques of Alzheimer's disease, and its expression is induced in reactive astrocytes by amyloid peptide (Moreno-Flores et al., 2001). Inducing astrocytes into the reactive state with application of basic FGF2 increases the production of fibronectin and neural cell adhesion molecules (NCAM) (Mahler et al., 1997). Furthermore, injured purkinje cells are unable to regenerate shortly after injury, but can regenerate at later time periods that correlate with an increase in NCAM (Dusart et al., 1999) indicating that increases in cell adhesion

molecules allow for aberrant neurite extension. Interestingly, either decreasing the amount of GFAP formed after injury using anti-sense technology (Costa et al., 2002) or blocking it entirely in a knockout (Menet et al., 2001) results in increases in adhesion molecule expression and enhanced neurite outgrowth. These findings indicate that adult reactive astrocytes provide some support to regenerating axons, but not enough to promote regeneration. The potential does exist to alter the balance towards regeneration by exploiting these growth promoting properties.

22.5 The glial scar and regenerating axons

Dystrophic axons in the glial scar: a balance of growth inhibition and promotion

When regenerating axons encounter the environment of the glial scar, so-called dystrophic end bulbs form, as first described by Ramón y Cajal (1928). For many years these unusually shaped end bulbs were considered sterile and thus, incapable of extending a growth cone through the lesion. These dystrophic endings come in a variety of bizarre shapes ranging from small globular clusters to huge multivesicular sacks (see Ramón y Cajal, 1928, p. 493). More recent research has indicated that axons with such endings do not lose their ability to regenerate following injury and that the dystrophic endings can, in fact, return to active growth states. Chronically injured axons in the spinal cord are capable of regenerating into implanted peripheral nerve grafts after 4 weeks of stagnating in the lesion environment (Houle, 1991). More importantly, even year old lesions of the adult rubrospinal tracts when treated with brain derived neurotrophic factor can result in restoration of the size of the soma (Kobayashi et al., 1997) or new axon growth into peripheral nerve grafts and upregulation of the growth associated protein GAP-43 (Kwon et al., 2002).

Li and Raisman (1995) examined dystrophic endings in the context of a chronic lesion and found that large varicosities and swollen endings of dystrophic endings persisted for 13 weeks. Furthermore, even at these lengthy time periods post-injury the so-called dystrophic sterile endings were capable of sprouting and many of the new sprouts were myelinated by migrating Schwann cells. Additional work has carefully examined the extent of axon retraction following spinal cord injury (Houle and Jin, 2001). Cervical cord hemisection produced numerous terminal end bulbs of dystrophic axons. With the use of more modern tracing techniques, Houle's experiments suggest that the majority of dystrophic endings actually remained very close to the lesion site, contradicting previous work indicating dieback. This presence of dystrophic growth cones in the glial scar for extended periods of time demonstrates that glial scars are inhibitory to regeneration, but also that they contain growth promoting molecules that balance inhibiting effects of the glial scar.

The significance of the interminable persistence of such unusual growth cones within the epicenter of the lesion also implies that some type of cytoskeletal and/or membrane plasticity must be occurring in order to maintain axonal viability and stability, even though they remain in one place over time. Recent work in our laboratory has begun to identify, in culture and *in vivo*, the behavior of dystrophic endings (Tom et al., 2002). Using a specially crafted gradient of aggrecan and laminin as a substrate for adult DRG's, classically shaped dystrophic endings are formed as the fibers struggle up the gradient. However, time-lapse analysis has revealed the surprising finding that "dystrophic" endings are not sterile at all. Rather, they are highly and continually active structures. They can remain stationary (i.e. running in place) for days as they constantly turn over their distal membranes, alter their cytoskeleton, and change the location of their complement of integrin receptors. We have evidence that these dynamic phenomena occur *in vivo* as well and, thus, it appears that the adult sensory neuron uses this form of aberrant growth cone to maintain itself in a hostile environment.

Regional differences in the glial scar: the penumbra versus the center

Fully adult sensory neurons placed into adult corpus callosum or lesioned spinal cord are capable of regenerating their axons in intact or degenerating white matter when minimal damage from cell transplant is created placing the cells far rostral to a lesion. Regeneration continues into the periphery of the glial scar, but ceases as axons reach the penumbra and epicenter of the lesion. Here proteoglycan upregulation occurs in a gradient, lowest in the lesion penumbra and increasing towards the lesion core, altering the balance of promotion and inhibition. As regenerating fibers pass through the lesion penumbra they alter their morphology and are strongly inhibited from moving further as they form ever greater numbers of dystrophic endings near the core of the lesion (Davies et al., 1997; 1999). Rather unexpectedly, transplanted adult sensory neurons were capable of extending axons very rapidly and robustly (they can regenerate at the rate of 1 mm per day) among oligodendrocytes, degenerating myelin, and astrocytes that are intensely reactive due to the accompanying Wallerian degeneration. However, once a critical level of CSPG was reached, regeneration ceased and dystrophic endings formed.

Thus, in addition to immature astrocytes, our experiments have revealed that reactive astroglia distal to a lesion are surprisingly growth supportive, at least to adult sensory axons, even within purportedly inhibitory white matter. Recent evidence from our lab, along with earlier described growth promoting molecules, suggests that extracellular fibronectin and astroglial geometric alignment may be two of several critical factors (Tom et al., 2003). The remarkable capacity for regeneration distal to the lesion can last for many, many months until the mechanically obstructive properties of glial hypertrophy come into play and block regeneration via more physical means.

Altering the balance: enhancing regeneration in the presence of inhibitory cues

Removal of extrinsic inhibitory cues from the glial scar with treatments such as the use of Ch'ase may aid regeneration; however, this may not be sufficient for long range regrowth. Neurotrophin-3 (NT-3) or nerve growth factor (NGF) delivered directly to transected neurons in the dorsal columns of animals treated with peripheral nerve graft transplants enhances growth into the graft, out the opposite end, and beyond the glial scar into host tissue (Oudega and Hagg, 1996; 1999). Exogenous NGF administration induces sprouting into the lesion of crushed dorsal columns as well (Bradbury et al., 1999). Intrathecal or adenoviral application of NT-3 or NGF to the injured DREZ induces DRG neurons to cross the peripheral nervous system/CNS barrier and enter some distance into the spinal cord (Zhang et al., 1998; Ramer et al., 2000; 2001; 2002; Romero et al., 2001) where the regenerating fibers restored nociceptive function. Thus, evidence from the injured spinal cord and DREZ indicates that regenerating axons can overcome proteoglycan barriers after neurotrophin stimulation, offering an additional therapeutic strategy.

One can alter intrinsic growth properties of mature neurons in other ways to enhance regeneration. For example, embryonic neurons are highly capable of regeneration and have the ability to upregulate integrin receptors for growth promoting molecules when mixed with inhibitory aggrecan. Mature neurons, on the contrary, are unable to do either in the presence of CSPGs (Condic, 2001). Overexpression of integrins via viral transduction engenders adult neurons with enhanced regenerative capability, on par with that of young neurons. Peripheral conditioning lesions also enhance the ability of CNS neurons to regenerate into a lesion site, and this occurs in part due to increases in cAMP levels in the neuron cell body (Qiu et al., 2002). Furthermore, this effect can be replicated without peripheral lesion by simply injected the cell bodies of sensory neurons with cAMP (Neumann et al., 2002), indicating that protein kinase A mediated pathways could be exploited to enhance the ability of a neuron to overcome scar inhibitors as well as myelin inhibitors following injury (see Volume I, Chapter 21).

CSPGs present in the glial scar impair neuron outgrowth by signaling through the Rho/ROCK pathway and specific inhibition of the Rho GTPase enhances process outgrowth (Dergham et al., 2002; Borisoff et al., 2003; Monnier et al., 2003) on proteoglycan containing substrates, as well as on myelin containing substrates. Pharmacologically blocking the downstream signaling from CSPGs may also enhance CNS regeneration (see Volume I, Chapter 24). Lastly, certain reparative states of the inflammatory cascade, which must be different from those that influence glial scar formation, may also have pro-regenerative effects on neurons. Activation of macrophages using the yeast cell wall extract Zymosan enhances retinal ganglion cell regeneration past the glial scar following optic nerve injury (Yin et al., 2003) and enhances process outgrowth of DRG neurons in a culture model of proteoglycan contained in the glial scar (Steinmetz et al., 2003). Interestingly, a simple sugar, mannose appears to be the mediator stimulating neurons to increase their ability to regenerate (Li et al., 2003).

22.6 Conclusions

Astrocytes play a critical role in the formation of the glial scar. They maintain the overall integrity of the CNS following injury, but inhibit regeneration to achieve this aim. Through the release of inhibitory proteoglycans and altered morphology, astrocytes prevent regenerating axons from extending through a lesion. However, the balance of these inhibitory proteoglycans along with growth promoting molecules produced by astrocytes enables dystrophic endings of axons to persist in the lesion vicinity.

Our discussion of the glial scar has led us to the conclusion that to best overcome the inhibitory environment of the glial scar combinatorial strategies will need to be employed. Treatments should include those that provide a growth supportive highway across the lesion cavity, those that intrinsically enhance the ability of neurons to elongate, as well as those that manipulate the extrinsic inhibitors that block growth in the immediate environment of the glial scar. With this approach to CNS injury, it may be possible to induce long distance and functional regeneration following injury.

REFERENCES

Asher, R.A., Morgenstern, D.A., Fidler, P.S., Adcock, K.H., Oohira, A., Braistead, J.E., Levine, J.M., Margolis, R.U.,

Rogers, J.H. and Fawcett, J.W. (2000). Neurocan is upregulated in injured brain and in cytokine-treated astrocytes. *J Neurosci*, **20**, 2427–2438.

Bahr, M., Przyrembel, C. and Bastmeyer, M. (1995). Astrocytes from adult rat optic nerves are nonpermissive for regenerating retinal ganglion cell axons. *Exper Neurol*, **131**, 211–220.

Barret, C.P., Guth, L., Donati, E.J. and Krikorian, J.G. (1981). Astroglial reaction in the gray matter of lumbar segments after midthoracic transection of the adult rat spinal cord. *Exper Neurol*, **73**, 365–377.

Becker, C.G. and Becker, T. (2002). Repellent guidance of regenerating optic axons by chondroitin sulfate glycosaminoglycans in zebrafish. *J Neurosci*, **22**, 842–853.

Bernstein, J.J., Getz, R., Jefferson, M. and Kelemen, M. (1985). Astrocytes secrete basal lamina after hemisection of rat spinal cord. *Brain Res*, **327**, 135–141.

Bignami, A. and Dahl, D. (1974). Astrocyte-specific protein and neuroglial differentiation. An immunofluorescence study with antibodies to the glial fibrillary acidic protein. *J Comp Neurol*, **153**, 27–38.

Bignami, A. and Dahl, D. (1976). The astroglial response to stabbing. Immunofluorscence studies with antibodies to astrocyte-specific protein (GFA) in mammalian and submammalian vertebrates. *Neuropathol Appl Neurobiol*, **2**, 99–110.

Borisoff, J.F., Chan, C.C.M., Hiebert, G.W., Oschipok, L., Robertson, G.S., Zamboni, R., Steeves, J.D. and Tetzlaff, W. (2003). Suppression of Rho-kinase activity promotes axonal growth on inhibitory CNS substrates. *Mol Cell Neurosci*, **22**, 405–416.

Bovolenta, P., Wandosell, F. and Nieto-Sampedro, M. (1993). Characterization of a neurite outgrowth inhibitor expressed after CNS injury. *Eur J Neurosci*, **5**, 454–465.

Bradbury, E.J., Khemani, S., King, V.R., Priestly, J.V. and McMahon, S.B. (1999). NT-3 promotes growth of lesioned adult rat sensory axons ascending in the dorsal columns of the spinal cord. *Eur J Neurosci*, **11**, 3873–3883.

Bradbury, E.J., Moon, L.D.F., Popat, R.J., King, V.R., Bennett, G.S., Patel, P.N., Fawcett, J.W. and McMahon, S.B. (2002). Chondroitinase ABC promotes functional recovery after spinal cord injury. *Nature*, **416**, 636–640.

Brittis, P.A., Canning, D.R. and Silver, J. (1992). Chondroitin sulfate as a regulator of neuronal patterning in the retina. *Science*, **255**, 733–736.

Brose, K. and Tessier-Lavigne, M. (2000). Slit proteins: key regulators of axon guidance, axonal branching, and cell migration. *Curr Opin Neurobiol*, **10**, 95–102.

Brückner, G., Bringmann, A., Härtig, W., Köppe, G., Delpech, B. and Brauer, K. (1998). Acute and long-lasting changes in extracellular-matrix chondroitin-sulphate proteoglycans induced by injection of chondroitinase ABC in the adult rat brain. *Exp Brain Res*, **121**, 300–310.

Bundeson, L.Q., Scheel, T.A., Bregman, B.S. and Kromer, L.F. (2003). Ephrin-B2 and EphB2 regulation of astrocyte-meningeal fibroblast interactions in response to spinal cord lesions in adult rats. *J Neurosci*, **23**, 7789–7800.

Bush, T.G., Puvanachandra, N., Horner, C.H., Polito, A., Ostenfeld, T., Svendson, C.N., Mucke, L., Johnson, M.H. and Sofroniew, M.V. (1999). Leukocyte infiltration, neuronal degeneration, and neurite outgrowth after ablation of scar-forming, reactive astrocytes in adult transgenic mice. *Neuron*, **23**, 297–308.

Caggiano, A.O., Zimber, M.P., Ganguly, A., Martinez, M., Blight, A.R. and Gruskin, E.A. (2003). Chondroitinase ABC I improves locomoter function after spinal cord contusion injury in the rat. Society for Neuroscience, Abstract No. 744.5.

Canning, D.R., McKeon, R.J., DeWitt, D.A., Perry, G., Wujek, J.R., Fredrickson, D.A. and Silver, J. (1993). β-Amyloid of Alzheimer's disease induces reactive gliosis that inhibits axonal outgrowth. *Exper Neurol*, **124**, 289–298.

Canning, D.R., Höke, A., Malemud, C.J. and Silver, J. (1996). A potent inhibitor of neurite outgrowth that predominates in the extracellular matrix of reactive astrocytes. *Int J Dev Neurosci*, **14**, 153–175.

Chauvet, N., Prieto, M. and Alonso, G. (1998). Tanycytes present in the adult rat mediobasal hypothalamus support the regeneration of monoaminergic axons. *Exp Neurol*, **151**, 1–13.

Chung, K., Shum, D.K. and Chan, S. (2000). Expression of chondroitin sulfate proteoglycans in the chiasm of mouse embryos. *J Comp Neurol*, **417**, 153–163.

Clemente, C.D. (1958). The regeneration of peripheral nerves inserted into the cerebral cortex and the healing of cerebral lesions. *J Comp Neurol*, **109**, 123–143.

Clemente, C.D. and Windle, W.F. (1954). Regeneration of severed nerve fibers in the spinal cord of the adult cat. *J Comp Neurol*, **101**, 691–731.

Cole, G.J. and McCabe, C.F. (1991). Identification of a developmentally regulated keratan sulfate proteoglycan that inhibits cell adhesion and neurite outgrowth. *Neuron*, **7**, 1007–1018.

Condic, M.L. (2001). Adult neuronal regeneration induced by transgenic integrin expression. *J Neurosci*, **21**, 4782–4788.

Costa, S., Planchenault, T., Charriere-Bertrand, C., Mouchel, Y., Fages, Ch., Juliano, S., Lefrançois, T., Barlovatz-Meimon, G. and Tardy, M. (2002). Astroglial permissivity for neuritic outgrowth in neuron-astrocyte cocultures depends on regulation of laminin bioavailability. *Glia*, **37**, 105–113.

Davies, S.J.A., Field, P.M. and Raisman, G. (1996). Regeneration of cut adult axons fails even in the presence of continuous aligned glial pathways. *Exper Neurol*, **142**, 203–216.

Davies, S.J.A., Fitch, M.T., Memberg, S.P., Hall, A.K., Raisman, G. and Silver, J. (1997). Regeneration of adult axons in white matter tracts of the central nervous system. *Nature*, **390**, 680–683.

Davies, S.J.A., Goucher, D.R., Doller, C. and Silver, J. (1999). Robust regeneration of adult sensory axons in degenerating white matter of the adult rat spinal cord. *J Neurosci*, **19**, 5810–5822.

De Winter, F., Oudega, M., Lankhorst, A.J., Hamers, F.P., Blits, B., Ruitenberg, M.J., Pasterkamp, R.J., Gispen, W.H. and Verhaagen, J. (2002). Injury-induced class 3 semaphorin expression in the rat spinal cord. *Exper Neurol*, **175**, 61–75.

Dergham, P., Ellezam, B., Essagian, C., Avedissian, H., Lubell, W.D. and McKerracher L. (2002). Rho signaling pathway targeted to promote spinal cord repair. *J Neurosci*, **22**, 6570–6577.

DiProspero, N.A., Meiners, S. and Geller, H.M. (1997). Inflammatory cytokines interact to modulate extracellular matrix and astrocytic support of neurite outgrowth. *Exper Neurol*, **148**, 628–639.

Dou, C.L. and Levine, J.M. (1994). Inhibition of neurite growth by the NG2 chondroitin sulfate proteoglycan. *J Neurosci*, **14**, 7616–7628.

Dusart, I., Morel, M.P., Wehrlé, R. and Sotelo, C. (1999). Late axonal sprouting of injured purkinje cells and its temporal correlation with permissive changes in the glial scar. *J Comp Neurol*, **408**, 399–418.

Eddleston, M. and Mucke, L. (1993). Molecular profile of reactive astrocytes – implications for their role in neurologic disease. *Neuroscience*, **54**, 15–36.

Eng, L.F. (1985). Glial fibrillary acidic protein (GFAP): the major protein of glial intermediate filaments in differentiated astrocytes. *J Neuroimmunol*, **8**, 203–214.

Faulkner, J.R., Herrmann, J.E., Woo, M.J., Tansey, K.E., Doan, N.B. and Sofroniew, M.V. (2004). Reactive astrocytes protect tissue and preserve function after spinal cord injury. *J Neurosci*, **24**, 2143–2155.

Fawcett, J.W. and Asher, R.A. (1999). The glial scar and central nervous system repair. *Brain Res Bull*, **49**, 377–391.

Fitch, M.T. and Silver, J. (1999). Beyond the glial scar: cellular and molecular mechanisms by which glial cells contribute to CNS regenerative failure. In: *CNS Regeneration: Basic Science and Clinical Advances* (eds Tuszynski, M.H. and Kordower, J.H.), Academic Press, San Diego, pp. 55–88.

Fitch, M.T., Doller, C., Combs, C.K., Landreth, G.E. and Silver, J. (1999). Cellular and molecular mechanisms of glial scarring and progressive cavitation: *in vivo* and *in vitro* analysis of inflammation-induced secondary injury after CNS trauma. *J Neurosci*, **19**, 8182–8198.

Frisén, J., Hægerstrand, A., Risling, M., Fried, K., Johansson, C.B., Hammarberg, H., Elde, R., Hökfelt, T. and Cullheim, S.

(1995). Spinal axons in central nervous system scar tissue are closely related to laminin-immunoreactive astrocytes. *Neurosci*, **65**, 293–304.

Gallo, V. and Bertolotto, A. (1990). Extracellular matrix of cultured glial cells: selective expression of chondroitin 4-sulfate by type-2 astrocytes and their progenitors. *Exp Cell Res*, **187**, 211–223.

Gallo, V., Bertolotto, A. and Levi, G. (1987). The proteoglycan chondroitin sulfate is present in a subpopulation of cultured astrocytes and in their precursors. *Dev Biol*, **123**, 282–285.

Geisert, E.E., Bidanest, D.J., Del Mar, N. and Robson, J.A. (1996). Up-regulation of a keratan sulfate proteoglycan following cortical injury in neonatal rats. *Int J Dev Neurosci*, **14**, 257–267.

Giulian, D., Woodward, J., Young, D.G., Krebs, J.F. and Lachman, L.B. (1988). Interleukin-1 injected into mammalian brain stimulates astrogliosis and neovascularization. *J Neurosci*, **8**, 2485–2490.

Grimpe, B. and Silver, J. (2002). The extracellular matrix in axon regeneration. *Prog Brain Res*, **137**, 333–349.

Grimpe, B. and Silver, J. (2004). A novel DNA enzyme reduces glycosaminoglycan chains in the glial scar and allows microtransplanted DRG axons to regenerate beyond lesions in the spinal cord. *J Neurosci*, **24**, 1393–1397.

Hagino, S., Iseki, K., Mori, T., Zhang, Y., Hikake, T., Yokoya, S., Takeuchi, M., Hasimoto, H., Kikuchi, S. and Wanaka, A. (2003). Slit and glypican-1 mRNAs are coexpressed in the reactive astrocytes of the injured adult brain. *Glia*, **42**, 130–138.

Hirsch, S. and Bähr, M. (1999). Immunocytochemical characterization of reactive optic nerve astrocytes and meningeal cells. *Glia*, **26**, 36–46.

Houle, J.D. (1991). Demonstration of the potential for chronically injured neurons to regenerate axons into intraspinal peripheral nerve grafts. *Exper Neurol*, **113**, 1–9.

Houle, J.D. and Jin, Y. (2001). Chronically injured supraspinal neurons exhibit only modest axonal dieback in response to a cervical hemisection lesion. *Exper Neurol*, **169**, 208–217.

Huber, A.B. and Schwab, M.E. (2000). Nogo-A, a potent inhibitor of neurite outgrowth and regeneration. *Biol Chem*, **381**, 407–419.

Hynds, D.L. and Snow, D.M. (1999). Neurite outgrowth inhibition by chondroitin sulfate proteoglycan stalling/stopping exceeds turning in human neuroblastoma growth cones. *Exper Neurol*, **160**, 244–255.

Inman, D.M. and Steward, O. (2003). Ascending sensory, but not other long-tract axons, regenerate into the connective tissue matrix that forms at the site of a spinal cord injury in mice. *J Comp Neurol*, **462**, 431–449.

Jhaveri, S. (1993). Midline glia of the tectum: a barrier for developing retinal axons. *Prespect Dev Neurobiol*, **1**, 237–243.

Johnson-Green, P.C., Dow, K.E. and Riopelle, R.J. (1991). Characterization of glycosaminoglycans produced by primary astrocytes *in vitro*. *Glia*, **4**, 314–321.

Jones, L.L., Yamaguchi, Y., Stallcup, W.B. and Tuszynski, M.H. (2002). NG2 is a major chondroitin sulfate proteoglycan produced after spinal cord injury and is expressed by macrophages and oligodendrocyte progenitors. *J Neurosci*, **22**, 2792–2803.

Jones, L.L., Margolis, R.U. and Tuszynski, M.H. (2003). The chondroitin sulfate proteoglycans neurocan, brevican, phosphacan, and versican are differentially regulated following spinal cord injury. *Exper Neurol*, **182**, 399–411.

Katoh-Semba, R., Matsuda, M., Kato, K. and Oohira, A. (1995). Chondroitin sulphate proteoglycans in the rat brain: candidates for axon barriers of sensory neurons and the possible modification by laminin of their actions. *Eur J Neurosci*, **7**, 613–621.

Kawaja, M.D. and Gage, F.H. (1991). Reactive astrocytes are substrates for the growth of adult CNS axons in the presence of elevated levels of nerve growth factor. *Neuron*, **7**, 1019–1030.

Kobayashi, N.R., Fan, D.P., Giehl, K.M., Bedard, A.M., Wiegand, S.J. and Tetzlaff, W. (1997). BDNF and NT-4/5 prevent atrophy of rat rubrospinal neurons after cervical axotomy, stimulate GAP-43 and Talpha1-tubulin mRNA expression, and promote axonal regeneration. *J Neurosci*, **17**, 9583–9595.

Kwon, B.K., Liu, J., Messerer, C., Kobayashi, N.R., McGraw, J., Oschipok, L. and Tetzlaff, W. (2002). Survival and regeneration of rubrospinal neurons 1 year after spinal cord injury. *Proc Natl Acad Sci USA*, **99**, 3246–3251.

Lagord, C., Berry, M. and Logan, A. (2002). Expression of TGFβ2 but not TGFβ1 correlates with the deposition of scar tissue in the lesioned spinal cord. *Mol Cell Neurosci*, **20**, 69–92.

Le Roux, P.D. and Reh, T.A. (1996). Reactive astroglia support primary dendritic but not axonal outgrowth from mouse cortical neurons *in vitro*. *Exp Neurol*, **137**, 49–65.

Li, Y. and Raisman, G. (1995). Sprouts from cut corticospinal axons persist in the presence of astrocytic scarring in long-term lesions of the adult rat spinal cord. *Exper Neurol*, **134**, 102–111.

Li, Y., Irwin, N., Yin, Y., Lanser, M. and Benowitz, L.I. (2003). Axon regeneration in goldfish and rat retinal ganglion cells: differential responsiveness to carbohydrates and cAMP. *J Neurosci*, **23**, 7830–7838.

Liesi, P., Kaakkola, S., Dahl, D. and Vaheri, A. (1984). Laminin is induced in astrocytes of adult brain by injury. *Embo J*, **3**, 683–686.

Logan, A., Frautschy, S.A., Gonzalez, A.M. and Baird, A. (1992). A time course for the focal elevation of synthesis of basic fibroblast growth factor and one if its high-affinity receptors (flg) following a localized cortical brain injury. *J Neurosci*, **12**, 3828–3837.

Mahler, M., Ben-Ari, Y. and Represa, A. (1997). Differential expression of fibronectin, tenascin-C and NCAMs in cultured hippocampal astrocytes activated by kainite, bacterial lipopolysaccharide or basic fibroblast growth factor. *Brain Res*, **775**, 63–73.

Margolis, R.K. and Margolis, R.U. (1993). Nervous tissue proteoglycans. *Experientia*, **49**, 429–446.

Mayes, D.A. and Houle, J.D. (2003). Combined use of matrix degrading enzymes and neurotrophic factors to facilitate axonal regeneration after spinal cord injury. Society for Neuroscience, Abstract No. 245.1.

McKeon, R.J., Schreiber, R.C., Rudge, J.S. and Silver, J. (1991). Reduction of neurite outgrowth in a model of glial scarring following CNS injury is correlated with the expression of inhibitory molecules on reactive astrocytes. *J Neurosci*, **11**, 3398–3411.

McKeon, R.J., Höke, A. and Silver, J. (1995). Injury-induced proteoglycan inhibit the potential for laminin-mediated axon growth on astrocytic scars. *Exper Neurol*, **136**, 32–43.

McKeon, R.J., Jurynec, M.J. and Buck, C.R. (1999). The chondroitin sulfate proteoglycans neurocan and phosphacan are expressed by reactive astrocytes in the chronic CNS glial scar. *J Neurosci*, **19**, 10778–10788.

Menet, V., Gimenéz y Ribotta, M., Chauvet, N., Drian, M.J., Lannoy, J., Colucci-Guyon, E. and Privat, A. (2001). Inactivation of the glial fibrillary acidic protein gene, but not that of vimentin, improves neuronal survival and neurite growth by modifying adhesion molecule expression. *J Neurosci*, **21**, 6147–6158.

Miyake, T., Hattori, T., Fukuda, M., Kitamura, T. and Fujita, S. (1988). Quantitative studies on proliferative changes of reactive astrocytes in mouse cerebral cortex. *Brain Res*, **451**, 133–138.

Mocchetti, I., Rabin, S.J., Colangelo, A.M., Whittemore, S.R. and Wrathall, J.R. (1996). Increased basic fibroblast growth factor expression following contusive spinal cord injury. *Exper Neurol*, **141**, 154–164.

Monnier, P.P., Sierra, A., Schwab, J.M., Henke-Fahle, S. and Mueller, B.K. (2003). The Rho/ROCK pathway mediates neurite growth-inhibitory activity associated with the chondroitin sulfate proteoglycans of the CNS glial scar. *Mol Cell Neurosci*, **22**, 319–330.

Monti Graziadei, G.A., Karlan, M.S., Bernstein, J.J. and Graziadei, P.P. (1980). Reinnervation of the olfactory bulb after section of the olfactory nerve in monkey (*Saimiri sciureus*). *Brain Res*, **189**, 343–354.

Moon, L.D.F. and Fawcett, J.W. (2001). Reduction in CNS scar formation without concomitant increase in axon regeneration following treatment of adult rat brain with a combination of antibodies to TGFβ1 and β2. *Eur J Neurosci*, **14**, 1667–1677.

Moon, L.D.F., Asher, R.A., Rhodes, K.E. and Fawcett, J.W. (2001). Regeneration of CNS axons back to their target following treatment of adult rat brain with chondroitinase ABC. *Nat Neurosci*, **4**, 465–466.

Moon, L.D.F., Asher, R.A., Rhodes, K.E. and Fawcett, J.W. (2002). Relationship between sprouting axons, proteoglycans and glial cells following unilateral nigrostriatal axotomy in the adult rat. *Neurosci*, **109**, 101–117.

Moreno-Flores, M.T., Martín-Aparicio, E., Salinero, O. and Wandosell, F. (2001). Fibronectin modulation by Aβ amyloid peptide (25–35) in cultured astrocytes of newborn rat cortex. *Neurosci Lett*, **314**, 87–91.

Morgenstern, D.A., Asher, R.A. and Fawcett, J.W. (2002). Chondroitin sulphate proteoglycans in the CNS injury response. *Prog Brain Res*, **137**, 313–332.

Morrison, E.E. and Costanzo, R.M. (1995). Regeneration of olfactory sensory neurons and reconnection in the aging hamster central nervous system. *Neurosci Lett*, **198**, 213–217.

Neumann, S., Bradke, F., Tessier-Lavigne, M. and Basbaum, A.I. (2002). Regeneration of sensory axons within the injured spinal cord induced by intraganglionic cAMP elevation. *Neuron*, **34**, 885–893.

Oudega, M. and Hagg, T. (1996). Nerve growth factor promotes regeneration of sensory axons into adult rat spinal cord. *Exper Neurol*, **140**, 218–229.

Oudega, M. and Hagg, T. (1999). Neurotrophins promote regeneration of sensory axons in the adult rat spinal cord. *Brain Res*, **818**, 431–438.

Pasterkamp, R.J., Giger, R.J., Ruitenberg, M.J., Holtmaat, A.J.G.D., De Wit, J., De Winter, F. and Verhaagen, J. (1999). Expression of the gene encoding the chemorepellent semaphoring III is induced in the fibroblast component of neural scar tissue formed following injuries of adult but not neonatal CNS. *Mol Cell Neurosci*, **13**, 143–166.

Pasterkamp, R.J., Anderson, P.N. and Verhaagen, J. (2001). Peripheral nerve injury fails to induce growth of lesioned ascending dorsal column axons into spinal cord scar tissue expressing the axon repellent Semaphorin3A. *Eur J Neurosci*, **13**, 457–471.

Pindzola, R.R., Doller, C. and Silver, J. (1993). Putative inhibitory extracellular matrix molecules at the dorsal root entry zone of the spinal cord during development and after root and sciatic nerve lesions. *Dev Biol*, **156**, 34–48.

Preston, E., Webster, J. and Small, D. (2001). Characteristics of sustained blood–brain barrier opening and tissue injury in a model for focal trauma in the rat. *J Neurotraum*, **18**, 83–92.

Qiu, J., Cai, D., Dai, H., McAtee, M., Hoffman, P.N., Bregman, B.S. and Filbin, M.T. (2002). Spinal axon regeneration induced by elevation of cyclic AMP. *Neuron*, **34**, 895–903.

Ramer, M.S., Priestly, J.V. and McMahon, S.B. (2000). Functional regeneration of sensory axons into the adult spinal cord. *Nature*, **403**, 312–316.

Ramer, M.S., Duraisingam, I., Priestley, J.V. and McMahon, S.B. (2001). Two-tiered inhibition of axon regeneration at the dorsal root entry zone. *J Neurosci*, **21**, 2651–2660.

Ramer, M.S., Bishop, T., Dockery, P., Mobarak, M.S., O'Leary, D., Fraher, J.P., Priestley, J.V. and McMahon, S.B. (2002). Neurotrophin-3-mediated regeneration and recovery of proprioception following dorsal rhizotomy. *Mol Cell Neurosci*, **19**, 239–249.

Ramón y Cajal. (1928). *Degeneration and Regeneration of the Nervous System*. (trans. May, R.M.), Oxford University Press, London.

Risling, M., Fried, K., Lindå, H., Carlstedt, T. and Cullheim, S. (1993). Regrowth of motor axons following spinal cord lesions: distribution of laminin and collagen in the CNS scar tissue. *Brain Res Bull*, **30**, 405–414.

Romero, M.I., Rangappa, N., Garry, M.G. and Smith, G.M. (2001). Functional regeneration of chronically injured sensory afferents into adult spinal cord after neurotrophin gene therapy. *J Neurosci*, **21**, 8408–8416.

Ronca, F., Anderson, J.S., Paech, V. and Margolis, R.U. (2001). Characterization of slit protein interactions with glypican-1. *J Biol Chem*, **276**, 29141–29147.

Rudge, J.S. and Silver, J. (1990). Inhibition of neurite outgrowth on astroglial scars *in vitro*. *J Neurosci*, **10**, 3594–3603.

Silver, J. and Miller, J.H. (2004). Regeneration beyond the glial scar. *Nat Rev Neurosci*, **5**, 146–156.

Smith, G. and Miller, R.H. (1991). Immature type-1 astrocytes suppress glial scar formation, are motile and interact with blood vessels. *Brain Res*, **543**, 111–122.

Smith, G. and Silver, J. (1988). Transplantation of immature and mature astrocytes and their effect on scar formation in the lesioned central nervous system. *Prog Brain Res*, **78**, 353–361.

Smith, G., Miller, R.H. and Silver, J. (1986). Changing role of forebrain astrocytes during development, regenerative failure, and induced regeneration upon transplantation. *J Comp Neurol*, **251**, 23–43.

Smith-Thomas, L.C., Fok-Seang, J., Stevens, J., Du, J.S., Muir, E., Faissner, A., Geller, H.M., Rogers, J.H. and Fawcett, J.W.

(1994). An inhibitor of neurite outgrowth produced by astrocytes. *J Cell Sci*, **107**, 1687–1695.

Snow, D.M. and Letourneau, P.C. (1992). Neurite outgrowth on a step gradient of chondroitin sulfate proteoglycan (CS-PG). *J Neurobiol*, **23**, 322–336.

Snow, D.M., Lemmon, V., Carrino, D.A., Caplan, A.I. and Silver, J. (1990a). Sulfated proteoglycans in astroglial barriers inhibit neurite outgrowth *in vitro*. *Exper Neurol*, **109**, 111–130.

Snow, D.M., Steindler, D.A. and Silver, J. (1990b). Molecular and cellular characterization of the glial roof plate of the spinal cord and optic tectum: a possible role for a proteoglycan in the development of an axon barrier. *Dev Biol*, **138**, 359–376.

Snow, D.M., Brown, E.M. and Letourneau, P.C. (1996). Growth cone behavior in the presence of soluble chondroitin sulfate proteoglycan (CSPG), compared to behavior on CSPG bound to laminin or fibronectin. *Int J Devl Neurosci*, **14**, 331–349.

Steinmetz, M.P., Tom, V.J., Miller, J.H., Horn, K.P., Grimpe, B. and Silver, J. (2003). A novel combinatorial strategy which dramatically influences axon regeneration across a model of the glial scar *in vitro*. Society for Neuroscience, Abstract No. 880.4.

Tang, X., Davies, J.E. and Davies, S.J.A. (2003). Changes in distribution, cell associations, and protein expression levels of NG2, neurocan, phosphacan, brevican, versican, V2, and tenascin-C during acute to chronic maturation of spinal cord scar tissue. *J Neurosci Res*, **71**, 427–444.

Tester, N.J., Plass, A.H. and Howland, D.R. (2003). Chondroitin sulfate glycosaminoglycans and the effects of chondroitinase ABC on behavioral and anatomical recovery following spinal cord injury in the adult cat. Society for Neuroscience, Abstract No. 744.17.

Tom, V.J., Doller, C.M. and Silver, J. (2002). Promoting regeneration of dystrophic axons. Society for Neuroscience, Abstract No. 635.14.

Tom, V.J., Doller, C.M. and Silver, J. (2003). Fibronectin is critical for axonal regeneration in white matter. Society for Neuroscience, Abstract No. 42.12.

Windle, W.F. (1956). Regeneration of axons in the vertebrate central nervous system. *Phys Rev*, **36**, 427–439.

Windle, W.F. and Chambers, W.W. (1950). Regeneration in the spinal cord of the cat and dog. *J Comp Neurol*, **93**, 241–258.

Windle, W.F., Clemente, C.D. and Chambers, W.W. (1952). Inhibition of formation of a glial barrier as a means of permitting a peripheral nerve to grow into the brain. *J Comp Neurol*, **96**, 359–369.

Wu, D.Y., Schneider, G.E., Silver, J., Poston, M. and Jhaveri, S. (1998). A role for tectal midline glia in the unilateral containment of retinocollicular axons. *J Neurosci*, **18**, 8344–8355.

Wyss-Coray, T., Feng, L., Masliah, E., Ruppe, M.D., Lee, H.S., Toggas, S.M., Rockenstein, E.M. and Mucke, L. (1995). Increased central nervous system production of extracellular matrix components and development of hydrocephalus in transgenic mice overexpressing transforming growth factor-beta 1. *Am J Pathol*, **147**, 53–67.

Xu, X.M., Guenard, V., Kleitman, N. and Bunge, M.B. (1995). Axonal regeneration into Schwann cell-seeded guidance channels grafted into transected adult rat spinal cord. *J Comp Neurol*, **351**, 145–160.

Yang, H.Y., Lieska, N., Shao, D., Kriho, V. and Pappas, G.D. (1994). Proteins of the intermediate filament cytoskeleton as markers for astrocytes and human astrocytomas. *Mol Chem Neuropathol*, **21**, 155–176.

Yin, Y., Cui, Q., Li, Y., Irwin, N., Fischer, D., Harvey, A.R. and Benowitz, L.I. (2003). Macrophage-derived factors stimulate optic nerve regeneration. *J Neurosci*, **23**, 2284–2293.

Yong, V.W., Moumdjian, R., Yong, F.P., Ruijs, T.C.G., Freedman, M.S., Cashman, N. and Antel, J.P. (1991). γ-Interferon promotes proliferation of adult human astrocytes *in vitro* and reactive gliosis in the adult mouse brain *in vivo*. *Proc Natl Acad Sci USA*, **88**, 7016–7020.

Zhang, Y., Dijkhuizen, P.A., Anderson, P.N., Lieberman, A.R. and Verhaagen, J. (1998). NT-3 delivered by an adenoviral vector induces injured dorsal root axons to regenerate into the spinal cord of adult rats. *J Neuroci Res*, **54**, 554–562.

23

Trophic factors and their influence on regeneration

Joel M. Levine and Lorne M. Mendell

Department of Neurobiology and Behavior, State University of New York at Stony Brook, Stony Brook, NY, USA

Developing neurons in both the central and peripheral nervous system face many challenges. They must migrate to their proper location, extend an axon towards their correct post-synaptic targets and survive a period of naturally occurring cell death. The neurotrophic hypothesis, a basic tenet of developmental neurobiology, states that as developing neurons extend axons to their target tissues, their survival becomes dependent on soluble factors released from the target tissues in limiting amounts. After injuries that sever axons, the damaged neurons face many of the same problems as developing axons, that is they must survive, extend an axon, and if function is to be restored, make synapses with correct target cells. Consequently, it has often been suggested that supplying exogenous neurotrophins (NTs) might have therapeutic value after traumatic injury to the nervous system. In this chapter, we review the biology of NTs and their receptors with an emphasis on their use to encourage nerve regeneration after damage to both the central and peripheral nervous system.

23.1 NT family and receptors

NTs are secreted growth and differentiation factors that bind directly to receptor complexes on their target cells and exert multiple downstream effects. The NT family consists of four highly conserved proteins that are found in all mammalian species: nerve growth factor (NGF), brain-derived neurotrophic factor (BDNF), neurotrophin-3 (NT3), and neurotrophin-4 (NT4). NTs are synthesized as pro-proteins that are cleaved intracellularly by furin proteases to generate the mature 13.5-kDa protein (for review, see Teng and Hempstead, 2004). Subunits form non-covalently linked dimers that are secreted. The structure of the biologically active dimer has been solved and it comprises a novel tertiary fold formed by 7 β-sheets organized into three anti-parallel strands and a cysteine knot. These structural motifs are not unique to the NT family as they are also found among members of the transforming growth factor β family as well as in platelet-derived growth factor. Although the prodomain is thought to promote the proper folding of the entire molecule and to help in sorting the molecule into secretory pathways, proNGF and proBDNF have been detected in mature mouse tissues (Lee et al., 2001). ProNGF can bind to the p75 receptor (see below) and this binding may lead to apoptosis.

NTs bind to a receptor complex comprised of two components: p75 and a tropomyosin-related kinase (Trk) transmembrane receptor protein tyrosine kinase. p75 is a member of the tumor necrosis factor (TNF) receptor superfamily and can bind all known NTs (for review, see Dechant and Barde, 2002). The Trk receptors, on the other hand, occur in three different forms that display a preference in their binding. TrkA binds only NGF (see Table 23. 1), TrkB binds both BDNF and NT4 and TrkC binds NT3. The extracellular domains of the different Trk receptors are similar in structure and contain an immunoglobulin-like domain that mediates ligand binding. They all contain a highly conserved intracellular tyrosine

Table 23.1. Summary of effects of NTs (Row 1) on different classes of injured neurons (Column 1). Details and reference citation in text.

	Trk receptors	NGF	BDNF/NT-4	*NT-3*
Motor axons	TrkB, TrkC		Enhances elongation via trkB; inhibits elongation via p75; enhanced conduction velocity	Enhanced conduction velocity-some species dependence
Sensory axons	TrkA, TrkB, TrkC	Enhanced nociceptor projections		Enhanced muscle spindle afferent projections/axonal conduction velocity
Corticospinal axons	TrkB, TrkC		Promotes survival; growth	Promotes sprouting
Rubrospinal axons	TrkB		Promotes survival; growth	
Vestibulospinal axons	TrkB		Promotes growth	
Reticulospinal axons	TrkB		Promotes growth	
Noradrenergic axons	TrkA		Promotes growth	
Serotonergic axons	TrkB		Promotes growth	

kinase domain. Although p75 is often described as a low-affinity receptor for NTs, it binds NTs with high affinity but with rapid kinetics. Its primary function is to augment NT binding to Trk receptors, but like other members of the TNF family, it also plays an important role in signaling apoptosis. These functions may be especially important when p75 is expressed without the Trk receptors. Ligand binding induces Trk subunit dimerization and the autophosphorylation of multiple tyrosine residues. This autophosphorylation initiates several different intracellular signaling cascades that are described below.

23.2 Cellular actions of neurotrophins and signal transduction

NGF was first identified and isolated using its ability to promote axon outgrowth as a bioassay (for a historical perspective, see Cowan, 2001; Levi-Montalcini, 1987). This neuritogenic property (the processes formed by a neuron in tissue culture are called neurites) remains a key hallmark of NT action. A second hallmark is cell survival. The initial proliferation and survival of sensory and sympathetic neurons is not dependent on NTs, but as axons reach their targets, these cells become dependent upon NTs for their survival. Removal of available NTs either with

antibodies or by genetic techniques increases naturally occurring cell death; conversely, over-expression of NTs leads to enhanced cell survival *in vivo*. Sympathetic neurons remain dependent on NGF throughout life but sensory neurons lose the requirement for NTs for survival as they mature. How these dual effects (neuritogenesis and cell survival) are initiated and maintained after ligand binding has been extensively studied. Here we briefly summarize those studies. Readers are referred to several recent reviews for a more detailed treatment of this subject (Huang and Reichardt, 2001; Segal, 2003). NT binding also leads to changes in gene expression but this topic is not considered further here.

Much of what we know about NT signaling comes from studies using the PC12 cell line. PC12 is an immortalized cell line derived from a spontaneously arising rat pheochromocytoma (Greene and Tischler, 1976). These cells proliferate indefinitely, but after the addition of NGF, they slowly cease dividing and begin to differentiate into neurite-bearing cells that closely resemble sympathetic neurons. Unlike cells from the embryonic peripheral nervous system (PNS), PC12 cells do not need NGF for survival. Therefore it is possible to study the signal transduction events initiated by NT binding.

NGF binding to TrkA receptors on PC12 cells activates three separate canonical signaling cascades.

While it is tempting to conjecture that each cascade results in different downstream effects (Markus et al., 2002), there is considerable cross-talk between each pathway and overlap in their physiological effects. The autophosphorylation of tyrosine785 on TrkA recruits phospholipase Cγ (PLCγ) to the membrane where it is phosphorylated by the activated Trk receptors. This activates the enzyme leading to increases in intracellular calcium and the activation of protein kinase C (PKC). A second major signaling pathway activated by NGF binding is the Ras-Raf-Mek-Erk pathway. Tyrosine phosphorylation of the intracellular domain of Trk receptors creates docking sites for adapter proteins including Shc, Grb-2, and SOS. The activation of SOS leads to the activation of Ras which in turn activates the Raf-Mek-Erk kinase cascade. Activated Erk in turn can trigger cAMP response element binding protein (CREB) resulting in changes in gene transcription. Lastly, the recruitment of Grb-2 by activated Trk receptors leads to the activation of PI3K. PI3K can also be activated by Ras. An important downstream target of PI3K is Akt/protein kinase B, which plays a major role in cell survival.

The functions of these three different signaling pathways in mediating the survival and differentiation effects of NTs have been investigated using pharmacological and genetic means. Several general principles have emerged from these studies. First, the activation of the Ras-Raf-Mek-Erk pathway is required for axon outgrowth (Cowley et al., 1994). Although this requirement for Ras has been demonstrated using both gain-of-function and loss-of-function approaches, the mechanism by which activated Ras influences the cytoskeletal organelles necessary for growth remains unknown. As there is considerable cross-talk between Ras and the Rho family GTPases that control cytoskeletal dynamics, this may be one means of regulating axon extension (Bar-Sagi and Hall, 2000). p75 may also participate in the regulation the cytoskeleton (see below). Second, the PI3K/Akt pathway mediates cell survival (Kaplan and Miller, 2000). Pre-apoptotic proteins such as Bad and caspase-9 are inactivated by Akt phosphorylation as is FKHRL1, a forkhead-family

transcription factor that regulates the expression of fas ligand (FasL). The PI3K pathway may also regulate the cytoskeletal reorganization necessary for axon turning and branching since phosphatidyl inositides regulate the rac GTPase. Lastly, although a direct role for the PLCγ pathway in either differentiation or survival has not yet been demonstrated, the downstream activation of PKC can lead to the activation of mek. Furthermore, the increases in intracellular calcium resulting from PLCγ activation in growth cones are likely to have diverse effects on cytoskeletal form and function (Doherty et al., 2000).

An important consideration in evaluating the action of NTs is the specific site on the neuron where signaling is activated. Classical studies using compartmentalized cultures of sympathetic and sensory neurons showed that the application of NTs to one axonal branch stimulated growth in that branch only, and that a signal travels retrogradely from the distal axon to the cell body to promote cell survival (Campenot, 1982a,b). This retrograde signal is likely to be a complex of ligand bound to activated Trk receptors contained within a signaling endosome (Grimes et al., 1996). Retrograde signaling activates PI3K and erk5 in the cell body leading to cell survival. NTs applied locally to the distal ends of axons may modify growth cone functions such as sprouting and turning (Gallo and Letourneau, 1998). Thus when considering the use of exogenous NTs to repair or protect damaged neurons, it is important to realize that *where* these agents are applied will have a direct bearing on possible therapeutic outcomes.

23.3 Negative effects of p75 on cell survival and growth

A major but not exclusive function of the p75 receptor subunit is to signal cell death (for review, see Hempstead, 2004). Because the intracellular domain of p75 does not have any known enzymatic or catalytic activities, cell death must be the result of ligand-induced protein-protein interactions. Ligand binding to p75 activates the well-known cell death pathway of c-jun N terminal kinase (JNK) which acts via p53 to activate cell death genes such as Bax. Ligand binding to p75 may also create docking sites for other cell death proteins (Hempstead, 2004). NT binding to Trk receptors silences the p75-mediated activation of the JNK-p53-Bax pathway while increasing the activation of the anti-apoptotic NF-κB transcription factor. Thus, survival or death is regulated by a balance between p75-mediated signaling and Trk mediated signaling. It is important to note, however, that proNTs that might be released after cell damage are preferential ligands for p75 and are more effective than fully processed NT dimers in activating cell death pathways (Lee et al., 2001).

p75 can also play an important role as a negative regulator of axon growth by virtue of its interactions with the rho GTPase (Yamashita et al., 1999). Rho is a key regulator of the structure of the actin-cytoskeleton that when activated, induces contraction of actin-myosin networks resulting in growth cone collapse and failure of axon extension (Hall, 1998). Myelin-associated growth inhibitory proteins found in the glial scar (see below) bind to a receptor complex comprising p75 and the nogo receptor protein (Wang et al., 2002). Ligand binding to this complex activates rho; however, NTs can reduce this activation and they do so as a result of their interactions with p75 not with Trk receptors (Yamashita and Tohyama, 2003). Thus, the binding of different ligands to p75 can activate different signaling pathways that have multiple consequences for the cells.

It is clear from this brief discussion that the effects of NTs on their target cells are complex and can vary according to the ligand being considered, according to the repertoire of receptors expressed by the cells, and according to the manner in which NTs are presented to the cells. These factors must be taken into account when considering the therapeutic use of these agents. For example, whilst exogenous NTs might stimulate terminal sprouting from damaged axon ends, they also have the potential to activate cell death pathways in neighboring neurons and glia that express p75 without the appropriate Trk receptor. Full recovery from spinal cord injury will require repair of both the damaged neuronal and glial elements and exogenous NTs can well affect both.

23.4 NTs and regeneration of peripheral axons

Damaged peripheral axons undergo a characteristic sequence of morphological and physiological changes. In very young animals or if the damage is close to the cell body, that is at the level of the roots, many cells die (see Hammarberg et al., 2000). If the cell survives in the immediate aftermath of the injury, the proximal stump of both sensory and motor or sympathetic axons retracts and there are a characteristic set of changes in the cell body known as chromatolysis. The cell body enlarges, the nucleus moves from a central to an eccentric position, and there are increases in RNA and protein content and in the number of free ribosomes. These changes indicate that the cell is now making the proteins and organelles necessary to reform and regrow an axon. The distal axonal segment undergoes Wallerian degeneration, leaving behind an endoneurial tube filled with Schwann cells. Most cells then display regeneration of the proximal portion of the axon at rates as high as 1 mm/day. Because of the role of target derived NTs in assuring survival of these axons during late stage development (Huang and Reichardt, 2001), it has been hypothesized that axotomy-induced deficits might be caused by a loss of neurotrophic support from the periphery, and that they might therefore be reversed by providing an exogenous source of NTs to the proximal stump. Indeed, disruption of the normal retrograde flow of NTs can lead to chromatolytic changes without cutting the axon, and if neuronal cell bodies are supplied exogenous NTs, they do not undergo chromatolysis after axonal injury (Nja and Purves, 1978). NTs also prevent cell death and can reverse the atrophy of cells in a NT-receptor specific manner (Verge et al., 1996; Terenghi, 1999; Boyd and Gordon, 2003). Furthermore, they can encourage elongation of the axon. Thus in evaluating the effect of NT replacement, it is necessary in some cases to consider the effects on both survival and regeneration whereas in other conditions survival is assured and regeneration is the only variable in play.

Motor neurons

The most complete studies of regeneration of peripheral neurons have been carried out on motor neurons. Motor neurons express TrkB, TrkC and p75 and the ability of both BDNF and NT3 to effect survival and regeneration has been studied extensively. Various models of injury have been used, including sciatic or tibial nerve transection in adults and in neonates, as well as ventral root (VR) avulsions.

Survival

The reduced survival of motor neurons that would normally occur after VR axotomy in neonates can be reversed by exogenously provided BDNF (Sendtner et al., 1992; Koliatsos et al., 1993; Yan et al., 1993; see Volume I, Chapter 16). However, this rescue is transient since the NT treated motor neurons do not survive beyond 4–5 weeks of age (Vejsada et al., 1998). NT-4/5, also acting through trkB been found to promote survival of neonatal motor neurons (Hughes et al., 1993). NT-3 has more varied effects on survival with some results indicating effects equal to those of BDNF, others indicating smaller effects (Hughes et al., 1993; Yan et al., 1993), and still others indicating no effect of NT-3 (Koliatsos et al., 1993). Although not discussed at length in this chapter, another trophic factor, glial derived neurotrophic factor (GDNF) also promotes survival of axotomized neonatal motor neurons (Vejsada et al., 1998), and when it is provided continuously after infection with engineered lentiviruses, survival can be prolonged up to 3 months (Hottinger et al., 2000). Treatment with either GDNF or BDNF prevents motor neuron cell death after spinal root avulsion in adult rats with this action being associated with upregulation of c-Jun and p75 and inhibition of neuronal nitric oxide synthase (nNOS) expression (Wu et al., 2003). The relevance of the increase in p75 is not clear since the BDNF-stimulated rescue from cell death does not occur in trkB$-/-$ mice suggesting that BDNF is acting through the trkB and not the p75 receptor (Alcantara et al., 1997).

Regeneration

When a peripheral nerve is damaged, NTs and their receptors undergo substantial changes in expression both peripherally in the distal stump and centrally in the motoneurons themselves. The motoneurons express enhanced levels of BDNF and trkB and p75 receptors, as do Schwann cells in the distal stump (Funakoshi et al., 1993; Hammarberg et al., 2000; see Volume I, Chapter 27). Motorneurons express a full length trkB receptor, whereas Schwann cells express a truncated form of trkB without the tyrosine kinase domain. This receptor binds BDNF but is unable to exert a cellular effect.

There is considerable evidence that BDNF enhances the regenerative potential of motor axons *in vivo* (Novikov, Novikova and Kellerth, 1997; Boyd and Gordon, 2001). To determine the relative contributions of TrkB and p75 receptors to this effect, Boyd and Gordon (2001) compared the kinetics of motor axon regeneration after nerve transection in p75$-/-$ and wild type mice. Careful analysis of the dose response relationship for regeneration in rats has revealed a biphasic relationship with low doses of BDNF (1–4 μg/day) facilitating regeneration and higher doses (>4 μg/day) inhibiting it (Boyd and Gordon, 2002). They observed more rapid onset and more extensive regeneration in the p75$-/-$ mice than in wild type suggesting an inhibitory effect of p75 activation. Another indication of the inhibitory effect associated with the p75 is the finding that blocking this receptor with the REX antibody eliminated the selective inhibitory effect of BDNF on axonal regeneration observed in response to administration of high doses of this NT (Boyd and Gordon, 2002). These effects are consistent with the idea that signaling through p75 can activate the Rho GTPase and negatively affect cytoskeletal dynamics in growth cones to compromise the ability of the axon to regenerate (see section on *Negative effects of p75 …*).

Axotomized motoneurons exhibit a substantial decline in axonal conduction velocity which recovers to normal values when they re-establish contact with the periphery (e.g., Mendell et al., 1995). A role for Trk receptors in this process was demonstrated by Munson et al. (1997). The activation of trkB improved recovery (or prevented decline) of conduction velocity of axotomized motor axons. Furthermore, these same investigators found that depriving *intact* motor axons of access to trkB ligands by provision of the immunoadhesin trkB-IgG reduced their conduction velocity in much the same way as axotomy.

NT-3 was found to enhance conduction velocity of axotomized motor axons in adult rat although not as effectively as trkB ligands (Munson et al., 1997). A similar series of experiments in cat revealed no effects of NT-3 on motor axons or properties of motor neurons (Mendell et al., 1999). Together, these experiments point to an important role for trkB ligands in the maintenance of motor axon properties in rats.

23.5 Sensory neurons

When a peripheral nerve is cut, sensory axons are also damaged and can undergo regeneration. The situation is more complex than in the case of the motor neurons since there are two processes (one centrally projecting and one peripheral) originating from the cell body that sits outside of the central nervous system (CNS) in the dorsal root ganglion (DRG). The regeneration of the peripherally directed process is well established but there is little long-distance growth of sensory axons within the CNS. The action of NTs on the regeneration of the peripherally projecting process of sensory neurons has not been examined, most likely because these processes are well known to normally regenerate. However, there is considerable evidence that NTs can enhance the regeneration of the centrally projecting axon branch. After a dorsal root (DR) crush injury, application by osmotic minipump of either NT3 or NGF but not BDNF to the dorsal root entry zone (DREZ) caused regenerating fibers to enter the spinal cord, something they do not do in the absence of NT support. Viral induction of NT3 expression was also effective (Zhang et al., 1998). In these cases, regenerating fibers grew within the spinal gray matter as

deep as lamina 5. The intrathecal application of NT3 to the crushed dorsal columns was able to stimulate large and medium diameter sensory axons to grow through and past the injury site for distances as long as 4 mm (Bradbury et al., 1999). Most of this growth was through the gray matter ventral to the normal pathway of these fibers although some axons did grow through the white matter of the dorsal columns, albeit in a highly disorganized fashion. As was the case after DR crush, BDNF was ineffective in this model although it is possible that the cholera toxin labeling methods used do not efficiently label the TrkB expressing afferents.

Because sensory fibers mediating different functional modalities (e.g., muscle stretch receptors, nociceptors) project to highly precise targets in the spinal cord (Willis and Coggeshall, 2004), they provide a valuable model system to investigate issues related to specificity of CNS regeneration, which is one of the crucial issues in re-establishing function after axonal damage. The specificity of individual NTs in assuring survival of selected classes of sensory afferents (e.g., NGF and nociceptors; NT-3 and muscle stretch afferents: Mendell, 1995; Lindsay, 1996) as well as the selective expression of trk receptors on sensory neurons (nociceptors express trkA; muscle stretch receptors express trkC: (McMahon et al., 1994)) has prompted considerable examination of their possible role in eliciting selective regeneration of sensory afferents into the spinal cord. Such treatments have been shown to result in the establishment of functional connections in the dorsal horn (measured electrophysiologically) and the recovery of sensory function, which is specific for the NT treatment. For example, treatment with intrathecally applied NGF or GDNF, but not BDNF or NT-3, resulted in recovery of thermal and mechanical nociception from the affected dermatomes (Ramer et al., 2000). More recently, this group (Ramer et al., 2002) has shown that intrathecal NT-3 results in recovery of proprioception after dorsal rhizotomy. Regenerating axons grow through the dorsal horn in a dorsolateral to ventromedial direction reaching as far as lamina X. Interestingly, some ectopic boutons were detected in laminae

Adult cat

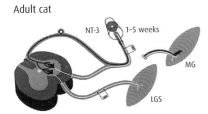

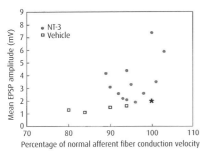

Figure 23.1. Experimental arrangement to demonstrate the effects of NT-3 applied to the cut end of the medial gastrocnemius (MG) nerve using an osmotic minipump. 1–5 weeks after axotomy and placement of the pump a terminal electrophysiological experiment was carried out on anesthetized cats where the treated axotomized medial gastrocnemious nerve was stimulated and intracellular recordings were made from intact motoneurons innervating the lateral gastrocnemius-soleus (LGS) muscles. Graph illustrates the results. The mean amplitude of the monosynaptic excitatory postsynaptic potential (EPSP) in controls in this system is 2 mV (*) and the afferent conduction velocity is 100% of normal (by definition). Axotomized MG nerves treated with vehicle in the osmotic minipump (□) exhibited a decline in conduction velocity to as low as 80% of normal and the mean EPSP amplitude across the motoneurons sampled in these experiments was always less than normal. However, if the nerve was treated with NT-3 (●), the decline in conduction velocity was less and the mean amplitude of the monosynaptic EPSP in these experiments was often substantially larger than the mean values in controls. Each square and circle represents mean data from up to 22 motoneurons in a single cat. Results adapted from Mendell et al. (1999).

I and II but pain behavior was not reported to be abnormal.

When a peripheral nerve is cut, the conduction velocity of the damaged fibers declines and the synapses made by their central terminals in the spinal

cord undergo a decrease in efficacy. This has been studied most carefully for synapses made by group Ia fibers on motoneurons (Eccles et al., 1959; Mendell et al., 1995). These fibers depend on the availability of NT-3 for survival during late fetal development (Kucera et al., 1995; Oakley et al., 1995) and continue to express trkC throughout adult life (Bergman et al., 1996). In line with this, the decrease in axonal conduction velocity in the proximal stump of the peripheral nerve and in the efficacy of central synapses of group Ia fibers on motoneurons can be prevented by providing NT-3 (but not NT-4) on the proximal stump of the transected peripheral nerve in the popliteal fossa (Munson et al., 1997; Mendell et al., 1999) (Fig. 23. 1). The effects associated with exogenous NT-3 disappear within about 1 week of its removal.

It is known that injured sensory and motor neurons increase their rate of axonal transport of NTs from the periphery via receptor-mediated mechanisms (Curtis et al., 1998) and it seems likely that these enhanced NT levels increase the ability of the cell body in the DRG to make proteins responsible for axon growth and synaptic machinery. Other evidence for this role for NT-3 comes from studies during development where it has been found that enhancement of NT-3 levels by intrathecal administration enhances the strength of the direct projection from intact segmental stretch afferents and descending fibers in the ventrolateral funiculus (VLF) to motoneurons (Arvanian et al., 2003) (Fig. 23. 2). Removal of NT-3 prevents normal development of spindle projections to motoneurons (Seebach et al., 1999).

23.6 Summary of NT effects on peripheral neurons

It is now clear that NTs can play several roles in promoting regeneration of peripheral neurons. They can accelerate the regenerative process of motor neurons into the distal stump of the peripheral nerve. But perhaps more importantly for their possible use in stimulating the regeneration of centrally projecting axons, they can apparently encourage peripheral axons to enter the CNS and grow for

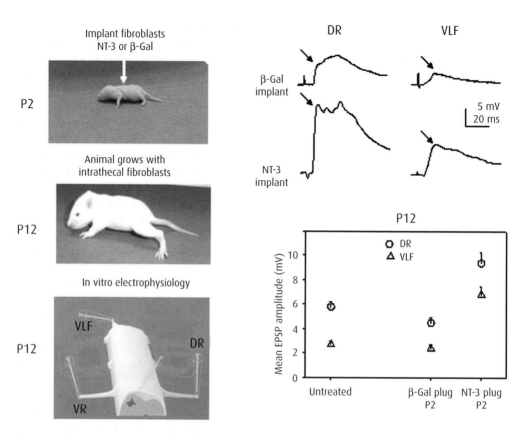

Figure 23.2. Experimental analysis of effects of intrathecally applied NT-3 on synaptic transmission in the spinal cord of neonatal rats. The fibroblast plugs engineered to secrete either β-Gal or NT-3 were inserted at P2 and the rats were prepared for electrophysiological recording at P12. The dissected left hemicord was placed in a dish with L5 (DR) and (VRs) and VLF drawn into suction electrodes for stimulation. Motoneurons impaled with sharp electrodes were identified by antidromic response to VR stimulation. Typical EPSPs are shown with arrows denoting the monosynaptic component (adapted from Arvanian et al., 2003). Graph documents the enlarged mean EPSPs from both DR and VLF in cords exposed to NT-3 compared to untreated or β-Gal-treated control rats.

some distance. Furthermore, the initial indication from electrophysiological and behavioral evidence is that regeneration into the spinal cord of sensory neurons encouraged by NTs is to targets that are appropriate for the modality of the peripheral receptor supplied by the regenerating fibers.

23.7 NTs and central axons

Unlike damaged peripheral axons, damaged CNS axons do not spontaneously regenerate. Rather the

ends of the damaged axons retract and then attempt to extend. This attempt is almost always unsuccessful and the cut ends enlarge forming characteristic end-bulbs (Ramon y Cajal, 1928). This failure is due to both the low intrinsic capacity of adult CNS neurons to regrow (see Volume I, Chapter 24) and the growth inhibitory conditions that develop at the site of injury (see Volume I, Chapters 21 and 22). Despite this low intrinsic capacity, studies carried out over the past 25 years or so have shown that central axons are able to elongate if an appropriate environment is provided (David and Aguayo, 1981). The most favorable environment is the Schwann cell tube that forms in the distal segment of a transected peripheral nerve although olfactory ensheathing glial may also provide a highly favorable substrate for regrowth. (Keyvan-Fouladi et al., 2003). The Schwann cells provide both a surface or substrate for growth and elevated levels of NTs. In this section, we summarize and evaluate attempts at using exogenous NTs to enhance axon regeneration and repair after spinal cord injury.

23.8 NTs and cell survival

After spinal cord injury, the cell bodies of cells whose axons form the rubrospinal or corticospinal tract (CST) atrophy but whether or not there is substantial cell death remains controversial. Injuries at the cervical level, which are close to neuronal cell bodies in the midbrain may induce cell death whereas injuries in the caudal regions of the cord may only induce cellular atrophy (Kwon et al., 2002). There is considerable evidence that the administration of exogenous NTs can promote the survival of neurons that would ordinarily die or atrophy after axonal injury (see Volume I, Chapter 16). For example, Kobayashi et al. (1997) found that red nucleus neurons, which express TrkB, could be rescued from axotomy-induced atrophy by the direct infusion of NT4/5 or BDNF into the midbrain. This atrophic state may be sustained for long periods of time and treatment with BDNF at intervals as long as 1 year after injury can still be an effective means of rescue (Kwon et al., 2002). The implication of this finding is that TrkB receptors remain functional on the soma of axotomized red nucleus neurons for some time after axotomy. This has been found for both rubrospinal (Liebl et al., 2001) and corticospinal (Lu et al., 2001) neuron cell bodies, although in both cases the TrkB expression on axons changes to a truncated form. NTs may therefore be effective when used at long intervals after the initial injury but may need to be delivered to the cell body where the full length receptor is expressed.

Although these studies suggest a role for NTs as survival factors after injury, it is important to note that in contrast to the PNS, the genetic deletion of NTs or their receptors has surprisingly few effects on the survival of populations of developing CNS neurons. For example, cholinergic neurons of the basal forebrain, whose differentiation is dependent upon NGF, survive well in the absence of NGF (Fagan et al., 1997). Apoptosis among cerebellar granule neurons is modestly increased in either BDNF−/− or TrkB−/− mice leading to abnormal foliation (Schwartz et al., 1997, Bates et al., 1999). BDNF and TrkB do play a substantial role in the development of cortical dendrites (McAllister et al., 1997) and in synaptic plasticity (Kang and Schuman, 1995). Little is known about the potential of NTs to influence either the survival or differentiation of the cells whose axons descend into the spinal cord and control motor function although there is evidence that NT3 enhances sprouting of developing corticospinal axons (Schnell et al., 1994).

23.9 Expression of NT receptors and release of NTs after injury

A consideration in evaluating the use of NTs is whether the expression of NTs and their receptors is changed by spinal cord injury. Changes in the levels of Trk and p75 receptors will alter the cellular response to exogenously applied NTs. Liebl et al. (2001) found significant declines in the expression of TrkA, TrkB and TrkC mRNA expression within 1 day of a contusion injury to the spinal cord. This decline was within the contusion itself; regions flanking the contusion site displayed no changes in Trk expression. At 42 days after the injury, the ependymal cells and astrocytes surrounding cysts at the contusion site expressed truncated TrkB transcripts lacking the intracellular tyrosine kinase domain. A similar decline in TrkB expression (as well as TrkA and TrkC) was found after a midthoracic hemisection (King et al., 2000). These investigators also found enhanced levels of truncated TrkB in regions surrounding the hemisection. In addition they detected elevated levels of p75 in the zone of injury reaching a peak 2 weeks after the hemisection.

While this may be due in part to the migration of Schwann cells into the injured region, it is also possible that p75 is expressed by any of the other cell types that populate the damaged site such as oligodendrocytes and their precursors. These data suggest that BDNF application at the contusion site might be ineffective, initially because of the absence of TrkB receptors, and later because the truncated receptors and p75 would bind the exogenously administered BDNF.

Another consideration is the possibility that endogenous NTs and proNTs can be released by cellular elements as a result of injury. Dougherty et al. (2000) demonstrated that an enhanced number of glia (astrocytes, oligodendrocytes and microglia) were immunoreactive for BDNF at the site of a compression injury. Immunoreactive glial, mostly oligodendrocytes, were found up to 20 mm rostral to the injury. In some cases, the number of BDNF-expressing glia remained elevated for up to 6 weeks after the injury. Although these findings suggest that these glia can be an endogenous source of NTs, there is presently no direct evidence that glial cells secrete or release NT in either the normal or injured spinal cord.

23.10 Effects after acute or chronic injury

An issue of both theoretical and practical significance concerns the ability of injured neurons to respond to NT treatment at different times after lesion. Since axotomized supraspinal cells can enter an inactive but non-degenerative state, it is possible that they can be rescued by delayed treatment with NTs. Such treatments usually involve resection or removal of the scar tissue that has formed around the lesion site and reinjuring any surviving axons. Removal of the scar may itself be beneficial since it could reduce inhibitory influences on axon regeneration. In general, delaying treatment after the injury reduces the extent of regeneration. NT-3 treatment in conjunction with antibodies that neutralize myelin-associated inhibitors of axon growth was more successful if initiated 2 weeks after the lesion than 8 weeks after the lesion

(von Meyenburg et al., 1998), but the effect of fibroblasts engineered to secrete NT-3 was found to be similar whether treatment was begun 1 or 3 months after injury (Grill et al., 1997). Coumans et al. (2001) reported that growth of axons into the distal stump is enhanced if the implantation of the fetal spinal cord and NT treatment is delayed for 2 or 4 weeks after the transection. Both BDNF and NT3 were able to encourage regeneration of red nucleus axons into growth-permissive peripheral nerve grafts 4–8 weeks after the initial injury (Ye and Houle, 1997). These studies suggest that individual growth factors may operate through different mechanisms, which are important only at certain windows of time after injury. It will be important to extend these experiments to longer times.

23.11 Administration of exogenous NTs

One must also consider how and where exogenous NTs are administered to the experimentally damaged spinal cord. Since NTs are large molecules, they cannot pass through the blood brain barrier (except possibly for a short time after the injury before the blood brain barrier is re-established) and thus must be introduced either to the lesion site or to the cell body of the damaged neurons. Tissue culture studies suggest that NTs can have differential effects depending on whether they are given to the cell body of developing neurons or to the tips of growing axons (Campeneot, 1982a, b) several delivery methods have proven effective *in vivo*. Some authors have inserted gelfoam soaked in NT (von Meyenburg et al., 1998; Novikova et al., 2002). Others have used osmotic minipumps to deliver the NT intrathecally (Xu et al., 1995; Jakeman et al., 1998). Fibroblasts (Grill et al., 1997) or stem cells (Liu et al., 1999; Blesch et al., 2002) genetically engineered to express a NT such as BDNF or NT-3 have been implanted with positive effects on axonal regeneration. Yet another approach has been to inject adeno-associated viruses (AAV) containing cDNAs encoding NT-3 or BDNF into the caudal stump of the transected spinal cord (Blits et al., 2003). The infected cells (mostly neurons) subsequently secrete the NTs over extended time courses. A more complex treatment has involved using short segments of intercostal nerve transduced with non replicating adenoviruses engineered to express NT-3 to serve as a bridge (Blits et al., 2000). Few studies have directly compared the effects of these different methods of NT administration but it seems important to do so.

23.12 How to analyze the effects of NTs

Before we consider the effects of different NTs on individual fiber tracts within the damaged spinal cord, we want to consider the question of how best to evaluate the effects of NT treatment. Given the many potential problems involved in demonstrating axon regeneration after spinal cord injury (Steward et al., 2003), the importance of this cannot be overstated. Axon regeneration can be studied anatomically using either the anterograde or retrograde transport of tracer substances. These methods allow for the labeling of specific neuronal populations such as corticospinal neurons originating in the cortex or rubrospinal neurons projecting from the midbrain. The injection of cholera toxin B subunit into the sciatic nerve has also been used effectively to label the centrally projecting axons of large diameter mechanosensory neurons. In the case of axons from the locus coeruleus or raphe, immunostaining for noradrenaline or serotonin could be carried out in the implant or in the distal stump to evaluate the density of innervation. In this case, however, the possibility that some of these fibers originate from local interneurons in the spinal gray matter cannot be excluded.

Axon regeneration should result in enhanced behavioral recovery (see Volume I, Chapter 30), and many studies have used the Basso, Beattie and Bresnahan (BBB) score to measure the effects of NT treatment. This test measures hindlimb locomotion in an open field environment (Basso et al., 1995). Although this test is considered a good measure of CST function and relatively free of motivational issues (Metz et al., 2000; Schucht et al., 2002), the scale is not a linear function of performance, but rather represents performance on increasingly complex tasks. Grid walking and footprint analysis are two commonly used tasks that are considered more quantitative than the BBB score. In the case of either transection or contusion injuries, behavioral improvement could depend on segmental or intersegmental reflexes wholly within the distal stump of the cord rather than on descending propriospinal or supraspinal fibers. NTs might affect these reflexes via direct effects on the function of spinal synapses (Mendell and Arvanian, 2002; Garraway et al., 2003) or by encouraging the remyelination of any spared axons (McTigue et al., 1998). Few if any studies have combined anatomy, behavior, and electrophysiological methods.

23.13 Specificity of effects: NTs; fiber tracts

The specificity of different NTs in promoting regeneration of different functional classes of DR fibers (see above) suggests that spinal axons should also be selectively responsive to different NTs. The ability of different NTs to promote the regeneration of different functional classes of spinal axons will depend on the Trk receptors expressed by those axons. For example, NGF has been found to affect the growth of sensory and noradrenergic axons but not corticospinal or raphespinal axons (Grill et al., 1997). Developing and adult corticospinal neurons express both TrkC and TrkB. NT3 acts as a sprouting factor for developing CST axons and it can induce the local sprouting of injured CST axons within the adult spinal cord. (Schnell and Schwab, 1993; Grill et al., 1997; von Meyenburg et al., 1998). Both a single injection of NT3 (Schnell et al., 1994) or continuous infusion from fibroblasts transfected to secrete NT3 (Tuszynski et al., 2003) have been shown to induce the sprouting of damaged CST fibers within the cord. NT3 has also been applied together with fetal spinal cord implants, Schwann cell containing minichannels, and denervated peripheral nerve grafts (Blits et al., 2000; Bamber et al., 2001; Coumans et al., 2001). Increased numbers of CST axons were found within the fetal grafts and Schwann cell mini-channels as compared to control treatments but not within peripheral nerve grafts. In some cases, there was also increased axonal growth around the lesion, through the gray matter, and into the distal cord for distances as long as 6 mm (Bamber et al., 2001). This growth may be sufficient to modify local circuits within the spinal cord since there were modest improvements in hindlimb function as assayed by the BBB and grid walking tests. Curiously, NT3 did not induce the sprouting of CST axons without a prior injury (Zhou et al., 2003). The failure of large numbers of axons to exit the distal graft/spinal cord interface and the growth through gray rather than white matter suggests that NT3 is acting locally to promote sprouting from damaged axons and that this stimulus is not sufficient to allow the axons to overcome the growth inhibitory environment of the glial scar.

Using similar methods, BDNF and NT4/5 have been shown to be an effective stimulus for the modest regrowth of reticulospinal, vestibulospinal and rubrospinal axons, all of which express TrkB (Menei et al., 1998; Jin et al., 2002). When applied to the cell body of lesioned rubrospinal neurons, BDNF promoted axon growth into peripheral nerve grafts. Application in the vicinity of the damaged axon ends also promoted growth into Schwann cell channels or into implants of fetal spinal cord cells. In this latter case, BDNF also enhanced the ingrowth of corticospinal axons (Bregman et al., 1997). The intrathecal infusion of BDNF for 28 days after contusion or transection injury to the spinal cord has been shown to lead to improvements in performance in open field locomotion tests. When Schwann cells were transfected to express BDNF and then implanted as trails, a small number of axons originating in the brainstem reticular and raphe nuclei were able to grow along the trails for as long as 5 mm. The effectiveness of BDNF when combined with a Schwann cell trail points to the need to provide damaged axons with a growth-permissive substrate as well as with trophic support.

These effects on specific descending tracts suggest that treatments with different NTs could have different motor effects. Vestibulospinal and reticulospinal tracts belong to the "medial" descending system and are largely concerned with mediating postural movements carried out by axial muscles (Lawrence and Kuypers, 1968a,b). The corticospinal and rubrospinal tracts belong to the lateral descending system and mediate voluntary movements carried out largely by distal muscles. The evaluation of the behavioral effects of NT treatments in spinal injured preparations may benefit from separate evaluation of postural and phasic movements rather than combining them into a single measure such as the BBB score.

23.14 Summary

In this chapter, we have tried to answer the question of *do exogenous NTs enhance repair and recovery after spinal cord injury*. As they do during development, exogeous NTs support the survival of damaged CNS neurons. In the well-studied case of motor neurons whose peripherally projecting axons have been damaged, BDNF acts as a survival factor and enhances the rate of nerve regeneration. Other trkB ligands (NT4/5) prevent the reduction in axon conduction velocity that is normally associated with peripheral nerve injury. After injury to the DR, the regrowth of the centrally projecting processes is also enhanced by exogenous NTs, which act in a modality-specific manner to restore segmental connections within the spinal cord. The role of NTs in supporting long-distance regeneration of damaged central axons, whether they originate in the cortex, brain-stem, or sensory ganglia, is less certain. Although NTs increase the extent of axon growth into permissive environments formed by either fetal implants or Schwann cell channels, growth out of the implant or graft and into the host is rarely observed, and if it occurs at all, is sparse at best. Consistent with this modest effect on axon regeneration, effects on functional recovery are also modest and could be due to a modification of existing circuits and synapses rather that the reformation of damaged connections.

As discussed elsewhere in this volume, the glial scar remains a formidable barrier to axon regeneration (see Volume I, Chapter 22). Much current research is aimed at understanding the nature of the molecules at the glial scar that create this growth non-permissive environment and to developing strategies to overcome these barriers. As discussed above, NT3 treatment results in axon sprouting within the gray matter. Axons grow around the scar but not through it. These results suggest that treatments with NTs alone may not be sufficient to allow CNS axons to overcome the inhibitory influences of the glial scar. Combining NT treatment with other agents that can reduce the barrier functions of the glial scar may be an important future direction.

ACKNOWLEDGEMENTS

The authors were supported by the NIH (JML, LMM), Christopher Reeve Paralysis Foundation (JML, LMM) and the New York State Spinal Cord Injury Board (JML).

REFERENCES

Alcantara, S., Frisen, J., del Rio, J.A., Soriano, E., Barbacid, M. Silos-Santiago, I. (1997). TrkB signaling is required for postnatal survival of CNS neurons and protects hippocampal and motor neurons from axotomy-induced cell death. *J Neurosci*, **17**, 3623–3633.

Arvanian, V.L., Horner, P.J., Gage, F.H. and Mendell, L.M. (2003). Intrathecal neurotrophin-3-secreting fibroblasts strengthen synaptic connections to motoneurons in the neonatal rat. *J Neurosci*, **23**, 8706–8712.

Bamber, N.I., Li, H., Lu, X., Oudega, M., Aebischer, P. and Xu, X.M. (2001). Neurotrophins BDNF and NT-3 promote axonal re-entry into the distal host spinal cord through Schwann cell-seeded mini-channels. *Eur J Neurosci*, **3**, 257–268.

Bar-Sagi, D. and Hall, A. (2000). Ras and Rho GTPases: a family reunion. *Cell*, **103**, 227–238.

Basso, D.M., Beattie, M.S. and Bresnahan, J.C. (1995). A sensitive and reliable locomotor rating scale for open field testing in rats. *J Neurotrauma*, **12**, 1–21.

Bates, B., Rios, M., Trumpp, A., Chen, C., Fan, C., Bishop, J.M. and Jaenisch, R (1999). Neurotrophin-3 is required for proper cerebellar development. *Nat Neurosci*, **2**, 115–117.

Bergman, E., Johnson, H., Zhang, X., Hokfelt, T. and Ulfhake, B. (1996). Neuropeptides and neurotrophin receptor mRNAs in primary sensory neurons of aged rats. *J Comp Neurol*, **375**, 303–319.

Blesch, A., Lu, P. and Tuszynski, M.H.(2002). Neurotrophic factors, gene therapy, and neural stem cells for spinal cord repair. *Brain Res Bull*, **57**, 833–838.

Blits, B., Dijkhuizen, P.A., Boer, G.J. and Verhaagen, J. (2000). Intercostal nerve implants transduced with an adenoviral vector encoding neurotrophin-3 promote regrowth of injured rat corticospinal tract fibers and improve hindlimb function. *Exp Neurol*, **164**, 25–37.

Blits, B., Oudega, M., Boer, G.J., Bartlett Bunge, M. and Verhaagen, J. (2003). Adeno-associated viral vector-mediated neurotrophin gene transfer in the injured adult rat spinal cord improves hind-limb function. *Neuroscience*, **118**, 271–281.

Boyd, J.G. and Gordon, T. (2001). The neurotrophin receptors, trkB and p75, differentially regulate motor axonal regeneration. *J Neurobiol*, **49**, 314–325.

Boyd, J.G. and Gordon, T. (2002). A dose-dependent facilitation and inhibition of peripheral nerve regeneration by brain-derived neurotrophic factor. *Eur J Neurosci*, **15**, 613–626.

Boyd, J.G. and Gordon T. (2003). Neurotrophic factors and their receptors in axonal regeneration and functional recovery after peripheral nerve injury. *Mol Neurobiol*, **27**, 277–324.

Bradbury, E.J., Khemani, S., King, V.R., Priestley, J.V. and McMahon, S.B. (1999). NT-3 promotes growth of lesioned adult rat sensory axons ascending in the dorsal columns of the spinal cord. *Eur J Neurosci*, **11**, 3873–3883.

Bregman, B.S., McAtee, M., Dai, H.N., Kuhn, P.L. (1997). Neurotrophic factors increase axonal growth after spinal cord injury and transplantation in the adult rat. *Exp Neurol*, **148**, 475–494.

Campenot, R.B. (1982a). Development of sympathetic neurons in compartmentalized cultures. I. Local control of neurite growth by nerve growth factor. *Dev Biol*, **93**, 1–12.

Campenot, R.B. (1982b). Development of sympathetic neurons in compartmentalized cultures. II. Local control of neurite survival by nerve growth factor. *Dev Biol*, **93**, 13–21.

Coumans, J.V., Lin, T.T-S., Dai, H.N., MacArthur, L., McAtee, M., Nash, C. and Bregman, B.S. (2001). Axonal regeneration and functional recovery after complete spinal cord transection in rats by delayed treatment with transplants and neurotrophins. *J Neurosci*, **21**, 9334–9344.

Cowan, W.M. (2001). Victor Hamburger and Rita Levi-Montalcini: The path to the discovery of nerve growth factor. *Ann Rev Neurosci*, **24**, 551–600.

Cowley, S., Paterson, H., Kemp, P. and Marshall, C.J. (1994). Activation of MAP kinase is necessary and sufficient for

PC12 differentiation and for transformation of NIH 3T3 cells. *Cell,* **77**, 841–852.

Curtis, R., Tonra, J.R., Stark, J.L., Adryan, K.M., Park, J.S., Cliffer, K.D., Lindsay, R.M. and DiStefano, P.S. (1998). Neuronal injury increases retrograde axonal transport of the neurotrophins to spinal sensory neurons and motor neurons via multiple receptor mechanisms. *Mol Cell Neurosci,* **12**, 105–118.

David, S. and Aguayo, A.J. (1981). Axonal elongation into peripheral nervous system bridges after central nervous system injury in adult rats. *Science,* **214**, 931–933.

Dechant, G. and Barde, Y.-A. (2002). The neurotrophin receptor p75ntr: novel functions and implications for diseases of the nervous system. *Nat Neurosci,* **5**, 1131–1136.

Doherty, P., Willimas, G. and Willimas, E.J. (2000). CAMs and axonal growth: a critical evaluation of the role of calcium and the MAPK cascade. *Mol Cell Neurosci,* **16**, 283–295.

Dougherty, K.D., Dreyfus, C.F. and Black, I.B. (2000). Brain-derived neurotrophic factor in astrocytes, oligodendrocytes, and microglia/macrophages after spinal cord injury. *Neurobiol Dis,* **7**, 574–585.

Eccles, J.C., Krnjevic, K. and Miledi, R. (1959). Delayed effects of peripheral severance of afferent nerve fibres on the efficacy of their central synapses. *J Physiol,* **145**, 204–220.

Funakoshi, H., Frisen, J., Barbany, G., Timmusk, T., Zachrisson, O., Verge, V.M. and Persson, H. (1993). Differential expression of mRNAs for neurotrophins and their receptors after axotomy of the sciatic nerve. *J Cell Biol,* **123**, 455–465.

Garraway, S., Petruska, J.C. and Mendell, L.M. (2003). BDNF modulates dorsal root evoked synaptic currents in substantia gelatinosa neurons. *Eur J Neurosci,* **18**, 2467–2476.

Gallo, G. and Letourneau, P.C. (1998). Localized sources of neurotrophins initiate axon collaterol sprouting. *J Neurosci,* **18**, 5403–5414.

Greene, L.S., Tischler, A.S. (1976). Establishment of a noradrenergic clonal line of rat adrenal pheochromocytoma cells which respond to nerve growth factor. *Proc Natl Acad Sci USA,* **73**, 2424–2428.

Grill, R.A., Blesch, A. and Tuszynski, M.H. (1997). Robust growth of chronically injured spinal cord axons induced by grafts of genetically modified NGF-secreting cells. *Exp Neurol,* **148**, 444–452.

Grimes, M.L., Zhou, J., Beattie, E.C., Yuen, E.C., Hall, D.E., Valletta, J.S., Topp, K.S., LaVail, J.H., Bunnett, N.W. and Mobley, W.C. (1996). Endocytosis of activated TrkA: evidence that nerve growth factor induces formation of signaling endosomes. *J Neurosci,* **16**, 7950–7964.

Hall, A. (1998). Rho GTPases and the actin cytoskeleton. *Science,* **279**, 509–514.

Hammarberg, H., Piehl, F., Risling, M. and Cullheim, S. (2000). Differential regulation of trophic factor receptor mRNAs in spinal motoneurons after sciatic nerve transection and ventral root avulsion in the rat. *J Comp Neurol,* **426**, 587–601.

Hempstead, B.L. (2002). The many faces of p75NTR. *Curr Opin Neurobiol,* **12**, 260–267.

Hottinger, A.F., Azzouz, M., Deglon, N., Aebischer, P. and Zurn, A.D. (2000). Complete and long-term rescue of lesioned adult motoneurons by lentiviral-mediated expression of glial cell line-derived neurotrophic factor in the facial nucleus. *J Neurosci,* **20**, 5587–5593.

Huang, E.J. and Reichardt, L.F. (2001). Neurotrophins: roles in neuronal development and function. *Ann Rev Neurosci,* **24**, 677–736.

Hughes, R.A., Sendtner, M. and Thoenen, H. (1993). Members of several gene families influence survival of rat motoneurons *in vitro* and *in vivo*. *J Neurosci Res,* **36**, 663–671.

Jakeman, L.B., Wei, P., Guan, Z. and Stokes, B.T. (1998). Brain-derived neurotrophic factor stimulates hindlimb stepping and sprouting of cholinergic fibers after spinal cord injury. *Exp Neurol,* **154**, 170–184.

Jin, Y., Tessler, A., Fischer, I. and Houle, J.D. (2002). Transplants of fibroblasts genetically modified to express BDNF promote axonal regeneration from supraspinal neurons following chronic spinal cord injury. *Exp Neurol,* **177**, 265–275.

Kang, H. and Schuman, E.C. (1995). Long-lasting neurotrophin-induced enhancement of synaptic transmission in the adult hippocampus. *Science,* **267**, 1658–1662.

Kaplan, D.R. and Miller, F.D. (2000). Neurotrophin signal; transduction in the nervous system. *Curr Opin Neurobiol,* **10**, 381–391.

Keyvan-Fouladi, N., Raisman, G. and Li, Y. (2003). Functional repair of the corticospinal tract by delayed transplantation of olfactory ensheathing cells in adult rats. *J Neurosci,* **23**, 9428–9434.

King, V.R., Bradbury, E.J., McMahon, S.B. and Priestley, J.V. (2000). Changes in truncated trkB and p75 receptor expression in the rat spinal cord following spinal cord hemisection and spinal cord hemisection plus neurotrophin treatment. *Exp Neurol,* **165**, 327–341.

Kobayashi, N.R., Fan, D., Giehl, K.M., Bedard, A.M., Wiegand, S.J. and Tetzlaff, W. (1997). BDNF and NT-4/5 prevent atrophy of rat rubrospinal neurons after cervical axotomy, stimulate GAP-43 and T_1-tubulin mRNA expression and promote axonal regeneration. *J Neurosci,* **17**, 9583–9595.

Koliatsos, V.E., Clatterbuck, R.E., Winslow, J.W., Cayouette, M.H. and Price, D.L. (1993). Evidence that brain-derived neurotrophic factor is a trophic factor for motor neurons *in vivo*. *Neuron,* **10**, 359–367.

Kucera, J., Fan, G., Jaenisch, R., Linnarsson, S. and Ernfors, P. (1995). Dependence of developing group Ia afferents on neurotrophin-3. *J Comp Neurol*, **363**, 307–320.

Kwon, B.W., Liu, J., Messerer, C., Kobayashi, N.R., McGraw, J., Oschipok, L. and Tetzlaff, W. (2002). Survival and regeneration of rubrospinal neurons 1 year after spinal cord injury. *Proc Natl Acad Sci USA*, **99**, 3246–3251.

Lawrence, D.G. and Kuypers, H.G. (1968a). The functional organization of the motor system in the monkey. I. The effects of bilateral pyramidal lesions. *Brain*, **91**, 1–14.

Lawrence, D.G. and Kuypers, H.G. (1968b). The functional organization of the motor system in the monkey. II. The effects of lesions of the descending brain-stem pathways. *Brain*, **91**, 15–36.

Lee, R., Kermani, P., Teng, K.K. and Hempstead, B.L. (2001). Regulation of cell survival by secreted proneurotrophins. *Science*, **294**, 1945–1948.

Levi-Montalcini, R. (1987). The nerve growth factor 35 years later. *Science*, **237**, 1154–1162.

Liebl, D.J., Huang, W., Young, W. and Parada, L.F. (2001). Regulation of trk receptors following contusion of the rat spinal cord. *Exp Neurol*, **167**, 15–26.

Lindsay, R.M. (1996). Role of neurotrophins and trk receptors in the development and maintenance of sensory neurons: an overview. *Philos Trans R Soc Lond B Biol Sci*, **351**, 365–373.

Liu, Y., Himes, B.T., Solowska, J., Moul, J., Chow, S.Y., Park, K.I., Tessler, A., Murray, M., Snyder, E.Y. and Fischer, I. (1999). Intraspinal delivery of neurotrophin-3 using neural stem cells genetically modified by recombinant retrovirus. *Exp Neurol*, **158**, 9–26.

Lu, P., Blesch, A. and Tuszynski, M.H. (2001). Neurotrophism without neurotropism: BDNF promotes survival but not growth of lesioned corticospinal neurons. *J Comp Neurol*, **436**, 456–470.

Markus, A., Patel, T.D. and Snider, W.D. (2002). Neurotrophic factors and axonal growth. *Curr Opin Neurobiol*, **12**, 523–531.

McAllister, A.K., Katz, L.C. and Lo, D.C. (1997). Opposing roles for endogenous BDNF and NT-3 in regulating cortical dendritic growth. *Neuron*, **18**, 767–778.

McMahon, S.B., Armanini, M.P., Ling, L.H. and Phillips, H.S. (1994). Expression and coexpression of trk receptors in subpopulations of adult primary sensory neurons projecting to identified peripheral targets. *Neuron*, **12**, 1161–1171.

McTigue, D.M., Horner, P.J., Stokes, B.T. and Gage, F.H. (1998). Neurotrophin-3 and brain-derived neurotrophic factor induce oligodendrocyte proliferation and myelination of regenerating axons in the contused adult rat spinal cord. *J Neurosci*, **18**, 5354–5365.

Mendell, L.M. (1995). Neurotrophic factors and the specification of neural function. *The Neuroscientist*, **1**, 26–34.

Mendell, L.M. and Arvanian, V.L. (2002). Diversity of neurotrophin action in the postnatal spinal cord. *Brain Res Rev*, **40**, 230–239.

Mendell, L.M., Taylor, J.S., Johnson, R.D. and Munson, J.B. (1995). Rescue of motoneuron and muscle afferent function in cats by regeneration into skin. II. Ia-motoneuron synapse. *J Neurophysiol*, **73**, 662–673.

Mendell, L.M., Johnson, R.D. and Munson, J.B. (1999). Neurotrophin modulation of the monosynaptic reflex after peripheral nerve transection. *J Neurosci*, **19**, 3162–3170.

Menei, P., Montero-Menei, C., Whittemore, S.R., Bunge, R.P. and Bunge, M.B. (1998). Schwann cells genetically modified to secrete human BDNF promote enhanced axonal regrowth across transected adult rat spinal cord. *Eur J Neurosci*, **10**, 607–621.

Metz, G.A., Merkler, D., Dietz, V., Schwab, M.E. and Fouad, K. (2000). Efficient testing of motor function in spinal cord injured rats. *Brain Res*, **883**, 165–177.

Munson, J.B., Shelton, D.L. and McMahon, S.B. (1997). Adult mammalian sensory and motor neurons: roles of endogenous neurotrophins and rescue by exogenous neurotrophins after axotomy. *J Neurosci*, **17**, 470–476.

Nja, A. and Purves, D. (1978). The effects of nerve growth factor and its antiserum on synapses in the superior cervical ganglion of the guinea-pig. *J Physiol*, **277**, 55–75.

Novikov, L., Novikova, L. and Kellerth, J.O. (1997). Brain-derived neurotrophic factor promotes axonal regeneration and long-term survival of adult rat spinal motoneurons *in vivo*. *Neurosci*, **79**, 765–774.

Novikova, L.N., Novikov, L.N. and Kellerth, J.O. (2002). Differential effects of neurotrophins on neuronal survival and axonal regeneration after spinal cord injury in adult rats. *J Comp Neurol*, **452**, 255–263.

Oakley, R.A., Garner, A.S., Large, T.H. and Frank, E. (1995). Muscle sensory neurons require neurotrophin-3 from peripheral tissues during the period of normal cell death. *Development*, **121**, 1341–1350.

Ramer, M.S., Priestley, J.V. and McMahon, S.B. (2000). Functional regeneration of sensory axons into the adult spinal cord. *Nature*, **403**, 312–316.

Ramer, M.S., Bishop, T., Dockery, P., Mobarak, M.S., O'Leary, D., Fraher, J.P., Priestley, J.V. and McMahon, S.B. (2002). Neurotrophin-3-mediated regeneration and recovery of proprioception following dorsal rhizotomy. *Mol Cell Neurosci*, **19**, 239–249.

Ramon y Cajal, S. (1928). *Degeneration and Regeneration of the Nervous System*, Oxford University Press, New York, NY.

Schnell, L. and Schwab, M.E. (1993). Sprouting and regeneration of lesioned corticospinal tract fibres in the adult rat spinal cord. *Eur J Neurosci*, **5**, 1156–1171.

Schnell, L., Schneider, R., Kolbeck, R., Barde, Y.-A. and Schwab, M.E. (1994). Neurotrophin-3 enhances sprouting of corticospinal tract during development and after adult spinal cord lesions. *Nature*, **367**, 170–173.

Schucht, P., Raineteau, O., Schwab, M.E. and Fouad, K. (2002). Anatomical correlates of locomotor recovery following dorsal and ventral lesions of the rat spinal cord. *Exp Neurol*, **176**, 143–153.

Schwartz, P.M., Borghesani, B.R., Levy, R.L., Pomeroy, S.L. and Segal, R.A. (1997). Abnormal cerebellar development and foliation in *BDNF-/-* mice reveals a role for neurotrophins in CNS patterning. *Neuron*, **19**, 269–281.

Seebach, B.S., Arvanov, V. and Mendell, L.M. (1999). Neurotrophin influence on the development of segmental reflexes in the rat. *J Neurophysiol*, **81**, 2398–2405.

Segal, R.A. (2003). Selectivity in neurotrophin signaling: theme and variations. *Ann Rev Neurosci*, **26**, 299–330.

Sendtner, M., Holtmann, B., Kolbeck, R., Thoenen, H. and Barde, Y.-A. (1992). Brain-derived neurotrophic factor prevents the death of motoneurons in newborn rats after nerve section. *Nature*, **360**, 757–759.

Steward, O., Zheng, B. and Tessier-Lavigne, M. (2003). False resurrections: distinguishing regenerated from spared axons in the injured central nervous system. *J Comp Neurol*, **459**, 1–8.

Teng, S. and Hempstead, B. (2004). Neurotrophins and their receptors: singaling trios in complex biological systems. *Cell Mol Life Sci*, **61**, 35–48.

Terenghi G. (1999). Peripheral nerve regeneration and neurotrophic factors. *J Anat*, **194**, 1–14.

Tuszynski, M.H., Grill, R., Jones, L.L., Brant, A., Blesch, A., Low, K., Lacroix, S. and Lu, P. (2003). NT-3 gene delivery elicits growth of chronically injured corticospinal axons and modestly improves functional deficits after chronic scar resection. *Exp Neurol*, **181**, 47–56.

Vejsada, R., Tseng, J.L., Lindsay, R.M., Acheson, A., Aebischer, P. and Kato, A.C. (1998). Synergistic but transient rescue effects of BDNF and GDNF on axotomized neonatal motoneurons. *Neuroscience*, **84**, 129–139.

Verge, V.M., Gratto, K.A., Karchewski, L.A. and Richardson, P.M. (1996). Neurotrophins and nerve injury in the adult. *Philos Trans R Soc Lond B Biol Sci*, **351**, 423–430.

von Meyenburg, J., Brosamle, C., Metz, G.A.S. and Schwab, M.E. (1998). Regeneration and sprouting of chronically injured corticospinal tract fibers in adult rats promoted by NT-3 and the mAb IN-1, which neutralizes myelin-associated neurite growth inhibitors. *Exp Neurol*, **154**, 583–594.

Wang, K.C., Kim, J.A., Sivasankaran, R., Segal, R. and He, Z. (2002). p75 interacts with the Nogo receptor as a co-receptor for Nogo, MAG and OMgp. *Nature*, **420**, 74–78.

Willis, Jr., W.D. and Coggeshall, R.E. (2004). *Sensory Mechanisms of the Spinal Cord*, 3rd edn., Kluwer Academic/Plenum Publishers, New York.

Wu, W., Li, L., Yick, L.W., Chai, H., Xie, Y., Yang, Y., Prevette, D.M. and Oppenheim, R.W. (2003). GDNF and BDNF alter the expression of neuronal NOS, c-Jun, and p75 and prevent motoneuron death following spinal root avulsion in adult rats. *J Neurotraum*, **20**, 603–612.

Xu, X.M., Guénard, V., Kleitman, N., Aebischer, P. and Bunge, M.B. (1995). A combination of BDNF and NT-3 promotes supraspinal axonal regeneration into Schwann cell grafts in adult rat throracic spinal cord. *Exp Neurol*, **134**, 261–272.

Yamashita, T. and Tohyama, M. (2003). The p75 receptor acts as a displacement factor that releases Rho from Rho-GDI. *Nat Neurosci*, **6**, 461–467.

Yamashita, T., Tucker, K.L. and Barde, Y.-A. (1999). Neurotrophin binding to the p75 receptor modulates Rho activity and axonal outgrowth. *Neuron*, **24**, 585–593.

Yan, Q., Elliott, J.L., Matheson, C., Sun, J., Zhang, L., Mu, X., Rex, K.L. and Snider, W.D. (1993). Influences of neurotrophins on mammalian motoneurons *in vivo*. *J Neurobiol*, **24**, 1555–1577.

Ye, J.H. and Houle, J.D. (1997). Treatment of the chronically injured spinal cord with neurotrophic factors can promote axonal regeneration from supraspinal neurons. *Exp Neurol*, **143**, 70–81.

Zhang, Y., Dijkhuizen, P.A., Anderson, P.N., Lieberman, A.R. and Verhaagen, J. (1998). NT-3 delivered by an adenoviral vector induces injured dorsal root axons to regenerate into the spinal cord of adult rats. *J Neurosci Res*, **54**, 554–562.

Zhou, L., Baumgartner, B.J., Hill-Felberg, S.J., McGowen, L.R. and Shine, H.D. (2003). Neurotrophin-3 expressed in situ induces axonal plasticity in the adult injured spinal cord. *J Neurosci*, **23**, 1424–1431.

Intraneuronal determinants of regeneration

Lisa J. McKerracher[1] and Michael E. Selzer[2]

[1]*Département de Pathologie et Biologie Cellulaire, Université de Montréal, Montréal, Québec, Canada and*
[2]*Department of Neurology, University of Pennsylvania Medical Center, Philadelphia, PA, USA*

24.1 Introduction

Neuronal damage in trauma to the central nervous system (CNS) results from interruption of axonal connections and from the death of neurons. Neuron loss may result from physical disruption at the lesion site and from local secondary responses, such as inflammation, which contribute to necrosis and to a complex series of molecular events that constitute a suicide program (apoptosis; Volume I, Chapter 16). Additionally, when an axon is transected, the portion that becomes detached from the cell body degenerates (Wallerian degeneration; Fig. 24.1; Volume I, Chapter 16). The proximal portion often retracts, sometimes long distances, and the neuron now deprived of its normal connections is vulnerable to retrograde death by apoptosis. However, if the neuron survives, its axon may regenerate. This is observed routinely in peripheral nerves but until the late 20th century, was thought impossible in the CNS.

Attempts of CNS axons to regrow soon after axon injury are suppressed by inhibitory signals in the injured axon tip (abortive sprouting). In the 1980s, Aguayo and colleagues inserted peripheral nerve grafts into the brain and spinal cord and showed that CNS axons have the capacity to regrow into a permissive environment (Aguayo et al., 1991). Schwab and colleagues demonstrated that CNS myelin contains proteins that block axon growth (Schwab, 2004) (see Volume I, Chapters 19 and 21). Removing myelin from the injured CNS promoted regeneration (Keirstead et al., 1995; Savio and

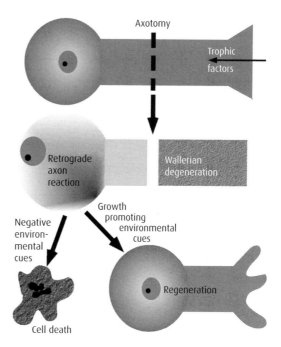

Figure 24.1. *Responses of neurons to axotomy.* Severing the axon results in degeneration of the axon distal to the injury (Wallerian degeneration). The proximal stump retracts for varying distances, while the cell body undergoes changes in morphology (chromatolysis) and metabolism collectively called the "retrograde axon reaction". This includes degenerative responses due in part to interruption of supply of target-derived trophic substances, which if severe enough, lead to the death of the neuron. If not, positive responses result in the activation of a regeneration program that leads to the formation of a growth cone and axon sprouting from the proximal stump.

Schwab, 1997). Another important barrier to regeneration is the glial scar that forms after CNS injury (Volume I, Chapter 22). Inhibitory proteins consisting mainly of proteoglycans contribute to the barrier of the glial scar (McKeon et al., 1991; Bradbury et al., 2002). These studies have led the way toward understanding the cellular and molecular basis of repair and recovery after CNS trauma.

Axons express receptors such as the Nogo receptor (NgR) that bind growth inhibitory proteins, as well as receptors for cytokines and for growth factors that promote growth and survival (e.g., the neurotrophin receptors (Trks) and guidance molecule receptors;

Volume I, Chapters 19, 21 and 23), both inhibitory and excitatory (Fig. 24.2). These receptors transmit intracellular signals that are integrated into signaling pathways both at the level of the growth cone, and retrogradely to the cell body. Tissue culture studies employing compartment chambers show that the site of exposure to a growth factor can determine the neuronal response (Campenot, 1994). Thus neurons located at a site of injury are affected differently than more remote neurons that project axons to injury sites.

Understanding the intraneuronal determinants of axon regeneration in the CNS should ultimately

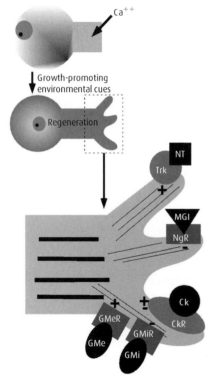

	Microtubule	MGI	Myelin-associated growth inhibitor	GMiR	Inhibitory guidance molecule receptor
	F-actin	NgR	Nogo receptor	GMe	Excitatory guidance molecule
NT	Neurotrophin	Ck	Cytokine		
Trk	Tyrosine kinase neurotrophin receptor	CkR	Cytokine receptor	GMeR	Excitatory guidance molecule receptor
		GMi	Inhibitory guidance molecule		

Figure 24.2. *Extracellular humoral influences on the growth cone.* Many substances exert positive or negative influences on the growth cone by binding to specific surface receptors and activating intracellular signaling pathways that lead to advance or retraction of the growth cone. Many of these signals act by activating the polymerization or depolymerization of F-actin in the filopodia and lamellipodium. Some of these molecular influences include neurotrophins (NT), which bind to receptors of the tyrosine kinase (Trk) family. At least three myelin-associated molecules cause growth cone collapse by binding to the Nogo receptor (NgR). Cytokines (Ck) released by non-neuronal cells at the site of an injury bind to cytokine receptors (CkR) and may be excitatory or inhibitory to growth. Several molecules that guide the growing axons during development are expressed in the mature CNS and may attract (Gme) or repel (Gmi) growing axons by binding to their respective receptors (GmeR and GmiR). Growth enhancement and inhibition are indicated by + and −, respectively.

help us attain functional regeneration after human CNS injury. This chapter will focus on the translation of extracellular cues to intracellular programs that are determinants of regenerative capacity.

24.2 Developmental loss of regenerative ability

In culture, primary embryonic neurons grow axons much faster than neurons from older animals. Thus, when grown on the same substrate (usually laminin) and in the same medium, sympathetic ganglion cell axons grow twice as fast when taken from 21-day rat embryos as from 30-day postnatal rats (Kleitman and Johnson, 1989). Retinal ganglion cell (RGC) axons also lose their ability to grow on a laminin substrate during embryonic life, in part due to a reduction in the neuronal content of laminin receptors (integrins) (Hall et al., 1987). Although axons of dorsal root ganglion (DRG) cells maintain their ability to grow into adulthood, there is a simplification and loss of F-actin staining in the growth cones of DRG neurons cultured from older (E14) compared with younger (E7) chick embryos, and grow 15% slower (Selzer et al., 2004). Similarly, optic nerve fibers regenerate in opossums until age 12 days, but not thereafter (MacLaren, 1996). Regeneration of spinal cord axons occurs in the tadpole but not in the post-metamorphic frog (Forehand and Farel, 1982; Beattie et al., 1990), and in mammals, axons regenerate into/through fetal spinal cord grafts and mediate functional recovery much more readily in early postnatal hosts than in adults (Bregman et al., 1993; Howland et al., 1995).

Dependence on neuron age

Although the inhibitory molecular environment contributes importantly to failure of axonal regeneration in the mature CNS (see Volume I, Chapters 21 and 22), much evidence suggests that as neurons mature, they become intrinsically less able to regenerate their axon. For example, when retinas and optic tecta taken from embryonic and postnatal hamsters were cultured together in different age combinations,

it was the age of the retina and not that of the tectum that determined whether retinal axons would regenerate into the tectum (Chen et al., 1995). Similarly, when combinations of embryonic and postnatal entorhinal cortex and hippocampus were co-cultured, embryonic entorhinal cortex neurons could regenerate axons into adult hippocampus but adult entorhinal neurons could not regenerate into embryonic hippocampus (Li et al., 1995). Moreover, experiments with dissociated neurons microinjected into adult CNS suggested that embryonic neurons can send out long axons when transplanted into myelinated axon tracts in several regions (Davies et al., 1994). However, with the exception of DRG neurons microinjected into the spinal cord (Davies et al., 1997), this has not worked with dissociated adult neurons. Thus, while the extracellular environment in the adult CNS contains molecules that act as growth inhibitors, both *in vitro* and *in vivo*, co-culture experiments suggest that much of the failure of axon regeneration seen in the adult CNS can be attributed to a developmental reduction in the intrinsic regenerative ability of neurons. An irreversible loss of regenerative ability occurs at birth in rat RGC. This change results from contact with amacrine cells (Goldberg et al., 2002) and persists even if the amacrine cells are subsequently removed.

24.3 Heterogeneity in neuronal regenerative ability

Another indication of the importance of neuron-intrinsic factors in determining the regenerative ability of axons is the heterogeneity in regenerative ability expressed by axons of different neurons growing through the same environment. For example, when axons belonging to identified reticulospinal neurons and cytoarchitectonically defined neuron groups of the lamprey brain are interrupted by a spinal cord transection, some regenerate with a very high probability, whereas others rarely regenerate, even though their axons travel in the same axon tracts (Jacobs et al., 1997). Similar heterogeneity has been observed in the regenerative ability of several spinal projecting axon tracts in zebrafish (Becker et al., 1998). In mammals, when offered a peripheral nerve graft to grow into, some neurons (e.g., those of the thalamic reticular nucleus, substantia nigra pars compacta, and deep cerebellar nuclei) regenerate axons robustly, while others (e.g., thalamocortical projection neurons, striatal projection neurons and cerebellar Purkinje cells) regenerate poorly (Anderson et al., 1998). These differences cannot be explained by differences in cell survival (Vidal-Sanz et al., 1987; Villegas-Perez et al., 1988). Not all RGCs that survive axotomy regenerate axons into peripheral nerve grafts. However, studies of chronic spinal cord injury show that even long-injured axons can regenerate, if given the appropriate simulus (Coumans et al., 2001).

24.4 Neuronal response to site of injury

One puzzling observation on regenerative potential is that the distance of the axonal injury from the prikaryon has a large impact on axon regrowth and cell survival. In neurons of the lamprey brain and spinal cord, axotomy close to the cell body results in sprouting of long axon-like neurites from the dendritic tree rather than from the cut axon tip (Mackler et al., 1986; Hall et al., 1989). When a hamster optic nerve is cut close to the eye and a peripheral nerve graft is inserted in the eye, axons extend from dendrites into the graft (Cho and So, 1989). Similarly, distal dendrites of neck motor neurons in adult cats can give rise to axon-like process that express (GAP-43) (Rose et al., 2001). The same phenomenon has been analyzed *in vitro* using rat hippocampal neurons (Goslin and Banker, 1989).

Neuronal survival is also affected by the site of axotomy. Optic nerve axons do not have "sustaining" collateral branches, but cutting the optic nerve progressively further from the eye leads to increasingly better RGC survival (Villegas-Perez et al., 1993). Paradoxically, axotomy near the cell body is correlated with *better* regeneration into peripheral nerve grafts (Vidal-Sanz et al., 1987; Lau et al., 1994) and upregulation of GAP-43 (Doster et al., 1991).

Observations about neuronal death can be difficult to interpret. An apparent loss of axotomized cholinergic medial septal neurons is reversed by infusing nerve growth factor (NGF), showing that many cells were simply atrophied (Hagg et al., 1989). Similarly, rat rubrospinal neurons thought to be dead a year after axotomy in the cervical spinal cord were able to regenerate into peripheral nerve grafts after application of growth factors (Kwon et al., 2002). Therefore, there is both cell death and neuronal atrophy after axotomy, and these encouraging results show that rescue of atrophied neurons is possible.

Relationship between survival and regeneration programs

A necessary prerequisite for axon regeneration is that the injured neuron survives. Studies in tissue culture suggested a link between some regenerative and cell survival pathways. For example, neurotrophins both promote cell survival and stimulate neurite outgrowth for embryonic neurons placed in culture (Volume I, Chapters 16 and 23). Studies in the adult CNS, however, show a clear separation between survival and regeneration. Many more RGCs survive axotomy than are able to extend axons in peripheral nerve grafts (Vidal-Sanz et al., 1987). Moreover, RGCs survive optic nerve injury in transgenic mice that overexpress *bcl-2*, an anti-apoptotic gene, but this does not confer an ability to regenerate better into the growth permissive environment of a peripheral nerve graft (Inoue et al., 2002).

24.5 Extrinsic molecular signaling of axon injury

The intrinsic growth capacity of an injured neuron is greatly influenced by its external environment. We have discussed several demonstrations of this, such as the ability of atrophied neurons to revive following exogenous application of growth factors, and the ability of growth inhibitory proteins in the CNS environment to suppress the regenerative potential

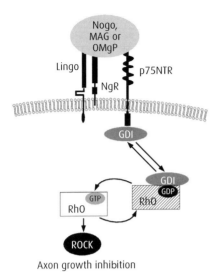

Figure 24.3. *Rock and Rho.* The growth-inhibiting effects of several molecules, including the myelin-associated growth inhibitors, converge on a common signaling mechanisms that involves activation of Rho GTPases and their activation of Rock, which leads to complex downstream effects, including the depolymerization of F-actin. It is likely that at least three receptor molecules are involved cooperatively in this process, Lingo, NgR and the low-affinity neurotrophin receptor p75 (Mi et al., 2004). The intracellular domain of p75 binds to the Rho-GDP dissociation inhibitor (GDI) (Yamashita and Tohyama, 2003), thus allowing dissociation of GDP from Rho, which is then activated by binding GTP.

of injured adult neurons. Figure 24.3 summarizes some known extracellular signals, and their affect on cytoskeletal dynamics. Ultimately, the translation of extracellular signals into intracellular signals increases cytoskeletal motility and axonal transport which drives axon growth and regeneration. Some of the important extrinsic signals are presented below, and the intrinsic drivers of regeneration are considered next.

Cytokines

After axonal injury *in vivo*, the inflammatory environment contributes substantially to the neuronal injury response. There are both beneficial and detrimental

aspects of the immune reaction and production of cytokines after traumatic injury. On one hand, it is clear that secondary tissue damage occurs following a pro-inflammatory response, and tissue damage is detrimental to recovery after traumatic injury. But some aspects of inflammation help promote axon regeneration, and there is a beneficial side for some inflammatory processes in spinal cord injury (Bethea and Dietrich, 2002). It has been shown that inflammation near the neuronal cell body can enhance axonal regeneration, as shown by provoking inflammation in rat DRG cells to elicit axon regeneration in crushed dorsal spinal roots (Lu and Richardson, 1991). After injury of the optic nerve, macrophage-derived factors produced in the eye following injection of zymosan promote RGC regeneration in the optic nerve (Yin et al., 2003). A separate experiment has shed light on the duality of macrophages. Transplanting macrophages stimulated by exposure to peripheral nerve can promote the clearance of myelin and regeneration of injured axons, while macrophages exposed to CNS myelin do not exhibit this potential (Lazarov-Spiegler et al., 1998).

Notwithstanding the demonstrated potential of growth factors from immune cells to promote regeneration, observations after spinal cord injury show the dark side of the pro-inflammatory response. Inflammation after injury evolves with time and causes secondary damage when invading inflammatory cells destroy injured tissue and contribute to necrosis (Popovich et al., 1999). One important pro-inflammatory cytokine released early after spinal cord injury is tumor necrosis factor (TNF). Elevated levels of TNF appear within hours of spinal cord injury and TNF is expressed by activated microglia, monocytes, and reactive astrocytes (Bethea and Dietrich, 2002; Neumann et al., 2002a). Cytokines and chemokines expressed by microglia signal invasion of hematogenous cells that express additional cytokines and chemokines (Babcock et al., 2003). The presence of TNF in the injured CNS may block axon regeneration through a mechanism that involves the activation of the small GTPase Rho. TNF has been shown to activate Rho in neurons expressing TNF receptors (Neumann et al., 2002a), and activation of

Rho is well known to block axon growth and regeneration (Tigyi et al., 1996; Lehmann et al., 1999; Bito et al., 2000). Surprisingly, however, recovery of function was not improved in mice where the TNF receptors were deleted (Bethea and Dietrich, 2002; Demjen et al., 2004). By contrast, other studies to block the inflammatory responses do improve functional recovery after spinal cord injury. Such strategies include the application of anti-integrin antibody to suppress the invasion of hematogenous macrophages (Gris et al., 2004), neutralization of the Fas receptor that is expressed by injured cells in the CNS (Demjen et al., 2004), and neutralization of the T-lymphocyte chemoattractant CXCL10 (Gonzalez et al., 2003).

Neurotrophins

Neurotrophins, and more broadly, neurotrophic factors, are peptide molecules that act on cells through specific receptors that activate intracellular signaling mechanism to promote the differentiation and survival of cells during development (Markus et al., 2002). The role of neurotrophic factors in promoting neuronal survival and axonal regeneration is considered in detail in Volume I, Chapter 23. However, as it is now clear that adult neurons are intrinsically less able to grow axons than embryonic neurons, interest has been shown in the possibility that the same molecules that promote neuronal survival and axon growth during development might be used to return neurons to their embryonic state and thus enhance the ability of their axons to regenerate. Moreover, low levels of trophic factors are known to be important in maintaining the integrity of neurons even in the adult. Neurons obtain some of their trophic support from the target tissues to which their axons project. When the axon is severed, the supply of trophic factors is interrupted. Thus after axotomy, neuronal survival and regenerative sprouting can be enhanced by supplying these factors exogenously. *Each type of neuron has its own requirement for a specific trophic factor or combination of factors.* When these are applied to models of spinal cord injury, the number of sprouts may increase but the distance of growth is small unless the trophic factors are combined with other manipulations, such as fetal tissue transplants (Coumans et al., 2001) or antibodies to Nogo (Schnell et al., 1994). However, after intrathecal application of NGF, neurotrophin-3 (NT-3), or glial cell-derived neurotrophic factor (GDNF) in the absence of additional manipulations, the crushed central axons of DRG cells, which ordinarily do not regenerate, regrew into the spinal cord, formed functional synapses with neurons in the dorsal horn and even partially reestablished sensory function (Ramer et al., 2000). Brain-derived neurotrophic factor (BDNF) was not effective. On the other hand, when fibroblasts modified to secrete BDNF were transplanted into a cervical partial hemisection, *rubrospinal* axons showed enhanced regeneration through and around the graft and some forelimb function was restored, with some axons reinvading the host spinal cord for long distances caudal to the graft (Liu et al., 1999). For example, fibroblasts have been genetically modified to produce NGF and injected into the spinal cord at the site of a chronic injury. This resulted in the growth of axons of DRG cells and coerulospinal neurons into the transplant. The effect was specific, since corticospinal, raphaespinal and motor axons did not respond (Blesch and Tuszynski, 1997). Regeneration of corticospinal axons was induced by fibroblasts that secreted leukemia inhibitory factor (LIF). The effects of neurotrophins in enhancing axonal regeneration is partly mediated by elevation of intracellular cAMP levels and consequent activation of protein kinase A (PKA) (Cai et al., 1999) (see below and Volume I, Chapters 21 and 23)

Excitotoxins

Release of the excitatory transmitter glutamate after CNS trauma results in the death of exposed neurons that express glutamate receptors (excitotoxicity). Chronic activation of N-methyl-D-aspartate (NMDA)-type glutamate receptors abnormally elevates intracellular calcium and may trigger apoptosis or necrosis, depending on the intensity of NMDA receptor activation and some animal studies suggest that blocking NMDA receptors can prevent cell death after neurotrauma (Hardingham and Bading, 2003). Oligodendrocytes are also vulnerable to glutamate toxicity, possibly involving AMPA receptors (McDonald et al., 1998).

In the context of regeneration, it is important to consider that growth cones exposed to an excitotoxic environment are also susceptible to growth cone collapse from elevated calcium, which disassembles the actin cytoskeleton. Calcium transients are important in the regulation of axon growth, and both too much and too little can arrest growth cone extension. However, glutamate added to neurons in culture can enhance rates of neurite outgrowth (Rashid and Cambray-Deakin, 1992) and glutamate can help steer axon turning (Zheng et al., 1996). There is strong evidence that glutamate receptor activity is required for dendritic growth of retinal neurons, together with inactivation of RhoA activity (Haas et al., 1998). Thus, glutamate may promote neurite outgrowth in development. The effects of glutamate on growth cone activity and axon regeneration after traumatic injury have not been as well investigated.

Growth inhibitors

The best characterized growth inhibitory molecules are concentrated in myelin: myelin-associated glycoprotein (MAG) (McKerracher et al., 1994; Mukhopadhyay et al., 1994), Nogo (Chen, 2000; GrandPré, 2000; Prinjha et al., 2000), and Oligodendrocyte-myelin glycoprotein (OmgP) (Kottis et al., 2002; Wang et al., 2002). A receptor that binds Nogo has been identified as the Nogo-66 receptor, NgR (Fournier et al., 2001). Surprisingly, MAG and OMgP also bind to the NgR. Thus all of the myelin-associated growth inhibitory proteins share a common signaling pathway in neurons (Fournier et al., 2001; Domeniconi et al., 2002; Wang et al., 2002). Other inhibitory proteins such as proteoglycans are expressed by cells that form the scar at the lesion site (McKeon et al., 1991; see Volume I, Chapter 22). The inhibitory role of myelin was for a time questioned because several studies showed that transplanted neurons grew axons on white matter (Bjorklund and Stenevi, 1984; Davies et al., 1994;

1997). There are age-related effects in the ability of growth inhibitory protein substrates to block axon regeneration, and therefore intrinsic differences contribute to the neuronal responsiveness to growth inhibitors (Cai et al., 2001). For additional discussion, see Volume I, Chapter 21.

Growth inhibitory proteins signal growth cone collapse by affecting intracellular signaling cascades (Volume I, Chapter 19). One component of the cascade is the small intracellular GTPase Rho, which is activated by growth inhibitory proteins (Niederost et al., 2002; Winton et al., 2002). Moreover, after spinal cord injury, there is an abnormally high activation of Rho observed in both neurons and glial cells, which prevents regeneration and contributes to apoptotic cell death (Dubreuil et al., 2003; Madura et al., 2004). Another key signaling molecule is cAMP. The elevation of cAMP can override the inhibitory response to NgR signaling (Cai et al., 1999). While Rho and cAMP act locally on the growth cone cytoskeleton to regulate regeneration, their effect on sustained axon elongation and the cell body response to injury are poorly understood. At the local level, single filopodial contact of growth cones with growth inhibitory proteins causes growth cone turning (Song et al., 1998), while contact with larger quantities, such as when neurons are placed on growth inhibitory substrates, causes the collapse of the growth cone and retraction of the neurite. Time lapse studies suggest that axons may attempt to grow around a growth inhibitory contact, such as an oligodendrocyte, but repeated contacts lead to failed neurite growth (Fawcett et al., 1989; Bandtlow et al., 1990).

24.6 Intrinsic signaling of axon injury

Calcium

Calcium acts as an intracellular signal in many functions, including growth cone guidance. Calcium enters the axon from the extracellular environment at the site of injury and local elevation in axoplasmic calcium concentration can trigger the rapid formation of a growth cone (Ziv and Spira, 1997). Once formed, however, the motility of the growth cone is inhibited by transient elevations of intracellular calcium in filopodia at sites of clusters of integrin molecules (Gomez et al., 2001), which serve as receptors for several extracellular matrix proteins, including laminin and fibronectin. Thus filopodial adhesion to substrate may be linked to growth cone turning because motility of filopodia in which calcium levels are high will be inhibited, while motility in those in which calcium is low will not. Inhibitory guidance molecules such as semaphorins and netrins also cause local elevations in intracellular calcium by activating L-type voltage-dependent calcium channels.

Cyclic nucleotides

The effects of neurotrophic factors, guidance molecules and myelin-associated growth inhibitors are dependent on the levels of cAMP. When levels are high the effect on the growth cone is chemoattraction, while when they are low, the effect is chemorepulsion (Ming et al., 1997; Song et al., 1998; Cai et al., 1999). In some cases, the effects of cGMP are the opposite of those of cAMP. Netrin can be chemoattractant or chemorepellant, depending on the receptor complex with which it interacts and on the intraneuronal ratio of cAMP/cGMP, a high ratio favoring chemoattraction and vice versa. Moreover, these cyclic nucleotides modulate the activity of L-type calcium channels in a way that is consistent with their effect on growth cone guidance (Nishiyama et al., 2003). Although axotomy increases cAMP levels in *Aplysia* motoneurons, which regenerate axons *in vitro* (Dash et al., 1998), spinal cord injury results in reduction of neuronal cAMP levels (Pearse et al., 2004). Raising cAMP levels *in vivo* enhance regeneration of the Mauthner axon (ordinarily a poor regenerator) in zebrafish (Bhatt et al., 2004), and could overcome growth inhibition and promote regeneration after spinal cord injury in rats (Neumann et al., 2002b; Qiu et al., 2002; Pearse et al., 2004). Injury-induced reduction in cAMP levels was prevented by administration of the phosphodiesterase IV inhibitor rolipram to rats with spinal cord contusions, while additionally injecting db-cAMP near the injury raised

cAMP levels above normal. When these two treatments were combined with transplants of Schwann cells into the injury, each treatment resulted in enhanced axonal regeneration (or preservation) and functional improvement, and the combination was more effective than any one alone (Pearse et al., 2004). Together, the emerging studies suggest that cAMP prepares the neuron for a regenerative response (see Volume I, Chapter 21).

Rho GTPases

Rho GTPases are a family of highly related proteins that are best characterized for their effect on the actin cytoskeleton, but they have entered the spotlight in the field of CNS regeneration for their key role in regulating the neuronal response to growth inhibitory proteins. The major members of the Rho family include Rho, Rac and Cdc42. In the CNS, Rho is the best understood for signaling axon growth inhibition in response to growth inhibitory proteins and CNS trauma. Isoforms of Rho exist, and in neurons RhoA is expressed at higher levels than RhoB and RhoC (Lehmann et al., 1999). Rho GTPases act as switches that cycle between a GDP-bound inactive state and a GTP-bound active state. The cellular response to growth inhibitory proteins is regulated by the Rho activity state. The first experiments to show the importance of Rho in neuronal response to growth inhibitors demonstrated that Rho inactivation could prevent growth cone collapse and promote neurite growth on myelin (Tigyi et al., 1996; Jin and Strittmatter, 1997; Lehmann et al., 1999). Additional evidence for the importance of Rho in growth inhibition was that inactivation of either Rho or Rho kinase could promote neurite growth on proteoglycan substrates that model inhibitory proteins of the glial scar (Dergham et al., 2002; Borisoff et al., 2003; Monnier et al., 2003). Inactivation of Rho with a cell permeable Rho antagonist, C3-07, allows axons to grow past an astrocyte/meningeal scar in a tissue culture model of the lesion scar (Shearer et al., 2003). Therefore, Rho is a key molecule for signaling by myelin growth inhibitors, as well as the different growth inhibitory proteins that make up the glial scar. Similarly, Rho regulates the neuronal response to chemorepulsive factors (Wahl, 2000).

After spinal cord injury, there is an abnormal, sustained activation of Rho, and highly activated Rho is correlated with upregulation of p75, a receptor that signals apoptosis of damaged neurons (Dubreuil et al., 2003; Madura et al., 2004). In situ assays demonstrated that Rho is highly activated in neurons, astrocytes and oligodendrocytes after spinal cord injury and that reversal of Rho activation was cell protective (Dubreuil et al., 2003). Inactivation of endothelial Rho is also protective in an animal model of stroke (Laufs et al., 2000).

Rho can be inactivated via ADP ribosylation by C3 transferase, a bacterial endotoxin. Several cell permeable versions have been constructed (Winton et al., 2002). Rho kinase (p160ROCK) is a downstream effector activated by Rho. After spinal cord injury, inactivation of Rho with C3, or of ROCK with Y-27632 or Fasudil, promoted axon regeneration and functional recovery (Dergham et al., 2002; Fournier et al., 2003). Activation states of Rho have not been investigated in development. It is possible that Rho GTPases and/or the exchange factors that regulate Rho activation may play a role in the age-dependent loss of intrinsic regenerative responses.

Transcription factors

Transcription factors are central to any coordinated molecular program, and several transcription factors are upregulated following axotomy and during axonal regeneration, including members of the Jun and Fos families, components of the transcription factor AP-1. Transgenic mice lacking the *c-jun* gene in the CNS showed deficient regeneration and sprouting of motor axons, atrophy of motoneurons, and failure of upregulation of several other regeneration-associated molecules such as CD-44 (Raivich et al., 2004).

The immediate early gene, nuclear factor-κB (NF-κB), exists in all cell types and has been implicated in the early control of the neuronal response to injury and regeneration. NF-κB is present in the cytoplasm in an inactive form bound to its inhibitor

IκB. Upon stimulation by an extracellular signal, NF-κB is released from its inhibitor, translocates to the nucleus and participates in many regulatory processes. NF-κB is activated as early as 30 min after CNS injury, is still present at 72 h, and is expressed by both macrophages/microglia and neurons (Bethea et al., 1998). Activation of NF-κB in neurons is a response to pro-inflammatory cytokines that are elevated after injury, and may be related to the apoptotic death of neurons that is part of the secondary inflammatory response. NF-κB is also activated during the excitotoxin-induced apoptosis of striatal neurons (Qin et al., 1998). NF-κB can be activated by Rho (Montaner et al., 1999), raising the possibility that the abnormal Rho activation after spinal cord injury (Dubreuil et al., 2003; Madura et al., 2004) may lead to activation of NF-κB and neuronal death.

Expression of the cAMP-responsive element binding protein (CREB) is associated with physiologic and anatomical plasticity in neurons. Given the importance of cAMP to axonal growth, it might be expected that CREB would participate in axon regeneration. Thus far, there is little evidence for this, although in *Aplysia* motoneurons, CREB enhanced axonal sprouting *in vitro* (Dash et al., 1998).

24.7 Intrinsic determinants of regeneration

After injury in the CNS, terminal enlargements form at the tips of cut axons, but their cytoskeleton may differ from growth cones in development (Volume I, Chapter 19). Damaged axons do not regenerate significant distances when the balance between positive and negative growth cues is unfavorable. Thus while many studies show that blocking growth-inhibiting molecules can promote regeneration in the injured spinal cord, axons do not typically grow further than a centimeter. Studies of axonal transport and the effect of conditioning lesions in promoting regeneration highlight that new protein synthesis and transport of the cytoskeleton are important intrinsic determinants of regeneration.

Axonal transport

Many neurons have long axons, which are dependent for their nourishment on the transport of substances from the cell body, a function that is performed by the microtubules (MTs). When a radio-labeled amino acid is injected in or near the cell body, and the time-course of movement of the labeled proteins down the axon determined, two types of forward transport are observed; rapid transport at 100–400 mm/day and slow transport at less than 6 mm/day. Rapid transport moves membranous organelles such as mitochondria and synaptic vescicles, while slow transport moves cytoskeletal and other proteins. The slow component has been subdivided into two overlapping components, SCa averaging 1.7 mm/day and SCb from 2–5 mm/day. Among cytoskeletal proteins, neurofilaments (NFs) is transported with SCa, whereas actin and tubulin are transported with SCb (Jacob and McQuarrie, 1991). The ultrastructural appearance of organelles attached to MTs by cross-linking structures eventually led to the isolation of a molecular motor, kinesin (Vale et al., 1985), which is a dimeric protein with ATPase activity. According to the current model, kinesin unbinds from the MT during the hydrolysis of ATP to ADP + Pi, analogous to myosin, the molecular motor of muscle (Fig. 24.4). Alternate binding and unbinding of the two monomers results in a hand-over-hand movement of kinesin along the MT, carrying its cargo with it (Yildiz et al., 2004). Different members of a kinesin-like family of molecules (KIFs) are now each thought to transport different organelles and molecules (Vale, 2003). For a long time, the mechanism of slow transport remained mysterious. Recently, however, it has been observed that slowly transported molecules such as NFs and MTs move rapidly but intermittently, so that they too are transported by the same mechanism as organelles, hopping on and off the MT fast transport system (Brown, 2003). MTs also transport substances retrogradely from the axon tip to the cell body at rates of approximately 300 μm/day. A molecular motor, dynein, has been identified for this fast retrograde transport system (Schnapp and

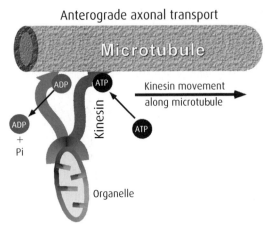

Anterograde axonal transport

Figure 24.4. *Kinesin is a molecular motor that transports cargo centrifugally along the MT.* Hydrolysis of ATP provides energy for a hand-over-hand movement of kinesin (see text for details).

Reese, 1989). Dyneins are cytoplasmic molecules that require complexing with other molecules, dynactins, in order to perform their transport function. Disruption of dynactin in motor neurons leads to blockage of retrograde transport and to motor neuronal degeneration (LaMonte et al., 2002). A slow retrograde transport system has not been observed. The ability of axons to regenerate must depend on the ability of the transport system to supply the growing tips with nutrients and structural components. Moreover, the retrograde transport system is critical in supplying the perikaryon with information about the state of the axon, including axotomy (see above and Volume I, Chapter 23). Thus in theory, heterogeneity in the efficiency of the retrograde transport system could contribute to heterogeneity in regenerative ability, although this has yet to be demonstrated. Pathologic processes that interrupt axonal transport will interrupt regeneration, although in the short run, growth cone motility can occur even in axon segments separated from the cell body.

Cytoskeletal proteins

During development, the growing tips of axons display growth cones, consisting of filopodia and

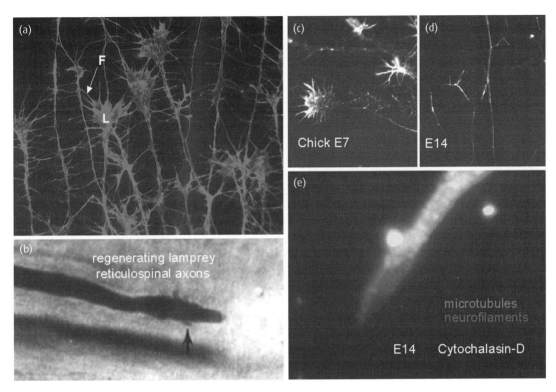

Figure 24.5. *An actin-independent mechanism of axon growth becomes more prominent with neuronal maturity and may be relevant to axon regeneration.* (a) The canonical form of embryonic growth cones in tissue culture labeled with phalloidin to show F-actin cytoskeleton (courtesy of J. Raper, University of Pennsylvania). Growth cones consist of a broad expanse, the lamellipodium (L) from which extend slender filopodia (F). (b) E7 chick DRG growth cones labeled for F-actin. (c) At E14, the growing axons have much less F-actin and less elaborate growth cones. (d) Axons regenerating in the transected lamprey spinal cord and labeled by intracellular injection of horseradish peroxidase have simple-shaped tips, lacking filopodia and extending only short, NF-containing processes (arrow; adapted with permission from (Lurie et al., 1994)). Other studies suggest that the growing tips have little F-actin (Hall et al., 1997). (e) in the presence of cytochalasin-D to depolymerize F-actin, E14 DRG axons regenerating in tissue culture lose their growth cones, but continue to grow with simplified axon tips, in which MTs (green) appear to extend further than NFs (red), possibly providing a protrusive force that underlies the axon extension (Selzer, M.E., Jones, S.L. and Gallo G., unpublished). The yellow/orange color indicates co-distribution of MTs and NFs.

lamellipodia (Fig. 24.5). These adhere to extracellular substrata and contain surface receptors for guidance and adhesion molecules that translate surface binding into intracellular signals serving many functions, including axon elongation and turning, as well as inhibition of axon growth. Filopodia contain F-actin, and elongate by polymerization of actin microfilaments at their distal (+) ends. Lamellipodia contain actin, myosin and MTs, but not NFs (see Volume I, Chapter 19). It is postulated that filopodia and lamellipodia exert tension on the axon through interactions among actin, myosin and the MTs, thus pulling the axon forward (Rochlin et al., 1996). The fastest growth seems to be associated with lamellipodial rather than filopodial action (Kleitman and Johnson, 1989), whereas filopodia are believed to be important in axon pathfinding and turning (Bentley and O'Connor, 1994). Experiments with low doses of actin- and MT-depolymerizing drugs suggest that both MTs and actin participate in growth cone responses to guidance molecules (Zhou and Cohan, 2004). In the absence of MT extension into the axon tip, the lamellipodium is motile but unable to turn. Bundles of actin filaments are required to coordinate MT organization in growth cones, and selective loss of an actin bundle causes repulsive growth cone turning.

The role of cytoskeletal elements in CNS regeneration is less clear. During CNS regeneration in mammals, growth cones are poorly formed, with a bullet-like appearance. Regeneration of peripheral nerve is accompanied by increased mRNA expression and synthesis of tubulin and actin, while NF is downregulated (Tetzlaff et al., 1991). This has led to the assumption that MTs and actin microfilaments participate in the mechanism of regeneration, but NFs do not. However, the mature CNS has relatively little of the extracellular matrix molecules (e.g., laminin, fibronectin and collagen) that support axon growth and regeneration in peripheral nerve. In many parts of the CNS, integrins, the receptors for these matrix molecules, are downregulated or inactivated late in development (de Curtis and Reichardt, 1993; Ivins et al., 2000; Yoshida et al., 2003).

Mature axons may also be more sensitive to some negative environmental cues than developing axons (Cai et al., 2001) (see above and Volume I, Chapter 21), and in the mammalian CNS there is a failure to upregulate tubulin, unless axons are successful in regenerating into a peripheral nerve graft (McKerracher et al., 1993). Some regenerating axons in CNS may not use the actin-based filopodial mechanism of elongation. After spinal cord transection in the lamprey, the large reticulospinal axons regenerate but their growing tips are simple in shape, lacking lamellipodia and filopodia (Lurie et al., 1994). This has been confirmed in the living spinal cord (Zhang et al., 2005). The tips are densely packed with NFs (Pijak et al., 1996) and contain MTs but very little F-actin (Hall et al., 1997). Moreover, the packing densitiy of NFs is increased in regenerating axons and most of all in their growing tips (Pijak et al., 1996) and the regenerative abilities of axons belonging to identified neurons is correlated

with recovery of NF mRNA expression following an initial downregulation (Jacobs et al., 1997). This suggested that transport of NFs into the axon tip might generate a protrusive force that pushes the axon forward. Similarly, in fish optic nerves during the early stages of regeneration, growth cones appear to lack filopodia and contain abundant NF (Lanners and Grafstein, 1980). Moreover, unlike the situation in peripheral nerve, NF mRNA and protein synthesis is increased during regeneration of fish optic nerve (Tesser et al., 1986). In mammals, when optic nerve axons are induced to regenerate into grafts of peripheral nerve, the rates of transport of both NF-M and β-tubulin are increased, while that for actin is decreased (McKerracher et al., 1990a).

A model for axon growth without growth cones is the chick DRG cell with cytochalasin used to block polymerization of F-actin. Growth cones collapse but axons continue to grow, albeit more slowly (Marsh and Letourneau, 1984), with tips that are simple in shape, lacking filopodia and lamellipodia. The residual growth is eliminated by the MT-depolymerizing drug colchicine, suggesting that MTs are essential to the residual growth. Preliminary data suggest that this is not due to their role in transporting structural elements such as NFs, but to MT polymerization itself (Selzer, M.E., Jones, S.L. and Gallo, G., unpublished). During embryonic development, growth cones become progressively simple in shape (Nordlander, 1987) and in chick DRG cell axons, they lose much of their F-actin (Selzer, M.E., Jones, S.L. and Gallo, G., unpublished), suggesting that growth in mature axons may rely less on actin than in early embryonic axons.

It may be that MTs and/or NFs play a larger role and actin a smaller role than they do in the growth of axons during development.

Conditioning lesions

It has long been known that after a second axon lesion closer to the cell body than the first lesion axon regeneration is accelerated. An important insight into the increase in intrinsic growth state produced by conditioning lesions was the demonstration that peripheral axotomy of DRG cells could promote subsequent regeneration of their central axons after dorsal column lesion in adult rats (Neumann and Woolf, 1999). Although the precise mechanism is still incompletely understood, the conditioning lesion results in an increase in cAMP levels in the DRG (Qiu et al., 2002). A conditioning lesion to peripheral nerve results in a modest increase in the rate of transport of proteins in SCb (e.g., tubulin and actin) but not SCa (e.g., NF) (Jacob and McQuarrie, 1991). However, after injury in the CNS there is a failure to maintain normal axonal transport of the cytoskeleton (McKerracher et al., 1990b), and axonal transport is accelerated (including NF) when RGC axons regenerate into peripheral nerve grafts (McKerracher et al., 1990a). Together these findings suggest that accelerated slow transport may be prerequisite for successful regeneration in the CNS.

Growth-associated proteins

A strategy that has been useful in identifying molecules that may be important in the mechanism of regeneration is to do protein electrophoresis on homogenates from nervous system tissues during regeneration of axons, and to compare the patterns of protein expression with that of the same tissue under control conditions. By this means several rapidly transported growth-associated proteins have been identified (Skene, 1989).

The best known growth-associated protein is G(rowth) A(ssociated) P(rotein) of 43 kDa (Skene and Willard, 1981; Doster et al., 1991). The precise function of this protein is not known but it is associated with the growth cone membrane, is phosphorylated by PKC and binds to calmodulin, inducing neurite sprouting and synaptic transmitter release (Oestreicher et al., 1997). GAP-43 is expressed constitutively in neurons during axon development and then downregulated. However, not all axon growth involves GAP-43. For example, the distal axons of DRG cells grow rapidly after peripheral nerve injury and this is associated with upregulation of GAP-43. However, the proximal axons of DRG cells can regenerate more slowly after dorsal root lesions and this is not associated with expression of GAP-43

(Andersen and Schreyer, 1999). Purkynje cells (Buffo et al., 1997) and thalamocortical neurons (Mason et al., 2000) ordinarily show little ability to regenerate axons even into Schwann cell, embryonic neural, or peripheral nerve grafts. Cell- type-specific overexpression of GAP-43 in transgenic mice did not induce axonal regeneration in these cells, although short-distance sprouting with growth cones did occur. These and other findings can be interpreted to imply that GAP-43 is important in the generation of growth cones but this is not sufficient to induce regeneration. However, when GAP-43 and cytoskeleton associated protein of 23 kDa (CAP-23) were overexpressed together, DRG axons were able to regenerate after spinal cord transection (Bomze et al., 2001). It was suggested that individually, GAP-43 and CAP-23 promote sprouting of the axon terminal by mobilizing subplasmalemmal actin accumulation, but that the two must act together to promote longer-distance regeneration. Whether actin is involved in the latter is not clear. In transgenic zebrafish, a GAP-43 promotor element that triggered expression of GAP-43 during axon development did not do so during regeneration of optic nerve (Udvadia et al., 2001). Thus the signaling pathways for axon elongation during regeneration may be different from those during axon development.

Another GAP, small proline-rich repeat protein 1A (SPRRP1A), is upregulated in DRG cells after peripheral axotomy. In DRG cells *in vitro*, overexpression of SPRRP1A resulted in enhanced neurite outgrowth, even on inhibitory substrates, and co-localization of the protein with F-actin in the ruffles of growth cones, whereas blocking SPRRP1A function inhibited axon growth (Bonilla et al., 2002). Thus SPRRP1A mimicked the effect of peripheral axotomy in DRG cells but its significance for regeneration in CNS is unknown.

Guidance molecule receptors

Of the molecules that have been identified as growth cone collapsing factors, some are associated with myelin (see Volume I, Chapter 21). Others are developmental guidance molecules, for example, netrins, semaphorins and ephrins (see Volume I, Chapter 19). These growth-inhibiting molecules will be effective only to the extent that axons bear receptors for them on their surfaces. Little is known about how axonal regeneration is influenced by expression of these receptors. In development, netrin exerts both chemoattractive and chemorepulsive effects. Chemoattraction is mediated by the receptor DCC, whereas chemorepulsion is mediated by a complex of DCC and Unc-5 (see Volume I, Chapter 19). In the lamprey, netrin is widely expressed by neurons and glia in the spinal cord and both DCC and Unc-5 are expressed by some reticulospinal neurons in the brainstem. Spinal cord transection resulted in upregulation of Unc-5 mRNA selectively in neurons that are known to regenerate poorly (Shifman and Selzer, 2000), suggesting that sensitivity to the chemorepulsive effects of netrin may influence the regenerative ability of some neurons. In the adult rat, RGCs express mRNAs for netrin-1 and for its receptors, DCC and Unc5h2. Following axotomy, both DCC and Unc5h2 were downregulated, regardless of whether the neuron's axon regenerated into a peripheral nerve graft (Ellezam et al., 2001). Thus the net effect of netrin signaling on regeneration of RGC axons is not clear. Although netrins were first discovered because of their chemoattractive effects (Kennedy et al., 1994), thus far evidence for an effect on axonal regeneration in CNS has suggested only chemorepulsion.

Semaphorins are almost exclusively growth inhibitory molecules. Following injuries in the CNS, fibroblasts of the glial scar express semaphorin III in the adult but not in the neonatal rat (Pasterkamp et al., 1999). In the rat spinal cord, injured corticospinal and rubrospinal tract axons express neuropilins and plexins, the receptors for semaphorins (De Winter et al., 2002). Thus semaphorin signaling may contribute to failure of regeneration in the injured spinal cord. Axotomy of olfactory neurons is normally followed by generation of new olfactory receptor neurons and regeneration of their axons into the olfactory bulb. Under these conditions, semaphorin III was only transiently expressed in cells at the lesion site. However, olfactory bulb ablation, which also leads to generation of new olfactory neurons, led to permanent expression of semaphorin III in cells at the lesion site and failure of olfactory axon regeneration past the lesion (Pasterkamp et al., 1998).

During development, the establishment of retinotopic projections on the optic tectum is guided by repulsive interactions between members of the ephrin-A family of membrane-bound ligands, which are expressed in gradients on the cells of the optic tectum, and Eph-A receptor tyrosine kinases, which are expressed in RGCs in gradients across the retina (O'Leary and Wilkinson, 1999). Ephrin-As are downregulated postnatally in mammals, chicks and fish, although Eph-As persist in most species. Ephrins were re-expressed in a correct gradient after lesions to the optic nerve in fish (Becker and Becker, 2000) and persisted into adulthood in frogs (Bach et al., 2003), which probably accounts for the accuracy with which retinotopic connectivity is reestablished in these species. A similar pattern of optic nerve section-induced expression has been noted in rat (Rodger et al., 2001), where regeneration does not normally occur.

In summary, correlative data suggest that embryonic guidance molecules may act to inhibit axonal regeneration in the CNS, but thus far, no evidence for a chemoattractive role has been seen.

Nogo receptor

The NgR signals growth inhibition by myelin-derived inhibitory proteins (Fournier et al., 2001; Wang et al., 2002; Wong et al., 2002). It seems likely that the level of expression of NgR by axons is a key determinant of regeneration because of its importance for signaling growth inhibition by MAG, OMgP and Nogo. Whether or not there is widespread expression of NgR in the CNS has been controversial, but now different NgR homologs have been identified, and expression of NgR in the CNS appears to be widespread (Lauren et al., 2003). The signaling by NgR has been well studied, and NgR has the potential to modify the actin cytoskeleton through its activation of Rho. NgR lacks a cytoplasmic domain and forms a receptor complex with the p75 neurotrophin receptor and a newly identified protein called Lingo (Yamashita et al., 1999; Mi et al., 2004; Fig. 24.3). When growth inhibitory proteins activate the receptor complex, Rho is activated (Yamashita and Tohyama, 2003). Plating neurons on growth inhibitory substrates activates Rho, and this blocks axon growth (Winton et al., 2002; Fournier et al., 2003). The role of Nogo and its receptor is discussed in Volume I, Chapter 21.

Cell adhesion molecules

The role of cell adhesion molecules in regeneration is discussed in detail in Volume I, Chapters 22 and 28. However, several strategies to promote regeneration involve transplantation of peripheral nerve grafts, Schwann cells or other growth promoting components of peripheral nerve, including fibroblasts genetically engineered to produce NGF. There is evidence that regeneration of CNS axons through these modified extracellular environments depends on the balance between permissive and inhibitory extracellular matrix molecules associated with these grafts (Jones et al., 2003). Therefore, the ability of neurons to express receptors or complimentary binding molecules on their surface could be important determinants of their intrinsic regenerative ability. Thus the ability of axons to regenerate through peripheral nerve grafts in mammalian experimental models correlated with their expression of L1 (Woolhead et al., 1998; Chaisuksunt et al., 2000b) and its close homolog CHL1 (Chaisuksunt et al., 2000a). In zebrafish, where axons regenerate spontaneously after spinal cord transection, the regenerative abilities of different supraspinal axon tracts correlated with the ability of their neurons to express the homophilic cell adhesion molecule L1 but not another homophilic member of the IgG superfamily, neural cell adhesion molecule (NCAM) (Becker et al., 1998). Moreover, morpholino-based inhibition of L1.1 synthesis caused inhibition of axon regeneration and locomotor recovery (Becker et al., 2004). After spinal cord injury in adult rats, treatment with soluble L1-Fc promoted axon regeneration and functional recovery (Roonprapunt et al.,

2003). Thus, adhesion molecules can help overcome an inhibitory environment and tip the balance to favor of axon regeneration.

24.8 Summary and conclusions

For over 100 years, the failure of axons in the CNS to regenerate has been considered the main factor limiting recovery from neural injury. The impressive gains in identification of growth-inhibitory molecules in the CNS led to expectations that their neutralization would lead to functional regeneration. However, results of therapeutic approaches based on this assumption have been mixed. More recent data suggest that neurons differ in their ability to regenerate through similar extracellular environments and moreover, they undergo a developmental loss of intrinsic regenerative ability. The factors mediating these intrinsic regenerative abilities include expression of: (a) receptors for inhibitory molecules such as the myelin-associated growth inhibitors and developmental guidance molecules, (b) surface molecules that permit axon adhesion to cells in the path of growth, (c) cytoskeletal proteins that mediate the mechanics of axon growth, and (d) molecules in the intracellular signaling cascades that mediate responses to chemoattractive and chemorepulsive cues. The tendency for growth cones to simplify progressively during development, with a reduced reliance on actin-driven growth cones, and the simple shapes of regenerating axon tips described in the lamprey and other animal models of CNS regeneration, suggest that axons may compensate for an abundance of inhibitory cues targeted at actin-based axon elongation by employing a second mechanism of growth (Fig. 24.6). In contrast to axon development, regeneration might involve internal protrusive forces generated by MTs, either through their own elongation, or by transporting other cytoskeletal elements such as NFs into the axon tip. Given the complexity of the regenerative program, it seems unlikely that a single approach will be sufficient to achieve functional restoration of neuronal circuits. Combination treatments will be increasingly prominent.

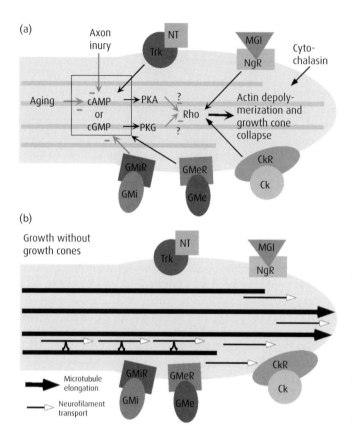

(a)

(b)

Growth without growth cones

Microtubule elongation

Neurofilament transport

Figure 24.6. *Hypothetical switch from an actin-based to MT-based growth in regeneration of injured mature axons.* (a) During development, there is a loss of intrinsic regenerative ability that is partially explained by a reduction in intraneuronal cAMP levels, which would thereby reduce the activation of PKA. It has been hypothesized that PKA inactivates Rho by phosphorylating it, thereby rendering the axon less susceptible to the effects of myelin-associated growth inhibitors and chemorepulsive guidance molecules. Thus the developmental changes, including a reduction in cAMP levels, lead to an increased sensitivity of the regenerating axon tip to several growth cone-collapsing influences in its extracellular environment. (b) Mature axons are capable of regenerating despite the absence of a conventional growth cone. The residual growth may be due to internal protrusive forces generated by MTs, either directly through their own elongation, or indirectly through their transport of other cytoskeletal elements such as NFs.

ACKNOWLEDGEMENTS

Dr. Lisa McKerracher is Chief Scientific Officer of BioAxone Therapeutic, which is investigating the effectiveness of a Rho inhibitor in enhancing regeneration. Dr. Selzer's research is supported by NIH grants R01-NS14837, R01-NS38537 and T32-HD07425.

REFERENCES

Aguayo, A.J., Rasminsky, M., Bray, G.M., Carbonetto, S., McKerracher, L., Villegas Pérez, M.P., Vidal Sanz, M. and Carter, D.A. (1991). Degenerative and regenerative responses of injured neurons in the central nervous system of adult mammals. *Philos Trans Roy Soc London (Biol)*, **331**, 337–343.

Andersen, L.B. and Schreyer, D.J. (1999). Constitutive expression of GAP-43 correlates with rapid, but not slow regrowth of injured dorsal root axons in the adult rat. *Exp Neurol*, **155**, 157–164.

Anderson, P.N., Campbell, G., Zhang, Y. and Lieberman, A.R. (1998). Cellular and molecular correlates of the regeneration of adult mammalian CNS axons into peripheral nerve grafts. *Prog Brain Res*, **117**, 211–232.

Babcock, A.A., Kuziel, W.A., Rivest, S. and Owens, T. (2003). Chemokine expression by glial cells directs leukocytes to sites of axonal injury in the CNS. *J Neurosci*, **23**, 7922–7930.

Bach, H., Feldheim, D.A., Flanagan, J.G. and Scalia, F. (2003). Persistence of graded EphA/ephrin-A expression in the adult frog visual system. *J Comp Neurol*, **467**, 549–565.

Bandtlow, C., Zachleder, T. and Schwab, M.E. (1990). Oligodendrocytes arrest neurite growth by contact inhibition. *J Neurosci*, **10**, 3837–3848.

Beattie, M.S., Bresnahan, J.C. and Lopate, G. (1990). Metamorphosis alters the response to spinal cord transection in Xenopus laevis frogs. *J Neurobiol*, **21**, 1108–1122.

Becker, C.G. and Becker, T. (2000). Gradients of ephrin-A2 and ephrin-A5b mRNA during retinotopic regeneration of the optic projection in adult zebrafish. *J Comp Neurol*, **427**, 469–483.

Becker, C.G., Lieberoth, B.C., Morellini, F., Feldner, J., Becker, T. and Schachner, M. (2004). L1.1 is involved in spinal cord regeneration in adult zebrafish. *J Neurosci*, **24**, 7837–7842.

Becker, T., Bernhardt, R.R., Reinhard, E., Wullimann, M.F., Tongiorgi, E. and Schachner, M. (1998). Readiness of zebrafish brain neurons to regenerate a spinal axon correlates with differential expression of specific cell recognition molecules. *J Neurosci*, **18**, 5789–5803.

Bentley, D. and O'Connor, T.P. (1994). Cytoskeletal events in growth cone steering. *Curr Opin Neurobiol*, **4**, 43–48.

Bethea, J.R. and Dietrich, W.D. (2002). Targeting the host inflammatory response in traumatic spinal cord injury. *Curr Opin Neurol*, **15**, 355–360.

Bethea, J.R., Castro, M., Keane, R.W., Lee, T.T., Dietrich, W.D. and Yezierski, R.P. (1998). Traumatic spinal cord injury induces nuclear factor-kappaB activation. *J Neurosci*, **18**, 3251–3260.

Bhatt, D.H., Otto, S.J., Depoister, B. and Fetcho, J.R. (2004). Cyclic AMP-induced repair of zebrafish spinal circuits. *Science*, **305**, 254–258.

Bito, H., Furuyashiki, T., Ishihara, H., Shibasaki, Y., Ohashi, K., Mizuno, K., Maekawa, M., Ishizaki, T. and Narumiya, S. (2000). A critical role for a Rho-associated kinase, p160ROCK, in determining axon outgrowth in mammalian CNS neurons. *Neuron*, **26**, 431–441.

Bjorklund, A. and Stenevi, U. (1984). Intracerebral neural implants: neuronal replacement and reconstruction of damaged circuitries. *Annu Rev Neurosci*, **7**, 279–308.

Blesch, A. and Tuszynski, M.H. (1997). Robust growth of chronically injured spinal cord axons induced by grafts of genetically modified NGF-secreting cells. *Exp Neurol*, **148**, 444–452.

Bomze, H.M., Bulsara, K.R., Iskandar, B.J., Caroni, P. and Skene, J.H. (2001). Spinal axon regeneration evoked by replacing two growth cone proteins in adult neurons. *Nat Neurosci*, **4**, 38–43.

Bonilla, I.E., Tanabe, K. and Strittmatter, S.M. (2002). Small proline-rich repeat protein 1A is expressed by axotomized neurons and promotes axonal outgrowth. *J Neurosci*, **22**, 1303–1315.

Borisoff, J.F., Chan, C.C., Hiebert, G.W., Oschipok, L., Robertson, G.S., Zamboni, R., Steeves, J.D. and Tetzlaff, W. (2003). Suppression of Rho-kinase activity promotes axonal growth on inhibitory CNS substrates. *Mol Cell Neurosci*, **22**, 405–416.

Bradbury, E.J., Moon, L.D., Popat, R.J., King, V.R., Bennett, G.S., Patel, P.N., Fawcett, J.W. and McMahon, S.B. (2002).

Chondroitinase ABC promotes functional recovery after spinal cord injury. *Nature*, **416**, 636–640.

Bregman, B.S., Kunkel-Bagden, E., Reier, P.J., Dai, H.N., McAtee, M. and Gao, D. (1993). Recovery of function after spinal cord injury: mechanisms underlying transplant-mediated recovery of function differ after spinal cord injury in newborn and adult rats. *Exp Neurol*, **123**, 3–16.

Brown, A. (2003). Axonal transport of membranous and non-membranous cargoes: a unified perspective. *J Cell Biol*, **160**, 817–821.

Buffo, A., Holtmaat, A.J., Savio, T., Verbeek, J.S., Oberdick, J., Oestreicher, A.B., Gispen, W.H., Verhaagen, J., Rossi, F. and Strata, P. (1997). Targeted overexpression of the neurite growth-associated protein B-50/GAP-43 in cerebellar Purkinje cells induces sprouting after axotomy but not axon regeneration into growth-permissive transplants. *J Neurosci*, **17**, 8778–8791.

Cai, D., Shen, Y., De Bellard, M., Tang, S. and Filbin, M.T. (1999). Prior exposure to neurotrophins blocks inhibition of axonal regeneration by MAG and myelin via a cAMP-dependent mechanism. *Neuron*, **22**, 89–101.

Cai, D., Qiu, J., Cao, Z., McAtee, M., Bregman, B.S. and Filbin, M.T. (2001). Neuronal cyclic AMP controls the developmental loss in ability of axons to regenerate. *J Neurosci*, **21**, 4731–4739.

Campenot, R.B. (1994). NGF and the local control of nerve terminal growth. *J Neurobiol*, **25**, 599–611.

Chaisuksunt, V., Campbell, G., Zhang, Y., Schachner, M., Lieberman, A.R. and Anderson, P.N. (2000a). The cell recognition molecule CHL1 is strongly upregulated by injured and regenerating thalamic neurons. *J Comp Neurol*, **425**, 382–392.

Chaisuksunt, V., Zhang, Y., Anderson, P.N., Campbell, G., Vaudano, E., Schachner, M. and Lieberman, A.R. (2000b). Axonal regeneration from CNS neurons in the cerebellum and brainstem of adult rats: correlation with the patterns of expression and distribution of messenger RNAs for L1, CHL1, c-jun and growth-associated protein-43. *Neuroscience*, **100**, 87–108.

Chen, D.F., Jhaveri, S. and Schneider, G.E. (1995). Intrinsic changes in developing retinal neurons result in regenerative failure of their axons. *Proc Natl Acad Sci USA*, **92**, 7287–7291.

Chen, M.S., Huber, A.B., van der Haar, M., Frank, M., Schnell, L., Spillmann, A.A., Christ, F. and Schwab, M.E. (2000). Nogo-A is a myelin-associated neurite outgrowth inhibitor and an antigen for monoclonal antibody IN-1. *Nature*, **403**, 434–438.

Cho, E.Y. and So, K.F. (1989). De novo formation of axon-like processes from axotomized retinal ganglion cells which exhibit long distance growth in a peripheral nerve graft in adult hamsters. *Brain Res*, **484**, 371–377.

Coumans, J.V., Lin, T.T., Dai, H.N., MacArthur, L., McAtee, M., Nash, C. and Bregman, B.S. (2001). Axonal regeneration and functional recovery after complete spinal cord transection in rats by delayed treatment with transplants and neurotrophins. *J Neurosci*, **21**, 9334–9344.

Dash, P.K., Tian, L.M. and Moore, A.N. (1998). Sequestration of cAMP response element-binding proteins by transcription factor decoys causes collateral elaboration of regenerating Aplysia motor neuron axons. *Proc Natl Acad Sci USA*, **95**, 8339–8344.

Davies, S.J., Field, P.M. and Raisman, G. (1994). Long interfascicular axon growth from embryonic neurons transplanted into adult myelinated tracts. *J Neurosci*, **14**, 1596–1612.

Davies, S.J., Fitch, M.T., Memberg, S.P., Hall, A.K., Raisman, G. and Silver, J. (1997). Regeneration of adult axons in white matter tracts of the central nervous system. *Nature*, **390**, 680–683.

de Curtis, I. and Reichardt, L.F. (1993). Function and spatial distribution in developing chick retina of the laminin receptor alpha 6 beta 1 and its isoforms. *Development*, **118**, 377–388.

De Winter, F., Holtmaat, A.J. and Verhaagen, J. (2002). Neuropilin and class 3 semaphorins in nervous system regeneration. *Adv Exp Med Biol*, **515**, 115–139.

Demjen, D., Klussmann, S., Kleber, S., Zuliani, C., Stieltjes, B., Metzger, C., Hirt, U.A., Walczak, H., Falk, W., Essig, M., Edler, L., Krammer, P.H. and Martin-Villalba, A. (2004). Neutralization of CD95 ligand promotes regeneration and functional recovery after spinal cord injury. *Nat Med*, **10**, 389–395.

Dergham, P., Ellezam, B., Essagian, C., Avedissian, H., Lubell, W.D. and McKerracher, L. (2002). Rho signaling pathway targeted to promote spinal cord repair. *J Neurosci*, **22**, 6570–6577.

Domeniconi, M., Cao, Z., Spencer, T., Sivasankaran, R., Wang, K.C., Nikulina, E., Kimura, N., Cai, H., Deng, K., Gao, Y., He, Z. and Filbin, M.T. (2002). Myelin-associated glycoprotein interacts with the Nogo66 receptor to inhibit neurite outgrowth. *Neuron*, **35**, 283–290.

Doster, S.K., Lozano, A.M., Aguayo, A.J. and Willard, M.B. (1991). Expression of the growth-associated protein GAP-43 in adult rat retinal ganglion cells following axon injury. *Neuron*, **6**, 635–647.

Dubreuil, C.I., Winton, M.J. and McKerracher, L. (2003). Rho activation patterns after spinal cord injury and the role of activated Rho in apoptosis in the central nervous system. *J Cell Biol*, **162**, 233–243.

Ellezam, B., Selles-Navarro, I., Manitt, C., Kennedy, T.E. and McKerracher, L. (2001). Expression of netrin-1 and its receptors DCC and UNC-5H2 after axotomy and during regeneration of adult rat retinal ganglion cells. *Exp Neurol*, **168**, 105–115.

Fawcett, J.W., Rokos, J. and Bakst, I. (1989). Oligodendrocytes repel axons and cause axonal growth cone collapse. *J Cell Sci*, **92(Pt 1)**, 93–100.

Forehand, C.J. and Farel, P.B. (1982). Anatomical and behavioral recovery from the effects of spinal cord transection: dependence on metamorphosis in anuran larvae. *J Neurosci*, **2**, 654–662.

Fournier, A.E., GrandPre, T. and Strittmatter, S.M. (2001). Identification of a receptor mediating Nogo-66 inhibition of axonal regeneration. *Nature*, **409**, 341–346.

Fournier, A.E., Takizawa, B.T. and Strittmatter, S.M. (2003). Rho kinase inhibition enhances axonal regeneration in the injured CNS. *J Neurosci*, **23**, 1416–1423.

Goldberg, J.L., Klassen, M.P., Hua, Y. and Barres, B.A. (2002). Amacrine-signaled loss of intrinsic axon growth ability by retinal ganglion cells. *Science*, **296**, 1860–1864.

Gomez, T.M., Robles, E., Poo, M. and Spitzer, N.C. (2001). Filopodial calcium transients promote substrate-dependent growth cone turning. *Science*, **291**, 1983–1987.

Gonzalez, R., Glaser, J., Liu, M.T., Lane, T.E. and Keirstead, H.S. (2003). Reducing inflammation decreases secondary degeneration and functional deficit after spinal cord injury. *Exp Neurol*, **184**, 456–463.

Goslin, K. and Banker, G. (1989). Experimental observations on the development of polarity by hippocampal neurons in culture. *J Cell Biol*, **108**, 1507–1516.

GrandPré, T., Nakamura, F., Vartanian, T. and Strittmatter, S.M. (2000). Identification of the Nogo inhibitor of axon regeneration as a reticulon protein. *Nature*, **403**, 439–444.

Gris, D., Marsh, D.R., Oatway, M.A., Chen, Y., Hamilton, E.F., Dekaban, G.A. and Weaver, L.C. (2004). Transient blockade of the CD11d/CD18 integrin reduces secondary damage after spinal cord injury, improving sensory, autonomic, and motor function. *J Neurosci*, **24**, 4043–4051.

Haas, K., Cline, H. and Malinow, R. (1998). No change in NMDA receptor-mediated response rise-time during development: evidence against transmitter spillover. *Neuropharmacology*, **37**, 1393–1398.

Hagg, T., Fass-Holmes, B., Vahlsing, H.L., Manthorpe, M., Conner, J.M. and Varon, S. (1989). Nerve growth factor (NGF) reverses axotomy-induced decreases in choline acetyltransferase, NGF receptor and size of medial septum cholinergic neurons. *Brain Res*, **505**, 29–38.

Hall, D.E., Neugebauer, K.M. and Reichardt, L.F. (1987). Embryonic neural retinal cell response to extracellular matrix proteins: developmental changes and effects of the cell substratum attachment antibody (CSAT). *J Cell Biol*, **104**, 623–634.

Hall, G.F., Poulos, A. and Cohen, M.J. (1989). Sprouts emerging from the dendrites of axotomized lamprey central neurons have axonlike ultrastructure. *J Neurosci*, **9**, 588–599.

Hall, G.F., Yao, J., Selzer, M.E. and Kosik, K.S. (1997). Cytoskeletal changes correlated with the loss of neuronal polarity in axotomized lamprey central neurons. *J Neurocytol*, **26**, 733–753.

Hardingham, G.E. and Bading, H. (2003). The Yin and Yang of NMDA receptor signalling. *Trend Neurosci*, **26**, 81–89.

Howland, D.R., Bregman, B.S., Tessler, A. and Goldberger, M.E. (1995). Transplants enhance locomotion in neonatal kittens whose spinal cords are transected: a behavioral and anatomical study. *Exp Neurol*, **135**, 123–145.

Inoue, T., Hosokawa, M., Morigiwa, K., Ohashi, Y. and Fukuda, Y. (2002). Bcl-2 overexpression does not enhance *in vivo* axonal regeneration of retinal ganglion cells after peripheral nerve transplantation in adult mice. *J Neurosci*, **22**, 4468–4477.

Ivins, J.K., Yurchenco, P.D. and Lander, A.D. (2000). Regulation of neurite outgrowth by integrin activation. *J Neurosci*, **20**, 6551–6560.

Jacob, J.M. and McQuarrie, I.G. (1991). Axotomy accelerates slow component b of axonal transport. *J Neurobiol*, **22**, 570–582.

Jacobs, A.J., Swain, G.P., Snedeker, J.A., Pijak, D.S., Gladstone, L.J. and Selzer, M.E. (1997). Recovery of neurofilament expression selectively in regenerating reticulospinal neurons. *J Neurosci*, **17**, 5206–5220.

Jin, Z. and Strittmatter, S.M. (1997). Rac1 mediates collapsin-1-induced growth cone collapse. *J Neurosci*, **17**, 6256–6263.

Jones, L.L., Sajed, D. and Tuszynski, M.H. (2003). Axonal regeneration through regions of chondroitin sulfate proteoglycan deposition after spinal cord injury: a balance of permissiveness and inhibition. *J Neurosci*, **23**, 9276–9288.

Keirstead, H.S., Dyer, J.K., Sholomenko, G.N., McGraw, J., Delaney, K.R. and Steeves, J.D. (1995). Axonal regeneration and physiological activity following transection and immunological disruption of myelin within the hatchling chick spinal cord. *J Neurosci*, **15**, 6963–6974.

Kennedy, T.E., Serafini, T., de la Torre, J.R. and Tessier-Lavigne, M. (1994). Netrins are diffusible chemotropic factors for commissural axons in the embryonic spinal cord. *Cell*, **78**, 425–435.

Kleitman, N. and Johnson, M.I. (1989). Rapid growth cone translocation on laminin is supported by lamellipodial not filopodial structures. *Cell Motil Cytoskel*, **13**, 288–300.

Kottis, V., Thibault, P., Mikol, D., Xiao, Z.C., Zhang, R., Dergham, P. and Braun, P.E. (2002). Oligodendrocyte-myelin glycoprotein (OMgp) is an inhibitor of neurite outgrowth. *J Neurochem*, **82**, 1566–1569.

Kwon, B.K., Liu, J., Messerer, C., Kobayashi, N.R., McGraw, J., Oschipok, L. and Tetzlaff, W. (2002). Survival and regeneration of rubrospinal neurons 1 year after spinal cord injury. *Proc Natl Acad Sci USA*, **99**, 3246–3251.

LaMonte, B.H., Wallace, K.E., Holloway, B.A., Shelly, S.S., Ascano, J., Tokito, M., Van Winkle, T., Howland, D.S. and Holzbaur, E.L. (2002). Disruption of dynein/dynactin inhibits axonal transport in motor neurons causing late-onset progressive degeneration. *Neuron*, **34**, 715–727.

Lanners, H.N. and Grafstein, B. (1980). Early stages of axonal regeneration in the goldfish optic tract: an electron microscopic study. *J Neurocytol*, **9**, 733–751.

Lau, K.C., So, K.F. and Tay, D. (1994). Intravitreal transplantation of a segment of peripheral nerve enhances axonal regeneration of retinal ganglion cells following distal axotomy. *Exp Neurol*, **128**, 211–215.

Laufs, U., Endres, M., Stagliano, N., Amin-Hanjani, S., Chui, D.S., Yang, S.X., Simoncini, T., Yamada, M., Rabkin, E., Allen, P.G., Huang, P.L., Bohm, M., Schoen, F.J., Moskowitz, M.A. and Liao, J.K. (2000). Neuroprotection mediated by changes in the endothelial actin cytoskeleton. *J Clin Invest*, **106**, 15–24.

Lauren, J., Airaksinen, M.S., Saarma, M. and Timmusk, T. (2003). Two novel mammalian Nogo receptor homologs differentially expressed in the central and peripheral nervous systems. *Mol Cell Neurosci*, **24**, 581–594.

Lazarov-Spiegler, O., Solomon, A.S. and Schwartz, M. (1998). Peripheral nerve-stimulated macrophages simulate a peripheral nerve-like regenerative response in rat transected optic nerve. *Glia*, **24**, 329–337.

Lehmann, M., Fournier, A., Selles-Navarro, I., Dergham, P., Sebok, A., Leclerc, N., Tigyi, G. and McKerracher, L. (1999). Inactivation of Rho signaling pathway promotes CNS axon regeneration. *J Neurosci*, **19**, 7537–7547.

Li, D., Field, P.M. and Raisman, G. (1995). Failure of axon regeneration in postnatal rat entorhinohippocampal slice coculture is due to maturation of the axon, not that of the pathway or target. *Eur J Neurosci*, **7**, 1164–1171.

Liu, Y., Kim, D., Himes, B.T., Chow, S.Y., Schallert, T., Murray, M., Tessler, A. and Fischer, I. (1999). Transplants of fibroblasts genetically modified to express BDNF promote regeneration of adult rat rubrospinal axons and recovery of forelimb function. *J Neurosci*, **19**, 4370–4387.

Lu, X. and Richardson, P.M. (1991). Inflammation near the nerve cell body enhances axonal regeneration. *J Neurosci*, **11**, 972–978.

Lurie, D.I., Pijak, D.S. and Selzer, M.E. (1994). Structure of reticulospinal axon growth cones and their cellular environment during regeneration in the lamprey spinal cord. *J Comp Neurol*, **344**, 559–580.

Mackler, S.A., Yin, H.S. and Selzer, M.E. (1986). Determinants of directional specificity in the regeneration of lamprey spinal axons. *J Neurosci*, **6**, 1814–1821.

MacLaren, R.E. (1996). Expression of myelin proteins in the opossum optic nerve: late appearance of inhibitors implicates an earlier non-myelin factor in preventing ganglion cell regeneration. *J Comp Neurol*, **372**, 27–36.

Madura, T., Yamashita, T., Kubo, T., Fujitani, M., Hosokawa, K. and Tohyama, M. (2004). Activation of Rho in the injured axons following spinal cord injury. *Embo Rep*, **5**, 412–417.

Markus, A., Patel, T.D. and Snider, W.D. (2002). Neurotrophic factors and axonal growth. *Curr Opin Neurobiol*, **12**, 523–531.

Marsh, L. and Letourneau, P.C. (1984). Growth of neurites without filopodial or lamellipodial activity in the presence of cytochalasin B. *J Cell Biol*, **99**, 2041–2047.

Mason, M.R., Campbell, G., Caroni, P., Anderson, P.N. and Lieberman, A.R. (2000). Overexpression of GAP-43 in thalamic projection neurons of transgenic mice does not enable them to regenerate axons through peripheral nerve grafts. *Exp Neurol*, **165**, 143–152.

McDonald, J.W., Althomsons, S.P., Hyrc, K.L., Choi, D.W. and Goldberg, M.P. (1998). Oligodendrocytes from forebrain are highly vulnerable to AMPA/kainate receptor-mediated excitotoxicity. *Nat Med*, **4**, 291–297.

McKeon, R.J., Schreiber, R.C., Rudge, J.S. and Silver, J. (1991). Reduction of neurite outgrowth in a model of glial scarring following CNS injury is correlated with the expression of inhibitory molecules on reactive astrocytes. *J Neurosci*, **11**, 3398–3411.

McKerracher, L., Vidal-Sanz, M. and Aguayo, A.J. (1990a). Slow transport rates of cytoskeletal proteins change during regeneration of axotomized retinal neurons in adult rats. *J Neurosci*, **10**, 641–648.

McKerracher, L., Vidal-Sanz, M., Essagian, C. and Aguayo, A.J. (1990b). Selective impairment of slow axonal transport after optic nerve injury in adult rats. *J Neurosci*, **10**, 2834–2841.

McKerracher, L., Essagian, C. and Aguayo, A.J. (1993). Marked increase in beta-tubulin mRNA expression during regeneration of axotomized retinal ganglion cells in adult mammals. *J Neurosci*, **13**, 5294.

McKerracher, L., David, S., Jackson, J.L., Kottis, V., Dunn, R. and Braun, P.E. (1994). Identification of myelin-associated glycoprotein as a major myelin-derived inhibitor of neurite outgrowth. *Neuron*, **13**, 805–811.

Mi, S., Lee, X., Shao, Z., Thill, G., Ji, B., Relton, J., Levesque, M., Allaire, N., Perrin, S., Sands, B., Crowell, T., Cate, R.L.,

McCoy, J.M. and Pepinsky, R.B. (2004). LINGO-1 is a component of the Nogo-66 receptor/p75 signaling complex. *Nat Neurosci*, **7**, 221–228.

Ming, G.L., Song, H.J., Berninger, B., Holt, C.E., Tessier-Lavigne, M. and Poo, M.M. (1997). cAMP-dependent growth cone guidance by netrin-1. *Neuron*, **19**, 1225–1235.

Monnier, P.P., Sierra, A., Schwab, J.M., Henke-Fahle, S. and Mueller, B.K. (2003). The Rho/ROCK pathway mediates neurite growth-inhibitory activity associated with the chondroitin sulfate proteoglycans of the CNS glial scar. *Mol Cell Neurosci*, **22**, 319–330.

Montaner, S., Perona, R., Saniger, L. and Lacal, J.C. (1999). Activation of serum response factor by RhoA is mediated by the nuclear factor-kappaB and C/EBP transcription factors. *J Biol Chem*, **274**, 8506–8515.

Mukhopadhyay, G., Doherty, P., Walsh, F.S., Crocker, P.R. and Filbin, M.T. (1994). A novel role for myelin-associated glycoprotein as an inhibitor of axonal regeneration. *Neuron*, **13**, 805–811.

Neumann, S. and Woolf, C.J. (1999). Regeneration of dorsal column fibers into and beyond the lesion site following adult spinal cord injury. *Neuron*, **23**, 83–91.

Neumann, H., Schweigreiter, R., Yamashita, T., Rosenkranz, K., Wekerle, H. and Barde, Y.A. (2002a). Tumor necrosis factor inhibits neurite outgrowth and branching of hippocampal neurons by a rho-dependent mechanism. *J Neurosci*, **22**, 854–862.

Neumann, S., Bradke, F., Tessier-Lavigne, M. and Basbaum, A.I. (2002b). Regeneration of sensory axons within the injured spinal cord induced by intraganglionic cAMP elevation. *Neuron*, **34**, 885–893.

Niederost, B., Oertle, T., Fritsche, J., McKinney, R.A. and Bandtlow, C.E. (2002). Nogo-A and myelin-associated glycoprotein mediate neurite growth inhibition by antagonistic regulation of RhoA and Rac1. *J Neurosci*, **22**, 10368–10376.

Nishiyama, M., Hoshino, A., Tsai, L., Henley, J.R., Goshima, Y., Tessier-Lavigne, M., Poo, M.M. and Hong, K. (2003). Cyclic AMP/GMP-dependent modulation of Ca2+ channels sets the polarity of nerve growth-cone turning. *Nature*, **424**, 990–995.

Nordlander, R.H. (1987). Axonal growth cones in the developing amphibian spinal cord. *J Comp Neurol*, **263**, 485–496.

Oestreicher, A.B., De Graan, P.N., Gispen, W.H., Verhaagen, J. and Schrama, L.H. (1997). B-50, the growth associated protein-43: modulation of cell morphology and communication in the nervous system. *Prog Neurobiol*, **53**, 627–686.

O'Leary, D.D. and Wilkinson, D.G. (1999). Eph receptors and ephrins in neural development. *Curr Opin Neurobiol*, **9**, 65–73.

Pasterkamp, R.J., De Winter, F., Holtmaat, A.J. and Verhaagen, J. (1998). Evidence for a role of the chemorepellent semaphorin III and its receptor neuropilin-1 in the regeneration of primary olfactory axons. *J Neurosci*, **18**, 9962–9976.

Pasterkamp, R.J., Giger, R.J., Ruitenberg, M.J., Holtmaat, A.J., De Wit, J., De Winter, F. and Verhaagen, J. (1999). Expression of the gene encoding the chemorepellent semaphorin III is induced in the fibroblast component of neural scar tissue formed following injuries of adult but not neonatal CNS. *Mol Cell Neurosci*, **13**, 143–166.

Pearse, D.D., Pereira, F.C., Marcillo, A.E., Bates, M.L., Berrocal, Y.A., Filbin, M.T. and Bunge, M.B. (2004). cAMP and Schwann cells promote axonal growth and functional recovery after spinal cord injury. *Nat Med*, **10**, 610–616.

Pijak, D.S., Hall, G.F., Tenicki, P.J., Boulos, A.S., Lurie, D.I. and Selzer, M.E. (1996). Neurofilament spacing, phosphorylation, and axon diameter in regenerating and uninjured lamprey axons. *J Comp Neurol*, **368**, 569–581.

Popovich, P.G., Guan, Z., Wei, P., Huitinga, I., van Rooijen, N. and Stokes, B.T. (1999). Depletion of hematogenous macrophages promotes partial hindlimb recovery and neuroanatomical repair after experimental spinal cord injury. *Exp Neurol*, **158**, 351–365.

Prinjha, R., Moore, S.E., Vinson, M., Blake, S., Morrow, R., Christie, G., Michalovich, D., Simmons, D.L. and Walsh, F.S. (2000). Inhibitor of neurite outgrowth in humans. *Nature*, **403**, 383–384.

Qin, Z.H., Wang, Y., Nakai, M. and Chase, T.N. (1998). Nuclear factor-kappa B contributes to excitotoxin-induced apoptosis in rat striatum. *Mol Pharmacol*, **53**, 33–42.

Qiu, J., Cai, D., Dai, H., McAtee, M., Hoffman, P.N., Bregman, B.S. and Filbin, M.T. (2002). Spinal axon regeneration induced by elevation of cyclic AMP. *Neuron*, **34**, 895–903.

Raivich, G., Bohatschek, M., Da Costa, C., Iwata, O., Galiano, M., Hristova, M., Nateri, A.S., Makwana, M., Riera-Sans, L., Wolfer, D.P., Lipp, H.P., Aguzzi, A., Wagner, E.F. and Behrens, A. (2004). The AP-1 transcription factor c-Jun is required for efficient axonal regeneration. *Neuron*, **43**, 57–67.

Ramer, M.S., Priestley, J.V. and McMahon, S.B. (2000). Functional regeneration of sensory axons into the adult spinal cord. *Nature*, **403**, 312–316.

Rashid, N.A. and Cambray-Deakin, M.A. (1992). *N*-methyl-D-aspartate effects on the growth, morphology and cytoskeleton of individual neurons *in vitro*. *Brain Res Dev Brain Res*, **67**, 301–308.

Rochlin, M.W., Wickline, K.M. and Bridgman, P.C. (1996). Microtubule stability decreases axon elongation but not axoplasm production. *J Neurosci*, **16**, 3236–3246.

Rodger, J., Lindsey, K.A., Leaver, S.G., King, C.E., Dunlop, S.A. and Beazley, L.D. (2001). Expression of ephrin-A2 in the superior colliculus and EphA5 in the retina following optic nerve section in adult rat. *Eur J Neurosci*, **14**, 1929–1936.

Roonprapunt, C., Huang, W., Grill, R., Friedlander, D., Grumet, M., Chen, S., Schachner, M. and Young, W. (2003). Soluble cell adhesion molecule L1-Fc promotes locomotor recovery in rats after spinal cord injury. *J Neurotraum*, **20**, 871–882.

Rose, P.K., MacDermid, V., Joshi, M. and Neuber-Hess, M. (2001). Emergence of axons from distal dendrites of adult mammalian neurons following a permanent axotomy. *Eur J Neurosci*, **13**, 1166–1176.

Savio, T. and Schwab, M.E. (1997). Lesioned corticospinal tract axons regenerate in myelin-free rat spinal cord. *Proc Natl Acad Sci*, **87**, 4130–4133.

Schnapp, B.J. and Reese, T.S. (1989). Dynein is the motor for retrograde axonal transport of organelles. *Proc Natl Acad Sci USA*, **86**, 1548–1552.

Schnell, L., Schneider, R., Kolbeck, R., Barde, Y.A. and Schwab, M.E. (1994). Neurotrophin-3 enhances sprouting of corticospinal tract during development and after adult spinal cord lesion. *Nature*, **367**, 170–173.

Schwab, M.E. (2004). Nogo and axon regeneration. *Curr Opin Neurobiol*, **14**, 118–124.

Shearer, M.C., Niclou, S.P., Brown, D., Asher, R.A., Holtmaat, A.J., Levine, J.M., Verhaagen, J. and Fawcett, J.W. (2003). The astrocyte/meningeal cell interface is a barrier to neurite outgrowth which can be overcome by manipulation of inhibitory molecules or axonal signalling pathways. *Mol Cell Neurosci*, **24**, 913–925.

Shifman, M.I. and Selzer, M.E. (2000). Expression of the netrin receptor UNC-5 in lamprey brain: modulation by spinal cord transection. *Neurorehabil Neural Repair*, **14**, 49–58.

Skene, J.H. and Willard, M. (1981). Characteristics of growth-associated polypeptides in regenerating toad retinal ganglion cell axons. *J Neurosci*, **1**, 419–426.

Skene, J.H.P. (1989). Axonal growth-associated proteins. *Annu Rev Neurosci*, **12**, 127–156.

Song, H., Ming, G., He, Z., Lehmann, M., Tessier-Lavigne, M. and Poo, M. (1998). Conversion of neuronal growth cone responses from repulsion to attraction by cyclic nucleotides. *Science*, **281**, 1515–1518.

Tesser, P., Jones, P.S. and Schechter, N. (1986). Elevated levels of retinal neurofilament mRNA accompany optic nerve regeneration. *J Neurochem*, **47**, 1235–1243.

Tetzlaff, W., Alexander, S.W., Miller, F.D. and Bisby, M.A. (1991). Response of facial and rubrospinal neurons to axotomy: changes in mRNA expression for cytoskeletal proteins and GAP-43. *J Neurosci*, **11**, 2528–2544.

Tigyi, G., Fischer, D.J., Sebok, A., Yang, C., Dyer, D.L. and Miledi, R. (1996). Lysophosphatidic acid-induced neurite retraction in PC12 cells: control by phosphoinositide – Ca^{2+} signaling and Rho. *J Neurochem*, **66**, 537–548.

Udvadia, A.J., Koster, R.W. and Skene, J.H. (2001). GAP-43 promoter elements in transgenic zebrafish reveal a difference in signals for axon growth during CNS development and regeneration. *Development*, **128**, 1175–1182.

Vale, R.D. (2003). The molecular motor toolbox for intracellular transport. *Cell*, **112**, 467–480.

Vale, R.D., Reese, T.S. and Sheetz, M.P. (1985). Identification of a novel force-generating protein, kinesin, involved in microtubule-based motility. *Cell*, **42**, 39–50.

Vidal-Sanz, M., Bray, G.M., Villegas-Perez, M.P., Thanos, S. and Aguayo, A.J. (1987). Axonal regeneration and synapse formation in the superior colliculus by retinal ganglion cells in the adult retina. *J Neurosci*, **7**, 2894–2909.

Villegas-Perez, M.P., Vidal-Sanz, M., Bray, G.M. and Aguayo, A.J. (1988). Influences of peripheral nerve grafts on the survival and regrowth of axotomized retinal ganglion cells in adult rats. *J Neurosci*, **8**, 265.

Villegas-Perez, M.P., Vidal-Sanz, M., Rasminsky, M., Bray, G.M. and Aguayo, A.J. (1993). Rapid and protracted phases of retinal ganglion cell loss follow axotomy in the optic nerve of adult rats. *J Neurobiol*, **24**, 23–36.

Wahl, S., Barth, H., Coiossek, T., Akoriess, K. and Mueller, B.K. (2000). Ephrin-A5 induces collapse of growth cones by activating Rho and Rho kinase. *J Cell Biol*, **149**, 263–270.

Wang, K.C., Koprivica, V., Kim, J.A., Sivasankaran, R., Guo, Y., Neve, R.L. and He, Z. (2002). Oligodendrocyte-myelin glycoprotein is a Nogo receptor ligand that inhibits neurite outgrowth. *Nature*, **417**, 941–944.

Winton, M.J., Dubreuil, C.I., Lasko, D., Leclerc, N. and McKerracher, L. (2002). Characterization of new cell permeable C3-like proteins that inactivate Rho and stimulate neurite outgrowth on inhibitory substrates. *J Biol Chem*, **277**, 226570–226577.

Wong, S.T., Henley, J.R., Kanning, K.C., Huang, K.H., Bothwell, M. and Poo, M.M. (2002). A p75(NTR) and Nogo receptor complex mediates repulsive signaling by myelin-associated glycoprotein. *Nat Neurosci*, **5**, 1302–1308.

Woolhead, C.L., Zhang, Y., Lieberman, A.R., Schachner, M., Emson, P.C. and Anderson, P.N. (1998). Differential effects of autologous peripheral nerve grafts to the corpus striatum of adult rats on the regeneration of axons of striatal and nigral neurons and on the expression of GAP-43 and the cell adhesion molecules N-CAM and L1. *J Comp Neurol*, **391**, 259–273.

Yamashita, T. and Tohyama, M. (2003). The p75 receptor acts as a displacement factor that releases Rho from Rho-GDI. *Nat Neurosci*, **6**, 461–467.

Yamashita, T., Tucker, K.L. and Barde, Y.A. (1999). Neurotrophin binding to the p75 receptor modulates Rho activity and axonal outgrowth. *Neuron*, **24**, 585–593.

Yildiz, A., Tomishige, M., Vale, R.D. and Selvin, P.R. (2004). Kinesin walks hand-over-hand. *Science*, **303**, 676–678.

Yin, Y., Cui, Q., Li, Y., Irwin, N., Fischer, D., Harvey, A.R. and Benowitz, L.I. (2003). Macrophage-derived factors stimulate optic nerve regeneration. *J Neurosci*, **23**, 2284–2293.

Yoshida, N., Hishiyama, S., Yamaguchi, M., Hashiguchi, M., Miyamoto, Y., Kaminogawa, S. and Hisatsune, T. (2003). Decrease in expression of alpha 5 beta 1 integrin during neuronal differentiation of cortical progenitor cells. *Exp Cell Res*, **287**, 262–271.

Zhang, G., Jin, L.-Q., Sul, J.-Y., Haydon, P.G. and Selzer, M.E. (2005). Live imaging of regenerating lamprey spinal axons. *Neurorehabil Neural Repair*, **19**, 46–57.

Zheng, J.Q., Wan, J.J. and Poo, M.M. (1996). Essential role of filopodia in chemotropic turning of nerve growth cone induced by a glutamate gradient. *J Neurosci*, **16**, 1140–1149.

Zhou, F.Q. and Cohan, C.S. (2004). How actin filaments and microtubules steer growth cones to their targets. *J Neurobiol*, **58**, 84–91.

Ziv, N.E. and Spira, M.E. (1997). Localized and transient elevations of intracellular Ca2+ induce the dedifferentiation of axonal segments into growth cones. *J Neurosci*, **17**, 3568–3579.

Promotion of regeneration in the injured nervous system

CONTENTS

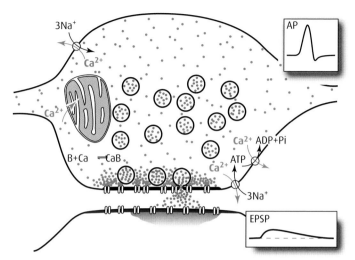

Plate 1 (figure 3.1). A schematic view of an axo-dendritic, or axo-somatic excitatory synapse formed by an hypothetical en passant bouton with a single active zone. An AP in the presynaptic terminal opens voltage-gated Ca^{2+} channels, which allow Ca^{2+} influx into the nerve terminal. After a brief period of a few milliseconds in small nerve terminals (Atluri and Regehr, 1996), Ca^{2+} will be spatially equilibrated, and most of the previously entered Ca^{2+} ions will be bound to endogenous Ca^{2+} buffers (Fig. 3.1b). Vesicles fusing with the plasma membrane (Jahn et al., 2003) release neurotransmitter, which acts on receptor-gated ion channels in the postsynaptic neuron to generate an EPSP. For further details, see text.

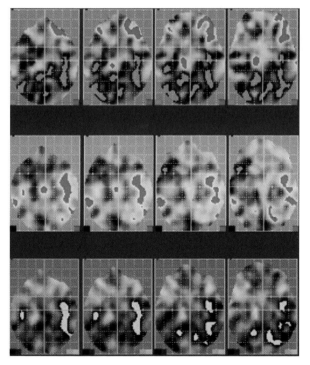

Plate 2 (figure 10.6b). Interregional analysis. Correlations of the right IPL with other parts of cortex are shown. Positive correlations are shown in **red**, negative correlations in **blue**. Auditory cortex in the superior temporal region is negatively correlated with the right IPL in sighted subjects (top panel) but positively in the blind (middle panel). Statistically significant differences are shown in the bottom panel with higher correlation in the blind in **yellow**. The increased correlation of the IPL with the superior temporal region is evident as is an increased correlation in prestriate cortex (Brodmann area 18). This amounts to a functional network for sound localization in the blind involving auditory, parietal and occipital regions.

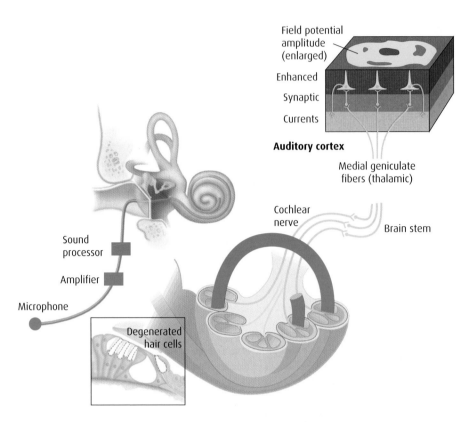

Plate 3 (figure 10.7). *CIs and auditory cortex.* CIs transform Environmental sounds into electrical signals by means of a microphone and digital signal processing. Stimulation of auditory nerve fibers in a tonotopic fashion induces activity in the auditory cortex, which leads to a strengthening of synaptic connections in young kittens (Klinke et al., 1999). The same process of auditory cortical plasticity is assumed to lead to excellent speech understanding in cochlear implant patients despite a highly incomplete signal (from Rauschecker, 1999b).

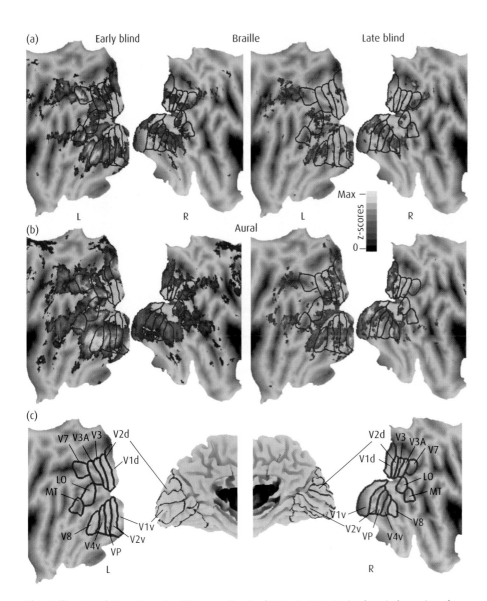

Plate 4 (figure 11.1). Two-dimensional flat maps showing fMRI activations in visual cortical areas in early and late blind subjects, during generation of verbs in response to nouns presented via (a) Braille or (b) aurally. Borders of visual areas are shown in sighted subjects (c). Reprinted, with permission of author and publisher, from Burton (2003); copyright 2003, Society for Neuroscience.

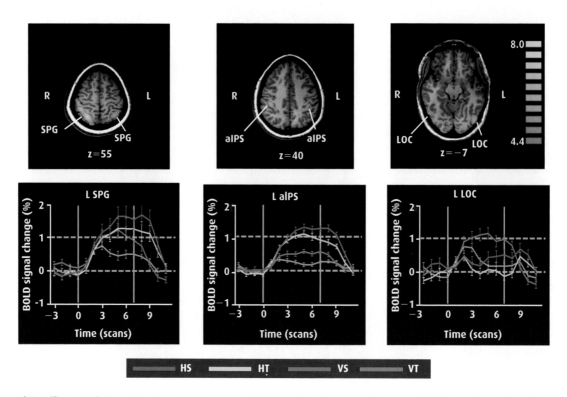

Plate 5 (figure 11.2). Bimodally shape-selective areas and fMRI activation time courses from areas in left hemisphere. Color scale at right represents *t* values. HS: haptic shape; HT: haptic texture; VS: visual shape; VT: visual texture. Modified from Zhang et al. (2004).

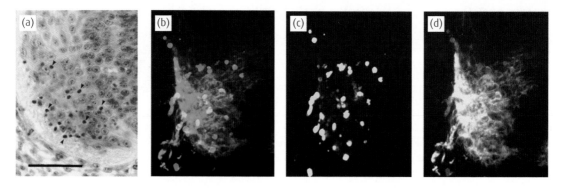

Plate 6 (figure 16.5). Photomicrographs of transverse sections through the cervical spinal cord of a 4-day-old chick embryo showing the distribution of dying neurons in the ventral horn. (a) Hematoxylin and eosin staining. (b–d) Labeling with the TUNEL method and spinal card-1 (SC-1) (a marker for ventral horn neurons) immunohistochemistry. (b) TUNEL + SC-1. (c) TUNEL (d) SCl. Scale bars. 50 μm *Arrows* in (a) indicate pyknotic profiles of degenerating neurons (from Yaginuma et al., 1996).

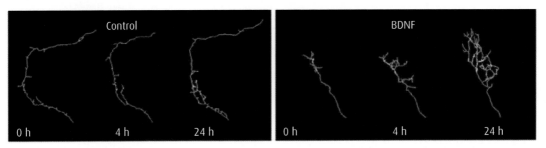

Plate 7 (figure 20.5). *BDNF increases RGC axon arborization and GFP-synaptobrevin puncta in vivo.* Tracings of three-dimensional arbors illustrate the effects of BDNF on axon arbor complexity and synapse number. Individual RGC axons double-labeled with GFP-synaptobrevin and DsRed were visualized by confocal microscopy in the live, developing tadpole after direct tectal injection of vehicle solution (control) or BDNF. BDNF not only increases axon arbor complexity but also increases the number and density of GFP-synaptobrevin clusters per axon terminal. Note the high proportion of branch points with synaptic clusters in these arbors (from Alsina et al. (2001)).

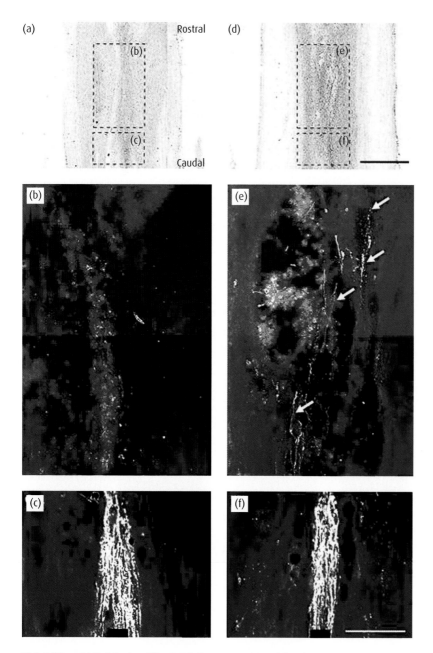

Plate 8 (figure 21.2). *Injection of db-cAMP induces regeneration of dorsal column axons in vivo*: Either saline (a–c) or 50 mM db-cAMP (d–f) was injected into L5 dorsal root ganglia and 1 week later dorsal column axons were lesioned. Axonal regeneration was assessed at 2 weeks post-injury. Darkfield images caudal to the lesion show that in both the control (c) and db-cAMP-injected (f) animals, regenerating axons approach the lesion site. However, the db-cAMP-treated (e) animals exhibit robust regeneration into and beyond the lesion site (arrows) as compared to the saline-injected controls (b). Scale bars: (a and d), 500 μm; (b, c, e and f), 150 μm (reprinted from Qui et al. (2002) *Neuron*, **34**, 895–903).

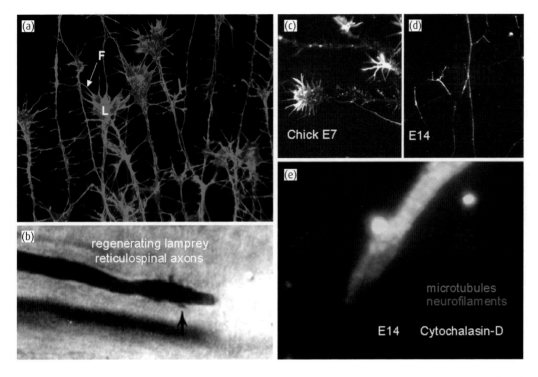

Plate 9 (figure 24.5). *An actin-independent mechanism of axon growth becomes more prominent with neuronal maturity and may be relevant to axon regeneration.* (a) The canonical form of embryonic growth cones in tissue culture labeled with phalloidin to show F-actin cytoskeleton (courtesy of J. Raper, University of Pennsylvania). Growth cones consist of a broad expanse, the lamellipodium (L) from which extend slender filopodia (F). (b) E7 chick DRG growth cones labeled for F-actin. (c) At E14, the growing axons have much less F-actin and less elaborate growth cones. (d) Axons regenerating in the transected lamprey spinal cord and labeled by intracellular injection of horseradish peroxidase have simple-shaped tips, lacking filopodia and extending only short, NF-containing processes (arrow; adapted with permission from (Lurie et al., 1994)). Other studies suggest that the growing tips have little F-actin (Hall et al., 1997). (e) in the presence of cytochalasin-D to depolymerize F-actin, E14 DRG axons regenerating in tissue culture lose their growth cones, but continue to grow with simplified axon tips, in which MTs (green) appear to extend further than NFs (red), possibly providing a protrusive force that underlies the axon extension (Selzer, M.E., Jones, S.L. and Gallo, G., unpublished). The yellow/orange color indicates co-distribution of MTs and NFs.

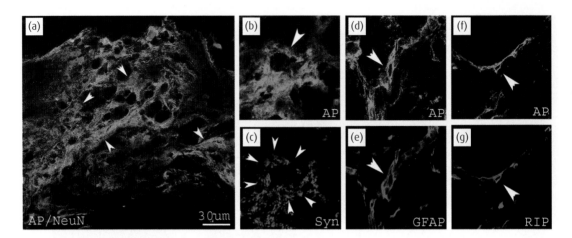

Plate 10 (figure 25.5). *NRP/GRP transplants differentiate in the injured spinal cord.* Graft-derived neurons are found at 5 weeks post-transplantation (a). Double immunofluorescence staining for AP (a, green) and NeuN (a, red), a marker of post-mitotic neurons, demonstrates graft-derived neurons. NRP/GRP grafts express synaptic markers at 5 weeks post-transplantation (b–c). Double immunofluorescence staining for AP (b, green) and the synaptic marker synaptophysin (c, red) suggests that grafted cells form synapses. Graft-derived astrocytes are present at 5 weeks post-transplantation (d–e). Double immunofluorescence staining for AP (d, green) and the astrocytic marker glial fibrillary acidic protein (GFAP) (e, red) shows graft-derived astrocytes. Graft-derived oligodendrocytes are present at 5 weeks post-transplantation (f–g). Double immunofluorescence staining for AP (f, green) with the oligodendrocytic marker RIP (g, red) shows graft-derived oligodendrocytes. Arrowheads denote double-labeled cells.

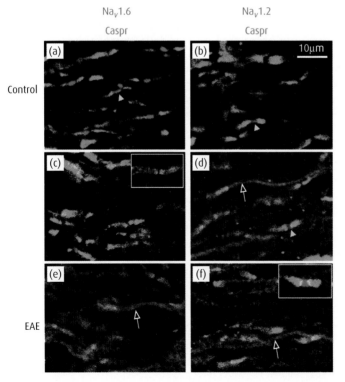

Plate 11 (figure 26.4). There is a switch in expression of sodium channels $Na_v1.6$ and $Na_v1.2$ in demyelinated axons within the CNS. Representative digital images of sections of optic nerve from control (a–b) and EAE (e–f) show immunostaining for $Na_v1.6$ and $Na_v1.2$ (red) and for Caspr (green). (a) and (b) demonstrate nodes with $Na_v1.6$ (a) and less commonly $Na_v1.2$ (b) immunostaining (yellow arrow heads) in healthy optic nerve. (c–e) and (d–f) demonstrate a pattern of progressive demyelination and nodal disruption in EAE, with weak and diffuse Caspr immunostaining at some nodes (inset, c). There is a loss of $Na_v1.6$ immunostaining (c and e) and increased frequency of nodes with $Na_v1.2$ immunostaining (d–f). Demyelinated axonal profiles with continuous $Na_v1.6$ (e, arrow) and, more commonly, $Na_v1.2$ (d, f, arrows) immunostaining are seen in EAE (modified from Craner et al. (2003a)).

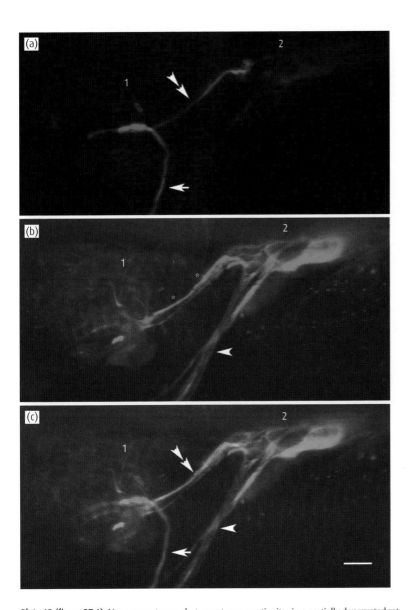

Plate 12 (figure 27.1). Nerve sprouts grow between two synaptic sites in a partially denervated rat muscle by following Schwann cell processes emerging from the denervated synaptic site. Two synaptic sites (labeled "1" and "2") in a rat soleus muscle 3 days after partial denervation. (a) Motor axon labeled by an anti-neurofilament antibody. The axon enters from the bottom of the panel (arrow), innervates site 1 and then "sprouts" to innervate site 2, a site denervated by the partial denervation. (b) Schwann cells labeled with an anti-nestin antibody. This antibody labels only Schwann cells that have lost axonal contact, that is "reactive" Schwann cells. Note the labeling of the old endoneurial tube that previously contained the axon innervating site 2 (arrowhead); the endoneurial tube of the axon innervating site 1 is unlabeled. Note also the association of the sprout in (a) with processes (asterisks) of the Schwann cells at site 2. (c) Merged image of the panels (a) & (b) with the axon in red and the Schwann cells in green. Scale bar indicates 10 μm. Modified from (Son and Thompson, 1995b).

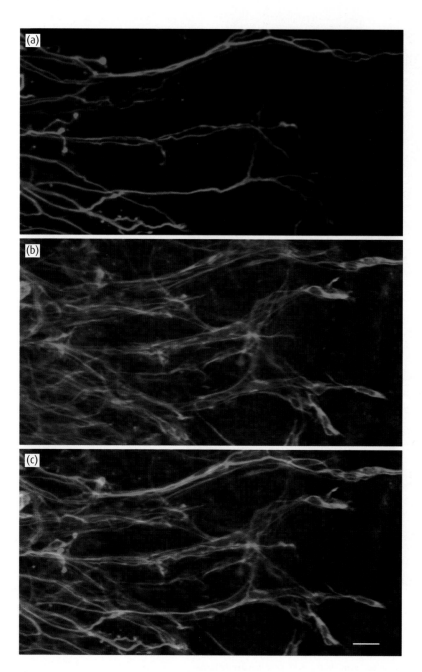

Plate 13 (figure 27.2). Nerve outgrowth across the surface of a muscle from the cut end of
a transplanted nerve. The transplant is located to the left of the panels. (a) Axons labeled by
anti-neurofilament antibody. (b) Reactive Schwann cells labeled with an anti-nestin antibody.
(c) Merged image of the upper panels with the axons in red and the Schwann cells in green. Growing
axons are clearly associated with Schwann cell processes extended from the transplant, although
there are Schwann cell processes that are not associated with axons. Scale bar indicates 40 μm.
Modified from (Son and Thompson, 1995a).

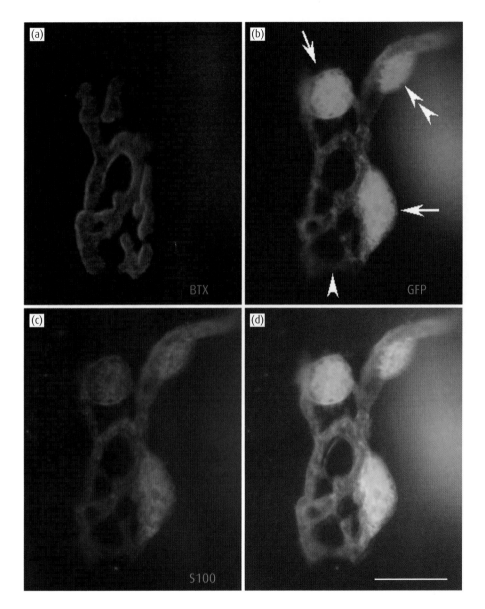

Plate 14 (figure 27.3). Schwann cells at the neuromuscular junction labeled by transgenic expression of green fluorescent protein. Junction of a sternomastoid muscle of an adult mouse. (a) Labeling of the acetylcholine receptors with BTX. (b) Fluorescence of green fluorescent protein (GFP). (c) Labeling of Schwann cells with an antibody to the protein S100B. (d) Merged image of panels (a–c) with each panel having the color shown. The promoter used to drive the GFP is the promoter for S100; not surprisingly the two labels appear in the same structures (compare b, c). The arrows indicate cell bodies of terminal Schwann cells. The double arrowhead indicates the cell body of a myelinating Schwann cell on the preterminal axon. As they cover the nerve terminal processes that occupy the synaptic gutters in panel (a), processes of the terminal Schwann cells match the receptor distribution except where they cover a nerve process traveling between two gutters (arrowhead). Scale bar indicates 20 μm. Modified from (Zuo et al., 2004).

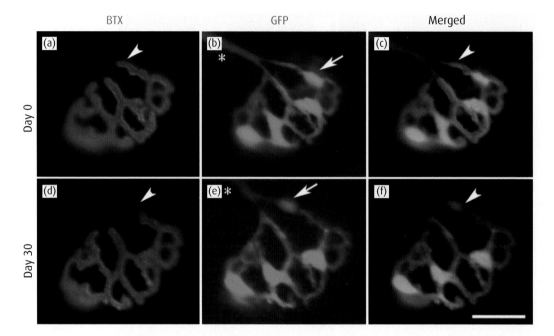

Plate 15 (figure 27.4). Vital images of terminal Schwann cells at a neuromuscular junction of a mouse sternomastoid muscle collected 30 days apart. Acetylcholine receptors (panels a, d) were labeled with non-blocking concentrations of rhodamine-conjugated alpha-BTX. Schwann cells (panels b, e) were visualized by their expression of green fluorescent protein. Images were merged in panels (c), (f). Panels (a)–(c) were collected at the first imaging session. Panels d–f were collected 30 days later. The synapse is remarkably stable except for some minor changes in acetylcholine receptors (arrowhead) and movement of one Schwann cell body (arrow). The synapse has the same number of Schwann cells (cell bodies are brighter ovals) at each time point. The asterisk indicates the site where the Schwann-cell wrapped axon enters the synaptic site. Scale bar indicates 30 μm. Modified from (Zuo et al., 2004).

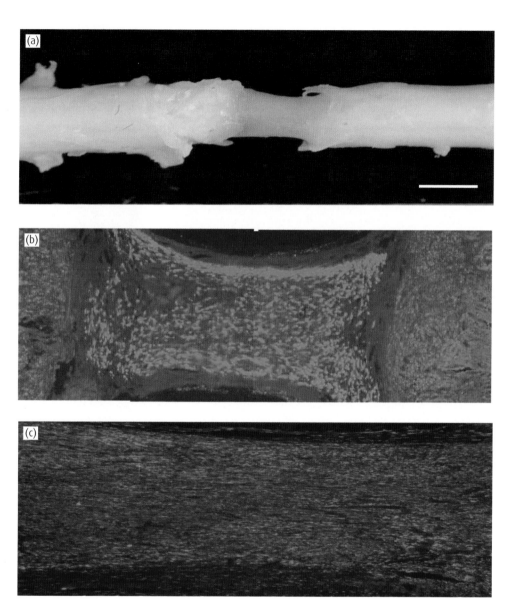

Plate 16 (figure 28.2). These panels illustrate a SC bridge inserted into a completely transected adult thoracic spinal cord. A 4 mm long SC/fibrin bridge was implanted a week before obtaining the picture in panel a. The SC/fibrin implant bridges the rostral (right) and caudal (left) spinal cord stumps. Panel b, horizontal paraffin section demonstrating by immunohistochemistry the presence of S100-positive SCs within the bridge a week after implantation. Panel c, a section stained at 4 weeks with an antibody that recognizes neurofilaments, showing the abundant presence of axons within the SC bridge at 8 weeks after implantation. Subsequent evaluation revealed that approximately 3000 axons were myelinated by SCs in the middle of the bridge, and the estimated total number of myelinated and unmyelinated axons in the bridge was 20,000. Bar represents 2 mm in a, 800 μm in (b), and 250 μm in (c). (Courtesy of Dr. Martin Oudega, The Miami Project to Cure Paralysis, Miami, FL, USA.)

25

Cellular replacement in spinal cord injury

Itzhak Fischer[1], Angelo C. Lepne[1], Steve Sang Woo Han[1] and Alan R. Tessler[1,2]

[1]*Department of Neurobiology and Anatomy, Drexel University College of Medicine and* [2]*Department of Veterans Affairs Hospital, Philadelphia, PA, USA*

Traumatic spinal cord injury (SCI) results in devastating and often permanent disability for which no effective biologic therapies exist. The injury initiates a cascade of complex, interrelated pathologic processes leading not only to cell death at the injury site and in higher brain centers but also to the severing, demyelination and physiologic inactivation of axons and the generation of an environment hostile to neural repair. Numerous studies have increased our understanding of why regeneration fails following SCI and documented promising experimental interventions to overcome this failure. Advances in our knowledge of stem cell biology over the past decade have raised hopes that grafts with the potential to differentiate into subsets or all the major cells of the spinal cord will be able to replace neurons and glial cells that have been destroyed or rendered dysfunctional by injury. The isolation and characterization of stem cells and lineage-restricted precursors from multiple regions in the developing and adult central nervous system (CNS), as well as from tissue outside the nervous system, bring these expectations closer to reality (see Volume I, Chapter 18). In addition, the discovery of endogenous precursor cells in the adult spinal cord revealed another source of cells that may be amenable to therapies. These ideas have captured the imagination because, although we are only beginning to understand the promises and pitfalls of this approach, the need for effective treatments for SCI is urgent (see Volume II, Chapter 37).

In this chapter, we summarize pioneering work on neural tissue transplantation that showed the feasibility of cell replacement as a treatment for SCI.

We then discuss the properties of distinct classes of stem cells and lineage-restricted precursors available for cell replacement, and present results of their transplantation into the spinal cord with respect to issues of fate, potential therapeutic properties and problems that need to be solved. We also consider strategies for activating endogenous stem cells in the adult spinal cord for repair. This chapter will focus on experimental strategies for cellular replacement in traumatic injury. Issues more specifically related to the repair of demyelinating spinal cord disease, chronic motor neuron degeneration and brain injury are covered elsewhere in this textbook.

Throughout this chapter we will use the term *neural stem cells (NSCs)* to describe multipotent cells like the neuroepithelial cells (NEPs) derived from the ventricular zone (VZ) of the developing CNS, which can self-renew and give rise to multiple classes of neurons and glial cells. The term *lineage-restricted precursor cells* will be reserved for the general description of cells with a more limited potential that are committed to either neuronal or glial lineages. The term *neural precursor cell (NPC)* will be used generally to refer to both multipotent stem cells and lineage-restricted cells. Finally, the term *pluripotent* will be used only for embryonic stem cells (ES).

25.1 Traumatic SCI

Traumatic injury to the human spinal cord, most commonly the result of falls, motor vehicle and sports accidents, and violence, induces a sequence of pathologic processes that begins within minutes and continues for years (reviewed in Houle and Tessler, 2003). Hemorrhage, edema, ischemia, metabolic derangements including increased intraneuronal calcium and extracellular potassium, and excessive production of free radicals and extracellular glutamate combine to produce a lesion that affects primarily gray matter and extends over several spinal cord segments. Neurons, astrocytes and oligodendrocytes in the damaged regions die primarily from necrosis but also from apoptosis. Axons originating in neurons located rostral and caudal to the injury are severed. Many of these axotomized neurons atrophy and die, among them rubrospinal (Mori et al., 1997), reticulospinal (Wu et al., 2003) and corticospinal neurons (Hains et al., 2003). After an abortive attempt to regenerate, surviving axons retract a short distance from the wound margins (Houle and Jin, 2001). The lesion eventually evolves over months and years into a multilobular cystic cavity whose walls are formed by reactive glia (Kakulas, 1999). Axons cannot grow across cavities or across the scar formed by reactive glia and connective tissue. The failure to regenerate is due to the limited capacity for growth of CNS neurons (Chen et al., 2000), and to inhibitory molecules present in the scar (Tang et al., 2003) and in degenerating CNS myelin beyond the scar (reviewed in Filbin, 2003). The limited regenerative capacity of CNS neurons and the inhibitory influences on regeneration exerted by the glial scar and CNS myelin proteins are discussed in other chapters in this textbook. Closed contusion injuries usually spare axons in the subpial white matter even in physiologically complete injuries (Kakulas, 1999), but damage to axons and oligodendrocytes strips axons of their myelin (Bunge et al., 1993) and exposure of voltage-gated potassium channels at the internodes (Nashmi and Fehlings, 2001) contributes to conduction failure in surviving axons (see Volume I, Chapter 26).

25.2 Strategies for SCI repair

The structural pathology of SCI suggests rational treatment strategies. Among these treatments are

the administration of neurotrophic factors (see Volume I, Chapters 23 and 29) and pharmacologic agents (see Volume I, Chapters 21 and 24), transplantation (see also Volume I, Chapters 28 and 34) and activity dependent training (cf. Volume I, Chapters 7 and 13; Volume II, Chapters 3 and 19). These interventions can reduce local tissue destruction and preserve axotomized neurons (Shibayama et al., 1998) (see Volume I, Chapters 16 and 17), mimic the actions of neurotransmitters depleted by the injury (reviewed by Rossignol et al. (2001)), reduce the glial scar (Bradbury et al., 2002) (see Volume I, Chapter 22) and increase conduction through demyelinated axons (Potter et al., 1998) (see also Volume I, Chapter 26). They are also designed to promote axon regeneration and sprouting and thereby encourage plasticity through reorganization of existing circuits and generation of new connections (McGee and Strittmatter, 2003; Bareyre et al., 2004) (cf. Volume I, Chapters 1 and 13). The effects of these treatments have been tested in several types of experimental injuries that provide useful models of the injury in humans. Standardized weight-drop contusion injuries of varying severity closely resemble closed human SCI (Metz et al., 2000). Contusion primarily damages gray matter and dorsal white matter while sparing a variable amount of white matter laterally and ventrally. The contusion model is useful for studying tissue rescue and functional recovery, but, because the injury is incomplete, regenerating axons cannot be reliably distinguished from sprouting axons and the mechanisms that account for recovery, particularly the role played by regenerating axons, are hard to define. Surgical lesions, including complete transections, dorsal or lateral hemisections and tract or funiculus sections, allow more precise identification of the pathways that have been cut and are therefore more useful for studying regeneration or sprouting of specific tracts and for defining the deficits and recovery associated with the interruption or growth of these pathways.

Transplants of neural and non-neural tissue have produced partial recovery of locomotor, sensory and autonomic function following both contusion and surgical injuries by reducing the glial scar, rescuing axotomized neurons and providing neuro-trophic factors and a substrate favorable for axon elongation (reviewed in Murray, 2004). Both neural and non-neural transplants may exert these actions if they express the appropriate molecules intrinsi-cally or after genetic modification, but only neural transplants have the potential to replace damaged tissue. The present review is therefore focused on neural transplants with emphasis on the poten-tial for NSCs and lineage-restricted precursors to replace damaged neurons and glia and to enhance regeneration.

25.3 Fetal tissue transplants for SCI

Fetal spinal cord (FSC) transplants

Whole pieces and homogenates of embryonic day (E) 11–14 rat spinal cord form durable transplants when grafted within a few hours of dissection into injured adult rat spinal cord without additional cul-turing (Theele et al., 1996). FSC transplants survive without immune suppression for many months in inbred and outbred strains of recipient rats. Their survival is robust even when they are transplanted acutely at the time of injury and are consequently exposed to the secondary phase of SCI, which includes a host inflammatory response that is toxic

to other types of graft. We now know that between E11 and E14 the number of multipotent NSC diminishes and the numbers of lineage-restricted precursor cells committed to neuronal or glial lineages increase (Kalyani and Rao, 1998). The FSC transplants have been reported to undergo extensive cell death during the first week following grafting into hemisection cavities, and their subsequent expan-sion may therefore arise from the small number of NSCs or lineage-restricted precursors that survive (Theele et al., 1996). The consistent appearance of fully differentiated neural cells in mature transplants grafted at different gestational ages (Reier et al., 1983; Bernstein et al., 1985) suggests that the grafts develop from similar types of lineage-restricted cells or from an NSC population. Recent observations in our labo-ratory (Lepore et al., unpublished data) suggest that, similar to FSC (Fig. 25.1), mixed neuronal- and glial-restricted precursors (NRP and GRP; Fig. 25.2), grafted into the injured adult spinal cord, survive, fill the lesion cavity and express markers for mature neu-rons, astrocytes and oligodendrocytes (Fig. 25.5). It is therefore plausible that both FSC and NRP/GRP transplants provide a microenvironment that retains some of the developmental cues of the embryonic environment and protects the grafted cells from the toxicity of the injured host.

FSC transplants grow in adult spinal cord as solid masses of cells that fill lesions up to 3 mm in length.

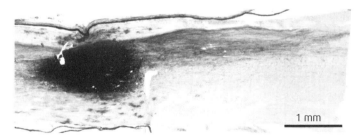

1 mm

Figure 25.1. *Intraspinal transplantation of E14/FSC.* Undissociated E14/FSC was grafted acutely into a lateral funiculus injury of the cervical spinal cord. Graft is derived from a transgenic rat embryo ubiquitously expressing the reporter gene, human placental alkaline phosphatase (AP), allowing for reliable identification of the transplanted cells and study of their differentiation profile (Mujtaba et al., 2002). By 3 weeks post-transplantation, the graft completely fills the lesion cavity and integrates with the adjacent host tissue. Graft-derived fibers project out of the transplant site into the host spinal cord. These fibers extend for distances greater than 5 mm in both the rostral and caudal direction.

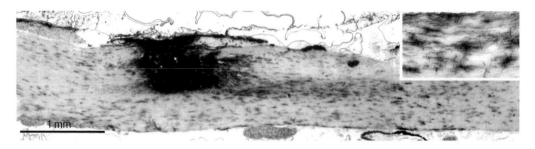

1 mm

Figure 25.2. *Intraspinal transplantation of NRP/GRP cells.* A mixed population of NRP and GRP was grafted acutely into a lateral funiculus injury in the cervical spinal cord. AP histochemistry was used to detect the presence of transplanted cells. NRP/GRP grafts fill the injury cavity at 3 weeks post-transplantation. Cells migrate robustly along white matter tracts in both rostral and caudal directions. Migrating cells elaborate mature morphologies (inset) by 3 weeks post-transplantation.

Grafts do not develop the characteristic butterfly appearance of normal spinal cord. They lack the corona of fully developed white matter tracts and motor neurons apparently do not survive, but they contain all of the neural elements that make up the neuropil of normal spinal cord (Reier et al., 1986; Itoh and Tessler, 1990b). Some relatively unmyelinated regions include concentrations of small neurons that express neuropeptides such as substance P and enkephalin, therefore resembling substantia gelatinosa (Jakeman et al., 1989). The FSC transplants integrate closely with host neuropil and are surrounded by an interrupted astrocytic scar, allowing axons to pass from host to graft and from graft to host (Reier et al., 1986). Most of the numerous synapses found within the grafts arise from donor neurons, and the cell bodies of host neurons that send axons into the grafts are generally located within 1 mm of the transplants (Jakeman and Reier, 1991). Host axons do not regenerate across the grafts to reenter host neuropil but recent studies indicated that axons of donor neurons can extend at least 5 mm into host spinal cord (Fig. 25.1). FSC transplants are therefore unlikely to serve as bridges for the regeneration of injured axons, but they may serve as functional relays where host axons establish connections with donor neurons whose axons extend into distal spinal cord. The presence of connections between host axons and neurons within transplants is best established for dorsal root ganglion neurons, whose regenerated axons form synapses with donor neurons that appear morphologically normal (Itoh and Tessler, 1990a) and that are functional by electrophysiologic criteria (Houle et al., 1996; Itoh et al., 1996). Regenerating primary afferent axons occupy only a small portion of the grafts, however, and do not traverse the grafts to reenter host spinal cord. Why FSC transplants fail to support more robust growth by host axons is unknown. One possibility is that growth is terminated by synapse formation. Indirect support for this idea comes from the observation that dorsal root axons grow for longer distances within grafts of fetal cortex than of FSC transplants but establish a much smaller number of synapses (Itoh and Tessler, 1990a). If this is true, then the most favorable transplants for supporting robust regeneration would include non-neuronal cells that guide the regenerating axons but do not form synapses. Indeed, FSC grafts generate glial cells that can provide trophic and guidance support, but the study of these cells has been limited by the difficulties of distinguishing graft from host glia. As discussed in the proceeding sections, it is possible to transplant purified glial precursors to produce immature astrocytes, which can provide guidance and trophic support, and oligodendrocytes to allow remyelination.

Additional mechanisms have been described by which FSC transplants may contribute to functional recovery. For example, transplants have been reported to prevent the loss of axotomized Clarke's nucleus (Himes et al., 2001) and red nucleus neurons (Mori et al., 1997) through retrograde cell death or atrophy, presumably by providing neurotrophic factors. Neurons that would be lost without a transplant can therefore remain as components of spinal cord circuits and even strengthen these circuits if they form axonal sprouts. FSC transplants have also been observed to reduce the extent of the astrocytic scar (Houle, 1992), which is thought to act as a physical and biochemical barrier to axon regrowth. In addition, probably also through the provision of neurotrophic factors, they have been reported to prevent the atrophy of hindlimb muscles (Houle et al., 1999) and to reverse the changes in motor neuron membrane properties that follow spinal cord transection (Beaumont et al., 2004). The available evidence provides examples of enhanced development of locomotor function supported by FSC transplants after transection of newborn rat (Iwashita et al., 1994; Miya et al., 1997) and cat (Howland et al., 1995) spinal cord, but the evidence for transplant-mediated recovery in adults is sparse. When, however, transplants are placed into a thoracic transection site after a 2–4 week delay and supplemental brain-derived neurotrophic factor (BDNF) or NT-3 is provided through a catheter, regenerated axons of serotonergic and other supraspinal neurons cross the grafts and continue to grow into caudal host spinal cord. Recipients recover weight-supported hindlimb plantar stepping when walking on a treadmill or on stairs (Coumans et al., 2001). Future clinical implementation of these strategies will require less invasive ways to deliver trophic factors and protocols that are effective at an earlier stage of injury. In addition, it is likely that the combination of FSC transplants with other interventions that increase axonal growth such as Nogo receptor inhibitors and elevation of cAMP will improve the functional outcome (Volume I, Chapter 21). One promising option is to use mixed NRP and GRP, the NPC types that comprise FSC transplants. These cells offer the capabilities of expansion, storage and genetic manipulation, without the problems associated with FSC tissue availability, cellular heterogeneity and logistics of harvesting. In addition, they can be derived from alternative sources such as NSC and ES cell cultures

(Mujtaba et al., 1999; Lee, S.H. et al., 2000) (see below).

Although FSC transplants in spinal cord are taken at or just after the time when motor neurons become post-mitotic (E11–E13) and first send axons into the ventral roots (E12), they contain few large ($>40 \mu m$) cholinergic neurons that resemble the motor neurons found in normal anterior horn (Reier et al., 1986). Several mechanisms may contribute to the paucity of demonstrable motor neurons. First, the intact or injured adult spinal cord differs dramatically from the spinal cord during embryogenesis, when precisely regulated concentration gradients of signaling factors, including sonic hedgehog (Shh), fibroblast growth factor (FGF) and retinoic acid, produce distinct patterns of expression of homeodomain transcription factors that direct the differentiation of motor neurons from ventral NPCs (reviewed by Harris (2003)). Second, many of the transplanted motor neurons are likely to die, either as the result of normally occurring programmed cell death or as the result of axotomy, to which immature neurons are extremely vulnerable (reviewed in Sieradzan and Vrbova, 1991). Incomplete maturation of the grafted cells may also be responsible. Survival during the period of programmed cell death and after axotomy, as well as the acquisition and maintenance of a mature motor neuronal phenotype, depend on the establishment of synaptic connections with target muscles that can provide trophic support and continuing interactions between muscle and nerve. Myelin present in the white matter of adult host spinal cord, however, prevents the growth of axons into ventral roots, where growing axons encounter a permissive peripheral nerve conduit towards skeletal muscles.

Several experimental strategies have been employed to circumvent the white matter barrier and to allow grafted FSC neurons access to peripheral nerve. For example, when suspensions of E14–15 ventral spinal cord cells are injected into the distal nerve stump of a cut tibial nerve, small numbers of neurons, which can be large ($<48 \mu m$) and multipolar, survive and establish functional connections with denervated medial gastrocnemius muscle (Erb et al., 1993;

Thomas et al., 2003). Whole pieces of the ventral portion of E12 spinal cord (Nogradi and Vrbova, 1996) or whole pieces of the entire E14 spinal cord (Duchossoy et al., 2001), transplanted into adult host spinal cord and apposed to an avulsed ventral root or peripheral nerve graft, also contain neurons that establish functional connections with denervated muscle and partially reverse muscle atrophy. Some of these multipolar neurons are as large as the small- and medium-sized motor neurons that normally innervate biceps brachii in intact rats and are immunoreactive for CGRP (Duchossoy et al., 2001), a phenotypic marker for motor neurons (Ramer et al., 2003). Even when their axons are provided with access to a ventral root or peripheral nerve, only a small number of motor neurons develop within the grafts. Moreover, there are no reports that these grafted motor neurons are integrated into functional circuits with either primary afferent or supraspinal axons that regenerate into intraspinal FSC grafts.

Transplants of embryonic bulbospinal neurons

An alternative treatment strategy is based on the idea that intraspinal transplants of brainstem monoaminergic neurons important for the control of locomotor and autonomic function can enhance recovery by replacing depleted neurotransmitters that activate intrinsic spinal cord circuits. A similar rationale led to treating patients with Parkinson's disease with fetal substantia nigra tissue transplanted into an ectopic location in the caudate or putamen. Exogenous administration of serotonin agonists to walking spinal cats has been shown to increase the duration and amplitude of hind limb flexor and extensor electromyographic (EMG) activity and noradrenergic agonists have been shown to initiate locomotion and increase the duration of the step cycle (reviewed by Barbeau and Rossignol (1991)) (see Volume I, Chapter 13). Evidence acquired over 15 years, has demonstrated that grafts of embryonic locus coeruleus cells, a source of noradrenergic neurons, and raphe cells, a source of serotonergic neurons, placed into the adult rat spinal cord caudal to transection, extend processes

into host spinal cord that reinnervate their normal targets and reverse the lesion-induced increase in receptor densities (reviewed in Gimenez y Ribotta et al., 1998a). The grafts promote recovery of hindlimb weight support and treadmill walking based on patterns of locomotor activity that EMG and kinematic analyses show to be similar to those of intact rats (Gimenez y Ribotta et al., 1998b). These transplants are therefore successful although they are placed into ectopic locations and can only incompletely restore the interrupted neural circuits.

25.4 Transplants of NSCs and lineage-restricted precursors for SCI

Development and properties of NSCs and lineage-restricted precursors

NPCs have considerable advantages over fetal tissue grafts for cellular replacement. Large numbers of well-characterized cells can be isolated and expanded from multiple sources including ES cells. These cells can be genetically modified *in vitro*, stored in quality-controlled cell banks and approved for clinical applications. Defined classes of NPC can be used to test specific hypotheses about cellular survival, migration, differentiation and potential for replacement following transplantation into the intact and injured spinal cord and to ultimately assess their therapeutic properties.

Stem cells can be operationally defined as cells with the capacity to divide, self-renew and differentiate into mature cell types (Gage, 2000). Multipotent NSCs have the potential to generate the three major cell types in the CNS, neurons, astrocytes and oligodendrocytes. Lineage-restricted precursor cells have a more limited differentiation potential and are committed to either neuronal or glial fates. Thus, cellular differentiation in the mammalian CNS may occur through sequential stages of lineage-restriction of NPC (Cai and Rao, 2002); however, this model remains a subject of debate (Anderson, 2001). The sequence of events that lead from NSC to restricted precursors and then to differentiated cell types is highly specified and regulated by well-balanced spatial and temporal cues in the environment and intrinsic determinants within the cells (Lillien, 1998; Temple, 2001). The process of differentiation has been demonstrated meticulously in the developing rodent spinal cord (Kalyani and Rao, 1998). We therefore focus on spinal cord-derived cells to illustrate the fundamental properties of NSC and lineage-restricted precursors, as well as their potential applications. Spinal cord NPC may indeed have the greatest potential for cellular replacement in the injured spinal cord. Analogous cells exist in the brain and perhaps even in regions outside the CNS, but, because cellular specification appears to occur at early stages in development (Temple, 2001), cells originating elsewhere may not be able to efficiently generate the appropriate subclasses of cells found in the spinal cord. Chapter 18 of this volume provides a more detailed survey of NPC isolated from other regions.

Multipotent NSCs

The caudal neural tube at E10.5 in rats consists of a uniform layer of proliferative, pseudostratified columnar NEP cells that line the ventricular cavity, forming the VZ. NEP cells (Kalyani et al., 1997) are multipotent NSC that give rise to dividing lineage-restricted precursor cells (Kalyani and Rao, 1998), both NRP (Mayer-Proschel et al., 1997) and GRP (Rao and Mayer-Proschel, 1997; Rao et al., 1998; Liu and Rao, 2004), which are the predominant cell types found in the developing spinal cord at E13.5. Thus, cellular differentiation in the embryonic spinal cord is believed to involve a gradual process of fate restriction that originates in NEP cells and proceeds along separate paths to NRP and GRP, which then migrate and differentiate at different stages of development into mature neurons, astrocytes and finally oligodendrocytes (Fig. 25.3). Although the terms NRP and GRP are used to describe lineage-restricted precursors, these cells represent complex populations in the embryonic and adult CNS with diverse properties and nomenclature, particularly for glial precursors (Liu and Rao, 2004).

NSC have been identified not only in the fetal CNS, but also at later stages of CNS development and in select regions of the brain and spinal cord throughout adult life (Weiss et al., 1996; Johansson et al., 1999; Pevny and Rao, 2003) (see Volume I, Chapter 18). In the developing spinal cord, NEP cells reside along the VZ. As development proceeds, the VZ becomes smaller but remnants remain throughout life and contain postnatal and adult NSC, although their precise location and identification are intensely debated. Recent studies have shown that NSC themselves are a heterogeneous population, with different classes of NSC described (Pevny and Rao, 2003). All of these cells appear multipotent, have the ability to form neurospheres, but differ in their initial state, bias in differentiation capacity and possibly degree of self-renewal. NSC populations may include astrocytic, radial glial-derived, ependymal and subventricular zone (SVZ) derived stem cell populations (Doetsch et al., 1999; Laywell et al., 2000; Johansson, 2003).

Populations of NPC are isolated at specific stages of differentiation based on characteristics such as antigen expression, growth factor requirements, proliferation ability and differentiation potential, but these stages only represent points along a continuum in the maturation of NPC. Depending on the developmental stage at which they are isolated and specific growth factor requirements, NSC are grown either as adherent cultures or as floating cell clusters termed "neurospheres". NEP cells isolated from the E10.5 rat spinal cord and grown as adherent cultures on a fibronectin substrate require FGF and unidentified factors in chick embryo extract to survive and maintain in their multipotent state (Kalyani et al., 1997). In differentiating culture conditions, NEP cells readily generate neurons, astrocytes and oligodendrocytes. NSC present at later stages of development (E14 onwards) and in the adult CNS are functionally similar in their ability to self-renew and to generate neurons, astrocytes and oligodendrocytes *in vitro* (Gage, 2000), but require epidermal growth factor (EGF) or both EGF and FGF for isolation and continued growth as neurospheres (Pevny and Rao, 2003). In addition to differences in culture

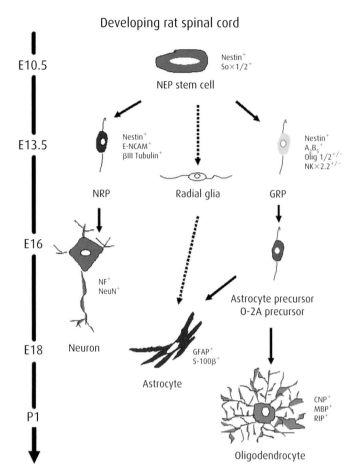

Developing rat spinal cord

E10.5

NEP stem cell — Nestin⁺ So×1/2⁺

E13.5

NRP — Nestin⁺ E-NCAM⁺ βIII Tubulin⁺

Radial glia

GRP — Nestin⁺ A₂B₅⁺ Olig 1/2⁺/⁻ NK×2.2⁺/⁻

E16

E18   Neuron — NF⁺ NeuN⁺

Astrocyte — GFAP⁺ S-100β⁺

Astrocyte precursor O-2A precursor

P1

Oligodendrocyte — CNP⁺ MBP⁺ RIP⁺

Figure 25.3. *Schematic diagram showing that differentiation into mature CNS phenotypes from NPCs occurs via a process of progressive fate restriction.* Mature cell types of the spinal cord derive from dividing multipotent VZ NSCs, termed NEP stem cells. NEP cells do not directly give rise to mature CNS phenotypes but first transition through NRP and GRP precursors, lineage-restricted progenitors with fate restrictions for neurons and glia, respectively. Fate restriction/differentiation occurs via a constantly evolving process; however, specific stages of this ongoing process can be isolated, based on characteristics such as antigen expression, growth factor requirements, proliferation ability and differentiation potential. Neurogenesis precedes astrogliogenesis, followed by oligodendrogenesis, which continues into the early postnatal period. Nevertheless, these processes also temporally overlap. The populations of NPCs depicted are heterogeneous. For example, various types of glial precursors have been described, including bipotential cells, astrocyte precursors, oligodendrocyte precursors and several subtypes of tri-potential GRP.

conditions and mitogen requirements, NSC from various regions and developmental ages differ in their inherent bias toward differentiated cell types. FGF-dependent NSC appear biased toward neuronal differentiation; EGF-dependent NSC, towards a glial fate (Qian et al., 2000).

NRP cells

Spinal cord-derived NRP are isolated either directly from the E13.5 rat spinal cord or from differentiating cultures of NEP cells using immunopanning or fluorescence-activated cell sorting (FACS), based on their cell surface expression of embryonic neural cell adhesion molecule (E-NCAM or PSA-NCAM). NRP

express the early neuronal-specific marker β-III tubulin, but when cultured under non-differentiating conditions, lack markers expressed by mature neurons (Mayer-Proschel et al., 1997). Even in culture conditions that favor glial cell differentiation, NRP remain committed to the neuronal lineage. Differentiated NRP form neurons capable of firing action potentials and can display multiple neurotransmitter phenotypes, including ones not normally present in the mature spinal cord, like dopaminergic neurons (Kalyani et al., 1998). Similar NRP exist in the human FSC (Li et al., 2000) and can be generated from both human (Carpenter et al., 2001) and mouse ES cells (Mujtaba et al., 1999). NRP have also been described in the postnatal and adult SVZ, a proliferative region lining the lateral ventricles of the forebrain (Luskin, 1993; Pencea et al., 2001), and have been isolated directly from the adult human hippocampus and SVZ (Roy et al., 2000; Wang et al., 2000). Thus, NPC restricted to neuronal lineage have been isolated using multiple methods from diverse locations within the CNS, including the embryonic spinal cord.

GRP cells

GRP differentiate into astrocytes and oligodendrocytes, but not neurons. Multiple classes of GRP have been described in the fetal and adult CNS (Liu and Rao, 2004). They can be distinguished from each other based on site of origin and age, culture methods used for isolation, response to cytokines, repertoire of marker expression and the types of glial cells they produce (Lee, J.C. et al., 2000). GRP can be directly isolated from the E13.5 rodent spinal cord as well as from multipotent NEP cells (Rao and Mayer-Proschel, 1997), based on their selective cell surface expression of A_2B_5 (Rao et al., 1998). Tripotential GRP that generate oligodendrocytes and both type-1 and type-2 astrocytes are a heterogeneous population that appear to represent the earliest GRP so far described (Rao et al., 1998; Gregori et al., 2002). Sorting strategies, based on the presence of A_2B_5 and the absence of E-NCAM, have generated functionally equivalent cells from human fetal brain tissue (Dietrich et al., 2002). A_2B_5-positive GRP are distinct from oligodendrocytes type-2 astrocytes (O2A) precursor cells. Originally isolated from rat optic nerves, O2A cells differentiate into oligodendrocytes and type-2 astrocytes *in vitro* (Raff et al., 1983) and into oligodendrocytes upon transplantation (Espinosa de los Monteros et al., 1993). Distinct oligodendrocyte (Keirstead et al., 1999) and astrocyte (Mi and Barres, 1999) precursor cells have also been described.

Transplants of stem cells and precursors

Candidate cell types for successful cellular replacement in the injured spinal cord should possess a

Table 25.1. Desired properties of cell replacement candidates: traumatic SCI.

Easily obtainable	Receive appropriate input (s)
Expandable (while maintaining properties)	Project to appropriate target (s)
Storable	Generate appropriate transmitter phenotype (s)
Replace some or all mature CNS cell types	Integrate functionally
Long-term survival and integration	Provide trophic support
Absence of uncontrolled proliferation	Restore balance of extracellular molecules
Amenable to genetic manipulation	Migrate to sites of pathology
Promote revascularization	Do not elicit pronounced immune response
Substrate for growth of endogenous fibers	Stimulate endogenous precursors
Ethical considerations	Amenable to alternative delivery protocols

Cell candidates will most likely be unable to fulfill all of these properties. The choice of an appropriate replacement candidate depends on the specific needs associated with the pathology.

number of advantageous properties (Table 25.1). These include straightforward isolation, expandability without a change in properties and capability of genetic modification. Transplanted cells should survive in a toxic environment, migrate where they are needed, differentiate into appropriate spinal cord cells, integrate into the host circuitry, restore or replace damaged neuronal circuits and contribute to functional recovery. These processes are complex and our understanding of the underlying mechanisms is still incomplete. Realistically, no single cell candidate is likely to possess all of these characteristics, nor will a single cell type be appropriate for all CNS pathologies. Instead, the appropriate cell type should be selected based on the characteristics of the specific CNS pathology. In many instances, multiple cell types, in conjunction with non-cell based therapy, may be most appropriate.

In comparison to studies employing FSC grafts, relatively few studies have examined the fate and efficacy of NPC transplanted into the spinal cord. In addition, the available studies can be difficult to compare because they differ from one another in many respects, including the starting populations and culture conditions of the cells and whether cells are grafted into the intact spinal cord or into one of several types of injury. A common finding, however, is that the adult spinal cord environment favors the survival and differentiation of glial cells, rather than neurons. For example, the adult spinal cord contains dividing cells that constitutively generate low numbers of new glial cells, but not neurons (Horner et al., 2000). When isolated and grown in culture with FGF, these cells have the characteristics of multipotent NSC-like cells *in vitro*, but, when transplanted back into the adult spinal cord, they express phenotypic markers of glial cells, but not of neurons (Shihabuddin et al., 2000; Yamamoto et al., 2001b). In contrast, when transplanted into a region of ongoing neurogenesis in the adult brain, the subgranular layer of the hippocampal dentate gyrus, they express neuronal markers, consistent with the idea that the adult spinal cord provides environmental cues that support differentiation only into glia. These studies illustrate an important concept in designing strategies for neural cell replacement: the fate of NPC *in vivo* is determined not by their intrinsic potential alone, but by their potential as expressed in the context of the host CNS environment. As the injured adult spinal cord limits both survival and differentiation into neurons, novel methods will be required to overcome these effects if NPC are to be useful for neuron replacement.

Multipotent NSC transplants

NSC would appear to be the most promising candidates for CNS cell replacement because of their potential to generate all damaged cell types, including neurons, astrocytes and oligodendrocytes. In addition, they can be prepared from the developing and adult CNS in large numbers as primary cells, derived from pluripotent ES cells, and passaged and expanded in culture. They are amenable to genetic manipulation and can be grafted in a relatively undifferentiated state, potentially allowing the host environment to push their fate towards appropriate phenotypes. NSC have been isolated from rodent and human CNS at all stages of development and grafted into the adult CNS (Rao and Mayer-Proschel, 2000), where they have been reported to promote recovery in models of degenerative disease and stroke (Snyder et al., 1995; Svendsen et al., 1997; Studer et al., 1998; Borlongan et al., 1999).

Several studies have assessed the fate of NSC following intraspinal transplantation. Cells isolated from embryonic and adult brain (Cao et al., 2001) or spinal cord (Ogawa et al., 2002; Vroemen et al., 2003) survived grafting into the intact or injured spinal cord with varying degrees of success and in some cases supported partial recovery of locomotor (Ogawa et al., 2002) or bladder (Mitsui et al., 2003) function. However, unless provided with instructional cues missing from the spinal cord, they differentiated overwhelmingly into glial cells (Cao et al., 2001; Ogawa et al., 2002; Vroemen et al., 2003). NSC prepared from E14 spinal cord and grown as neurospheres do not survive in the injured adult spinal cord when transplanted within 24 h of injury (Chow et al., 2000). Delayed transplantation of cells until 1 week following injury, combined with bolus administration of methylprednisolone and continuous immunosuppression with cyclosporine A, allowed ~50% of the grafted cells to survive for at least 2 months. Some of the transplanted cells differentiated into astrocytes and oligodendrocytes, but none generated neurons, unless exogenous BDNF was administered at the time of transplantation. Wu, P. et al. (2002) have demonstrated efficient region-specific generation of neurons from fetal human NSC that had been primed *in vitro* with a differentiation cocktail consisting of basic FGF (bFGF), heparin and laminin, with or without Shh. When grafted into regions of the brain and spinal cord that contain endogenous cholinergic neurons, these transplants differentiated into cholinergic neurons, a neuronal phenotype that has proven especially difficult to obtain from grafted NPC. In uninjured spinal cord, the primed cells resembled large endogenous motor neurons morphologically, but whether they form functional connections with muscles or survive in injured spinal cord has not been studied. Cells that had not been primed expressed astrocytic markers or remained undifferentiated when grafted into the spinal cord or into non-neurogenic regions of brain. NSC derived from mouse ES cells have been reported to enhance locomotor recovery when grafted into a thoracic contusion injury 9 days after injury (McDonald et al., 1999). As the transplanted cells differentiated predominantly into glia, most of the recovery was attributed to remyelination and sparing of host tissue. Grafted NSC have also been reported to remyelinate spinal cord axons in several different models of myelin loss (Hammang et al., 1997; Akiyama et al., 2001). In addition to primary NSC cultures, transplantation of NSC that have

been derived from ES cells has also been documented (reviewed in Lang et al., 2004).

NSC have usually been transplanted as a component of neurospheres (Reynolds and Weiss, 1996; Weiss et al., 1996; Svendsen et al., 1997; Ogawa et al., 2002; Pluchino et al., 2003). Undifferentiated NSC are a small (~5%) component of neurospheres, however, and the bulk of cells are lineage-restricted precursors or mature cell types (Tropepe et al., 1999; Suslov et al., 2002; Kim and Morshead, 2003; Seaberg and van der Kooy, 2003). To examine the features of a pure NSC population, we isolated NEP cells from E10.5 spinal cord and grafted them into the adult spinal cord and brain. NEP cells can be isolated as a near homogenous population by dissection at the appropriate developmental stage (Kalyani et al., 1997). Recently, spinal cord-derived NEP cells failed to survive in the intact adult striatum, hippocampus or spinal cord (Fig. 25.4), suggesting that most CNS regions do not support the survival of this specific population of multipotent cells (Lepore et al., 2004);

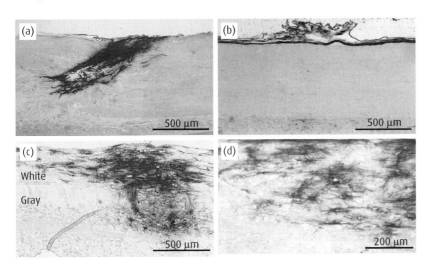

Figure 25.4. *Intraspinal transplantation of NEP cells (a–b) and mixed NRP/GRP cells (c–d).* NEP cells and mixed populations of NRP/GRP cells were grafted into the intact spinal cord of adult rats under identical transplantation conditions, yielding distinct fates *in vivo*. AP histochemistry was used to detect transplanted cells. Grafted NEP cells are present in the spinal cord 3 days post-transplantation and appear morphologically immature (a). NEP cells are not detected at 7 days post-engraftment (b). In contrast to NEP cells, mixed NRP/GRP transplants are detected in both the gray and white matter 3 weeks after engraftment (c–d). Migration occurs preferentially along white matter tracts (c–d). Cells acquire several mature morphologies (d).

however, the value of other types of NSC cannot be excluded. Therefore, lineage-restricted precursor cells, NRP and GRP, which are derived from NEP cells (Mayer-Proschel et al., 1997; Rao and Mayer-Proschel, 1997; Mujtaba et al., 1999), may be more promising, as described below.

Glial precursor transplants

Several different types of glial precursor cells have been used as intraspinal transplants. Oligodendrocyte precursor cells, for example, have been shown to remyelinate denuded host axons after differentiating into myelin-producing oligodendrocytes (Zhang et al., 1999) or into both oligodendrocytes and Schwann cells (Keirstead et al., 1999). O2A cells (Groves et al., 1993) and oligospheres derived from ES cells (Liu et al., 2000) have also been reported to differentiate into functionally competent oligodendrocytes. Spinal cord-derived GRP survived transplantation into the adult uninjured spinal cord and acquired mature morphologies both in gray matter and white matter (Han et al., 2004). GRP migrated selectively along white matter tracts in both rostral and caudal directions over several spinal cord segments, and differentiated into mature astrocytes and oligodendrocytes, but not neurons. Survival, migration and differentiation were similar when these same GRP were transplanted into injured cord (Han et al., 2004). The wide migration of glial precursor cells through white matter may offer additional therapeutic advantages over NSC and neuronal precursors. They have the potential to replace cells over a large region of the injured spinal cord and to provide disseminated trophic support for regenerating axons and for remyelination. On the other hand, astrocytes produced from glial precursor cell transplants may contribute to glial scar formation (Bradbury et al., 2002), and transplant-derived oligodendrocytes may inhibit the regeneration of host axons if they express growth inhibitory molecules such as Nogo and myelin-associated glycoprotein (MAG) (Merkler et al., 2001; GrandPre et al., 2002; Liu et al., 2002; see Volume I, Chapter 21). These properties may vary depending on the developmental age at which the glial precursors are isolated. It will be important to determine if in fact glial precursor cell-derived astrocytes and oligodendrocytes contribute to these undesirable effects. The potential of other types of glial cells, Schwann cells and olfactory ensheathing cells, as intraspinal transplants is discussed in Volume I, Chapter 28.

Neuronal precursor transplants

Since the adult spinal cord environment lacks the requisite signals or possesses inhibitory factors that prevent the production of new neurons from endogenous or transplanted multipotent cells, various strategies have emerged to encourage neuronal replacement, including transplantation of NRP cells. The hope is that graft-derived neurons will contribute to repair by the same mechanisms as discussed above for FSC grafts (see above). They might function as a neuronal relay, as a bridge for the regrowth of endogenous fibers, or as a source of trophic or growth-promoting factors. The difficulties involved in replacing lost neurons and rewiring their connections while avoiding aberrant connections that can result in undesirable outcomes such as neuropathic pain are evident.

The inability of the adult spinal cord to generate neurons may reflect a failure of multipotent cells to transition to the neuronal precursor stage or a failure to support the survival and differentiation of neuronal precursors. To distinguish between these two mechanisms, purified populations of FSC-derived NRP have been transplanted into adult uninjured spinal cord (Han et al., 2002). NRP survived in both white and gray matter, elaborated long processes, migrated selectively in white matter and expressed markers of differentiated neurons, but not of astrocytes or oligodendrocytes. Grafted cells also expressed neurotransmitter phenotypes and the synaptic protein synaptophysin, suggesting that synapses may have been formed with transplanted and/or host neurons. NRP-derived neurons extended processes in white matter, despite the axonal growth inhibitory environment present in the adult CNS. Similarly, telomerase immortalized NRP from human

FSC have been reported to survive in injured rat spinal cord for up to 6 months and to differentiate into mature GABAergic neurons (Roy et al., 2004).

These studies therefore raise hopes that transplanting cells committed to the neuronal lineage will provide a strategy for neuronal replacement in CNS areas that do not normally undergo neurogenesis. It is not yet clear whether these approaches are directly applicable to the traumatically injured spinal cord, where fetal rat NRP, for example, survived poorly and failed to differentiate into neurons (Cao et al., 2002). Neuronal differentiation appears to be inhibited as most cells express immature neuronal markers but not markers of fully differentiated neurons. Interestingly, NRP co-transplanted into the injured adult spinal cord with GRP (Fig. 25.5) express markers for mature neurons, suggesting that glial precursors (and/or their differentiated glial progeny) provide a microenvironment that is both protective and instructive (Lepore et al., 2004). Mixed NRP/GRP grafts also show selective migration out of the injury site into the white matter of the intact host CNS (Fig. 25.2). The migratory capabilities of NRP and GRP in the injured spinal cord are particularly attractive for CNS repair. NRP, which by and large remain at the grafting site, have the potential of becoming relays for reconstructing circuits and creating a permissive environment at the injury site. The migration stream, consisting mostly of grafted GRP and subsequently glial cells, can potentially guide and myelinate growing axons. If NRP/GRP grafts can survive for long periods of time (as suggested by preliminary unpublished findings in our laboratory), transplantation of lineage-restricted precursors might prove an effective and safe therapeutic strategy.

Alternative sources of stem and precursor cells

NPC can not only be directly isolated from CNS tissue, but also derived from cultures of rodent and human ES cells (reviewed in Lang et al., 2004). ES cells, which have been identified in several species

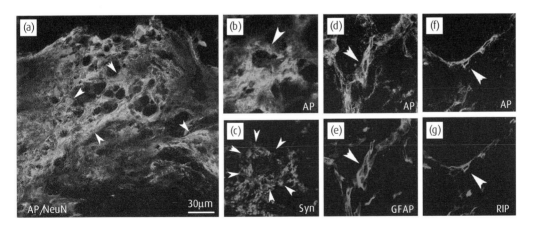

Figure 25.5. *NRP/GRP transplants differentiate in the injured spinal cord.* Graft-derived neurons are found at 5 weeks post-transplantation (a). Double immunofluorescence staining for AP (a, green) and NeuN (a, red), a marker of post-mitotic neurons, demonstrates graft-derived neurons. NRP/GRP grafts express synaptic markers at 5 weeks post-transplantation (b–c). Double immunofluorescence staining for AP (b, green) and the synaptic marker synaptophysin (c, red) suggests that grafted cells form synapses. Graft-derived astrocytes are present at 5 weeks post-transplantation (d–e). Double immunofluorescence staining for AP (d, green) and the astrocytic marker glial fibrillary acidic protein (GFAP) (e, red) shows graft-derived astrocytes. Graft-derived oligodendrocytes are present at 5 weeks post-transplantation (f–g). Double immunofluorescence staining for AP (f, green) with the oligodendrocytic marker RIP (g, red) shows graft-derived oligodendrocytes. Arrowheads denote double-labeled cells.

(Thomson et al., 1995; 1998), offer the advantages of extensive *in vitro* expansion in an undifferentiated state, the potential to generate all desired cell types, as well as ease in genetic manipulation. Furthermore, because transplants of ES-derived cells have not been subjected to regional specification, as during *in vivo* development, they may have the potential to respond appropriately to local signals at the injury site. Several different selection strategies, based on expression of cell surface antigens, promoter-driven selection or differences in culture conditions, have allowed various classes of NPC to be obtained from ES cell cultures, including NSC (McDonald et al., 1999), NRP and GRP (Mujtaba et al., 1999) and midbrain dopaminergic precursors (Lee, S.H. et al., 2000). Nevertheless, better understanding of the events that normally regulate the generation of NPC during CNS development will be necessary to optimize strategies for obtaining them from ES cells.

Understanding the developmental cues that normally specify cell fate *in vivo* has already allowed cells with specific phenotypes to be generated from cultures of ES cells and embryonic germ cells, primordial cells of the gonadal ridge (Shamblott et al., 1998). For example, *in vitro* exposure of mouse ES cells to factors that specify motor neuron fate has been used to successfully derive motor neurons and motor neuron precursors. Following engraftment into the E15–17 chick spinal cord, a stage when motor neurons begin to differentiate, both motor neuron precursors and post-mitotic motor neurons survive, differentiate, extend axons into the periphery and make synapses with muscles (Wichterle et al., 2002). Similarly, ES cells committed to a motor neuronal fate have been shown to survive transplantation into the ventral gray matter of adult rats and extend axons into ventral roots of animals treated with a cAMP analog or Rho kinase inhibitor (Harper et al., 2004). NSC derived from human germ cell cultures and grafted into rat spinal cord inoculated with Sindbis virus to kill motor neurons, survive and migrate, but only inefficiently differentiate into mature motor neurons or send axons into the sciatic nerve (Kerr et al., 2003). The partial recovery

observed in transplant recipients was attributed to rescue of endogenous motor neurons and maintenance of synaptic input to endogenous motor neurons, rather than to differentiation of grafted cells into functional neurons.

Non-neural cells may also be a source of neural phenotypes. For example, bone marrow stromal cells, multipotent mesenchymal stem cells resident in adult bone marrow, have been reported to differentiate into neural stem-like cells (Hermann et al., 2004) and mature CNS cell types, including neurons (Brazelton et al., 2000; Mezey et al., 2000; Jiang et al., 2002). However, recent work has brought some of these findings into question. *In vitro* transdifferentiation protocols have been shown to non-specifically induce a "neuronal-like" phenotype in stromal cells in culture that was mistakenly interpreted as evidence of neuronal differentiation (Lu et al., 2004a; Neuhuber et al., 2004). Findings initially interpreted as evidence of *in vivo* transdifferentiation have been suggested to be due to fusion of grafted stromal cells and endogenous neural cells (Alvarez-Dolado et al., 2003), and some *in vivo* studies could not be replicated (Castro et al., 2002). Bone marrow stromal cells are therefore unlikely to contribute to spinal cord repair by cell replacement, although they may do so by delivering trophic factors or by producing myelin that can partially restore axonal conduction (Akiyama et al., 2002a, b; Hofstetter et al., 2002).

25.5 Mobilization of endogenous neural precursors for replacement

Endogenous NPC also represent a potential resource that can be mobilized for repair. Bromodeoxyuridine (BrdU) analysis has shown that the adult spinal cord contains a population of slowly dividing stem cells (Adrian and Walker, 1962) that produces an exclusively glial progeny (Horner et al., 2000). These cells are found in and near the central canal ependymal layer (Johansson et al., 1999; Martens et al., 2002), in white matter tracts and substantia gelatinosa (Horner et al., 2000) and they have been isolated from both lateral and medial regions (Yamamoto et al., 2001b).

Infusions of EGF, FGF and heparin into the fourth ventricle (Martens et al., 2002) or EGF and FGF intrathecally (Kojima and Tator, 2000) increase the numbers of proliferating cells. Resident precursor cells also proliferate following injury, but they form astrocytes and oligodendrocytes rather than neurons (Yamamoto et al., 2001b; Han et al., 2004), and, despite their proliferation (Lipson and Horner, 2002), spontaneous recovery is poor.

Resident cells in the adult spinal cord have the capacity to generate neurons given the right environment. They differentiate into neurons *in vitro* and following transplantation into neurogenic regions of the hippocampus, but not when grafted back into the adult spinal cord (Shihabuddin et al., 2000). Identifying the mechanisms responsible for neurogenic failure may lead to better strategies for endogenous neuronal replacement. Notch signaling, which plays an important role in cell specification during development, may be partly responsible for the failure of neuronal differentiation. Notch inhibits neurogenesis by inhibiting pro-neuronal basic helix–loop-helix (bHLH) factors. Spinal cord NPC that proliferate following injury have been shown to upregulate Notch1, a member of the Notch receptor family, and do not express bHLH such as Ngn2, Mash1 or NeuroD. However, forced expression of Ngn2 or inhibition of Notch signaling using a dominant-negative ligand for Notch1 promotes neurogenesis *in vitro* (Yamamoto et al., 2001a). Spinal cord astrocytes may also contribute to the lack of neurogenesis because astrocytes derived from neurogenic regions of the hippocampus promote neurogenesis in cultured adult NPC to a much greater extent than astrocytes derived from the spinal cord (Song et al., 2002). Astrocytes from neonatal spinal cord promoted neurogenesis to a greater extent than adult spinal cord astrocytes, suggesting developmental down-regulation of a putative neurogenesis-promoting factor.

25.6 Practical considerations

Important practical issues will have to be resolved before cell replacement therapy can be successful. These include choosing the best methods and timing of cell delivery, and deciding whether to use non-cellular scaffolds.

Cell delivery methods

Most studies have delivered intraspinal transplants by direct parenchymal injection. If transferred to the clinic, this would be an expensive, invasive technique that would probably require general anesthesia and would have the potential to inflict additional damage on the already injured spinal cord. In addition, many diseases that are candidates for NPC transplantation therapy are diffuse (e.g., multiple sclerosis (MS)) and would require delivery of engrafted cells over extensive, non-contiguous areas (Pluchino et al., 2003). Transplantation of NPC directly into the cerebrospinal fluid offers a potential alternative to intraparenchymal injection. Previous work has demonstrated that NSC can be delivered to SCI sites and MS plaques via intraventricular injection (Wu, S. et al., 2002; Bai et al., 2003; Ben-Hur et al., 2003b; Pluchino et al., 2003). Intrathecal injection (De la Calle and Paino, 2002; De la Calle et al., 2002) at lumbar levels (lumbar puncture; spinal tap) is a very promising strategy because of its minimal invasiveness, simplicity and low cost, and because it would allow multiple injections at desired intervals. NPC may be well suited for lumbar puncture delivery because of their responsiveness to signals expressed in the injured CNS. They have been shown not only to proliferate and differentiate following injury, but also to migrate towards sites of injury (Ishii et al., 2001; Yamamoto et al., 2001b; Han et al., 2004). *In vitro* studies have demonstrated that they migrate in response to factors found at SCI sites (Wang et al., 1996; Bartholdi and Schwab, 1997), including microglia (Aarum et al., 2003), chemokines (Ehtesham et al., 2004; Ji et al., 2004; Peng et al., 2004; Tran et al., 2004) and inflammatory cytokines such as TNFα and IFNγ (Ben-Hur et al., 2003a) and PDGF (Armstrong et al., 1990; Forsberg-Nilsson et al., 1998). In preliminary studies, NRP and GRP, grafted via lumbar puncture, localized to an injury site in the cervical spinal cord, where they expressed markers for mature neurons, astrocytes and oligo-dendrocytes (Bakshi et al., 2004; Lepore et al., unpublished data).

Time of engraftment

The best time for engraftment following injury will also have to be determined and it may differ among transplant types. The early environment following injury is toxic to the survival of some types of transplanted cells and inhibits their differentiation. Transplants of FSC (Coumans et al., 2001), NSC (Ogawa et al., 2002), olfactory-ensheathing glia (Keyvan-Fouladi et al., 2003) and bone marrow stromal cells (Hofstetter et al., 2002) performed after the first week post-injury have been reported to enhance regenerative and behavioral efficacy over that observed when transplants are performed acutely after injury. Grafting at long intervals after injury confronts additional obstacles to repair beyond the already formidable difficulties presented by an acute injury (reviewed by Houle and Tessler (2003)). Early grafting is advantageous because transplants may be able to decrease secondary cell death and glial scar formation, and because impediments to axon sprouting and regeneration, including the glial scar, have not yet become established. Transplants of NPC such as NRP and GRP that survive and differentiate robustly in the acutely injured adult spinal cord may obviate the need for delayed engraftment and consequently may promote the greatest benefit if transplanted at the earliest possible time point.

Non-cellular scaffolds/matrices

Non-cellular scaffolds/matrices may also make an important contribution to engraftment of cells in the injured spinal cord (reviewed in Friedman et al., 2002; Geller and Fawcett, 2002). These materials are designed for implantation into the CNS, are made of biocompatible materials and are fabricated to mimic the consistency and topography of the spinal cord. They can be seeded with cells and modified to increase their efficacy, including treatments that

allow them to supply exogenous growth factors. Snyder and colleagues (Teng et al., 2002), for example, have demonstrated that implantation of a polymer scaffold seeded with NSCs (C17.2) into the hemisected rat spinal cord results in reduced tissue loss, axonal regrowth and recovery of function. Guidance cable scaffolds, seeded with olfactory ensheathing glia or Schwann cells, have also been reported to promote regeneration and recovery in the complete transection model (Ramon-Cueto et al., 1998; Xu et al., 1999; Oudega et al., 2001).

25.7 Combination therapy

NPC transplantation is a promising treatment strategy, but the complexity of SCI will likely require a multi-faceted approach that combines replacement therapy with other strategies that have proven useful in experimental models. These therapies include but are not limited to administration of pharmacologic agents that mimic neurotransmitters (Kim et al., 1999), delivery of factors that reduce secondary tissue loss, minimize glial scar formation and enhance regeneration (GrandPre et al., 2002), application of scaffolds that direct axon growth (Teng et al., 2002) and training regimens that modify intrinsic spinal cord circuitry (reviewed in Fouad and Pearson, 2004). Synergistic strategies that have promoted regeneration and recovery after experimental injuries illustrate this concept. For example, exogenous administration of neurotrophic factors in combination with E14 FSC transplant following complete mid-thoracic transection results in regenerative and behavioral benefits that exceed those produced by the transplants alone (Coumans et al., 2001). Supraspinal axons regenerated into and through transplants to reenter host neuropil, and regeneration was associated with partial recovery of motor function. Transplantation of Schwann cells (Pearse et al., 2004) or bone marrow stromal cells (Lu et al., 2004b) in conjunction with agents that elevate intra-spinal cAMP levels, has resulted in some of the most dramatic benefits seen in models of SCI to date. Engineering of grafted cells themselves has also proven to be a beneficial therapeutic approach. NPC that have been modified to produce and secrete neurotrophic factors have also resulted in increased host axonal growth following transplantation into a hemisection injury (Lu et al., 2003). These examples represent the important trend toward combination therapy and the integrated approach that builds on the exciting recent advances in cellular transplantation and is likely to be the most effective strategy for successful treatment of patients with SCI.

ACKNOWLEDGEMENTS

We acknowledge all the members of our group for their assistance. A.C.L. recognizes the support of the Neuroscience graduate program. S.S.W.H. acknowledges the support of the MD/PhD and Neuroscience graduate programs. I.F. is supported by NIH grant NS37515. A.T. is supported by the Research Service of the Department of Veterans Affairs. The Spinal Cord Program is supported by NIH grant NS24707, the Eastern Paralyzed Veterans Association and the Spinal Cord Research Center of Drexel University College of Medicine. We also acknowledge the contribution of our collaboration with Dr. Mahendra Rao at the NIA.

REFERENCES

Aarum, J., Sandberg, K., Haeberlein, S.L. and Persson, M.A. (2003). Migration and differentiation of neural precursor cells can be directed by microglia. *Proc Natl Acad Sci USA*, **100**, 15983–15988.

Adrian Jr., E.K. and Walker, B.E. (1962). Incorporation of thymidine-H3 by cells in normal and injured mouse spinal cord. *J Neuropathol Exp Neurol*, **21**, 597–609.

Akiyama, Y., Honmou, O., Kato, T., Uede, T., Hashi, K. and Kocsis, J.D. (2001). Transplantation of clonal neural precursor cells derived from adult human brain establishes functional peripheral myelin in the rat spinal cord. *Exp Neurol*, **167**, 27–39.

Akiyama, Y., Radtke, C., Honmou, O. and Kocsis, J.D. (2002a). Remyelination of the spinal cord following intravenous delivery of bone marrow cells. *Glia*, **39**, 229–236.

Akiyama, Y., Radtke, C. and Kocsis, J.D. (2002b). Remyelination of the rat spinal cord by transplantation of identified bone marrow stromal cells. *J Neurosci*, **22**, 6623–6630.

Alvarez-Dolado, M., Pardal, R., Garcia-Verdugo, J.M., Fike, J.R., Lee, H.O., Pfeffer, K., Lois, C., Morrison, S.J. and Alvarez-Buylla, A. (2003). Fusion of bone-marrow-derived cells with Purkinje neurons, cardiomyocytes and hepatocytes. *Nature*, **425**, 968–973.

Anderson, D.J. (2001). Stem cells and pattern formation in the nervous system: the possible versus the actual. *Neuron*, **30**, 19–35.

Armstrong, R.C., Harvath, L. and Dubois-Dalcq, M.E. (1990). Type 1 astrocytes and oligodendrocyte-type 2 astrocyte glial progenitors migrate toward distinct molecules. *J Neurosci Res*, **27**, 400–407.

Bai, H., Suzuki, Y., Noda, T., Wu, S., Kataoka, K., Kitada, M., Ohta, M., Chou, H. and Ide, C. (2003). Dissemination and proliferation of neural stem cells on the spinal cord by injection into the fourth ventricle of the rat: a method for cell transplantation. *J Neurosci Methods*, **124**, 181–187.

Bakshi, A., Hunter, C., Swanger, S., Lepore, A. and Fischer, I. (2004). Minimally invasive delivery of stem cells for spinal cord injury: advantages of the lumbar puncture technique. *J Neurosurg Spine*, **1**, 330–337.

Barbeau, H. and Rossignol, S. (1991). Initiation and modulation of the locomotor pattern in the adult chronic spinal cat by noradrenergic, serotonergic and dopaminergic drugs. *Brain Res*, **546**, 250–260.

Bareyre, F.M., Kerschensteiner, M., Raineteau, O., Mettenleiter, T.C., Weinmann, O. and Schwab, M.E. (2004). The injured spinal cord spontaneously forms a new intraspinal circuit in adult rats. *Nat Neurosci*, **7**, 269–277.

Bartholdi, D. and Schwab, M.E. (1997). Expression of proinflammatory cytokine and chemokine mRNA upon experimental spinal cord injury in mouse: an in situ hybridization study. *Eur J Neurosci*, **9**, 1422–1438.

Beaumont, E., Houle, J.D., Peterson, C.A. and Gardiner, P.F. (2004). Passive exercise and fetal spinal cord transplant both help to restore motoneuronal properties after spinal cord transection in rats. *Muscle Nerve*, **29**, 234–242.

Ben-Hur, T., Ben-Menachem, O., Furer, V., Einstein, O., Mizrachi-Kol, R. and Grigoriadis, N. (2003a). Effects of proinflammatory cytokines on the growth, fate, and motility of multipotential neural precursor cells. *Mol Cell Neurosci*, **24**, 623–631.

Ben-Hur, T., Einstein, O., Mizrachi-Kol, R., Ben-Menachem, O., Reinhartz, E., Karussis, D. and Abramsky, O. (2003b). Transplanted multipotential neural precursor cells migrate into the inflamed white matter in response to experimental autoimmune encephalomyelitis. *Glia*, **41**, 73–80.

Bernstein, J.J., Hoovler, D.W. and Turtil, S. (1985). Initial growth of transplanted E11 fetal cortex and spinal cord in adult rat spinal cord. *Brain Res*, **343**, 336–345.

Borlongan, C.V., Sanberg, P.R. and Freeman, T.B. (1999). Neural transplantation for neurodegenerative disorders. *Lancet*, **353**(Suppl. 1), SI29–SI30.

Bradbury, E.J., Moon, L.D., Popat, R.J., King, V.R., Bennett, G.S., Patel, P.N., Fawcett, J.W. and McMahon, S.B. (2002). Chondroitinase ABC promotes functional recovery after spinal cord injury. *Nature*, **416**, 636–640.

Brazelton, T.R., Rossi, F.M., Keshet, G.I. and Blau, H.M. (2000). From marrow to brain: expression of neuronal phenotypes in adult mice. *Science*, **290**, 1775–1779.

Bunge, R.P., Puckett, W.R., Becerra, J.L., Marcillo, A. and Quencer, R.M. (1993). Observations on the pathology of human spinal cord injury. A review and classification of 22 new cases with details from a case of chronic cord compression with extensive focal demyelination. *Adv Neurol*, **59**, 75–89.

Cai, J. and Rao, M.S. (2002). Stem cell and precursor cell therapy. *Neuromol Med*, **2**, 233–249.

Cao, Q.L., Zhang, Y.P., Howard, R.M., Walters, W.M., Tsoulfas, P. and Whittemore, S.R. (2001). Pluripotent stem cells engrafted into the normal or lesioned adult rat spinal cord are restricted to a glial lineage. *Exp Neurol*, **167**, 48–58.

Cao, Q.L., Howard, R.M., Dennison, J.B. and Whittemore, S.R. (2002). Differentiation of engrafted neuronal-restricted precursor cells is inhibited in the traumatically injured spinal cord. *Exp Neurol*, **177**, 349–359.

Carpenter, M.K., Inokuma, M.S., Denham, J., Mujtaba, T., Chiu, C.P. and Rao, M.S. (2001). Enrichment of neurons and neural precursors from human embryonic stem cells. *Exp Neurol*, **172**, 383–397.

Castro, R.F., Jackson, K.A., Goodell, M.A., Robertson, C.S., Liu, H. and Shine, H.D. (2002). Failure of bone marrow cells to transdifferentiate into neural cells *in vivo*. *Science*, **297**, 1299.

Chen, M.S., Huber, A.B., van der Haar, M.E., Frank, M., Schnell, L., Spillmann, A.A., Christ, F. and Schwab, M.E. (2000). Nogo-A is a myelin-associated neurite outgrowth inhibitor and an antigen for monoclonal antibody IN-1. *Nature*, **403**, 434–439.

Chow, S.Y., Moul, J., Tobias, C.A., Himes, B.T., Liu, Y., Obrocka, M., Hodge, L., Tessler, A. and Fischer, I. (2000). Characterization and intraspinal grafting of EGF/bFGF-dependent neurospheres derived from embryonic rat spinal cord. *Brain Res*, **874**, 87–106.

Coumans, J.V., Lin, T.T., Dai, H.N., MacArthur, L., McAtee, M., Nash, C. and Bregman, B.S. (2001). Axonal regeneration and functional recovery after complete spinal cord transection in rats by delayed treatment with transplants and neurotrophins. *J Neurosci*, **21**, 9334–9344.

De la Calle, J.L. and Paino, C.L. (2002). A procedure for direct lumbar puncture in rats. *Brain Res Bull*, **59**, 245–250.

De la Calle, J.L., Mena, M.A., Gonzalez-Escalada, J.R. and Paino, C.L. (2002). Intrathecal transplantation of neuroblastoma cells decreases heat hyperalgesia and cold allodynia in a rat model of neuropathic pain. *Brain Res Bull*, **59**, 205–211.

Dietrich, J., Noble, M. and Mayer-Proschel, M. (2002). Characterization of $A_2B_5^+$ glial precursor cells from cryopreserved human fetal brain progenitor cells. *Glia*, **40**, 65–77.

Doetsch, F., Garcia-Verdugo, J.M. and Alvarez-Buylla, A. (1999). Regeneration of a germinal layer in the adult mammalian brain. *Proc Natl Acad Sci USA*, **96**, 11619–11624.

Duchossoy, Y., Kassar-Duchossoy, L., Orsal, D., Stettler, O. and Horvat, J.C. (2001). Reinnervation of the biceps brachii muscle following cotransplantation of fetal spinal cord and autologous peripheral nerve into the injured cervical spinal cord of the adult rat. *Exp Neurol*, **167**, 329–340.

Ehtesham, M., Yuan, X., Kabos, P., Chung, N.H., Liu, G., Akasaki, Y., Black, K.L. and Yu, J.S. (2004). Glioma tropic neural stem cells consist of astrocytic precursors and their migratory capacity is mediated by CXCR4. *Neoplasia*, **6**, 287–293.

Erb, D.E., Mora, R.J. and Bunge, R.P. (1993). Reinnervation of adult rat gastrocnemius muscle by embryonic motoneurons transplanted into the axotomized tibial nerve. *Exp Neurol*, **124**, 372–376.

Espinosa de los Monteros, A., Zhang, M. and De Vellis, J. (1993). O2A progenitor cells transplanted into the neonatal rat brain develop into oligodendrocytes but not astrocytes. *Proc Natl Acad Sci USA*, **90**, 50–54.

Filbin, M.T. (2003). Myelin-associated inhibitors of axonal regeneration in the adult mammalian CNS. *Nat Rev Neurosci*, **4**, 703–713.

Forsberg-Nilsson, K., Behar, T.N., Afrakhte, M., Barker, J.L. and McKay, R.D. (1998). Platelet-derived growth factor induces chemotaxis of neuroepithelial stem cells. *J Neurosci Res*, **53**, 521–530.

Fouad, K. and Pearson, K. (2004). Restoring walking after spinal cord injury. *Prog Neurobiol*, **73**, 107–126.

Friedman, J.A., Windebank, A.J., Moore, M.J., Spinner, R.J., Currier, B.L. and Yaszemski, M.J. (2002). Biodegradable polymer grafts for surgical repair of the injured spinal cord. *Neurosurgery*, **51**, 742–751; discussion 751–752.

Gage, F.H. (2000). Mammalian neural stem cells. *Science*, **287**, 1433–1438.

Geller, H.M. and Fawcett, J.W. (2002). Building a bridge: engineering spinal cord repair. *Exp Neurol*, **174**, 125–136.

Gimenez y Ribotta, M., Orsal, D., Feraboli-Lohnherr, D. and Privat, A. (1998a). Recovery of locomotion following transplantation of monoaminergic neurons in the spinal cord of paraplegic rats. *Ann NY Acad Sci*, **860**, 393–411.

Gimenez y Ribotta, M., Orsal, D., Feraboli-Lohnherr, D., Privat, A., Provencher, J. and Rossignol, S. (1998b). Kinematic analysis of recovered locomotor movements of the hindlimbs in paraplegic rats transplanted with monoaminergic embryonic neurons. *Ann NY Acad Sci*, **860**, 521–523.

GrandPre, T., Li, S. and Strittmatter, S.M. (2002). Nogo-66 receptor antagonist peptide promotes axonal regeneration. *Nature*, **417**, 547–551.

Gregori, N., Proschel, C., Noble, M. and Mayer-Proschel, M. (2002). The tripotential glial-restricted precursor (GRP) cell and glial development in the spinal cord: generation of bipotential oligodendrocyte-type-2 astrocyte progenitor cells and dorsal–ventral differences in GRP cell function. *J Neurosci*, **22**, 248–256.

Groves, A.K., Barnett, S.C., Franklin, R.J., Crang, A.J., Mayer, M., Blakemore, W.F. and Noble, M. (1993). Repair of demyelinated lesions by transplantation of purified O-2A progenitor cells. *Nature*, **362**, 453–455.

Hains, B.C., Black, J.A. and Waxman, S.G. (2003). Primary cortical motor neurons undergo apoptosis after axotomizing spinal cord injury. *J Comp Neurol*, **462**, 328–341.

Hammang, J.P., Archer, D.R. and Duncan, I.D. (1997). Myelination following transplantation of EGF-responsive neural stem cells into a myelin-deficient environment. *Exp Neurol*, **147**, 84–95.

Han, S.S., Kang, D.Y., Mujtaba, T., Rao, M.S. and Fischer, I. (2002). Grafted lineage-restricted precursors differentiate exclusively into neurons in the adult spinal cord. *Exp Neurol*, **177**, 360–375.

Han, S.S., Liu, Y., Tyler-Polsz, C., Rao, M.S. and Fischer, I. (2004). Transplantation of glial-restricted precursor cells into the adult spinal cord: survival, glial-specific differentiation, and preferential migration in white matter. *Glia*, **45**, 1–16.

Harper, J.M., Krishnan, C., Darman, J.S., Deshpande, D.M., Peck, S., Shats, I., Backovic, S., Rothstein, J.D. and Kerr, D.A. (2004). Axonal growth of embryonic stem cell-derived motoneurons *in vitro* and in motoneuron-injured adult rats. *Proc Natl Acad Sci USA*, **101**, 7123–7128.

Harris, W.A. (2003). Specifying motor neurons: up and down and back to front. *Nat Neurosci*, **6**, 1247–1249.

Hermann, A., Gastl, R., Liebau, S., Popa, M.O., Fiedler, J., Boehm, B.O., Maisel, M., Lerche, H., Schwarz, J., Brenner, R. and Storch, A. (2004). Efficient generation of neural stem cell-like cells from adult human bone marrow stromal cells. *J Cell Sci*, **117**, 4411–4422.

Himes, B.T., Liu, Y., Solowska, J.M., Snyder, E.Y., Fischer, I. and Tessler, A. (2001). Transplants of cells genetically modified to express neurotrophin-3 rescue axotomized Clarke's nucleus neurons after spinal cord hemisection in adult rats. *J Neurosci Res*, **65**, 549–564.

Hofstetter, C.P., Schwarz, E.J., Hess, D., Widenfalk, J., El Manira, A., Prockop, D.J. and Olson, L. (2002). Marrow stromal cells form guiding strands in the injured spinal cord and promote recovery. *Proc Natl Acad Sci USA*, **99**, 2199–2204.

Horner, P.J., Power, A.E., Kempermann, G., Kuhn, H.G., Palmer, T.D., Winkler, J., Thal, L.J. and Gage, F.H. (2000). Proliferation and differentiation of progenitor cells throughout the intact adult rat spinal cord. *J Neurosci*, **20**, 2218–2228.

Houle, J. (1992). The structural integrity of glial scar tissue associated with a chronic spinal cord lesion can be altered by transplanted fetal spinal cord tissue. *J Neurosci Res*, **31**, 120–130.

Houle, J.D. and Jin, Y. (2001). Chronically injured supraspinal neurons exhibit only modest axonal dieback in response to a cervical hemisection lesion. *Exp Neurol*, **169**, 208–217.

Houle, J.D. and Tessler, A. (2003). Repair of chronic spinal cord injury. *Exp Neurol*, **182**, 247–260.

Houle, J.D., Skinner, R.D., Garcia-Rill, E. and Turner, K.L. (1996). Synaptic evoked potentials from regenerating dorsal root axons within fetal spinal cord tissue transplants. *Exp Neurol*, **139**, 278–290.

Houle, J.D., Morris, K., Skinner, R.D., Garcia-Rill, E. and Peterson, C.A. (1999). Effects of fetal spinal cord tissue transplants and cycling exercise on the soleus muscle in spinalized rats. *Muscle Nerve*, **22**, 846–856.

Howland, D.R., Bregman, B.S., Tessler, A. and Goldberger, M.E. (1995). Transplants enhance locomotion in neonatal kittens whose spinal cords are transected: a behavioral and anatomical study. *Exp Neurol*, **135**, 123–145.

Ishii, K., Toda, M., Nakai, Y., Asou, H., Watanabe, M., Nakamura, M., Yato, Y., Fujimura, Y., Kawakami, Y., Toyama, Y. and Uyemura, K. (2001). Increase of oligodendrocyte progenitor cells after spinal cord injury. *J Neurosci Res*, **65**, 500–507.

Itoh, Y. and Tessler, A. (1990a). Regeneration of adult dorsal root axons into transplants of fetal spinal cord and brain: a comparison of growth and synapse formation in appropriate and inappropriate targets. *J Comp Neurol*, **302**, 272–293.

Itoh, Y. and Tessler, A. (1990b). Ultrastructural organization of regenerated adult dorsal root axons within transplants of fetal spinal cord. *J Comp Neurol*, **292**, 396–411.

Itoh, Y., Waldeck, R.F., Tessler, A. and Pinter, M.J. (1996). Regenerated dorsal root fibers form functional synapses in embryonic spinal cord transplants. *J Neurophysiol*, **76**, 1236–1245.

Iwashita, Y., Kawaguchi, S. and Murata, M. (1994). Restoration of function by replacement of spinal cord segments in the rat. *Nature*, **367**, 167–170.

Jakeman, L.B. and Reier, P.J. (1991). Axonal projections between fetal spinal cord transplants and the adult rat spinal cord: a neuroanatomical tracing study of local interactions. *J Comp Neurol*, **307**, 311–334.

Jakeman, L.B., Reier, P.J., Bregman, B.S., Wade, E.B., Dailey, M., Kastner, R.J., Himes, B.T. and Tessler, A. (1989). Differentiation of substantia gelatinosa-like regions in intraspinal and intracerebral transplants of embryonic spinal cord tissue in the rat. *Exp Neurol*, **103**, 17–33.

Ji, J.F., He, B.P., Dheen, S.T. and Tay, S.S. (2004). Expression of chemokine receptors CXCR4, CCR2, CCR5 and CX3CR1 in neural progenitor cells isolated from the subventricular zone of the adult rat brain. *Neurosci Lett*, **355**, 236–240.

Jiang, Y., Jahagirdar, B.N., Reinhardt, R.L., Schwartz, R.E., Keene, C.D., Ortiz-Gonzalez, X.R., Reyes, M., Lenvik, T., Lund, T., Blackstad, M., Du, J., Aldrich, S., Lisberg, A., Low, W.C., Largaespada, D.A. and Verfaillie, C.M. (2002). Pluripotency of mesenchymal stem cells derived from adult marrow. *Nature*, **418**, 41–49.

Johansson, C.B. (2003). Mechanism of stem cells in the central nervous system. *J Cell Physiol*, **196**, 409–418.

Johansson, C.B., Momma, S., Clarke, D.L., Risling, M., Lendahl, U. and Frisen, J. (1999). Identification of a neural stem cell in the adult mammalian central nervous system. *Cell*, **96**, 25–34.

Kakulas, B.A. (1999). A review of the neuropathology of human spinal cord injury with emphasis on special features. *J Spinal Cord Med*, **22**, 119–124.

Kalyani, A.J. and Rao, M.S. (1998). Cell lineage in the developing neural tube. *Biochem Cell Biol*, **76**, 1051–1068.

Kalyani, A., Hobson, K. and Rao, M.S. (1997). Neuroepithelial stem cells from the embryonic spinal cord: isolation, characterization, and clonal analysis. *Dev Biol*, **186**, 202–223.

Kalyani, A.J., Piper, D., Mujtaba, T., Lucero, M.T. and Rao, M.S. (1998). Spinal cord neuronal precursors generate multiple neuronal phenotypes in culture. *J Neurosci*, **18**, 7856–7868.

Keirstead, H.S., Ben-Hur, T., Rogister, B., O'Leary, M.T., Dubois-Dalcq, M. and Blakemore, W.F. (1999). Polysialylated neural cell adhesion molecule-positive CNS precursors generate both oligodendrocytes and Schwann cells to remyelinate the CNS after transplantation. *J Neurosci*, **19**, 7529–7536.

Kerr, D.A., Llado, J., Shamblott, M.J., Maragakis, N.J., Irani, D.N., Crawford, T.O., Krishnan, C., Dike, S., Gearhart, J.D. and Rothstein, J.D. (2003). Human embryonic germ cell derivatives facilitate motor recovery of rats with diffuse motor neuron injury. *J Neurosci*, **23**, 5131–5140.

Keyvan-Fouladi, N., Raisman, G. and Li, Y. (2003). Functional repair of the corticospinal tract by delayed transplantation of olfactory ensheathing cells in adult rats. *J Neurosci*, **23**, 9428–9434.

Kim, M. and Morshead, C.M. (2003). Distinct populations of forebrain neural stem and progenitor cells can be isolated using side-population analysis. *J Neurosci*, **23**, 10703–10709.

Kim, D., Adipudi, V., Shibayama, M., Giszter, S., Tessler, A., Murray, M. and Simansky, K.J. (1999). Direct agonists for serotonin receptors enhance locomotor function in rats that received neural transplants after neonatal spinal transection. *J Neurosci*, **19**, 6213–6224.

Kojima, A. and Tator, C.H. (2000). Epidermal growth factor and fibroblast growth factor 2 cause proliferation of ependymal precursor cells in the adult rat spinal cord *in vivo*. *J Neuropathol Exp Neurol*, **59**, 687–697.

Lang, K.J., Rathjen, J., Vassilieva, S. and Rathjen, P.D. (2004). Differentiation of embryonic stem cells to a neural fate: a route to re-building the nervous system? *J Neurosci Res*, **76**, 184–192.

Laywell, E.D., Rakic, P., Kukekov, V.G., Holland, E.C. and Steindler, D.A. (2000). Identification of a multipotent astrocytic stem cell in the immature and adult mouse brain. *Proc Natl Acad Sci USA*, **97**, 13883–13888.

Lee, J.C., Mayer-Proschel, M. and Rao, M.S. (2000). Gliogenesis in the central nervous system. *Glia*, **30**, 105–121.

Lee, S.H., Lumelsky, N., Studer, L., Auerbach, J.M. and McKay, R.D. (2000). Efficient generation of midbrain and hindbrain neurons from mouse embryonic stem cells. *Nat Biotechnol*, **18**, 675–679.

Lepore, A.C., Han, S.S., Tyler-Polsz, C., Cai, J., Rao, M.S. and Fischer, I. (2004). Differential fate of multipotent and lineage-restricted neural precursors following transplantation into the adult CNS. *Neuron Glia Biol*, **1**, 113–126.

Li, R., Thode, S., Zhou, J., Richard, N., Pardinas, J., Rao, M.S. and Sah, D.W. (2000). Motoneuron differentiation of immortalized human spinal cord cell lines. *J Neurosci Res*, **59**, 342–352.

Lillien, L. (1998). Neural progenitors and stem cells: mechanisms of progenitor heterogeneity. *Curr Opin Neurobiol*, **8**, 37–44.

Lipson, A.C. and Horner, P.J. (2002). Potent possibilities: endogenous stem cells in the adult spinal cord. *Prog Brain Res*, **137**, 283–297.

Liu, Y. and Rao, M.S. (2004). Glial progenitors in the CNS and possible lineage relationships among them. *Biol Cell*, **96**, 279–290.

Liu, S., Qu, Y., Stewart, T.J., Howard, M.J., Chakrabortty, S., Holekamp, T.F. and McDonald, J.W. (2000). Embryonic stem cells differentiate into oligodendrocytes and myelinate in culture and after spinal cord transplantation. *Proc Natl Acad Sci USA*, **97**, 6126–6131.

Liu, B.P., Fournier, A., GrandPre, T. and Strittmatter, S.M. (2002). Myelin-associated glycoprotein as a functional ligand for the Nogo-66 receptor. *Science*, **297**, 1190–1193.

Lu, P., Jones, L.L., Snyder, E.Y. and Tuszynski, M.H. (2003). Neural stem cells constitutively secrete neurotrophic factors and promote extensive host axonal growth after spinal cord injury. *Exp Neurol*, **181**, 115–129.

Lu, P., Blesch, A. and Tuszynski, M.H. (2004a). Induction of bone marrow stromal cells to neurons: differentiation, transdifferentiation, or artifact? *J Neurosci Res*, **77**, 174–191.

Lu, P., Yang, H., Jones, L.L., Filbin, M.T. and Tuszynski, M.H. (2004b). Combinatorial therapy with neurotrophins and cAMP promotes axonal regeneration beyond sites of spinal cord injury. *J Neurosci*, **24**, 6402–6409.

Luskin, M.B. (1993). Restricted proliferation and migration of postnatally generated neurons derived from the forebrain subventricular zone. *Neuron*, **11**, 173–189.

Martens, D.J., Seaberg, R.M. and van der Kooy, D. (2002). *In vivo* infusions of exogenous growth factors into the fourth ventricle of the adult mouse brain increase the proliferation of neural progenitors around the fourth ventricle and the central canal of the spinal cord. *Eur J Neurosci*, **16**, 1045–1057.

Mayer-Proschel, M., Kalyani, A.J., Mujtaba, T. and Rao, M.S. (1997). Isolation of lineage-restricted neuronal precursors from multipotent neuroepithelial stem cells. *Neuron*, **19**, 773–785.

McDonald, J.W., Liu, X.Z., Qu, Y., Liu, S., Mickey, S.K., Turetsky, D., Gottlieb, D.I. and Choi, D.W. (1999). Transplanted embryonic stem cells survive, differentiate and promote recovery in injured rat spinal cord. *Nat Med*, **5**, 1410–1412.

McGee, A.W. and Strittmatter, S.M. (2003). The Nogo-66 receptor: focusing myelin inhibition of axon regeneration. *Trends Neurosci*, **26**, 193–198.

Merkler, D., Metz, G.A., Raineteau, O., Dietz, V., Schwab, M.E. and Fouad, K. (2001). Locomotor recovery in spinal cord-injured rats treated with an antibody neutralizing the myelin-associated neurite growth inhibitor Nogo-A. *J Neurosci*, **21**, 3665–3673.

Metz, G.A., Curt, A., van de Meent, H., Klusman, I., Schwab, M.E. and Dietz, V. (2000). Validation of the weight-drop contusion model in rats: a comparative study of human spinal cord injury. *J Neurotraum*, **17**, 1–17.

Mezey, E., Chandross, K.J., Harta, G., Maki, R.A. and McKercher, S.R. (2000). Turning blood into brain: cells bearing neuronal antigens generated *in vivo* from bone marrow. *Science*, **290**, 1779–1782.

Mi, H. and Barres, B.A. (1999). Purification and characterization of astrocyte precursor cells in the developing rat optic nerve. *J Neurosci*, **19**, 1049–1061.

Mitsui, T., Kakizaki, H., Tanaka, H., Shibata, T., Matsuoka, I. and Koyanagi, T. (2003). Immortalized neural stem cells transplanted into the injured spinal cord promote recovery of voiding function in the rat. *J Urol*, **170**, 1421–1425.

Miya, D., Giszter, S., Mori, F., Adipudi, V., Tessler, A. and Murray, M. (1997). Fetal transplants alter the development of function after spinal cord transection in newborn rats. *J Neurosci*, **17**, 4856–4872.

Mori, F., Himes, B.T., Kowada, M., Murray, M. and Tessler, A. (1997). Fetal spinal cord transplants rescue some axotomized rubrospinal neurons from retrograde cell death in adult rats. *Exp Neurol*, **143**, 45–60.

Mujtaba, T., Piper, D.R., Kalyani, A., Groves, A.K., Lucero, M.T. and Rao, M.S. (1999). Lineage-restricted neural precursors can be isolated from both the mouse neural tube and cultured ES cells. *Dev Biol*, **214**, 113–127.

Mujtaba, T., Han, S.S., Fischer, I., Sandgren, E.P. and Rao, M.S. (2002). Stable expression of the alkaline phosphatase marker gene by neural cells in culture and after transplantation into the CNS using cells derived from a transgenic rat. *Exp Neurol*, **174**, 48–57.

Murray, M. (2004). Cellular transplants: steps toward restoration of function in spinal injured animals. *Prog Brain Res*, **143**, 133–146.

Nashmi, R. and Fehlings, M.G. (2001). Mechanisms of axonal dysfunction after spinal cord injury: with an emphasis on the role of voltage-gated potassium channels. *Brain Res Brain Res Rev*, **38**, 165–191.

Neuhuber, B., Gallo, G., Howard, L., Kostura, L., Mackay, A. and Fischer, I. (2004). Reevaluation of *in vitro* differentiation protocols for bone marrow stromal cells: disruption of actin cytoskeleton induces rapid morphological changes and mimics neuronal phenotype. *J Neurosci Res*, **77**, 192–204.

Nogradi, A. and Vrbova, G. (1996). Improved motor function of denervated rat hindlimb muscles induced by embryonic spinal cord grafts. *Eur J Neurosci*, **8**, 2198–2203.

Ogawa, Y., Sawamoto, K., Miyata, T., Miyao, S., Watanabe, M., Nakamura, M., Bregman, B.S., Koike, M., Uchiyama, Y., Toyama, Y. and Okano, H. (2002). Transplantation of *in vitro*-expanded fetal neural progenitor cells results in neurogenesis and functional recovery after spinal cord contusion injury in adult rats. *J Neurosci Res*, **69**, 925–933.

Oudega, M., Gautier, S.E., Chapon, P., Fragoso, M., Bates, M.L., Parel, J.M. and Bunge, M.B. (2001). Axonal regeneration into

Schwann cell grafts within resorbable poly(alpha-hydroxy-acid) guidance channels in the adult rat spinal cord. *Biomaterials*, **22**, 1125–1136.

Pearse, D.D., Pereira, F.C., Marcillo, A.E., Bates, M.L., Berrocal, Y.A., Filbin, M.T. and Bunge, M.B. (2004). cAMP and Schwann cells promote axonal growth and functional recovery after spinal cord injury. *Nat Med*, **10**, 610–616.

Pencea, V., Bingaman, K.D., Freedman, L.J. and Luskin, M.B. (2001). Neurogenesis in the subventricular zone and rostral migratory stream of the neonatal and adult primate forebrain. *Exp Neurol*, **172**, 1–16.

Peng, H., Huang, Y., Rose, J., Erichsen, D., Herek, S., Fujii, N., Tamamura, H. and Zheng, J. (2004). Stromal cell-derived factor 1-mediated CXCR4 signaling in rat and human cortical neural progenitor cells. *J Neurosci Res*, **76**, 35–50.

Pevny, L. and Rao, M.S. (2003). The stem-cell menagerie. *Trends Neurosci*, **26**, 351–359.

Pluchino, S., Quattrini, A., Brambilla, E., Gritti, A., Salani, G., Dina, G., Galli, R., Del Carro, U., Amadio, S., Bergami, A., Furlan, R., Comi, G., Vescovi, A.L. and Martino, G. (2003). Injection of adult neurospheres induces recovery in a chronic model of multiple sclerosis. *Nature*, **422**, 688–694.

Potter, P.J., Hayes, K.C., Segal, J.L., Hsieh, J.T., Brunnemann, S.R., Delaney, G.A., Tierney, D.S. and Mason, D. (1998). Randomized double-blind crossover trial of fampridine-SR (sustained release 4-aminopyridine) in patients with incomplete spinal cord injury. *J Neurotraum*, **15**, 837–849.

Qian, X., Shen, Q., Goderie, S.K., He, W., Capela, A., Davis, A.A. and Temple, S. (2000). Timing of CNS cell generation: a programmed sequence of neuron and glial cell production from isolated murine cortical stem cells. *Neuron*, **28**, 69–80.

Raff, M.C., Miller, R.H. and Noble, M. (1983). A glial progenitor cell that develops *in vitro* into an astrocyte or an oligodendrocyte depending on culture medium. *Nature*, **303**, 390–396.

Ramer, M.S., Bradbury, E.J., Michael, G.J., Lever, I.J. and McMahon, S.B. (2003). Glial cell line-derived neurotrophic factor increases calcitonin gene-related peptide immunoreactivity in sensory and motoneurons *in vivo*. *Eur J Neurosci*, **18**, 2713–2721.

Ramon-Cueto, A., Plant, G.W., Avila, J. and Bunge, M.B. (1998). Long-distance axonal regeneration in the transected adult rat spinal cord is promoted by olfactory ensheathing glia transplants. *J Neurosci*, **18**, 3803–3815.

Rao, M.S. and Mayer-Proschel, M. (1997). Glial-restricted precursors are derived from multipotent neuroepithelial stem cells. *Dev Biol*, **188**, 48–63.

Rao, M.S. and Mayer-Proschel, M. (2000). Precursor cells for transplantation. *Prog Brain Res*, **128**, 273–292.

Rao, M.S., Noble, M. and Mayer-Proschel, M. (1998). A tripotential glial precursor cell is present in the developing spinal cord. *Proc Natl Acad Sci USA*, **95**, 3996–4001.

Reier, P.J., Perlow, M.J. and Guth, L. (1983). Development of embryonic spinal cord transplants in the rat. *Brain Res*, **312**, 201–219.

Reier, P.J., Bregman, B.S. and Wujek, J.R. (1986). Intraspinal transplantation of embryonic spinal cord tissue in neonatal and adult rats. *J Comp Neurol*, **247**, 275–296.

Reynolds, B.A. and Weiss, S. (1996). Clonal and population analyses demonstrate that an EGF-responsive mammalian embryonic CNS precursor is a stem cell. *Dev Biol*, **175**, 1–13.

Rossignol, S., Giroux, N., Chau, C., Marcoux, J., Brustein, E. and Reader, T.A. (2001). Pharmacological aids to locomotor training after spinal injury in the cat. *J Physiol*, **533**, 65–74.

Roy, N.S., Benraiss, A., Wang, S., Fraser, R.A., Goodman, R., Couldwell, W.T., Nedergaard, M., Kawaguchi, A., Okano, H. and Goldman, S.A. (2000). Promoter-targeted selection and isolation of neural progenitor cells from the adult human ventricular zone. *J Neurosci Res*, **59**, 321–331.

Roy, N.S., Nakano, T., Keyoung, H.M., Windrem, M., Rashbaum, W.K., Alonso, M.L., Kang, J., Peng, W., Carpenter, M.K., Lin, J., Nedergaard, M. and Goldman, S.A. (2004). Telomerase immortalization of neuronally restricted progenitor cells derived from the human fetal spinal cord. *Nat Biotechnol*, **22**, 297–305.

Seaberg, R.M. and van der Kooy, D. (2003). Stem and progenitor cells: the premature desertion of rigorous definitions. *Trends Neurosci*, **26**, 125–131.

Shamblott, M.J., Axelman, J., Wang, S., Bugg, E.M., Littlefield, J.W., Donovan, P.J., Blumenthal, P.D., Huggins, G.R. and Gearhart, J.D. (1998). Derivation of pluripotent stem cells from cultured human primordial germ cells. *Proc Natl Acad Sci USA*, **95**, 13726–13731.

Shibayama, M., Hattori, S., Himes, B.T., Murray, M. and Tessler, A. (1998). Neurotrophin-3 prevents death of axotomized Clarke's nucleus neurons in adult rat. *J Comp Neurol*, **390**, 102–111.

Shihabuddin, L.S., Horner, P.J., Ray, J. and Gage, F.H. (2000). Adult spinal cord stem cells generate neurons after transplantation in the adult dentate gyrus. *J Neurosci*, **20**, 8727–8735.

Sieradzan, K. and Vrbova, G. (1991). Factors influencing survival of transplanted embryonic motoneurones in the spinal cord of adult rats. *Exp Neurol*, **114**, 286–299.

Snyder, E.Y., Taylor, R.M. and Wolfe, J.H. (1995). Neural progenitor cell engraftment corrects lysosomal storage throughout the MPS VII mouse brain. *Nature*, **374**, 367–370.

Song, H., Stevens, C.F. and Gage, F.H. (2002). Astroglia induce neurogenesis from adult neural stem cells. *Nature*, **417**, 39–44.

Studer, L., Tabar, V. and McKay, R.D. (1998). Transplantation of expanded mesencephalic precursors leads to recovery in parkinsonian rats. *Nat Neurosci*, **1**, 290–295.

Suslov, O.N., Kukekov, V.G., Ignatova, T.N. and Steindler, D.A. (2002). Neural stem cell heterogeneity demonstrated by molecular phenotyping of clonal neurospheres. *Proc Natl Acad Sci USA*, **99**, 14506–14511.

Svendsen, C.N., Caldwell, M.A., Shen, J., ter Borg, M.G., Rosser, A.E., Tyers, P., Karmiol, S. and Dunnett, S.B. (1997). Long-term survival of human central nervous system progenitor cells transplanted into a rat model of Parkinson's disease. *Exp Neurol*, **148**, 135–146.

Tang, X., Davies, J.E. and Davies, S.J. (2003). Changes in distribution, cell associations, and protein expression levels of NG2, neurocan, phosphacan, brevican, versican V2, and tenascin-C during acute to chronic maturation of spinal cord scar tissue. *J Neurosci Res*, **71**, 427–444.

Temple, S. (2001). The development of neural stem cells. *Nature*, **414**, 112–117.

Teng, Y.D., Lavik, E.B., Qu, X., Park, K.I., Ourednik, J., Zurakowski, D., Langer, R. and Snyder, E.Y. (2002). Functional recovery following traumatic spinal cord injury mediated by a unique polymer scaffold seeded with neural stem cells. *Proc Natl Acad Sci USA*, **99**, 3024–3029.

Theele, D.P., Schrimsher, G.W. and Reier, P.J. (1996). Comparison of the growth and fate of fetal spinal iso- and allografts in the adult rat injured spinal cord. *Exp Neurol*, **142**, 128–143.

Thomas, C.K., Sesodia, S., Erb, D.E. and Grumbles, R.M. (2003). Properties of medial gastrocnemius motor units and muscle fibers reinnervated by embryonic ventral spinal cord cells. *Exp Neurol*, **180**, 25–31.

Thomson, J.A., Kalishman, J., Golos, T.G., Durning, M., Harris, C.P., Becker, R.A. and Hearn, J.P. (1995). Isolation of a primate embryonic stem cell line. *Proc Natl Acad Sci USA*, **92**, 7844–7848.

Thomson, J.A., Itskovitz-Eldor, J., Shapiro, S.S., Waknitz, M.A., Swiergiel, J.J., Marshall, V.S. and Jones, J.M. (1998). Embryonic stem cell lines derived from human blastocysts. *Science*, **282**, 1145–1147.

Tran, P.B., Ren, D., Veldhouse, T.J. and Miller, R.J. (2004). Chemokine receptors are expressed widely by embryonic and adult neural progenitor cells. *J Neurosci Res*, **76**, 20–34.

Tropepe, V., Sibilia, M., Ciruna, B.G., Rossant, J., Wagner, E.F. and van der Kooy, D. (1999). Distinct neural stem cells proliferate in response to EGF and FGF in the developing mouse telencephalon. *Dev Biol*, **208**, 166–188.

Vroemen, M., Aigner, L., Winkler, J. and Weidner, N. (2003). Adult neural progenitor cell grafts survive after acute spinal cord injury and integrate along axonal pathways. *Eur J Neurosci*, **18**, 743–751.

Wang, C.X., Nuttin, B., Heremans, H., Dom, R. and Gybels, J. (1996). Production of tumor necrosis factor in spinal cord following traumatic injury in rats. *J Neuroimmunol*, **69**, 151–156.

Wang, S., Roy, N.S., Benraiss, A. and Goldman, S.A. (2000). Promoter-based isolation and fluorescence-activated sorting of mitotic neuronal progenitor cells from the adult mammalian ependymal/subependymal zone. *Dev Neurosci*, **22**, 167–176.

Weiss, S., Dunne, C., Hewson, J., Wohl, C., Wheatley, M., Peterson, A.C. and Reynolds, B.A. (1996). Multipotent CNS stem cells are present in the adult mammalian spinal cord and ventricular neuroaxis. *J Neurosci*, **16**, 7599–7609.

Wichterle, H., Liebram, I., Porter, J.A. and Jessell, T.M. (2002). Directed differentiation of embryonic stem cells into motor neurons. *Cell*, **110**, 385–397.

Wu, K.L., Chan, S.H., Chao, Y.M. and Chan, J.Y. (2003). Expression of pro-inflammatory cytokine and caspase genes promotes neuronal apoptosis in pontine reticular formation after spinal cord transection. *Neurobiol Dis*, **14**, 19–31.

Wu, P., Tarasenko, Y.I., Gu, Y., Huang, L.Y., Coggeshall, R.E. and Yu, Y. (2002). Region-specific generation of cholinergic neurons from fetal human neural stem cells grafted in adult rat. *Nat Neurosci*, **5**, 1271–1278.

Wu, S., Suzuki, Y., Noda, T., Bai, H., Kitada, M., Kataoka, K., Nishimura, Y. and Ide, C. (2002). Immunohistochemical and electron microscopic study of invasion and differentiation in spinal cord lesion of neural stem cells grafted through cerebrospinal fluid in rat. *J Neurosci Res*, **69**, 940–945.

Xu, X.M., Zhang, S.X., Li, H., Aebischer, P. and Bunge, M.B. (1999). Regrowth of axons into the distal spinal cord through a Schwann-cell-seeded mini-channel implanted into hemisected adult rat spinal cord. *Eur J Neurosci*, **11**, 1723–1740.

Yamamoto, S., Nagao, M., Sugimori, M., Kosako, H., Nakatomi, H., Yamamoto, N., Takebayashi, H., Nabeshima, Y., Kitamura, T., Weinmaster, G., Nakamura, K. and Nakafuku, M. (2001a). Transcription factor expression and Notch-dependent regulation of neural progenitors in the adult rat spinal cord. *J Neurosci*, **21**, 9814–9823.

Yamamoto, S., Yamamoto, N., Kitamura, T., Nakamura, K. and Nakafuku, M. (2001b). Proliferation of parenchymal neural progenitors in response to injury in the adult rat spinal cord. *Exp Neurol*, **172**, 115–127.

Zhang, S.C., Ge, B. and Duncan, I.D. (1999). Adult brain retains the potential to generate oligodendroglial progenitors with extensive myelination capacity. *Proc Natl Acad Sci USA*, **96**, 4089–4094.

26

Dysfunction and recovery in demyelinated and dysmyelinated axons

Stephen G. Waxman

Department of Neurology and Center for Neuroscience Research, Yale University School of Medicine,
New Haven and Rehabilitation Research Center, VA Connecticut Healthcare System, West Haven, CT, USA

Since information is transmitted from site to site within the nervous system via the conduction of sequences of action potentials, it is not surprising that the need to optimize the conduction time has shaped the evolution of nerve fibers. In axons without myelin, which are present both in lower species and in phylogenetically old tracts in higher species, action potentials travel at a speed (the conduction velocity) that is proportional to diameter$^{1/2}$. Thus, in order to achieve a faster speed of conduction, species that lack myelin have to substantially enlarge their axons. In the squid which lacks myelin, axons evolved to be as large as 400–900 μm in diameter, a fortuitous specialization which enabled early electrophysiologists to study the ionic basis for nerve impulses conduction through the first recordings from within single nerve fibers. Increased conduction speed in these axons comes at a price: an increase in size. In higher species, on the other hand, high conduction velocities are achieved in some axons by ensheathment with myelin. Myelinated fibers are subject to several types of pathology including dysmyelination (failure to form normal myelin) and demyelination (loss of myelin after it has been formed). This chapter will discuss the organization and function of normal myelinated axons and of demyelinated and dysmyelinated axons.

26.1 The myelinated axon and its sheath

The myelinated fiber consists of an axon and its surrounding myelin sheaths. Schwann cells in the peripheral nervous system (PNS), and oligodendrocytes in the central nervous system (CNS), produce myelin. While a single Schwann cell myelinates one axon, one oligodendrocyte myelinates a family of axons; there are from 1–2 to nearly 100 axons per oligodendrocyte (Bjartmar et al., 1994). The oligodendrocyte cell body does not surround its myelin sheaths as a Schwann cell does but, on the contrary, maintains contact with its myelin sheaths via thin cytoplasmic bridges (Bunge et al., 1961; Hirano, 1968). It has been speculated that the tenuous connection between the genomic and biosynthetic machinery within the oligodendrocyte cell body and the myelin underlies the paucity of remyelination within the CNS. However, there is evidence for local synthesis of myelin membrane in distal parts of the oligodendroglial processes which contain polyribosomes (Waxman and Sims, 1984), close to the myelin sheaths (Waxman et al., 1988).

As a result of its high electrical resistance and low capacitance, the myelin functions as an insulator which prevents current loss during action potential conduction. The myelin is periodically punctuated by nodes of Ranvier. Internode distances range from less than 100 μm (small-diameter fibers) to slightly over 1 mm (larger-diameter fibers), and optimize conduction velocity. As noted below, sodium channels (which provide the inward transmembrane current necessary for the generation of action potentials) are clustered in high density within the axon membrane at the nodes. Due to this, myelinated fibers conduct action potentials in a discontinuous, or saltatory manner, unlike non-myelinated fibers which usually conduct impulses in a slower continuous manner (Huxley and Stämpfli, 1949). Conduction velocity is approximately proportional to fiber diameter in myelinated fibers. Thus, above a critical diameter where the conduction velocity–diameter relationships intersect, myelinated fibers conduct action potentials more rapidly than non-myelinated fibers of the same diameter; this critical diameter is approximately 0.2 μm, a size which corresponds with the diameter at which myelination is first seen within the CNS (Waxman and Bennett, 1972).

26.2 Molecular organization of the myelinated axon

In contrast to non-myelinated axons which generally display a uniform membrane structure which does not vary substantially from one region to another (Black et al., 1981), the membrane of the myelinated axon is highly specialized, with several types of voltage-sensitive ion channels and other proteins distributed along it in a non-uniform manner (Fig. 26.1). Na$^+$ channels are aggregated in high density (approximately 1000/μm^2) in the axon membrane at the node of Ranvier (Ritchie and Rogart, 1977; Waxman, 1977). The density of Na$^+$ channels is much lower (<25/μm^2) in the internodal axon membrane beneath the myelin sheath (Ritchie and Rogart, 1977; Waxman, 1977), too low to support secure conduction under most circumstances.

Nine different sodium channel subtypes (see Table 26.1) have been identified thus far, with distinct molecular structures superimposed on an invariant overall motif (four similar domains, each containing six membrane-spanning segments). Na$_v$ 1.6 is known to be a major nodal sodium channel (Caldwell et al., 2000) but other sodium channel subtypes (e.g. Na$_v$1.2, Na$_v$1.8) are also present at some nodes (Craner et al., 2003a; 2004a); moreover, Na$_v$1.6 is also present along non-myelinated axons where it contributes to the continuous conduction of action potentials (Black et al., 2002).

Most sodium channel isoforms are sensitive to low (nanomolar) concentrations of tetrodotoxin (TTX). Two TTX-resistant (TTX-R) sodium channels, termed Na$_v$1.8/SNS (Akopian et al., 1996) and Na$_v$ 1.9/NaN (Dib-Hajj et al., 1998) have, however, been cloned from dorsal root ganglion (DRG) neurons. Na$_v$1.8/SNS (where SNS is Sensory Neuron Specific) produces a slowly inactivating current (Akopian et al., 1996) which recovers rapidly from inactivation (Dib-Hajj et al., 1997) and contributes to the upstroke of the action potential in cells in which it is present (Renganathan et al., 2001). Na$_v$1.9/NaN is non-inactivating; because of substantial overlap between activation and steady-state inactivation, it contributes a depolarizing influence at resting potential, boosts sub-threshold inputs, and lowers the threshold for action potential generation (Cummins et al., 1999; Herzog et al., 2001; Baker et al., 2003). These TTX-R channel isoforms are expressed preferentially in small DRG neurons and their non-myelinated and small myelinated axons (Fjell et al., 1997; Liu et al., 2001), with Na$_v$1.9/NaN expressed exclusively in nociceptive units (Fang et al., 2002). Na$_v$1.8/SNS and Na$_v$1.9/NaN are both present at nociceptive nerve terminals, suggesting that they play roles in nociceptive sensory transduction as well as impulse transmission (Black and Waxman, 2002).

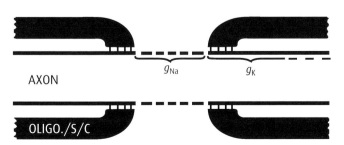

Figure 26.1. The normal myelinated axon displays a complex ion channel organization, as shown in this schematic. g^{Na^+}: sodium channels; g_{K^+} fast: potassium channels. Sodium channels are clustered at the node of Ranvier. Fast potassium channels, responsible for repolarization of the action potential, are present in the axon membrane under the myelin.

Intra-axonal recordings indicate the presence of at least three types of physiologically distinct voltage-gated potassium K^+ channels in myelinated axons: a "fast" K^+ channel, a "slow" K^+ channel, and an inward rectifier which is permeable to both K^+ and Na^+. Fast K^+ channels can be blocked with external 4-aminopyridine (4-AP) and are localized in relatively low densities in the nodal axon membrane and in highest density in the axon membrane beneath the myelin (Chiu and Ritchie, 1980; 1981; Ritchie et al., 1981; Foster et al., 1982; Kocsis et al., 1982; Eng et al., 1988; Zhou et al., 1998). Voltage-clamp studies on myelinated axons have been interpreted as indicating that the fast K^+ channel density is highest in the paranode, falling to one-sixth of paranodal density in the node and internode (Röper and Schwarz, 1989), but the resolution of this technique may not be adequate to differentiate paranodal from juxtaparanodal regions. Molecular analysis has demonstrated $K_v1.1$ and $K_v1.2$ potassium channel subunits at the juxtaparanode (Wang et al., 1993; Rasband et al., 1998; Vabnick and Shrager 1998).

The complementary distribution of Na^+ channels and fast K^+ channels in the axon membrane contributes to the pathophysiology of demyelinated axons. The low density of Na^+ channels within the exposed axon membrane after damage to the myelin results in a low density of inward Na^+ current which can impair conduction (Waxman, 1982). Loss of myelin also unmasks fast K^+ channels which tend to clamp the demyelinated axon membrane close to the K^+ equilibrium potential Ek, opposing depolarization and further interfering with the conduction of action potentials (Chiu and Ritchie, 1981).

The expression of fast K^+ channels in the axon membrane under the myelin also suggests the possibility of increasing the safety factor for conduction in demyelinated axons via pharmacological blockade of the fast K^+ channels that are unmasked by demyelination (Bowe et al., 1987; Kocsis et al., 1987).

26.3 Action potential conduction in myelinated, demyelinated and dysmyelinated axons

In mammalian myelinated axons at 37°C, the internodal conduction time (time between excitation of one node and the next) is brief, approximately 20 μs

Table 26.1. Voltage-gated sodium channels.

Name	Former name	Primary sites of distribution	Relevance to demyelinating diseases	References
$Na_v1.1$	Type I	Neurons	–	–
$Na_v1.2$	Type II	Neurons, including premyelinated axons, non-myelinated axons	Expressed along dysmyelinated and some demyelinated axons	Craner et al., 2003; Craner et al., 2004a, b
$Na_v1.3$	Type III	Embryonic neurons	–	–
$Na_v1.4$	μ1	Skeletal muscle	–	–
$Na_v1.5$	–	Cardiac muscle	–	–
$Na_v1.6$	Type VI	Nodes in myelinated axons; initial segments; non-myelinated axons	Expressed along some demyelinated axons; co-localizes with markers of axonal injury	Craner et al., 2004a; Craner et al., 2004b
$Na_v1.7$	PN1	DRG neurons	–	–
$Na_v1.8$	SNS, PN3	DRG neurons	Upregulated in Purkinje neurons in EAE and MS	Black et al., 2000; Saab et al., 2004
$Na_v1.9$	NaN	DRG neurons	–	–

(Rasminsky and Sears, 1972). Action potential conduction is rapid, and occurs in a unidirectional manner because sodium channels close soon after activation and remain refractory (as a result of inactivation) for a short time.

In healthy myelinated axons the high resistance, low capacitance myelin shunts the action current from each active node of Ranvier to subsequent nodes through the relatively low-resistance axoplasm (Fig. 26.2a). In normal myelinated fibers, the safety factor (the ratio between current available to stimulate a node of Ranvier and current required to stimulate the node) is 5–7 (Tasaki, 1953).

This situation is disrupted in demyelinated and dysmyelinated axons. Following loss of the myelin there is a decreased density of action current as a result of capacitative and resistive shunting through the bared axon membrane (Fig. 26.2b). Therefore, the charging time for the nodal membrane is increased and it takes longer than normal for the axon to reach threshold. In axons where the safety factor is reduced but is still greater than 1.0, conduction will continue but conduction velocity will be reduced. Internodal conduction time can be increased under these

circumstances more than 20-fold, to nearly 500 μs (Rasminsky and Sears, 1972). In more severely demyelinated axons, the safety factor can fall to less than 1.0; in these axons threshold is not reached; and conduction block ensues (Waxman, 1982).

Figure 26.3 illustrates the spectrum of conduction abnormalities that produce clinical signs and symptoms in demyelinated and dysmyelinated axons. Some of these abnormalities are negative in the Jacksonian sense. *Slowed conduction* (Fig. 26.3b) appears to have less of an effect than conduction block in producing clinical deficits (McDonald, 1963; McDonald and Sears, 1970). *Temporal dispersion* (loss of synchrony in tracts in which different fibers exhibit unequal degrees of conduction slowing) occurs in demyelinated nerves and tracts as a corollary of decreased conduction velocity (see Fig. 26.3c), and can produce clinical abnormalities by interfering with functions such as the stretch reflex that require synchronous discharge.

Conduction block is produced in demyelinated fibers by multiple mechanisms, including capacitative current loss through damaged myelin sheaths and impedance mismatch in focally demyelinated

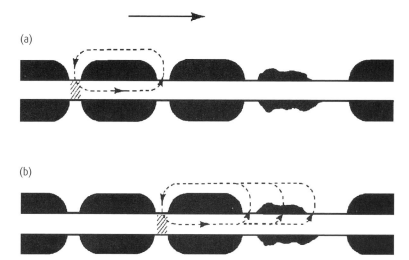

Figure 26.2. As a result of its low capacitance and higher resistance, myelin focuses transmembrane current on the nodes of Ranvier. (a) The action potential is conducted from left to right (arrow). In normal parts of the fiber the myelin functions as an insulator. (b) Dashed arrows illustrate current flow resulting from an action potential that is located at the cross-hatched node. Current is lost in demyelinated regions as a result of capacitative and resistive shunting.

axons (Sears et al., 1978; Waxman and Brill, 1978). The low Na$^+$ channel density in the demyelinated axon membrane contributes to conduction block. In addition, fast K$^+$ channels (normally covered by the myelin) are unmasked after demyelination and tend to hold the demyelinated membrane close to the potassium equilibrium potential Ek, thus impeding action potential electrogenesis (Bostock et al., 1981; Ritchie and Chiu, 1981).

Hyperpolarization produced by electrogenic pump (Na$^+$K$^+$-ATPase) activity may contribute to conduction block of high-frequency impulse trains (Bostock and Grafe, 1985). Elevated intracellular Na$^+$ at an upstream "driving node" (Rasminsky and Sears, 1972) and axonal depolarization due to increases in extracellular K$^+$ concentration (Brismar, 1981) may also contribute to high-frequency conduction failure.

In *frequency-related conduction block*, high-frequency impulse trains fail to propagate while low-frequency impulse trains traverse the lesion (Fig. 26.3d). *Total conduction block* ensues in more severely affected fibers, with single action potentials failing to propagate beyond the zone of demyelination (Fig. 26.3e).

Conduction abnormalities that are positive in a Jacksonian sense (Fig. 26.3f–i) include *ectopic impulse generation* (Fig. 26.3f) (Smith and McDonald, 1980) and *pathological cross-talk* (see Fig. 26.3h). *Increased mechanosensitivity* (Fig. 26.3g) probably underlies clinical phenomena such as Tinel's and Lhermitte's

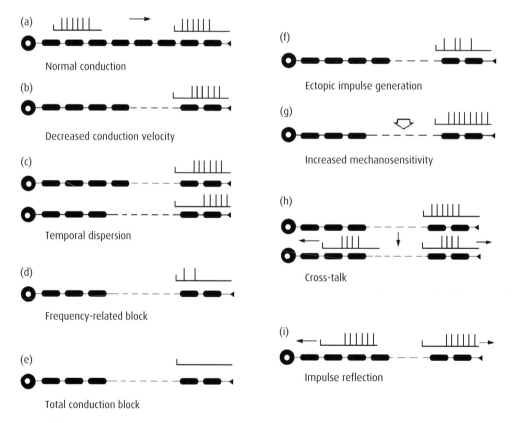

Figure 26.3. A spectrum of conduction abnormalities occurs in demyelinated axons. Demyelinated regions of the axon are diagrammatically shown as dashed lines. Cell bodies are located to the left, and axon terminals to the right. The direction of normal conduction is indicated by the arrow (see text for further explanation).

sign (Smith and McDonald 1980; Vollmer et al., 1991). *Impulse reflection* (Fig. 26.3i) may also occur in some focally demyelinated fibers (Burchiel, 1980). The reflected (antidromic) impulses can collide with and abolish orthodromic impulses, thus interfering with normal impulse traffic.

26.4 Blocking factors?

While occasional reports have purported that "neuro-electric blocking factors" or "sodium channel blocking factors" may contribute to axonal conduction block in neuro-inflammatory disorders, these reports in general have not been substantiated by subsequent studies (see, e.g. Bornstein and Crain, 1965; Cerf and Carels, 1966; Lumdsen et al., 1975; Seil et al., 1976; Schauf and Davis, 1981; Seil, 1981). Recently, it has been suggested that paralysis in Guillain–Barre' syndrome may be due to a Na^+ channel blocking factor in the cerebrospinal fluid (Brinkmeier, 1992) and that the cerebrospinal fluid of multiple sclerosis (MS) patients contains the same factor (Brinkmeier et al., 1993). A recent report has purported to identify this blocking factor as a pentapeptide with the sequence Gln-Tyr-Asn-Ala-Asp (QYNAD) (Brinkmeier et al., 2000), and suggested that QYNAD blocks sodium channels at concentrations as low as $10\,\mu M$, by shifting steady-state inactivation to more negative potentials (Weber et al., 1999; Brinkmeier et al., 2000). Multiple investigators, however, have not been able to replicate these results, and have not observed a sodium channel blocking effect of QYNAD even at concentrations as high as $500\,\mu M$ (Cummins et al., 2003). Thus the suggestion that Na^+ channel blocking factors contribute to the pathophysiology of Guillain–Barre' syndrome or MS, remains speculative and unsubstantiated.

26.5 Restoration of conduction following loss of myelin: continuous conduction

While normal myelinated fibers conduct impulses in a saltatory manner with action potential electrogenesis essentially confined to the nodes of Ranvier where Na^+ channels are aggregated (Rasminsky and Sears, 1972), some demyelinated axons display continuous action potential conduction (Bostock and Sears, 1976; 1978) which reflects more widespread distribution of Na^+ channels (Foster et al., 1980). Conduction can proceed over continuous lengths of demyelination exceeding 2 mm (several internodes) with a velocity as low as 5% of the normal, saltatory conduction velocity (Felts et al., 1977).

Given that sodium channels are sequestered at nodes along normal myelinated axons, what are the pre-requisites for continuous conduction along previously internodal parts of the axon following demyelination? Computer simulations indicate that, in some small-caliber demyelinated axons in which input impedance is high, a relatively low density of Na^+ channels, similar to the density in acutely demyelinated regions, may support conduction (Waxman and Brill, 1978; Waxman et al., 1989). The reduction in diameter of some demyelinated axons (Prineas and Connell, 1978; Smith et al., 1983a, b), which possibly occurs as a result of decreased neurofilament phosphorylation and increased neurofilament packing density (De Waegh et al., 1992), may thus be an adaptive change. This consideration does not apply, however, to larger axons, which have a lower input impedance. Due to this, the acquisition of a higher-than-normal Na^+ channel density appears to be required for restoration of conduction after loss of the myelin sheath.

Ultrastructural studies on experimentally demyelinated axons provided the first evidence for the development of regions of high sodium channel densities within the bare axon membrane after demyelination (Foster et al., 1980; Black et al., 1987). More recent evidence for the acquisition of increased Na^+ channel densities in the demyelinated axon membrane has been provided by immunocytochemical studies. For example, studies on demyelinated lateral line nerves in fish demonstrated the development of relatively high densities of Na^+ channels in previously internodal regions (England et al., 1991). Immunocytochemical observations several weeks following injection of the demyelinating toxin doxorubicin provided evidence for the expression of sodium channels at newly formed nodes along mammalian remyelinated axons (Dugandzija-Novakovic et al., 1995).

The early immunocytochemical studies utilized generic sodium channel antibodies that could not differentiate between channel subtypes, and thus did not reveal the identity of the sodium channels that are deployed in demyelinated axons. A clue was provided by early studies, which suggested that demyelinated parts of the axon can acquire higher-than-normal densities of Na^+ channels due to a dedifferentiation to an earlier developmental stage. Although the mature internodal membrane does not support secure conduction (Ritchie and Rogart, 1977; Waxman, 1977), the premyelinated axon membrane (including regions destined to develop into internodal membrane), is electrically excitable and conducts impulses (Foster et al., 1982; Waxman et al., 1989). Studies on developing axons (Black et al., 1986) indicate that suppression of Na^+ channel expression, after axons are covered by myelin, reduces excitability within the internodal regions of mature myelinated axons. Loss of the myelin might thus be expected to result in loss of suppression of Na^+ channel expression.

Studies at the molecular level provide evidence that that there is, in fact, a dedifferentiation of the axon membrane in some demyelinated axons. Dysmyelinatal axons in the shiverer brain continue to express $Na_v1.2$ channel (Westenbroek et al., 2002), which are expressed along premyelinatal axons during unusual development (Boiko et al., 2001). Craner et al. (2003; 2004a, b) used subtype-specific antibodies for immunocytochemical analysis of demyelinated CNS axons in experimental allergic encephalomyelitis (EAE) and in multiple sclerosis (MS; see Volume II, Chapter 38. Their results demonstrate that, in demyelinated CNS axons, there is a switch from $Na_v1.6$ to $Na_v1.2$ expression at nodes (Fig. 26.4). Some demyelinated axons exhibit immunostaining for $Na_v1.2$ and, less frequently for $Na_v1.6$ channels which extends continuously for tens of micrometers along the fiber trajectory (i.e. as far as the axons can be followed within sections) (Fig. 26.4d–f). A similar pattern of diffuse $Na_v1.2$ immunostaining is seen in premyelinated axons (Boiko et al., 2001) and may provide a basis for continuous impulse conduction prior to

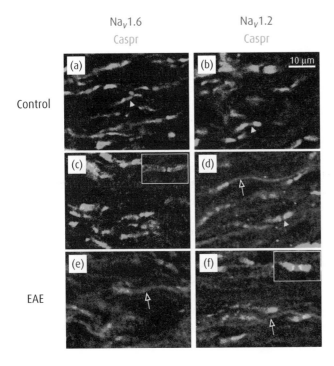

Figure 26.4. There is a switch in expression of sodium channels $Na_v1.6$ and $Na_v1.2$ in demyelinated axons within the CNS. Representative digital images of sections of optic nerve from control (a–b) and EAE (e–f) show immunostaining for $Na_v1.6$ and $Na_v1.2$ (red) and for Caspr (green). (a) and (b) demonstrate nodes with $Na_v1.6$ (a) and less commonly $Na_v1.2$ (b) immunostaining (yellow arrow heads) in healthy optic nerve. (c–e) and (d–f) demonstrate a pattern of progressive demyelination and nodal disruption in EAE, with weak and diffuse Caspr immunostaining at some nodes (inset, c). There is a loss of $Na_v1.6$ immunostaining (c and e) and increased frequency of nodes with $Na_v1.2$ immunostaining (d–f). Demyelinated axonal profiles with continuous $Na_v1.6$ (e, arrow) and, more commonly, $Na_v1.2$ (d, f, arrows) immunostaining are seen in EAE (modified from Craner et al. (2003a)).

myelination. The functional implications of a switch to $Na_v1.2$ expression (rather than $Na_v1.6$) are not entirely understood. Some evidence from patch-clamp studies (Zhou and Goldin, 2002; Herzog et al., 2003) suggests that different kinetic properties may permit $Na_v1.6$ channels to support higher firing rates. $Na_v1.2$ channels show greater accumulation of inactivation at high frequencies of stimulation (>20 Hz) compared to $Na_v1.6$ (Rush et al., 2005). $Na_v1.2$ channels may thus permit conduction to continue in demyelinated axons, albeit with a lower safety factor for high-frequency impulse trains.

26.6 Discontinuous conduction following loss of myelin

Non-uniform (but not necessarily saltatory) conduction of action potentials may also contribute, at least transiently, to recovery of conduction in some demyelinated axons. In this type of conduction, the action potential propagates between separate foci of inward current generation ("phi-nodes"), which appear to be scattered aggregations of Na^+ channels (Smith et al., 1982). Phi-nodes develop several days before remyelination, consistent with the suggestion (Smith et al., 1982) that they are the precursors of nodes. Consistent with the idea that these membrane foci are clusters of Na^+ channels, freeze-fracture electron microscopy demonstrates patches of E-face intramembranous particles with a particle size similar to those in the nodal axon at phi-nodes (Rosenbluth and Blakemore, 1984). Moreover, the number of intramembranous particles in each patch is approximately the same as a mature node (Black et al., 1986). Whether this mode of conduction can occur in a stable manner, over many months, or is a transient prelude to remyelination, is not known.

26.7 Molecular remodeling of the demyelinated axon

How does the demyelinated axon acquire a higher-than-normal density of sodium channels? Although the acquisition of additional sodium channels by the demyelinated axon membrane could, in theory, reflect the redistribution of pre-existing Na^+ channels which diffuse from nearby nodes into the demyelinated (previously internodal) membrane, the available evidence suggests that this is not the case. When studied by patch-clamp, the vestiges of nodes of Ranvier in demyelinated axons display sharp gradients in channel density, which suggest that Na^+ channels do not diffuse away in large numbers following demyelination (Shrager, 1989). A three-fold increase in Na^+ channel concentration per weight of tissue has been observed radioimmunoassay studies at 21–28 days after peripheral nerve demyelination, supporting the idea that new Na^+ channels are inserted into the demyelinated axon membrane (England et al., 1991). A four-fold increase in saxitoxin (STX)-binding sites has been observed in demyelinated white matter in MS patients, compared with normal white matter (Moll et al., 1991). The switch from expression of $Na_v1.6$ to $Na_v1.2$ channels, which includes upregulation of transcription of the $Na_v1.2$ gene (Craner et al., 2003a), also indicates that new channels are produced in neurons that give rise to demyelinated axons.

Increased production of sodium channels in neurons after demyelination or other types of injury does not necessarily imply that the appropriate types of sodium channels are added to the axon membrane. As shown in Fig. 26.5, DRG neurons express abnormal combinations of sodium channels after their axons are transected, with downregulation of the expression of sodium channels $Na_v1.8$ and $Na_v1.9$ and an attenuation of their currents (Dib-Hajj et al., 1996; 1999; Sleeper et al., 2000). This is accompanied by upregulated expression of $Na_v1.3$ (Waxman et al., 1994; Black et al., 1999a). Since $Na_v1.3$ produces a rapidly repriming sodium current, these changes in channel expression result in an altered pattern of firing (Cummins and Waxman, 1997; Cummins et al., 2001).

26.8 A channelopathy associated with demyelinating disease

Altered sodium channel expression which appears to be maladaptive has been observed within one particular type of neuron, the cerebellar Purkinje

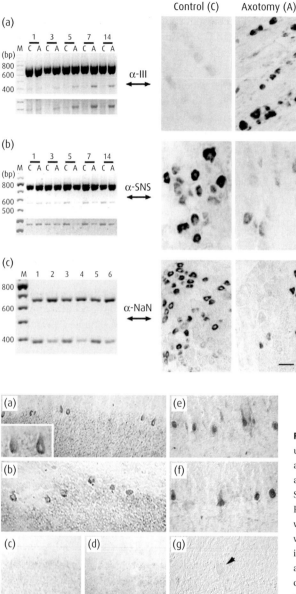

Control (C)   Axotomy (A)

Figure 26.5. Na$^+$ channel expression changes strikingly in DRG neurons following axonal transection. mRNA for Na$^+$ channel Na$_v$1.3 (a) is upregulated, and mRNA for Na$_v$1.8/SNS (b) and Na$_v$1.9/NaN (c) are downregulated, in DRG neurons following transection of their axons within the sciatic nerve. The in situ hybridizations (right side) show α-III, SNS and NaN mRNA in control DRG, and at 5–7 days post-axotomy. RT-PCR (left side) shows products of co-amplification of α-III and SNS together with β-actin transcripts in control (C) and axotomized (A) DRG (days post-axotomy indicated above gels), with computer-enhanced images of amplification products shown below gels. Co-amplification of NaN (392 bp) and GAPDH (6076 bp) shows decreased expression of NaN mRNA at 7 days post-axotomy (lanes 2, 4 and 6) compared to controls (lanes 1, 3 and 5). (a and b panels modified from Dib-Hajj et al., 1996) (c modified from Dib-Hajj et al., 1998).

Figure 26.6. Expression of sodium channel Na$_v$1.8/SNS is upregulated within cerebellar Purkinje cells in MS. Panels at left show in situ hybridization with Na$_v$1.8-specific antisense riboprobes, and demonstrates the absence of SNS mRNA in control cerebellum (c) and its presence in Purkinje cells in post-mortem tissue from two patients with MS (a, b). No signal is present following hybridization with sense riboprobe (d). Panels on the right show immunostaining with antibody directed against Na$_v$1.8, and illustrate absence of Na$_v$1.8 protein in control cerebellum (g, arrow indicates Purkinje cell) and its presence in MS (e, f) (modified from Black et al. (2000)).

cell, in animal models of demyelination and in tissue from MS patients (Fig. 26.6). The Na$_v$1.8 sodium channel (also termed SNS), is normally expressed only in spinal sensory and trigeminal neurons (Akopian et al., 1996). Black et al. (2000) showed that expression of Na$_v$1.8 is upregulated in Purkinje cells

in rodent models of CNS dysmyelination (Black et al., 1999b) and in the Purkinje cells of mice with chronic relapsing experimental allergic encephalomyelitis (CR-EAE), an inflammatory model of MS. The expression of Na$_v$1.8 is also upregulated in Purkinje cells in post-mortem tissue from patients with MS who had exhibited cerebellar deficits on neurological examination (Black et al., 2000). There is some evidence suggesting that the up-regulation of $Na_v1.8$ is triggered by NGF receptors which are known to up-regulated within Purkinje cells in experimental autoimmune encephalomyelitis and MS (Damarjian et al., 2004).

$Na_v1.8$ contributes a substantial fraction of the inward transmembrane current underlying action potential electrogenesis in cells in which it is normally present (Renganathan et al., 2001). The expression of $Na_v1.8$ does not appear to be an adaptive change because $Na_v1.8$ is not deployed along demyelinated Purkinje cell axons. Evidence supporting the idea that it is maladaptive (perturbing the pattern of impulse activity in Purkinje cells) has been provided by patch-clamp studies which demonstrate markedly different patterns of impulse activity in $Na_v1.8 +/+$, as compared to $Na_v1.8 -/-$ (DRG) neurons (Renganathan et al., 2001) and from the observation that transfection with $Na_v1.8$ can substantially distort the pattern of impulse activity in cultured Purkinje neurons (Renganathan et al., 2003). In both of these situations the presence of $Na_v1.8$ channels is associated with larger amplitude action potentials and with sustained, pacemaker-like activity, which is not seen in the absence of $Na_v1.8$, in response to sustained depolarizing stimuli. Renganathan et al. (2003) also observed that expression of $Na_v1.8$ results in disruption of the stereotyped, composite groups of action potentials normally produced by Purkinje neurons. Saab et al. (2004) demonstrated similar changes in Purkinje neurons *in vivo* in mice with experimental autoimmune encephalomyelitis. If these changes occur within Purkinje cells in MS, they would be expected to distort the pattern of Purkinje cell firing, and thus perturb cerebellar function.

26.9 Transfer of channels from glia to axons?

Ritchie and his colleagues have made the speculative proposal, that sodium channels are synthesized in glial cells, with subsequent transfer to the axon after demyelination (Bevan et al., 1985; Gray and Ritchie, 1985). There is some data that is consistent with this speculation. For example, the axon membrane at the node is contacted by perinodal astrocyte processes and Schwann cell microvilli in a highly specific manner, with precise alignment of sodium channel clusters and apposing glial cell processes (Hildebrand, 1971; Waxman and Black, 1984); similar glial processes contact demyelinated axons at sites of Na^+ channel clustering (Black et al., 1984; Rosenbluth and Blakemore, 1984; Rosenbluth, 1985). These observations suggest that axon-glial cell contact may be involved in some aspect of the development of Na^+ channel clusters in the axon membrane. There is also substantial evidence for sodium channel production by astrocytes. The mRNAs for neuronal-type Na^+ channel α- and β-subunits are present in astrocytes (Oh and Waxman, 1994; Black et al., 1994a, b) and patch-clamp has demonstrated voltage-sensitive Na^+ currents in these cells (Bevan et al., 1985; Barres et al., 1989; Sontheimer et al., 1992). It should be emphasized, however, that transfer of ion channels from glial cells to axons has not been demonstrated. Arguing against the "glial cell transfer" hypothesis, England et al. (1991) have noted that there are increased numbers of Na^+ channels along demyelinated axons in fish lateral line nerves after injection of doxorubicin which kills Schwann cells (England et al., 1991). Alternative functions have been proposed for astrocyte Na^+ channels (e.g., providing a return pathway for Na^+ ions that maintains astrocyte Na^+ and K^+-ATPase activity (Sontheimer et al., 1994)). It is possible that astrocytes participate in some other aspect of sodium channel deployment along axons, e.g. by presenting membrane-associated molecules or secreting extracellular molecules that target or anchor Na^+ channels at specific axonal loci (Waxman, 1992).

26.10 Impedance mismatch and impedance matching in demyelinated axons

Although an increased Na^+ channel density in demyelinated axon regions can contribute to

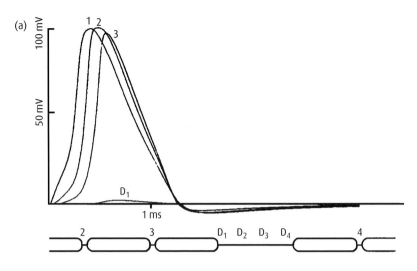

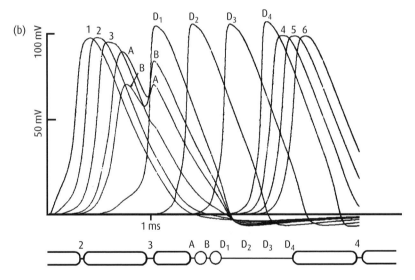

Figure 26.7. Impedance mismatch contributes to conduction block in focally demyelinated axons. (a) Computer simulations showing conduction through a focally demyelinated axon. Even in the presence of an adequate density of sodium channels in the demyelinated zone (D_1–D_4), conduction fails as a result of impedance mismatch. (b) Interposition of two short internodes, just proximal to the demyelinated zone, provides impedance matching that facilitates conduction into, and then through, the demyelinated zone (from Waxman and Brill (1978)).

restoration of action potential electrogenesis, it does not, in itself insure secure conduction. Impedance mismatch (which is largely a result of increased membrane capacitance after loss of myelin shielding) is another factor that can contribute to conduction block at sites of axonal inhomogeneity, such as the transition between myelinated and demyelinated regions (Waxman, 1978). Figure 26.7(a) shows computer-simulated action potentials (Waxman

and Brill, 1978) in a focally demyelinated (between nodes D1 and D4) fiber, in which the demyelinated axon membrane has acquired a high Na$^+$ channel density (similar to that at nodes). There is conduction block at the junction between normal and demyelinated axon region (D1), despite the high Na$^+$ channel density in the demyelinated area, because impedance mismatch prevents threshold from being reached.

Impedance mismatch must be reversed in order for action potentials to successfully traverse the demyelinated zone. Impedance matching can be achieved by the development of relatively short myelinated segments proximal to the demyelinated area (Waxman and Brill, 1978), decrease in axon diameter of the demyelinated region (Sears and Bostock, 1981), the development of an increased Na^+ channel density at the node upstream to the demyelinated area, or the development of a specialized transition zone (with relatively high Na^+ channel densities or relatively low K^+ channel densities) at the border of the region of demyelination (Waxman and Wood, 1984). As shown in Fig. 26.7(b) these mechanisms can facilitate the conduction of impulses along focally demyelinated axons.

26.11 Remyelination

Remyelination with even thin, or short, myelin sheaths is predicted by computer modeling to provide a capacitative shield that promotes conduction through previously demyelinated fibers, assuming that the newly formed nodes of Ranvier develop sodium channel densities similar to those in normal fibers, and impedance mismatch is corrected. Early evidence for acquisition of a high density of sodium channels at newly formed nodes was provided by cytochemical studies (Weiner et al., 1980). Experimentally demyelinated–remyelinated axons display an increase in STX binding that is proportional to the increase in nodal membrane area imposed by the closer nodal spacing, again suggesting that the new nodes develop a high sodium channel density (Ritchie, 1982), and immunocytochemical studies of newly formed nodes along remyelinated axons reveal foci of sodium channels (Shrager, 1989).

As expected from these observations, oligodendrocyte and Schwann cell-mediated remyelination of CNS axons can both enhance conduction along CNS axons (see Smith et al., 1981). Remyelination of dorsal column axons by Schwann cells, for example, restores secure action potential conduction, characterized by a normal refractory period of transmission

(but with decreased conduction velocity) and improves the conduction of high-frequency impulse trains in these fibers (Blight and Young, 1989; Felts and Smith, 1991). These results provide a rationale for studies on the transplantation of myelin-forming cells to the demyelinated CNS.

In the first physiological study of conduction properties in axons myelinated by transplanted cells, Utzschneider et al. (1994) transplanted oligodendrocytes to the *md* rat spinal cord and demonstrated a four-fold increase in conduction velocity, which approached myelinated control values after formation of myelin around myelin-deficient axons by transplanted glial cells. Refractory period was restored to normal and the ability to follow high-frequency stimulation was enhanced. In addition, action potentials could be initiated outside the transplant region, could invade and propagate into the region of demyelination, and could then propagate beyond the demyelinated region. Kocsis and colleagues have demonstrated similar enhancement of action potential conduction following transplantation of Schwann cells (Honmou et al., 1996), olfactory ensheathing cells (Imaizumi et al., 1998), "humanized" olfactory ensheathing cells from the pig (Imaizumi et al., 2000) and bone marrow stromal cells (Akiyama et al., 2002) to demyelinated lesions within the spinal cord of adult rats. Thus it may be possible to restore action potential conduction in demyelinated and dysmyelinated axons within the CNS by transplantation of myelin-forming cells. Cell transplantation is discussed elsewhere in this volume.

26.12 Neuroprotection of axons in the demyelinating diseases

Studies on demyelination have been confounded by the fact that there is at least some axonal degeneration in most "demyelinating" disorders. Numerous studies suggest that there is substantial axonal loss in MS (see, e.g., McDonald et al., 1992; Davie et al., 1995; Ferguson et al., 1997; Trapp et al., 1999). The loss of axons appears to contribute significantly to

(a) CONT + Phen   (b)   EAE   (c) EAE + Phen

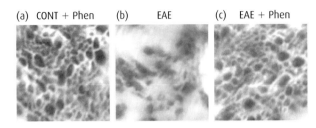

Figure 26.8. Protection of optic nerve axons in EAE by phenytoin. Neurofilament-stained axons within optic nerves from control (a), untreated EAE (b) and phenytoin-treated EAE (c). There was 49% loss of axons in untreated EAE, but only 12% loss in phenytoin treated EAE. See Lo et al. (2002) for quantitation. (From Lo et al., 2002).

permanent neurological disability in animal models of MS and in human MS (Losseff et al., 1996; Bjartmar et al., 2000; Wujeck et al., 2002).

Although the relationship of axonal degeneration to demyelination is not yet clear, neuroprotection of axons has emerged as a major theme in recent MS research. Studies in a representative white matter tract, the optic nerve, have demonstrated that persistently activated sodium channels can trigger Ca^{2+}-mediated axonal degeneration, by providing a route for persistent sodium current that drives reverse Na^+/Ca^{2+} exchange (Stys et al., 1992b). Craner et al. (2004a) have demonstrated the presence of both $Na_v1.6$ sodium channels and the Na/Ca^{2+} exchanger which are co-localized at sites of axonal damage in EAE, a model of MS. Block of sodium channels prevents axonal injury within the optic nerve when it is exposed to insults as injurious as 60 min of anoxia *in vitro* (Stys et al., 1992a, b). The early studies (Stys et al., 1992b) on axonal neuroprotection utilized TTX, a potent sodium channel blocker that cannot be used in the clinical domain. More recent studies, however, have explored the use of sodium channel blockers that can be used clinically. Lo et al. (2002; 2003) recently studied the effect of phenytoin (which is known to block persistent as well as transient sodium currents; Chao and Alzheimer, 1995) on axonal degeneration in a rodent model of MS, EAE, and observed robust protection of axons (Fig. 26.8). In untreated EAE they observed reproducible and severe axonal injury (e.g. loss of 49% of axons within the optic nerve and 63% loss of axons within corticospinal tract). Oral administration of phenytoin, at doses which resulted in serum levels within the human therapeutic range, reduced the loss of optic nerve axons from 49% to 12% of the

total fiber population (Lo et al., 2002; 2003), and reduced the loss of corticospinal tract axons from 63% to 28%. Importantly, there was also significant improvement in clinical status in phenytoin-treated EAE (Lo et al., 2002; 2003). This study provides proof-of-principle that is possible to protect axons, so that they do not degenerate with sodium channel blockers in a model of MS.

26.13 Conclusion and overview

As discussed above, myelin plays a crucial role in action potential conduction, but the myelinated fiber is more than a naked axon with myelin wrapped around it. Within the membrane of the myelinated axon there are nodal aggregations of sodium channels which produce action potentials and support saltatory conduction, and under the myelin there are potassium channels which tend to retard electrogenesis. The presence of multiple channel sodium subtypes adds another layer of complexity. The intricate organization of the myelinated fiber is matched by the complexity of demyelination, in which passive and active properties of the axon interact to shape conduction properties. The presence of degenerating axons within most demyelinated tracts further complicates the picture.

The multiple determinants of altered axonal conduction after demyelination and the occurrence of axonal degeneration have made the dysmyelinating and demyelinating disorders more difficult to study, but may also provide multiple therapeutic opportunities to enhance the function of demyelinated and dysmyelinated axons. These include promotion of Na^+ channel expression at sites where myelin is absent, pharmacological manipulation of K^+ channels, correction of impedance mismatch at the edge of demyelinated regions, transplantation of myelin-forming cells, and protection of axons so that they do not degenerate. Progress on these avenues will almost certainly open up new therapeutic opportunities, and is proceeding at a rapid pace.

ACKNOWLEDGEMENTS

Research in the author's laboratory has been supported in part by grants from the National Multiple Sclerosis Society and the Rehabilitation Research Service and Medical Research Service, Department of Veterans Affairs and by gifts from the Eastern Paralyzed Veterans Association, the Paralyzed Veterans of America, the Nancy Davis Foundation, and Destination Cure.

REFERENCES

Akiyama, Y., Radtke, C. and Kocsis, J.D. (2002). Remyelination of the rat spinal cord by transplantation of identified bone marrow stromal cells. *J Neurosci*, **22**, 6623–6630.

Akopian, A.N., Sivilotti, L. and Wood, J.N. (1996). A tetrodotoxin-resistant voltage-gated sodium channel expressed by sensory neurons. *Nature*, **379**, 257–262.

Baker, M., Chandra, S., Ding, Y., Waxman, S. and Wood, J. (2003). GTP-induced TTX-resistant Na+ current regulates excitability in mouse and rat small diameter sensory neurons. *J Physiol*, **548.2**, 373–383.

Barres, B.A., Chun, L.L.Y. and Corey, D.P. (1989). Glial and neuronal forms of the voltage-dependent sodium channels: characteristics and cell-type distribution. *Neuron*, **2**, 1375–1388.

Bevan, S., Chiu, S.Y., Gray, P.T.A. and Ritchie, J.M. (1985). The presence of voltage-gated sodium, potassium and chloride channels in rat cultured astrocytes. *Proc Roy Soc London B*, **225**, 229–313.

Bjartmar, C., Hildebrand, C. and Loinder, K. (1994). Morphological heterogeneity of rat oligodendrocytes: electron microscopic studies on serial sections. *Glia*, **11**, 235–244.

Bjartmar, C., Kidd, G., Mork, S., Rudnick, R. and Trapp, B. (2000). Neurological disability correlates with spinal cord axonal loss and reduced *N*-acetyl aspartate in chronic MS patients. *Ann Neurol*, **48**, 893–901.

Black, J.A. and Waxman, S.G. (2002). Molecular identities of two tetrodotoxin-resistant sodium channels in corneal axons. *Exp Eye Res*, **75**, 193–199.

Black, J.A., Foster, R.E. and Waxman, S.G. (1981). Freeze-fracture ultrastructure of rat C.N.S. and P.N.S. nonmyelinated axolemma. *J Neurocytol*, **10**, 981–993.

Black, J.A., Waxman, S.G. and Hildebrand, C. (1984). Membrane specialization and axo-glial association in the rat retinal nerve fibre layer: freeze-fracture observations. *J Neurocytol*, **13**, 417–430.

Black, J.A., Waxman, S.G., Sims, T.J. and Gilmore, S.A. (1986). Effects of delayed myelination by oligodendrocytes and Schwann cells on the macromolecular structure of axonal membrane in rat spinal cord. *J Neurocytol*, **15**, 745–762.

Black, J.A., Waxman, S.G. and Smith, M.E. (1987). Macromolecular structure of axonal membrane during acute experimental allergic encephalomyelitis in rat and guinea pig spinal cord. *J Neuropath Exp Neurol*, **46**, 167–184.

Black, J.A., Westenbroek, R., Ransom, B.R., Catterall, W.A. and Waxman, S.G. (1994a). Type II sodium channels in spinal cord astrocytes in situ: immunocytochemical observations. *Glia*, **12**, 219–227.

Black, J.A., Yokoyama, S., Waxman, S.G., Oh, Y., Zur, K.B., Sontheimer, H., Higashida, H. and Ransom, B.R. (1994b). Sodium channel mRNAs in cultured spinal cord astrocytes: in situ hybridization in identified cell types. *Mol Brain Res*, **23**, 235–245.

Black, J.A., Cummins, T.R., Plumpton, C., Chen, Y.H., Hormuzdiar, W., Clare, J.J. and Waxman, S.G. (1999a). Upregulation of a silent sodium channel after peripheral, but not central, nerve injury in DRG neurons. *J Neurophysiol*, **82**, 2776–2785.

Black, J.A., Fjell, J., Dib-Hajj, S., Duncan, I.D., O'Connor, L.T., Fried, K., Gladwell, Z., Tate, S. and Waxman, S.G. (1999b). Abnormal expression of SNS/PN3 sodium channel in cerebellar Purkinje cells following loss of myelin in the taiep rat. *Neuroreport*, **10**, 913–918.

Black, J.A., Dib-Hajj, S., Baker, D., Newcombe, J., Cuzner, M.L. and Waxman, S.G. (2000). Sensory neuron-specific sodium channel SNS is abnormally expressed in the brains of mice with experimental allergic encephalomyelitis and humans with multiple sclerosis. *Proc Natl Acad Sci USA*, **97**, 11598–11602.

Black, J.A., Renganathan, M. and Waxman, S.G. (2002). Sodium channel Nav1.6 is expressed along nonmyelinated axons and it contributes to conduction. *Mol Brain Res*, **105**, 19–28.

Blight, A.R. and Young, W. (1989). Central axons in injured cat spinal cord recover electrophysiological function following remyelination by Schwann cells. *J Neurol Sci*, **91**, 15–34.

Boiko, T., Rasband, M.N., Levinson, S.R., Caldwell, J.H., Mandel, G., Trimmer, J.S. and Mattews, G. (2001). Compact myelin dictates the differential targeting of two sodium channel isoforms in the same axon. *Neuron*, **30**, 91–104.

Bornstein, M.B. and Crain, S.M. (1965). Functional studies of cultured brain tissues as related to "demyelinative disorders." *Science*, **148**, 1242–1244.

Bostock, H. and Sears, T.A. (1976). Continuous conduction in demyelinated mammalian nerve fibres. *Nature*, **263**, 786–787.

Bostock, H. and Sears, T.A. (1978). The internodal axon membrane: electrical excitability and continuous conduction in segmental demyelination. *J Physiol (Lond)*, **280**, 273–301.

Bostock, H. and Grafe, P. (1985). Activity–dependent excitability changes in normal and demyelinated rat spinal root axons. *J Physiol (Lond)*, **365**, 239–257.

Bostock, H., Sears, T.A. and Sherratt, R.M. (1981). The effects of 4-aminopyridine and tetraethylammonium ions on normal and demyelinated mammalian nerve fibers. *J Physiol (Lond)*, **313**, 301–315.

Bowe, C.M., Kocsis, J.D., Targ, E.F. and Waxman, S.G. (1987). Physiological effects of 4-aminopyridine on demyelinated mammalian motor and sensory fibers. *Ann Neurol* **22**, 264–268.

Brinkmeier, H., Wollinsky, K.H., Hulser, P.-J., Seewald, M.J., Mehrkens H.H. and Kornhuber, H.H. (1992). The acute paralysis in Guillain–Barre syndrome is related to Na+ channel blocking factor in the cerebrospinal. *Euro J Physiol*, **421**, 552–557.

Brinkmeier, H., Wollinsky, K.H., Seewald, M.J., Hulser, P.J., Mehrkens, H.H., Kornhuber, H.H. and Rudel, R. (1993). Factors in the cerebrospinal fluid of MS patients interfering with voltage-dependent sodium channels. *Neurosci Lett*, **156**, 172–175.

Brinkmeier, H., Aulkemeyer, P., Wollinsky, K.H. and Rudel, R. (2000). An endogenous pentapeptide acting as a sodium channel blocker in inflammatory autoimmune disorders of the CNS. *Nat Med*, **6**, 808–811.

Brismar, T. (1981). Specific permeability properties of demyelinated rat nerve fibers. *Acta Physiol Scand*, **113**, 167–176.

Bunge, M.B., Bunge, R.P. and Pappas, G.D. (1961). Electron microscope demonstration of connections between glia and myelin sheaths in the developing mammalian central nervous system. *J Cell Biol*, **12**, 448–453.

Burchiel, K. (1980). Abnormal impulse generation in focally demyelinated trigeminal roots. *J Neurosurg*, **53**, 674–683.

Caldwell, J.H., Schaller, K.L., Lasher, R.S., Peles, E. and Levinson, S.R. (2000). Sodium channel Na(v)1.6 is localized at nodes of ranvier, dendrites, and synapses. *Proc Natl Acad Sci*, **97**, 5616–5620.

Cerf, J.A. and Carels, G. (1966). Multiple sclerosis: serum factor producing reversible alterations in bioelectric responses. *Science*, **152**, 1066–1068.

Chao, T.I. and Alzheimer, C. (1995). Effects of phenytoin on the persistent Na+ current of mammalian CNS neurones. *Neuroreport*, **6**, 1778–1780.

Chiu, S.Y. and Ritchie, J.M. (1980). Potassium channels in nodal and internodal axonal membrane in mammalian myelinated fibers. *Nature*, **284**, 170–171.

Chiu, S.Y. and Ritchie, J.M. (1981). Evidence for the presence of potassium channels in the paranodal region of acutely demyelinated nerve fibres. *J Physiol (Lond)*, **313**, 415–437.

Craner, M.J., Lo, A.C., Black, J.A. and Waxman, S.G. (2003). Abnormal sodium channel distribution in optic nerve axons in a model of inflammatory demyelination. *Brain*, **126**, 1552–1561.

Craner, M.J., Hains, B.C., Lo, A.C., Black, J.A. and Waxman, S.G. (2004a). Colocalization of sodium channel Na$_v$1.6 and the sodium–calcium exchanger at sites of axonal injury in the spinal cord in EAE. *Brain*, **127**, 294–303.

Craner, M.J., Newcombe, J., Black, J.A., Hartle, C., Cuzner, M.L. and Waxman, S.G. (2004b). Molecular changes in neurons in MS: altered axonal expression of Na$_v$1.2 and Na$_v$1.6 sodium channels and Na+/Ca^{2+} exchanger. *Proc Natl Acad Sci*, **101**, 8168–8173.

Cummins, T.R. and Waxman, S.G. (1997). Downregulation of tetrodotoxin-resistant sodium currents and upregulation of rapidly repriming tetrodotoxin-sensitive sodium current in small spinal sensory neurons after nerve injury. *J Neurosci*, **17**, 3503–3514.

Cummins, T.R., Dib-Hajj, S.D., Black, J.A., Akopian, A.N., Wood, J.N. and Waxman, S.G. (1999). A novel persistent tetrodotoxin-resistant sodium current in SNS-null and wild-type small primary sensory neurons. *J Neurosci*, **19**, RC43, 1–6.

Cummins, T.R., Aglieco, F., Renganathan, M., Herzog, R.I., Dib-Hajj, S.D. and Waxman, S.G. (2001). Na$_v$1.3 sodium channels: rapid repriming and slow closed-state inactivation display quantitative differences after expression in a mammalian cell line and in spinal sensory neurons. *J Neurosci*, **21**, 5952–5961.

Cummins, T.R., Renganathan, M., Stys, P.K., Herzog, M.D., Scarfo, B.S., Horn, R., Dib-Hajj, S.D. and Waxman, S.G. (2003). The pentapeptide QYNAD does not block voltage-gated sodium channels. *Neurology*, **60**, 224–229.

Damarjian, T.G., Craner, M.J., Black, J.A. and Waxman, S.G. (2004). Upregulation and colocalization of p75 and Na$_v$1.8 in Purkinje neurons in EAE. *Neurosci Lett*, **369**, 186–190.

Davie, C., Barker, G.J., Webb, S., Tofts, P.S., Thompson, A.J., Harding, A.E., McDonald, W.I. and Miller, D.H. (1995). Persistent functional deficit in MS and autosomal dominant cerebellar ataxia is associated with axon loss. *Brain*, **118**, 1583–1592.

De Waegh, S.M., Lee, V.M. and Brady, S.T. (1992). Local modulation of neurofilament phosphorylation, axonal caliber, and slow axonal transport by myelinating Schwann cells. *Cell*, **68**, 451–463.

Dib-Hajj, S., Black, J.A., Felts, P. and Waxman, S.G. (1996). Down-regulation of transcripts for Na channel alpha-SNS in spinal sensory neurons following axotomy. *Proc Natl Acad Sci*, **93**, 14950–14954.

Dib-Hajj, S.D., Ishikawa, I., Cummins, T.R. and Waxman, S.G. (1997). Insertion of a SNS-specific tetrapeptide in the S3–S4 linker of D4 accelerates recovery from inactivation of skeletal muscle voltage-gated Na channel μ1 in HEK293 cells. *FEBS Lett*, **416**, 11–14.

Dib-Hajj, S.D., Tyrrell, L., Black, J.A. and Waxman, S.G. (1998). NaN, a novel voltage-gated Na channel, is expressed preferentially in peripheral sensory neurons and down-regulated after axotomy. *Proc Natl Acad Sci*, **95**, 8963–8968.

Dib-Hajj, S.D., Fjell, J., Cummins, T.R., Zheng, Z., Fried, K., LaMotte, R., Black, J.A. and Waxman, S.G. (1999). Plasticity of sodium channel expression in DRG neurons in the chronic constriction injury model of neuropathic pain. *Pain*, **83**, 591–600.

Dugandzija-Novakovic, S., Koszowski, A.G., Levinson, S.R. and Shrager, P. (1995). Clustering of Na+ channels and node of Ranvier formation in remyelinating axons. *J Neurosci*, **15**, 492–503.

Eng, D.L., Gordon, T.R., Kocsis, J.D. and Waxman, S.G. (1988). Development of 4-AP and TEA sensitivities in mammalian myelinated nerve fibers. *J Neurophysiol*, **60**, 2168–2179.

England, J.D., Gamboni, F. and Levinson, S.R. (1991). Increased numbers of sodium channels form along demyelinated axons. *Brain Res*, **548**, 334–337.

Fang, X., Djouhri, L., Black, J.A., Dib-Hajj, S.D., Waxman, S.G. and Lawson, S.N. (2002). The presence and role of the TTX resistant sodium channel Nav1.9 (NaN) in nociceptive primary afferent neurons. *J Neurosci*, **22**(17), 7425–7433.

Felts, P. and Smith, K.J. (1991). Conduction properties of central nerve fibers remyelinated by Schwann cells. *Brain Res*, **574**, 178–192.

Felts, P., Baker, T.A. and Smith, K.J. (1977). Conduction in segmentally demyelinated mammalian central axons. *J Neurosci*, **17**, 7267–7277.

Ferguson, B., Matyszak, M.K., Esiri, M.M., et al. (1997). Axonal damage in acute multiple sclerosis lesions. *Brain*, **120**, 393–399.

Fjell, J., Dibhajj, S., Fried, K., Black, J.A. and Waxman, S.G. (1997). Differential expression of sodium channel genes in retinal ganglion cells. *Mol Brain Res*, **50**, 197–204.

Foster, R.E., Whalen, C.C. and Waxman, S.G. (1980). Reorganization of the axonal membrane of demyelinated nerve fibers: morphological evidence. *Science*, **210**, 661–663.

Foster, R.E., Connors, B.W. and Waxman, S.G. (1982). Rat optic nerve: electrophysiological, pharmacological, and anatomical studies during development. *Dev Brain Res*, **3**, 361–376.

Gray, P.T. and Ritchie, J.M. (1985). Ion channels in Schwann and glial cells. *Trend Neurosci*, **8**, 411–415.

Herzog, R.I., Cummins, T.R. and Waxman, S.G. (2001). Persistent TTX-resistant Na$^+$ current affects resting potential and response to depolarization in simulated spinal sensory neurons. *J Neurophysiol*, **86**, 1351–1364.

Herzog, R.I., Cummins, T.R., Ghassemi, F., Dib-Hajj, S.D. and Waxman, S.G. (2003). Distinct repriming and closed-state inactivation kinetics of Na$_v$1.6 and Na$_v$1.7 sodium channels in spinal sensory neurons. *J Physiol (Lond)*, **551.3**, 741–751.

Hildebrand, C. (1971). Ultrastructural and light-microscopic studies of the developing feline spinal cord white matter. I. The nodes of Ranvier. *Acta Physiol Scand Suppl*, **364**, 81–101.

Hirano, A. (1968). A confirmation of the oligodendroglial origin of myelin in the adult rat. *J Cell Biol*, **38**, 337–340.

Honmou, O., Felts, P.A., Waxman, S.G. and Kocsis, J.D. (1996). Restoration of normal conduction properties in demyelinated spinal cord axons in the adult rat by transplantation of exogenous Schwann cells. *J Neurosci*, **16**, 3199–3208.

Huxley, A.F. and Stämpfli, R. (1949). Evidence for saltatory conduction in peripheral myelinated nerve fibres. *J Physiol (Lond)*, **108**, 315–339.

Imaizumi, T., Lankford, K.L., Waxman, S.G., Green, C.A. and Kocsis, J.D. (1998). Transplanted olfacotry ensheathing cells remyelinate and enhance axonal conduction in the demyelinated dorsal columns of the rat spinal cord. *J Neurosci*, **18**, 6176–6185.

Imaizumi, T., Lankford, K.L., Burton, W.V., Foder, W.L. and Kocsis, J.D. (2000). Xenotransplantation of transgenic pig olfactory ensheathing cells promotes axonal regeneration in rat spinal cord. *Nat Biotechnol*, **18**, 949–953.

Kocsis, J.D., Waxman, S.G., Hildebrand, C. and Ruiz, J.A. (1982). Regenerating mammalian nerve fibres: changes in action potential waveform and firing characteristics following blockage of potassium conductance. *Proc Roy Soc Lond,* **B217**, 277–287.

Kocsis, J.D., Eng, D.L., Gordon, T.R. and Waxman, S.G. (1987). Functional differences between 4-aminopyridine and tetraethylammonium-sensitive potassium channels in myelinated axons. *Neurosci Lett,* **75**, 193–198.

Losseff, N., Webb, S. and O'Riordan, J. (1996). Spinal cord atrophy and disability in MS – a new MRI method with potential to monitor disease progression. *Brain,* **119**, 701–708.

Liu, C.J., Dib-Hajj, S.D., Black, J.A., Greenwood, J., Lian, Z. and Waxman, S.G. (2001). Direct interaction with contactin targets voltage-gated sodium channel Nav1.9/NaN to the cell membrane. *J Biol Chem,* **276**, 46553–46561.

Lo, A., Black, J. and Waxman, S. (2002). Neuroprotection of axons with phenytoin in EAE. *NeuroReport,* **13**, 1909–1912.

Lo, A.C., Saab, C.J., Black, J.A. and Waxman, S.G. (2003). Phenytoin protects spinal cord axons and preserves axonal conduction and neurological function in a model of neuroinflammation *in vivo. J Neurophysiol,* **90**, 3566–3572.

Lumsden, C.E., Howard, L., Aparicio, S.R. and Bradbury, M. (1975). Anti-synaptic antibody in allergic encephalomyelitis: II: the synapse-blocking effects in tissue culture of demyelinating sera from experimental allergic encephalomyelitis. *Brain Res,* **93**, 283–299.

McDonald, W., et al. (1992). Pathological evolution of MS. *Neuropathol Appl Neurobiol,* **18**, 319–334.

McDonald, W.I. (1963). The effects of experimental demyelination on conduction in peripheral nerve: a histological and electrophysiological study. Electrophysiological observations. *Brain,* **86**, 501–524.

McDonald, W.I. and Sears, T.A. (1970). The effects of experimental demyelination on conduction in the central nervous system. *Brain,* **93**, 583–598.

Moll, C., Mourre, C., Lazdunski, M. and Ulrich, J. (1991). Increase of sodium channels in demyelinated lesions of multiple sclerosis. *Brain Res,* **556**, 311–316.

Oh, Y. and Waxman, S.G. (1994). The beta 1 subunit mRNA of the rat brain Na$^+$ channel is expressed in glial cells. *Proc Natl Acad Sci USA,* **91**, 9985–9989.

Prineas, J. and Connell, F. (1978). Fine structure of chronically active multiple sclerosis plaques. *Neurology,* **28**, 68–75.

Rasband, M., Trimmer, J.S., Schwarz, T.L., Levinson, S.R., Ellisman, M.H., Schachner, M. and Shrager, P. (1998). Potassium channel distribution, clustering, and function in remyelinating rat axons. *J Neurosci,* **18**, 36–47.

Rasminsky, M. and Sears, T.A. (1972). Internodal conduction in undissected demyelinated nerve fibers. *J Physiol (Lond),* **227**, 323–350.

Renganathan, M., Cummins, T.R. and Waxman, S.G. (2001). Contribution of Na(v)1.8 sodium channels to action potential electrogenesis in DRG neurons. *J Neurophysiol,* **86**, 629–640.

Renganathan, M., Gelderblom, M., Black, J.A. and Waxman, S.G. (2003). Expression of Nav 1.8 sodium channels perturbs the firing patterns of cerebellar Purkinje cells. *Brain Res,* **959**, 235–242.

Ritchie, J.M. (1982). Sodium and potassium channels in regenerating and developing mammalian myelinated nerves. *Proc Roy Soc London,* **B215**, 273–287.

Ritchie, J.M. and Rogart, R.B. (1977). The density of sodium channels in mammalian myelinated nerve fibers and the nature of the axonal membrane under the myelin sheath. *Proc Natl Acad Sci,* **74**, 211–215.

Ritchie, J.M. and Chiu, S.Y. (1981). Distribution of sodium and potassium channels in mammalian myelinated nerve. In: *Demyelinating Diseases, Basic and Clinical Electrophysiology* (eds Waxman, S.G. and Ritchie, J.M.),. Raven Press, New York, pp. 329–342

Ritchie, J.M., Rang, H.P. and Pellegrino, R. (1981). Sodium and potassium channels in demyelinated and remyelinated mammalian nerve. *Nature,* **294**, 257–259.

Röper, J. and Schwarz, J.R. (1989). Heterogeneous distribution of fast and slow potassium channels in myelinated rat nerve fibers. *J Physiol (Lond),* **416**, 93–110.

Rosenbluth, J. (1985). Intramembranous particle patches in myelin-deficient rat mutant. *Neurosci Lett,* **62**, 19–24.

Rosenbluth, J. and Blakemore, W.F. (1984). Structural specializations in cat of chronically demyelinated spinal cord axons as seen in freeze-fracture replicas. *Neurosci Lett,* **48**, 171–177.

Rush, A.M., Dib-Hajj, S.D. and Waxman, S.G. (2003). Electrophysiological properties of two axonal sodium channels, Na$_v$1.2 and Na$_v$1.6, expressed in spinal sensory neurons. *J Physiol,* **564.3**, 803–815.

Saab, C.Y., Craner, M.J., Kataoka, Y. and Waxman, S.G. (2004). Abnormal Purkinje cell activity *in vivo* in experimental allergic encephalomyelitis. *Exp Brain Res,* **158**, 1–8.

Schauf, C.L. and Davis, F.A. (1981). Circulating toxic factors in multiple sclerosis: a perspective. In: *Demyelinating Disease: Basic and Clinical Electrophysiology* (eds Waxman, S.G. and Ritchie, J.M.), Raven Press, New York, pp. 267–280.

Sears, T.A. and Bostock, H. (1981). Conduction failure in demyelination: is it inevitable? In: *Demyelinating Diseases: Basic and Clinical Electrophysiology* (eds Waxman, S.G. and Ritchie, J.M.), Raven Press, New York, pp. 357–375.

Sears, T.A., Bostock, H. and Sherratt, M. (1978). The pathophysiology of demyelination and its implications for the symptomatic treatment of multiple sclerosis. *Neurology*, **28**, 21–26.

Seil, F.J. (1981). Tissue culture studies of neuroelectric blocking factors. In: *Demyelinating Disease: Basic and Clinical Electrophysiology* (eds Waxman, S.G. and Ritchie, J.M.), Raven Press, New York, pp. 281–288.

Seil, F.J., Leiman, A.L. and Kelly, J.M. (1976). Neuroelectric blocking factors in multiple sclerosis and normal human sera. *Arch Neurol*, **33**, 418–422.

Shrager, P. (1989). Sodium channels in single demyelinated mammalian axons. *Brain Res*, **483**, 149–154.

Sleeper, A.A., Cummins, T.R., Dib-Hajj, S.D., Hormuzdiar, W., Tyrrell, L., Waxman, S.G. and Black, J.A. (2000). Changes in expression of two tetrodotoxin-resistant sodium channels and their currents in dorsal root ganglion neurons after sciatic nerve injury but not rhizotomy. *J Neurosci*, **20**, 7279–7289.

Smith, K.J. and McDonald, W.I. (1980). Spontaneous and mechanically evoked activity due to central demyelinating lesions. *Nature*, **286**, 154–155.

Smith, K.J., Blakemore, W.F. and McDonald, W.I. (1981). The restoration of conduction by central remyelination. *Brain*, **104**, 383–404.

Smith, K.J., Bostock, H. and Hall, S.M. (1982). Saltatory conduction precedes remyelination in axons demyelinated with lysophosphatidyl choline. *J Neurol Sci*, **54**, 13–31.

Smith, K.J., Blakemore, W.F. and McDonanld, W.I. (1983a). Central remyelination restores secure conduction. *Nature*, **280**, 395–396.

Smith, M.E., Kocsis, J.D. and Waxman, S.G. (1983b). Myelin protein metabolism in demyelination and remyelination in sciatic nerve. *Brain Res*, **270**, 37–44.

Sontheimer, H., Black, J.A., Ransom, B.R. and Waxman, S.G. (1992). Ion channels in spinal cord astrocytes *in vitro*. I. Transient expression of high levels of Na+ and K+ channels. *J Neurophysiol*, **68**, 985–1000.

Sontheimer, H., Fernandez-Marques, E., Ullrich, N., Pappas, C.A. and Waxman, S.G. (1994). Astrocyte Na+ channels are required for maintenance of Na+/K(+)-ATPase activity. *J Neurosci*, **14**, 2464–2475.

Stys, P., Ransom, B. and Waxman, S. (1992a). Tertiary and quaternary local anesthetics protect CNS white matter from anoxic injury at concentrations that do not block excitability. *J Neurophysiol*, **67**, 236–240.

Stys, P., Waxman, S. and Ransom, B. (1992b). Ionic mechanisms of anoxic injury in mammalian CNS white matter: role of Na+ channels and Na$^+$–Ca^{2+} exchanger. *J Neurosci*, **12**, 430–439.

Tasaki, I. (1953). *Nervous Transmission*. C. Thomas Publication, Springfield, I11.

Trapp, B.D., Ransohoff, R. and Rudick, R. (1999). Axonal pathology in multiple sclerosis: relationship to neurologic disability. *Curr Opin Neurol*, **12**, 295–302.

Utzschneider, D.A., Archer, D.R., Kocsis, J.D., Waxman, S.G. and Duncan, I.D. (1994). Transplantation of glial cells enhances action potential conduction of amyelinated spinal cord axons in the myelin-deficient rat. *Proc Natl Acad Sci*, **91**, 53–57.

Vabnick, I. and Shrager, P. (1998). Ion channel redistribution and function during development of the myelinated axon. *J Neurobiol*, **37**, 80–96.

Vollmer, T.L., Brass, L.M. and Waxman, S.G. (1991). Lhermitte's sign in a patient with herpes zoster. *J Neurol Sci*, **106**, 153–157.

Wang, H., Kunkel, D.D., Martin, T.M., Schwartkroin, P.A. and Tempel, B.L. (1993). Heteromultimeric K+ channels in terminal juxtaparanodal regions of neurons. *Nature*, **365**, 75–79.

Waxman, S.G. (1977). Conduction in myelinated, unmyelinated, and demyelinated fibers. *Arch Neurol*, **34**, 585–590.

Waxman, S.G. (1978). Prerequisites for conduction in demyelinated fibers. *Neurology*, **28**, 27–34.

Waxman, S.G. (1982). Membranes, myelin and the pathophysiology of multiple sclerosis. *New Engl J Med*, **306**, 1529–1533.

Waxman, S.G. (1987). Molecular organization of the cell membrane in normal and pathological axons: relation to glial contact. In: *Glial-Neuronal Communication in Development and Regeneration* (eds Althaus, H. and Seifert, W.), Springler-Verlag, Germany, pp. 711–736.

Waxman, S.G. (1992). The perinodal astrocyte: functional and developmental considerations. In: *Biology and Pathobiology of Astrocyte–Neuron Interactions* (eds Fedoroff, S., Doucette, R. and Juurlink, B.H.), Plenum Publishing Corp., New York, pp. 15–26.

Waxman, S.G. and Bennett, M.V.L. (1972). Relative conduction velocities of small myelinated and non-myelinated fibers in the central nervous system. *Nat New Biol*, **238**, 217–219.

Waxman, S.G. and Black, J.A. (1984). Freeze-fracture ultrastructure of the perinodal astrocyte and associated glial junctions. *Brain Res*, **308**, 77–87.

Waxman, S.G. and Brill, M.H. (1978). Conduction through demyelinated plaques in multiple sclerosis: computer simulations of facilitation by short internodes. *J Neurol Neurosurg Psychiat*, **41**, 408–417.

Waxman, S.G. and Sims, T.J. (1984). Specificity in central myelination: evidence for local regulation of myelin thickness. *Brain Res*, **292**, 179–185.

Waxman, S.G. and Wood, S.L. (1984). Impulse conduction in inhomogeneous axons: Effects of variation in voltage-sensitive ionic conductances on invasion of demyelinated axon segments and preterminal fibers. *Brain Res*, **294**, 111–122.

Waxman, S.G., Sims, T.J. and Gilmore, S.A. (1988). Cytoplasmic membrane elaborations in oligodendrocytes during myelination of spinal motoneuron axons. *Glia*, **1**, 286–291.

Waxman, S.G., Black, J.A., Kocsis, J.A. and Ritchie, J.M. (1989). Low density of sodium channels supports conduction in axons of neonatal rat optic nerve. *Proc Natl Acad Sci*, **86**, 1406–1410.

Waxman, S.G., Kocsis, J.D. and Black, J.A. (1994). Type III sodium channel mRNA is expressed in embryonic but not adult spinal sensory neurons, and is reexpressed following axotomy. *J Neurophysiol*, **72**, 466–470.

Weber, F., Brinkmeier, H., Aulkemeyer, P., Wollinsky, K.H. and Rudel, R. (1999). A small sodium channel blocking factor in the CSF is preferentially found in Guillain–Barre syndrome. *J Neurol*, **246**, 955–960.

Weiner, L.P., Waxman, S.G., Stohlman, S.A. and Kwan, A. (1980). Remyelination following viral-induced demyelination: ferric ion-ferrocyanide staining of nodes of Ranvier within the CNS. *Ann Neurol*, **8**, 580–583.

Westenbroek, R.E., Noebels, J.L. and Catterall, W.A. (1992). Elevated expression of type II Na^+ channels in hypomyelinated axons of shiverer mouse brain. *J Neurosci*, **12**, 2259–2267.

Wujeck, J., Bjartmar, C., Richer, E., Ransohoff, R.M., Yu, M., Tuohy, V.K. and Trapp, B.D. (2002). Axon loss in spinal cord determines neurological disability in model of MS. *J Neuropathol Exp Neurol*, **61**, 23–32.

Zhou, W. and Goldin, A.L. (2004). Use-dependent potentiation of the $Na_v1.6$ sodium channel. *Biophys J*, **87**, 3862–3872.

Zhou, L., Zhang, C.L., Messing, A. and Chiu, S.Y. (1998). Temperature-sensitive neuromuscular transmission in Kv1.1-null mice: role of potassium channels under the myelin in young nerves. *J Neurosci*, **18**, 7200–7215.

Role of Schwann cells in peripheral nerve regeneration

Wesley J. Thompson

Section of Neurobiology, School of Biological Sciences, Institutes for Cell and Molecular Biology and Neuroscience, University of Texas, Austin, TX 78712, USA

27.1 Introduction

The objective of this review is to consider evidence that Schwann cells, the glial cells of the peripheral nervous system, play a crucial role in guiding and supporting the regeneration of peripheral axons. The presentation is biased by the author's own research perspective. It is certainly not encyclopedic and, for the inevitable slighting of important contributions, apologies are offered. The interest in peripheral nerve regeneration comes from its history, the substantial body of knowledge already obtained, and from its clinical import (see Volume II, Chapter 40). This interest is shown by the large number of reviews of the topic that have appeared, many in the last few years (cf. Hall, 1989; Fawcett and Keynes, 1990; Welcher et al., 1991; Bunge, 1993; 1994; Reynolds and Woolf, 1993; Brecknell and Fawcett, 1996; Ide, 1996; Scherer and Salzer, 1996; Fu and Gordon, 1997; Scherer, 1997; Taylor and Suter, 1997; Anderson et al., 1998; Frostick et al., 1998; Stoll and Muller, 1999; Terenghi, 1999; Hall, 2001; Jones et al., 2001; Fenrich and Gordon, 2004).

Schwann cells are derived embryologically from the neural crest (cf. Lobsiger et al., 2002). These cells associate with developing peripheral axons, migrate along these axons as they extend to their peripheral targets, and ultimately separate and wrap these axons (Peters and Muir, 1959; Lubinska, 1961; Speidel, 1964). Schwann cells provide two distinct types of axonal wrappings, one for larger axons that contains myelin and one for smaller axons that does not. These two types of Schwann cells are termed myelinating and non-myelinating and they have distinctly different patterns of gene expression (cf. Jessen and Mirsky, 1991; Zorick and Lemke, 1996). Additionally, Schwann cells that are of the non-myelinating phenotype cover motor axon terminals and are associated with sensory nerve endings and with the cell bodies and/or synapses of peripheral neurons. On the basis of the ability of non-myelinating cells to form myelin when these cells come in contact with axons that are normally myelinated (Aguayo et al., 1976), as well as upon the dedifferentiation of myelinating cells following axonal degeneration, most investigators consider these types of Schwann cells to be dictated by axonal contact and inter-convertible (cf. Zorick and Lemke, 1996).

Schwann cells have long been believed to provide trophic support of axons. Indeed, recent evidence indicates that these cells are crucial for the maintenance of developing axons. Fetal motor neurons withdraw their nerve terminals from muscle and die following the ablation of genes necessary for early Schwann cell development (Riethmacher et al., 1997; Morris et al., 1999; Woldeyesus et al., 1999; Wolpowitz et al., 2000; Britsch et al., 2001). These experiments have resolved a long-standing controversy about the role of Schwann cells in navigation of developing axons to targets (cf. Keynes, 1987): Schwann cells are dispensable, since, even though axons die in these cases, they initially make it to their targets in the absence of Schwann cells. Interestingly, the dependence of motor axons on Schwann cells probably even extends to adult animals, since many Schwann cell pathologies lead to axon pathology and "die-back" of axons (Scherer, 1999; Martini, 2001; Yin et al., 2004). Even though they are not responsible for axon extension in early development, Schwann cells still might be needed for growth of axons in the adult when cues present in tissues that promote axon extension might no longer be present. In addressing some recent work in this area, this review will make prominent use of studies of nerve regeneration and sprouting in rodent muscle.

27.2 Historical note

That Schwann cells might play some special role in the growth of nerve fibers in the periphery was an attractive idea from the time of the discovery and description of cells located along the course of peripheral axons by Schwann (1839). These cells were subsequently referred to by other investigators as "cells of Schwann" but are now known simply as "Schwann cells". Schwann proposed that the strings of cells he observed along developing nerves, like those he observed along developing muscle fibers, fused together to form nerve fibers and muscle fibers, respectively. He was correct about the latter, but wrong about the former. The issue of the origin of axons generated considerable controversy near the end of the 19th century, and this controversy was perpetuated by disagreements over how nerves regenerated. Some investigators claimed that strings of Schwann cells that proliferated within the sheaths of the distal nerve stump (forming the so-called "bands of Büngner") fused to form the new axons. Ramon y Cajal (1928) reports that these proponents of a "syncytial" origin of axons claimed that axons reformed within the distal nerve stump even if a gap continued to separate the distal from the central stump; muscle contractions evoked by stimulation of such distal stumps were offered as evidence of such regeneration independent of "central centers". Such ideas were debunked only when more careful experiments showed that axons formed as protoplasmic extensions of nerve cell bodies and that, in cases where functional axons could be demonstrated in what

were believed to be isolated distal stumps, axons from the central stump had entered the distal stump by a circuitous route (Ramon y Cajal, 1906).

27.3 Promotion of regeneration by endoneurial tubes

Even though it was shown that Schwann cells do not fuse to generate peripheral axons, it appeared that they played an important role in promoting axon growth/regrowth. In the 1800s and early 1900s, Waller, Nageotte, Marinesco, Ranvier, and Cajal examined stained preparations of regenerating peripheral nerves with their microscopes (citations in Ramon y Cajal, 1928). They saw that axons and their myelin coatings distal to a lesion site underwent rapid degeneration. This degeneration was accompanied by activation and proliferation of Schwann cells in the distal nerve stump, as well as the infiltration of immune cells. Moreover, the "endoneurial tubes" consisting of the basal lamina deposited by Schwann cells at the perimeter of each axon and the perineurium surrounding axon fascicles (cf. Salzer, 1999) persisted. These tubes, filled with Schwann cells and immune cells, remained in the distal parts of the injured nerve and served as conduits through which axons, after crossing the lesion site, re-grew. Ramon y Cajal (1928) advanced the idea that these endoneurial tubes and their contents provided "neurotrophic" support for the advancement of the regenerating axons. Recent experiments suggest that cues that persist in the distal stump of the nerve can even selectively influence which types of axons regenerate along these pathways (Brushart, 1993; Brushart et al., 1998; Le et al., 2001; Mears et al., 2003; see however Robinson and Madison, 2004).

The importance of the old nerve sheaths in directing the growth of axons has recently been elegantly demonstrated (Nguyen et al., 2002). Muscles of mice expressing a genetically encoded fluorescent protein in their motor axons were vitally imaged. The paths that individual motor axons took to form neuromuscular junctions on the fibers were noted. The nerve to the muscle was then crushed and the muscle re-imaged a second time following nerve regeneration and reinnervation of the muscle fibers. Fluorescent axons were found to have retraced the old pathways and terminated on the same set of muscle fibers at the ends of these pathways. Similar experiments were conducted imaging fluorescent cutaneous axons through the skin, examining their pathways and rates of regeneration (Pan et al., 2003). A role of the endoneurial tubes in guiding regenerating axons to synaptic sites in muscles was also indicated by earlier vital imaging experiments. A motor axon commonly regenerates to denervated synaptic sites by growing along the same pathway as the axon that previously innervated this muscle fiber (Rich and Lichtman, 1989; but see exceptions of innervation by escaped fibers and sprouts described below).

Experiments implanting peripheral nerves into the central nervous system showing that neurons that were otherwise refractory to regeneration could be coaxed to grow within the endoneurial tubes of these nerves excited more interest in the role of these tubes and their Schwann cells (Benfey and Aguayo, 1982; Bray et al., 1987; Anderson et al., 1998). It was shown that living Schwann cells were required to promote this growth (Berry et al., 1988; Smith and Stevenson, 1988) and that the axons grew in contact with Schwann cells (Kleitman et al., 1988b). Some studies report that living Schwann cells are likewise needed for efficient regeneration in the peripheral nervous system, as inhibition of Schwann cell mitosis (Hall, 1986; Enver and Hall, 1994) or killing the Schwann cells in a nerve inhibits regeneration (cf. Nadim et al., 1990). Other studies seem to indicate a supportive role for Schwann cells but report that the growth of axons actually occurs on the Schwann cell basal lamina rather than on the surface of living Schwann cells (Ide et al., 1983; Scherer and Easter, 1984; Schwab and Thoenen, 1985; Kuffler, 1986; Sketelj et al., 1989; Osawa et al., 1990; Fugleholm et al., 1994). Still other electron microscopic studies clearly show that the leading tip of mammalian motor axons regenerate within endoneurial tubes in association with the membranes of Schwann cells (Derron Bishop, personal communication; Cook and Bishop, 2004). The discrepancies between the observations of growth on Schwann cell basal lamina versus growth on Schwann cells are presently unresolved, but both sets of observations may describe the growth preferences of axons encountering endoneurial tubes and Schwann cells after different degrees of denervation- or transplantation-induced modification (cf. Ferguson and Muir, 2000).

27.4 Growth across the lesion site

Even if axons regenerate within endoneurial tubes on the distal side of a nerve lesion, how they cross the lesion site is so far left unexplained. It is well known that simple crush lesions that do not interrupt these tubes lead to more rapid regeneration across the lesion site as well as a more accurate, selective reinnervation by axons of their original targets (cf. Westerfield and Powell, 1983; Farel and Bemelmans, 1986). Such a result is not surprising since the tubes act as conduits, guiding the course of the growth of any axon that enters them. Lesions that leave these tubes intact while interrupting the axons within them are likely to result in axons regenerating down their original endoneurial tubes and reinnervating their original targets. But how do axons behave when they have to cross a gap between the nerve ends?

This issue arose quite early in the study of regeneration. Some of Cajal's contemporaries (Nageotte and Marinesco, as cited by Ramon y Cajal, 1928) believed that their microscopic observations showed that Schwann cells or some similar cell type extended in association with axons that grew to bridge a gap between the central and distal stumps. These investigators even claimed the formation of glial "syncytium" that grew from the distal stump towards the central stump. While recognizing the presence of some kind of "nutritive plasma" between the ends of the nerve, Cajal rejected these claims, arguing that the cells having similar staining to the Schwann cells in the central stump were absent from the axons and, although the axons grew to the distal stump through some kind of neurotrophic influence emanating from it, these axons grew naked. Since this early period several investigations have shown that Schwann cells extend as bands or chains of cells both in culture and *in vivo*, even in the absence of axons (Abercrombie and Johnson, 1942; Holmes and Young, 1942; Thomas, 1966; Crang and Blakemore, 1987; Anderson et al., 1991; Feneley et al., 1991; Williams et al., 1993; Tseng et al., 2003; and see below). It has been shown that the distal nerve stump exerts a tropic effect on the extension of axons from a central stump by inserting this central stump into one arm of a Y-shaped tube (Abernethy et al., 1992). Axons extended preferentially to a second arm of the tube in which a distal nerve stump was sutured rather than the arm in which other tissue was placed. Using a similar assay, it could be shown that a Schwann cell cable formed preferentially between two axonless nerve segments (Abernethy et al., 1994; Madison and Archibald, 1994; see also Williams et al., 1984). However, understanding the role of the glia in bridging the gap between the central and distal stumps of a damaged nerve and promoting nerve regeneration has been impeded by the lack of good markers for both cell types, and by the inability to follow the regeneration in real time.

Procedures used for repair of nerve injuries in human patients also demonstrate the importance of bridging gaps in nerves (see review by Chiu (1999)). Several methods have been used to try to repair cases of extensive nerve damage or evulsions, including suturing the proximal and distal ends of the nerve to each end of a vein taken from the patient. The most effective method of encouraging regeneration across such a gap appears to be transplantation of a nerve segment with its endoneurial tubes to the site of damage (an autograft) and its apposition to each of the cut ends. More recently, investigators have tried to design synthetic nerve guides that will facilitate nerve regeneration (see review by Schmidt and Leach (2003)). One of the approaches is to infuse these guides with Schwann cells (cf. Guénard et al., 1992; Komiyama et al., 2004; Nishiura et al., 2004).

27.5 Reinnervation of muscle

The author's own laboratory began investigating the involvement of Schwann cells in regeneration unintentionally, during experiments of immunostaining of neuromuscular preparations in the rat. An unexpected growth of Schwann cells at neuromuscular junctions was found following muscle denervation. Antibodies against neurofilament and synaptic vesicle proteins were used to identify axons and nerve terminals in the muscle and an antibody against the protein S100B, a small calcium binding protein of uncertain function, was used to mark the Schwann cells. By applying these primary antibodies followed by fluorophore-conjugated secondary antibodies, nerve terminals and axons could be visualized in one color and the Schwann cells in a second color. Further, by applying a third fluorophore conjugated to bungarotoxin (BTX), the acetylcholine receptors in the muscle fiber's postsynaptic apparatus could labeled as well. Thus, all three cellular components of the synapse could be visualized by changing filters on a fluorescence microscope. Particularly advantageous for these experiments was a whole mount procedure (Froehner et al., 1987) that enabled viewing not only of the junction in its entirety but also of the surrounding muscle fibers and nerve segments. Crushing the muscle nerve was used to denervate the muscle (Son and Thompson, 1995a). Axons however regenerate quickly following such lesions, returning to the muscle beginning ca. 6 days after the denervation. This allowed the study of muscle reinnervation after only a short period of denervation. By sacrificing animals at various stages of denervation and examining the neuromuscular junctions, inferences were made about the events that were transpiring during denervation and reinnervation.

Several conclusions resulted from this kind of study:

1 Within the first few days of denervation, the terminal Schwann cells (i.e. those Schwann cells that cover the nerve terminal) began to extend processes into the spaces between the muscle fibers surrounding the synaptic sites (Astrow et al., 1994). These processes became longer and more elaborate the longer the period of denervation. These findings duplicated those of a prior study (Reynolds and Woolf, 1992). Schwann cells inside

the endoneurial tubes probably extend similar processes after the removal of axons but these are confined by the tubes (cf. Payer, 1979).

2 When the axons regenerated to synaptic sites, the most common pathway they took (with the exceptions noted below) was through the old endoneurial tube/sheath (Son and Thompson, 1995a). This tube could be identified by the labeled Schwann cells it contained. The returning axon appeared to grow into the old synaptic site, that is over the acetylcholine receptors identified by their labeling with BTX. However, the nerve growth did not stop at the boundaries of the previous synaptic site. Indeed, many axonal processes were found extending from the synapse into the spaces between the muscle fibers. Such "overshooting" of the old synaptic site was reported in the drawings of Tello (1907) and were noted by Gutmann and Young (1944) in their study of muscle reinnervation. The latter investigators named these overshooting axons "escaped fibers". The availability of the anti-S100 antibody marker for Schwann cells enabled the demonstration that such escaped fibers were always associated with Schwann cell processes. The inference was drawn that these Schwann cell processes were those extended during the period of denervation. The Schwann cell processes were frequently longer than the axonal growths, but the axons were never longer than the Schwann cells. These results suggested that the axons were following Schwann cell processes that had been extended during the period of denervation. A similar conclusion was reached by investigators who examined the extensions of motor terminals in frog muscles; here also terminal extension occurs in concert with extension of Schwann cell coverings (Koirala et al., 2000).

3 With longer times following reinnervation, these escaped fibers and Schwann cell processes were withdrawn, except for cases where the escaped fibers grew to and entered a synaptic site on an adjoining muscle fiber (Son and Thompson, 1995a). Thus, in many cases, the escaped fibers had actually innervated adjacent muscle fibers at their old synaptic sites, before these sites had

become reinnervated by axons arriving over the endoneurial tubes leading to these synaptic sites. Similar observations had been reported much earlier by investigators who had excellent methods for nerve staining but who lacked the ability to simultaneously label Schwann cells (Tello, 1907; Gutmann and Young, 1944). Other investigators (Letinsky et al., 1976; Wernig et al., 1981a; Ko and Chen, 1996) had noted escaped fibers that were associated with Schwann cells in electron micrographs of frog neuromuscular junctions during reinnervation or seasonal remodeling. Schwann cell-directed nerve growth like this offers an obvious explanation for one of the prominent changes in the innervation of muscles that follows denervation and reinnervation: it is well known that the location within the muscle of the fibers innervated by individual motor axons (i.e. single motor units) changes a scattered distribution across large cross-sections of the muscle to one where fibers in single units are clustered into large, contiguous groups within the muscle (Kugelberg et al., 1970).

27.6 Terminal Schwann cells mediate sprouting of the nerve terminal

The observations that suggested regenerating axons grew to adjacent synaptic sites by following the processes extended by Schwann cells raised the issue of whether Schwann cells played a similar role in another type of nerve growth that had been extensively described and studied, the phenomenon of "terminal sprouting". Many investigators had examined the response to damage of only a portion of the motor axons supplying a muscle, that is a "partial denervation" (Edds, 1950; Thompson and Jansen, 1977; Brown and Ironton, 1978; Brown et al., 1981). Such a partial denervation results in denervated muscle fibers scattered amongst muscle fibers whose innervation remains intact. These experiments had shown that the remaining axons often sprout from their nerve terminals and grow to innervate many of the denervated muscle fibers. In electron micrographs, other investigators had noted that the sprouts were associated with Schwann cells (Duchen, 1971; Wernig et al., 1981a; Gorio et al., 1983), but whether the Schwann cells led or followed the sprouts was unclear. An examination of the role of the Schwann

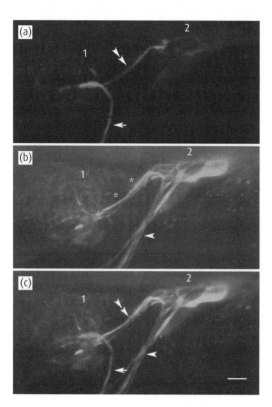

Figure 27.1. Nerve sprouts grow between two synaptic sites in a partially denervated rat muscle by following Schwann cell processes emerging from the denervated synaptic site. Two synaptic sites (labeled "1" and "2") in a rat soleus muscle 3 days after partial denervation. (a) Motor axon labeled by an anti-neurofilament antibody. The axon enters from the bottom of the panel (arrow), innervates site 1 and then "sprouts" to innervate site 2, a site denervated by the partial denervation. (b) Schwann cells labeled with an anti-nestin antibody. This antibody labels only Schwann cells that have lost axonal contact, that is "reactive" Schwann cells. Note the labeling of the old endoneurial tube that previously contained the axon innervating site 2 (arrowhead); the endoneurial tube of the axon innervating site 1 is unlabeled. Note also the association of the sprout in (a) with processes (asterisks) of the Schwann cells at site 2. (c) Merged image of the panels (a) & (b) with the axon in red and the Schwann cells in green. Scale bar indicates 10 μm. Modified from (Son and Thompson, 1995b).

cells was made possible by production of a monoclonal antibody (Astrow et al., 1992) that recognizes an epitope on the intermediate filament nestin (Kopp and Thompson, 1998). This antibody does not label Schwann cells at innervated neuromuscular junctions but does label them following the degeneration of the motor axon. Thus, this antibody labeled Schwann cells that are usually called "reactive". A similar labeling of reactive terminal Schwann cells by antibodies to nestin has been reported (Carlsson et al., 1999; Vaittinen et al., 1999). When this antibody was used to label partially denervated muscles, the Schwann cells at innervated junctions remained unlabeled while those present at junctions lacking innervation were brightly labeled. Such labeled muscles were scanned for nerve sprouts that had grown to innervate denervated synaptic sites. In most of the cases, the sprouts were associated with Schwann cell processes that were labeled with the antibody (Son and Thompson, 1995b) (Fig. 27.1). Since the Schwann cells above the innervated synaptic sites remained un-reactive and unlabeled by the antibody, this suggested that the sprout had grown in association with a Schwann cell that had extended processes from the denervated synaptic site. The teleological interpretation of these findings is that the Schwann cells at the denervated site had extended processes in search of a nearby axon in attempt to induce this axon to grow to the denervated site. If true, this would represent an inversion of how most investigators thought about the induction of sprouting: it had been proposed that factors produced by denervated fibers induced and guided the growth of nearby nerves.

27.7 Another example of nerve growth along a novel path

The observations above suggested that the axons that grow along novel paths in skeletal muscle (e.g., between synaptic sites) might be following pathways consisting of living Schwann cells. What about the growth between cut ends of nerves? Several experiments indirectly addressed this question. The cut end of a nerve in the leg of a rat was transplanted to the surface of the soleus muscle (Son and

Thompson, 1995a). Nerves had been shown to grow from such transplants and axons in these nerves could be induced to innervate the muscle onto which they were transplanted following the denervation or paralysis of this muscle (Jansen et al., 1973). It was also known that these axons grew in association with Schwann cells (Saito and Zacks, 1969; Korneliussen and Sommerschild, 1976). However, the relationship between the extension of Schwann cells and axons was not known. Immunostaining revealed that axons emerged from the ends of the transplant, but bands and fascicles of Schwann cells and their processes grew as well (Fig. 27.2). All the growing axons were associated with Schwann cell processes but some Schwann cell processes were devoid of axons. If, instead of transplanting a nerve with axons, a nerve was transplanted that had been crushed proximally to temporarily remove its axons, fascicles of Schwann cells and their processes emerged and grew across the muscle. This showed, in agreement with earlier findings, that Schwann cells do not need axons to grow from the cut ends of a nerve (see discussion above). It appeared that the Schwann cells might set the limit to the rate of axon extension when axons were present because axons grew out across the surface of the muscle more slowly than axons grew within nerves and their endoneurial tubes following denervations by crush (Son and Thompson, 1995a). This hypothesis was supported by performing an experiment where Schwann cells were allowed to grow from the cut end of the nerve across the muscle in the absence of axons (achieved by crushing the nerve more proximally). In this case, once the axons regenerated to the site of the implant, they extended across the muscle surface more rapidly in the presence of the Schwann cells that had gone before them. These observations suggested that the pathways laid down by the Schwann cells during the absence of axons facilitated the rate of axonal growth.

27.8 Limitations to the interpretation of these findings

There are several unanswered questions from the observations reported above. First, are Schwann cells

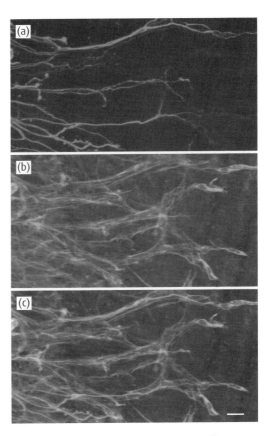

Figure 27.2. Nerve outgrowth across the surface of a muscle from the cut end of a transplanted nerve. The transplant is located to the left of the panels. (a) Axons labeled by anti-neurofilament antibody. (b) Reactive Schwann cells labeled with an anti-nestin antibody. (c) Merged image of the upper panels with the axons in red and the Schwann cells in green. Growing axons are clearly associated with Schwann cell processes extended from the transplant, although there are Schwann cell processes that are not associated with axons. Scale bar indicates 40 μm. Modified from (Son and Thompson, 1995a).

really necessary for this type of nerve growth? The correlations made during these observations do not prove causation. What would happen if Schwann cells were not present? A related question is whether the Schwann cells might be the preferred substrate for growth, but in their absence, other substrates would be found by axons to be acceptable replacements. For example, Stolz et al. (1991) have reported that macrophages can act as a scaffold for nerve growth.

Still another issue is how well static images obtained at intervals from different animals show the sequence of events that actually occur at any single junction (Lichtman and Sanes, 2003). One should be cautious inferring the temporal sequence of events from such static images.

27.9 Evidence that Schwann cells are required for sprouting

To test if Schwann cells are necessary for axons to grow within muscles requires an examination of the consequences of their removal in the living animal. Such Schwann cell ablations have been achieved in frog muscle by applying *in vivo* an antibody that recognizes a component on the surface of Schwann cells and then using complement to lyse the cells to which the antibody bound (Reddy et al., 2003). Since the nerve sheaths prevent access of the antibody to the Schwann cells in the nerve, the ablation is confined to terminal Schwann cells. At established, adult junctions, such ablations result in a retraction of some of the nerve terminal so that these terminals become smaller and less efficacious in synaptic transmission. At developing junctions in tadpoles, ablation of terminal Schwann cells results in a dramatic suppression of the normal growth of nerve terminals, growth that had previously been shown to be correlated with the growth of the synaptic glia (Herrera et al., 2000). The consequences of ablation for reinnervation have not yet been reported.

Experiments also on frogs have shown that axons can regenerate to muscles even after killing the Schwann cells at the neuromuscular junctions and along the muscle nerve by freezing (Kuffler, 1986). However, in these cases the regenerating axons are commonly accompanied by Schwann cells. At the junction, however, these experiments suggest that components of the synaptic basal lamina are responsible for the growth of the axon, because nerve terminals reoccupy synaptic areas devoid of Schwann cells.

In mammals, observations to date have been limited to the neonatal rat. Here, in contrast to the extension of cell processes that follows denervation in the adult, denervation results in the rapid, apoptotic death of terminal Schwann cells (Trachtenberg and Thompson, 1996). These experiments together with those by others (Grinspan et al., 1996; Syroid et al., 1996) show that neonatal Schwann cells are trophically dependent upon motor axons. Not surprisingly, partial denervation results in the death of terminal Schwann cells above the denervated junctions (Lubischer and Thompson, 1999). The terminal sprouting that would be expected to give rise to innervation of denervated junctions is rare in these neonatal animals. Such a result would be expected if the terminal Schwann cells above the denervated synaptic sites were required for terminal sprouts to grow and innervate these sites. However, since the experiments are conducted in neonates, other developmental differences could account for the lack of terminal sprouting. More experiments employing Schwann cell ablation are needed.

27.10 Examining the role of Schwann cells with vital imaging

Several laboratories have examined muscle reinnervation by collecting repeated, vital images of axons, postsynaptic acetylcholine receptors, and Schwann cells.

The first effort in mammals (O'Malley et al., 1999) used a blue fluorescent dye (calcein blue) that, when applied as an acetoxymethyl (AM) ester to mouse muscle, gave selective labeling of Schwann cells. In combination with the red fluorescent mitochondrial dye 4-Di-2-Asp that labels nerve terminals, they examined neuromuscular junctions during the course of reinnervation and reported that axons grew beyond the junction by following Schwann cell process that had extended from the junction.

Fluorescent lectins that bind to components of the extracellular matrix of Schwann cells have been used to image the cells and their matrix in living frogs (Chen et al., 1991; Chen and Ko, 1994; Koirala et al., 2000). The regeneration of fluorescently labeled axons was found to induce the frog Schwann cells to extend processes that the axons then followed, in some cases to reinnervate denervated synaptic sites on adjacent muscle fibers.

For our own imaging experiments we undertook a different approach to label the cellular components. Transgenic mice were prepared using the promoter

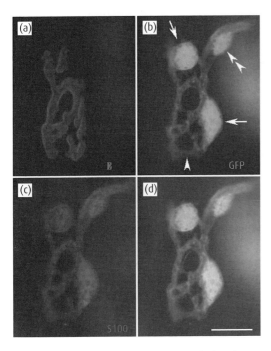

Figure 27.3. Schwann cells at the neuromuscular junction labeled by transgenic expression of green fluorescent protein. Junction of a sternomastoid muscle of an adult mouse. (a) Labeling of the acetylcholine receptors with BTX. (b) Fluorescence of green fluorescent protein (GFP). (c) Labeling of Schwann cells with an antibody to the protein S100B. (d) Merged image of panels (a–c) with each panel having the color shown. The promoter used to drive the GFP is the promoter for S100; not surprisingly the two labels appear in the same structures (compare b, c). The arrows indicate cell bodies of terminal Schwann cells. The double arrowhead indicates the cell body of a myelinating Schwann cell on the preterminal axon. As they cover the nerve terminal processes that occupy the synaptic gutters in panel (a), processes of the terminal Schwann cells match the receptor distribution except where they cover a nerve process traveling between two gutters (arrowhead). Scale bar indicates 20 μm. Modified from (Zuo et al., 2004).

for a Schwann cell marker, the protein S100B, linked to sequences coding for a fluorescent protein (Zuo et al., 2004). Fluorescent Schwann cells were seen along peripheral nerves and at neuromuscular junctions in several of these lines of mice. The cell bodies of the terminal Schwann cells and their processes overlying the neuromuscular junction were brightly labeled (Fig. 27.3). As expected, the processes covered each of the nerve terminal branches that were positioned above the synaptic gutters as well as the nerve processes that ran between these gutters. By using short exposures to low intensity light of the wavelengths necessary to excite the fluorophores, a sensitive charge coupled device (CCD) camera, and image processing software, vital images of these junctions could be collected from a living mouse (Fig. 27.4). As first shown in the experiments of Magrassi et al. (1987), neuromuscular junctions can be individually identified on the basis of the pretzel-like pattern of their acetylcholine receptors, labeled by concentrations of a fluorochrome-conjugated BTX insufficient to alter synaptic transmission. This receptor pattern serves as a "fingerprint" for each junction. These same junctions can be found and re-imaged hours to months later. As reported previously (O'Malley et al., 1999), the terminal Schwann cells were remarkably constant in the positions and numbers of their cell bodies. However, the fluorescent-protein-labeled Schwann cells were observed to extend and retract short processes in a dynamic fashion reminiscent of earlier observations (Ogata and Yamasaki, 1985; Robbins and Polak, 1988).

Upon crushing the muscle nerve, Schwann cells began to extend processes from the junction into the surrounding muscle, as reported previously (Reynolds and Woolf, 1992; Astrow et al., 1994). These processes were dynamic, mostly extending but occasionally retracting. Motor axons could be imaged in these same preparations by using double transgenic animals that expressed not only a green fluorescent protein in their Schwann cells as described above but also a blue fluorescent protein driven by a neuronal promotor in their motor neurons (Feng et al., 2000). As expected from previous studies, a motor axon commonly returned to a denervated

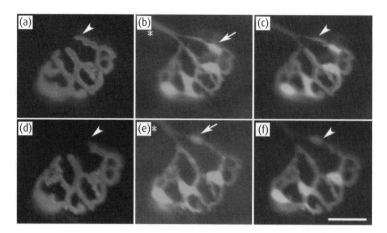

Figure 27.4. Vital images of terminal Schwann cells at a neuromuscular junction of a mouse sternomastoid muscle collected 30 days apart. Acetylcholine receptors (panels a, d) were labeled with non-blocking concentrations of rhodamine-conjugated alpha-BTX. Schwann cells (panels b, e) were visualized by their expression of green fluorescent protein. Images were merged in panels (c), (f). Panels (a)–(c) were collected at the first imaging session. Panels d–f were collected 30 days later. The synapse is remarkably stable except for some minor changes in acetylcholine receptors (arrowhead) and movement of one Schwann cell body (arrow). The synapse has the same number of Schwann cells (cell bodies are brighter ovals) at each time point. The asterisk indicates the site where the Schwann-cell wrapped axon enters the synaptic site. Scale bar indicates 30 μm. Modified from (Zuo et al., 2004).

synaptic site by growing through the endoneurial tube that contained fluorescent glial cells. The regenerating axons escaped from the confines of synaptic sites by following the Schwann cells (Kang and Thompson, 2002), as expected from the previous, non-vital (Son and Thompson, 1995a) and vital (O'Malley et al., 1999) observations. These escaped fibers and their associated Schwann cell processes appeared to be retained only for a short period unless they became connected to a second synaptic site on an adjoining muscle fiber. If such a connection did not form, then the escaped fiber was withdrawn. Withdrawal of the escaped fiber preceded the withdrawal of the glial process. Frequently an escaped fiber followed Schwann cell process and reached the synaptic site on an adjacent muscle fiber. Here it commonly made a synaptic connection. Moreover, in many cases this escaped fiber entered the endoneurial tube of this second synaptic site and grew in the retrograde direction. This axon then turned to grow orthogradely down the branches of this endoneurial tube to innervate additional denervated synaptic sites located at the ends of these endoneurial tubes. This type of growth is illustrated in the cartoon of (Fig. 27.5). Such a result is not surprising considering the guidance that endoneurial tubes and their Schwann cells provide regenerating axons entering the distal stump after a nerve lesion. This result, together with the observations of escaped fibers growing in association with Schwann cells, argues that Schwann cells play a prominent role in promoting rapid, efficient reinnervation of muscle fibers.

27.11 Schwann cells guide the formation of nerve sprouts

Transgenic mice expressing fluorescent proteins in Schwann cells and axons have also been used to examine the growth of sprouts in partially denervated muscle (Tian and Thompson, 2002,

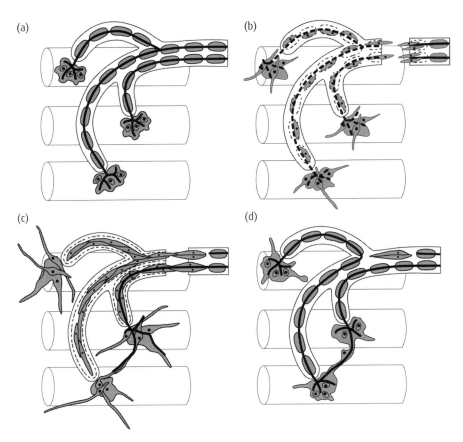

Figure 27.5. Cartoon illustrating the role of Schwann cells in the reinnervation of neuromuscular junctions. Three synaptic sites on three muscle fibers are shown at successive times. (a) Two axons (black lines) innervating these sites. One axon branches to innervate the lower and upper muscle fiber. Both axons have myelinating and terminal Schwann cells shown in grey. (b) Degeneration of these axons following injury to the nerve. The myelinating Schwann cells begin to dedifferentiate and the terminal Schwann cells begin to extend processes from the denervated synaptic sites. (c) Early stages of reinnervation. Only one of the axons has returned. This axon follows the lower endoneurial tube and is led, by growth on Schwann cells, to the middle synaptic site. Here it finds Schwann cells extending from the site and grows along their processes, forming escaped fibers. One of these escaped fibers follows the Schwann cells towards the lower synaptic site. (d) Growth of one of the escaped fibers in panel (c) to innervate the lower synaptic site. This axon continues to grow retrogradely in the endoneurial tube of this lower site and comes to innervate the upper synaptic site as well. As synaptic sites begin to be reoccupied, the Schwann cell processes are withdrawn and the axons begin to re-myelinate. From (Kang et al., 2003).

unpublished data). Images collected from these mice clearly show that the Schwann cells at denervated synaptic sites grow processes to contact neighboring, innervated synaptic sites. Such contacts are followed by growth of axons from the nerve terminals that then form synapses at the denervated sites. Thus, this scenario, originally proposed from static images of partially denervated muscles, has been confirmed by vital imaging.

27.12 Is there a tropic guidance of Schwann cell growth during nerve sprouting in muscle?

One of the central conclusions from earlier studies of terminal sprouting in muscle (Brown et al., 1981) was that factors arising from denervated or inactive muscle promote the growth of nearby nerve terminals and attract this growth towards the denervated fibers. Considering observations above and the possible role of Schwann cells at denervated sites, is there some attractive influence guiding the growth of Schwann cells to nearby innervated synaptic sites? It appears that Schwann cell growth from denervated synaptic sites in a completely denervated muscle is random until the time motor axons begin to return to the muscle. Upon the return of the axons, Schwann cell processes often connect synaptic sites that are not yet reinnervated with those that have been reinnervated. These Schwann cell processes connecting adjacent endplates have been called "bridges" (Love and Thompson, 1999). Is it possible that these bridges form as a consequence of some attraction by the innervated synaptic sites? Inhibiting synaptic transmission at reinnervated sites by topical application of botulinum toxin or BTX, inhibited the formation of such bridges, suggesting that there might be a tropism that depends upon active synapses (Love and Thompson, 1999). In several vital observations of terminal sprouting it appeared that Schwann cells grew in an directed fashion to nearby innervated synaptic sites (Tian and Thompson, 2002, unpublished data). These results suggest there is a tropism, but its nature remains unknown. However, the issue here is reminiscent of the studies of the bridging of gaps in nerves. A number of previous studies have suggested tropic influences in Schwann cell growth and migration (cf. Politis et al., 1982; Nachemson et al., 1988; Dubovy and Svizenska, 1994; Gu et al., 1995), although these tropic influences do not arise from synaptic sites.

An ability of newly generated muscle fibers to attract axons capable of innervating them would be advantageous, especially during development when different generations of muscle fibers arise sequentially. How do newly generated muscle fibers become innervated? Electron microscopic evidence suggests that axons extend from muscle fibers that are already innervated (cf. Kelly and Zacks, 1969), possibly in association with Schwann cells. Interestingly, growth factors involved in the generation of new muscle fibers appear to serve as chemoattractants for nerves (Ebens et al., 1996) and mitogens for Schwann cells (Krasnoselsky et al., 1994). The role of Schwann cells here has not been investigated. Experiments in adult animals suggest similar tropic influences remain. The consequences of ablation of a single muscle fiber have been followed by vitally imaging the surrounding nerve fibers (Van Mier and Lichtman, 1994). Nerve terminals located on the surrounding muscle fibers began to sprout as the ablated fiber regenerated within its basal lamina. These sprouts grew preferentially towards the regenerating fiber. A study of the involvement of Schwann cells in this growth utilizing vital imaging has begun (Li and Thompson, 2004). Muscle fiber ablation can induce the growth of Schwann cell processes from nearby junctions even in the absence of nerve growth. These findings suggest that Schwann cells could be a component of the response bringing innervation to muscle fibers following their injury.

27.13 Role of Schwann cells in the reoccupation of synaptic sites on muscle

Observations of the reinnervation of frog neuromuscular junctions ultimately lead to the discovery of the crucial synapse-organizing-protein agrin (McMahan, 1990). These same experiments have given us information about the role of Schwann cells in the reinnervation process. Regenerating frog motor neurons were found to precisely reoccupy the very same synaptic areas previously occupied by nerve terminals (Letinsky et al., 1976). A series of elegant experiments then analyzed the likely source of the cue for this preference for the old synaptic site by ablating its cellular components, the muscle fiber and Schwann cells. Ultimately these experiments led to the conclusion that the cue was some molecule(s) present in the basal lamina of the synapse that was absent from the non-synaptic basal lamina surrounding the muscle fiber (McMahan et al., 1980; Nitkin et al., 1983). The muscle fiber could be ablated and the basal lamina was still reoccupied by regenerated nerve terminals, although, if the muscle fiber was present, the extent and stability of such reoccupation was increased. Similarly, it was observed that terminal Schwann cells, which occupied the synaptic site at the time of the denervation and shortly thereafter, gradually abandoned portions of these sites, and yet, the great majority of the synaptic site was reoccupied by the regenerating nerve (Letinsky et al., 1976). In some experiments Schwann cells were killed and synaptic sites were still recognized by regenerating axons in the absence of Schwann cells (Kuffler, 1986). Even though the frequency and the persistence of such Schwann-cell-less contacts was low, these experiments suggested that the motor axon could still recognize the old synaptic site in the absence of Schwann cells.

On the other hand, a number of studies have clearly shown that frog neuromuscular junctions undergo considerable remodeling, including regression/retraction of nerve terminals followed by their re-extension, in correlation with seasonal changes (Wernig et al., 1980). Examination of the morphology of these junctions has revealed that Schwann cells and terminals abandon synaptic sites during the regression phase and reoccupy these areas or new areas during periods of expansion. A number of observations have suggested that Schwann cells might be involved in these expansions and retractions, including observations of Schwann cell processes in advance of axons in the gutters during periods of regrowth (Wernig et al., 1981b; Anzil et al., 1984; Macleod et al., 2001). Further, vital imaging experiments in which terminal areas were imaged both before and after regeneration of nerves to the sartorius muscle showed that there was a surprising degree of imprecision in reoccupation of old synaptic sites often resulting in a loss of receptor areas in the muscle (Astrow et al., 1996). Schwann cell bodies were observed to change their positions within the junctions during reinnervation but their role in

determining the reinnervation pattern remained unclear.

Just as in the frog, Schwann cells initially remain above denervated synaptic sites in rodents but gradually abandon portions of these sites (Miledi and Slater, 1968; 1970; Wernig et al., 1984). Transgenic mice with fluorescent-protein-tagged Schwann cells have been used to show that an increasingly large portion of the acetylcholine-rich receptor areas in the synaptic sites lose coverage by Schwann cell processes with increasing periods of denervation (Kang and Thompson, 2002, unpublished data). When nerves regenerate to synaptic sites having portions of that site abandoned by Schwann cells, their path of growth over the site is predicted by the remaining Schwann cell processes (Kang and Thompson, 2002; Tian and Thompson, 2002, unpublished data). The regenerating axon ignored receptor areas that were devoid of Schwann cell processes. In many cases these abandoned sites were never reoccupied by the regenerating nerve and the acetylcholine receptors at these sites disappeared, presumably as the resumption of neuromuscular transmission at the reoccupied sites initiated their displacement (Balice-Gordon and Lichtman, 1994). In other cases both nerve processes and Schwann cell processes reoccupied some of these areas and in these cases the areas persisted. These experiments together argue that the guidance of regenerating nerve processes by Schwann cells in the mouse extends to the reinnervation of the synaptic site and suggests that, in the absence of Schwann cells, some of the old synaptic site is never reoccupied and its receptors are lost. Whether Schwann cells are required for reoccupation and persistence of nerve terminals at sites contacted during reinnervation is a question that remains unanswered.

27.14 A role for terminal Schwann cells in synaptic remodeling?

One interesting case where it appears that Schwann cells can explain remodeling of neuromuscular synapses comes from a mutant mouse in which a particular laminin isoform located in the synaptic basal lamina (laminin-beta-2) is genetically ablated (Noakes et al., 1995). These mice show gradual reduction in the efficacy of neuromuscular transmission, and electron microscopic examination shows that Schwann cells begin to intrude into the synaptic cleft between the nerve terminal and muscle, effectively reducing the area of synaptic contact. This laminin isoform containing laminin-beta-2 appears to be repulsive for Schwann cells and may normally prevent their intrusion into the junction (Patton et al., 1998; Sanes, 1998; Miner and Patton, 1999). Instances of this kind of glial separation of presynaptic terminals from their postsynaptic targets termed "synaptic stripping" have also been reported for neuron–neuron synapses (Matthews and Nelson, 1975).

Muscle innervation undergoes considerable remodeling during development. Initially muscle fibers are polyneuronally innervated. All but one motor neuronal input is lost from the single area of synaptic contact on each muscle fiber during late fetal and early postnatal development. This "synapse elimination" corrects for the initial over connection of the motoneurons to the muscle fibers; it involves no death of motoneurons but rather a reduction in the number of muscle fibers each innervates (Brown et al., 1976). Recent studies of mice expressing fluorescent proteins in their motor axons have given us a great deal of information about the competition among the axons at each site. The inputs appear to compete for synaptic territory and the loser(s) in the competition withdraws from the synaptic site (Walsh and Lichtman, 2003). Several electron microscopic studies have suggested that Schwann cells might interpose themselves between nerve terminals and muscle fibers during this process (Korneliussen and Jansen, 1976; Bixby, 1981) as they do during the degeneration of nerve terminals following damage to motor nerves (Miledi and Slater, 1968; 1970; Jirmanová, 1975). Other studies have shown that the losing axon that withdraws from the synaptic site ends in a swelling, called a retraction bulb, that is surrounded by Schwann cell wrappings (Riley, 1981). Recent vital imaging experiments have been conducted during this elimination. Time-lapse images of these retraction bulbs, combined with serial electron microscopic reconstructions, have shown that Schwann cells actively partition/divide the withdrawing process into small pieces and engulf these pieces (Bishop et al., 2004). Whether Schwann cells might participate in a similar manner in removal of synaptic terminals in contact with the muscle fiber target remains unclear at present.

27.15 How do Schwann cells perform the tasks they accomplish during regeneration?

The presentation above emphasizes the cellular events involving Schwann cells and regeneration and does not deal with the issue of the molecules involved. Previous reviews, including those cited at the beginning, have dealt extensively with these aspects of the molecular biology of Schwann cells. Clearly, Schwann cells interact with each other, components of the immune system, cells and matrices along their pathways, and axons. These interactions involve a large array of molecules. This contention is supported by the large number of molecules already identified as well as those implicated by the recent application of expression microarrays (cf. Kubo et al., 2002; Cameron et al., 2003; Schworer et al., 2003; Birge et al., 2004). The types of molecules that are likely to play a role include those in the list below

1 Molecules involved in cell adhesion and cell migration. Schwann cells extend processes and migrate as they lay down the pathways that axons follow. Molecules that promote Schwann cell process extension by modulating their adhesion to the substrates they encounter as well as the molecules that promote axonal growth on Schwann cell surfaces will be crucially important. Experiments in tissue culture have analyzed the hierarchical preference of nerves for growth on different cell types (Fallon, 1985; Tomaselli et al., 1986; Ard et al., 1987; Bixby et al., 1988). These experiments have shown that Schwann cells are preferred by axons over other cell surfaces. Use of blocking antibodies has helped

in the identification of some of the important molecules (Bixby et al., 1988; Kleitman et al., 1988a). These molecules include L1 and N-cadherin, homophilic adhesion molecules that interact with the same molecules present on axons or other Schwann cells (Martini and Schachner, 1988; Moos et al., 1988; Letourneau et al., 1990; 1991; Cifuentes-Diaz et al., 1994; Takeda et al., 1996; Kamiguchi and Lemmon, 1997). Other adhesion molecules identified on Schwann cells include N-CAM (Rieger et al., 1988) and ninjurin (Araki and Milbrandt, 1996). The expression of many of these molecules is up-regulated in reactive Schwann cells (cf. Nieke and Schachner, 1985; Daniloff et al., 1986; Seilheimer and Schachner, 1988). Thus, these molecules are available to promote both Schwann cell and axon extension following nerve degeneration. Molecules in the extracellular matrix, in particular laminin (cf. Anton et al., 1994a; Probstmeier et al., 2001) and the integrin receptors for these matrix molecules are important for the extension of Schwann cells. Molecules that promote the migration of reactive Schwann would likewise promote regeneration. Molecules identified with this function include nerve growth factor (NGF), L1, neuregulin, the low-affinity NGF receptor (p75-NGFR), galectin-1, CD-9, sphingosine 1-phosphate (S1P), lysophosphatidic acid (LPA), insulin-like growth factor-1 (IGF-1), and glial-derived neurotrophic factor (cf. Anton et al., 1994b; 1995; Mahanthappa et al., 1996; Cheng et al., 2000; Paratcha et al., 2003; Yamauchi et al., 2003; 2004; Barber et al., 2004; Horie et al., 2004; see also Sanes et al., 1986).

2 Molecules involved in removing/modifying barriers to growth. Schwann cells are confronted with physical barriers to their growth following the degeneration of their associated axon or terminal. Upon nerve damage, Schwann cells must remove the axonal and myelin debris from within the endoneurial tubes (cf. Stoll et al., 1989). They express cytokines that attract macrophages to assist in this task (cf. Toews et al., 1998; Rutkowski et al., 1999; Subang and Richardson, 2001; Shamash et al., 2002; Tofaris et al., 2002; Horie et al., 2004). Within a nerve, Schwann cells are constrained by

the basal lamina and perineurial cells that form the endoneurial tubes. At the neuromuscular junction, terminal Schwann cells are presumably constrained by the basal lamina that these cells produce just outside their processes that cover the nerve terminal. This basal lamina is continuous with the basal lamina of the muscle fiber and the basal lamina that is located between the nerve terminal and the muscle fiber (Birks et al., 1960). If Schwann cells are to break out of the confines of their sheaths to lay down pathways for escaped fibers or sprouts or to promote the formation of axonal sprouts that leave endoneurial tubes (so-called "nodal sprouts"), then they must be able to puncture these sheaths. Similarly, if they are to navigate through intercellular spaces, they may need to open a path for themselves, breaking down material between the cells. Interestingly, Schwann cells have been shown to express and secrete proteases that could play such a role as well as protease inhibitors that modulate this type of function (cf. Kalderon, 1979; Krystosek et al., 1988; Clark et al., 1991; Rogister et al., 1993; Kioussi et al., 1995; La Fleur et al., 1996; Bosse et al., 2000; Ferguson and Muir, 2000; Krekoski et al., 2002; Asundi et al., 2003; Demestre et al., 2004).

3 Molecules involved in trophic, chemotropic, and other cell–cell signaling interactions. Schwann cells undergo dramatic changes in their differentiation and their interaction with other cell types following lesions to axons and during regeneration. The exchange of trophic factors among Schwann cells, axons, perineurial cells, fibroblasts, macrophages, and even muscle fibers is clearly important in these changes and in regeneration. Schwann cells produce and respond to a large number of trophic factors, cytokines, and other signaling molecules, many of which are up-regulated in reactive Schwann cells. A partial list would include neuregulin, NGF, brain-derived neurotrophic factor (BDNF), leukemia inhibitory factor (LIF), ciliary neurotrophic factor (CNTF), glial-derived neurotrophic factor (GDNF), insulin-like growth factor (IGF-1 and -2), neurotrophin-3, platelet-derived growth factor (PDGF-B),

fibroblast growth factor (FGF), desert hedgehog, tumor necrosis factor (TNF), transforming growth factor-beta (TGF-beta), lysophosphatidic acid (Hansson et al., 1986; Taniuchi et al., 1986; Heumann et al., 1987; Cohen et al., 1992; Meyer et al., 1992; Marchionni et al., 1993; Rogister et al., 1993; Henderson et al., 1994; Einheber et al., 1995; Guenard et al., 1995; Dowsing et al., 1999; Parmantier et al., 1999; Lisak et al., 2001; Oya et al., 2002; Li et al., 2003; Paratcha et al., 2003; Yamauchi et al., 2003). Some of these molecules can be shown to affect motor neuron survival and regeneration. Many of them are involved in promoting the reactive state of Schwann cells. Many have multiple roles. For example, axonally supplied neuregulin is involved in the early differentiation and survival of Schwann cells (cf. Jessen and Mirsky, 1997), becomes an autocrine/paracrine factor after removal of axons (cf. Raabe et al., 1996; Carroll et al., 1997; Rosenbaum et al., 1997), and a factor that promotes migration (cf. Mahanthappa et al., 1996; Meintanis et al., 2001) and Schwann cell mitosis upon the return of axons (Morrissey et al., 1995). Neuregulin release from axons also appears to be rapidly induced following release of trophic factors from Schwann cells (Esper and Loeb, 2004). Several actions of axons on Schwann cells appear to involve neural activity and molecules released in an activity-dependent fashion (Jahromi et al., 1992; Reist and Smith, 1992; Esper and Loeb, 2004).

4 Molecules involved in remodeling the cytoskeleton and promoting growth of Schwann cell processes. Cytoskeletal changes occur in Schwann cells as they respond to signaling molecules by extending processes and migrating (Neuberger and Cornbrooks, 1989; Cheng et al., 2000; Weiner et al., 2001; Li et al., 2003; Barber et al., 2004). For example, the intermediate filament glial fibrilliary acidic protein (GFAP) is up-regulated in frog terminal Schwann cells following denervation of neuromuscular junctions, an upregulation that appears to result at least in part from the loss of neurotransmitters normally released from the nerve terminal that interact with receptors on the Schwann cells (Georgiou et al., 1994). Reactive Schwann cells up-regulate their expression of nestin (Kopp and Thompson, 1998; Vaittinen et al., 1999). Schwann cells can also express proteins normally found in neuronal growth cones (Curtis et al., 1992; Woolf et al., 1992; Plantinga et al., 1993).

5 Molecules involved in cell proliferation. Proliferation of Schwann cells occurs during the initial phases of nerve denervation (during the infiltration of immune cells and the degradation of myelin) (Pellegrino et al., 1986) and during the return of axons (Wood and Bunge, 1975; Salzer et al., 1980; Pellegrino and Spencer, 1985). The mitogenic signals (Davis and Stroobant, 1990; Rogister et al., 1993; Krasnoselsky et al., 1994; Cheng et al., 1995; Einheber et al., 1995; Levi et al., 1995; Morrissey et al., 1995; Minghetti et al., 1996; Rosenbaum et al., 1997) probably play a crucial role in regeneration as anti-mitotic agents can inhibit regeneration (Hall, 1986).

27.16 Molecules that Schwann cells produce that promote synaptogenesis

Recently, culture experiments have been conducted to show that Schwann cells produce diffusible molecules that can promote synaptogenesis by neurons (Peng et al., 2003; Taylor and Bampton, 2004; Ullian et al., 2004). These experiments make possible assays to identify molecules that are important in promoting synaptogenesis.

27.17 Concluding statement

The roles that Schwann cells play in the regeneration and sprouting of axons continue to intrigue many investigators. With the development of new tools in molecular biology, cell biology and imaging, our appreciation of the intricate, elegant but also complex involvement of Schwann cells will continue to expand.

ACKNOWLEDGEMENTS

None of the work conducted in my own lab would have been possible without the excellent pre- and postdoctoral students who have done work on muscle reinnervation and sprouting. Some of their experiments and, most importantly, their ideas that led to these experiments, are described in this review. I therefore wish to acknowledge: Stephanie Astrow, Christopher Hayworth, Hyuno Kang, Yue Li, Jane Lubischer, Young-jin Son, Lee Sutton, Le Tian, Joshua Trachtenberg, Yi Zuo. The imaging experiments would also be deficient without the fluorescent-protein-expressing transgenic mice prepared by Guoping Feng, Joshua Sanes, and Jeff Lichtman.

REFERENCES

Abercrombie, M. and Johnson, M.L. (1942). The outwandering of cells in tissue cultures of nerves undergoing Wallerian degeneration. *J Exp Biol*, **19**, 266–283.

Abernethy, D.A., Rud, A. and Thomas, P.K. (1992). Neurotropic influence of the distal stump of transected peripheral nerve on axonal regeneration: absence of topographic specificity in adult nerve. *J Anat*, **180**, 395–400.

Abernethy, D.A., Thomas, P.K., Rud, A. and King, R.H. (1994). Mutual attraction between emigrant cells from transected denervated nerve. *J Anat*, **184**, 239–249.

Aguayo, A.J., Charron, L. and Bray, G.M. (1976). Potential of Schwann cells from unmyelinated nerves to produce myelin: a quantitative ultrastructural and radiographic study. *J Neurocytol*, **5**, 565–573.

Anderson, P.N., Nadim, W. and Turmaine, M. (1991). Schwann cell migration through freeze-killed peripheral nerve grafts without accompanying axons. *Acta Neuropathol (Berl)*, **82**, 193–199.

Anderson, P.N., Campbell, G., Zhang, Y. and Lieberman, A.R. (1998). Cellular and molecular correlates of the regeneration of adult mammalian CNS axons into peripheral nerve grafts. *Prog Brain Res*, **117**, 211–232.

Anton, E.S., Sandrock, A.W.J. and Matthew, W.D. (1994a). Merosin promotes neurite growth and Schwann cell migration *in vitro* and nerve regeneration *in vivo*: evidence using an antibody to merosin, ARM-1. *Dev Biol*, **164**, 133–146.

Anton, E.S., Weskamp, G., Reichardt, L.F. and Matthew, W.D. (1994b). Nerve growth factor and its low-affinity receptor promote Schwann cell migration. *Proc Natl Acad Sci USA*, **91**, 2795–2799.

Anton, E.S., Hadjiargyrou, M., Patterson, P.H. and Matthew, W.D. (1995). CD9 plays a role in Schwann cell migration *in vitro*. *J Neurosci*, **15**, 584–595.

Anzil, A.P., Bieser, A. and Wernig, A. (1984). Light and electron microscopic identification of nerve terminal sprouting and retraction in normal adult frog muscle. *J Physiol*, **350**, 393–399.

Araki, T. and Milbrandt, J. (1996). Ninjurin, a novel adhesion molecule, is induced by nerve injury and promotes axonal growth. *Neuron*, **17**, 353–361.

Ard, M.D., Bunge, R.P. and Bunge, M.B. (1987). Comparison of the Schwann cell surface and Schwann cell extracellular matrix as promoters of neurite growth. *J Neurocytol*, **16**, 539–555.

Astrow, S.H., Sutton, L.A. and Thompson, W.J. (1992). Developmental and neural regulation of a subsarcolemmal component of the rat neuromuscular junction. *J Neurosci*, **12**, 1602–1615.

Astrow, S.H., Son, Y.-J. and Thompson, W.J. (1994). Differential neural regulation of a neuromuscular junction-associated antigen in muscle fibers and Schwann cells. *J Neurobiol*, **25**, 937–952.

Astrow, S.H., Pitaevski, V. and Herrera, A.A. (1996). Precision of reinnervation and synaptic remodeling observed in neuromuscular junctions of living frogs. *J Neurosci*, **16**, 5130–5140.

Asundi, V.K., Erdman, R., Stahl, R.C. and Carey, D.J. (2003). Matrix metalloproteinase-dependent shedding of syndecan-3, a transmembrane heparan sulfate proteoglycan, in Schwann cells. *J Neurosci Res*, **73**, 593–602.

Balice-Gordon, R.J. and Lichtman, J.W. (1994). Long-term synapse loss induced by focal blockade of postsynaptic receptors. *Nature*, **372**, 519–524.

Barber, S.C., Mellor, H., Gampel, A. and Scolding, N.J. (2004). S1P and LPA trigger Schwann cell actin changes and migration. *Eur J Neurosci*, **19**, 3142–3150.

Benfey, M. and Aguayo, A. (1982). Extensive elongation of axons from rat brain into peripheral nerve grafts. *Nature*, **296**, 150–153.

Berry, M., Rees, L., Hall, S., Yiu, P. and Sievers, J. (1988). Optic axons regenerate into sciatic nerve isografts only in the presence of Schwann cells. *Brain Res Bull*, **20**, 223–231.

Birge, R.B., Wadsworth, S., Akakura, R., Abeysinghe, H., Kanojia, R., MacIelag, M., Desbarats, J., Escalante, M., Singh, K., Sundarababu, S., Parris, K., Childs, G., August, A., Siekierka, J. and Weinstein, D.E. (2004). A role for Schwann cells in the neuroregenerative effects of a non-immunosuppressive fk506 derivative, jnj460. *Neuroscience*, **124**, 351–366.

Birks, R., Huxley, H.E. and Katz, B. (1960). The fine structure of the neuromuscular junction of the frog. *J Physiol*, **150**, 134–144.

Bishop, D.L., Misgeld, T., Walsh, M.K., Gan, W.B. and Lichtman, J.W. (2004). Axon branch removal at developing synapses by axosome shedding. *Neuron*, **44**, 651–661.

Bixby, J.L. (1981). Ultrastructural observations on synapse elimination in neonatal rabbit skeletal muscle. *J Neurocytol*, **10**, 81–100.

Bixby, J.L., Lilien, J. and Reichardt, L.F. (1988). Identification of the major proteins that promote neuronal process outgrowth on Schwann cells *in vitro*. *J Cell Biol*, **107**, 353–361.

Bosse, F., Petzold, G., Greiner-Petter, R., Pippirs, U., Gillen, C. and Muller, H.W. (2000). Cellular localization of the disintegrin CRII-7/rMDC15 mRNA in rat PNS and CNS and regulated expression in postnatal development and after nerve injury. *Glia*, **32**, 313–327.

Bray, G.M., Villegas-Perez, M.P., Vidal-Sanz, M. and Aguayo, A.J. (1987). The use of peripheral nerve grafts to enhance neuronal survival, promote growth and permit terminal reconnections in the central nervous system of adult rats. *J Exp Biol*, **132**, 5–19.

Brecknell, J.E. and Fawcett, J.W. (1996). Axonal regeneration. *Biol Rev Camb Philos Soc*, **71**, 227–255.

Britsch, S., Goerich, D.E., Riethmacher, D., Peirano, R.I., Rossner, M., Nave, K.A., Birchmeier, C. and Wegner, M. (2001). The transcription factor Sox10 is a key regulator of peripheral glial development. *Genes Dev*, **15**, 66–78.

Brown, M.C. and Ironton, R. (1978). Sprouting and regression of neuromuscular synapses in partially denervated mammalian muscles. *J Physiol*, **278**, 325–348.

Brown, M.C., Jansen, J.K.S. and Van Essen, D. (1976). Polyneuronal innervation of skeletal muscle in new-born rats and its elimination during maturation. *J Physiol*, **261**, 387–422.

Brown, M.C., Holland, R.L. and Hopkins, W.G. (1981). Motor nerve sprouting. *Ann Rev Neurosci*, **4**, 17–42.

Brushart, T.M. (1993). Motor axons preferentially reinnervate motor pathways. *J Neurosci*, **13**, 2730–2738.

Brushart, T.M., Gerber, J., Kessens, P., Chen, Y.G. and Royall, R.M. (1998). Contributions of pathway and neuron to preferential motor reinnervation. *J Neurosci*, **18**, 8674–8681.

Bunge, R.P. (1993). Expanding roles for the Schwann cell: ensheathment, myelination, trophism and regeneration. *Curr Opin Neurobiol*, **3**, 805–809.

Bunge, R.P. (1994). The role of the Schwann cell in trophic support and regeneration. *J Neurol*, **242**, S19–S21.

Cameron, A.A., Vansant, G., Wu, W., Carlo, D.J. and Ill, C.R. (2003). Identification of reciprocally regulated gene modules in regenerating dorsal root ganglion neurons and activated peripheral or central nervous system glia. *J Cell Biochem*, **88**, 970–985.

Carlsson, L., Li, Z., Paulin, D. and Thornell, L.E. (1999). Nestin is expressed during development and in myotendinous and neuromuscular junctions in wild type and desmin knockout mice. *Exp Cell Res*, **251**, 213–223.

Carroll, S.L., Miller, M.L., Frohnert, P.W., Kim, S.S. and Corbett, J.A. (1997). Expression of neuregulins and their putative receptors, erbB2 and erbB3, is induced during Wallerian degeneration. *J Neurosci*, **17**, 1642–1659.

Chen, L. and Ko, C.-P. (1994). Extension of synaptic extracellular matrix during nerve terminal sprouting in living frog neuromuscular junctions. *J Neurosci*, **14**, 796–808.

Chen, L., Folsom, D.B. and Ko, C.-P. (1991). The remodeling of synaptic extracellular matrix and its dynamic relationship with nerve terminals at living frog neuromuscular junctions. *J Neurosci*, **11**, 2920–2930.

Cheng, H.L., Steinway, M.L., Russell, J.W. and Feldman, E.L. (2000). GTPases and phosphatidylinositol 3-kinase are critical for insulin-like growth factor-I-mediated Schwann cell motility. *J Biol Chem*, **275**, 27197–27204.

Cheng, L., Khan, M. and Mudge, A.W. (1995). Calcitonin gene-related peptide promotes Schwann cell proliferation. *J Cell Biol*, **129**, 789–796.

Chiu, D.T. (1999). Autogenous venous nerve conduits. A review. *Hand Clin*, **15**, 667–671.

Cifuentes-Diaz, C., Nicolet, M., Goudou, D., Rieger, F. and Mege, R.M. (1994). *N*-cadherin expression in developing, adult and denervated chicken neuromuscular system: accumulations at both the neuromuscular junction and the node of Ranvier. *Development*, **120**, 1–11.

Clark, M.B., Zeheb, R., White, T.K. and Bunge, R.P. (1991). Schwann cell plasminogen activator is regulated by neurons. *Glia*, **4**, 514–528.

Cohen, J.A., Yachnis, A.T., Arai, M., Davis, J.G. and Scherer, S.S. (1992). Expression of the *neu* proto-oncogene by Schwann cells during peripheral nerve development and Wallerian degeneration. *J Neurosci Res*, **31**, 622–634.

Cook, M.R. and Bishop, D.L. (2004). Structural correlates to synapse reoccupation and axon regeneration at the neuromuscular junction. Society for Neuroscience, Abstract 30, 618.610.

Crang, A.J. and Blakemore, W.F. (1987). Observations on the migratory behaviour of Schwann cells from adult peripheral nerve explant cultures. *J Neurocytol*, **16**, 423–431.

Curtis, R., Stewart, H.J.S., Hall, S.M., Wilkin, G.P., Mirsky, R. and Jessen, K.R. (1992). GAP-43 is expressed by nonmyelin-forming Schwann cells of the peripheral nervous system. *J Cell Biol*, **116**, 1455–1464.

Daniloff, J.K., Levi, G., Grumet, M., Rieger, F. and Edelman, G.M. (1986). Altered expression of neuronal cell adhesion molecules induced by nerve injury and repair. *J Cell Biol*, **103**, 929–945.

Davis, J.B. and Stroobant, P. (1990). Platelet-derived growth factors and fibroblast growth factors are mitogens for rat Schwann cells. *J Cell Biol*, **110**, 1353–1360.

Demestre, M., Wells, G.M., Miller, K.M., Smith, K.J., Hughes, R.A., Gearing, A.J. and Gregson, N.A. (2004). Characterisation of matrix metalloproteinases and the effects of a broad-spectrum inhibitor (BB-1101) in peripheral nerve regeneration. *Neuroscience*, **124**, 767–779.

Dowsing, B.J., Morrison, W.A., Nicola, N.A., Starkey, G.P., Bucci, T. and Kilpatrick, T.J. (1999). Leukemia inhibitory factor is an autocrine survival factor for Schwann cells. *J Neurochem*, **73**, 96–104.

Dubovy, P. and Svizenska, I. (1994). Denervated skeletal muscle stimulates migration of Schwann cells from the distal stump of transected peripheral nerve: an *in vivo* study. *Glia*, **12**, 99–107.

Duchen, L.W. (1971). An electron microscopic study of the changes induced by botulinum toxin in the motor end-plates of slow and fast skeletal muscle fibres of the mouse. *J Neurol Sci*, **14**, 47–60.

Ebens, A., Brose, K., Leonardo, E.D., Hanson, M.G.J., Bladt, F., Birchmeier, C., Barres, B.A. and Tessier-Lavigne, M. (1996). Hepatocyte growth factor/scatter factor is an axonal chemoattractant and a neurotrophic factor for spinal motor neurons. *Neuron* **17**, 1157–1172.

Edds Jr., M.V. (1950). Collateral regeneration of residual motor axons in partially denervated muscles. *J Exp Zool*, **113**, 517–551.

Einheber, S., Hannocks, M.J., Metz, C.N., Rifkin, D.B. and Salzer, J.L. (1995). Transforming growth factor-β 1 regulates axon/Schwann cell interactions. *J Cell Biol*, **129**, 443–458.

Enver, M.K. and Hall, S.M. (1994). Are Schwann cells essential for axonal regeneration into muscle autografts? *Neuropathol Appl Neurobiol*, **20**, 587–598.

Esper, R.M. and Loeb, J.A. (2004). Rapid axoglial signaling mediated by neuregulin and neurotrophic factors. *J Neurosci*, **24**, 6218–6227.

Fallon, J.R. (1985). Neurite guidance by non-neuronal cells in culture: Preferential outgrowth of peripheral neurites on glial as compared to nonglial cell surfaces. *J Neurosci*, **5**, 3169–3177.

Farel, P.B. and Bemelmans, S.E. (1986). Restoration of neuromuscular specificity following ventral rhizotomy in the bullfrog tadpole, Rana catesbeiana. *J Comp Neurol*, **254**, 125–132.

Fawcett, J.W. and Keynes, R.J. (1990). Peripheral nerve regeneration. *Ann Rev Neurosci*, **13**, 43–60.

Feneley, M.R., Fawcett, J.W. and Keynes, R.J. (1991). The role of Schwann cells in the regeneration of peripheral nerve axons through muscle basal lamina grafts. *Exp Neurol*, **114**, 275–285.

Feng, G., Mellor, R.H., Bernstein, M., Keller-Peck, C., Nguyen, Q.T., Wallace, M., Nerbonne, J.M., Lichtman, J.W. and Sanes, J.R. (2000). Imaging neuronal subsets in transgenic mice expressing multiple spectral variants of GFP. *Neuron*, **28**, 41–51.

Fenrich, K. and Gordon, T. (2004). Canadian Association of Neuroscience review: axonal regeneration in the peripheral and central nervous systems – current issues and advances. *Can J Neurol Sci*, **31**, 142–156.

Ferguson, T.A. and Muir, D. (2000). MMP-2 and MMP-9 increase the neurite-promoting potential of Schwann cell basal laminae and are upregulated in degenerated nerve. *Mol Cell Neurosci*, **16**, 157–167.

Froehner, S.C., Murnane, A.A., Tobler, M., Peng, H.B. and Sealock, R. (1987). A postsynaptic Mr 58,000 (58K) protein concentrated at acetylcholine receptor-rich sites in Torpedo electroplaques and skeletal muscle. *J Cell Biol*, **104**, 1633–1646.

Frostick, S.P., Yin, Q. and Kemp, G.J. (1998). Schwann cells, neurotrophic factors, and peripheral nerve regeneration. *Microsurgery*, **18**, 397–405.

Fu, S.Y. and Gordon, T. (1997). The cellular and molecular basis of peripheral nerve regeneration. *Mol Neurobiol*, **14**, 67–116.

Fugleholm, K., Schmalbruch, H. and Krarup, C. (1994). Early peripheral nerve regeneration after crushing, sectioning, and freeze studied by implanted electrodes in the cat. *J Neurosci*, **14**, 2659–2673.

Georgiou, J., Robitaille, R., Trimble, W.S. and Charlton, M.P. (1994). Synaptic regulation of glial protein expression *in vivo*. *Neuron*, **12**, 443–455.

Gorio, A., Carmignoto, G., Finesso, M., Polato, P. and Nunzi, M.G. (1983). Muscle reinnervation-II. Sprouting, synapse formation and repression. *Neuroscience*, **8**, 403–416.

Grinspan, J.B., Marchionni, M.A., Reeves, M., Coulaloglou, M. and Scherer, S.S. (1996). Axonal interactions regulate Schwann cell apoptosis in developing peripheral nerve: neuregulin receptors and the role of neuregulins. *J Neurosci*, **16**, 6107–6118.

Gu, X., Thomas, P.K. and King, R.H. (1995). Chemotropism in nerve regeneration studied in tissue culture. *J Anat*, **186**, 153–163.

Guénard, V., Kleitman, N., Morrissey, T.K., Bunge, R.P. and Asebischer, P. (1992). Syngeneic Schwann cells derived from adult nerves seeded in semipermeable guidance channels enhance peripheral nerve regeneration. *J Neurosci*, **12**, 3310–3320.

Guénard, V., Gwynn, L.A. and Wood, P.M. (1995). Transforming growth factor-beta blocks myelination but not ensheathment of axons by Schwann cells *in vitro*. *J Neurosci*, **15**, 419–428.

Gutmann, E. and Young, J.Z. (1944). The re-innervation of muscle after various periods of atrophy. *J Anat*, **78**, 15–43.

Hall, S. (2001). Nerve repair: a neurobiologist's view. *J Hand Surg (Brit)*, **26**, 129–136.

Hall, S.M. (1986). The effect of inhibiting Schwann cell mitosis on the re-innervation of acellular autografts in the peripheral nervous system of the mouse. *Neuropathol Appl Neurobiol*, **12**, 401–414.

Hall, S.M. (1989). Regeneration in the peripheral nervous system. *Neuropathol Appl Neurobiol*, **15**, 513–529.

Hansson, H.A., Dahlin, L.B., Danielsen, N., Fryklund, L., Nachemson, A.K., Polleryd, P., Rozell, B., Skottner, A., Stemme, S. and Lundborg, G. (1986). Evidence indicating trophic importance of IGF-I in regenerating peripheral nerves. *Acta Physiol Scand*, **126**, 609–614.

Henderson, C.E., Phillips, H.S., Pollock, R.A., Davies, A.M., Lemeulle, C., Armanini, M., Simpson, L.C., Moffet, B., Vandlen, R.A., Koliatsos, V.E. and Rosenthal, A. (1994). GDNF: a potent survival factor for motoneurons present in peripheral nerve and muscle. *Science*, **266**, 1062–1064.

Herrera, A.A., Qiang, H. and Ko, C.P. (2000). The role of perisynaptic Schwann cells in development of neuromuscular junctions in the frog (Xenopus laevis). *J Neurobiol*, **45**, 237–254.

Heumann, R., Korsching, S., Bandtlow, C. and Thoenen, H. (1987). Changes of nerve growth factor synthesis in non-neuronal cells in response to sciatic nerve transection. *J Cell Biol*, **104**, 1623–1631.

Holmes, W. and Young, J.Z. (1942). Nerve regeneration after immediate and delayed suture. *J Anat*, **77**, 63–96.

Horie, H., Kadoya, T., Hikawa, N., Sango, K., Inoue, H., Takeshita, K., Asawa, R., Hiroi, T., Sato, M., Yoshioka, T. and Ishikawa, Y. (2004). Oxidized galectin-1 stimulates macrophages to promote axonal regeneration in peripheral nerves after axotomy. *J Neurosci*, **24**, 1873–1880.

Ide, C. (1996). Peripheral nerve regeneration. *Neurosci Res*, **25**, 101–121.

Ide, C., Tohyama, K., Yokota, R., Nitatori, T. and Onodera, S. (1983). Schwann cell basal lamina and nerve regeneration. *Brain Res*, **288**, 61–75.

Jahromi, B.S., Robitaille, R., Charlton, M.P. (1992). Transmitter release increases intracellular calcium in perisynaptic Schwann cells in situ. *Neuron*, **8**, 1069–1077.

Jansen, J.K., Lømo, T., Nicolaysen, K. and Westgaard, R.H. (1973). Hyperinnervation of skeletal muscle fibers: dependence on muscle activity. *Science*, **181**, 559–561.

Jessen, K.R. and Mirsky, R. (1991). Schwann cell precursors and their development. *Glia*, **4**, 185–194.

Jessen, K.R. and Mirsky, R. (1997). Embryonic Schwann cell development: the biology of Schwann cell precursors and early Schwann cells. *J Anat*, **191**(Pt 4), 501–505.

Jirmanová, I. (1975). Ultrastructure of motor end-plates during pharmacologically-induced degeneration and subsequent regeneration of skeletal muscle. *J Neurocytol*, **4**, 141–155.

Jones, L.L., Oudega, M., Bunge, M.B. and Tuszynski, M.H. (2001). Neurotrophic factors, cellular bridges and gene therapy for spinal cord injury. *J Physiol*, **533**, 83–89.

Kalderon, N. (1979). Migration of Schwann cells and wrapping of neurites *in vitro*: a function of protease activity (plasmin) in the growth medium. *Proc Natl Acad Sci USA*, **76**, 5992–5996.

Kamiguchi, H. and Lemmon, V. (1997). Neural cell adhesion molecule L1: signaling pathways and growth cone motility. *J Neurosci Res*, **49**, 1–8.

Kang, H. and Thompson, W.J. (2002). Schwann cell processes guide axons reinnervating the neuromuscular junction. Society of Neuroscience, Abstract 28, 234.216.

Kang, H., Tian, L. and Thompson, W. (2003). Terminal Schwann cells guide the reinnervation of muscle after nerve injury. *J Neurocytol*, **32**, 975–985.

Kelly, A.M. and Zacks, S.I. (1969). The fine structure of motor endplate morphogenesis. *J Cell Biol*, **42**, 154–169.

Keynes, R.J. (1987). Schwann cells during neural development and regeneration: leaders or followers? *TINS*, **10**, 137–139.

Kioussi, C., Mamalaki, A., Jessen, K., Mirsky, R., Hersh, L.B. and Matsas, R. (1995). Expression of endopeptidase-24.11 (common acute lymphoblastic leukaemia antigen CD10) in the sciatic nerve of the adult rat after lesion and during regeneration. *Eur J Neurosci*, **7**, 951–961.

Kleitman, N., Simon, D.K., Schachner, M. and Bunge, R.P. (1988a). Growth of embryonic retinal neurites elicited by contact with Schwann cell surfaces is blocked by antibodies to L1. *Exp Neurol*, **102**, 298–306.

Kleitman, N., Wood, P., Johnson, M.I. and Bunge, R.P. (1988b). Schwann cell surfaces but not extracellular matrix organized by Schwann cells support neurite outgrowth from embryonic rat retina. *J Neurosci*, **8**, 653–663.

Ko, C.-P. and Chen, L. (1996). Synaptic remodeling revealed by repeated *in vivo* observations and electron microscopy of identified frog neuromuscular junctions. *J Neurosci*, **16**, 1780–1790.

Koirala, S., Qiang, H. and Ko, C.P. (2000). Reciprocal interactions between perisynaptic Schwann cells and regenerating nerve terminals at the frog neuromuscular junction. *J Neurobiol*, **44**, 343–360.

Komiyama, T., Nakao, Y., Toyama, Y., Vacanti, C.A., Vacanti, M.P. and Ignotz, R.A. (2004). Novel technique for peripheral nerve reconstruction in the absence of an artificial conduit. *J Neurosci Methods*, **134**, 133–140.

Kopp, D.M. and Thompson, W.J. (1998). Innervation-dependent expression of nestin at the mammalian neuromuscular junction. Society for Neuroscience, Abstract 24, 1038.

Korneliussen, H. and Jansen, J.K.S. (1976). Morphological aspects of the elimination of polyneuronal innervation of skeletal muscle fibres in newborn rats. *J Neurocytol*, **5**, 591–604.

Korneliussen, H. and Sommerschild, H. (1976). Ultrastructure of the new neuromuscular junctions formed during reinnervation of rat soleus muscle by a "foreign" nerve. *Cell Tiss Res*, **167**, 439–452.

Krasnoselsky, A., Massay, M.J., DeFrances, M.C., Michalopoulos, G., Zarnegar, R. and Ratner, N. (1994). Hepatocyte growth factor is a mitogen for Schwann cells and is present in neurofibromas. *J Neurosci*, **14**, 7284–7290.

Krekoski, C.A., Neubauer, D., Graham, J.B. and Muir, D. (2002). Metalloproteinase-dependent predegeneration *in vitro* enhances axonal regeneration within a cellular peripheral nerve grafts. *J Neurosci*, **22**, 10408–10415.

Krystosek, A., Verrall, S. and Seeds, N.W. (1988). Plasminogen activator secretion in relation to Schwann cell activities. *Int J Dev Neurosci*, **6**, 483–493.

Kubo, T., Yamashita, T., Yamaguchi, A., Hosokawa, K. and Tohyama, M. (2002). Analysis of genes induced in peripheral nerve after axotomy using cDNA microarrays. *J Neurochem*, **82**, 1129–1136.

Kuffler, D.P. (1986). Accurate reinnervation of motor end plates after disruption of sheath cells and muscle fibers. *J Comp Neurol*, **250**, 228–235.

Kugelberg, E., Edström, L. and Abbruzzese, M. (1970). Mapping of motor units in experimentally reinnervated rat muscle: interpretation of histochemical and atrophic fibre patterns in neurogenic lesions. *J Neurol Neurosurg Psychiat*, **33**, 319–329.

La Fleur, M., Underwood, J.L., Rappolee, D.A. and Werb, Z. (1996). Basement membrane and repair of injury to peripheral nerve: defining a potential role for macrophages, matrix metalloproteinases, and tissue inhibitor of metalloproteinases-1. *J Exp Med*, **184**, 2311–2326.

Le, T.B., Aszmann, O., Chen, Y.G., Royall, R.M. and Brushart, T.M. (2001). Effects of pathway and neuronal aging on the specificity of motor axon regeneration. *Exp Neurol*, **167**, 126–132.

Letinsky, M.S., Fischbeck, K.H. and McMahan, U.J. (1976). Precision of reinnervation of original postsynaptic sites in frog muscle after a nerve crush. *J Neurocytol*, **5**, 691–718.

Letourneau, P.C., Shattuck, T.A., Roche, F.K., Takeichi, M. and Lemmon, V. (1990). Nerve growth cone migration onto Schwann cells involves the calcium-dependent adhesion molecule, N-cadherin. *Dev Biol*, **138**, 430–442.

Letourneau, P.C., Roche, F.K., Shattuck, T.A., Lemmon, V. and Takeichi, M. (1991). Interactions of Schwann cells with neurites and with other Schwann cells involve the calcium-dependent adhesion molecule, N-cadherin. *J Neurobiol* **22**, 707–720.

Levi, A.D., Bunge, R.P., Lofgren, J.A., Meima, L., Hefti, F., Nikolics, K. and Sliwkowski, M.X. (1995). The influence of heregulins on human Schwann cell proliferation. *J Neurosci*, **15**, 1329–1340.

Li, Y. and Thompson, W.J. (2004). Terminal Schwann cells extend processes in response to the presence of regenerating muscle fibers. Society for Neuroscience, Abstract 30, 618.611.

Li, Y., Gonzalez, M.I., Meinkoth, J.L., Field, J., Kazanietz, M.G. and Tennekoon, G.I. (2003). Lysophosphatidic acid promotes survival and differentiation of rat Schwann cells. *J Biol Chem*, **278**, 9585–9591.

Lichtman, J.W. and Sanes, J.R. (2003). Watching the neuromuscular junction. *J Neurocytol*, **32**, 767–775.

Lisak, R.P., Bealmear, B., Benjamins, J.A. and Skoff, A.M. (2001). Interferon-gamma, tumor necrosis factor-alpha, and transforming growth factor-beta inhibit cyclic AMP-induced Schwann cell differentiation. *Glia*, **36**, 354–363.

Lobsiger, C.S., Taylor, V. and Suter, U. (2002). The early life of a Schwann cell. *Biol Chem*, **383**, 245–253.

Love, F.M. and Thompson, W.J. (1999). Glial cells promote muscle reinnervation by responding to activity-dependent postsynaptic signals. *J Neurosci*, **19**, 10390–10396.

Lubinska, L. (1961). Sedentary and migratory states of Schwann cells. *Exp Cell Res* (**Suppl. 8**), 74–99.

Lubischer, J.L. and Thompson, W.J. (1999). Neonatal partial denervation results in nodal but not terminal sprouting and a decrease in efficacy of remaining neuromuscular junctions in rat soleus muscle. *J Neurosci*, **19**, 8931–8944.

Macleod, G.T., Dickens, P.A. and Bennett, M.R. (2001). Formation and function of synapses with respect to Schwann cells at the end of motor nerve terminal branches on mature amphibian (Bufo marinus) muscle. *J Neurosci*, **21**, 2380–2392.

Madison, R.D. and Archibald, S.J. (1994). Point sources of Schwann cells result in growth into a nerve entubulation repair site in the absence of axons: effects of freeze-thawing. *Exp Neurol*, **128**, 266–275.

Magrassi, L., Purves, D. and Lichtman, J.W. (1987). Fluorescent probes that stain living nerve terminals. *J Neurosci*, **7**, 1207–1214.

Mahanthappa, N.K., Anton, E.S. and Matthew, W.D. (1996). Glial growth factor 2, a soluble neuregulin, directly increases Schwann cell motility and indirectly promotes neurite outgrowth. *J Neurosci*, **16**, 4673–4683.

Marchionni, M.A., Goodearl, A.D.J., Chen, M.S., Bermingham-McDonogh, O., Kirk, C., Hendricks, M., Danehy, F., Misumi, D., Sudhalter, J., Kobayashi, K., Wroblemski, D., Lynch, C., Baldassare, M., Hiles, I., Davis, J.B., Hsuan, J.J., Totty, N.F., Otsu, M., McBurney, R.N., Waterfield, M.D., Stroobant, P. and Gwynne, D. (1993). Glial growth factors are alternatively spliced erbB2 ligands expressed in the nervous system. *Nature*, **362**, 312–318.

Martini, R. (2001). The effect of myelinating Schwann cells on axons. *Mus Nerve*, **24**, 456–466.

Martini, R. and Schachner, M. (1988). Immunoelectron microscopic localization of neural cell adhesion molecules (L1, N-CAM, and myelin-associated glycoprotein) in regenerating adult mouse sciatic nerve. *J Cell Biol*, **106**, 1735–1746.

Matthews, M.R. and Nelson, V.H. (1975). Detachment of structurally intact nerve endings from chromatolytic neurones of rat superior cervical ganglion during the depression of synaptic transmission induced by post-ganglionic axotomy. *J Physiol*, **245**, 91–135.

McMahan, U.J. (1990). The agrin hypothesis. *Cold Spring Harb Symp Quant Biol*, **55**, 407–418.

McMahan, U.J., Edgington, D.R. and Kuffler, D.P. (1980). Factors that influence regeneration of the neuromuscular junction. *J Exp Biol*, **89**, 31–42.

Mears, S., Schachner, M. and Brushart, T.M. (2003). Antibodies to myelin-associated glycoprotein accelerate preferential motor reinnervation. *J Peripher Nerv Syst*, **8**, 91–99.

Meintanis, S., Thomaidou, D., Jessen, K.R., Mirsky, R. and Matsas, R. (2001). The neuron-glia signal beta-neuregulin promotes Schwann cell motility via the MAPK pathway. *Glia*, **34**, 39–51.

Meyer, M., Matsuoka, I., Wetmore, C., Olson, L. and Thoenen, H. (1992). Enhanced synthesis of brain-derived neurotrophic factor in the lesioned peripheral nerve: different mechanisms are responsible for the regulation of BDNF and NGF mRNA. *J Cell Biol*, **119**, 45–54.

Miledi, R. and Slater, C.R. (1968). Electrophysiology and electron-microscopy of rat neuromuscular junctions after nerve degeneration. *Proc Roy Soc B*, **169**, 289–306.

Miledi, R. and Slater, C.R. (1970). On the degeneration of rat neuromuscular junctions after nerve section. *J Physiol*, **207**, 507–528.

Miner, J.H. and Patton, B.L. (1999). Laminin-11. *Int J Biochem Cell Biol*, **31**, 811–816.

Minghetti, L., Goodearl, A.D., Mistry, K. and Stroobant, P. (1996). Glial growth factors I–III are specific mitogens for glial cells. *J Neurosci Res*, **43**, 684–693.

Moos, M., Tacke, R., Scherer, H., Teplow, D., Fruh, K. and Schachner, M. (1988). Neural adhesion molecule L1 as a member of the immunoglobulin super family with binding domains similar to fibronectin. *Nature*, **334**, 701–703.

Morris, J.K., Lin, W., Hauser, C., Marchuk, Y., Getman, D. and Lee, K.F. (1999). Rescue of the cardiac defect in ErbB2 mutant mice reveals essential roles of ErbB2 in peripheral nervous system development. *Neuron*, **23**, 273–283.

Morrissey, T.K., Levi, A.D., Nuijens, A., Sliwkowski, M.X. and Bunge, R.P. (1995). Axon-induced mitogenesis of human Schwann cells involves heregulin and p185erbB2. *Proc Natl Acad Sci USA*, **92**, 1431–1435.

Nachemson, A.K., Hansson, H.A. and Lundborg, G. (1988). Neurotropism in nerve regeneration: an immunohistochemical study. *Acta Physiol Scand*, **133**, 139–148.

Nadim, W., Anderson, P.N. and Turmaine, M. (1990). The role of Schwann cells and basal lamina tubes in the regeneration of axons through long lengths of freeze-killed nerve grafts. *Neuropathol Appl Neurobiol*, **16**, 411–421.

Neuberger, T.J. and Cornbrooks, C.J. (1989). Transient modulation of Schwann cell antigens after peripheral nerve transection and subsequent regeneration. *J Neurocytol*, **18**, 695–710.

Nguyen, Q.T., Sanes, J.R. and Lichtman, J.W. (2002). Pre-existing pathways promote precise projection patterns. *Nat Neurosci*, **5**, 861–867.

Nieke, J. and Schachner, M. (1985). Expression of the neural cell adhesion molecules L1 and N-CAM and their common carbohydrate epitope L2/HNK-1 during development and after transection of the mouse sciatic nerve. *Differentiation*, **30**, 141–151.

Nishiura, Y., Brandt, J., Nilsson, A., Kanje, M. and Dahlin, L.B. (2004). Addition of cultured Schwann cells to tendon autografts and freeze-thawed muscle grafts improves peripheral nerve regeneration. *Tissue Eng*, **10**, 157–164.

Nitkin, R.M., Wallace, B.G., Spria, M.E., Godfrey, E.W. and McMahan, U.J. (1983). Molecular components of the synaptic basal lamina that direct differentiation of regenerating neuromuscular junctions. *Cold Spring Harb Symp Quant Biol*, **48**, 653–665.

Noakes, P.G., Gautam, M., Mudd, J., Sanes, J.R. and Merlie, J.P. (1995). Aberrant differentiation of neuromuscular junctions in mice lacking s-laminin/laminin β2. *Nature*, **374**, 258–262.

Ogata, T. and Yamasaki, Y. (1985). The three-dimensional structure of motor endplates in different fiber types of rat intercostal muscle. A scanning electron-microscopic study. *Cell Tissue Res*, **241**, 465–472.

O'Malley, J.P., Waran, M.T. and Balice-Gordon, R.J. (1999). *In vivo* observations of terminal Schwann cells at normal, denervated, and reinnervated mouse neuromuscular junctions. *J Neurobiol*, **38**, 270–286.

Osawa, T., Tohyama, K. and Ide, C. (1990). Allogeneic nerve grafts in the rat, with special reference to the role of Schwann cell basal laminae in nerve regeneration. *J Neurocytol*, **19**, 833–849.

Oya, T., Zhao, Y.L., Takagawa, K., Kawaguchi, M., Shirakawa, K., Yamauchi, T. and Sasahara, M. (2002). Platelet-derived growth factor-b expression induced after rat peripheral nerve injuries. *Glia*, **38**, 303–312.

Pan, Y.A., Misgeld, T., Lichtman, J.W. and Sanes, J.R. (2003). Effects of neurotoxic and neuroprotective agents on peripheral nerve regeneration assayed by time-lapse imaging *in vivo*. *J Neurosci*, **23**, 11479–11488.

Paratcha, G., Ledda, F. and Ibanez, C.F. (2003). The neural cell adhesion molecule NCAM is an alternative signaling receptor for GDNF family ligands. *Cell*, **113**, 867–879.

Parmantier, E., Lynn, B., Lawson, D., Turmaine, M., Namini, S.S., Chakrabarti, L., McMahon, A.P., Jessen, K.R. and Mirsky, R. (1999). Schwann cell-derived Desert hedgehog controls the development of peripheral nerve sheaths. *Neuron*, **23**, 713–724.

Patton, B.L., Chiu, A.Y. and Sanes, J.R. (1998). Synaptic laminin prevents glial entry into the synaptic cleft. *Nature*, **393**, 698–701.

Payer, A.F. (1979). An ultrastructural study of Schwann cell response to axonal degeneration. *J Comp Neurol*, **183**, 365–384.

Pellegrino, R.G. and Spencer, P.S. (1985). Schwann cell mitosis in response to regenerating peripheral axons *in vivo*. *Brain Res*, **341**, 16–25.

Pellegrino, R.G., Politis, M.J., Ritchie, J.M. and Spencer, P.S. (1986). Events in degenerating cat peripheral nerve: induction of Schwann cell S phase and its relation to nerve fibre degeneration. *J Neurocytol*, **15**, 17–28.

Peng, H.B., Yang, J.F., Dai, Z., Lee, C.W., Hung, H.W., Feng, Z.H. and Ko, C.P. (2003). Differential effects of neurotrophins and Schwann cell-derived signals on neuronal survival/growth and synaptogenesis. *J Neurosci*, **23**, 5050–5060.

Peters, A. and Muir, A.R. (1959). The relationship between axons and Schwann cells during development of peripheral nerves in the rat. *J Exp Physiol*, **44**, 117–130.

Plantinga, L.C., Verhaagen, J., Edwards, P.M., Hol, E.M., Bar, P.R. and Gispen, W.H. (1993). The expression of B-50/GAP-43 in Schwann cells is upregulated in degenerating peripheral nerve stumps following nerve injury. *Brain Res*, **602**, 69–76.

Politis, M.J., Ederle, K. and Spencer, P.S. (1982). Tropism in nerve regeneration *in vivo*. Attraction of regenerating axons by diffusible factors derived from cells in distal nerve stumps of transected peripheral nerves. *Brain Res*, **253**, 1–12.

Probstmeier, R., Nellen, J., Gloor, S., Wernig, A. and Pesheva, P. (2001). Tenascin-R is expressed by Schwann cells in the peripheral nervous system. *J Neurosci Res*, **64**, 70–78.

Raabe, T.D., Clive, D.R., Neuberger, T.J., Wen, D. and DeVries, G.H. (1996). Cultured neonatal Schwann cells contain and secrete neuregulins. *J Neurosci Res*, **46**, 263–270.

Ramon y Cajal, S. (1906). The structure and connexions of neurons. In: *Nobel Lectures, Physiology or Medicine*, Elsevier, Amsterdam, pp. 1901–1921.

Ramon y Cajal, S. (1928) *Degeneration and Regeneration of the Nervous System* (trans. May, R.M.), Hafner, New York.

Reddy, L.V., Koirala, S., Sugiura, Y., Herrera, A.A. and Ko, C.P. (2003). Glial cells maintain synaptic structure and function and promote development of the neuromuscular junction *in vivo*. *Neuron*, **40**, 563–580.

Reist, N.E. and Smith, S.J. (1992). Neurally evoked calcium transients in terminal Schwann cells at the neuromuscular junction. *Proc Natl Acad Sci USA*, **89**, 7625–7629.

Reynolds, M.L. and Woolf, C.J. (1992). Terminal Schwann cells elaborate extensive processes following denervation of the motor endplate. *J Neurocytol*, **21**, 50–66.

Reynolds, M.L. and Woolf, C.J. (1993). Reciprocal Schwann cell-axon interactions. *Curr Opin Neurobiol*, **3**, 683–693.

Rich, M.M. and Lichtman, J.W. (1989). *In vivo* visualization of pre- and postsynaptic changes during synapse elimination in reinnervated mouse muscle. *J Neurosci*, **9**, 1781–1805.

Rieger, F., Nicolet, M., Pincon-Raymond, M., Murawsky, M., Levi, G. and Edelman, G.M. (1988). Distribution and role in regeneration of N-CAM in the basal laminae of muscle and Schwann cells. *J Cell Biol*, **107**, 707–719.

Riethmacher, D., Sonnenberg-Riethmacher, E., Brinkman, V., Yamaai, T., Lewin, G.R. and Birchmeier, C. (1997). Severe neuropathies in mice with target mutations in the ErbB3 receptor. *Nature*, **389**, 725–730.

Riley, D.A. (1981). Ultrastructural evidence for axon retraction during the spontaneous elimination of polyneuronal innervation of the rat soleus muscle. *J Neurocytol*, **10**, 425–440.

Robbins, N. and Polak, J. (1988). Filopodia, lamellipodia and retractions at mouse neuromuscular junctions. *J Neurocytol*, **17**, 545–561.

Robinson, G.A. and Madison, R.D. (2004). Motor neurons can preferentially reinnervate cutaneous pathways. *Exp Neurol*, **190**, 407–413.

Rogister, B., Delree, P., Leprince, P., Martin, D., Sadzot, C., Malgrange, B., Munaut, C., Rigo, J.M., Lefebvre, P.P., Octave, J.N., et al. (1993). Transforming growth factor beta as a neuronoglial signal during peripheral nervous system response to injury. *J Neurosci Res*, **34**, 32–43.

Rosenbaum, C., Karyala, S., Marchionni, M.A., Kim, H.A., Krasnoselsky, A.L., Happel, B., Isaacs, I., Brackenbury, R. and Ratner, N. (1997). Schwann cells express NDF and SMDF/n-ARIA mRNAs, secrete neuregulin, and show constitutive activation of erbB3 receptors: evidence for a neuregulin autocrine loop. *Exp Neurol*, **148**, 604–615.

Rutkowski, J.L., Tuite, G.F., Lincoln, P.M., Boyer, P.J., Tennekoon, G.I. and Kunkel, S.L. (1999). Signals for proinflammatory cytokine secretion by human Schwann cells. *J Neuroimmunol*, **101**, 47–60.

Saito, A. and Zacks, S.I. (1969). Fine structure of neuromuscular junctions after nerve section and implantation of nerve in denervated muscle. *Exp Mol Pathol*, **10**, 256–273.

Salzer, J.L. (1999). Creating barriers: a new role for Schwann cells and Desert hedgehog. *Neuron*, **23**, 627–629.

Salzer, J.L., Williams, A.K., Glaser, L. and Bunge, R.P. (1980). Studies of Schwann cell proliferation. II. Characterization of the stimulation and specificity of the response to a neurite membrane fraction. *J Cell Biol*, **84**, 753–766.

Sanes, J.R. (1998). Synaptic laminin prevents glial entry into the synaptic cleft. *Nature*, **393**, 698–701.

Sanes, J.R., Schachner, M. and Covault, J. (1986). Expression of several adhesive macromolecules N-CAM, L1, J1, NILE, uvomorulin, laminin, fibronectin, and a heparan sulfate proteoglycan in embryonic, adult, and denervated adult skeletal muscle. *J Cell Biol*, **102**, 420–431.

Scherer, S. (1999). Axonal pathology in demyelinating diseases. *Ann Neurol*, **45**, 6–7.

Scherer, S.S. (1997). The biology and pathobiology of Schwann cells. *Curr Opin Neurol*, **10**, 386–397.

Scherer, S.S. and Easter Jr., S.S. (1984). Degenerative and regenerative changes in the trochlear nerve of goldfish. *J Neurocytol*, **13**, 519–565.

Scherer, S.S. and Salzer, J.L. (1996). Axon–Schwann cell interactions during peripheral nerve degeneration and regeneration. In: *Glial Cell Development* (ed. Richardson, K.R. Ja.W.D.), BIOS Scientific Publishers, Oxford, pp. 165–196.

Schmidt, C.E. and Leach, J.B. (2003). Neural tissue engineering: strategies for repair and regeneration. *Annu Rev Biomed Eng*, **5**, 293–347.

Schwab, M.E. and Thoenen, H. (1985). Dissociated neurons regenerate into sciatic but not optic nerve explants in culture irrespective of neurotrophic factors. *J Neurosci*, **5**, 2415–2423.

Schwann, T. (1839). *Microscopical Researches into the Accordance in the Structure and Growth of Animals and Plants*. Sydenham Society, London.

Schworer, C.M., Masker, K.K., Wood, G.C. and Carey, D.J. (2003). Microarray analysis of gene expression in proliferating Schwann cells: synergistic response of a specific subset of genes to the mitogenic action of heregulin plus forskolin. *J Neurosci Res*, **73**, 456–464.

Seilheimer, B. and Schachner, M. (1988). Studies of adhesion molecules mediating interactions between cells of peripheral nervous system indicate a major role for L1 in mediating sensory neuron growth on Schwann cells in culture. *J Cell Biol*, **107**, 341–351.

Shamash, S., Reichert, F. and Rotshenker, S. (2002). The cytokine network of Wallerian degeneration: tumor necrosis factor-alpha, interleukin-1alpha, and interleukin-1beta. *J Neurosci*, **22**, 3052–3060.

Sketelj, J., Bresjanac, M. and Popovic, M. (1989). Rapid growth of regenerating axons across the segments of sciatic nerve devoid of Schwann cells. *J Neurosci Res*, **24**, 153–162.

Smith, G.V. and Stevenson, J.A. (1988). Peripheral nerve grafts lacking viable Schwann cells fail to support central nervous system axonal regeneration. *Exp Brain Res*, **69**, 299–306.

Son, Y.-J. and Thompson, W.J. (1995a). Schwann cell processes guide regeneration of peripheral axons. *Neuron*, **14**, 125–132.

Son, Y.-J. and Thompson, W.J. (1995b). Nerve sprouting in muscle is induced and guided by processes extended by Schwann cells. *Neuron*, **14**, 133–141.

Speidel, C.C. (1964). *In vivo* studies of myelinated nerve fibers. *Int Rev Cytol*, **16**, 173–231.

Stoll, G. and Muller, H.W. (1999). Nerve injury, axonal degeneration and neural regeneration: basic insights. *Brain Pathol*, **9**, 313–325.

Stoll, G., Griffin, J.W., Li, C.Y. and Trapp, B.D. (1989). Wallerian degeneration in the peripheral nervous system: participation of both Schwann cells and macrophages in myelin degradation. *J Neurocytol*, **18**, 671–683.

Stolz, B., Erulkar, S.D. and Kuffler, D.P. (1991). Macrophages direct process elongation from adult frog motorneurons in culture. *Proc Roy Soc London B*, **244**, 227–231.

Subang, M.C. and Richardson, P.M. (2001). Influence of injury and cytokines on synthesis of monocyte chemoattractant protein-1 mRNA in peripheral nervous tissue. *Eur J Neurosci*, **13**, 521–528.

Syroid, D.E., Maycox, P.R., Burrola, P.G., Liu, N., Wen, D., Lee, K.F., Lemke, G. and Kilpatrick, T.J. (1996). Cell death in the Schwann cell lineage and its regulation by neuregulin. *Proc Natl Acad Sci USA*, **93**, 9229–9234.

Takeda, Y., Asou, H., Murakami, Y., Miura, M., Kobayashi, M. and Uyemura, K. (1996). A nonneuronal isoform of cell adhesion molecule L1: tissue-specific expression and functional analysis. *J Neurochem*, **66**, 2338–2349.

Taniuchi, M., Clark, H.B. and Johnson, E.M. (1986). Induction of nerve growth factor receptor in Schwann cells after axotomy. *PNAS*, **83**, 4094–4098.

Taylor, J.S. and Bampton, E.T. (2004). Factors secreted by Schwann cells stimulate the regeneration of neonatal retinal ganglion cells. *J Anat*, **204**, 25–31.

Taylor, V. and Suter, U. (1997). Molecular biology of axon-glia interactions in the peripheral nervous system. *Prog Nucleic Acid Res Mol Biol*, **56**, 225–256.

Tello, F. (1907). Degeneration et regeneration des plagues motrices. *Travaux du Laboratorire de Recherches Biologiques de l'Universit'e de Madrid*, **5**, 117–149.

Terenghi, G. (1999). Peripheral nerve regeneration and neurotrophic factors. *J Anat*, **194(Pt 1)**, 1–14.

Thomas, P.K. (1966). The cellular response to nerve injury. 1. The cellular outgrowth from the distal stump of transected nerve. *J Anat*, **100**, 287–303.

Thompson, W. and Jansen, J.K.S. (1977). The extent of sprouting of remaining motor units in partly denervated immature and adult rat soleus muscle. *Neuroscience*, **2**, 523–535.

Tian, L. and Thompson, W.J. (2002). Schwann cells induce and guide nerve growth during sprouting in reinnervated soleus muscles *in vivo*. Society for Neuroscience, Abstract 28, 234.214.

Toews, A.D., Barrett, C. and Morell, P. (1998). Monocyte chemoattractant protein 1 is responsible for macrophage recruitment following injury to sciatic nerve. *J Neurosci Res*, **53**, 260–267.

Tofaris, G.K., Patterson, P.H., Jessen, K.R. and Mirsky, R. (2002). Denervated Schwann cells attract macrophages by secretion of leukemia inhibitory factor (LIF) and monocyte chemoattractant protein-1 in a process regulated by interleukin-6 and LIF. *J Neurosci*, **22**, 6696–6703.

Tomaselli, K.J., Reichardt, L.F. and Bixby, J.L. (1986). Distinct molecular interactions mediate neuronal process outgrowth on non-neuronal cell surfaces and extracellular matrices. *J Cell Biol*, **103**, 2659–2672.

Trachtenberg, J.T. and Thompson, W.J. (1996). Schwann cell apoptosis at developing neuromuscular junctions is regulated by glial growth factor. *Nature*, **379**, 174–177.

Tseng, C.Y., Hu, G., Ambron, R.T. and Chiu, D.T. (2003). Histologic analysis of Schwann cell migration and peripheral nerve regeneration in the autogenous venous nerve conduit (AVNC). *J Reconstr Microsurg*, **19**, 331–340.

Ullian, E.M., Harris, B.T., Wu, A., Chan, J.R. and Barres, B.A. (2004). Schwann cells and astrocytes induce synapse formation by spinal motor neurons in culture. *Mol Cell Neurosci*, **25**, 241–251.

Vaittinen, S., Lukka, R., Sahlgren, C., Rantanen, J., Hurme, T., Lendahl, U., Eriksson, J.E. and Kalimo, H. (1999). Specific and innervation-regulated expression of the intermediate filament protein nestin at neuromuscular and myotendinous junctions in skeletal muscle. *Am J Pathol*, **154**, 591–600.

Van Mier, P. and Lichtman, J.W. (1994). Regenerating muscle fibers induce directional sprouting from nearby nerve terminals: Studies in living mice. *J Neurosci*, **14**, 5672–5686.

Walsh, M.K. and Lichtman, J.W. (2003). *In vivo* time-lapse imaging of synaptic takeover associated with naturally occurring synapse elimination. *Neuron*, **37**, 67–73.

Weiner, J.A., Fukushima, N., Contos, J.J., Scherer, S.S. and Chun, J. (2001). Regulation of Schwann cell morphology and adhesion by receptor-mediated lysophosphatidic acid signaling. *J Neurosci*, **21**, 7069–7078.

Welcher, A.A., Suter, U., De-Leon, M., Bitler, C.M. and Shooter, E.M. (1991). Molecular approaches to nerve regeneration. *Philos Trans Roy Soc London Biol*, **331**, 295–301.

Wernig, A., Pécot-Dechavassine, M. and Stöver, H. (1980). Sprouting and regression of the nerve at the frog neuromuscular junction in normal conditions and after prolonged paralysis with curare. *J Neurocytol*, **9**, 277–303.

Wernig, A., Anzil, A.P. and Bieser, A. (1981a). Light and electron microscopic identification of a nerve sprout in muscle of normal adult frog. *Neurosci Lett*, **21**, 261–266.

Wernig, A., Anzil, A.P., Bieser, A. and Schwarz, U. (1981b). Abandoned synaptic sites in muscles of normal adult frog. *Neurosci Lett*, **23**, 105–110.

Wernig, A., Carmody, J.J., Anzil, A.P., Hansert, E., Marciniak, M. and Zucker, H. (1984). Persistence of nerve sprouting with features of synapse remodelling in soleus muscles of adult mice. *Neuroscience*, **11**, 241–253.

Westerfield, M. and Powell, S.L. (1983). Selective reinnervation of limb muscles by regenerating frog motor axons. *Dev Brain Res*, **10**, 301–304.

Williams, L.R., Powell, H.C., Lundborg, G. and Varon, S. (1984). Competence of nerve tissue as distal insert promoting nerve regeneration in a silicone chamber. *Brain Res*, **293**, 201–211.

Williams, L.R., Azzam, N.A., Zalewski, A.A. and Azzam, R.N. (1993). Regenerating axons are not required to induce the formation of a Schwann cell cable in a silicone chamber. *Exp Neurol*, **120**, 49–59.

Woldeyesus, M.T., Britsch, S., Riethmacher, D., Xu, L., Sonnenberg-Riethmacher, E., Abou-Rebyeh, F., Harvey, R., Caroni, P. and Birchmeier, C. (1999). Peripheral nervous system defects in erbB2 mutants following genetic rescue of heart development. *Genes Dev*, **13**, 2538–2548.

Wolpowitz, D., Mason, T.B., Dietrich, P., Mendelsohn, M., Talmage, D.A. and Role, L.W. (2000). Cysteine-rich domain isoforms of the neuregulin-1 gene are required for maintenance of peripheral synapses. *Neuron*, **25**, 79–91.

Wood, P.M. and Bunge, R.P. (1975). Evidence that sensory axons are mitogenic for Schwann cells. *Nature*, **256**, 662–664.

Woolf, C.J., Reynolds, M.L., Chong, M.S., Emson, P., Irwin, N. and Benowitz, L.I. (1992). Denervation of the motor endplate results in the rapid expression by terminal Schwann cells of the growth-associated protein GAP-43. *J Neurosci*, **12**, 3999–4010.

Yamauchi, J., Chan, J.R. and Shooter, E.M. (2003). Neurotrophin 3 activation of TrkC induces Schwann cell migration through the c-Jun N-terminal kinase pathway. *Proc Natl Acad Sci USA*, **100**, 14421–14426.

Yamauchi, J., Chan, J.R. and Shooter, E.M. (2004). Neurotrophins regulate Schwann cell migration by activating divergent signaling pathways dependent on Rho GTPases. *Proc Natl Acad Sci USA*, **101**, 8774–8779.

Yin, X., Kidd, G.J., Pioro, E.P., McDonough, J., Dutta, R., Feltri, M.L., Wrabetz, L., Messing, A., Wyatt, R.M., Balice-Gordon, R.J. and Trapp, B.D. (2004). Dysmyelinated lower motor neurons retract and regenerate dysfunctional synaptic terminals. *J Neurosci*, **24**, 3890–3898.

Zorick, T.S. and Lemke, G. (1996). Schwann cell differentiation. *Curr Opin Cell Biol*, **8**, 870–876.

Zuo, Y., Lubischer, J.L., Kang, H., Tian, L., Mikesh, M., Marks, A., Scofield, V.L., Maika, S., Newman, C., Krieg, P. and Thompson, W.J. (2004). Fluorescent proteins expressed in mouse transgenic lines mark subsets of glia, neurons, macrophages, and dendritic cells for vital examination. *J Neurosci*, **24**, 10999–11009.

28

Transplantation of Schwann cells and olfactory ensheathing cells to promote regeneration in the CNS

Mary Bartlett Bunge and Patrick M. Wood

The Miami Project to Cure Paralysis, University of Miami Miller School of Medicine, Miami, FL, USA

The goal of this chapter is to provide an overview of the efficacy of Schwann cell (SC) and olfactory ensheathing cell (OEC) transplantation to repair the central nervous system (CNS). A transplanted bridge of cells to span the site of injury is a promising strategy to provide a permissive scaffold for axonal growth (reviewed in Bunge, 2001; Geller and Fawcett, 2002). Both cell types have been shown to be effective; both cell types offer advantages. SCs may be easily extricated from peripheral nerve and placed into culture to generate far larger numbers than OECs; they effectively myelinate regenerated fibers or remyelinate denuded axons *in vivo*. Because they do not invade astrocyte territory, they are not as migratory as OECs and additional strategies are needed to lure the regenerated fibers from the SC implant, unlike OECs. OECs are less accessible and are not yet available in large numbers, but they have been demonstrated to be reparative, including improving functional outcome, in certain lesion paradigms. They normally occupy an area of the mammalian CNS that undergoes continuous nerve fiber growth throughout adult life. Repair of the spinal cord receives most attention in this chapter because the constraints on page length and reference number preclude a more inclusive review. SC and OEC transplantation have been compared earlier (Plant et al., 2001b).

28.1 SCs

Rationale for using SCs in spinal cord repair

Normally, SCs are absent from the CNS parenchyma. Because it was known for a long time that axonal regeneration occurred naturally in the peripheral nervous system (PNS), strategies to place the favorable peripheral milieu into the non-regenerating CNS were devised by numerous investigators, starting successfully with Tello (1911). Pieces of degenerating peripheral nerve were inserted into rabbit cerebral cortex that had been deeply cut. In his mentor's words (Ramón y Cajal, 1991), "... the piece of nerve [was] assailed by thick bundles of fibers which [were] in continuity with the axons of the white and gray matter. These newly-formed fibers [converged] from various points of the cortex, as though they were attracted by an irresistible force." This result led Ramón y Cajal (1991) to speculate that CNS axons will regenerate if provided a suitable environment. This suggestion was proven in the early 1980s by the seminal work of the Aguayo group (Richardson et al., 1980; David and Aguayo, 1981), demonstrating that the peripheral nerve environment did, indeed, foster regeneration of axons from neurons in the CNS.

In the mammalian PNS, SCs ensheathe or myelinate all axons. After nerve damage, successfully regenerating axons generally extend into the tubes of SCs that survive within their basal lamina encasement (bands of Bungner). Experiments have shown that it is the SC that is primarily responsible for axonal regeneration (Berry et al., 1988; Smith and Stevenson, 1988; Volume I, Chapter 27). Thus, another strategy has been to transplant purified populations of SCs rather than pieces of peripheral nerve into the CNS to promote repair. When, in the 1970s, techniques to obtain purified populations of these cells in tissue culture became available, Richard Bunge (1975) raised the possibility that these preparations could be constructed into cellular bridges as a type of cellular therapy for the vertebrate, including human, CNS.

Advantages of using SC rather than peripheral nerve implants are: (i) the availability of large numbers of cells after their extraction from peripheral nerve and proliferation in culture, (ii) the lessened complexity of using a homogeneous population of cells without perineurium and extracellular matrix, (iii) the possibility of transducing them with growth-promoting genes while in culture, and (iv) autologous transplantation in humans. A piece of nerve could be removed from a person requiring CNS repair, the SCs then isolated to generate large numbers in culture. Techniques are now available to generate adequate numbers of SCs from adult humans for transplantation (Casella et al., 1996 and references therein).

Many studies have demonstrated that SCs survive in the CNS. Moreover, they function in the CNS to ensheathe or myelinate axons (including long-projecting axons; e.g., Gilmore and Sims, 1993), depending upon axonal diameter. Tissue culture work has shown that SCs support axonal growth from CNS neurons. SCs produce growth factors, express cell adhesion molecules and surface integrins, and generate extracellular matrix components, all known to promote axonal growth. Interestingly, SCs are able to survive in the human spinal cord; it has been known since 1893 that SCs (and accompanying nerve fibers, termed schwannosis) are present in spinal cord lesions (reviewed in Adelman and Aronson, 1972). Schwannosis is observed in 82% of human spinal

cords by 4 months after injury and up to 24 years after injury, the longest period examined (Bruce et al., 2000).

The presence of SC myelin in the CNS is most easily recognized in 1 μm toluidine-blue stained plastic sections (e.g., Bunge et al., 1994; Honmou et al., 1996; Olby and Blakemore, 1996; Li et al., 1999; Lankford et al., 2002). In contrast to oligodendrocyte-generated myelin, the SC nucleus is observed next to the myelin sheath, the SC-myelinated axons are more separated from one another by extracellular matrix, and often the SC-myelin sheaths are grouped into fascicles that may be related to perineurium (Fig. 28.1). In these stained plastic sections, SC myelin is darker than CNS myelin after staining.

Endogenous SC migration into the spinal cord

SCs enter the spinal cord following photochemical, contusion, compression, transection, X-irradiation, or demyelinating lesions (references in Bunge et al., 1994, and below). It is striking that by 6–10 days following a photochemical thrombosis lesion (with no transplantation), fascicles of SCs and axons are visible in the dorsal rim of the cord at the epicenter where tissue may be destroyed (Bunge et al., 1994; Olby and Blakemore, 1996; see also Beattie et al., 1997; Brook et al., 1998). By 10–14 days, the SCs start to myelinate ingrown fibers or remyelinate spared fibers. Over weeks, fascicles of SCs and axons increase dramatically in the lesion area, usually in longitudinal array; these are sometimes associated with perineurium and meningeal cells (Bunge et al., 1994). In two recent studies of moderately contused rat spinal cord (Takami et al., 2002; Pearse et al., 2004), mean counts of 2125 and 1580 SC-myelinated axons, respectively, were found in control non-transplanted animals compared to 5212 and 4540 after SC transplantation.

Localized electrolytic lesions of the rat corticospinal tract (CST) destroy all tissue elements in a small circumscribed area (Li et al., 1999). In a zone of partial damage surrounding this lesion, corticospinal axons become demyelinated and occasional SCs are

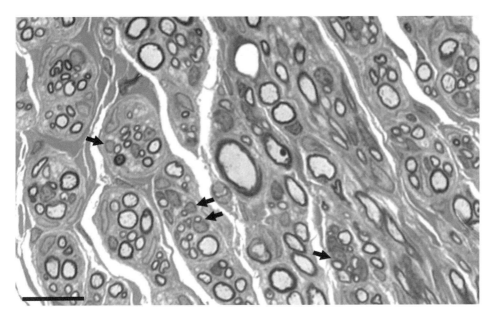

Figure 28.1. This photomicrograph of a 1 μm thick, stained plastic section shows a transverse view of the interior of a bridge similar to the bridges illustrated in Fig. 28.2. Many myelin sheaths, formed by the Schwann cells in the bridge, are shown. A characteristic that enables identification of this myelin as peripheral rather than central is the presence of a Schwann cell nucleus adjacent to the myelin sheath (arrows). Fasciculation of myelinated axons is another clue for identifying peripheral myelin. This Schwann cell-bridge was transplanted into a completely transected adult rat thoracic spinal cord and the recipient animal was maintained for 12 weeks. Bar, 15 μm. (Courtesy of Dr. Lawrence Moon, The Miami Project to Cure Paralysis, Miami, FL, USA).

found along blood vessels and incoming dorsal root fibers. After 3 weeks, large numbers of SCs have accumulated along the lesion track, and have infiltrated only the white matter of this penumbra region, where they remyelinate the demyelinated axons.

Normally, there is a sharp transition between SCs in the root and oligodendrocytes and astrocytes at the point of entry of axons into the spinal cord; here the astrocytes in combination with basal lamina form an impenetrable barrier to SCs, the glia limitans. After damage, there is a clear association of loss of astrocytes constituting the glia limitans, the presence of demyelinated axons once myelinated by oligodendrocytes, and SC remyelination of CNS axons (reviewed in Franklin and Blakemore, 1993). SCs enter cord parenchyma from the dorsal roots, from the subarachnoid space via gaps in the glia limitans or in association with blood vessels, or from nerves accompanying the parenchymal vasculature. Many

studies have observed invading SCs in the dorsal cord, close to or in apparent continuity with dorsal roots (e.g., reviewed in Blight and Young, 1989; Franklin and Blakemore, 1993; Bunge et al., 1994; Beattie et al., 1997; Gilmore and Sims, 1997; Brook et al., 1998; Li et al., 1999; Bruce et al., 2000). Consequently, invading SCs usually are present in the dorsal but not the ventral cord. SC ingress may be prevented ventrally by a more complex glia limitans barrier at the ventral roots than at the dorsal roots (Sims et al., 1985).

A valuable model to study SC ingress is irradiation of the neonatal rat spinal cord which leads to loss of oligodendrocytes and astrocytes, reducing central myelination and causing loss of barrier function of the glia limitans (reviewed in Gilmore and Sims, 1997). By 3 weeks following irradiation, SCs first appear in the dorsal funiculi near the dorsal root entry zone and then, at a distance from the roots or regions of SCs in the cord, migrating through radiation-induced gaps in the dorsal glial limitans or entering in association with the blood vessels penetrating the dorsal surface of the cord. Despite the initial loss of glia throughout the cord, SCs do not appear in ventral white matter at this time. The discontinuities in the dorsal surface glia limitans are not seen ventrally, correlating with SC entry only dorsally (Sims et al., 1998).

However, 2 months after irradiation SCs begin to appear in the ventral cord, in a different distribution than dorsally. Occurring principally in the gray matter, they do not enter from ventral roots, but are associated with blood vessels that are devoid of their usual astrocytic covering. In all likelihood the SCs are entering the cord by migration along blood vessels (such as the ventral spinal artery) that penetrate the cord surface (Sims et al., 1998). The Virchow-Robinson spaces, lined by astrocytic processes and surrounding the large arteries entering the spinal cord, have been considered conduits for SC migration following transplantation (Baron-Van Evercooren et al., 1996). In the studies of human spinal cord injury (SCI) cited above (Adelman and Aronson, 1972), schwannosis occurs predominantly in association with intramedullary branches of the anterior spinal artery. SCs are observed near parenchymal blood vessels in many studies (e.g., Baron-Van Evercooren et al., 1993; 1996; Brook et al., 1993; 1994; reviewed in Franklin and Blakemore, 1993; Bunge et al., 1994; Li et al., 1999; Bruce et al., 2000).

SC invasion usually occurs when axons which should or could be myelinated by oligodendrocytes are present (Franklin and Blakemore, 1993). In localized electrolytic lesions of the CST, SCs enter not the primary lesion, but only the partially damaged penumbra where demyelinated axons are extant (Li et al., 1999). That SCs migrate towards an area of demyelination is seen frequently (e.g., Blakemore, 1976; Baron-Van Evercooren et al., 1993; 1996). Possible diffusible chemotactic signals released by demyelinated axons have not yet been identified.

Normal intact white matter tracts generally are not a favorable migratory substratum for SC migration. Areas of demyelination do not attract significant numbers of SCs when they are implanted into

normal white matter a few millimeters from the demyelinated zone (Iwashita and Blakemore, 2000). On the basis of many studies, an apparent cause is the presence of astrocytes and their associated basement membrane (e.g., Blakemore, 1976). When axons are demyelinated in the myelin deficient rat due to oligodendrocyte degeneration, astrocytes are present (contributing to an intact glia limitans) and SCs do not invade the cord. If astrocytes are no longer present after irradiation of this animal, however, SCs enter the cord and myelinate the demyelinated axons (Duncan et al., 1988). In human spinal cord lesions, the degree of schwannosis is inversely related to the extent of astrogliosis (Bruce et al., 2000).

28.2 SCs remyelinate axons and restore conduction

Remyelination of CNS axons by SCs has been observed in many studies of experimentally induced and naturally occurring pathologic processes (see Blakemore, 1976; Duncan et al., 1981; Blight and Young, 1989; Honmou et al., 1996 for references). Axons are remyelinated by either endogenous SCs that have migrated into the demyelinated site, as described in the previous section, or by transplanted SCs. Cultured SCs from a wide range of donor ages and prepared by many different procedures lead to relatively extensive remyelination of CNS axons when transplanted into areas of demyelination.

Studies have been done to determine if remyelination by *host* SCs restores axonal conduction after demyelination. The extent of SC remyelination is related to the severity of a contusion lesion, as assessed by the extent of axon loss; when only 4% of the original population of axons (~10,000 axons) in the dorsal cord survive, essentially all axons in the dorsal columns are remyelinated by SCs (Blight and Young, 1989). By 30 min after contusion, cortical somatosensory evoked potentials (CSEPs) from hindlimb (tibial nerve) stimulation vanish. By 3 weeks, when remyelination is well advanced, near normal CSEPs are again found (despite the survival of only 6800 myelinated axons dorsally in one case). Thus, endogenous SCs can restore conduction in the mammalian spinal cord sensory pathways (Blight and Young, 1989). Near normal conduction through an ethidium bromide-induced demyelinating lesion in the dorsal columns also returns following endogenous SC remyelination in the rat (Felts and Smith, 1992).

SC transplantation experiments to achieve remyelination began by applying teased crushed peripheral nerve on areas of the rat or cat spinal cord demyelinated by a combination of X-irradiation (to prevent endogenous SC or oligodendrocyte remyelination) and lysolecithin (to induce demyelination); remyelination occurred only when a source of SCs was provided (Blakemore, 1977; see also Harrison, 1980). The first transplantation experiments with purified populations of rat SCs generated in tissue culture were reported in 1981 (Duncan et al., 1981). Remyelination was evident 2–18 weeks after injection of SCs into lysolecithin-demyelinated mouse dorsal columns. That the transplanted SCs formed the myelin was proven by their rejection upon removal of immune suppression. Thus, SCs prepared *in vitro* retain their potential to form myelin in the CNS and, moreover, are capable of myelinating central axons of a xenogenic host.

Restoration of conduction properties has been studied following remyelination by *transplanted* SCs. Demyelination and prevention of prompt host myelinating cell invasion are achieved by using the X-irradiation/ethidium bromide strategy (Honmou et al., 1996); the dorsal columns remain glial cell-free for 5–6 weeks. If cultured SC suspensions are injected at 3 days after ethidium bromide treatment, the demyelinated axons are remyelinated 3–4 weeks later. Whereas the demyelinated axons exhibit conduction slowing and block and reduced ability to follow high-frequency stimulation, SC remyelination leads to restoration of near normal conduction properties. Thus, transplanted SCs repair functional deficits caused by demyelination in the adult mammalian CNS. Another role of SCs is thereby implied, that of causing nodal clustering of Na+ channels that is essential for normal conduction (Honmou et al., 1996).

28.3 SCs integrate into spinal cord structure

Limited suspensions of about 10,000 cultured SCs may be introduced into spinal cord white matter tracts by a minimally traumatic air pressure microinjection technique that severs a small number of axons, but prevents distortion of the tract (Li and Raisman, 1997). In this paradigm, prominent blood vessels radiating from the transplant are accompanied by SCs that disperse from these perivascular spaces and the transplant to insert themselves into the CST in strict rostrocaudal alignment where they myelinate the axons (Li and Raisman, 1997). The introduction of SCs engenders an astrocytic response, but the longitudinal astrocyte alignment along the CST is normal and does not impede SC migration; the transplanted SCs appear to be able to counteract the disruptive effects of the lesion on the glial alignment in the tract (Li and Raisman, 1997). Thus, this microtransplantation technique leads to the formation of a mosaic of peripheral and central tissue in which the complex and regular host glial arrangement is retained.

28.4 SCs induce axonal branching and terminal arborizations

Using the microtransplantation technique mentioned above to minimize disturbance of the tract architecture, cultured SCs placed into either the cervical corticospinal or ascending dorsal column tracts cause sprouting of both types of axons by 2 days (Li and Raisman, 1994). Both severed and neighboring uncut axons branch and extend for considerable distances and, when the fibers enter SC territory, form arborizations with small bouton-like expansions.

28.5 SCs direct axonal growth

When SCs are deposited in the thalamus in a 4 mm-long column from a micropipette, they induce aligned axon growth into these columns (Brook et al., 1994).

Axons extend in the columns through the thalamus and the dorsal surface of the thalamus, across the extracellular space of the choroid fissure, and into the brain by penetrating the ventral pial surface of the hippocampus (Brook et al., 1994). Because this is not a normal trajectory, it is clear that the SCs not only induce axonal growth, but also guide this growth from one area to another. The SCs used in this study were of adult rat nerve origin, relevant to future clinical potential. When SCs are deposited as a trail into the caudal stump of a completely transected rat spinal cord, the axons that regenerate across the transection site and enter the caudal stump are tightly bundled as they extend along the length of the trail, not leaving the confines of the trail (Menei et al., 1998).

28.6 SC transplants promote axonal regeneration

SCs prepared in culture began to be tested in *in vivo* CNS injury paradigms in the early 1980s. At 1 week after compression injury in the adult cat cord, an autologous predegenerated piece of nerve was placed into the injury site followed by SCs cultured from adult cat ganglia at either end of the nerve (Wrathall et al., 1982). By 7 days, SC-ensheathed axons bridge the interface and also are observed 1–2 mm into rostral stumps and nerve grafts. Animals receiving only nerve had not reached this stage at 14 days. Thus, the addition of SCs hastens the elongation of axons into the nerve graft.

A few years later, a study reported that, within 14 days of transplantation, cultured SCs in association with their extracellular matrix and the supporting collagen substratum on which they were prepared, promote regeneration of cholinergic axons from the host septum, across a 2–3 mm gap, and into the denervated hippocampus (Kromer and Cornbrooks, 1985). The regrowing fibers traverse the lesion in close association with the cell layer on the collagen strip. Cultured acellular collagen substratum does not support axonal regrowth. These two types of grafts had been positioned in the adult rat intracephalic cavity to bridge the gap between the lesioned surfaces of the septum and hippocampus.

The efficacy of SC transplantation to repair the spinal cord has been tested in a number of lesion models: photochemical, compression, contusion, dorsal hemisection, lateral hemisection, and complete transection. Transplantation of limited numbers of SCs into highly focal lesions has been discussed above. When SCs are injected into a cavity created by an inflatable balloon, the cells survive better when implanted immediately or at 10 days than at 3 days (Martin et al., 1991; 1996). The gliotic reaction is less with immediate injections. The grafts contain numerous axons, mainly sensory from nearby dorsal roots; corticospinal and monoaminergic fibers are not detectable. Purified populations of SCs also have been placed into dorsal cavities created by photochemical lesioning in adult rat cord. The cells were transplanted inside a spiraled roll of the collagen substratum on which the SCs were cultured (Paino and Bunge 1991; Paino et al., 1994). There is a robust response; thousands of axons enter the rolls and are related to the SCs. Acellular collagen rolls do not contain axons.

More recently, SCs have been injected into thoracic contusion sites (that develop into cavities) a week after injury (Takami et al., 2002) by the multicenter animal spinal cord injury study (MASCIS) Impactor (Young, 2002). It is important to study contusion injury due to its relevance to human SCI, although it is difficult to distinguish between spared and sprouting fibers and regenerated fibers after repair. SCs in this contusion study and in the complete transection paradigm (see below) are prepared from adult animals for clinical relevance. Prefatory work with OECs indicated that transplantation is more effective at 7 days rather than at the time of contusion and that grafting in fluid medium is better than in a fibrin matrix (Plant et al., 2003); because a comparison of SC and OEC transplantation was planned, it was decided to transplant SCs as well as OECs at 7 days after contusion in medium. (The OEC results are presented in the OEC section below.) After injection of two million SCs into the contusion site (Takami et al., 2002), at 12 weeks there is diminished cavitation, reduced injury-induced tissue loss, more than twice as many myelinated axons (predominantly in longitudinal array) in the SC transplant compared to an injection of medium, significant axonal sparing and/or regeneration of spinal and supraspinal axons, and a modest, though significant, improvement in gross locomotor behavior as assessed by the BBB rating scale (Basso et al., 1995).

Bridges of purified SCs (3 to 5 mm long) unite completely transected adult rat thoracic spinal cord stumps (see Fig. 28.2); fibers grow from both stumps onto the bridge (Xu et al., 1997). A complete transection model is valuable because the recognition of regenerated fibers beyond the transection is unambiguous. The SCs in matrigel, a commercial preparation of basal lamina components, are confined inside a polymer channel into which each cord stump is inserted. The channel reduces invasion of scar tissue and leads to a more parallel array of ingrowing nerve fibers (Guest et al., 1997). Both rat and human SC implants promote axonal regeneration (Xu et al., 1995a; 1997; Guest et al., 1997). With rat SCs, spinal neurons as far away as levels C3 and S4 extend descending and ascending fibers onto the bridge; myelinated axons and eight times more unmyelinated, but ensheathed, axons are present, primarily from spinal cord and sensory neurons (Xu et al., 1997). Electrical stimulation of axons in these bridges produces measurable evoked responses (Pinzon et al., 2001). In this SC bridge/transection paradigm there is little growth from brain stem neurons, and regenerated fibers on the bridge do not exit to enter the spinal cord (Xu et al., 1997). These findings have spurred the development of combination strategies to be described below.

One reason that axons fail to leave SC grafts may be due to a gauntlet of chondroitin sulfate proteoglycan (CSPG) at the caudal SC graft/host cord interface (Plant et al., 2001a). CSPGs, upregulated in CNS injury, have been implicated in failure of neurite growth in many *in vitro* and *in vivo* studies (reviewed in Fawcett and Asher, 1999; Silver and Miller, 2004). The intraparenchymal infusion of an enzyme, chondroitinase ABC, to digest CSPGs near the caudal SC graft/host spinal cord interface enables substantially more axons to leave the SC bridge (Chau et al., 2003).

Polymer channels containing rat SCs, but only half the diameter of the spinal cord to fit into a lateral hemisection lesion, foster axonal regeneration (Xu et al., 1999). A mean of 1000 myelinated axons and nine times more unmyelinated axons are found in this "hemi-bridge," comparable to the work with SC-filled channels bridging a complete transection (Xu et al., 1997). But, besides propriospinal and sensory axons, neurons from a number of brain stem regions extend fibers into the SC hemi-bridge. Moreover, some regenerating axons leave the graft to extend into the caudal spinal cord as far as 3.5 mm. These axons grow toward the gray matter, where they form bouton-like structures (Xu et al., 1999). This improved response compared to SC bridges spanning a complete transection, may result, at least in part, from restoration of cerebrospinal fluid circulation and relatively more stable graft/cord interfaces due to the more limited laminectomy than that required for the complete transection/SC bridge model. SC-filled polycarbonate channels placed into the dorsal spinal cord elicit ingrowth of fascicles of SC-myelinated and ensheathed axons as well (Montgomery et al., 1996).

The provision of neurotrophic factors in combination with SC bridges improves the regenerative response. The infusion of brain derived neurotrophic factor (BDNF) and NT-3 into the cord beyond the graft/host cord interface in the hemi-channel paradigm does not significantly increase the number of myelinated axons in the SC bridge, but more axons penetrate the interface and grow as much as 6 mm in the spinal cord beyond (Bamber et al., 2001). In the caudal cord, the axons extend preferentially towards and in gray matter. When glial cell line-derived neurotrophic factor (GDNF) is added to the SC/matrigel bridge in this hemi-channel model, propriospinal axon regeneration is promoted eight-fold, myelin formation is enhanced six-fold, and the graft/host interfaces are improved in that reactive gliosis, infiltration of macrophages, and cavitation are diminished (Iannotti et al., 2003).

The efficacy of BDNF and NT-3 has also been tested in the complete transection/SC transplantation model. The two neurotrophins were delivered together into the channel for 14 days after transplantation; the animals were maintained for another 14 days (Xu et al., 1995b). One month later, the myelinated axon number in the graft is doubled

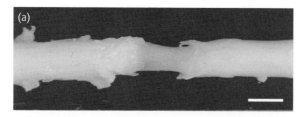

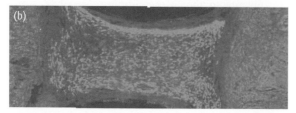

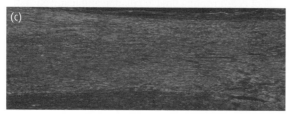

Figure 28.2. These panels illustrate a SC bridge inserted into a completely transected adult thoracic spinal cord. A 4 mm long SC/fibrin bridge was implanted a week before obtaining the picture in panel a. The SC/fibrin implant bridges the rostral (right) and caudal (left) spinal cord stumps. Panel b, horizontal paraffin section demonstrating by immunohistochemistry the presence of S100-positive SCs within the bridge a week after implantation. Panel c, a section stained at 4 weeks with an antibody that recognizes neurofilaments, showing the abundant presence of axons within the SC bridge at 8 weeks after implantation. Subsequent evaluation revealed that approximately 3000 axons were myelinated by SCs in the middle of the bridge, and the estimated total number of myelinated and unmyelinated axons in the bridge was 20,000. Bar represents 2 mm in a, 800 μm in (b), and 250 μm in (c). (Courtesy of Dr. Martin Oudega, The Miami Project to Cure Paralysis, Miami, FL, USA.)

and the number of neuronal somata that extended axons onto the bridge is tripled. There is another important difference from the SC implant alone. There are axons in the graft from brain stem neurons, distant from the thoracic implant. Thus, regeneration of some neuronal populations distant from the injury/ implant site can be elicited by a combination of trophic factors and a favorable cellular substrate. Not all growth factors, however, exhibit the same effect in this transection/SC paradigm. The provision of neurotrophic factors, IGF-1 and platelet-derived growth factor (PDGF), mixed initially into the SC transplant, does not promote axonal regeneration onto the bridge. With these factors, axonal regrowth into the transplant is diminished by up to 63% although SC myelination of ingrowing axons is promoted (Oudega et al., 1997).

SCs have been genetically modified to deliver the neurotrophins, nerve growth factor (NGF), BDNF, and NT-3. When SCs are thus prepared to provide high levels of NGF in a cord not damaged other than

that occurring during the transplantation procedure, the transplants are more densely penetrated by sensory nociceptive axons from the dorsolateral fasiculus than after non-transduced SC transplantation (Tuszynski et al., 1998). Over time, the SC grafts also contain coeruleospinal axons, unlike control SC grafts. The expression of the NGF transgene is observed for at least six months (Tuszynski et al., 1998). In a subsequent study, rats received a dorsal hemisection lesion before receiving transplants of transduced, again for NGF, or non-transduced SC grafts (Weidner et al., 1999). This type of lesion interrupted many descending tracts. Again, overexpression of NGF robustly increases axonal growth. Compared with non-transduced SC implants, the numbers of coeruleospinal and sensory axons increase 90-fold and 20-fold, respectively, in transduced cell grafts. Moreover, SCs appropriately remyelinate coeruleospinal axons and appropriately ensheathe the nociceptive sensory axons extending into grafts, mirroring the normal situation *in vivo*. A difference between NGF-producing fibroblast and

NGF-producing SC transplants is not in the degree of ingrowth of axons, but in the lack of orientation of axons into linear bundles in fibroblast grafts.

SCs have also been transduced to carry the human BDNF gene and secrete higher than normal amounts of the neurotrophin (Menei et al., 1998). Untreated or transduced SCs were transplanted into a complete transection site and also as a 5 mm long trail that extended into the caudal stump. The trails remain largely intact for at least a month, the duration of the experiment, and axons are found in close alignment with the trail. When the animals with engineered SCs are compared with those receiving untreated SCs, more serotonergic and some adrenergic axons reach the end of the trail beyond the transection site. Tracing also provided evidence that reticulospinal and raphespinal fibers cross the transection site and grow the length of the trail. No such evidence is found when the animals do not receive SCs. In sum, when SCs are transplanted with the capacity to provide augmented levels of neurotrophins, axonal regeneration is substantially improved.

SC bridges have been tested with other strategies to improve repair after SCI. Combining the complete transection/SC bridge model with intravenous administration of methylprednisolone, a number of improvements are seen compared to animals in which only SCs are transplanted: more cord stump tissue inserted into the polymer channel survives, scar formation at the graft/host interface is lessened, myelinated axons in the bridge are nearly doubled, the number of cord neurons extending axons onto the bridge doubles, and axons from brain stem neurons regenerate onto the bridge (Chen et al., 1996; Bunge, 2001). In addition, there is modest fiber growth into the distal cord from the bridge. This is significant because when peripheral nerve is inserted at the same level as the SC bridge, a brain stem neuronal response is not observed in contrast to insertion at the high cervical level (Richardson et al., 1984). Thus, the administration of methylprednisolone overcomes, to some degree, the distance between graft and brain stem. Another combination strategy involved the transplantation of OECs into the stumps beside the SC bridge after complete transection

(Ramón-Cueto et al., 1998). This study is described in the OEC section below.

In very recent work, the elevation of cyclic adenosine monophosphate (AMP) in combination with SC implantation into contusion injury has led to substantial repair (Pearse et al., 2004). The best results were obtained with the triple combination of SC implantation, a one-time injection of dibutyryl-cyclic AMP fore and aft of the transplant, and a 2-week subcutaneous infusion of a phosphodiesterase 4 inhibitor (to prevent the breakdown of cyclic AMP). The use of both injection and subcutaneous infusion prevents a drop in the cyclic AMP levels in the cord and brain stem that occurs after this injury, then increases levels above uninjured controls. With the triple combination, lateral white matter sparing is improved by 230%, the number of myelinated axons in grafts is increased by 500%, serotonergic fibers grow into the SC graft and also beyond, and more fibers from the reticular formation and red and raphe nuclei are present below the injury/transplant site. In addition, a number of functional tests show that the BBB rating scale is improved by 4.5 points, there are significantly fewer footfall errors on a gridwalk, base of support is improved, and foot exorotation is more normal as determined by footprint analysis (Pearse et al., 2004).

28.7 OECs

Rationale for using OECs in CNS repair

The mammalian olfactory epithelium and the axon tracts projecting from the epithelium to the olfactory bulb undergo continuous renewal throughout life. If axons are severed along the olfactory tract, the injured neurons die rather than regenerate and are replaced by new neurons (Monti Graziadei and Graziadei, 1979; Graziadei and Monti Graziadei, 1980; Doucette et al., 1983; Calof and Chikaraisha, 1989) that project their axons through channels formed by OECs (Doucette, 1984). The new axons are ensheathed by OECs as they cross the meningeal boundary of the olfactory bulb, grow through the nerve fiber layer and arrive at target sites in individual glomeruli within the olfactory bulb (Barber and Lindsay, 1982; Raisman, 1985; Doucette, 1991). Remarkably, following olfactory neuron-induced death and ensuing axonal degeneration, OECs do not appear to proliferate but retain the configuration that their processes manifest before injury (Fig. 28.3, Williams et al., 2004). These very recent findings indicate that preformed OEC pathways survive after injury and guide and support the growth of new replacement axons. The ability of the new olfactory axons to grow into regions containing astrocytes suggests that OECs might possess special properties that would promote regeneration of axons in other parts of the CNS as well (Raisman, 1985; Ramón-Cueto and Nieto-Sampedro, 1992).

Is it actually true that OECs enable olfactory axons to grow into regions of the bulb containing astrocytes? The available evidence indicates that new olfactory axons may have very few encounters with astrocyte processes en route to their targets in the glomeruli. After entering the bulb, the axons run parallel to the surface in a region where most of the cells are OECs (Barber and Lindsay, 1982; Doucette, 1991; Valverde and Lopez-Mascaraque, 1991; Franceschini and Barnett, 1996; Au et al., 2002). Both OEC and astrocyte processes may contribute to the glia limitans (Doucette, 1984; 1991; Raisman, 1985) but, at the region where the olfactory nerve rootlets merge with the nerve fiber layer, the glia limitans is formed almost exclusively by OECs, with a relatively minor contribution by astrocytes (Doucette, 1991). Immunocytochemical studies show that glial fibrillary acidic protein (GFAP) is much more intense in the glomerular layer of the bulb than in the nerve fiber layer (Barber and Lindsay, 1982; Franceschini and Barnett, 1996; Au et al., 2002). This evidence suggests that, contrary to the prevailing view, intermingling of OECs and astrocytes is limited and that there is little interaction of new axons with astrocyte processes until they arrive in the vicinity of the glomeruli.

Does the presence of OECs moderate the formation of an astroglial scar in the olfactory bulb, thereby allowing entry of new axons? After axotomy of the nerve fiber layer, the lesion site contains reactive astrocytes and microglia, despite the presence of OECs (Doucette et al., 1983). Both electron microscopic (EM) observations and anterograde tracing indicate that new axons grow around, not through, lesions in the bulb, in contrast to orderly growth through nerve lesions at the cribiform plate (Monti Graziadei and Graziadei, 1979; Graziadei and Monti Graziadei, 1980; Doucette et al., 1983). Thus, the presence of OECs may not necessarily ensure axonal or glial penetration of an astrocytic scar.

Recent studies, however, have suggested that OECs may interact with astrocytes more favorably than SCs. OECs, but not SCs, when confronted with a co-cultured astrocyte monolayer, migrate freely into the area containing astrocytes (Lakatos et al., 2000). Also in contrast to SCs, OECs induce less astrocyte hypertrophy and immunoreactivity with GFAP and CSPG antibodies. In agreement with these results, the injection of OECs into uninjured spinal cord tissue results in less GFAP immunoreactivity than observed with SCs (Lakatos et al., 2003a). But can transplanted OECs actually reduce astrogliosis after injury? This may depend on injury severity. Reduced GFAP immunostaining intensity is observed in OEC-transplanted rats after photochemical (Verdu et al., 2001) or contusion (Takami et al., 2002) injury but not after complete cord transection (Ramón-Cueto et al., 1998; 2000). The facile migration of OECs within non-permissive astrocyte populations and the tempering of astrocyte hyper-reactivity, would be expected to promote axonal regeneration through the non-permissive terrain surrounding a lesion but verification of these properties by quantitative biochemical methods, and in different injury environments, is still needed to establish their general validity.

28.8 Are OECs a single cell type or a mixture of cell types?

An important determinant of the success of transplanted OECs in promoting repair may be the cellular composition of the OEC preparation. Cultures derived from either olfactory nerves (i.e. the lamina propria) or olfactory bulb contain cells exhibiting

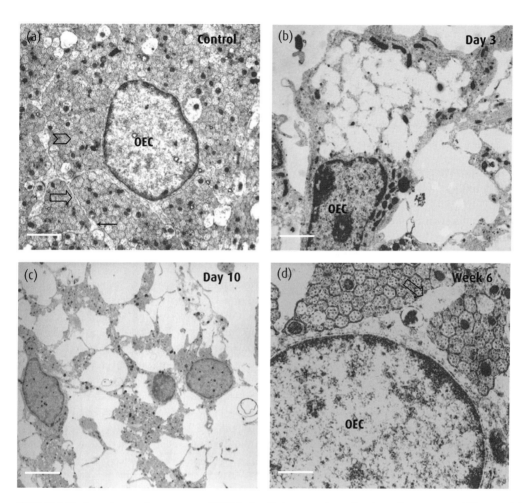

Figure 28.3. Electron microscopic appearance of OECs in the olfactory nerve layer after zinc sulfate treatment. (a) In control tissue, OECs were visible throughout the olfactory nerve layer and had a characteristic appearance of medium electron density, slightly clumpy chromatin beneath the nuclear envelope, and scattered intermediate filaments. Individual OECs extended thin cytoplasmic processes around bundles of the small-diameter axons of the olfactory neurons. (arrow, OEC process; arrowhead, olfactory receptor axon) (b) By day 3, axons exhibited signs of degeneration, and many had disappeared, but OECs remained in position with their processes seemingly retaining their original configuration. (c) Ten days after treatment, all evidence of olfactory receptor axons had gone, leaving a lattice of OEC processes, defining areas where the axons had been. (d) Six weeks after treatment, the compact arrangement of olfactory receptor axons had returned, and they were once again visible in a characteristic honeycomb configuration ensheathed by OEC processes. Scale bars, 1 μm in (a); 1.5 μm in (b); 2.7 μm in (c); 0.5 μm in (d). Figure 28.3 is taken from "Response of OECs to the Degeneration and Regeneration of the Peripheral Olfactory System and the Involvement of Neuregulins," by Sarah K. Williams, Robin J. Franklin and Susan C. Barnett, *J. Comp. Neurol*, **170**, 50–62 (2004). This figure is reprinted with permission from the authors and from Wiley-Liss, Inc., a subsidiary of John Wiley and Sons, Inc.

a flat, polygonal astrocyte-like ("A cells") morphology as well as cells exhibiting SC-like ("S cells") morphology (Barber and Lindsay, 1982; Pixley, 1992; Franceschini and Barnett, 1996; Li et al., 1997; Au and Roskams, 2003). Recently, it has been suggested that A cells, which also express fibronectin (a protein generally considered to be a fibroblast marker), are actually fibroblasts (Li et al., 2003). Fibroblasts are not resident within the olfactory bulb, but could derive from residual fragments of the olfactory bulb meninges or nerve rootlets, which are usually stripped off during bulb dissection. The presence of variable proportions of A cells and S cells in a transplant population could lead to differing outcomes following transplantation (see Lakatos et al., 2003a,b).

28.9 OECs promote regeneration of injured CNS axons

Enthusiasm for the strategy of OEC transplantation into the injured CNS was generated by an early experiment in which purified OECs, pre-labeled with a nuclear dye (Hoechst) were injected into the spinal cord at the dorsal root entry zone following transection of the dorsal root (Ramón-Cueto and Nieto-Sampedro, 1994). All animals receiving OECs, but not controls, exhibited regeneration of axons across the dorsal root entry zone and into the contra-lateral dorsal horn. Hoechst positive cells, assumed to be the transplanted OECs, were observed along the pathway of regeneration. In a similar injury model, the transplantation of frozen and thawed OECs led to recovery of spinal H-wave and withdrawal reflexes (Navarro et al., 1999). In more recent studies, however, enhanced regrowth of axons following transection of dorsal roots and transplantation of Hoechst- labeled OECs into either the dorsal root or the dorsal horn was not found (Gomez et al., 2003; Barnett and Riddell, 2004).

Improved regeneration of injured CST axons and improved performance in a test of forelimb function following transplantation of adult OECs has been reported (Li et al., 1997; 1998). The OECs, including both S cells and fibronectin + A cells, were transplanted into a small lesion in the CST in rats. In the OEC recipients only, CST axons traversed the grafts and entered the cord caudal to the lesion. Axons encased in SC-like myelin were observed within the graft. Although none of the control rats with complete lesions of the CST could perform the forelimb reaching test, OEC-transplanted rats with complete lesions were able to perform the test. The clinical

relevance of OEC-mediated repair of the CST has been further supported by a recent study in which delayed transplantation of the OECs led to improved performance in the forelimb reaching test (Keyvan-Fouladi et al., 2003).

Following transplantation of OECs (A and S cells) with accompanying extracellular matrix, improved breathing and climbing abilities were observed in rats with dorsal cervical hemisection injuries to the spinal cord (Li et al., 2003). OEC-transplanted animals with lesions as large or larger than control non-breathing animals were able to breathe and exhibited recovery of electrical activity in the phrenic nerve, although this did not achieve complete normality. The OEC-transplanted animals made markedly fewer errors in the climbing test. It was acknowledged that several mechanisms could contribute to this recovery. Furthermore, persistent deficits often remained in the OEC-transplanted rats.

OEC transplants have been shown to promote axonal regeneration even after a complete transection injury to the spinal cord (Ramón-Cueto et al., 1998). In this study a 4 mm segment of cord was removed, SCs within a matrigel-filled polymer channel were placed between the cord stumps and Hoechst-labeled OECs, purified by immunopanning with anti-p75 antibody, were injected into the cord stumps next to the channel. Extensive migration of the transplanted OECs was deduced from the presence of many Hoechst-labeled nuclei within the cord. Interestingly, a connective tissue shell formed around the polymer channel and OECs also migrated into this shell. In rats with OECs, many serotonergic axons grew longitudinally through the connective tissue shell instead of through the SC bridge; some of these fibers grew, through both gray and white matter, for a distance of up to 1.5 cm into the caudal cord stump. Numerous descending axons, anterogradely labeled from the rostral cord stump, traversed the graft, and extended for up to 0.8 cm into the caudal stump. Injured ascending spinal axons regenerated for distances of up to 2.5 cm, traversing the graft and crossing both graft/cord interfaces. Axonal regeneration into the caudal stump was not observed in rats with SC grafts without accompanying OECs.

Remarkable improvements in hindlimb locomotion and sensory tests have been reported in rats with complete cord transections tested 8 months after acute transplantation of purified OECs alone (Ramón-Cueto et al., 2000). Prior to injury, all rats were trained to climb an inclined grid placed at increasing angles and then onto a platform at the top of the grid; the ability to perform this task was lost after injury. All OEC-transplanted animals showed some degree of motor and sensory recovery, whereas non-transplanted animals showed no recovery in the tests performed. Nearly one fourth of the rats with OEC transplants were able to climb a vertical (90°) grid and onto the horizontal platform at the top. In OEC rats, tissue was preserved at the injury site, whereas large cavities were found at the lesion site in controls. Notably, persistent, intensely GFAP+, astrocytic scars were present in both OEC and control rats. In rats with OEC transplants, serotonergic and noradrenergic axons grew for long distances into the cord stump caudal to the injury, through both gray and white matter. Both these fiber types distributed into the dorsal and ventral horns, delineating neurons. CST axons regenerated along the surface of the spinal cord before entering the cord caudal to the injury site. In controls, no axons re-entered the caudal stump.

In a partial replication of this promising study, rats that received unpurified olfactory cells or tissue fragments from olfactory lamina propria demonstrated modestly higher BBB test scores than controls (~5 in OEC rats compared to ~2 in controls, Lu et al., 2001). In all rats receiving olfactory cells or tissue (but not controls), suppression of the H-reflex was observed, indicating a recovery of spinal reflex inhibition, and some reticulospinal and raphespinal axons grew into the cord caudal to the lesion. To establish the potential clinical relevance of this strategy, in a separate experiment olfactory tissue was transplanted after a 4-week delay (Lu et al., 2002). Again, regeneration of raphespinal axons into the cord caudal to the lesion was observed and BBB test scores recovered from 1 to 4.5 in rats receiving olfactory tissue, but not in controls.

The efficacy of OECs and SCs in spinal cord repair has been directly compared in a clinically relevant contusion model of SCI (Takami et al., 2002; see SC section above). Purified SCs and/or OECs were injected into the contusion site a week after injury and repair was assessed 11 weeks later. Significant tissue sparing, diminished cavitation, and promotion of axonal growth into grafts result from SC and OEG grafts alike. Also, all grafts resulted in modest sparing and/or sprouting of corticospinal axons. But grafts containing SCs, in contrast to OEC transplants, exhibited twice as many myelinated axons, promoted more axonal sparing and/or regeneration of spinal and supraspinal axons and led to an improvement in hindlimb movement (from ~10.5 to ~12 on the BBB scale). In this study, OECs were less effective in promoting repair than SCs. Possibly the OECs did not survive as well as SCs.

28.10 Do OECs produce myelin?

Although OECs do not normally form myelin in the olfactory system, numerous studies have demonstrated that SC-like myelin is produced following the transplantation of OECs (Franklin et al., 1996; Li et al., 1997; 1998; Imaizumi et al., 1998; 2000; Barnett et al., 2000; Kato et al., 2000; Smith et al., 2002; Radtke et al., 2003). Myelination is observed in both demyelinated lesions produced by ethidium bromide/X-irradiation and after traumatic injury. In most experiments, myelination is achieved with transplants of mixed A cells and S cells; however, myelination is also observed after transplantation of a reversibly transformed clonal OEC cell line (Franklin et al., 1996). A recent study has shown that the amount of myelin produced after transplantation of highly purified OECs is substantially increased (three-fold) with co-transplantation of meningeal fibroblasts, underscoring a possible need of accessory cells for full myelinating function (Lakatos et al., 2003b; see also Li et al., 2003). Transplantation of OECs also lead to recovery of electrophysiologic function following demyelination due to X-irradiation/ethidium bromide (Imaizumi et al., 1998).

Although the evidence that SC-like myelin is formed following OEC transplantation is compelling, there was, until very recently, little conclusive evidence that it is actually the transplanted OECs that generate the myelin. In three new studies, the capacity of OECs to produce myelin has been tested using OECs pre-labeled with genetic markers or magnetic beads. When OECs expressing the *lacZ* transgene were transplanted into a clip compression model of SCI, SC-like myelin was formed by *lacZ* negative cells, as seen clearly by EM (Boyd et al., 2004); SC-axon units were closely surrounded by perineurial-like processes containing *lacZ* reaction product. In a dorsal hemisection injury model, however, myelin was formed by the transplanted OECs, as shown by immuno-EM detection of green-fluorescent protein (Sasaki et al., 2004). Nonetheless, some of the new myelin was formed by cells negative for the marker. Thus, in both studies, host SCs enter the transplant site and contribute to new myelination. In a third study, OECs pre-labeled with magnetic beads formed myelin in focal regions of demyelination (Dunning et al., 2004). The ability of transplanted OECs to produce myelin may depend, therefore, on a number of still undefined factors, including transplant composition and injury parameters.

SC immigration occurs rapidly and spontaneously following many types of spinal cord injury. (e.g. Bunge et al., 1994; Brook et al., 1998; see SC section above). In addition, a rapid angiogenic response is induced by the injection of OECs and other cell types into the lesioned CST (Li et al., 1998); ingrowth of new vessels clothed in basal lamina could promote the migration of SCs into the lesion. Rapid migration of host SCs into spinal cord transplant sites containing genetically labeled OECs was reported recently (Ramer et al., 2004). These results suggest that transplanted OECs may actually facilitate migration of host SCs into a transplant.

Some of the SC-like myelin seen after OEC transplantation could also derive from SCs present as contaminants in the OEC preparations. Small peripheral nerve fascicles, containing unmyelinated axons ensheathed by SCs, and lying between the meningeal membrane and the glia limitans of the olfactory bulb, or beneath the glia limitans at the surface of the nerve fiber layer, have been described

(Doucette, 1991). These nerves could be fascicles of sympathetic axons that are known to innervate smooth muscle in the walls of larger diameter blood vessels in the spinal cord (McNicholas et al., 1980; Amenta et al., 1990).

If myelination is consistently obtained following OEC transplantation, why is it important to understand which cell (host SC or transplanted OEC) is actually producing the myelin? One reason is that, if this strategy is to be used clinically in humans, it is prudent to proceed with the most accurate knowledge about the mechanism by which the strategy exerts its effect. An approach that works in animals may not succeed in humans, where individual variability is a well-established phenomenon that often interferes with specific treatments. Secondly, the most clinically relevant source of autologous OECs is the lamina propria and there is both a high risk of infection with this material, considering intended use in the CNS, and uncertainty whether enough cells could be obtained for grafting, especially in a diffuse demyelinating disease such as multiple sclerosis. Finally, if it is true that OECs facilitate myelination by SCs, it might be possible to replace the OECs with either a drug or other device that achieves the same result without subjecting an injured patient to another invasive procedure.

28.11 Concluding remarks

Based on the encouraging results of OEC transplantation in injured rats, clinical studies in persons with SCI have been initiated in China, Australia, and Portugal; definitive outcomes of these trials have not yet emerged. In the meantime, more information is needed to resolve issues related to the cellular and molecular mechanisms by which OECs promote regeneration. What is the explanation for OEC heterogeneity and the basis of the requirement for meningeal fibroblasts for optimal function? Will the long-term survival and extensive migration of transplanted OECs, deduced from Hoechst labeling, be confirmed by new experiments with genetically labeled OECs? How do OECs aid regenerating axons to extend through regions of intense astrogliosis? How do OECs modify axonal growth cone behavior?. By what mechanisms do transplanted OECs elicit favorable responses from host cells (e.g. angiogenesis, ingress of host SCs) (Ramer et al., 2004), thereby optimizing conditions for effective repair?

More than ample evidence has accumulated to demonstrate that SCs promote axonal regeneration and provide myelin for spared or regenerated fibers in the CNS. A key question is how to foster growth of regenerated axons from the peripheral nerve environment, the SC bridge, into the spinal cord. What accompanying strategies will be required? Elevation of cyclic AMP? Administration of neurotrophic factors? Use of both SCs and OECs? Although SC populations have not yet been tested in SCI clinical trials, peripheral nerve in combination with a neurotrophic factor cocktail is being examined in spinal cord injured persons in Taiwan. Cellular bridge prostheses to span the injury may be an important strategy for future interventions. Restoring function by activating neurons in one or two additional spinal segments could improve the quality of life for a spinal cord injured person (see Volume II, Chapter 37). A cellular bridge may enable axonal extension into contiguous segments to where propriospinal circuits remain intact after SCI (Jordan and Schmidt, 2002). Evidence exists that propriospinal neurons access locomotor neurons in distal segments. The possibility exists, therefore, that re-establishment of connections to neurons in the propriospinal pathways may be sufficient to relay commands to initiate locomotion.

ACKNOWLEDGMENTS

The authors are supported by the Christopher Reeve Paralysis and Hollfelder Foundations, NINDS grants N09923 and 38665, The Miami Project to Cure Paralysis, and the Buoniconti Fund. We are grateful to Drs. Sarah K. Williams and Susan C. Barnett, University of Glasgow, Glasgow, UK, and Dr. Robin J. Franklin, University of Cambridge, Cambridge, UK, for providing Figure 28.3. We thank Diana Masella for word processing.

REFERENCES

Adelman, L.S. and Aronson, S.M. (1972). Intramedullary nerve fiber and Schwann cell proliferation within the spinal cord (schwannosis). *Neurology*, **22**, 726–731.

Amenta, F., Bronzetti, E., Ferrante, F. and Ricci, A. (1990). The noradrenergic innervation of spinal blood vessels in old rats. *Neurobiol Aging*, **11**, 47–50.

Au, E. and Roskams, A.J. (2003). Olfactory ensheathing cells of the lamina propria *in vivo* and *in vitro*. *Glia*, **41**, 224–236.

Au, W.W., Treloar, H.B. and Greer, C.A. (2002). Sublaminar organization of the mouse olfactory bulb nerve fiber layer. *J Comp Neurol*, **446**, 68–70.

Bamber, N.I., Li, H., Lu, X., Oudega, M., Aebischer, P. and Xu, X.M. (2001). Neurotrophins BDNF and NT-3 promote axonal re-entry into the distal host spinal cord through Schwann cell-seeded mini-channels. *Europ J Neurosci*, **13**, 257–268.

Barber, P.C. and Lindsay, R.M. (1982). Schwann cells of the olfactory nerve contain glial fibrillary acidic protein and resemble astrocytes. *Neuroscience*, **7**, 3077–3090.

Barnett, S.C. and Riddell, J.S. (2004). Olfactory ensheathing cells (OECs) and the treatment of CNS injury: advantages and possible caveats. *J Anat*, **204**, 57–67.

Barnett, S.C., Alexander, C.L., Iwashita, Y., Gilson, J.M., Crowther, J., Clark, L., Dunn, L.T., Papanastassiou, V., Kennedy, P.G.E. and Franklin, R.J.M. (2000). Identification of a human olfactory ensheathing cell that can effect transplant-mediated remyelination of demyelinated CNS axons. *Brain*, **123**, 1581–1588.

Baron-Van Evercooren, A., Duhamel-Clerin, E., Boutry, J.M., Hauw, J.J. and Gumpel, M. (1993). Pathways of migration of transplanted Schwann cells in the demyelinated mouse spinal cord. *J Neurosci Res*, **35**, 428–438.

Baron-Van Evercooren, A., Avellana-Adalid, V., Ben Younes-Chennoufi, A., Gansmuller, A., Nait-Oumesmar, B. and Vignais, L. (1996). Cell–cell interactions during the migration of myelin-forming cells transplanted in the demyelinated spinal cord. *Glia*, **16**, 147–164.

Basso, D.M., Beattie, M.S. and Bresnahan, J.C. (1995). A sensitive and reliable locomotor rating scale for open field testing in rats. *J Neurotraum*, **12**, 1–21.

Beattie, M.S., Bresnahan, J.C., Komon, J., Tovar, C.A., Van Meter, M., Anderson, D.K., Faden, A.I., Hsu, C.Y., Noble, L.J., Salzman, S. and Young, W. (1997). Endogenous repair after spinal cord contusion injuries in the rat. *Exp Neurol*, **148**, 453–463.

Berry, M., Rees, L., Hall, S., Yiu, P. and Sievers, J. (1988). Optic axons regenerate into sciatic nerve isografts only in the presence of Schwann cells. *Brain Res Bull*, **20**, 223–231.

Blakemore, W.F. (1976). Invasion of Schwann cells into the spinal cord of the rat following local injections of lysolecithin. *Neuropathol Appl Neurobiol*, **2**, 21–39.

Blakemore, W.F. (1977). Remyelination of CNS axons by Schwann cells transplanted from the sciatic nerve. *Nature*, **266**, 68–69.

Blight, A.R. and Young, W. (1989). Central axons in injured cat spinal cord recover electrophysiological function following remyelination by Schwann cells. *J Neurol Sci*, **91**, 15–34.

Boyd, J.G., Lee, J., Skihar, V., Doucette, R. and Kawaja, M.D. (2004). *LacZ*-expressing olfactory ensheathing cells do not associate with myelinated axons after implantation into the compressed spinal cord. *Proc Natl Acad Sci USA*, **101**, 2162–2166.

Brook, G.A., Lawrence, J.M. and Raisman, G. (1993). Morphology and migration of cultured Schwann cells transplanted into the fimbria and hippocampus in adult rats. *Glia*, **9**, 292–304.

Brook, G.A., Lawrence, J.M., Shah, B. and Raisman, G. (1994). Extrusion transplantation of Schwann cells into the adult rat thalamus induces directional host axon growth. *Exp Neurol*, **126**, 31–43.

Brook, G.A., Plate, D., Franzen, R., Martin, D., Moonen, G., Schoenen, J., Schmitt, A.B., Noth, J. and Nacimiento, W. (1998). Spontaneous longitudinally oriented axonal regeneration is associated with the Schwann cell framework within the lesion site following spinal cord compression injury of the rat. *J Neurosci Res*, **53**, 51–65.

Bruce, J.H., Norenberg, M.D., Kraydieh, S., Puckett, W., Marcillo, A. and Dietrich, D. (2000). Schwannosis: role of gliosis and proteogycan in human spinal cord injury. *J Neurotraum*, **9**, 781–788.

Bunge, M.B. (2001). Bridging areas of injury in the spinal cord. *Neuroscientist*, **7**, 325–339.

Bunge, M.B., Holets, V.R., Bates, M.L., Clarke, T.S. and Watson, B.D. (1994). Characterization of photochemically induced spinal cord injury in the rat by light and electron microscopy. *Exp Neurol*, **127**, 76–93.

Bunge, R.P. (1975). Changing uses of nerve tissue culture 1950–1975. In: *The Nervous System, Volume 1, The Basic Neurosciences* (ed. Tower, D.B.), Raven Press, NY, pp. 31–42.

Calof, A.L. and Chikaraisha, D.M. (1989). Analysis of neurogenesis in a mammalian neuroepithelium: proliferation and differentiation of an olfactory neuron precursor *in vitro*. *Neuron*, **3**, 115–127.

Casella, G.T.B., Bunge, R.P. and Wood, P.M. (1996). Improved method for harvesting human Schwann cells from mature peripheral nerve and expansion *in vitro*. *Glia*, **17**, 327–338.

Chau, C.H., Shum, D.K.Y., Li, H., Pei, J., Lui, Y.Y., Wirthlin, L., Chan, Y.S. and Xu, X.-M. (2003). Chondroitinase ABC enhances axonal regrowth through Schwann cell-seeded guidance channels after spinal cord injury. *FASEB J Exp Art*, **18**, 194–196. http://www.fasebj.org/cgi/doi/1096/fj.03–0196fje

Chen, A., Xu, X.M., Kleitman, N. and Bunge, M.B. (1996). Methylprednisolone administration improves axonal regeneration into Schwann cell grafts in transected adult rat thoracic spinal cord. *Exp Neurol*, **138**, 261–276.

David, S. and Aguayo, A.J. (1981). Axonal elongation into peripheral nervous system "bridges" after central nervous system injury in adult rats. *Science*, **214**, 931–933.

Doucette, R. (1984). The glial cells in the nerve fiber layer of the olfactory bulb. *Anat Rec*, **210**, 385–391.

Doucette, R. (1991). PNS–CNS transitional zone of the first cranial nerve. *J Comp Neurol*, **312**, 451–466.

Doucette, J.R., Kiernan, J.A. and Flumerfelt, B.A. (1983). The re-innervation of olfactory glomeruli following transection of primary olfactory axons in the central or peripheral nervous system. *J Anat*, **137**, 1–19.

Duncan, I.D., Aguayo, A.J., Bunge, R.P. and Wood, P.M. (1981). Transplantation of rat Schwann cells grown in tissue culture into the mouse spinal cord. *J Neuro Sci*, **49**, 241–252.

Duncan, I.D., Hammang, J.P. and Gilmore, S.A. (1988). Schwann cell myelination of the myelin deficient rat spinal cord following X-irradiation. *Glia*, **1**, 233–239.

Dunning, M.D., ffrench-Constant, C., Brindle, K.M. and Franklin, J.M.F. (2004). Detection of transplanted Schwann cells and olfactory ensheathing cells by magnetic resonance imaging. *ISRT 7th Research Network Meeting*, London [abstract].

Fawcett, J.W. and Asher, R.A. (1999). The glial scar and central nervous system repair. *Brain Res Bull*, **49**, 377–391.

Felts, P.A. and Smith, K.J. (1992). Conduction properties of central nerve fibers remyelinated by Schwann cells. *Brain Res*, **574**, 178–192.

Franceschini, I.A. and Barnett, S.C. (1996). Low affinity NGF-receptor and E-N-CAM expression define two types of olfactory nerve ensheathing cells that share a common lineage. *Dev Biol*, **173**, 327–343.

Franklin, R.J. and Blakemore, W.F. (1993). Requirements for Schwann cell migration within CNS environments: a view point. *Int J Dev Neurosci*, **11**, 641–649.

Franklin, R.J., Gilson, J.M., Franceschini, I.A. and Barnett, S.C. (1996). Schwann cell-like myelination following transplantation of an olfactory bulb-ensheathing cell line into areas of demyelination in the adult CNS. *Glia*, **17**, 217–224.

Geller, H.M. and Fawcett, J.W. (2002). Building a bridge: engineering spinal cord repair. *Exp Neurol*, **174**, 125–136.

Gilmore, S.A. and Sims, T.J. (1993). Patterns of Schwann cell myelination of axons within the spinal cord. *J Chem Neuroanat*, **6**, 191–199.

Gilmore, S.A. and Sims, T.J. (1997). Glial–glial and glial–neuronal interfaces in radiation-induced, glia-depleted spinal cord. *J Anat*, **190**, 5–21.

Gomez, V.M., Averill, S., King, V., Yang, Q., Pérez, E.D., Chacón, S.C., Ward, R., Nieto-Sampedro, M., Priestly, J. and Taylor, J. (2003). Transplantation of olfactory ensheathing cells fails to promote significant axonal regeneration from dorsal roots into the rat cervical cord. *J Neurocytol*, **32**, 53–70.

Graziadei, P.P.C. and Monti Graziadei, G.A. (1980). Neurogenesis and neuron regeneration in the olfactory system of mammals. III. Deafferentation and reinnervation of the olfactory bulb following section of the *fila olfactoria* in rat. *J Neurocytol*, **9**, 145–162.

Guest, J.D., Rao, A., Olson, L., Bunge, M.B. and Bunge, R.P. (1997). The ability of human Schwann cell grafts to promote regeneration in the transected nude rat spinal cord. *Exp Neurol*, **148**, 502–522.

Harrison, B.M. (1980). Remyelination by cells introduced into a stable demyelinating lesion in the central nervous system. *J Neurol Sci*, **46**, 63–81.

Honmou, O., Felts, P.A., Waxman, S.G. and Kocsis, J.D. (1996). Restoration of normal conduction properties in demyelinated spinal cord axons in the adult rat by transplantation of exogenous Schwann cells. *J Neurosci*, **16**, 3199–3208.

Iannotti, C., Li, H., Yan, P., Lu, X., Wirthlin, L. and Xu, X.-M. (2003). Glial cell line-derived neurotrophic factor-enriched bridging transplants promote propriospinal axonal regeneration and enhance myelination after spinal cord injury. *Exp Neurol*, **183**, 379–393.

Imaizumi, T., Lankford, K.L., Waxman, S.G., Greer, C.A. and Kocsis, J.D. (1998). Transplanted olfactory ensheathing cells remyelinate and enhance axonal conduction in the demyelinated dorsal columns of the rat spinal cord. *J Neurosci*, **18**, 6176–6185.

Imaizumi, T., Lankford, K.L. and Kocsis, J.D. (2000). Transplantation of olfactory ensheathing cells or Schwann cells restores rapid and secure conduction across the transection spinal cord. *Brain Res*, **854**, 70–78.

Iwashita, Y. and Blakemore, W.F. (2000). Areas of demyelination do not attract significant numbers of Schwann cells transplanted into normal white matter. *Glia*, **31**, 232–240.

Jordan, L.M. and Schmidt, B.J. (2002). Propriospinal neurons involved in the control of locomotion: potential targets for repair strategies? *Prog Brain Res*, **137**, 125–139.

Kato, T., Honmou, O., Uede, T., Hashi, K. and Kocsis, J. (2000). Transplantation of human olfactory ensheathing cells elicits remyelination of demyelinated rat spinal cord. *Glia*, **30**, 209–218.

Keyvan-Fouladi, N., Raisman, G. and Li, Y. (2003). Functional repair of the corticospinal tract by delayed transplantation of olfactory ensheathing cells in adult rats. *J Neurosci*, **23**, 9428–9434.

Kromer, L.F. and Cornbrooks, C.J. (1985). Transplants of Schwann cell cultures promote axonal regeneration in the adult mammalion brain. *Proc Natl Acad Sci USA*, **82**, 6330–6334.

Lakatos, A., Franklin, R.J.M. and Barnett, S.C. (2000). Olfactory ensheathing cells and Schwann cells differ in their *in vitro* interactions with astrocytes. *Glia*, **32**, 214–225.

Lakatos, A., Barnett, S.C. and Franklin, R.J.M. (2003a). Olfactory ensheathing cells induce less host astrocyte response and chondroitin sulfate proteoglycan expression than Schwann cells following transplantation into adult CNS white matter. *Exp Neurol*, **184**, 237–246.

Lakatos, A., Smith, P.M., Barnett, S.C. and Franklin, R.J. (2003b). Meningeal cells enhance limited CNS remyelination by transplanted olfactory ensheathing cells. *Brain*, **126**, 598–609.

Lankford, K.L., Imaizumi, T., Honmou, O. and Kocsis, J.D. (2002). A quantitative morphometric analysis of rat spinal cord remyelination following transplantation of allogenic Schwann cells. *J Comp Neurol*, **443**, 259–274.

Li, Y. and Raisman, G. (1994). Schwann cells induce sprouting in motor and sensory axons in the adult rat spinal cord. *J Neurosci*, **14**, 4050–4063.

Li, Y. and Raisman, G. (1997). Integration of transplanted cultured Schwann cells into the long myelinated fiber tracts of the adult spinal cord. *Exp Neurol*, **145**, 396–411.

Li, Y., Field, P.M. and Raisman, G. (1997). Repair of adult rat corticospinal tract by transplants of olfactory ensheathing transplants. *Science*, **277**, 2000–2002.

Li, Y., Field, P.M. and Raisman, G. (1998). Regeneration of adult rat corticospinal axons induced by transplanted olfactory ensheathing cells. *J Neurosci*, **18**, 10514–10524.

Li, Y., Field, P.M. and Raisman, G. (1999). Death of oligodendrocytes and microglial phagocytosis of myelin precede immigration of Schwann cells into the spinal cord. *J Neurocytol*, **28**, 417–427.

Li, Y., Decherchi, P. and Raisman, G. (2003). Transplantation of olfactory ensheathing cells into spinal cord lesions restores breathing and climbing. *J Neurosci*, **23**, 727–731.

Lu, J., Féron, F., Ho, S.M., Mackay-Sim, A. and Waite, P.M.E. (2001). Transplantation of nasal olfactory tissue promotes partial recovery in paraplegic adult rats. *Brain Res*, **889**, 344–357.

Lu, J., Féron, F., Ho, S.M., Mackay-Sim, A. and Waite, P.M.E. (2002). Olfactory ensheathing cells promote locomotor recovery after delayed transplantation into transected spinal cord. *Brain*, **125**, 14–21.

Martin, D., Schoenen, J., Delrée, P., Leprince, P., Rogister, B. and Moonen, G. (1991). Grafts of syngenic cultured, adult dorsal root ganglion-derived Schwann cells to the injured spinal cord of adult rats: preliminary morphological studies. *Neurosci Lett*, **124**, 44–48.

Martin, D., Robe, P., Franzen, R., Delrée, P., Schoenen, J., Stevenaert, A. and Moonen, G. (1996). Effects of Schwann cell transplantation in a contusion model of rat spinal cord injury. *J Neurosci Res*, **45**, 588–597.

McNicholas, L.F., Martin, W.R., Sloan, J.W. and Nozaki, M. (1980). Innervation of the spinal cord by sympathetic fibers. *Exp Neurol*, **69**, 383–394.

Menei, P., Montero-Menei, C., Whittemore, S.R., Bunge, R.P. and Bunge, M.B. (1998). Schwann cells genetically modified to secrete human BDNF promote enhanced axonal regrowth across transected adult rat spinal cord. *Eur J Neurosci*, **10**, 607–621.

Montgomery, C.T., Tenaglia, E.A. and Robson, J.A. (1996). Axonal growth into tubes implanted within lesions in the spinal cords of adult rats. *Exp Neurol*, **137**, 277–290.

Monti Graziadei, G.A. and Graziadei, P.P.C. (1979). Neurogenesis and neuron regeneration in the olfactory system of mammals. II. Degeneration and reconstitution of the olfactory sensory neurons after axotomy. *J Neurocytol*, **8**, 197–213.

Navarro, X., Valero, A., Gudiño, G., Forés, J., Rodriguez, F.J., Verdú, E., Pascual, R., Cuadras, J. and Nieto-Sampedro, M. (1999). Ensheathing glia transplants promote dorsal root regeneration and spinal reflex restitution after multiple lumbar rhizotomy. *Ann Neurol*, **45**, 207–215.

Olby, N.J. and Blakemore, W.F. (1996). Primary demyelination and regeneration of ascending axons in the dorsal funiculus of the rat spinal cord following photochemically induced injury. *J Neurocytol*, **25**, 465–480.

Oudega, M., Xu, X.-M., Guénard, V., Kleitman, N. and Bunge, M.B. (1997). A combination of insulin-like growth factor-1 and platelet-derived growth factor enhances myelination but diminishes axonal regeneration into Schwann cell grafts in the adult rat spinal cord. *Glia*, **19**, 247–258.

Paino, C.L. and Bunge, M.B. (1991). Induction of axon growth into Schwann cell implants into lesioned adult rat spinal cord. *Exp Neurol*, **114**, 254–257.

Paino, C.L., Fernandez-Valle, C., Bates, M.L. and Bunge, M.B. (1994). Regrowth of axons in lesioned adult rat spinal cord: promotion by implants of cultured Schwann cells. *J Neurocytol*, **23**, 433–452.

Pearse, D.D., Pereira, F.C., Marcillo, A.E., Bates, M.L., Berrocal, Y.A. and Bunge, M.B. (2004). cAMP and Schwann cells promote axonal growth and functional recovery after spinal cord injury. *Nat Med*, **10**, 610–616.

Pinzon, A., Calancie, B., Oudega, M. and Noga, B.R. (2001). Conduction of impulses by axons regenerated in a Schwann cell graft in the transected adult rat thoracic spinal cord. *J Neurosci Res*, **64**, 533–541.

Pixley, S.K. (1992). The olfactory nerve contains two populations of glia, identified both *in vivo* and *in vitro*. *Glia*, **5**, 269–284.

Plant, G.W., Bates, M.L. and Bunge, M.B. (2001a). Inhibitory proteoglycan immunoreactivity is higher at the caudal than the rostral Schwann cell graft-transected spinal cord interface. *Mol Cell Neurosci*, **17**, 471–487.

Plant, G.W., Ramón-Cueto, A. and Bunge, M.B. (2001b). Transplantation of Schwann cells and ensheathing glia to improve regeneration in adult spinal cord. In: *Axonal Regeneration in the Central Nervous System* (eds Ingoglia, N.A. and Murray, M.), Marcel Dekker, New York, pp. 529–561

Plant, G.W., Christensen, C.L., Oudega, M. and Bunge, M.B. (2003). Delayed transplantation of olfactory ensheathing glia promotes sparing/regeneration of supraspinal axons in the contused adult rat spinal cord. *J Neurotraum*, **20**, 1–16.

Radtke, C., Yukinori, A., Brokaw, J., Lankford, K.L., Wewetzer, K., Fodor, W.L. and Kocsis, J.D. (2003). Remyelination of the nonhuman primate spinal cord by transplantation of H-transferase transgenic adult pig olfactory ensheathing cells. *FASEB J Exp Art*, **18**, 335–337. http://www.fasebj.org/cgi/doi:10.1096/fj.03–0214fje

Raisman, G. (1985). Specialized neuroglial arrangement may explain the capacity of vomeronasal axons to reinnervate central neurons. *Neuroscience*, **14**, 237–254.

Ramer, L.M., Au, E., Richter, M., Liu, J., Tetzlaff, W. and Roskams, A.J. (2004). Peripheral olfactory ensheathing cells reduce scar and cavity formation and promote regeneration following spinal cord injury. *J Comp Neurol*, **473**, 1–15.

Ramón y Cajal, S. (1991). In: *Cajal's Degeneration and Regeneration of the Nervous System* (trans. May, R.M.) (eds De Felipe, J. and Jones, E.G.), Oxford University Press, New York, p. 769.

Ramón-Cueto, A. and Nieto-Sampedro, M. (1992). Glial cells from adult rat olfactory bulb: immunocytochemical properties of pure cultures of ensheathing cells. *Neuroscience*, **47**, 213–220.

Ramón-Cueto, A. and Nieto-Sampedro, M. (1994). Regeneration into the spinal cord of transected dorsal root axons is promoted by ensheathing glia transplants. *Exp Neurol*, **127**, 232–244.

Ramón-Cueto, A., Plant, G.W., Avila, J. and Bunge, M.B. (1998). Long-distance axonal regeneration in the transected adult rat spinal cord is promoted by olfactory ensheathing glia transplants. *J Neurosci*, **18**, 3803–3815.

Ramón-Cueto, A., Cordero, M.I., Santos-Benito, F.F. and Avila, J. (2000). Functional recovery of paraplegic rats and motor axon regeneration in their spinal cords by olfactory ensheathing cells. *Neuron*, **25**, 425–435.

Richardson, P.M., McGuinness, U.M. and Aguayo, A.J. (1980). Axons from CNS neurons regenerate into PNS grafts. *Nature*, **284**, 264–265.

Richardson, P.M., Issa, V.M. and Aguayo, A.J. (1984). Regeneration of long spinal axons in the rat. *J Neurocytol*, **13**, 165–182.

Sasaki, M., Lankford, K.L., Zemedkun, M. and Kocsis, J.D. (2004). Identified olfactory ensheathing cells transplanted into the transected dorsal funiculus bridge the lesion and form myelin. *J Neurosci*, **24**, 8485–8493.

Silver, J. and Miller, J.H. (2004). Regeneration beyond the glial scar. *Nature Rev/Neurosci*, **5**, 146–156.

Sims, T.J., Gilmore, S.A., Waxman, S.G. and Klinge, E. (1985). Dorsal-ventral differences in the glia limitans of the spinal cord: an ultrastructural study in developing normal and irradiated rats. *J Neuropath Exp Neurol*, **44**, 415–429.

Sims, T.J., Durgun, M.B. and Gilmore, S.A. (1998). Schwann cell invasion of ventral spinal cord: the effect of irradiation on astrocyte barriers. *J Neuropath Exp Neurol*, **57**, 866–873.

Smith, G.V. and Stevenson, J.A. (1988). Peripheral nerve grafts lacking viable Schwann cells fail to support nervous system regeneration. *Exp Brain Res*, **69**, 299–306.

Smith, P.M., Lakatos, A., Barnett, S.C., Jeffery, N.D. and Franklin, R.J.M. (2002). Cryopreserved cells isolated from the adult canine olfactory bulb are capable of extensive remyelination following transplantation into the adult rat CNS. *Exp Neurol*, **176**, 402–406.

Takami, T., Oudega, M., Bates, M.L., Wood, P.M., Kleitman, N. and Bunge, M.B. (2002). Schwann cell but not olfactory ensheathing glia transplants improve hindlimb locomotor performance in the moderately contused adult rat thoracic spinal cord. *J Neurosci*, **22**, 6670–6681.

Tello, F. (1911). La influencia del neurotropismo en la regeneración de los centros nerviosos. *Trab del Lab de Invest Univ Madrid*, **9**, 123–159.

Tuszynski, M.H., Weidner, N., McCormack, M., Miller, I., Powell, H. and Conner, J. (1998). Grafts of genetically modified Schwann cells for the spinal cord; survival, axon growth, and myelination. *Cell Transplant*, **7**, 187–196.

Valverde, F. and Lopez-Mascaraque, L. (1991). Neuroglial arrangements in the olfactory glomeruli of the hedgehog. *J Comp Neurol*, **307**, 658–674.

Verdu, E., Garcia-Alias, G., Fores, J., Gudino-Cabrera, G., Muneton, V.C., Nieto-Sampedro, M. and Navarro, X. (2001). Effects of ensheathing cells transplanted into photochemically damaged spinal cord. *NeuroReport*, **12**, 2303–2309.

Weidner, N., Blesch, A., Grill, R.J. and Tuszynski, M.H. (1999). Nerve growth factor-hypersecreting Schwann cell grafts augment and guide spinal cord axonal growth and remyelinate central nervous system axons in a phenotypically appropriate manner that correlates with expression of L1. *J Comp Neurol*, **413**, 495–506.

Williams, S.K., Franklin, R.J.M. and Barnett, S.C. (2004). Response of olfactory ensheathing cells to the degeneration and regeneration of the peripheral olfactory system and the involvement of the neuregulins. *J Comp Neurol*, **470**, 50–62.

Wrathall, J.R., Rigamonti, D.D., Braford, M.R. and Kao, C.C. (1982). Reconstruction of the contused cat spinal cord by the delayed nerve graft technique and cultured peripheral non-neuronal cells. *Acta Neuropathol*, **57**, 59–69.

Xu, X.-M., Guénard, V., Kleitman, N. and Bunge, M.B. (1995a). Axonal regeneration into Schwann cell-seeded guidance channels grafted into transected adult rat spinal cord. *J Comp Neurol*, **351**, 145–160.

Xu, X.-M., Guénard, V., Kleitman, N., Aebischer, P. and Bunge, M.B. (1995b). A combination of BDNF and NT-3 promotes supraspinal axonal regeneration into Schwann cell grafts in adult rat thoracic spinal cord. *Exp Neurol*, **134**, 261–272.

Xu, X.-M., Chen, A., Guénard, V., Kleitman, N. and Bunge, M.B. (1997). Bridging Schwann cell transplants promote axonal regeneration from both the rostral and caudal stumps of transected adult rat spinal cord. *J Neurocytol*, **26**, 1–16.

Xu, X.-M., Zhang, S.-X., Li, H., Aebischer, P. and Bunge, M.B. (1999). Regrowth of axons into the distal spinal cord through a Schwann cell-seeded mini-channel implanted into hemisected adult rat spinal cord. *Eur J Neurosci*, **11**, 1723–1740.

Young, W. (2002). Spinal cord contusion models. (eds McKerracher, L., Doucet, G. and Rossignol, S.). *Prog Brain Res*, **137**, 231–255.

Trophic factor delivery by gene therapy

Ken Nakamura[1] and Un Jung Kang[2]

[1]Department of Neurology, University of California, San Francisco, CA and [2]Department of Neurology, University of Chicago, Chicago, IL, USA

29.1 Introduction

Neurotrophic factors were initially discovered as critical molecules in the growth and survival of developing neurons (Levi-Montalcini, 1966). They have subsequently been shown to enhance certain neuronal phenotypes, and to promote the survival and regeneration of damaged adult neurons. For these reasons, neurotrophic factors have tremendous therapeutic potential for a wide range of neurologic diseases. However, supplementation of neurotrophic factors can also have undesirable side effects. Therefore, successful clinical application depends on a thorough understanding of the endogenous functions and effects of neurotrophic factors. In addition, an efficient means of delivering appropriate concentrations of neurotrophic factors to target cells is required. Systemic therapy is not a viable option, given that neurotrophic factors generally have short half-lives, do not cross the blood–brain barrier, and have a wide range of effects on various targets. Intraventricular delivery also lacks anatomic and cellular specificity (Nutt et al., 2003). Intraparenchymal delivery (Gill et al., 2003) could overcome some of these limitations, although certain neurotrophic factors have limited diffusion from the injection site. Therefore, gene therapy represents the most promising means of providing continuous delivery of neurotrophic factors to specific anatomic and cellular targets.

A variety of gene therapy approaches have been considered for neurologic diseases. These include the replacement of missing neurotransmitters, augmenting the phenotypes of remaining neurons, promotion of neuronal regeneration, and prevention of further degeneration by delivering genes that impede cell death pathways. Although the replacement of missing transmitters has been an effective approach for diseases such as Parkinson's disease (PD; Volume II, Chapter 35), the underlying degenerative process is not impeded. In many cases, our understanding of disease pathophysiology is insufficient to allow more direct interventions. In other diseases such as stroke (see Volume II, Chapter 36) and spinal cord injury (see Volume II, Chapter 37), the primary insult has already occurred at the time of clinical presentation. This chapter examines the rational, therapeutic potential, strategies, and obstacles to the delivery of neurotrophic factors using gene therapy for the treatment of neurologic diseases.

29.2 Gene therapy methodologies

Vehicles of central nervous system gene therapy

Gene therapy methods have developed remarkably over the last decade, and continue to evolve rapidly. There is no single gene therapy vehicle that is optimal for all purposes. Instead, the specific requirements of each situation must be considered when selecting a vector. Two general approaches are used for gene therapy. In ex *vivo* approaches, cells are genetically modified *in vitro* to express relevant genes, and then delivered to target areas. For ex *vivo* therapy, choosing the optimal cell type is critical. As most cell lines have the potential to form tumors, primary cell types such as fibroblasts, myoblasts, astrocytes, Schwann cells (Weidner et al., 1999), olfactory ensheathing glia (OEG) (Ruitenberg et al., 2003), and stem cells have been explored as cellular vehicles. Other approaches include the use of encapsulated cell grafts (Bachoud-Levi et al., 2000), so as to provide a physical barrier restricting further growth and limiting immunologic reactions. Cells may also be chosen based on their endogenous production of trophic factors and ability to provide substrates that are conducive for neurite growth (Weidner et al., 1999; Ruitenberg et al., 2003). To genetically modify various cell types, retroviruses derived from the Moloney murine leukemia virus (MLV) are commonly used because of their high efficiency in transducing cells by integrating into the cellular genome of dividing cells. As integration can occur at sites that are important for normal cellular function, there is a small risk of insertional mutagenesis. Other vectors such as adenovirus (AdV) (Barkats et al., 1997) or adeno-associated virus (AAV) (Lehtonen et al., 2002) have been utilized for genetically modifying primary neurons that do not divide prior to implantation.

In vivo gene therapy involves the direct delivery of genes to target cells. In most central nervous system (CNS) applications, this requires that the vector be capable of infecting non-dividing cells. AdV is a double stranded DNA virus that is associated with human respiratory infections, conjunctivitis, and gastroenteritis. AdV has been shown to infect both neurons and glia after direct intracerebral injection (Akli et al., 1993; Davidson et al., 1993). First generation vectors were made replication defective by deleting the early E1 gene from its 36 kb genome. However, residual expression of wild-type viral genes produces host immune responses that contributed to problems in early clinical trials (Marshall, 1999). "Gutless" adenoviral vectors that lack all of the viral genome have been developed, and show promise for diminished immune response with increased transgene capacity (Thomas et al., 2000; Sakhuja et al., 2003).

AAV is a small and non-pathogenic single stranded DNA virus that has become an efficient and safe delivery tool to neurons (Kaplitt et al., 1994). Recent studies have found that different serotypes of AAV have preferential tropisms for distinct neuronal populations (Davidson et al., 2000; Tenenbaum et al., 2004). Wild-type AAV has been shown to integrate into a specific site on chromosome 19, but recombinant vectors tend to exist mainly episomally (Tenenbaum et al., 2003).

Herpes simplex virus (HSV) is a large neurotrophic double stranded DNA virus that can accommodate inserts up to 150 kb in size. HSV has a natural tendency to enter latent states within the CNS. It is also readily transported retrogradely, anterogradely, and transsynaptically, and therefore has been used for tracing anatomic pathways within the CNS (Norgren and Lehman, 1998). Two types of herpes virus vectors have been used. Recombinant herpes virus vector contains the transgene incorporated into the viral genome by homologous recombination (Burton et al., 2002). Amplicon vectors are plasmids consisting of a viral origin of replication and a packaging signal, and therefore require a helper virus for viral replication and production (Wang, S. et al., 2002). Active investigations to improve long-term expression of the transgene and to minimize immune responses are in progress (Bowers et al., 2003).

Retroviral vectors derived from MLV have limited roles for *in vivo* gene therapy in the CNS. In contrast, lentiviral vectors have the ability to transduce non-dividing neurons *in vivo* with great efficiency (Blomer et al., 1997). Lentiviruses are derived from human or feline immunodeficiency viruses and can accommodate inserts that are up to 8 kb in size (Poeschla et al., 1998). Given their origin, safety issues have been of particular concern for lentiviruses. To address this, vectors with most viral genes deleted combined with helper cells (Dull et al., 1998), and self-inactivating constructs disabling the virus' ability to replicate independently (Miyoshi et al., 1998) have been developed.

Selection of gene therapy vehicles for clinical application

An important clinical requirement of gene therapy is the ability to sustain long-term transgene expression.

This is particularly important for neurodegenerative diseases, which develop gradually over years. Unfortunately, long-term expression has been difficult to achieve using ex *vivo* paradigms. For instance, despite extensive research including the use of constitutive promoters, long-term expression of transgenes by leukemia retroviruses has remained elusive. In contrast, long-term expression has been demonstrated with minimal immunologic reaction using a variety of *in vivo* gene therapy vectors such as AAV (Tenenbaum et al., 2004) and lentivirus (Blomer et al., 1997).

Another issue facing gene therapy is the ability to generate sufficient quantities of protein to exert intended biologic effects. The level of expression depends on many factors including the proportion of target cells infected, the number of viral particles entering each cell, the transcriptional activities of the transgenes that are usually driven by viral promoters, and properties of the protein including its half-life. On the other hand, too much gene product may also be detrimental. As a result, the ability to regulate gene expression is important for therapeutic and safety purposes. The most extensively studied regulation system uses tetracycline-responsive transcriptional elements derived from the original Gossen and Bujard construct (Gossen and Bujard, 1992). Problems such as the toxicity of the transcriptional protein (tTA), its potential immunogenicity, and leaky expression of transgenes are being actively investigated (Kafri et al., 2000). Other regulatory systems include ecdysone-responsive elements (Suhr et al., 1998) and a rapamycin-dimerizing system (Ye et al., 1999).

A third issue concerns the ability to deliver transgenes to all target areas, while minimizing non-specific delivery. For certain disorders, such as diffuse metabolic diseases, the global delivery of viral vectors may be necessary. Intracarotid injection of virus can be combined with disruption of the blood–brain barrier using agents such as mannitol, so as to maximize intraparenchymal diffusion (Bourgoin et al., 2003). For many diseases, such as Alzheimer's disease (AD) and Huntington's disease (HD), neuronal degeneration is limited to specific areas of the brain and involves only certain cell types. Currently, stereotaxic injection of viruses is the method of choice for these diseases. However, the areas over which injected viruses and their gene products can diffuse are limited. For instance, nerve growth factor (NGF) diffuses no more than 1–2 mm from genetically modified cells (Tuszynski, 2002). Therefore, multiple injections are necessary to cover large target areas. This carries the risk of bleeding and damage to other unintended areas. Another means of delivering vectors to specific neuronal populations relies on the ability of some viruses to be transported either retrogradely or anterogradely. For instance, HSV infects nerve terminals with high efficiency prior to retrograde transport to the sensory neurons in the dorsal ganglia, and subsequent anterograde transport to the spinal cord. Lentivirus, AAV, and AdV have also been shown to undergo retrograde transport. Robust expression of protein can be obtained in CNS motor and sensory neurons following the intramuscular delivery of recombinant viruses (Ghadge et al., 1995; Kaspar et al., 2003). In the future, the synaptic transfer of recombinant genes, as might be achieved by delivering recombinant proteins conjugated to the non-toxic tetanus toxin C-fragment (Kissa et al., 2002) may also help access central targets from peripheral injection sites. Yet another approach is to capitalize on the endogenous ability of viruses to disseminate by using live attenuated viruses, whose growth is regulated either by tetracycline regulatable transgenes (Berkhout et al., 2002) or drugs such as ganciclovir to control viral proliferation (Fukuda et al., 2003). Clearly, such an approach would require tremendous efforts to ensure patient safety.

Choice of viral vector may also be guided by the natural tropism of certain viruses. For instance, wild-type HSV targets sensory neurons of dorsal root ganglia (DRG) or trigeminal ganglia with high efficiency following skin inoculation (Mata et al., 2004). In contrast, adenoviruses tend to infect glia with higher efficacy (e.g., Tai et al., 2003), while AAVs have a variety of transduction patterns in the CNS depending on the specific serotype (Davidson et al., 2000; Tenenbaum et al., 2004). Some cell types such as stem cells also have the ability to migrate within the CNS, and may be used to target ex *vivo* gene therapy approaches in the future. Stem cells have been shown to migrate toward ischemia, tumors, or other damaged areas (Hoehn et al., 2002). Additional levels of selective transgene expression may be achieved using cell type-specific promoters, although these promoters have shown weaker transcriptional activities than corresponding viral promoters to this point (Li et al., 1999). The use of synthetic promoters with strong transcriptional activity is also being investigated (Li et al., 1999).

29.3 Rationale and progress in the delivery of neurotrophic factors using gene therapy for neurologic diseases

An earlier chapter (Volume I, Chapter 23) discusses the basic biology of neurotrophic factors in greater detail. The best known neurotrophic factors belong to the neurotrophin (NT) family and include NGF, brain-derived neurotrophic factor (BDNF), NT-3, and NT-4/5 (Thoenen and Sendtner, 2002). All NTs bind to P75^{NTR}, which is a member of the tumor necrosis superfamily of receptors that contain a cytoplasmic death domain. NTs also bind to transmembrane tyrosine kinase receptors (Trks) that mediate signal transduction pathways leading to neuronal survival and neurite growth. NGF acts at TrkA, BDNF and NT-4/5 at TrkB, and NT-3 predominantly at TrkC. Truncated forms of TrkB on the ependymal cells surface limits the diffusion of BDNF into the parenchyma, whereas NGF diffuses more readily (Biffo et al., 1995).

Glial cell line-derived neurotrophic factor (GDNF) is a distant member of the transforming growth factor (TNF)-β superfamily of trophic factors that also includes neurturin, artemin (neublastin), and persephin. GDNF family ligands bind to glycosylphosphatidylinositol (GPI)-anchored GDNF family receptors α (GFRα1–4), which then stimulate autophosphorylation of a transmembrane Trk, Ret. GDNF can also signal via GFRα1 in the absence of Ret. (Saarma, 2000). The neurotrophic effect of GDNF, except in motorneurons, requires the presence of TNF-β to activate the transport of GFRα1 to the cell membrane (Saarma, 2000; Peterziel et al., 2002).

Ciliary neurotrophic factor (CNTF) is a member of the interleukin (IL)-6 cytokine family that also includes leukemia inhibitory factor (LIF), IL-11, cardiotrophin-1, and oncostatin M. CNTF binds to the high-affinity trimeric CNTF receptor consisting of CNTFRα, LIFRβ, and gp130, which activates intracellular Jak/Tyk tyrosine kinases (Auguste et al., 1996). A variety of other growth factors show therapeutic potential for neurologic diseases includes acidic fibroblast growth factor, basic fibroblast growth factor (bFGF), insulin-like growth factor 1 (IGF-1), and hepatocyte growth factor. This section reviews the application of neurotrophic factor gene therapy to animal models of selected neurologic diseases, in which clinical applications are being investigated.

AD

AD is the most common cause of dementia, and is characterized by an inexorable decline in short-term memory and other cognitive functions. The etiology of AD is unknown, although converging evidence suggests that the accumulation of amyloid β-protein (Aβ) due to an imbalance between production and degradation plays a central role (Sisodia and St George-Hyslop, 2002). Ultimately, this results in widespread neuronal loss in the hippocampus and neocortex, along with extracellular deposits of amyloid plaques and intracellular deposition of tangles consisting of hyperphosphorylated tau. Early in AD, decreased cholinergic expression and shrinkage of neurons in the nucleus basalis of Meynart (NBM), the major cholinergic projection to the neocortex, plays a prominent role in the pathogenesis (Dawbarn and Allen, 2003). Basal forebrain cholinergic neurons (BFCN) express NGF receptors, and retrogradely transport NGF released from innervation targets to their cell bodies (Alberch et al., 2004). In patients with AD, levels of NGF are increased in the cortex and hippocampus, but decreased in the NBM, suggesting a defect in retrograde transport (Scott et al., 1995). In addition, transgenic mice lacking NGF and TrkA show loss of cholinergic neurons in the basal forebrain (Capsoni et al., 2000). Cholinergic deficits are thought to be responsible for memory loss and attention problems, and drug therapy with acetylcholinesterase inhibitors is modestly beneficial (Mesulam, 2004).

A variety of animal models have been studied to characterize the therapeutic potential of NGF for AD (Table 29.1). The ability of NGF delivered by gene therapy to protect against cholinergic degeneration following fimbria/fornix lesions was first shown by Rosenberg et al., who transplanted rat fibroblasts that were engineered to express human NGF using the MLV (Rosenberg et al., 1988). The protective effects of NGF have since been replicated using a multitude of other ex *vivo* and *in vivo* gene therapy paradigms (Kawaja et al., 1992; Klein et al., 2000), and also extended to primates (Tuszynski, 2002). NGF has also been found to restore age-related atrophy in rats and monkeys (Chen and Gage, 1995; Smith et al., 1999). Given the protective effects of NGF on BFCN, intraventricular delivery of NGF was attempted in several AD patients, but was limited by non-specific side effects such as weight loss and back pain (Eriksdotter Jonhagen et al., 1998). A recently published phase 1 clinical trial of NGF-expressing antologous fibroblasts in patients with AD noted no long-term adverse effects, reduction in the rate of cognitive decline, increase in cortical metabolism measured by serial 18-fluorodeoxyglucose PET scan, and evidence of growth response in one patient (Tuszynski et al., 2005). Future studies in humans may provide insight into whether NGF's protective effects for BFCNs extend to the processes causing degeneration in AD (Mesulam, 2004).

PD

PD is the second most common neurodegenerative disorder, and is characterized by the relatively selective degeneration of dopaminergic neurons in the substantia nigra pars compacta (Bernheimer et al., 1973). As in AD, most cases of PD are sporadic, although a small number of genetic cases have been described (Dawson and Dawson, 2003). The etiology of PD remains unknown, and mitochondrial dysfunction, oxidative stress, and abnormal protein processing have all been implicated in the pathogenesis (Dawson and Dawson, 2003). Gene therapy approaches for PD have focused on either reconstituting the dopamine synthetic machinery, or using neurotrophic factors to augment dopaminergic function and protect against further degeneration (Kang and Nakamura, 2003). Although there is no evidence that neurotrophic factor deficiency plays a major role in the pathogenesis of PD, levels of GDNF are known to be decreased by approximately 20% in surviving neurons (Chauhan et al., 2001).

Many factors including NGF, BDNF, NT-3, NT-4/5, GDNF, TGFβ, platelet-derived growth factor (PDGF), bFGF, and CNTF have been shown to promote the survival of dopaminergic neurons in culture and experimental models of dopaminergic neuronal death (Knusel et al., 1990; Hyman et al., 1991; Lin et al., 1993; Hyman et al., 1994; Hynes et al., 1994). Of note, the effects of GDNF have been most robust in *in vivo* models. In normal animals, GDNF increases dopaminergic markers (Hudson et al., 1995). In addition, GDNF delivered to the substantia nigra using *in vivo* paradigms with AdV (Choi-Lundberg et al., 1997; Lapchak et al., 1997), AAV (Mandel et al., 1997, Kirik et al., 2000; Georgievska et al., 2002), lentivirus (Kordower et al., 2000), and herpes virus (Hao et al., 2003) vectors, and ex *vivo* paradigms using neural stem cells (Akerud et al., 2001) and encapsulated cells (Lindner et al., 1995) has been found to protect dopaminergic neurons and terminals from 6-hydroxydopamine (6-OHDA) toxicity in rodents and 1-methyl-4-phenyl-1,2,3,6-tetrahydropyridine (MPTP) in primates. The timing of GDNF gene therapy is important, since delaying the delivery of GDNF following 6-OHDA lesions in rats results in limited regrowth and sprouting of axons into the striatum (Bjorklund et al., 2000). Although both anterograde (Kordower et al., 2000) and retrograde (Tomac et al., 1995) transport of GDNF have been demonstrated, the site of GDNF delivery is also of critical importance. GDNF introduced into the substantia nigra protects cell bodies but not terminals

Table 29.1. Gene therapy experiments in models of neurologic diseases.

Neurologic disease model	Neurotrophic factor	Delivery vehicle	References
Alzheimer's disease			
Fimbria/fornix transection in rat	NGF	AAV, fibroblasts, neural progenitor cells	Rosenberg et al. (1988), Kawaja et al. (1992), Mandel et al. (1999)
Fimbria/fornix transection in monkey	NGF	Encapsulated fibroblasts	Kordower et al. (1994)
NBM lesions in rat (ibotenic acid)	NGF	Fibroblasts	Winkler et al. (1998)
Aging rat	NGF	AAV, fibroblasts, neural progenitor cells	Chen and Gage (1995), Klein et al. (2000), Martinez-Serrano et al. (1995)
Aging monkey	NGF	Fibroblasts	Smith et al. (1999)
Human AD	NGF	Fibroblasts	Tuszynski (2002)
Parkinson's disease			
6-OHDA model in rodents	BDNF	Fibroblasts	Lucidi-Phillipi et al. (1995), Levivier et al. (1995)
	GDNF	AdV, AAV, HSV lentivirus, neural stem cell	Lapchak et al. (1997), Choi-Lundberg et al. (1997), Mandel et al. (1997), Kirik et al. (2000), Georgievska et al. (2002), Akerud et al. (2001), Hao et al. (2003)
	Neurturin	Fibroblast	Akerud et al. (1999), Rosenblad et al. (2000)
	Artemin	Lentivirus	Rosenblad et al. (2000)
	Persephin	Neural stem cell	Akerud et al. (2002)
Intrastriatal MPP$^+$ in rat	BDNF	Fibroblasts	Frim et al. (1994)
MPTP model in monkey	GDNF	Lentivirus, encapsulated cells	Kordower et al. (2000), Kishima et al. (2004)
Huntington's disease			
Quinolinic acid/kainic acid lesions in rat striatum	NGF	Stem cells, fibroblasts	Martinez-Serrano and Bjorklund (1996), Schumacher et al. (1991)
	BDNF	Fibroblasts, stem cells, AAV, AdV	Perez-Navarro et al. (2000b), Martinez-Serrano and Bjorklund (1996), Kells et al. (2004), Bemelmans et al. (1999)
	NT-3	Fibroblasts	Perez-Navarro et al. (2000b)
	NT-4	Fibroblasts	Perez-Navarro et al. (2000b)
	GDNF	AAV, fibroblasts	Perez-Navarro et al. (1999), Perez-Navarro et al. (1996), Kells et al. (2004)
	Neurturin	Fibroblasts	Marco et al. (2002), Perez-Navarro et al. (2000a)
	CNTF	Encapsulated fibroblasts, lentivirus	Regulier et al. (2002), de Almeida et al. (2001)
Quinolinic acid striatal lesions in monkey	CNTF	Encapsulated fibroblasts	Emerich et al. (1997)
3-nitroproprionic acid in rat	CNTF	AdV	Mittoux et al. (2002)
3-nitroproprionic acid in monkey	GDNF	AAV	McBride et al. (2003)
	CNTF	Encapsulated fibroblasts	Mittoux (2000)
Transgenic mutant huntingtin mouse	CNTF	Lentivirus	Zala et al. (2004)

(*cont.*)

Table 29.1. (*continued*).

Neurologic disease model	Neurotrophic factor	Delivery vehicle	References
Human HD	CNTF	Encapsulated fibroblasts	Bachoud-Levi et al. (2000)
Amyotrophic lateral sclerosis			
G93A SOD1 mutant mouse	GDNF	AAV, myoblasts, AdV, lentivirus	Kaspar et al. (2003), Mohajeri et al. (1999), Wang, L.J. et al. (2002), Acsadi et al. (2002), Guillot et al. (2004)
	IGF-1	AAV, lentivirus	Kaspar et al. (2003)
Mouse mutant progressive motor neuronopathy (pmn)	NT-3	AdV	Haase et al. (1997)
	GDNF	Encapsulated fibroblasts	Sagot et al. (1996)
	CNTF	AdV	Haase et al. (1999)
Spinal cord injury			
Transection or crush injury models in rat	NGF	Fibroblasts	Jones et al. (2001), Grill, R.J. et al. (1997)
	BDNF	Fibroblasts, OEG	Liu et al. (1999), Jones et al. (2001), Menei et al. (1998), Jin et al. (2002), Ruitenberg et al. (2003)
	NT-3	Fibroblasts, AdV, OEG	Blits et al. (2000), Grill, R. et al. (1997), Ruitenberg et al. (2003)
	GDNF	Fibroblasts, AdV, HSV	Blesch and Tuszynski (2003), Tai et al. (2003), Natsume et al. (2003)
Neuropathy			
Metabolic/toxic neuropathy models in rat	NGF	HSV	Goss et al. (2002)
	NT-3	AdV, HSV, IM/electroporation of plasmid DNA	Pradat et al. (2001), Chattopadhyay et al. (2002), Pradat et al. (2002)
	VEGF	IM of plasmid DNA	Schratzberger et al. (2001)
Diabetic neuropathy in human	VEGF	IM of plasmid DNA	Isner et al. (2001)

Representative list of major models of selected neurologic diseases for which gene therapy experiments have been attempted. Gene delivery methods with selected references are listed for each neurotrophic factor. IM is intramuscular injection.

from 6-OHDA lesions (Choi-Lundberg et al., 1997; Mandel et al., 1997), while introduction of GDNF into the striatum protects both terminals and cell bodies (Choi-Lundberg et al., 1998). Behavioral recovery is only observed when striatal fibers are preserved (Bilang-Bleuel et al., 1997; Bjorklund et al., 2000; Kirik et al., 2000). A primate study showed that delivery of GDNF to both the nigra and striatum a week following MPTP treatment provided both functional and anatomic protection (Kordower et al., 2000).

Given these promising results, intraventricular delivery of GDNF was attempted in PD patients (Nutt et al., 2003). However, no significant regeneration of nigrostriatal neurons or intraparenchymal diffusion of the intracerebroventricular GDNF was found (Kordower et al., 1999). Intraparechymal delivery of GDNF to the putamen of five patients with PD was also attempted, and some clinical improvements and an increase in [^{18}F]dopa uptake were noted (Gill et al., 2003). A larger and controlled study is in progress.

A variety of other GDNF family ligands have also been shown to protect against dopaminergic toxins (Table 29.1). For instance, fibroblasts-expressing neurturin, lentivirus-expressing artemin, and neuronal-stem-cells-expressing persephin all protect against 6-OHDA neurotoxicity (Akerud et al., 1999; Rosenblad et al., 2000). BDNF has also been delivered by a variety of ex *vivo* and *in vivo* gene therapy paradigms. Implants of BDNF-producing fibroblast cells protect against the toxicities of 6-OHDA (Levivier et al., 1995) and 1-methyl-4-phenylpyridinium (MPP$^+$) (Frim et al., 1994). In addition, implantation of BDNF-expressing fibroblasts into the substantia nigra induced sprouting of dopaminergic fibers into grafts (Lucidi-Phillipi et al., 1995).

HD

HD is an autosomal dominant disease in which an expansion of trinucleotide CAG repeats results in abnormally long polyglutamine tracts in the huntingtin protein (Alberch et al., 2002). HD is characterized by abnormal involuntary movements including chorea, dystonia, and parkinsonism as well as cognitive deficits and psychiatric manifestations. Early in the disease, there is a preferential degeneration of medium spiny neurons in the striatum that project to the external segment of the globus pallidus and express gamma amino butyric acid (GABA) and enkephalin. As the disease progresses, there is also degeneration of neurons that express GABA and substance P, and project via the direct pathway to the substantia nigra pars reticulata and the internal segment of the globus pallidus (Alberch et al., 2002). Atrophy and loss of cortical neurons also occurs with disease progression.

A variety of neurotrophic factors have been investigated for their role in the pathogenesis of HD, and their potential to protect against striatal neuronal degeneration (Table 29.1). BDNF is expressed in cortical neurons, and medium spiny neurons in the striatum express TrkB receptors. BDNF levels are decreased by 45% in the fronto-parietal cortex of HD brains (Zuccato et al., 2001). Wild-type huntingtin up-regulates the transcription of BDNF by inhibiting the neuron restrictive silencer element (Zuccato et al., 2003) and mutations in the HD protein result in a loss of this inhibitory function, and may lead to decreased production of cortical BDNF (Zuccato et al., 2001). BDNF and CNTF have been shown to prevent huntingtin-induced cell death in culture (Saudou et al., 1998). BDNF delivered by ex *vivo* gene therapy using fibroblasts or *in vivo* gene therapy using AdV has been shown to protect a wide range of striatal projection neurons against quinolinic acid lesions (Perez-Navarro et al., 2000b; Alberch et al., 2002).

GDNF has also been studied for its potential to protect striatal neurons. mRNA of GDNF and GFRα-1 increase after intrastriatal injections of quinolinic or kainic acid (Alberch et al., 2002). In addition, GDNF-expressing fibroblast cell lines protect GABA/substance P positive neurons that project to the substantia nigra pars reticulata and the globus pallidus internus in the direct pathway, but do not protect striatal projection neurons in the indirect pathway (Perez-Navarro et al., 1999) or striatal parvalbumin-positive neurons (Perez-Navarro et al., 1996) following quinolinic acid lesions. Interestingly, neurturin-expressing cell lines have the opposite effect, protecting striatal neurons in the indirect but not direct pathway (Perez-Navarro et al., 2000a; Marco et al., 2002).

CNTF has also been extensively investigated as a potential neuroprotective agent in HD. Delivery of CNTF to the striata of rats using minipumps (Anderson et al., 1996), engineered lentiviral vectors (Regulier et al., 2002), or polymer-encapsulated baby hamster kidney (BHK) fibroblast cells (Emerich et al., 1997), protects against the toxicity of intrastriatal quinolinic acid injections. In the latter study, CNTF not only protected GABAergic, cholinergic, and diaphorase-positive striatal neurons, but also preserved projections into the globus pallidus and substantia nigra pars reticulata and prevented secondary cortical neuronal atrophy, suggesting both anterograde and retrograde effects. Delivery of CNTF using AdV to rats (Mittoux et al., 2002), or encapsulated CNTF-expressing BHK cells in monkeys (Mittoux et al., 2000), also protects striatal neurons against the toxicity of 3-nitropropionic acid. A phase I gene therapy study for HD involving the transplantation of encapsulated CNTF-expressing BHK cells into the lateral ventricles of patients with HD is underway (Bachoud-Levi et al., 2000).

Amyotrophic lateral sclerosis

Amyotrophic lateral sclerosis (ALS) is a devastating disease involving the progressive degeneration of motor neurons. The etiology remains unknown, but 5–10% of cases are inherited in an autosomal dominant pattern, with 20% of these involving mutations in the SOD1 gene. In ALS, levels of mRNA for GDNF are elevated in muscle samples (Yamamoto et al., 1999), but GDNFR-α are unchanged (Mitsuma et al., 1999). Both ex *vivo* therapy using myoblasts-expressing GNDF (Mohajeri et al., 1999) and *in vivo* gene therapy of AAV-expressing GDNF delivered intramuscularly result in retrograde transport of GDNF and prolong the survival of G93A SOD1 mutant mice (Wang, L.J. et al., 2002).

Recent experiments have focused attention on IGF-1 as a potential disease modifying therapy for ALS (Table 29.1). In one particularly promising study (Kaspar et al., 2003), AAV-expressing either IGF-1 or GDNF was injected intramuscularly into G93A SOD1 mutant mice. When given before disease onset, IGF-1 and GDNF prolonged median survival by 37 and 11 days, respectively (normal death at approximately 120 days). Of even greater clinical relevance, IGF-1 delivered after disease onset increased median survival by 22 days, while GDNF increased survival by 7 days. In contrast, intramuscular delivery of IGF-1-expressing lentivirus (which is not transported retrogradely) offered significantly less protection, indicating that retrograde transport to the cell body was critical. Based on these promising results, a clinical trial of IGF-1 gene therapy is currently being planned. Although, the subcutaneous delivery of IGF-1 to patients with ALS was only marginally successful in one of two randomized trials (Mitchell et al., 2002), lack of effect was likely a result of insufficient drug delivery to target cells.

Spinal cord injury

Spinal cord injury is a major source of morbidity affecting patients of all ages. The initial cellular damage and disruption of axonal pathways is followed by secondary ischemic injury. Progressive cell death and demyelination, as well as a glial scar that can impede axonal regrowth also occur. Neurotrophic factors are particularly promising in that they have both neuroprotective and regenerative effects, which may help to overcome the growth inhibiting environment at the injury site.

A variety of growth factors have been studied in animal models of spinal cord injury including GDNF (Henderson et al., 1994), NT-3, BDNF, and NGF, with the optimal factor depending on the neuronal population studied (Table 29.1). For instance, following cholera-toxin induced lesions of the rat dorsal root entry zone (DREZ), intrathecal GDNF was more effective than NGF, BDNF, or NT3 in stimulating axonal growth of all types of DRG neurons across the DREZ and into spinal cord white matter (Ramer et al., 2000). Fibroblasts-expressing GDNF also promoted significant regeneration of dorsal column sensory, propriospinal, and local motor axons when grafted into transected spinal rat spinal cord (Blesch and Tuszynski, 2003), but did not affect corticospinal, raphae-spinal, and coerulospinal axons. Schwann cells expressing GDNF also promoted propriospinal axonal regeneration and myelination (Iannotti et al., 2003).

Corticospinal tract axons, however, are particularly resistant to the regenerative properties of a variety of neurotrophic factors. In fact, NT-3 is the only known neurotrophic factor that promotes the growth of this cell population in animal models of spinal cord injury (Grill, R. et al., 1997). Grafting of fibroblasts genetically modified to express NT-3 into rats following acute dorsal spinal cord hemisection, resulted in partial functional recovery and growth of corticospinal axons through host gray matter and distal to lesion sites (Grill, R. et al., 1997).

BDNF has also been shown to protect certain neuronal types in models of spinal cord injury. For instance, grafting of BDNF-expressing fibroblasts into a partial cervical hemisection model resulted in the regeneration of 7% of axons in the rubrospinal tract (Liu et al., 1999). These axons extended through fibroblast grafts and caudal white matter to terminate in normal targets. In another study (Jin et al., 2002), BDNF-expressing fibroblasts increased the growth of rubrospinal, reticulospinal, and vestibulospinal tract (VST) axons when transplanted 4 weeks following unilateral hemisection of rats at C3. However, only VST axons extended into host spinal cord caudal to grafts. BDNF- and NT-3-expressing fibroblasts also partially rescued axotomized red nucleus neurons from loss and atrophy (Tobias et al., 2003), and delivery of BDNF using OEG as a cell vehicle improved hind limb performance (Ruitenberg et al., 2003).

NGF also acts as a potent stimulus for sensory axon growth following spinal cord injury. NGF-expressing fibroblasts grafted 1–3 months after bilateral dorsal hemisection resulted in dense growth of ceruraspinal and primary sensory axons of the dorsolateral fasciculus into the grafted lesion site. In contrast, no growth from corticospinal, raphae spinal, or local motor neurons was detected (Grill, R.J. et al., 1997).

Despite relative success in the initiation of axonal growth, stimulating axons to grow beyond neurotrophic factor secreting grafts has proven to be much more difficult (Blesch and Tuszynski, 2003). This may be a result of chemotropic effects that direct axonal growth to areas of highest growth factor concentration. Therefore, although the injury site may represent the optimal location for growth factor production initially, it may also restrict further axonal extension. In order to promote further growth, it may be necessary to turn off growth factor expression at the injury site, while initiating expression at more distal sites (Jones et al., 2001). One solution is to deliver a trail of growth-factor-expressing cells, extending from the transection site to the distal spinal cord (Menei et al., 1998). Alternatively, multiple sequential grafts could be implanted, either at different stages of recovery or with different regulatable elements. The delineation of the optimal targets and growth factor combinations for spinal cord injury is an area of active research that will most likely form the basis for clinical trials within the next several years.

Peripheral neuropathy

It was initially hoped that the systemic delivery of neurotrophic factors might be effective for peripheral neuropathies, since target nerves can be reached without crossing the blood–brain barrier. However, the success of systemic approaches has been limited (Wellmer et al., 2001), most likely due to the induction of systemic side effects at therapeutic doses. To overcome these complications, gene therapy has been extensively investigated for its potential therapeutic applications to peripheral neuropathies.

The importance of NGF in peripheral nerve development has been demonstrated by congenital pain insensitivity and anhidrosis in patients with mutations of TrkA, the high-affinity NGF receptor (Indo et al., 1996). Supplementation with NGF is protective in a variety of animal models of peripheral neuropathy. For instance, systemic NGF protects peripheral nerves against cisplatin toxicity (Apfel et al., 1992). Herpes virus is particularly well suited for gene transfer into sensory neurons since the latent life cycle of the wild-type virus occurs in the sensory ganglia of peripheral nerves. NGF-expressing HSV decreases electrophysiologic abnormalities in streptozotocin-induced diabetic neuropathy (Goss et al., 2002), and results in electrophysiologic, histologic, and behavioral protection against cisplatin neuropathy (Chattopadhyay et al., 2004). Despite these and other promising findings in animal models, treatment with subcutaneous NGF failed to protect in a phase III study of diabetic neuropathy (Apfel et al., 2000).

Delivery of NT-3 also protects in a variety of animal models of peripheral neuropathy. For instance, subcutaneous injection of NT3-expressing HSV resulted in expression in the DRG, and protected sensory neurons against pyridoxine (Chattopadhyay et al., 2002) and cisplatin toxicity (Chattopadhyay et al., 2004) by electrophysiologic, histologic, and behavioral measures of proprioception. Similarly, intramuscular injection of NT-3-expressing AdV protects against both streptozotocin and acrylamide-induced neuropathies (Pradat et al., 2001).

In diabetic neuropathy, the primary pathology may be destruction of the vas nervosum. In order to improve vascularity and blood flow, gene therapy delivering vascular endothelial growth factor (VEGF) has been attempted and found to restore large and small fiber peripheral nerve function in the streptozotocin rat model of diabetes (Schratzberger et al., 2001). A clinical trial delivering recombinant VEGF to patients with diabetic neuropathy has been initiated (Isner et al., 2001).

29.4 Using combinations of growth factors and other treatment modalities

In some instances, the delivery of multiple growth factors simultaneously might enhance protective effects. One approach is to deliver multiple neurotrophic factors to a single target. In a model of brachial plexus injury in neonatal rats, the co-delivery of BDNF and GDNF using polymer implants promoted motor neuron survival and functional recovery, while neither growth factor was effective alone (Aszmann et al., 2002). In another example, co-infection with adenoviruses-expressing CNTF and NT-3 enhanced the survival of mutant progressive motor neuronopathy mice when compared to either alone (Haase et al., 1997). In other instances, it may be most effective to selectively deliver specific growth factors to different cell types. The choice of growth factors could be based on specific target characteristics. For instance, in models of HD, neurturin only protects striatal neurons in the indirect pathway (Marco et al., 2002), while GDNF protects neurons in the direct pathway (Perez-Navarro et al., 1999). Similarly, following spinal cord injury, NGF promotes the regeneration of primary sensory and supraspinal cerulospinal axons, while NT-3 stimulates the regeneration of corticospinal tract axons (Grill, R. et al., 1997).

In order to maximize the effectiveness of neurotrophic factors, other components of growth factor signaling pathways such as receptor expression can also be targeted. For instance, following optic nerve transection, TrkB mRNA decreases in retinal ganglion cells, and the co-administration of AAV-expressing TrkB and exogenous BDNF synergistically increases survival (Cheng et al., 2002). Delivery of neurotrophic factors can also be combined with other therapeutic modalities that are not directly related to the primary signaling pathway. For example, in spinal cord injury, axonal regeneration is impeded by local scar tissue formation and inhibitory factors from myelin (Jones et al., 2001). Here, one strategy is to use matrigel or peripheral nerve bridges in conjunction with gene therapy delivering neurotrophic factors (Iannotti et al., 2003).

29.5 Limitations of neurotrophic factor gene therapy

With the exception of diseases such as ALS and spinal cord injury, most animal models of neurologic disorders reproduce anatomic deficits, but fail to recapitulate the underlying disease pathophysiology. As a result, it is particularly difficult to predict the clinical efficacy of these therapies. For example, levels of BDNF in the cerebral cortex increase after quinolinic acid lesions of the striatum (Canals et al., 2001; Zuccato et al., 2001), but are decreased in HD. As a result, one might predict that BDNF therapy will be much less effective in treating HD than it is for excitotoxic models. Overall, there is a paucity of published literature regarding the efficacy of neurotrophic factor therapy in transgenic mouse models expressing human mutations.

Even if neurotrophic factors are found to protect against degenerative processes in humans, these protective effects may be unrelated to underlying disease pathophysiology. As a result, there may be continued degeneration that negates any protective effects over time. In addition, in advanced disease, multiple neuronal populations are frequently involved that may require the concurrent delivery of different neurotrophic factors. For instance, in advanced PD, in addition to nigral dopaminergic neurons, there is also degeneration of noradrenergic neurons in the locus ceruleus, cholinergic neurons in the dorsal motor nucleus of the vagus and dopaminergic neurons in the ventral tegmental area, all of which contribute to disabling clinical symptoms.

Patient safety is critical to the clinical application of gene therapy. As discussed in Section 29.2, adverse effects could result from the uncontrolled proliferation of viral vectors or transplanted cells. In addition, the delivered gene product itself could also have deleterious effects. Some of these side effects, such as weight loss (Williams, 1991) and Schwann cell hyperplasia seen following intraventricular NGF (Winkler et al., 1997), may not occur with gene therapy approaches that allow more localized delivery of neurotrophic factors (Tuszynski, 2002). However, in other instances, growth factors may have unexpected adverse effects on the underlying disease process. For instance, AAV-mediated delivery of either GDNF (Arvidsson et al., 2003) or BDNF to the striatum (Gustafsson et al., 2003), through anterograde transport from the substantia nigra, was unexpectedly found to increase cell death following middle cerebral artery occlusion. In another example, striatal delivery of GDNF resulted in aberrant sprouting of tyrosine hydroxylase (TH)-immunoreactive fibers in other basal ganglia structures that are not normally innervated by nigral dopaminergic neurons, presumably due to anterograde transportation of GDNF protein (Georgievska et al., 2002). Potential functional consequences of this aberrant sprouting, such as the development of dyskinesias, should be addressed prior to clinical application. AdV-mediated NGF gene delivery in the spinal cord also resulted in aberrant sprouting of nociceptive fibers and the development of hyperalgesia (Romero et al., 2000).

29.6 Conclusions

Gene therapy has the potential to effectively deliver neurotrophic factors in a wide range of neurologic diseases. However, in many instances, significant research is still required to determine the optimal neurotrophic factors and targets for delivery. In a few select diseases, experimental results from animal models are either particularly convincing or unable to provide additional useful information. In these cases, immediate progression to clinical trials may be warranted. Although gene therapy has failed to provide the miracle medical cures that were originally envisioned, and continues to face numerous obstacles, it remains an exceedingly promising therapeutic modality.

Abbreviations

Amyloid β-protein (Aβ), Alzheimer's disease (AD), adenovirus (AdV), adeno-associated virus (AAV), Amyotrophic lateral sclerosis (ALS), baby hamster kidney (BHK), brain-derived neurotrophic factor (BDNF), basic fibroblast growth factor (bFGF), basal forebrain cortical neurons (BFCN), ciliary neurotrophic factor (CNTF), dorsal root entry zone (DREZ), herpes simplex virus (HSV), 6-hydroxydopamine (6-OHDA), insulin-like growth factor 1 (IGF-1), glycosylphosphatidylinositol (GPI), glial cell line-derived neurotrophic factor (GDNF), GDNF family receptors (GFR), Huntington's disease (HD), 1-methyl-4-phenylpyridinium (MPP$^+$), 1-methyl-4-phenyl-1,2,3,6-tetrahydropyridine (MPTP), neurotrophin (NT), nerve growth factor (NGF), nucleus basalis of Meynart (NBM), olfactory ensheathing glia (OEG), Parkinson's disease (PD), platelet-derived growth factor (PDGF), transforming growth factor β (TGFβ), tyrosine hydroxylase (TH), tyrosine kinase receptor (Trk), vascular endothelial growth factor (VEGF), vestibulospinal tract (VST).

REFERENCES

Acsadi, G., Anguelov, R.A., Yang, H., Toth, G., Thomas, R., Jani, A., Wang, Y., Ianakova, E., Mohammad, S., Lewis, R.A. and Shy, M.E. (2002). *Hum Gene Ther*, **13**, 1047–1059.

Akerud, P., Alberch, J., Eketjall, S., Wagner, J. and Arenas, E. (1999). *J Neurochem*, **73**, 70–78.

Akerud, P., Canals, J.M., Snyder, E.Y. and Arenas, E. (2001). *J Neurosci*, **21**, 8108–8118.

Akli, S., Caillaud, C., Vigne, E., Stratford-Perricaudet, L.D., Poenaru, L., Perricaudet, M., Kahn, A. and Peschanski, M.R. (1993). *Nat Genet*, **3**, 224–228.

Alberch, J., Perez-Navarro, E. and Canals, J.M. (2002). *Brain Res Bull*, **57**, 817–822.

Alberch, J., Perez-Navarro, E. and Canals, J.M. (2004). *Prog Brain Res*, **146**, 195–229.

Anderson, K.D., Panayotatos, N., Corcoran, T.L., Lindsay, R.M. and Wiegand, S.J. (1996). *Proc Natl Acad Sci USA*, **93**, 7346–7351.

Apfel, S.C., Arezzo, J.C., Lipson, L. and Kessler, J.A. (1992). *Ann Neurol*, **31**, 76–80.

Apfel, S.C., Schwartz, S., Adornato, B.T., Freeman, R., Biton, V., Rendell, M., Vinik, A., Giuliani, M., Stevens, J.C., Barbano, R. and Dyck, P.J. (2000). *JAMA*, **284**, 2215–2221.

Arvidsson, A., Kirik, D., Lundberg, C., Mandel, R.J., Andsberg, G., Kokaia, Z. and Lindvall, O. (2003). *Neurobiol Dis*, **14**, 542–556.

Aszmann, O.C., Korak, K.J., Kropf, N., Fine, E., Aebischer, P. and Frey, M. (2002). *Plast Reconstr Surg*, **110**, 1066–1072.

Auguste, P., Robledo, O., Olivier, C., Froger, J., Praloran, V., Pouplard-Barthelaix, A. and Gascan, H. (1996). *J Biol Chem*, **271**, 26049–26056.

Bachoud-Levi, A.C., Deglon, N., Nguyen, J.P., Bloch, J., Bourdet, C., Winkel, L., Remy, P., Goddard, M., Lefaucheur, J.P., Brugieres, P., Baudic, S., Cesaro, P., Peschanski, M. and Aebischer, P. (2000). *Hum Gene Ther*, **11**, 1723–1729.

Barkats, M., Nakao, N., Grasbon-Frodl, E.M., Bilang-Bleuel, A., Revah, F., Mallet, J. and Brundin, P. (1997). *Neuroscience*, **78**, 703–713.

Bemelmans, A.P., Horellou, P., Pradier, L., Brunet, I., Colin, P. and Mallet, J. (1999). *Hum Gene Ther*, **10**, 2987–2997.

Berkhout, B., Verhoef, K., Marzio, G., Klaver, B., Vink, M., Zhou, X. and Das, A.T. (2002). *J Neurovirol*, **8**(**Suppl. 2**), 134–137.

Bernheimer, H., Birkmayer, W., Hornykiewicz, O., Jellinger, K. and Seitelberger, F. (1973). *J Neurol Sci*, **20**, 415–455.

Biffo, S., Offenhauser, N., Carter, B.D. and Barde, Y.A. (1995). *Development*, **121**, 2461–2470.

Bilang-Bleuel, A., Revah, F., Colin, P., Locquet, I., Robert, J.J., Mallet, J. and Horellou, P. (1997). *Proc Natl Acad Sci USA*, **94**, 8818–8823.

Bjorklund, A., Kirik, D., Rosenblad, C., Georgievska, B., Lundberg, C. and Mandel, R.J. (2000). *Brain Res*, **886**, 82–98.

Blesch, A. and Tuszynski, M.H. (2003). *J Comp Neurol*, **467**, 403–417.

Blits, B., Dijkhuizen, P.A., Boer, G.J. and Verhaagen, J. (2000). *Exp Neurol*, **164**, 25–37.

Blomer, U., Naldini, L., Kafri, T., Trono, D., Verma, I.M. and Gage, F.H. (1997). *J Virol*, **71**, 6641–6649.

Bourgoin, C., Emiliani, C., Kremer, E.J., Gelot, A., Tancini, B., Gravel, R.A., Drugan, C., Orlacchio, A., Poenaru, L. and Caillaud, C. (2003). *Gene Ther*, **10**, 1841–1849.

Bowers, W.J., Olschowka, J.A. and Federoff, H.J. (2003). *Gene Ther*, **10**, 941–945.

Burton, E.A., Bai, Q., Goins, W.F. and Glorioso, J.C. (2002). *Curr Opin Biotechnol*, **13**, 424–428.

Canals, J.M., Checa, N., Marco, S., Akerud, P., Michels, A., Perez-Navarro, E., Tolosa, E., Arenas, E. and Alberch, J. (2001). *J Neurosci*, **21**, 117–124.

Capsoni, S., Ugolini, G., Comparini, A., Ruberti, F., Berardi, N. and Cattaneo, A. (2000). *Proc Natl Acad Sci USA*, **97**, 6826–6831.

Chattopadhyay, M., Wolfe, D., Huang, S., Goss, J., Glorioso, J.C., Mata, M. and Fink, D.J. (2002). *Ann Neurol*, **51**, 19–27.

Chattopadhyay, M., Goss, J., Wolfe, D., Goins, W.C., Huang, S., Glorioso, J.C., Mata, M. and Fink, D.J. (2004). *Brain*, **127**, 929–939.

Chauhan, N.B., Siegel, G.J. and Lee, J.M. (2001). *J Chem Neuroanat*, **21**, 277–288.

Chen, K.S. and Gage, F.H. (1995). *J Neurosci*, **15**, 2819–2825.

Cheng, L., Sapieha, P., Kittlerova, P., Hauswirth, W.W. and Di Polo, A. (2002). *J Neurosci*, **22**, 3977–3986.

Choi-Lundberg, D.L., Lin, Q., Chang, Y.N., Chiang, Y.L., Hay, C.M., Mohajeri, H., Davidson, B.L. and Bohn, M.C. (1997). *Science*, **275**, 838–841.

Choi-Lundberg, D.L., Lin, Q., Schallert, T., Crippens, D., Davidson, B.L., Chang, Y.N., Chiang, Y.L., Qian, J., Bardwaj, L. and Bohn, M.C. (1998). *Exp Neurol*, **154**, 261–275.

Davidson, B.L., Allen, E.D., Kozarsky, K.F., Wilson, J.M. and Roessler, B.J. (1993). *Nat Genet*, **3**, 219–223.

Davidson, B.L., Stein, C.S., Heth, J.A., Martins, I., Kotin, R.M., Derksen, T.A., Zabner, J., Ghodsi, A. and Chiorini, J.A. (2000). *Proc Natl Acad Sci USA*, **97**, 3428–3432.

Dawbarn, D. and Allen, S.J. (2003). *Neuropathol Appl Neurobiol*, **29**, 211–230.

Dawson, T.M. and Dawson, V.L. (2003). *Science*, **302**, 819–822.

de Almeida, L.P., Zala, D., Aebischer, P. and Deglon, N. (2001). *Neurobiol Dis*, **8**, 433–446.

Dull, T., Zufferey, R., Kelly, M., Mandel, R.J., Nguyen, M., Trono, D. and Naldini, L. (1998). *J Virol*, **72**, 8463–8471.

Emerich, D.F., Winn, S.R., Hantraye, P.M., Peschanski, M., Chen, E.Y., Chu, Y., McDermott, P., Baetge, E.E. and Kordower, J.H. (1997). *Nature*, **386**, 395–399.

Eriksdotter Jonhagen, M., Nordberg, A., Amberla, K., Backman, L., Ebendal, T., Meyerson, B., Olson, L., Seiger, S.M., Theodorsson, E., Viitanen, M., Winblad, B. and Wahlund, L.O. (1998). *Dement Geriatr Cogn Disord*, **9**, 246–257.

Frim, D.M., Uhler, T.A., Galpern, W.R., Beal, M.F., Breakefield, X.O. and Isacson, O. (1994). *Proc Natl Acad Sci USA*, **91**, 5104–5108.

Fukuda, Y., Yamamura, J., Uwano, T., Nishijo, H., Kurokawa, M., Fukuda, M., Ono, T. and Shiraki, K. (2003). *Neurosci Res*, **45**, 233–241.

Georgievska, B., Kirik, D. and Bjorklund, A. (2002). *Exp Neurol*, **177**, 461–474.

Ghadge, G., Roos, R.P., Kang, U.J., Wollmann, R., Fishman, P.S., Kalynych, A.M., Barr, E. and Leiden, J.M. (1995). *Gene Ther*, **2**, 132–137.

Gill, S.S., Patel, N.K., Hotton, G.R., O'Sullivan, K., McCarter, R., Bunnage, M., Brooks, D.J., Svendsen, C.N. and Heywood, P. (2003). *Nat Med*, **9**, 589–595.

Goss, J.R., Goins, W.F., Lacomis, D., Mata, M., Glorioso, J.C. and Fink, D.J. (2002). *Diabetes*, **51**, 2227–2232.

Gossen, M. and Bujard, H. (1992). *Proc Natl Acad Sci USA*, **89**, 5547–5551.

Grill, R., Murai, K., Blesch, A., Gage, F.H. and Tuszynski, M.H. (1997). *J Neurosci*, **17**, 5560–5572.

Grill, R.J., Blesch, A. and Tuszynski, M.H. (1997). *Exp Neurol*, **148**, 444–452.

Guillot, S., Azzouz, M., Deglon, N., Zurn, A. and Aebischer, P. (2004). *Neurobiol Dis*, **16**, 139–149.

Gustafsson, E., Andsberg, G., Darsalia, V., Mohapel, P., Mandel, R.J., Kirik, D., Lindvall, O. and Kokaia, Z. (2003). *Eur J Neurosci*, **17**, 2667–2678.

Haase, G., Kennel, P., Pettmann, B., Vigne, E., Akli, S., Revah, F., Schmalbruch, H. and Kahn, A. (1997). *Nat Med*, **3**, 429–436.

Haase, G., Pettmann, B., Bordet, T., Villa, P., Vigne, E., Schmalbruch, H. and Kahn, A. (1999). *Ann Neurol*, **45**, 296–304.

Hao, S., Mata, M., Wolfe, D., Huang, S., Glorioso, J.C. and Fink, D.J. (2003). *Mol Ther*, **8**, 367–375.

Henderson, C.E., Phillips, H.S., Pollock, R.A., Davies, A.M., Lemeulle, C., Armanini, M., Simpson, L.C., Moffet, B., Vandlen, R.A., Koliatsos, V.E. and Rosenthal, A. (1994). *Science*, **266**, 1062–1064.

Hoehn, M., Kustermann, E., Blunk, J., Wiedermann, D., Trapp, T., Wecker, S., Focking, M., Arnold, H., Hescheler, J., Fleischmann, B.K., Schwindt, W. and Buhrle, C. (2002). *Proc Natl Acad Sci USA*, **99**, 16267–16272.

Hudson, J., Granholm, A.C., Gerhardt, G.A., Henry, M.A., Hoffman, A., Biddle, P., Leela, N.S., Mackerlova, L., Lile, J.D. and Collins, F. (1995). *Brain Res Bull*, **36**, 425–432.

Hyman, C., Hofer, M., Barde, Y.A., Juhasz, M., Yancopoulos, G.D., Squinto, S.P. and Lindsay, R.M. (1991). *Nature*, **350**, 230–232.

Hyman, C., Juhasz, M., Jackson, C., Wright, P., Ip, N.Y. and Lindsay, R.M. (1994). *J Neurosci*, **14**, 335–347.

Hynes, M.A., Poulsen, K., Armanini, M., Berkemeier, L., Phillips, H. and Rosenthal, A. (1994). *J Neurosci Res*, **37**, 144–154.

Iannotti, C., Li, H., Yan, P., Lu, X., Wirthlin, L. and Xu, X.M. (2003). *Exp Neurol*, **183**, 379–393.

Indo, Y., Tsuruta, M., Hayashida, Y., Karim, M.A., Ohta, K., Kawano, T., Mitsubuchi, H., Tonoki, H., Awaya, Y. and Matsuda, I. (1996). *Nat Genet*, **13**, 485–488.

Isner, J.M., Ropper, A. and Hirst, K. (2001). *Hum Gene Ther*, **12**, 1593–1594.

Jin, Y., Fischer, I., Tessler, A. and Houle, J.D. (2002). *Exp Neurol*, **177**, 265–275.

Jones, L.L., Oudega, M., Bunge, M.B. and Tuszynski, M.H. (2001). *J Physiol*, **533**, 83–89.

Kafri, T., van Praag, H., Gage, F.H. and Verma, I.M. (2000). *Mol Ther*, **1**, 516–521.

Kang, U.J. and Nakamura, K. (2003). *Ann Neurol*, **54(Suppl. 6)**, S103–S109.

Kaplitt, M.G., Leone, P., Samulski, R.J., Xiao, X., Pfaff, D.W., O'Malley, K.L. and During, M.J. (1994). *Nat Genet*, **8**, 148–154.

Kaspar, B.K., Llado, J., Sherkat, N., Rothstein, J.D. and Gage, F.H. (2003). *Science*, **301**, 839–842.

Kawaja, M.D., Rosenberg, M.B., Yoshida, K. and Gage, F.H. (1992). *J Neurosci*, **12**, 2849–2864.

Kells, A.P., Fong, D.M., Dragunow, M., During, M.J., Young, D. and Connor, B. (2004). *Mol Ther*, **9**, 682–688.

Kirik, D., Rosenblad, C., Bjorklund, A. and Mandel, R.J. (2000). *J Neurosci*, **20**, 4686–4700.

Kishima, H., Poyot, T., Bloch, J., Dauguet, J., Conde, F., Dolle, F., Hinnen, F., Pralong, W., Palfi, S., Deglon, N., Aebischer, P. and Hantraye, P. (2004). *Neurobiol Dis*, **16**, 428–439.

Kissa, K., Mordelet, E., Soudais, C., Kremer, E.J., Demeneix, B.A., Brulet, P. and Coen, L. (2002). *Mol Cell Neurosci*, **20**, 627–637.

Klein, R.L., Hirko, A.C., Meyers, C.A., Grimes, J.R., Muzyczka, N. and Meyer, E.M. (2000). *Brain Res*, **875**, 144–151.

Knusel, B., Michel, P.P., Schwaber, J.S. and Hefti, F. (1990). *J Neurosci*, **10**, 558–570.

Kordower, J.H., Winn, S.R., Liu, Y.T., Mufson, E.J., Sladek Jr., J.R., Hammang, J.P., Baetge, E.E. and Emerich, D.F. (1994). *Proc Natl Acad Sci USA*, **91**, 10898–10902.

Kordower, J.H., Palfi, S., Chen, E.Y., Ma, S.Y., Sendera, T., Cochran, E.J., Mufson, E.J., Penn, R., Goetz, C.G. and Comella, C.D. (1999). *Ann Neurol*, **46**, 419–424.

Kordower, J.H., Emborg, M.E., Bloch, J., Ma, S.Y., Chu, Y., Leventhal, L., McBride, J., Chen, E.Y., Palfi, S., Roitberg, B.Z., Brown, W.D., Holden, J.E., Pyzalski, R., Taylor, M.D., Carvey, P., Ling, Z., Trono, D., Hantraye, P., Deglon, N. and Aebischer, P. (2000). *Science*, **290**, 767–773.

Lapchak, P.A., Araujo, D.M., Hilt, D.C., Sheng, J. and Jiao, S. (1997). *Brain Res*, **777**, 153–160.

Lehtonen, E., Bonnaud, F., Melas, C., Lubansu, A., Malgrange, B., Chtarto, A., Velu, T., Brotchi, J., Levivier, M., Peschanski, M. and Tenenbaum, L. (2002). *NeuroReport*, **13**, 1503–1507.

Levi-Montalcini, R. (1966). *Harvey Lect*, **60**, 217–259.

Levivier, M., Przedborski, S., Bencsics, C. and Kang, U.J. (1995). *J Neurosci*, **15**, 7810–7820.

Li, X., Eastman, E.M., Schwartz, R.J. and Draghia-Akli, R. (1999). *Nat Biotechnol*, **17**, 241–245.

Lin, L.F.H., Doherty, D.H., Lile, J.D., Bektesh, S. and Collins, F. (1993). *Science*, **260**, 1130–1132.

Lindner, M.D., Winn, S.R., Baetge, E.E., Hammang, J.P., Gentile, F.T., Doherty, E., McDermott, P.E., Frydel, B., Ullman, M.D., Schallert, T. and Emerich, D.F. (1995). *Exp Neurol*, **132**, 62–76.

Liu, Y., Kim, D., Himes, B.T., Chow, S.Y., Schallert, T., Murray, M., Tessler, A. and Fischer, I. (1999). *J Neurosci*, **19**, 4370–4387.

Lucidi-Phillipi, C.A., Gage, F.H., Shults, C.W., Jones, K.R., Reichardt, L.F. and Kang, U.J. (1995). *J Comp Neurol*, **354**, 361–376.

Mandel, R.J., Spratt, S.K., Snyder, R.O. and Leff, S.E. (1997). *Proc Natl Acad Sci USA*, **94**, 14083–14088.

Mandel, R.J., Gage, F.H., Clevenger, D.G., Spratt, S.K., Snyder, R.O. and Leff, S.E. (1999). *Exp Neurol*, **155**, 59–64.

Marco, S., Perez-Navarro, E., Tolosa, E., Arenas, E. and Alberch, J. (2002). *J Neurobiol*, **50**, 323–332.

Marshall, E. (1999). *Science*, **286**, 2244–2245.

Martinez-Serrano, A. and Bjorklund, A. (1996). *J Neurosci*, **16**, 4604–4616.

Martinez-Serrano, A., Lundberg, C., Horellou, P., Fischer, W., Bentlage, C., Campbell, K., McKay, R.D.G., Mallet, J. and Bjorklund, A. (1995). *J Neurosci*, **15**, 5668–5680.

Mata, M., Glorioso, J.C. and Fink, D.J. (2004). *Curr Neurol Neurosci Rep*, **4**, 1–2.

McBride, J.L., During, M.J., Wuu, J., Chen, E.Y., Leurgans, S.E. and Kordower, J.H. (2003). *Exp Neurol*, **181**, 213–223.

Menei, P., Montero-Menei, C., Whittemore, S.R., Bunge, R.P. and Bunge, M.B. (1998). *Eur J Neurosci*, **10**, 607–621.

Mesulam, M. (2004). *Learn Mem*, **11**, 43–49.

Mitchell, J.D., Wokke, J.H. and Borasio, G.D. (2002). *Cochrane Database System Review*, CD002064.

Mitsuma, N., Yamamoto, M., Li, M., Ito, Y., Mitsuma, T., Mutoh, T., Takahashi, M. and Sobue, G. (1999). *Brain Res*, **820**, 77–85.

Mittoux, V., Joseph, J.M., Conde, F., Palfi, S., Dautry, C., Poyot, T., Bloch, J., Deglon, N., Ouary, S., Nimchinsky, E.A., Brouillet, E., Hof, P.R., Peschanski, M., Aebischer, P. and Hantraye, P. (2000). *Hum Gene Ther*, **11**, 1177–1187.

Mittoux, V., Ouary, S., Monville, C., Lisovoski, F., Poyot, T., Conde, F., Escartin, C., Robichon, R., Brouillet, E., Peschanski, M. and Hantraye, P. (2002). *J Neurosci*, **22**, 4478–4486.

Miyoshi, H., Blomer, U., Takahashi, M., Gage, F.H. and Verma, I.M. (1998). *J Virol*, **72**, 8150–8157.

Mohajeri, M.H., Figlewicz, D.A. and Bohn, M.C. (1999). *Hum Gene Ther*, **10**, 1853–1866.

Natsume, A., Wolfe, D., Hu, J., Huang, S., Puskovic, V., Glorioso, J.C., Fink, D.J. and Mata, M. (2003). *Exp Neurol*, **184**, 878–886.

Norgren Jr., R.B. and Lehman, M.N. (1998). *Neurosci Biobehav Rev*, **22**, 695–708.

Nutt, J.G., Burchiel, K.J., Comella, C.L., Jankovic, J., Lang, A.E., Laws Jr., E.R., Lozano, A.M., Penn, R.D., Simpson Jr., R.K., Stacy, M. and Wooten, G.F. (2003). *Neurology*, **60**, 69–73.

Perez-Navarro, E., Arenas, E., Reiriz, J., Calvo, N. and Alberch, J. (1996). *Neuroscience*, **75**, 345–352.

Perez-Navarro, E., Arenas, E., Marco, S. and Alberch, J. (1999). *Eur J Neurosci*, **11**, 241–249.

Perez-Navarro, E., Akerud, P., Marco, S., Canals, J.M., Tolosa, E., Arenas, E. and Alberch, J. (2000a). *Neuroscience*, **98**, 89–96.

Perez-Navarro, E., Canudas, A.M., Akerund, P., Alberch, J. and Arenas, E. (2000b). *J Neurochem*, **75**, 2190–2199.

Peterziel, H., Unsicker, K. and Krieglstein, K. (2002). *J Cell Biol*, **159**, 157–167.

Poeschla, E.M., Wong-Staal, F. and Looney, D.J. (1998). *Nat Med*, **4**, 354–357.

Pradat, P.F., Kennel, P., Naimi-Sadaoui, S., Finiels, F., Orsini, C., Revah, F., Delaere, P. and Mallet, J. (2001). *Hum Gene Ther*, **12**, 2237–2249.

Pradat, P.F., Kennel, P., Naimi-Sadaoui, S., Finiels, F., Scherman, D., Orsini, C., Delaere, P., Mallet, J. and Revah, F. (2002). *Gene Ther*, **9**, 1333–1337.

Ramer, M.S., Priestley, J.V. and McMahon, S.B. (2000). *Nature*, **403**, 312–316.

Regulier, E., Pereira de Almeida, L., Sommer, B., Aebischer, P. and Deglon, N. (2002). *Hum Gene Ther*, **13**, 1981–1990.

Romero, M.I., Rangappa, N., Li, L., Lightfoot, E., Garry, M.G. and Smith, G.M. (2000). *J Neurosci*, **20**, 4435–4445.

Rosenberg, M.B., Friedmann, T., Robertson, R.C., Tuszynski, M., Wolff, J.A., Breakefield, X.O. and Gage, F.H. (1988). *Science*, **242**, 1575–1578.

Rosenblad, C., Gronborg, M., Hansen, C., Blom, N., Meyer, M., Johansen, J., Dago, L., Kirik, D., Patel, U.A., Lundberg, C., Trono, D., Bjorklund, A. and Johansen, T.E. (2000). *Mol Cell Neurosci*, **15**, 199–214.

Ruitenberg, M.J., Plant, G.W., Hamers, F.P., Wortel, J., Blits, B., Dijkhuizen, P.A., Gispen, W.H., Boer, G.J. and Verhaagen, J. (2003). *J Neurosci*, **23**, 7045–7058.

Saarma, M. (2000). *Eur J Biochem*, **267**, 6968–6971.

Sagot, Y., Tan, S.A., Hammang, J.P., Aebischer, P. and Kato, A.C. (1996). *J Neurosci*, **16**, 2335–2341.

Sakhuja, K., Reddy, P.S., Ganesh, S., Cantaniag, F., Pattison, S., Limbach, P., Kayda, D.B., Kadan, M.J., Kaleko, M. and Connelly, S. (2003). *Hum Gene Ther*, **14**, 243–254.

Saudou, F., Finkbeiner, S., Devys, D. and Greenberg, M.E. (1998). *Cell*, **95**, 55–66.

Schratzberger, P., Walter, D.H., Rittig, K., Bahlmann, F.H., Pola, R., Curry, C., Silver, M., Krainin, J.G., Weinberg, D.H., Ropper, A.H. and Isner, J.M. (2001). *J Clin Invest*, **107**, 1083–1092.

Schumacher, J.M., Short, M.P., Hyman, B.T., Breakefield, X.O. and Isacson, O. (1991). *Neuroscience*, **45**, 561–570.

Scott, S.A., Mufson, E.J., Weingartner, J.A., Skau, K.A. and Crutcher, K.A. (1995). *J Neurosci*, **15**, 6213–6221.

Sisodia, S.S. and St George-Hyslop, P.H. (2002). *Nat Rev Neurosci*, **3**, 281–290.

Smith, D.E., Roberts, J., Gage, F.H. and Tuszynski, M.H. (1999). *Proc Natl Acad Sci USA*, **96**, 10893–10898.

Suhr, S.T., Gil, E.B., Senut, M.C. and Gage, F.H. (1998). *Proc Natl Acad Sci USA*, **95**, 7999–8004.

Tai, M.H., Cheng, H., Wu, J.P., Liu, Y.L., Lin, P.R., Kuo, J.S., Tseng, C.J. and Tzeng, S.F. (2003). *Exp Neurol*, **183**, 508–515.

Tenenbaum, L., Lehtonen, E. and Monahan, P.E. (2003). *Curr Gene Ther*, **3**, 545–565.

Tenenbaum, L., Chtarto, A., Lehtonen, E., Velu, T., Brotchi, J. and Levivier, M. (2004). *J Gene Med*, **6(Suppl. 1)**, S212–S222.

Thoenen, H. and Sendtner, M. (2002). *Nat Neurosci*, **5(Suppl.)**, 1046–1050.

Thomas, C.E., Schiedner, G., Kochanek, S., Castro, M.G. and Lowenstein, P.R. (2000). *Proc Natl Acad Sci USA*, **97**, 7482–7487.

Tobias, C.A., Shumsky, J.S., Shibata, M., Tuszynski, M.H., Fischer, I., Tessler, A. and Murray, M. (2003). *Exp Neurol*, **184**, 97–113.

Tomac, A., Widenfalk, J., Lin, L.F.H., Kohno, T., Ebendal, T., Hoffer, B.J. and Olson, L. (1995). *Proc Natl Acad Sci USA*, **92**, 8274–8278.

Tuszynski, M.H., Thal, L., Pay, M., Salmon, D.P., U.H.S., Bakay, R., Patel, P., Blesch, A., Vahlsing, H.L., Ho, G., Tong, G., Potkin, S.G., Fallon, J., Hansen, L., Mufson, E.J., Kordower, J.H.,

Gall, C. and Conner, J. (2005). A phase 1 clinical trial of nerve growth factor gene therapy for Alzheimer disease. *Nat Med*, **11(5)**, 551–555.

Wang, L.J., Lu, Y.Y., Muramatsu, S., Ikeguchi, K., Fujimoto, K., Okada, T., Mizukami, H., Matsushita, T., Hanazono, Y., Kume, A., Nagatsu, T., Ozawa, K. and Nakano, I. (2002). *J Neurosci*, **22**, 6920–6928.

Wang, S., Fraefel, C. and Breakefield, X. (2002). *Method Enzymol*, **346**, 593–603.

Weidner, N., Blesch, A., Grill, R.J. and Tuszynski, M.H. (1999). *J Comp Neurol*, **413**, 495–506.

Wellmer, A., Misra, V.P., Sharief, M.K., Kopelman, P.G. and Anand, P. (2001). *J Peripher Nerv Syst*, **6**, 204–210.

Williams, L.R. (1991). *Exp Neurol*, **113**, 31–37.

Winkler, J., Ramirez, G.A., Kuhn, H.G., Peterson, D.A., Day-Lollini, P.A., Stewart, G.R., Tuszynski, M.H., Gage, F.H. and Thal, L.J. (1997). *Ann Neurol*, **41**, 82–93.

Winkler, J., Thal, L.J., Gage, F.H. and Fisher, L.J. (1998). *J Mol Med*, **76**, 555–567.

Yamamoto, M., Mitsuma, N., Inukai, A., Ito, Y., Li, M., Mitsuma, T. and Sobue, G. (1999). *Neurochem Res*, **24**, 785–790.

Ye, X., Rivera, V.M., Zoltick, P., Cerasoli Jr., F., Schnell, M.A., Gao, G., Hughes, J.V., Gilman, M. and Wilson, J.M. (1999). *Science*, **283**, 88–91.

Zala, D., Bensadoun, J.C., Pereira de Almeida, L., Leavitt, B.R., Gutekunst, C.A., Aebischer, P., Hayden, M.R. and Deglon, N. (2004). *Exp Neurol*, **185**, 26–35.

Zuccato, C., Ciammola, A., Rigamonti, D., Leavitt, B.R., Goffredo, D., Conti, L., MacDonald, M.E., Friedlander, R.M., Silani, V., Hayden, M.R., Timmusk, T., Sipione, S. and Cattaneo, E. (2001). *Science*, **293**, 493–498.

Zuccato, C., Tartari, M., Crotti, A., Goffredo, D., Valenza, M., Conti, L., Cataudella, T., Leavitt, B.R., Hayden, M.R., Timmusk, T., Rigamonti, D. and Cattaneo, E. (2003). *Nat Genet*, **35**, 76–83.

Assessment of sensorimotor function after spinal cord injury and repair

Ronaldo M. Ichiyama[1], Roland R. Roy[2] and V. Reggie Edgerton[1,2,3]

Departments of [1]Physiological Science and [2]Neurobiology and [3]Brain Research Institute, UCLA, Los Angeles, CA, USA

30.1 Introduction

This chapter focuses on methods to assess postural and locomotor performance in laboratory animals. The main purpose is to identify the specific neuro-motor deficits resulting from spinal cord injury (SCI) and those interventions that may be used to improve the level of recovery (see Volume I, Chapters 21–26, 28 and 29). Furthermore, we have focused on methods that reflect *in vivo* function. The methods include not only those which demonstrate the degree of motor dysfunction, but also those which provide some insight into the specific neural deficits that could account for the level of postural and locomotor performance.

In selecting methods to assess motor performance, the experimental design and the specific questions being addressed should be carefully considered. In the literature related to SCI over the past few years there has been the perception that there is a single test that can be used to define motor performance levels. In addition, there seems to have evolved the concept that the primary criteria for selecting a method of measurement of performance are that they can be easily and quickly administered, as well as inexpensive. Although such criteria can be rationalized in the clinical environment, in most cases this is not acceptable for drawing clear scientific conclusions. The view that a meaningful "measurement" can be validly and reliably derived from a visual impression to generate a rating of the performance of an animal in a minimally controlled environment has become pervasive in the area of SCI.

Another commonly expressed misconception about the significance of a particular motor test is related to whether the motor task is "voluntary". Furthermore, the implication is that if the task is voluntary then it is an indication of control from the motor cortex. Often when adjustments in foot placement during a movement are made (e.g. in a ladder climb), this is assumed to be voluntary and cortically derived. Whether this is actually the case is questionable. Very complex adjustments are usually assessed to be voluntary in nature, when in fact the spinal cord can generate many corrective tasks without any supraspinal input. The issue becomes even less clear in regards to whether the motor task is controlled by neural networks in the brainstem rather than the cerebral motor cortex.

Accurate interpretations of movements being voluntary and centrally driven are further questionable in light of the fact that full weight-bearing overground locomotion can be performed in cats after the cerebral cortex has been removed (Bard and Macht, 1958). Even in non-human primates, it is clear that the corticospinal tract (CST) does not have to be intact for an animal to generate locomotion (Vilensky et al., 1992). On the other hand it is quite clear that the descending input from the brainstem plays a very critical role in the control of posture and locomotion (Orlovsky et al., 1999). However, the brainstem is not an essential source of control to stand or to step, even in humans.

A general concept that is useful in selecting neuromotor performance assays is that there are many ways to perform a given motor task, including stepping. It is possible, for example, that an animal can fully recover in performing a motor task by using a strategy that completely bypasses the neural circuitry one is interested in studying. This is often possible when the challenge of the motor task is insufficient. At the same time it is often difficult to categorize the recovery clearly as a compensatory versus a repair strategy. In many cases even when there is neural reorganization underlying the basis for the recovery, the repair process is not likely to be one that completely re-establishes the original neural circuitry. On the other hand, it is likely that when there is some neural repair and reorganization occurring, there will be still some compensatory strategies that underlie the apparent recovery of the behavior.

To establish the impact of interventions such as cellular implants, factors which inhibit or stimulate growth, or pharmacological agents that modulate the spinal and supraspinal neural circuitries, a series of assays should be administered to determine the success of re-establishing new connectivity across a spinal cord lesion. There is extensive coordination that occurs between the forelimbs and hindlimbs simply from the mechanical linkage of the upper and lower body, independent of any neural control that might mediate interlimb coordination. To establish the presence of new functional connectivity, supraspinal and intraspinal stimulation and recordings from the specific circuits of interest should be demonstrated electrophysiologically. Even this test of connectivity, however, does not establish whether the newly developed synapses are behaviorally functional. In fact, the newly established synaptic connections could further disrupt the motor control or even cause additional pain. Detailed analysis of the activation patterns of the different motor pools and quantitative kinematic analyses during well-controlled motor tasks can help to determine the *in vivo* functional significance of the new connectivity. To clearly establish the functional significance, further experiments such as temporarily anesthetizing or surgically eliminating the new connections may be necessary. One cannot conclude renewed functional connectivity with any reasonable level of certainty based on subjective visual observations of

the movement of an animal, and from these observations generate a score that purports to reflect intralimb or interlimb coordination.

To summarize some of the general principles in selecting neuromotor assays to be studied are as follows:

1 Select tests which match the specific question being proposed.
2 The administration of a single motor task for a wide variety of types of injuries in multiple species severely limits one's ability to discriminate the effects of a lesion or post-injury intervention.
3 Define the nature of the hypothesized new connectivity by establishing the synaptic efficacy and its level of contribution to the performance of the motor task *in vivo*.
4 Avoid subjective rating scales unless a large number of animals are being tested and the intention is to obtain a gross indication of some generalized effect of an intervention.
5 Selecting a motor task based on convenience of use is likely to limit the impact of a study.

30.2 Posture

Following SCI the ability to stand and maintain equilibrium is a highly desirable accomplishment. It is somewhat surprising that this motor task has received relatively little attention given the clear demonstration of the ability of the spinal cord to sustain a standing position simply by placing pressure on the plantar surface of the foot (Sherrington, 1906). When pressure is placed on the bottom of the foot of a complete spinal animal the hindlimbs can extend sufficiently to support the weight of the hindquarters. After an initial extensor response, the level of activation of the extensor motor pools will subside and the hindlimbs will collapse. If the animal is trained daily by initiating the extensor thrust repeatedly, the length of time that the extension is sustained increases. Complete spinal cats have been trained to stand for as much as 20 continuous minutes without any stimulation imposed by the experimenter (de Leon

(a)

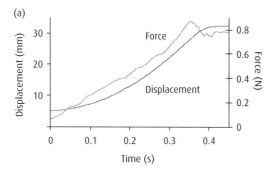

(b)

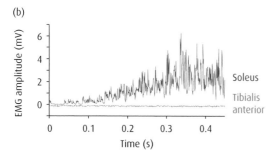

(c)

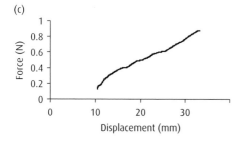

Figure 30.1. Standing is one mode of sensorimotor training used to test the performance of spinal cats and rats. The *in vivo* functional properties of the neuromuscular system that contribute to the thrust reflex can be used as a measure of the effectiveness of the stand training. A robotic arm with an attached bar is programmed to elevate the paw of one hindlimb resting on the bar. With the body weight of the rat supported, the resistance to raising the paw is recorded as the bar is pushing upward on the plantar surface of the paw. (a) Shows the lifting phase of the test; (b) shows the relative activation level (rectified and filtered EMG) of the soleus and tibialis anterior muscles from chronically implanted electrodes; (c) illustrates the stiffness of the hindlimb from the relationship between displacement and force (Bigbee et al., 2002).

et al., 1998a). Also the extensor response becomes greater, resulting in a stiffer limb (Fig. 30.1) (Bigbee et al., 2002). Thompson and co-workers (Bose et al., 2002) also have devised a means to assess stiffness of the ankle plantarflexors.

During standing it is apparent that the spinal cord control strategy is very dynamic. The spinal cord is basically receiving sensory information associated with weight bearing and, in response, modulating the levels of activation of the appropriate motor pools necessary to sustain some level of equilibrium and full weight support. Standing is not simply a result obtained by "locking the knees" in a hyperextended position. In effect the complete spinal animal cannot only maintain equilibrium, but it can also learn to stand (de Leon et al., 1998a) as well as to step (Lovely et al., 1986; Barbeau and Rossignol, 1987; de Leon et al., 1998b). Some quantitative methods of measurement of standing ability can include the following:

1 The length of time that full weight bearing can be sustained without external stimuli (de Leon et al., 1998a).
2 The strength of the extensor thrust measured by assessing the stiffness of the limbs to a given force imposed either downward on the hips or upward from the plantar surface of the feet (Bigbee et al., 2002).
3 Comparing the magnitude of corrective responses relative to the magnitude and direction of the perturbation similar to that described by Beloozerova et al. (2003).

30.3 Locomotion

In SCI research recovery of locomotion is a commonly stated or implied goal. In fact, more often than not recovery of stepping-like actions is the only function assessed after different neural repair strategies. A given treatment is termed effective if some improvement in some measure of mobility is observed. A plethora of tests of motor performance have been developed in animal models and new ones are implemented regularly. As noted previously, the specific objective of each study will dictate the most appropriate motor assay. For example, is the objective to demonstrate supraspinal–spinal connectivity, segmental circuitries that can generate standing and stepping in the absence of supraspinal or afferent input, or the ability of spinal circuitries that have intact sensory input to generate a locomotor pattern? Or is the question related to the level of ipsilateral–contralateral coordination that can be manifested. In many instances it is desirable to differentiate whether the issue is to determine what an animal can do versus what it wants or chooses to do. In most cases, measures of recovery of locomotion should include quantifiable data related to the kinematics of stepping (stride length; height and duration; swing and stance duration), segmental and joint angular kinematics, intralimb joint dynamics and interlimb coordination. These measures should reflect the capacity of the animal to step when adequately challenged by the experimental conditions.

Treadmill locomotion

Treadmill locomotion has a number of advantages in assessing stepping ability. It requires the animal to remain within a specified space, which is ideal for collecting video and electromyographic (EMG) data concomitantly. Stepping on a treadmill belt provides a means of observing more consistent locomotor activity, thus minimizing variations in the speed and continuity of stepping and at the same time challenges the animal's stepping ability over a range of controlled speeds. The performance of spinal animals on the treadmill seems to peak at a certain speed and shows more variability at both slower and faster speeds (Lovely et al., 1986). Therefore, impairments in locomotor performance can be detected more easily during treadmill locomotion than during open-field or walkway tasks, where the animal chooses the direction and speed of locomotion and when to step or stand.

Using body weight support systems provides another advantage of performing locomotion on a treadmill (de Leon et al., 2002a). An animal can be tested with varying amounts of weight-bearing assistance needed to perform the task. The percent of body weight that can be supported while generating successful steps also can be used as a measure of locomotor performance. Providing support during locomotion is a very important component of step training programs as well as in testing motor performance ability (see Table 30.1).

Kinematics

Detailed kinematic analysis of the step cycle can be obtained using cinematographic or videographic techniques (Metz et al., 2000b; Muir and Webb, 2000; Shumsky et al., 2003). Several commercially available systems can capture and reconstruct limb movements three-dimensionally (3-D). Commonly, visual markers are placed over bony landmarks to allow for reconstruction of body segments. These 3-D reconstructions provide extensive linear and angular displacement, velocity and acceleration information. Intralimb and interlimb coordination can be defined in all three planes of rotation. No other analysis technique to date can provide this amount of kinematic detail about motion. Kinematic data can be obtained using this method regardless of the level, type or severity of the SCI. However, the cost of the equipment and the amount of training and time necessary to collect and analyze corresponding kinematic data are significant. Another limitation of this approach is the difficulty in reliably tracking external markers that represent the knee and shoulder because of skin movement. X-ray cinematography is one method which can be used to increase the accuracy of identifying specific bony landmarks (Kuhtz-Buschbeck et al., 1996) when more detailed kinematics are needed.

EMG Recording

The EMG activity of muscles recruited during specific tasks has been a reliable indicator of functionality at the motor pool and, in some cases, the motor unit level (Lovely et al., 1986; Gregor et al., 1988; Thomas and Noga, 2003). EMG activity patterns

Table 30.1. Tools for assessing motor function after SCI[a].

Functional parameters	Posture/locomotion (Treadmill)[b]							Electrophysiology						Other Motor Tests						
	Speed	Distance	Weight support	Kinematics	EMG	Pharmacological interventions	Robotics	Fictive locomotion	TMS stimulation	SSEP stimulation	MLR stimulation	Spinal cord physiology	Muscle physiology	Limb force-displacement	Grasping strength	Footfall pattern	Grid, ladder and beam walking	Swimming	Rope climbing	Food retrieval
Motor unit recruitment level	X		X	X	X		X	X			X			X	X	X	X	X	X	X
Motor pool coordination	X	X	X	X	X		X	X			X				X	X			X	X
Corticospinal control														X				X[c]	X[c]	X[c]
Weight bearing	X	X	X	X	X	X	X							X		X	X			
FL–HL coordination	X			X	X		X									X				
Bilateral coordination	X			X	X		X	X								X	X			
Interjoint coordination				X	X		X										X			
Limb adduction, abduction, rotation	X			X												X	X			
Plantar placement	X			X	X											X				
Stepping ability	X	X	X	X	X	X	X									X	X			
Fatigue	X	X					X								X			X		
Sensorimotor correction				X			X										X			
Limb stiffness			X	X	X									X						
Functional synaptic connectivity				X[d]	X[d]				X	X	X	X			X					X
Muscle force													X							

FL–HL, forelimb–hindlimb; TMS, transcranial magnetic stimulation; SSEP, somatosensory-evoked potentials; MLR, mesencephalic locomotor region.

[a] This table represents a series of functions that are tested or inferred to be tested by different motor assessment tools. It is subdivided into those motor assessment tools that can (1) best be applied with a motor driven treadmill belt (*in vivo*); (2) reflect a range of electrophysiological tests usually applied in terminal experiments; and (3) those which represent a range of behavioral skills requiring specialized mechanisms of neural control. The blocks within this matrix marked by an X imply that a given assessment tool can be used as a quantitative assessment of the relevant function listed on the far left.

[b] These tools can also be used to assess overground locomotion, but can be more easily controlled during treadmill locomotion (see text).

[c] Some features of these motor tasks probably require some corticospinal input.

[d] Detailed analysis of limb kinematics combined with EMG analysis are needed to assess FL–HL coordination after a spinal cord lesion.

indicate the level and timing of output from a specific motor pool (Roy et al., 1991). The relationship of the pattern of activity of one muscle relative to other muscles provides a measure of coordination of the motor pools, a critical element that defines the quality of locomotion. EMG patterns from the same motor pool can be compared over a period of months when electrodes are implanted appropriately. In SCI research and in the clinical setting EMG techniques are commonly used to determine the level and pattern of activity within and among specific muscles and motor pools. Both intramuscular and surface EMG electrodes have been used. The number of muscles studied at one time is limited by the costs and availability of equipment, in addition to anatomical issues, that is, the location of the muscles. Muscle synergies can be studied with EMG techniques when recordings are made from multiple muscles (motor pools) during the performance of specific behavioral tasks. The EMG signals, however, cannot be directly translated into the force or displacement generated by the muscle. For example, the same level of activation of a muscle can generate a high force output and low velocity or vice versa depending on the loading conditions. This relationship between force and velocity is well characterized and is a function of the intrinsic properties of skeletal muscle (Gregor et al., 1988).

Robotics

We have used a rodent robotic device to train rats and mice to walk bipedally after a complete spinal cord transection (de Leon et al., 2002a, b; Timoszyk et al., 2002; Fong et al., 2003). Animals are placed in an upper body harness, which is attached to an automated body weight support system (Timoszyk et al., 2005). Robotic arms are attached to the ankles using neoprene bracelets. These robotic arms can work both in an active mode, that is, actively moving the legs, or in a passive mode, that is, recording ankle displacement. Using this device step kinematics based on ankle position can be obtained, and measurements such as the number of steps, step height and length, swing and stance duration, interlimb

coordination, etc. can be extrapolated (Fig. 30.2). An advantage of this method is that a large amount of data can be collected and analyzed quickly. However, animals need to be trained to walk with the robotic arms attached to their ankles. Although this method currently does not provide data on individual joint kinematics, other biomechanical sensors, such as accelerometers, goniometers and/or simultaneous video analyses, can be used to characterize the joint kinematics when this level of detail is desired (Weytjens et al., 1992).

Overground locomotion

Overground locomotion also has been widely used to assess recovery of motor function after SCI. Most overground locomotor tasks involve some sort of walkway, for example, wide and narrow beam walk (Kunkel-Bagden et al., 1993; Cheng et al., 1997) and the Cat Walk (Hamers et al., 2001), which the animal is trained to traverse for a reward. There is no experimental control over the speed and consistency at which the animal traverses the walkway. The variable speed can make it more difficult to interpret the significance of EMG amplitude changes over time. Using this method, the preferred locomotor pattern and speed at that particular instant can sometimes be determined. Many environmental and motivational factors, such as fear and the level of practice, can affect the assessment of motor performance when the animal is placed in an environment that allows for multiple motor strategies. For example, in this task the motivation of the animal must be sufficient to elicit the desired behavior. Does the task represent a test of psychological state traits rather than the physiological capacity of the nervous system to control locomotion? To alter the difficulty of the task, the width of the walkway can be varied, for example, using a wide or a narrow beam. Each of these tests reflects the ability to execute a different task and, in most cases these different tasks may be accomplished using different neural control mechanisms and circuitries.

Recently, footprint analysis has become increasingly popular. Several methods have been developed

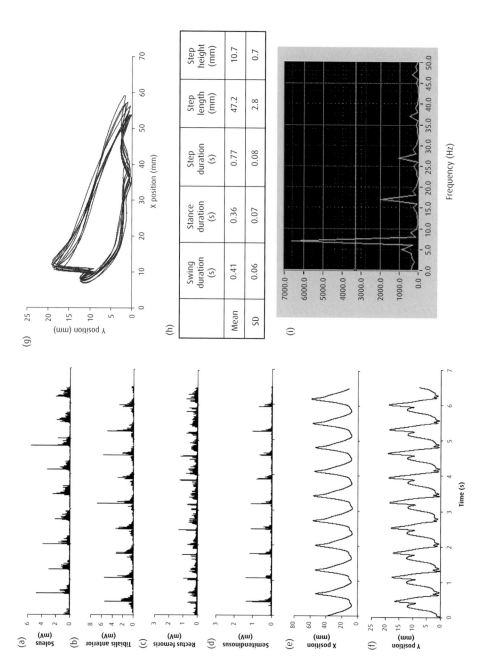

	Swing duration (s)	Stance duration (s)	Step duration (s)	Step length (mm)	Step height (mm)
Mean	0.41	0.36	0.77	47.2	10.7
SD	0.06	0.07	0.08	2.8	0.7

Figure 30.2. In a complete spinal rat, the rectified EMG activity recorded from electrodes implanted chronically in four muscles during nine consecutive steps is shown (a–d). Movement of the ankle in the X (horizontal) and Y (vertical) directions are shown in (e) and (f). The X–Y trajectory of the ankle movement (g) illustrates a consistent trajectory over these nine steps. Some basic step characteristics can be derived from these steps (h). The FFT (fast Fourier transform) frequency spectrum analysis from the robotic arm (i) can be used as a measure of consistency and smoothness of the movement, which can be compared across animals on repeated tests. The FFT frequency spectrum in (i) was derived from the horizontal movement.

based on the premise that the footprint analysis provides an indirect assessment of stepping kinematics. Traditionally, the forepaws and the hindpaws are inked with different colors and the animal is placed either on a treadmill or on a walkway over white recording paper (Kunkel-Bagden et al., 1993; Metz et al., 2000b). The ink marks provide information on the number of steps, stride length, toe spread, paw rotation, width of the base of support, interlimb coordination, etc. To circumvent some potential problems associated with the use of ink on the animal's paws and the lack of timing information, video images collected through the bottom of a plexiglass walkway have been used (Cheng et al., 1997). More recently, an automated footprint analysis system (the "Cat Walk") using an illumination method that only allows light through the glass floor of the walkway when the paw contacts its surface has been developed (Hamers et al., 2001).

Following severe SCI, footprint analysis is limited because a useful level of successful foot placements cannot be executed. It is virtually impossible to analyze recovery of function in the hindlimbs using footprint analysis under those conditions. In addition, intralimb joint coordination cannot be assessed, and, therefore, the resultant potential foot deviations cannot be linked to the status of the other limb segments.

30.4 Skilled sensorimotor tests

Ladder and grid walking

Several other tests have been implemented to measure the recovery of locomotor tasks requiring fine and sudden adjustments. Most of these tests challenge the animal to walk on uneven surfaces, e.g. grid walk (Kunkel-Bagden and Bregman, 1990; Kunkel-Bagden et al., 1993), ladder beam (von Euler et al., 1996; Soblosky et al., 1997), and inclined grid climb (Ramon-Cueto and Avila, 1999). Theoretically, these tests require the animal to process, integrate and predict afferent information and then make corrections effectively for successful completion of the task. Animals are trained to cross a walkway and the number of failures (e.g. footfalls), and the time it

takes them to cross are recorded. The ladder rung walking test has been used to assess both hindlimb and forelimb function. In this test the spacing of the rungs is variable and is periodically changed, thus preventing the animals from learning the absolute and relative location of the rungs and allows the test to be used repeatedly (Metz and Whishaw, 2002).

It has been claimed that these more complex tasks can be used to define deficits in descending fine motor control and that CST function reflects voluntary control. However, the ability of an injured animal to appropriately adjust the limb during these tests cannot be directly linked with any specific ascending or descending neuromotor tract, neither can it clearly differentiate control from supraspinal versus spinal neural networks. For example, cats with a complete spinal cord transection can successfully accomplish complex motor tasks, such as stepping over obstacles (Forssberg et al., 1975; Hodgson et al., 1994; Nakata et al., 1994) (see Table 30.1).

Rope climbing

For this test, rats are trained to climb up a thick rope using both the forelimbs and hindlimbs to reach the top of a platform for a food reward. The time it takes the rat to reach the goal is recorded. The rope climbing test (Carlini et al., 1967; Z'Graggen et al., 1998) has been used to assess forelimb function after SCI. However, it is difficult to interpret the results of rope climbing with respect to a given SCI. In the case of either a cervical or a thoracic lesion, function of both the forelimbs and hindlimbs may be affected and, therefore, it will not be clear as to how much of the compensatory action will be due to the forelimbs or hindlimbs in either of these lesions. Certainly the results from this test alone cannot be interpreted with reasonable assurance to represent a measure of recovery of motor performance that can be attributable to some regenerative mechanism.

Swimming

Several versions of swimming tests have been used to assess motor performance in SCI animals

(Gruner and Altman, 1980; Kerasidis et al., 1987). In general, a rodent is placed in a swimming pool that is filled with enough water to force the animal to swim without touching the bottom of the pool (usually 30 cm in depth). Different types of measurements can be taken, such as the time required to swim across the pool or to reach a platform or escape ladder. In addition, the movement of the limbs can be assessed, particularly in plexiglass swimming pools. One important aspect of this test is the dissociation between limb motion and body weight support, unlike overground or treadmill locomotion. There are a number of seemingly subtle features of the test procedure that can have a major effect on the reliability of the test as well as its validity as a measure of a given type of motor performance. The water temperature can have a major effect on the animal, physiologically and psychologically. Also the amount of bubbles that accumulate in the coating has a major impact on the intensity of the swimming task. Again, the investigators must examine carefully the specific question being asked relative to the specific procedures used in administering swimming tests.

30.5 Fine motor control

The CST has been a popular target in regenerative studies after SCI. This is the case in spite of the fact that in several mammalian species the CST is relatively unimportant and even unnecessary for locomotion. An assessment of fine motor control of the forelimbs would be more appropriate to test following a CST lesion. Food retrieval tasks for rats (Kartje-Tillotson and Castro 1980; Z'Graggen et al. 1998; Ballermann et al., 2000, 2001) have been developed to specifically assess recovery of fine motor control. Animals are trained to retrieve a food pellet from a small box attached to the cage through a small aperture. The entire apparatus is constructed with plexiglass and the animal's performance is video taped for analysis. Generally, the number of successful attempts is computed. An important issue to consider is how much the completion of a task can be attributed to grasping reflexes of spinal origin

versus grasping mediated by cortical control. In neonatal rats grasping is considered a spinal reflex when the animal is unable to cease the grip once an object is placed in their hands (Diener and Bregman, 1998).

Another test used is the removal of a sticker placed on the nose. The number of times the animal removes the sticker in a certain time period is recorded in addition to a qualitative assessment of the extent of forelimb movement during removal (Diener and Bregman, 1998). A potential limitation of these types of tasks is the motivational component. Animals need to be trained extensively to accomplish the food pellet task. Failure to execute this task correctly may not necessarily mean impairment of CST. No analysis can be performed if the animal is not motivated enough to retrieve the reward. It is also possible to analyze the kinematics of hand or paw movement using video techniques, but this is extremely time consuming.

30.6 Stimulation of the mesencephalic locomotor region

The basic locomotor pattern in mammals can be elicited from the brainstem and largely from the mesencephalic locomotor region (MLR). Therefore, it seems prudent to place emphasis on its role in the recovery of locomotion following regenerative interventions. Based on a series of experiments performed by Shik and Orlovsky (1976), it is clear that stimulation of selected sites within the brainstem can initiate and sustain locomotion on a treadmill. Decerebrated animals maintained over a period of days can execute full weight-bearing stepping, demonstrating that cortical input to the spinal cord is not essential for basic postural and locomotor tasks. Yet, there continues to be an emphasis on the role of the CST as the primary supraspinal descending system that controls locomotion. When an intervention is being used to re-establish connectivity, a demonstration of the initiation of locomotion by stimulating the MLR following the intervention would be extremely convincing. This test would not only demonstrate the re-establishment of descending and perhaps ascending synaptic function, but also would demonstrate that the newly developed synapses formed in a way that could mediate significant behavioral effects. It is also possible that any restored synaptic function could be counterproductive with respect to movement. For example, one could imagine that the new connectivity could activate flexors and extensors in a temporal pattern that would be counterproductive, that is, the system would be activated, but poorly coordinated. Assuming that locomotion could be initiated by stimulating the MLR in a decerebrated preparation, it would then be desirable to conduct further experiments to demonstrate the efficacy of the intervention in an intact *in vivo* model of posture and locomotion.

30.7 Fictive locomotion

Fictive locomotion is the generation of alternating phases of motor efferent patterns from the spinal cord that approximates those occurring during locomotion (Grillner, 1975). Experimentally fictive locomotion can be demonstrated in a mammal when all supraspinal input to the spinal circuitry and all rhythmic afferent input to the spinal cord segments in question are eliminated. By definition, fictive locomotion is assessed based on the motor axon output from central pattern generation. Fictive locomotion can be used as a measure of the ability of the neural circuitry intrinsic to the spinal cord to generate locomotor-like activity after an SCI or application of some interventional strategy. It is possible that one could successfully establish connectivity across a lesion, but the animal remains unable to successfully step because of a persistent impairment of the spinal neural circuits.

Fictive locomotion used in combination with other assays can be an important tool in identifying a mechanism that may underlie any behavioral change that is observed. The spinal circuitry alone, that is, without brain and sensory input, cannot generate effective locomotion because it has no means of adapting to the instantaneous mechanical and kinematic state of the musculoskeletal component that it normally

innervates (Edgerton et al., 2001). However, if the afferent information to the circuits is intact, then the spinal circuitry is able to generate effective locomotion and adapt to different speeds of stepping, different loads and even to sudden disruptions in the step cycle so that stepping can be continued uninterrupted (Forssberg et al., 1975). There are a number of experimental interventions designed to improve posture and locomotion being tested for which studies of fictive locomotion could provide considerable insight into the nature of any change in locomotor potential (Baker et al., 1984; Gossard et al., 1991).

30.8 Rating scales for assessing motor performance

Rating scales have been used clinically for many years to assess motor performance in humans (Ditunno, 1992). In addition, some rating scales have been used in animal experimentation (Tarlov, 1954; Tarlov and Herz, 1954; Basso et al., 1995). Their application can be useful under some circumstances; for example, when testing large numbers of animals and when it is impractical to perform precise measurements. Subjective rating scales have become more popular and even generally used indiscriminately in spite of their limitations. In experiments in which the question being asked is whether an intervention designed to enhance recovery from SCI is effective, direct and precise quantitative parameters are essential.

30.9 Electrophysiological measurements

Motor-evoked potentials

Transcranial magnetic stimulation (TMS) of the motor cortex and recording motor-evoked potentials (MEPs) via EMG electrodes can be used to assess synaptic connectivity between the motor cortex and a motor pool. The procedure is routinely used to study the conduction properties of the corticospinal pathways (Lewko et al., 1995; Cariga et al., 2002). Advantages of this procedure are that it is non-invasive and that it can be performed in awake human subjects and animals. In some cases, it has been shown to be a more sensitive indicator of preserved corticospinal innervation than visible contractions alone (Calancie et al., 1999). However, TMS can be unpleasant, for example it can cause headaches. In addition, its usefulness in assessing locomotor ability is questionable, since the CST may not be essential for locomotion even in non-human primates. In animals either TMS or stimulation via electrodes placed over the surface of the motor cortex can be used to produce MEPs generated in a peripheral nerve, in the spinal cord, as well as in muscles (Thomas and Noga, 2003). Stimulation of specific regions of the brain can be used to study different descending tracts. For example, the connectivity of pure extrapyramidal motor pathways has been studied by stimulating the red nucleus (rubrospinal pathways) and recording MEPs from extremity muscles or the spinal cord in animals. These procedures provide information related to functional differences that are not apparent with behavioral tests (van de Meent et al., 1996) (Table 30.1).

Somatosensory-evoked potentials

One established electrophysiological test for sensory function is the stimulation of the tibial nerve in the popliteal fossa and recording somatosensory-evoked potentials (SSEPs) in the sensorimotor cortex via needle electrodes in the scalp. This provides information on the connectivity of any sensory pathways to the cortex. A method used to evaluate the spinal circuitry is the stimulation of the tibial nerve at the politeal fossa and recording of the H-reflex elicited in the triceps surae muscles (Lewko et al., 1995). As with TMS advantages of these procedures include their non-invasiveness and repeatability, thus making follow-up studies feasible. A limitation is that the question remains open as to what specific tracts are involved in the transmission of SSEP, as well as MEP, responses (Metz et al., 2000a). There also is a question as to how MEPs or SSEPs are correlated with outcome measures of motor function *in vivo* (Nashmi et al., 1997; Metz et al., 2000a).

30.10 Epidural spinal cord stimulation

Numerous experiments have demonstrated that non-patterned electrical stimulation (ES) (Ichiyama et al., 2005; Iwahara et al., 1992) of the lumbosacral enlargement can induce locomotor patterns and even hindlimb stepping in acute and chronic low-spinal kittens and acute spinalized rats (Iwahara et al., 1992), cats (Edgerton et al., 1976; Grillner and Zangger, 1979) and humans (Dimitrijevic et al., 1998; Gerasimenko et al., 2002, 2003). Dimitrijevic et al. (1998) showed that bilateral or unilateral epidural spinal cord ES can elicit step-like EMG activity bilaterally or unilaterally, respectively, in chronic, complete paraplegic subjects (ASIA A). Herman et al. (2002) reported that a combination of treadmill training and spinal cord ES markedly improved the quality and quantity of stepping during the training session and resulted in immediate improvement in the quality of overground walking. Therefore, ES of the spinal cord can be used as a measure of the functionality of the intrinsic spinal cord in the studies noted above circuitry after SCI. Stimulation of the dorsum of the spinal cord differs from the demonstration of fictive locomotion in that the afferent input is intact when stimulating the cord dorsum. On the other hand, stimulation of the dorsum of the spinal cord differs from MLR stimulation in that any specificity in the control from descending sources is bypassed.

30.11 Monosynaptic and polysynaptic reflexes

A wide variety of monosynaptic and polysynaptic reflexes have been used to test some aspects of neuromotor connectivity after SCI. A commonly used assay is the placing reaction test: for example, contact and proprioceptive placing responses. Several versions of this response have been used as measures of postural reflexes (Prendergast and Shusterman, 1982; Kunkel-Bagden et al., 1992, 1993; Helgren and Goldberger, 1993; Suresh Babu et al., 2000). It has been proposed that these responses are associated with the CST pathway and tracts running in the ventral portion of the spinal cord (Webb and Muir, 2002) or by descending vestibulospinal pathways activated by acceleration of otolith receptors (Gruner et al., 1996). There are, however, severe limitations with the interpretation of these tests. For example, there is a poor correlation of the placing response to the performance of more complex motor tasks and the placing response is highly variable within and between animals. In addition, the response is highly dependent on the excitability level of the spinal cord; for example, after SCI the paralyzed animals often show a clearer placing response than normal animals (Metz et al., 2000b).

A host of other reflexes such as monopedal hopping (Helgren and Goldberger, 1993; Kunkel-Bagden et al., 1993; Suresh Babu et al., 2000; Webb and Muir, 2002) positive supporting reflex (Helgren and Goldberger, 1993), paw shake response (Kuhtz-Buschbeck et al., 1996), flexor reflex (Kuhtz-Buschbeck et al., 1996), grasping reflex (Suresh Babu et al., 2000), righting reflex (Suresh Babu et al., 2000), air stepping (Ankeny et al., 2001), vibratory reflex (Gildenberg et al., 1985), etc., have been assessed after SCI. Although these tests may indicate some level of connectivity between central and peripheral elements in the neuromuscular unit, they do not necessarily provide any indication of the locomotor potential of the subject.

General concepts

1 There is no single test of motor function performance that can be used to answer all questions related to the level of sensorimotor recovery following SCI. It is critical to select the tests that enable one to test the specific hypotheses formulated.

2 There are many neural control strategies that can be used to perform a motor task, even for the more stereotypical tasks of stepping and maintaining standing posture. Therefore, it is crucial when the effectiveness of an intervention is being tested that the changes in performance can be attributed directly to that intervention and not simply to an alternative way to accomplish the same task.

3 Ideally the tests of sensorimotor performance will enable one to determine whether any recovery observed after an intervention following an SCI can be attributed to one or more of the following factors:
  – enables the recruitment of more motor units within one or more motor pools;
  – enables the neural control networks to more effectively coordinate the level and pattern of recruitment of the motor pools needed to perform the task; and/or
  – improves the muscle output by enhancing muscle mass and/or its intrinsic structural organization to enhance force generation.

4 The test must be of high enough difficulty to reveal the deficits.

5 The test should be helpful in defining whether the performance can be attributed to supraspinal versus spinal mechanisms. This is particularly critical in models designed to achieve functional connectivity across a complete lesion or to improve supraspinal–spinal connectivity after an incomplete lesion.

6 The relative importance of supraspinal and spinal levels of neural control varies markedly depending on the motor task: for example, locomotion versus fine motor control, and to some degree on the animal model being studied.

7 The relative importance among the supraspinal sources of control of sensorimotor tasks varies considerably depending on the specific motor tasks being performed. Furthermore, the relative level of importance of these sources of control can change markedly after SCI and the application of interventions designed to induce new axonal growth and connectivity.

REFERENCES

Acosta, C.N., Nelson, K., Timoszyk, B., Reinkensmeyer, D., Roy, R.R., Edgerton, V.R. and de Leon, R. (2003). Robotic control of hindlimb weight bearing during locomotor training improves stepping in spinal transected rats. Society for Neuroscience, Washington, DC. *Abstract Viewer/Itinerary Planner*, 2003.

Ankeny, D.P., McTigue, D.M., Guan, Z., Yan, Q., Kinstler, O., Stokes, B.T. and Jakeman, L.B. (2001). Pegylated brain-derived neurotrophic factor shows improved distribution into the spinal cord and stimulates locomotor activity and morphological changes after injury. *Exp Neurol*, **170**, 85–100.

Baker, L.L., Chandler, S.H. and Goldberg, L.J. (1984). L-dopa-induced locomotor-like activity in ankle flexor and extensor nerves of chronic and acute spinal cats. *Exp Neurol*, **86**, 515–526.

Ballermann, M., Tompkins, G. and Whishaw, I.Q. (2000). Skilled forelimb reaching for pasta guided by tactile input in the rat as measured by accuracy, spatial adjustments, and force. *Behav Brain Res*, **109**, 49–57.

Ballermann, M., McKenna, J. and Whishaw, I.Q. (2001). A grasp-related deficit in tactile discrimination following dorsal column lesion in the rat. *Brain Res Bull*, **54**, 237–242.

Barbeau, H. and Rossignol, S. (1987). Recovery of locomotion after chronic spinalization in the adult cat. *Brain Res*, **412**, 84–95.

Bard, P. and Macht, M.B. (1958). The behavior of chronically decerebrate cats. In: *Neurological Basis of Behavior* (eds Wolstenholme, G.E.W. and O'Connor, C.M.), Churchill, London, pp. 55–71.

Basso, D.M., Beattie, M.S. and Bresnahan, J.C. (1995). A sensitive and reliable locomotor rating scale for open field testing in rats. *J Neurotraum*, **12**, 1–21.

Beloozerova, I.N., Zelenin, P.V., Popova, L.B., Orlovsky, G.N., Grillner, S. and Deliagina, T.G. (2003). Postural control in the rabbit maintaining balance on the tilting platform. *J Neurophysiol*, **90**, 3783–3793.

Bigbee, A.J., Tillakaratne, N.J.K., Hodgson, J., Roy, R.R., Zhong, H., Shah, R., Oliva, A., Tobin, A.J. and Edgerton, V.R. (2002). Quantitative analysis of standing ability following stand training in rats after spinal cord transection. Society for Neuroscience, Orlando, FL.

Bose, P., Parmer, R. and Thompson, F.J. (2002). Velocity-dependent ankle torque in rats after contusion injury of the midthoracic spinal cord: time course. *J Neurotraum*, **19**, 1231–1249.

Calancie, B., Alexeeva, N., Broton, J.G., Suys, S., Hall, A. and Klose, K.J. (1999). Distribution and latency of muscle responses to transcranial magnetic stimulation of motor cortex after spinal cord injury in humans. *J Neurotraum*, **16**, 49–67.

Cariga, P., Catley, M., Nowicky, A.V., Savic, G., Ellaway, P.H. and Davey, N.J. (2002). Segmental recording of cortical motor evoked potentials from thoracic paravertebral myotomes in complete spinal cord injury. *Spine*, **27**, 1438–1443.

Carlini, E.A., Teresa, M., Silva, A., Cesare, L.C. and Endo, R.M. (1967). Effects of chronic administration of beta-(3,4-dimethoxyphenyl)-ethylamine and beta-(3,4,5-trimethoxy-phenyl)-ethylamine on the climbing rope performance of rats. *Med Pharmacol Exp Int J Exp Med*, **17**, 534–542.

Cheng, H., Almstrom, S., Gimenez-Llort, L., Chang, R., Ove Ogren, S., Hoffer, B. and Olson, L. (1997). Gait analysis of adult paraplegic rats after spinal cord repair. *Exp Neurol*, **148**, 544–557.

de Leon, R.D., Hodgson, J.A., Roy, R.R. and Edgerton, V.R. (1998a). Full weight-bearing hindlimb standing following stand training in the adult spinal cat. *J Neurophysiol*, **80**, 83–91.

de Leon, R.D., Hodgson, J.A., Roy, R.R. and Edgerton, V.R. (1998b). Locomotor capacity attributable to step training versus spontaneous recovery after spinalization in adult cats. *J Neurophysiol*, **79**, 1329–1340.

de Leon, R.D., Kubasak, M.D., Phelps, P.E., Timoszyk, W.K., Reinkensmeyer, D.J., Roy, R.R. and Edgerton, V.R. (2002a). Using robotics to teach the spinal cord to walk. *Brain Res Rev*, **40**, 267–273.

de Leon, R.D., Reinkensmeyer, D.J., Timoszyk, W.K., London, N.J., Roy, R.R. and Edgerton, V.R. (2002b). Use of robotics in assessing the adaptive capacity of the rat lumbar spinal cord. In: *Progress in Brain Research* (eds McKerracher, L., Doucet, G. and Rosignol, S.), Elsevier Science, The Netherlands, pp. 141–149.

Diener, P.S. and Bregman, B.S. (1998). Fetal spinal cord transplants support the development of target reaching and coordinated postural adjustments after neonatal cervical spinal cord injury. *J Neurosci*, **18**, 763–778.

Dimitrijevic, M.R., Gerasimenko, Y. and Pinter, M.M. (1998). Evidence for a spinal central pattern generator in humans. *Ann NY Acad Sci*, **860**, 360–376.

Ditunno, Jr., J.F. (1992). Functional assessment measures in CNS trauma. *J Neurotrauma*, **9(Suppl. 1)**, S301–S305.

Edgerton, V.R., Grillner, S., Sjostrom, A. and Zangger, P. (1976). Central generation of locomotion in vertebrates. In: *Neural Control of Locomotion* (eds Herman, R.M., Grillner, S., Stein, P.S.G. and Stuart, D.G.), Plenum Publishing Corporation, New York, NY, pp. 439–464.

Edgerton, V.R., de Leon, R.D., Harkema, S.J., Hodgson, J.A., London, N., Reinkensmeyer, D.J., Roy, R.R., Talmadge, R.J., Tillakaratne, N.J., Timoszyk, W. and Tobin, A. (2001). Retraining the injured spinal cord. *J Physiol*, **533**, 15–22.

Fong, A.J., Edgerton, V.R., Cai, L.L., Otoshi, C.K., Timoszyk, W.K., Merlo, M., Bigbee, A.J., Zhong, V., Roy, R.R., Reinkensmeyer, D.J. and Burdick, J.W. (2003). Effects of quipazine and robotic training spinal mice. Society for Neuroscience, Washington, DC. *Abstract Viewer/Itinerary Planner*, 2003.

Forssberg, H., Grillner, S. and Rossignol, S. (1975). Phase dependent reflex reversal during walking in chronic spinal cats. *Brain Res*, **85**, 103–107.

Gerasimenko, Y.P., Makarovskii, A.N. and Nikitin, O.A. (2002). Control of locomotor activity in humans and animals in the absence of supraspinal influences. *Neurosci Behav Physiol*, **32**, 417–423.

Gerasimenko, Y.P., Avelev, V.D., Nikitin, O.A. and Lavrov, I.A. (2003). Initiation of locomotor activity in spinal cats by epidural stimulation of the spinal cord. *Neurosci Behav Physiol*, **33**, 247–254.

Gildenberg, P.L., Campos, R.J. and Dimitrijevic, M.R. (1985). Characteristics of the tonic stretch reflex in spastic spinal cord and head-injured patients. *Appl Neurophysiol*, **48**, 106–110.

Gossard, J.P., Cabelguen, J.M. and Rossignol, S. (1991). An intracellular study of muscle primary afferents during fictive locomotion in the cat. *J Neurophysiol*, **65**, 914–926.

Gregor, R.J., Roy, R.R., Whiting, W.C., Lovely, R.G., Hodgson, J.A. and Edgerton, V.R. (1988). Mechanical output of the cat soleus during treadmill locomotion: *in vivo* vs in situ characteristics. *J Biomech*, **21**, 721–732.

Grillner, S. (1975). Locomotion in vertebrates: central mechanisms and reflex interaction. *Physiol Rev*, **55**, 247–304.

Grillner, S. and Zangger, P. (1979). On the central generation of locomotion in the low spinal cat. *Exp Brain Res*, **34**, 241–261.

Gruner, J.A. and Altman, J. (1980). Swimming in the rat: analysis of locomotor performance in comparison to stepping. *Exp Brain Res*, **40**, 374–382.

Gruner, J.A., Yee, A.K. and Blight, A.R. (1996). Histological and functional evaluation of experimental spinal cord injury: evidence of a stepwise response to graded compression. *Brain Res*, **729**, 90–101.

Hamers, F.P., Lankhorst, A.J., van Laar, T.J., Veldhuis, W.B. and Gispen, W.H. (2001). Automated quantitative gait analysis during overground locomotion in the rat: its application to spinal cord contusion and transection injuries. *J Neurotraum*, **18**, 187–201.

Helgren, M.E. and Goldberger, M.E. (1993). The recovery of postural reflexes and locomotion following low thoracic hemisection in adult cats involves compensation by undamaged primary afferent pathways. *Exp Neurol*, **123**, 17–34.

Herman, R., He, J., D'Luzansky, S., Willis, W. and Dilli, S. (2002). Spinal cord stimulation facilitates functional walking in a chronic, incomplete spinal cord injured. *Spinal Cord*, **40**, 65–68.

Hodgson, J.A., Roy, R.R., de Leon, R., Dobkin, B. and Edgerton, V.R. (1994). Can the mammalian lumbar spinal cord learn a motor task? *Med Sci Sports Exer*, **26**, 1491–1497.

Ichiyama, R.M., Gerasimenko, Y.P., Zhong, H., Roy, R.R. and Edgerton, V.R. (2005). Hindlimb stepping movements in complete spinal rats induced by epidural spinal cord stimulation. *Neurosci Lett*, **383**, 339–344.

Iwahara, T., Atsuta, Y., Garcia-Rill, E. and Skinner, R.D. (1992). Spinal cord stimulation-induced locomotion in the adult cat. *Brain Res Bull*, **28**, 99–105.

Kartje-Tillotson, G. and Castro, A.J. (1980). Limb preference after unilateral pyramidotomy in adult and neonatal rats. *Physiol Behav*, **24**, 293–296.

Kerasidis, H., Wrathall, J.R. and Gale, K. (1987). Behavioral assessment of functional deficit in rats with contusive spinal cord injury. *J Neurosci Meth*, **20**, 167–179.

Kuhtz-Buschbeck, J.P., Boczek-Funcke, A., Mautes, A., Nacimiento, W. and Weinhardt, C. (1996). Recovery of locomotion after spinal cord hemisection: an X-ray study of the cat hindlimb. *Exp Neurol*, **137**, 212–224.

Kunkel-Bagden, E. and Bregman, B.S. (1990). Spinal cord transplants enhance the recovery of locomotor function after spinal cord injury at birth. *Exp Brain Res*, **81**, 25–34.

Kunkel-Bagden, E., Dai, H.N. and Bregman, B.S. (1992). Recovery of function after spinal cord hemisection in newborn and adult rats: differential effects on reflex and locomotor function. *Exp Neurol*, **116**, 40–51.

Kunkel-Bagden, E., Dai, H.N. and Bregman, B.S. (1993). Methods to assess the development and recovery of locomotor function after spinal cord injury in rats. *Exp Neurol*, **119**, 153–164.

Lewko, J.P., Tarkka, I.M. and Dimitrijevic, M.R. (1995). Neurophysiological assessment of the motor and sensory spinal pathways in chronic spinal cord injury. *Restor Neurol Neurosci*, **7**, 225–234.

Lovely, R.G., Gregor, R.J., Roy, R.R. and Edgerton, V.R. (1986). Effects of training on the recovery of full-weight-bearing stepping in the adult spinal cat. *Exp Neurol*, **92**, 421–435.

Metz, G.A. and Whishaw, I.Q. (2002). Cortical and subcortical lesions impair skilled walking in the ladder rung walking test: a new task to evaluate fore- and hindlimb stepping, placing, and co-ordination. *J Neurosci Meth*, **115**, 169–179.

Metz, G.A., Curt, A., van de Meent, H., Klusman, I., Schwab, M.E. and Dietz, V. (2000a). Validation of the weight-drop contusion model in rats: a comparative study of human spinal cord injury. *J Neurotraum*, **17**, 1–17.

Metz, G.A., Merkler, D., Dietz, V., Schwab, M.E. and Fouad, K. (2000b). Efficient testing of motor function in spinal cord injured rats. *Brain Res*, **883**, 165–177.

Muir, G.D. and Webb, A.A. (2000). Mini-review: assessment of behavioural recovery following spinal cord injury in rats. *Eur J Neurosci*, **12**, 3079–3086.

Nakata, K., Hodgson, J.A., de Leon, R., Roy, R.R. and Edgerton, V.R. (1994). Prolonged modification of the mechanics of the step cycle by single and repetitive mechanical stimuli in chronic spinal cats. Society for Neuroscience.

Nashmi, R., Imamura, H., Tator, C.H. and Fehlings, M.G. (1997). Serial recording of somatosensory and myoelectric motor evoked potentials: role in assessing functional recovery after graded spinal cord injury in the rat. *J Neurotraum*, **14**, 151–159.

Orlovsky, G.N., Deliagina, T.G. and Grillner, S. (1999). *Neuronal Control of Locomotion from Mollusc to Man*. Oxford University Press, New York.

Prendergast, J. and Shusterman, R. (1982). Normal development of motor behavior in the rat and effect of midthoracic spinal hemisection at birth on that development. *Exp Neurol*, **78**, 176–189.

Ramon-Cueto, A. and Avila, J. (1999). Two modes of microtubule-associated protein 1B phosphorylation are differentially regulated during peripheral nerve regeneration. *Brain Res*, **815**, 213–226.

Roy, R.R., Hutchison, D.L., Pierotti, D.J., Hodgson, J.A. and Edgerton, V.R. (1991). EMG patterns of rat ankle extensors and flexors during treadmill locomotion and swimming. *J Appl Physiol*, **70**, 2522–2529.

Sherrington, C.S. (1906). *The Integrative Action of the Nervous System*. Yale University Press, New Haven, CT.

Shik, M.L. and Orlovsky, G.N. (1976). Neurophysiology of locomotor automatism. *Physiol Rev*, **56**, 465–501.

Shumsky, J.S., Tobias, C.A., Tumolo, M., Long, W.D., Giszter, S.F. and Murray, M. (2003). Delayed transplantation of fibroblasts genetically modified to secrete BDNF and NT-3 into a spinal cord injury site is associated with limited recovery of function. *Exp Neurol*, **184**, 114–130.

Soblosky, J.S., Colgin, L.L., Chorney-Lane, D., Davidson, J.F. and Carey, M.E. (1997). Ladder beam and camera video recording system for evaluating forelimb and hindlimb deficits after sensorimotor cortex injury in rats. *J Neurosci Meth*, **78**, 75–83.

Suresh Babu, R., Muthusamy, R. and Namasivayam, A. (2000). Behavioural assessment of functional recovery after spinal cord hemisection in the bonnet monkey (*Macaca radiata*). *J Neurol Sci*, **178**, 136–152.

Tarlov, I.M. (1954). Spinal cord compression studies. III. Time limits for recovery after gradual compression in dogs. *AMA Arch Neurol Psychiatr*, **71**, 588–597.

Tarlov, I.M. and Herz, E. (1954). Spinal cord compression studies. IV. Outlook with complete paralysis in man. *AMA Arch Neurol Psychiatr*, **72**, 43–59.

Thomas, C.K. and Noga, B.R. (2003). Physiological methods to measure motor function in humans and animals with spinal cord injury. *J Rehab Res Dev*, **40**, 25–34.

Timoszyk, W.K., De Leon, R.D., London, N., Roy, R.R., Edgerton, V.R. and Reinkensmeyer, D.J. (2002). The rat lumbosacral spinal cord adapts to robotic loading applied during stance. *J Neurophysiol*, **88**, 3108–3117.

Timoszyk, W.K., Nessler, J.A., Acosta, C., Roy, R.R., Edgerton, V.R., Reinkensmeyer, D.J. and de Leon, R. (2005). Hindlimb loading determines stepping quantity and quality following spinal cord transection. *Brain Res*, **1050(1–2)**, 180–189.

van de Meent, H., Hamers, F.P., Lankhorst, A.J., Buise, M.P., Joosten, E.A. and Gispen, W.H. (1996). New assessment techniques for evaluation of posttraumatic spinal cord function in the rat. *J Neurotraum*, **13**, 741–754.

Vilensky, J.A., Moore, A.M., Eidelberg, E. and Walden, J.G. (1992). Recovery of locomotion in monkeys with spinal cord lesions. *J Motor Behav*, **24**, 288–296.

von Euler, M., Akesson, E., Samuelsson, E.B., Seiger, A. and Sundstrom, E. (1996). Motor performance score: a new algorithm for accurate behavioral testing of spinal cord injury in rats. *Exp Neurol*, **137**, 242–254.

Webb, A.A. and Muir, G.D. (2002). Compensatory locomotor adjustments of rats with cervical or thoracic spinal cord hemisections. *J Neurotraum*, **19**, 239–256.

Weytjens, J.L., Viberg, D.A., Caputi, A.A., Kallesoe, K. and Hoffer, J.A. (1992). New transducers for measuring muscle length in unrestrained animals. *J Neurosci Meth*, **45**, 217–225.

Z'Graggen, W.J., Metz, G.A., Kartje, G.L., Thallmair, M. and Schwab, M.E. (1998). Functional recovery and enhanced corticofugal plasticity after unilateral pyramidal tract lesion and blockade of myelin-associated neurite growth inhibitors in adult rats. *J Neurosci*, **18**, 4744–4757.

Translational research: application to human neural injury

CONTENTS

Alzheimer's disease, model systems and experimental therapeutics

Donald L. Price[1,2,3,4], Tong Li[1,4], Huaibin Cai[5] and Philip C. Wong[1,3,4]

Departments of [1]Pathology, [2]Neurology, [3]Neuroscience and [4]the Division of Neuropathology, The Johns Hopkins University School of Medicine, Baltimore and [5]The National Institute on Aging, Laboratory of Neurogenetics, Bethesda, MD, USA

31.1 Introduction

Alzheimer's Disease (AD), the most common disease manifesting as memory loss and dementia in the elderly, affects more than 4 million elderly individuals in the United States (Brookmeyer et al., 1998; Mayeux, 2003; Cummings, 2004). Due to increased life expectancy and the baby boom, the elderly are the most rapidly growing segment of our society. Thus, over the next several decades, the number of persons with AD in the United States will triple. Because of its prevalence, costs, lack of mechanism-based treatments, and impact on individuals and caregivers, AD is one of the most challenging diseases in medicine (Price et al., 1998; Wong et al., 2002; Citron, 2004; Walsh and Selkoe, 2004). The development of effective new therapies will have a significant impact on the health and care of the elderly. This review focuses on important research relevant to AD, including: the diagnosis of clinical syndrome; value of laboratory studies, particularly new imaging efforts; advances in genetics and neuropathology/biochemistry; knowledge of pathogenesis; and development of experimental models of value for understanding disease mechanisms and for developing experimental therapeutics.

The classical clinical syndrome of AD (i.e. progressive memory loss, altered cognition, and dementia) (Cummings, 2004) results from abnormalities associated with dysfunction and death of specific populations of neurons in neural systems involved in memory and cognition (Price et al., 1998). A variety of laboratory approaches and imaging methods are useful for diagnosis, for predicting the clinical course and for assessing outcomes of therapy. The pathology in these brain regions/circuits is characterized by intracellular and extracellular protein aggregates (i.e. the tau and Aβ-related abnormalities, respectively) that comprise the neurofibrillary tangles (NFT) and neuritic plaques, long recognized as hallmarks of this illness (Lee et al., 2001; Morris and Price, 2001; Wong et al., 2002). Genetic evidence indicates that the inheritance of mutations in several genes causes autosomal dominant familial AD (fAD), while the presence of certain alleles of other genes, particularly *ApoE4*, are significant risk factors for putative sporadic disease (Price et al., 1998; Tanzi and Bertram, 2001; Sisodia and George-Hyslop, 2002). The information from genetics, pathology, and biochemistry has been critical for defining disease mechanisms and for creating models of disease (i.e. mice expressing mutant transgenes). In parallel, results of targeting genes encoding proteins hypothesized to play key roles in disease pathways have provided new understanding of the contributions of these proteins for AD. Some of these proteins are therapeutic targets. The values of these targets for new treatment strategies are being tested in model systems. As safety and efficacy are assured, some of these approaches will be used in human trials (Citron, 2004).

To illustrate some of these concepts, we first describe clinical and laboratory studies that enhance diagnostic accuracy, followed by discussion of genetic, pathological, and biochemical features of the human illness. Subsequently, we review selected aspects of: the biology of proteins implicated in pathogenesis of disease; selected transgenic and gene targeted models; the identification of several therapeutic targets; and results of several experimental treatments in models.

31.2 Clinical features

Mild cognitive impairment and AD-type dementia

AD is the most common cause of memory loss and cognitive impairments occurring in the elderly (Price et al., 1998; Morris et al., 2001; Peterson et al., 2001; 2003; Wong et al., 2002; Mayeux, 2003; Nestor et al., 2004). The disease often initially manifests as a syndrome termed mild cognitive impairment (MCI), which is usually characterized by: a memory complaint (corroborated by informant); memory impairments on formal testing; intact general cognition; preserved activities of daily living; and absence of overt dementia (Petersen, 2003). MCI is regarded by many as a transitional stage between normal aging and early AD (Morris et al., 2001; Petersen et al., 2001; Petersen, 2003). The clinical manifestations of symptomatic AD include difficulties in memory and in other domains of cognitive functions (executive functions, language, attention, judgment, etc.) (Price and Morris, 1999; Albert et al., 2001; Morris and Price, 2001; Morris et al., 2001; Petersen et al., 2001; Killiany et al., 2002; Cummings, 2004; Nestor et al., 2004). Some patients develop psychotic symptoms, such as depression/hallucinations and delusions (Lyketsos et al., 2002). Over time, mental functions and activities of daily living are increasingly impaired, and, in the late stages, these individuals become profoundly demented, bedridden, and usually die of intercurrent illnesses. For additional clinical details, see Volume II, Chapter 31.

Diagnosis laboratory studies and imaging

In making a diagnosis of AD, clinicians rely on histories from patients and informants, results of physical, neurological, and psychiatric examinations, levels of performance on neuropsychological tests (Albert et al., 2001; Silverman et al., 2001; Cummings, 2004; Nestor et al., 2004), and outcomes of laboratory studies (Sunderland et al., 2003), including neuroimaging (Jack et al., 2000; Killiany et al., 2002; Klunk et al., 2004). These investigations help to exclude other disorders that can mimic AD.

In AD, the cerebrospinal fluid (CSF) levels of $A\beta$ peptide are often low and levels of tau may be higher than controls (Sunderland et al., 2003). Values vary between individuals and single measures may not be great diagnostic assistance. However, future research should disclose whether serial measures of CSF markers have diagnostic utility. Over several examinations, the clinical profile, in concert with laboratory assessments, allows the clinician to make a diagnosis of possible or probable AD (McKhann et al., 1984).

Magnetic resonance imaging (MRI) often discloses AD-related regional brain atrophy, particularly involving hippocampus (Jack et al., 2000) and entorhinal cortex (Killiany et al., 2002; Cummings, 2004; Nestor et al., 2004). Rates of hippocampal atrophy appear to correlate with changes in clinical status (Jack et al., 2000) and may have predictive value for diagnosis of AD. Positron emission tomography (PET) with ^{18}F doxyglucose and single photon emission computerized tomography (SPECT), commonly demonstrate decreased glucose utilization and reduced regional blood flow in the parietal and temporal lobes with involvement of other cortical areas at later stages (Jack et al., 2000; Silverman et al., 2001). PET can also be used to quantitatively map the distributions of a variety of different radiolabeled tracers (Nestor et al., 2004).

Of great interest are the investigations carried out by a Pittsburgh-Swedish consortium who used Pittsburgh Compound-B (PIB) to assess $A\beta$ amyloid burden *in vivo*. PIB is a brain penetrant ^{11}C-labeled uncharged thioflavin derivative, which binds to $A\beta$ with high affinity (Klunk et al., 2004). In comparison with controls, subjects with AD have a marked retention of label in several areas of brain that often accumulate amyloid. The PET patterns of labeled PIB are thought to reflect the $A\beta$ burden in the brains of these individuals (Klunk et al., 2004). This approach should eventually prove useful for enhancing accuracy of diagnosis of early AD and for assessing the efficacies of anti-amyloid therapeutics. At present, only symptomatic treatments are available for affected individuals (Lyketsos et al., 2002; Petersen, 2003; Cummings, 2004). However, new mechanism-based therapies are on the horizon (Wong et al., 2002; Monsonego and Weiner, 2003; Selkoe and Schenk, 2003; Citron, 2004; Cummings, 2004; Walsh and Selkoe, 2004), and, in the future, the ability to make early and accurate diagnoses of AD will become increasingly important for identifying the clinical populations most likely to respond to specific treatments.

31.3 Genetics

Genetic risk factors for AD include: mutations in *APP* (chromosome 21); mutations in *presenilin 1* (*PS1*) (chromosome 14) and *PS2* (chromosome 1); and different susceptibility alleles of *ApoE* (chromosome 19) (Price et al., 1998; Tanzi and Bertram, 2001; Sisodia and George-Hyslop, 2002; Mayeux, 2003; Ghiso and Wisniewski, 2004). The presence of autosomal dominant mutations in *APP, PS1,* or *PS2* usually causes disease earlier than occurs in sporadic cases. Genetic testing can identify individuals with these mutations. Individuals with trisomy 21 or Down's Syndrome (DS) have an extra copy of *APP* (and other genes) in the obligate DS region; these individuals develop AD pathology relatively early in life. The presence of A*poE* 4, in a dose dependent fashion, predisposes to later onset AD (Strittmatter et al., 1993; Corder et al., 1994). The proteins encoded by mutant genes and the alleles of *ApoE* are discussed below. Significantly, other loci that confer risk have been identified (Bertram et al., 2000; Ertekin-Taner et al., 2000; Myers et al., 2000; Tanzi and Bertram 2001; Mayeux, 2003).

Amyloid precursor protein

Encoded by a member of the *APP* gene family, including the genes encoding the APP like proteins (APLPs) (Heber et al., 2000), APP is a type I transmembrane protein existing as several isoforms (Sisodia and George-Hyslop, 2002). It is abundant in the nervous system, but its specific functions remain to be fully defined (Cao and Sudhof, 2001; Sisodia and George-Hyslop, 2002; Kamenetz et al., 2003). Expressed in many different cell types, APP is particularly abundant in neurons and is transported anterograde in axons to terminals (Koo et al., 1990; Sisodia et al., 1993; Buxbaum et al., 1998). The protein is cleaved by activities of BACE1 (*β-site APP cleaving enzyme 1*) and the γ-secretase complex (see below), which generate the N- and C-termini of Aβ peptides, respectively and release the APP ectodomain and C-terminal cytoplasmic domain (Vassar et al., 1999; Vassar and Citron, 2000; Cai et al., 2001; Sisodia and George-Hyslop, 2002; De Strooper, 2003; Selkoe and Kopan, 2003; Citron, 2004; Haass, 2004; Iwatsubo, 2004; Marjaux et al., 2004). The majority of mutations in *APP, PS1* and *PS2* influence these cleavages to increase the levels of all Aβ species or the relative amounts of toxic Aβ42 (Tanzi and Bertram, 2001; Sisodia and George-Hyslop, 2002; Ghiso and Wisniewski, 2004). For example, *APPswe*, a double mutation involving codons 670 and 671, enhances many-fold the BACE1 cleavage at the N-terminus of Aβ; the result is substantial elevation in levels of all Aβ 1–40, 42 peptides. In several families, the normally occurring Valine residue at position 717 (of APP-770) is replaced with Ile, Gly, or Phe; these mutations promote γ-secretase activities and lead to increased secretion of longer and more toxic forms of Aβ (i.e. Aβ1–42 and 11–42, 43). A hereditary disease associated with Aβ deposition around blood vessels and with cerebral hemorrhages is linked with an *APP* mutation at position 693 (Glu–Gln substitution, corresponding to amino acid 22 of Aβ), which is associated with formation of Aβ peptide species that are more prone to aggregate into fibrils (Ghiso and Wisniewski, 2004; Herzig et al., 2004). Thus, some of the *APP* mutations linked to fAD can influence the processing of APP and the biology of Aβ by increasing the production of Aβ peptides or the amounts of the longer, more toxic Aβ42; other mutations may promote fibril formation.

PS1 and PS2

PS1 and *PS2* encode two highly homologous and conserved 43- to 50-kD multipass transmembrane proteins (Sherrington et al., 1995; Doan et al., 1996; Price et al., 1998; Sisodia and George-Hyslop, 2002) that are key participants in γ-secretase activity involved in generation of Aβ from APP and in cleavages essential for Notch1 signaling involved in cell-fate decisions (Kopan and Goate, 2002; Sisodia and George-Hyslop, 2002; Selkoe and Kopan, 2003). PS1 and PS2 are endoproteolytically cleaved by a hypothetical "presenillinase" to form a N-terminal ~28-kDa fragment and a C-terminal ~18-kDa fragments (Doan et al., 1996; Thinakaran et al., 1997), both of which (along with several other proteins described below) are critical components of the γ-secretase complex (Sisodia and George-Hyslop, 2002; Wolfe, 2002; De Strooper, 2003; Selkoe and Kopan, 2003; Haass, 2004; Iwatsubo, 2004; Marjaux et al., 2004).

Nearly 50% of cases of early-onset cases of fAD are linked to mutations in *PS1* which has been reported to harbor >90 different mutations (Sherrington et al., 1995; Price et al., 1998; Tanzi and Bertram, 2001; Sisodia and George-Hyslop, 2002). A small number of *PS2* mutations cause autosomal dominant disease in fAD pedigrees (Price et al., 1998; Tanzi and Bertram, 2001). The majority of abnormalities in *PS* genes are missense mutations that result in single amino acid substitutions, which enhance γ-secretase activities and increase the levels of the Aβ42 peptides.

ApoE

At the single *ApoE* locus, there are three alleles (*ApoE2, ApoE3,* and *ApoE4*), encoding three ApoE isoforms, all of which carries cholesterol and other lipids in the blood (Corder et al., 1994). In human brain, ApoE is expressed predominantly in astrocytes. The *ApoE3* allele is most common in the general population (frequency of 0.78), whereas the allelic frequency of *ApoE4* is 0.14. However, in clinic-based studies, patients with late-onset disease (>65 years of age) have an *ApoE4* allelic frequency of 0.50; the risk for AD is increased in a dose dependent fashion by the presence of *ApoE4* (Strittmatter et al., 1993; Corder et al., 1994; Tanzi and Bertram, 2001; Mayeux, 2003). The mechanisms whereby the *ApoE allele* type elevates the risk for late-onset disease are not known. This glycoprotein has no effect on Aβ synthesis (DeMattos et al., 2002b). Because significant differences exist in the abilities of ApoE isoforms to bind Aβ, it has been hypothesized that they can differentially influence aggregation, deposition and/or clearance of Aβ. Although the presence of the *ApoE4* allele confers risk in late-onset disease (Tanzi and Bertram, 2001), *ApoE* genotyping, a useful research tool, does not appear helpful for routine diagnostic purposes.

31.4 Neuropathology and biochemistry

Abnormalities involving brain regions/ neural systems

The clinical signs reflect the distribution of abnormalities among different populations of neurons in brain regions/systems critical for memory, learning, and cognitive performance. Circuits damaged by the disease include: the basal forebrain cholinergic system, amygdala, hippocampus, entorhinal cortex, limbic cortex, and neocortex (Whitehouse et al., 1981; Hyman et al., 1984; Braak and Braak, 1991; Gomez-Isla et al., 1996; Price and Morris, 1999; Beach et al., 2000). In these regions/circuits, abnormalities include: fibrillary alterations in tangles and neurites; the presence of conformational alterations in phospho-tau present in both of these lesions (Lee et al., 2001); neuritic Aβ-containing plaques (sites of synaptic disconnection) in brain regions receiving inputs from affected neurons (Price and Morris, 1999; Sisodia and George-Hyslop, 2002); reductions in both generic and transmitter-specific synaptic markers in the target fields of these neurons (Terry et al., 1991; Masliah et al., 1994; Sze et al., 1997; Price and Sisodia, 1998; Beach et al., 2000; Minger et al., 2001); evidence of death of neurons in these regions (Whitehouse et al., 1981; Gomez-Isla et al., 1996; Mattson, 2001; Gastard et al., 2003); and local glial/inflammatory reactions, particularly associated with plaques (Akiyama et al., 2000). Disruption of synaptic communication in these circuits has profound clinical consequences (Sze et al., 1997; Price and Sisodia, 1998). Abnormalities that damage circuits in the entorhinal cortex, medial temporal cortex, and hippocampus, contribute significantly to memory impairments. Pathology in the neocortex is reflected by deficits in higher cognitive functions, such as disturbances in language, calculation, problem solving, and judgment. Alterations in the basal forebrain cholinergic system may contribute to difficulties in memory, arousal, and attention, while involvement of the limbic cortex, amygdala, thalamus, and monoaminergic systems is thought to give rise to the behavioral and emotional disturbances occurring in some individuals (Price et al., 1998; Cummings, 2004).

Aβ Amyloid and neuritic plaques

Aβ, a 4-kD peptide, is derived by β- and γ-secretase cleavages of APP to generate Aβ1–40, 42 and 11–40, 42 amyloid peptides (Iwatsubo et al., 1994; Price et al., 1998; Cai et al., 2001; Sisodia and George-Hyslop, 2002). In cases of AD, these Aβ peptides accumulate in the extracellular space of the neuropil of the cortex and hippocampus. In neurons, APP is rapidly transported in axons to synapses (Koo et al., 1990; Sisodia et al., 1993; Buxbaum et al., 1998) and amyloid deposits occur in proximity to neurites (swollen axons/terminals containing filamentous and membranous organelles) (Price et al., 1998; Sisodia and George-Hyslop, 2002). Available evidence suggests that extracellular monomeric Aβ 40 and 42, 43 peptides are principally produced at terminals by β- and γ-secretase cleavage activities (Buxbaum et al., 1998; Wong et al., 2001; Sisodia and George-Hyslop, 2002). In the neuropil, these peptides adopt β-pleated sheet conformations and assemble into protofilaments and amyloid fibrils (Caughey and Lansbury, 2003); these aggregates are birefringent when stained with Congo Red or thioflavin dyes and viewed in polarized light or under fluorescence illumination, respectively. Over the years, there has been considerable discussion concerning the nature of Aβ species and the peptide conformational states exhibiting the greatest toxicity, with plaques, fibrils, protofibrils, and oligomers all proposed as candidate offenders

(Lambert et al., 1998; Hartley et al., 1999; McLean et al., 1999; Walsh et al., 1999; 2002; Klein et al., 2001; Wang et al., 2002; Caughey and Lansbury, 2003; Gong et al., 2003). It now is believed that oligomers and multimers, which some term Aβ-derived difusable ligands (ADDL's), are the principle toxic entities (Iwatsubo et al., 1994; Hartley et al., 1999; Lue et al., 1999; McLean et al., 1999; Walsh et al, 1999; 2002; Wang et al., 2002; Gong et al., 2003).

In this model, APP and pro-amyloidogenic secretases transported to synapses and terminals, are thought to be a major source of the APP that gives rise to Aβ (Wong et al., 2001). Released at terminals, Aβ may influence synaptic functions. It has been hypothesized that Aβ may act as a modulator depressing activity at excitatory, glutaminergic synapses via interactions with the N-methyl-D-aspartate (NMDA) receptor (Kamenetz et al., 2003). When levels of Aβ42 peptide multimers are increased, terminals are damaged and become disconnected from targets, forming the swollen neurites which surround amyloid deposits in plaques. This hypothesis is supported by: axonal transport studies of labeled APP; demonstration of C-terminal fragments in the target fields of labeled neurons; immunocytochemical studies which have been interpreted to show colocalization of APP with several secretase proteins in neurites around Aβ deposits (Lesuisse et al., 2001; Sheng et al., 2004); and lesion studies (involving damage to entorhinal cortex or perforant pathway) which reduce levels of APP and Aβ in target fields (Lazarov et al., 2002; Sheng et al., 2002). Thus, at synapses, BACE1 cleaves APP to form amyloidogenic C-terminal derivatives (Buxbaum et al., 1998), which are cleaved subsequently by γ-secretase to generate Aβ 40, 42, 43 peptides. The Aβ oligomers act as toxins and disrupt synaptic functions, including long-term potentiation (LTP) (Hsia et al., 1999; Walsh et al., 2002). Thus, neuritic amyloid plaques, a classical feature of AD, are complex structures, representing sites of Aβ synaptic toxicity associated with degenerative changes in terminals forming neurites, and disconnection of inputs from targets. Surrounding plaques are astrocytes and microglia which produce cytokines, chemokines, and other factors (including complement components) involved in inflammatory processes (Akiyama et al., 2000).

Neurofibrillary pathology

The NFT are fibrillar intracytolplasmic inclusions in cell bodies/proximal dendrites of affected neurons, while neuropil threads and neurites are swollen filament-containing dendrites and distal axons/terminals, respectively (Lee et al., 2001). The principal intracellular component of these lesions are paired helical filaments (PHF) comprised of poorly soluble hyperphosphorylated isoforms of tau, a low molecular weight microtubule-associated protein (Lee et al., 2001). In human brain, alternative splicing from a single *tau* gene leads to formation of six tau isoforms, consisting of three isoforms of three repeat (3-R) tau and three isoforms of four repeat (4-R) tau, the latter derived by inclusion of exon 10 in the transcript (Lee et al., 2001; Edbauer et al., 2002). Normally, tau is synthesized in neuronal cell bodies and transported anterograde in axons, where it acts, via repeat regions that interact with tubulin, to stabilize tubulin polymers critical for microtubule assembly and stability (Lee et al., 2001; Edbauer et al., 2002). The post-translationally modified tau manifest as the neurofibrillary pathology in some neurodegenerative disorders differs somewhat in the different tauopathies: in cases of AD, the PHF of tangles are comprised of six isoforms of tau; in contrast, the fibrillary inclusions occurring in cases of progressive supranuclear palsy (PSP) and cortical basal degeneration (CBD) are characterized by 4-R tau, while the inclusions seen in individuals with Pick Disease (PD) are enriched in 3-R tau (Lee et al., 2001).

All of the AD-linked fibrillar inclusions (NFT, neurites and threads) are thought to result from common mechanisms (Lee et al., 2001). However, in spite of considerable clinical, pathological, and experimental research, the links between tau pathology and Aβ are not fully defined (Busciglio et al., 1995; Lee et al., 2001; Mattson, 2001). In one hypothetical model, Aβ42 damages synapses leading to synaptic disconnections which, perhaps preferentially in primates with six isoforms of tau, leads a retrograde signal that ultimately triggers tau phosphorylation, conformational changes in this protein, and formation of PHF. Since the cytoskeleton is essential for maintaining cell geometry and for the intracellular trafficking and motor driven transport of proteins and organelles, disturbances of the cytoskeleton can lead to alterations in axonal transport, which, in turn can compromise the functions and viabilities of neurons. Eventually, affected nerve cells die (possibly by apoptosis) (Whitehouse et al., 1981; Mattson, 2001; Gastard et al., 2003; Koo and Kopan, 2004), and extracellular NFT are left behind as "tombstones" of the nerve cells destroyed by disease.

31.5 APP processing by secretases

As indicated above, APP is processed by activities of secretase enzymes resulting in release of the soluble ectodomain of APP (APPs), the production of a cytosolic fragment termed the *APP intracellular domain* (AICD), and the generation of several Aβ peptides. In the central nervous system (CNS), Aβ peptides are formed by sequential endoproteolytic cleavages of neuronal APP by two membrane-bound enzyme activities: BACE1 cleaves APP at the Aβ + 1 and +11 sites to generate APP C-terminal fragments (APP-βCTFs) (Cai et al., 2001; Luo et al., 2001); and the γ-secretase complex cleaves, via regulated intramembranous proteolysis, APP-βCTFs at several sites including Aβ 40 and 42, 43 to form Aβ peptides (De Strooper, 2003; Li et al., 2003; Selkoe and Schenk, 2003; Citron, 2004; Haass, 2004; Iwatsubo, 2004; Koo and Kopan, 2004; Ma et al., 2004; Marjuax et al., 2004). Moreover, emerging evidence indicates that γ-secretase cleavages of APP-β CTF or α CTF release the AICD, which forms a multimeric complex with Fe 65, a nuclear adaptor protein (Cao and Sudhof, 2001). This complex or Fe 65 alone (in a new conformation) appears to enter the nucleus and bind to the histone acetyltransferase, Tip60, to influence gene transcription (Cao and Sudhof, 2001). This signaling pathway, although not fully established for APP/AICD, is analogous to the signal generated by the S3 cleavage to produce *Notch1 intracellular domain* (NICD) in the Notch1 signaling pathway (Selkoe and Kopan, 2003; Iwatsubo, 2004). In other cells, APP can also be cleaved endoproteolytically within the Aβ sequence through alternative, non-amyloidogenic pathways involving α-secretase (TACE, *T*NF-*a*lpha *c*onverting *e*nzyme) or BACE2 (Farzan et al., 2000; Haass, 2004). The α-secretase and BACE2 cleavages (at positions 16 and 17, 19 and 20, and 20–21 of Aβ), which occur in non-neural tissues, preclude the formation of Aβ peptides and are thought to protect these organs from Aβ amyloidosis. The physiological roles of APP and its derivatives (APPs, APP-CTFs, Aβ, and AICD) are not well understood. As mentioned above, it has been suggested that Aβ modulates (depresses) synaptic transmission at excitatory synapses via the NMDA receptor, and that excessive levels of toxic Aβ42 damage synapses and eventually lead to neurodegeneration. Much current research focuses on: the roles of APP, Aβ, AICD, and Fe65 in the biology of neurons; the proteins that influence processing of APP and levels/lengths of Aβ species in neural tissues; the ways of selectively modulating secretase activities or cleavage sites; the approaches that have the potential to protect against toxic Aβ species, including Aβ oligomers or ADDLs; and the factors that influence metabolism/clearance of the amyloid peptide (Iwata et al., 2000; 2004; Vekrellis et al., 2000; Demattos et al., 2002a; 2004; Cirrito et al., 2003; Farris et al., 2003; Marjuax et al., 2004; Tanzi et al., 2004). The secretases and their enzyme activities are discussed below.

β-secretases

BACE1 and BACE2, encoded by genes on chromosomes 11 and 21, respectively, are transmembrane aspartyl proteases that are directly involved in the cleavages of APP (Sinha et al., 1999; Vassar et al., 1999; Bennett et al., 2000; Farzan et al., 2000; Cai et al., 2001; Luo et al., 2001; Haass, 2004). Levels of BACE1 mRNA levels are readily detectable in many regions of brain; BACE1 protein is demonstrable in the CNS where BACE1 immunoreactivity is demonstrable in some synaptic regions. BACE1 preferentially cleaves APP at the +11 > +1 sites of Aβ in APP (Cai et al., 2001) and

this enzyme is essential for the generation of Aβ (Cai et al., 2001; Luo et al., 2001). Significantly, APP*swe* is cleaved perhaps 100 fold more efficiently at the +1 site than occurs with wild-type APP. Thus, the presence of this mutation greatly increases BACE1 cleavage and accounts for the elevation of all Aβ species in the presence of this mutation. It has been suggested that expression of BACE1 appears to be increased in brains from some cases of sporadic AD (Fukumoto et al., 2002; Yang et al., 2003; Li R. et al., 2004).

Analyses of cells and brains from *BACE1−/−* mice, which show no overt developmental phenotype (Cai et al., 2001; Luo et al., 2001), disclose that Aβ1–40/42 and Aβ11–40/42 are not secreted in these samples (Cai et al., 2001; Luo et al., 2001). Thus, BACE1 is the principal neuronal β-secretase and is responsible for the penultimate pro-amyloidogenic cleavages. In the CNS, BACE1, APP, and, presumably, components of γ-secretase complex are present at some, if not all synaptic terminals. While it has proved challenging to detect BACE1 in PNS, BACE1 immunoreactivity has been demonstrated in swollen neurites of *APPswe PS1ΔE9* mice with amyloid deposits (Sheng et al., 2004). Although BACE1 mRNA is present in a variety of tissues (particularly the pancreas), levels of this protein are low in most non-neural tissues. Significantly, in the pancreas, levels of BACE1 mRNA are high, in this organ, but the transcript is alternatively spliced to produce a smaller protein incapable of cleaving APP (Bodendorf et al., 2002).

BACE2 mRNA, present in a variety of systemic organs, is very low in neural tissues, except for scattered nuclei in the hypothalamus and brainstem (Bennett et al., 2000). Moreover, BACE2 activity appears to be virtually undetectable in brain regions involved in AD. BACE2 is responsible, along with α-secretase (Sisodia et al., 1990), for anti-amyloidogenic cleavages (in the case of BACE2 at +19/+20 and +20/21 of Aβ) (Farzan et al., 2000). Thus, BACE2 acts like α-secretase (Sisodia et al., 1990; Sisodia and George-Hyslop, 2002). We have suggested that the high levels of BACE1, combined with low levels of BACE2 and TACE in brain, contribute to the vulnerability of CNS to Aβ amyloidosis (Wong et al., 2001).

γ-secretase

γ-Secretase activities, essential for the regulated intramembraneous proteolysis of a variety of transmembrane proteins, are dependent upon a multi-protein catalytic complex, which includes PS (Sisodia and George-Hyslop, 2002; De strooper, 2003; Li et al., 2003; Selkoe and Kopan, 2003; Haass, 2004; Hartmann and De Strooper, 2004; Iwatsubo, 2004; Ma et al., 2004; Marjaux et al., 2004); Nicastrin (Nct), a type I transmembrane glycoprotein (Yu et al., 2000; Edbauer et al., 2002; Kopan and Goate, 2002; Sisodia and George-Hyslop, 2002; De Strooper, 2003; Li et al., 2003) and Aph-1 and Pen-2 two multipass transmembrane proteins (Francis et al., 2002; Goutte et al., 2002; Steiner et al., 2002).

Significantly, γ-secretase cleaves both Notch1 and APP, generating intracellular peptides termed the NICD and the AICD (Cao and Sudhof, 2001; Kopan and Goate, 2002; Selkoe and Kopan, 2003). These intracellular peptides are involved in activation of transcription in the nucleus (Cao and Sudhof, 2001; Selkoe and Kopan, 2003). As described above, the AICD interacts with FE65, a cytosolic adapter; this interaction, either directly or indirectly leads an intracellular signal which influences transcription (Cao and Sudhof, 2001; Selkoe and Kopan, 2003).

Studies of targeting of *PS1, Nct* and *Aph-1* in mice (Shen et al., 1997; Wong et al., 1997; Kopan and Goate, 2002; Li et al., 2003; Ma et al., 2004), which are described below, are consistent with the concept that PS1 and Nct are, along with Aph-1 and Pen-2 (De Strooper, 2003; Haass, 2004), critical components of the γ-secretase complex. As discussed below, the phenotypes of targeted *PS1, Nct,* and *Aph-1* mice are the result of impaired Notch1 signaling.

The exact functions of each protein and their interaction with regard to enzyme activity are not yet fully defined. PS1 may: act as an aspartyl protease itself; function as a co-factor critical for the activity of γ-secretase; or play a role in trafficking of APP or proteins critical for enzyme activity to the proper compartment for γ-secretase cleavage (De Strooper et al., 1998; Naruse et al., 1998; Wolfe et al., 1999; Esler et al., 2000; Wolfe, 2002). These concepts are supported by several observations: PS1 is isolated with γ-secretase under specific detergent soluble conditions (Li et al., 2000a); PS1 is selectively cross-linked or photoaffinity-labeled by transition-state inhibitors (Esler et al., 2000; Li et al., 2000b); substitutions of aspartate residues at D257 in TM 6 and at D385 in TM 7 have been reported to reduce secretion of Aβ and cleavage of Notch1 *in vitro* (Wolfe et al., 1999); and cells in which *PS1* has been targeted show decreased levels of secretion of Aβ (Naruse et al., 1998; De Strooper, 2003; Li et al., 2003).

Nct, Aph-1, and Pen-2 also play roles in the multi-protein catalytic complex (Yu et al., 2000; Edbauer et al., 2002; Francis et al., 2002; Li et al., 2003). Studies of *Nct−/−* mice and *Nct−/−* fibroblasts have shown that Nct is an integral member of the γ-secretase complex (Li et al., 2003), and partial decreases in the level of Nct significantly reduce the secretion of Aβ (Li et al., 2003). Aph-1 and Pen-2 (Francis et al., 2002; Goutte et al., 2002; De Strooper, 2003) are novel transmembrane proteins: Aph-1 has seven predicted transmembrane domains; while Pen-2 has two predicted transmembrane regions (De Strooper, 2003). Targeting of Aph-1a discloses that it is the major mammalian APH-1 homolog during embryogenesis. *Aph-1a−/−* mouse embryo exhibits a Notch1−/− like phenotype (Ma et al., 2004). Aph-1 and Pen-2 are now recognized to be critical components of γ-secretase complex (Francis et al., 2002; Haass, 2004). The levels and distributions of γ-secretase subunits has begun to be clarified by determining binding sites of γ-secretase inhibitors (Yan et al., 2004) and by immunocytochemistry.

31.6 Models of Aβ amyloidosis in CNS

Mutant *APP* and *PS1* mice

Transgenic approaches have been used to model features of autosomal dominant neurodegenerative diseases in mice. In mice, expression of *APPswe* or *APP₇₁₇* minigenes (with or without mutant *PS1*) leads to an Aβ amyloidosis in the murine CNS

(Sturchler-Pierrat et al., 1997; Mucke et al., 2000). The nature and levels of the expressed transgene and the specific mutations influence the severity of the pathology. Mice expressing both mutant *PS1* and mutant *APP* develop accelerated disease. In these animals, levels of Aβ (particularly Aβ42) in brain are increased significantly, and diffuse Aβ deposits and neuritic plaques appear in the hippocampus and cortex. In transgenic mice generated at Johns Hopkins by Dr. David Borchelt and colleagues (Borchelt et al., 1996; 1997; Lesuisse et al., 2001), the pathology evolves in stages: levels of Aβ in brain increase with age; later, diffuse Aβ deposits become detectable in brain; swollen neurites develop in proximity to Aβ deposits; mature neuritic plaques increase in numbers; and plaques are associated with glial responses. In these mice, aggregated tau and NFT are not detectable. The density of synaptic terminals may be reduced (Boncristiano et al., 2002) as are levels of several neurotransmitter markers. In some cases, these abnormalities appear linked to a deficiency in synaptic transmission (Chapman et al., 1999; Hsia et al., 1999) which has been described in some lines of mice. Although amyloid has been detected *in vivo* by several methods in limited brain regions (Bacskai et al., 2003), it has proved more difficult to detect amyloid with whole brain imaging. However, recent advances in imaging amyloid in models look promising (Wadghiri et al., 2003; Jack et al., 2004; Zhang et al., 2004).

Learning deficits, problems in object recognition memory, and difficulties performing tasks assessing spatial reference and working memory have been identified in some of the lines of mice with high levels of mutant transgene expression (Chapman et al., 1999; Chen et al., 2000; Savonenko et al., 2003). Behavioral deficits have been correlated with physiological properties identified in hippocampal circuits (Chapman et al., 1999). Although the mutant mice do not recapitulate the complete phenotype of AD, these animals are very useful subjects for research designed to examine disease mechanisms and to test novel therapies designed to ameliorate the amyloid-related pathology and behavioral abnormalities.

Tau mice

Mice normally express three copies of the murine variant of 4-R tau while humans express three copies of both 3-R tau and 4-R tau (Lee et al., 2001). The paucity of tau abnormalities in these various lines of mutant *APP* or *APP/PS1* mice described above may be related to differences in tau isoforms expressed in different species (mouse versus human). Early efforts to express mutant *tau* transgenes in mice did not lead to striking clinical phenotypes or pathology. More recently generated mice overexpressing *tau* show clinical signs (Higuchi et al., 2002). For example, overexpression of *tau* in some lines of mice leads to weakness thought to reflect high levels of the transgene product in motor neurons with subsequent degeneration of these cells. Consistent with the idea is the evidence of accumulation of hyperphosphorylated tau in neurons of the spinal cord, brainstem, and cortex of these mice. When the prion or Thy1 promoters are used to drive tau_{P301L} (a mutation linked to autosomal dominant frontotemporal dementia with parkinsonism), NFT-like lesions develop in neurons of the brain and spinal cord (Lewis et al., 2000; Gotz et al., 2001). Mice expressing $APPswe/tau_{P301L}$ exhibit enhanced fibrillary pathology in neurons of limbic system and olfactory cortex (Lewis et al., 2001). Moreover, when Aβ42 fibrils are injected into specific brain regions of tau_{P301L} mice, the number of tangles is increased in those neurons projecting to sites of injection (Götz et al., 2001).

Mutant *APP, PS1* and *tau* mice

A triple-transgenic mouse (3xTg-AD) was created by microinjecting *APPswe* and $tau_{P301}L$ into single cells derived from monozygous $PS1_{M146V}$ in mice (Oddo et al., 2003). These mice develop age-related plaques and tangles. Deficits in LTP appear to antedate overt pathology (Oddo et al., 2003). However, mice bearing both mutant *tau* and *APP* (or *APP/PS1*) or mutant *tau* mice injected with Aβ are not fully satisfactory models of fAD because the presence of the mutant *tau* alone is associated with the development of tangles.

31.7 Targeting genes in amyloid pathways

To better understand the functions of some of the proteins playing roles in AD, investigators have targeted genes encoding these proteins, including: *APP; amyloid precursor-like protein* genes *(APLPs); BACE1; PS1; Nct;* and *Aph-1.*

APP and APLPs−/− mice

Homozygous *APP−/−* mice are viable and fertile, but appear to have subtle alterations in locomotor activity and forelimb grip strength (Zheng et al., 1995). The absence of substantial phenotypes in *APP−/−* mice is thought to be related to functional redundancy of two amyloid precursor-like proteins, APLP1 and APLP2, homologous to APP. *APLP2−/−* mice appear relatively normal (von Koch et al., 1997), while *APLP1−/−* mice exhibit postnatal growth deficits (Heber et al., 2000). *APLP1−/−* mice are viable, but *APP−/−/APLP2−/−* mice and *APLP1−/−/APLP2−/−* mice do not survive the perinatal period (Heber et al., 2000). These observations support the concept that some redundancy exists between members of this interesting family of proteins (Heber et al., 2000).

BACE1−/− mice

BACE1−/− mice are viable and healthy, have no obvious phenotype or pathology, and can mate successfully (Vassar and Citron, 2000; Cai et al., 2001; Luo et al., 2001). Importantly, cortical neurons cultured from *BACE1−/−* embryos do not show cleavages at the +1 and +11 sites of Aβ, and, in these cells, the secretion of Aβ peptides is abolished even in the presence of elevated levels of exogenous wildtype or mutant APP (Cai et al., 2001). The brains of *BACE1−/−* mice appear morphologically normal and Aβ peptides are not produced (Cai et al., 2001; Luo et al., 2001). These results establish that BACE1 is the neuronal β-secretase required to cleave APP to generate the N-termini of Aβ (Cai et al., 2001). At present, a consensus has not been reached with regards to other substrates cleaved by BACE1 (Haass, 2004). Preliminary behavioral studies of the *BACE1−/−* mice indicate that the animals

manifest alterations of some tests of cognition and emotion (Savonenko, Laird, Cai, Price and Wong, personal observations). Nevertheless, BACE1 appears to be an outstanding target for development of an anti-amyloidogenic therapy.

PS1 and PS2−/− mice

In contrast to *BACE1−/−* mice, *PS1−/−* mice do not survive beyond the early postnatal period and show severe developmental abnormalities involving the axial skeleton, ribs and spinal ganglia: their features resemble those seen in a Notch1−/− mouse (Shen et al., 1997; Wong et al., 1997). Abnormalities occur because PS1 (along with Nct, Aph-1 and Pen-2) are components of the γ-secretase complex that carry out the S3 intramembranous cleavage of Notch1, a receptor protein involved in critical cell-fate decisions during development (Huppert et al., 2000; Edbauer et al., 2002; Francis et al., 2002; De Strooper, 2003; Li et al., 2003; Selkoe and Kopan, 2003). Without this cleavage, the NICD is not released from the plasma membrane and does not reach the nucleus to initiate transcriptional processes essential for proper development. In cell culture, absence of *PS1* or substitutions at particular aspartate residues leads to reduced levels of γ-secretase cleavage products and levels of Aβ (De Strooper et al., 1998; Wolfe et al., 1999). *PS2−/−* mice are viable and fertile, though they develop age-associated mild pulmonary fibrosis and hemorrhage. Mice lacking *PS1* and *PS2* die midway through gestation showing a full *Notch1−/−* like phenotype. To study the role of PS1 *in vivo* in adult mice, investigators have generated conditional *PS1*-targeted mice lacking postnatal PS1 expression in the forebrain (Feng et al., 2001; Yu et al., 2001). As expected, the absence of PS1 results in decreased generation of Aβ in this region of brain, providing support for the concept that PS1 is critical for γ-secretase activity in the CNS.

Nct−/− mice

Another critical member of the γ-secretase complex is Nct, a type I transmembrane glycoprotein, which forms high-molecular weight complexes with PS (Yu et al., 2000) and binds to the membrane-tethered form of Notch1, and participates in Notch1 signaling and processing of *APP* (Yu et al., 2000; Edbauer et al., 2002; De Strooper, 2003; Li et al., 2003). To determine whether Nct is required for proteolytic processing of Notch1 and APP in mammals and to clarify the role of Nct in the assembly of the γ-secretase complex, Nct-deficient (*Nct−/−*) mice were generated and fibroblasts were derived from *Nct−/−* embryos (Li et al., 2003). *Nct−/−* embryos die by embryonic day 10.5 and exhibit several defects in developmental patterning, including abnormal somite segmentation; the phenotype closely resembles that seen in embryos lacking *Notch1* or both *PS*. Importantly, secretion of Aβ peptides is abolished in *Nct−/−* fibroblasts, whereas it is reduced by ~50% in *Nct+/−* cells (Li et al., 2003). The failure to generate Aβ peptides in *Nct−/−* cells is accompanied by destabilization of the PS/γ-secretase complex and accumulation of APP C-terminal fragments. Moreover, analysis of APP trafficking in *Nct−/−* fibroblasts reveals a significant delay in the rate of APP reinternalization compared with that of control cells. Thus, Nct, along with Aph-1 and Pen-2 (see below) is a critical component of the γ-secretase complex.

Aph-1−/− mice

Aph-1, along with Nct and Pen-2, are essential components of the PS-dependent γ-secretase complex. The three murine *Aph-1* alleles are termed *Aph-1a*, *Aph-1b* and *Aph-1c;* they encode four distinct Aph-1 isoforms: Aph-1aL and Aph-1aS derived from differential splicing of *Aph-1a*, Aph-1b and Aph-1c (Ma et al., 2004). To determine the contributions of mammalian Aph-1 homolog in formation of functional γ-secretase complexes, we generated *Aph-1a −/−* mice and derived immortalized fibroblasts from these embryos (Ma et al., 2004). As compared to littermate controls, the development of *Aph-1a −/−* embryos are dramatically retarded by embryonic day 9.5; these embryos exhibit patterning defects that resemble, but are not identical to those of *Notch1, Nct* or *PS−/−* embryos. Moreover, in immortalized

Aph-1a−/− fibroblasts, the levels of Nct, PS fragments and Pen-2 are dramatically decreased. Consequently, deletion of *Aph-1a* results in significant reduction in levels of the high-molecular weight γ-secretase complex and secretion of Aβ. Importantly, complementation analysis of *Aph-1a−/−* cells reveals that all mammalian Aph-1 isoforms are capable of restoring the levels of Nct, PS and Pen-2 (Ma et al., 2004; Li, T. et al., 2004). Taken together, the findings establish that Aph-1a is the major mammalian Aph-1 homolog present in PS-dependent γ-secretase complexes during embryogenesis, and support the view that the various mammalian Aph-1 isoforms define a set of distinct functional γ-secretase complexes critical for generation of Aβ (Edbauer et al., 2002; Francis et al., 2002; De Strooper 2003; Li et al., 2003). These mammalian proteins should be valuable therapeutic targets for anti-amyloidogenic treatments (De Strooper, 2003; Li et al., 2003).

Influences of *ApoE−/−* and *ApoJ−/−* genotypes on Aβ Amyloidosis in mutant mice

ApoE and clusterin, two abundant high-density apolipoproteins in the CNS (Holtzman et al., 2000; DeMattos et al., 2004) are present at similar concentrations in brain and are expressed by glial cells. Immunoreactivities for both proteins are present in association with plaques and levels may be increased in brains of cases of AD. These apolipoproteins bind Aβ with high affinity, are associated with Aβ in the CSF, and facilitate transport of Aβ across the blood–brain barrier (Holtzman et al., 2000; DeMattos et al., 2004). They influence Aβ aggregation *in vitro* and promote Aβ uptake and degradation. In APP_{717} ApoE−/− mice, non-fibrillar Aβ deposits develop in the brain, but there is virtually no evidence of neuritic degeneration (Bales et al., 1997). Expression of human *ApoE3* or *ApoE4* restores fibrillar deposition with *ApoE4* leading to a more dramatic increase of formation of neuritic plaques (Sun et al., 1998). In subsequent experiments, DeMattos and colleagues mated PD*APP* mice with *ApoJ−/−* mice and found that the progeny exhibit levels of Aβ equivalent to the

PDAPP mice, but show fewer fibrillar Aβ deposits and less neuritic dystrophy (DeMattos et al., 2004). This outcome was interpreted to suggest that ApoJ influences Aβ structure and neuritic toxicity *in vivo*. More specifically, clusterin (or ApoJ) is thought to increase fibrillar deposits and neuritic damage. To examine the influences of ApoE and clusterin, DeMattos and colleagues (DeMattos et al., 2004) generated PD*APP* mice, which lack ApoE or clusterin or both apolipoproteins. *ApoE−/−* clusterin−/− *PDAPP* mice accumulate equivalent levels of Aβ, but exhibit less fibrillar Aβ(DeMattos et al., 2004). In contrast, the *PDAPP ApoE−/−/clusterin−/−* mice show an earlier onset and marked increase in Aβ and amyloid deposits (DeMattos et al., 2004). *ApoE−/−* and *ApoE−/−/clusterin−/−* mice exhibit elevated levels of Aβ in the CSF as well as differences in the elimination half life of Aβ in interstitial fluid measured by microdialysis (DeMattos et al., 2004). The findings were interpreted to indicate that ApoE and clusterin have additive effects on Aβ deposition and that ApoE plays a role in regulating Aβ metabolism and its influence is independent of Aβ synthesis (DeMattos et al., 2004).

31.8 Experimental therapeutics

Many experimental therapeutic efforts have focused on influencing Aβ production (by inhibiting or modulating secretase activities), aggregation, clearance, and downstream neurotoxicity (Monsonego and Weiner, 2003; Citron, 2004; Walsh and Selkoe, 2004). As indicated above, although mutant-transgenic mice do not recapitulate the full phenotype of AD, they represent excellent models of Aβ amyloidosis and are highly suitable for identification of therapeutic targets and for testing new treatments *in vitro*. In this short review, it is not possible to discuss all of these therapeutic efforts in mice. Instead, we focus on several highly selected examples which illustrate the vaule (and potential downsides) of extrapolating these approaches in model systems.

Many pharmaceutical and biotechnology companies and some academic laboratories are using high throughput screening and molecular modeling strategies to discover compounds that inhibit these enzyme activities (Vassar and Citron, 2000; Wolfe, 2002; Citron, 2004; Marjaux et al., 2004; Walsh and Selkoe, 2004). Once lead compounds are identified, medicinal chemists will try to modify the compounds and agents to enhance efficacy, permit passage through the blood–brain barrier, and reduce any potential toxicities.

Strategies influencing β- and γ- secretase activities

Both β- and γ-secretase activities represent therapeutic targets for the development of novel protease inhibitors.

BACE1

BACE1−/− mice are viable and live a normal life span without developing an obvious phenotype (Cai et al., 2001). *In vitro*, BACE1-deficient neurons fail to secrete Aβ even when co-expressing the *APPswe* and mutant *PS1* genes (Cai et al., 2001; Luo et al., 2001). *BACE1−/−; APPswe; PS1ΔE9* mice do not develop the Aβ deposits and age-associated abnormalities in working memory that occur in the *APPswe; PS1ΔE9* model of Aβ amyloidosis. Similarly, *BACE1−/−* TG2576+ mice appear to be rescued from age-dependent memory deficits and physiological abnormalities (Ohno et al., 2004). As these data indicate, BACE1 is a very attractive therapeutic target. However, although initial behavioral studies suggested that *BACE1−/−* mice show no abnormalities, more recent investigations have disclosed abnormalities in performance of tasks assessing cognition and emotional responsiveness. These abnormalities do not occur if mutant *APP* is overexpressed in brain. Intriguingly, the *BACE1−/−* phenotype resembles that seen in *Fe 65−/−* mice. These observations raise the question of a role for defective AICD signaling in the behavioral phenotype of *BACE1−/−* and *Fe 65−/−* mice. Thus, reductions of BACE1 activity (and possibly decreases in AICD signaling) may lead to cognitive problems. This discovery should be kept in mind by investigators trying to identify potential mechanism-based toxicities associated with the use of BACE1 inhibitors.

γ-secretase

γ-secretase substrates, other than APP, include: Notch family members; Notch ligands; ErbB4; CD44; and E Cadherin (Sisodia and George-Hyslop, 2002; Selkoe and Kopan, 2003; Koo and Kopan 2004). As demonstrated by gene targeting strategies, this complex is critically dependent upon the presence of PS1 and 2, Nct, Aph-1, and Pen-2. Because reductions in these components decrease levels of Aβ *in vitro* or *in vivo*, γ-secretase activity is a target for therapy. Thus, reductions in activity of γ-secretase decreases production of Aβ in cell free and cell-based systems and in mutant mice with Aβ amyloidosis (De Strooper, 2003; Li et al., 2003; Citron 2004; Haass, 2004; Iwatsubo, 2004; Ma et al., 2004; Marjaux et al., 2004; Walsh and Selkoe, 2004). However, γ-secretase activities are also critical for a variety of biological processes, and γ-secretase inhibitors can influence these activities. In a recent publication, one of these inhibitors, LY-411, -575, was shown to reduce Aβ production, but it also had significant effects on T- and B-cell development and on properties of the intestinal mucosa (proliferation of goblet cells, increased mucin in gut lumen and crypt necrosis). Thus, several problems could become manifest following inhibition of this enzyme.

γ-secretase cleavage modulation

Epidemiological studies have demonstrated that the prevalence of AD is reduced among persons who have previously used non-steroidal anti-inflammatory drugs (NSAIDs) (Petersen, 2003; Cummings, 2004). Moreover, short-term treatment of mutant *APP* mice with ibuprofen reduces Aβ levels and plaques (Lim et al., 2000). These effects were initially interpreted to reflect anti-inflammatory activities of NSAIDS (Akiyama et al., 2000). However, more recent *in vitro* investigations have suggested that NSAIDS can modulate γ-secretase cleavages *in vitro* (Weggen

et al., 2001). At very high doses, a subset of NSAIDs (ibuprofen and indomethacin but not naproxen) can modulate the γ-secretase cleavage specificities for APP (favoring cleavage at Aβ 38 versus 42) and possibly other substrates. The molecular target(s) leading to this cleavage shift are unknown. As no direct inhibition of enzyme activity occurs, Notch signaling does not appear to be disrupted, presumably reducing the potential mechanism-based liabilities of this approach.

Immunotherapy for Aβ Amyloidosis

In both prevention and treatment trials in mutant *APP* and *APP/PS1* mice, both Aβ immunization with Freund's adjuvant vaccination and passive transfer of Aβ antibodies reduce levels of Aβ and plaque burden (Schenk et al., 1999; Bard et al., 2000; Morgan et al., 2000; DeMattos et al., 2001; 2002a; Dodart et al., 2002; Kotilinek et al., 2002; Monsonega and Weiner, 2003; Selkoe and Schenk, 2003). Efficacy seems to be related to antibody titer. The mechanisms of enhanced clearance are not certain, but two hypotheses have been suggested: (1) a small amount of Aβ antibody reaches the brain, binds to Aβ peptides, promotes the disassembly of fibrils, and, via the Fc antibody domain, encourages activated microglia to enter the affected region and remove Aβ (Schenk et al., 1999); and/or (2) serum antibodies serve as a sink to draw the amyloid peptides from the brain into the circulation, thus changing the equilibrium of Aβ in different compartments and promoting removal of Aβ from the brain (Morgan et al., 2000; Demattos et al., 2001; 2002a; Dodart et al., 2002; Cirrito et al., 2003; Oddo et al., 2004). These are not mutually exclusive mechanisms. Thus, active or passive immunotherapy in the mutant mice can partially clear Aβ, attenuate learning and behavioral deficits in at least two cohorts of mutant *APP* mice (Morgan et al., 2000; Dodart et al., 2002; Kotilinek et al., 2002), and reduce tau abnormalities in the triple-transgenic mice (Oddo et al., 2004). In immunized mice, adverse events were not reported.

In humans, although Phase 1 trials with Aβ peptide and adjuvant were not associated with any adverse events, Phase 2 trials were suspended because of severe adverse reactions (meningoencephalitis) in a subset of patients (Monsonego and Weiner, 2003; Nicoll et al., 2003). The pathology in this case, consistent with T-cell meningitis (Nicoll et al., 2003), was interpreted to show some clearance of Aβ deposits (Nicoll et al., 2003). Specifically, some areas of cortex contained very few plaques, yet these regions exhibited a relatively high density of tangles, neuropil threads and vascular amyloid deposits. There was paucity of plaque-associated dystrophic neurites and astrocytic clusters. In some regions with low plaque densities, Aβ immunoreactivity was associated with microglia. T-cells were conspicuous in subarachnoid space and around some vessels (Nicoll et al., 2003). The adverse events occurring in the subset of patients illustrate the challenges of extrapolating outcomes in mice to trials with humans.

Interestingly, assessment of cognitive functions in a small subset of patients (30) who received vaccination and booster immunizations disclosed that patients who generated Aβ antibodies (as measured of a new assay), had a slower decline in several functional measures (Hock et al., 2003). Investigators have continued to pursue the passive immunization approach and are attempting to make a vaccine with antigens that do not stimulate T-cell mediated immunologic attacks (Monsonego and Weiner, 2003).

31.9 Perspective

Presently available therapies for patients include: cholinesterase inhibitors; neuroprotective approaches; drugs that interact with glutamate receptors; pharmacological agents for behavioral disturbances, etc. (Lyketsos et al., 2002; Cummings, 2004). These treatments do not directly influence the disease process and new disease-modifying treatments are the major unmet need in this field. The identification of genes mutated in the inherited forms of AD has allowed investigators to create *in vitro* and *in vivo* model systems relevant to AD and to pursue novel approaches to therapy.

After reviewing the clinical syndrome, the laboratory studies, the genetics and biochemistry, and the neurobiology of AD, we emphasized the value of transgenic and gene targeted models, the study of which has provided extraordinary new information about: the mechanisms of Aβ amyloidogenesis; the reasons for vulnerability of brain to amyloidosis; and the proteins that are potential therapeutic targets. New models using conditional expression systems will allow investigators to examine some of the mechanisms by which mutant proteins cause dysfunction of neurons and to delineate pathogenic pathways that can be further tested by breeding strategies and by RNAi injection methods. The results of these approaches will provide a better understanding of the mechanisms leading to diseases, help us to design new treatments, and allow us to assess the brain following amyloid mediated imaging.

Summary

Investigations of a variety of neurodegenerative diseases and genetically engineered (transgenic or gene targeted) models have reproduced some of the features of human neurodegenerative disorders in animals, have provided important new information about the disease mechanisms and participants in pathogenic pathways, and have allowed identification of new therapeutic targets. This information has provided the basis for new therapeutic strategies that are being tested in models. These lines of research have made spectacular progress over the past few years, and we anticipate that future discoveries will lead to design of promising mechanism-based therapies that can be tested in models of AD and other devastating illnesses of humans.

ACKNOWLEDGEMENTS

The authors wish to thank the many colleagues who have worked at JHMI as well as those at other institutions for their contributions to some of the original work cited in this review and for their helpful discussions. Aspects of this work were supported by grants from the U.S. Public Health Service (AG05146, NS41438, NS45150, AG14248) as well as the Metropolitan Life Foundation, Adler Foundation, Alzheimer's Association, CART Fund, and Bristol-Myers Squibb Foundation.

REFERENCES

Akiyama, H., Barger, S.W., Barnum, S., Bradt, B., Bauer, J., Cole, G.M., Cooper, N.R., Eikelenboom, P., Emmerling, M., Fiebich, B.L., Finch, C.E., Frautschy, S., Griffin, W.S., Hampel, H., Hull, M., Landreth, G., Lue, L., Mrak, R., Mackenzie, I.R., McGeer, P.L., O'Banion, M.K., Pachter, J., Pasinetti, G., Plata-Salaman, C., Rogers, J., Rydel, R., Shen, Y., Streit, W., Strohmeyer, R., Tooyoma, I., Van Muiswinkel, F.L., Veerhuis, R., Walker, D., Webster, S., Wegrzyniak, B., Wenk, G. and Wyss-Coray, T. (2000). Inflammation and Alzheimer's disease. *Neurobiol Aging*, **21**(3), 383–421.

Albert, M.S., Moss, M.B., Tanzi, R. and Jones, K. (2001). Preclinical prediction of AD using neuropsychological tests. *J Int Neuropsychol Soc*, **7**(5), 631–639.

Bacskai, B.J., Hickey, G.A., Skoch, J., Kajdasz, S.T., Wang, Y., Huang, G.F., Mathis, C.A., Klunk, W.E. and Hyman, B.T. (2003). Four-dimensional multiphoton imaging of brain entry, amyloid binding, and clearance of an amyloid-beta ligand in transgenic mice. *Proc Natl Acad Sci USA*, **100**(21), 12462–12467.

Bales, K.R., Verina, T., Dodel, R.C., Du, Y., Altstiel, L.D., Bender, M., Hyslop, P., Johnstone, E.M., Little, S.P., Cummins, D.J., Piccardo, P., Ghetti, B. and Paul, S.M. (1997). Lack of apolipoprotein E dramatically reduces amyloid-peptide deposition. *Nat Genet*, **17**, 263–264.

Bard, F., Cannon, C., Barbour, R., Burke, R.L., Games, D., Grajeda, H., Guido, T., Hu, K., Huang, J., Johnson-Wood, K., Khan, K., Kholodenko, D., Lee, M., Lieberburg, I., Motter, R., Nguyen, M., Soriano, F., Vasquez, N., Weiss, K., Welch, B., Seubert, P., Schenk, D. and Yednock, T. (2000). Peripherally administered antibodies against amyloid beta-peptide enter the central nervous system and reduce pathology in a mouse model of Alzheimer disease. *Nat Med*, **6**(8), 916–919.

Beach, T.G., Kuo, Y.-M., Spiegel, K., Emmerling, M.R., Sue, L.I., Kokjohn, K. and Roher, A.E. (2000). The cholinergic deficit coincides with A-beta deposition at the earliest histopathologic stages of Alzheimer disease. *J Neuropathol Exp Neurol*, **59**, 308–313.

Bennett, B.D., Babu-Khan, S., Loeloff, R., Louis, J.C., Curran, E., Citron, M. and Vassar, R. (2000). Expression analysis of BACE2 in brain and peripheral tissues. *J Biol Chem*, **275**(27), 20647–20651.

Bertram, L., Blacker, D., Mullin, K., Keeney, D., Jones, J., Basu, S., Yhu, S., McInnis, M.G., Go, R.C.P., Vekrellis, K., Selkoe, D.J., Saunders, A.J. and Tanzi, R.E. (2000). Evidence for genetic linkage of Alzheimer's disease to chromosome 10q. *Science*, **290**, 2302–2303.

Bodendorf, U., Danner, S., Fischer, F., Stefani, M., Sturchler-Pierrat, C., Wiederhold, K.H., Staufenbiel, M. and Paganetti, P. (2002). Expression of human beta-secretase in the mouse brain increases the steady-state level of beta-amyloid. *J Neurochem*, **80**(5), 799–806.

Boncristiano, S., Calhoun, M.E., Kelly, P.H., Pfeifer, M., Bondolfi, L., Stalder, M., Phinney, A.L., Abramowski, D., Sturchler-Pierrat, C., Enz, A., Sommer, B., Staufenbiel, M. and Jucker, M. (2002). Cholinergic changes in the APP23 transgenic mouse model of cerebral amyloidosis. *J Neurosci*, **22**(8), 3234–3243.

Borchelt, D.R., Thinakaran, G., Eckman, C.B., Lee, M.K., Davenport, F., Ratovitsky, T., Prada, C.M., Kim, G., Seekins, S., Yager, D., Slunt, H.H., Wang, R., Seeger, M., Levey, A.I., Gandy, S.E., Copeland, N.G., Jenkins, N.A., Price, D.L., Younkin, S.G. and Sisodia, S.S. (1996). Familial Alzheimer's disease-linked presenilin 1 variants elevate Abeta1–42/1–40 ratio *in vitro* and *in vivo*. *Neuron*, **17**(5), 1005–1013.

Borchelt, D.R., Ratovitski, T., Van Lare, J., Lee, M.K., Gonzales, V., Jenkins, N.A., Copeland, N.G., Price, D.L. and Sisodia, S.S. (1997). Accelerated amyloid deposition in the brains of transgenic mice coexpressing mutant presenilin 1 and amyloid precursor proteins. *Neuron*, **19**(4), 939–945.

Braak, H. and Braak, E. (1991). Neuropathological staging of Alzheimer-related changes. *Acta Neuropathol*, **82**, 239–259.

Brookmeyer, R., Gray, S. and Kawas, C. (1998). Projections of Alzheimer's disease in the United States and the public health impact of delaying disease onset. *Am J Public Health*, **88**(9), 1337–1342.

Busciglio, J., Lorenzo, A., Yeh, J. and Yankner, B.A. (1995). β-amyloid fibrils induce tau phosphorylation and loss of microtubule binding. *Neuron*, **14**, 879–888.

Buxbaum, J.D., Thinakaran, G., Koliatsos, V., O'Callahan, J., Slunt, H.H., Price, D.L. and Sisodia, S.S. (1998). Alzheimer amyloid protein precursor in the rat hippocampus: transport and processing through the perforant path. *J Neurosci*, **18**(23), 9629–9637.

Cai, H., Wang, Y., McCarthy, D., Wen, H., Borchelt, D.R., Price, D.L. and Wong, P.C. (2001). BACE1 is the major beta-secretase for generation of Abeta peptides by neurons. *Nat Neurosci,* **4**(3), 233–234.

Calhoun, M.E., Wiederhold, K.H., Abramowski, D., Phinney, A.L., Probst, A., Sturchler-Pierrat, C., Staufenbiel, M., Sommer, B. and Jucker, M. (1998). Neuron loss in APP transgenic mice. *Nature,* **395**, 755–756.

Cao, X. and Sudhof, T.C. (2001). A transcriptionally [correction of transcriptively] active complex of APP with Fe65 and histone acetyltransferase Tip60. *Science,* **293**(**5527**), 115–120.

Caughey, B. and Lansbury, P.T. (2003). Protofibrils, pores, fibrils, and neurodegeneration: separating the responsible protein aggregates from the innocent bystanders. *Annu Rev Neurosci,* **26**, 267–298.

Chapman, P.F., White, G.L., Jones, M.W., Cooper-Blacketer, D., Marshall, V.J., Irizarry, M., Younkin, L., Good, M.A., Bliss, T.V.P., Hyman, B.T., Younkin, S.G. and Hsiao, K.K. (1999). Impaired synaptic plasticity and learning in aged amyloid precursor protein transgenic mice. *Nat Neurosci,* **2**, 271–276.

Chen, G., Chen, K.S., Knox, J., Inglis, J., Bernard, A., Martin, S.J., Justice, A., McConlogue, L., Games, D., Freedman, S.B. and Morris, R.G.M. (2000). A learning deficit related to age and β-amyloid plaques in a mouse model of Alzheimer's disease. *Nature,* **408**, 975–979.

Cirrito, J.R., May, P.C., O'Dell, M.A., Taylor, J.W., Parsadanian, M., Cramer, J.W., Audia, J.E., Nissen, J.S., Bales, K.R., Paul, S.M., DeMattos, R.B. and Holtzman, D.M. (2003). *In vivo* assessment of brain interstitial fluid with microdialysis reveals plaque-associated changes in amyloid-beta metabolism and half-life. *J Neurosci,* **23**(**26**), 8844–8853.

Citron, M. (2004). Strategies for disease modification in Alzheimer's disease. *Nat Rev Neurosci,* **5**(9), 677–685.

Corder, E.H., Saunders, A.M., Risch, N.J., Strittmatter, W.J., Schmechel, D.E., Gaskell Jr., P.C., Rimmler, J.B., Locke, P.A., Conneally, P.M., Schmader, K.E., Small, G.W., Roses, A.D., Haines, J.L. and Pericak-Vance, M.A. (1994). Protective effect of apolipoprotein E type 2 allele for late onset Alzheimer disease. *Nat Genet,* **7**, 180–184.

Cummings, J.L. (2004). Alzheimer's disease. *N Engl J Med,* **351**(1), 56–67.

De Strooper, B. (2003). Aph-1, pen-2, and nicastrin with presenilin generate an active gamma-secretase complex. *Neuron,* **38**(1), 9–12.

De Strooper, B., Saftig, P., Craessaerts, K., Vanderstichele, H., Guhde, G., Annaert, W.G., Von Figura, K. and Van Leuven, F. (1998). Deficiency of presenilin-1 inhibits the normal cleavage of amyloid precursor protein. *Nature,* **391**(**6665**), 387–390.

DeMattos, R.B., Bales, K.R., Cummins, D.J., Dodart, J.C., Paul, S.M. and Holtzman, D.M. (2001). Peripheral anti-Aβ antibody alters CNS and plasma Aβ clearance and decreases brain Aβ burden in a mouse model of Alzheimer's disease. *Proc Natl Acad Sci USA,* **98**, 8850–8855.

DeMattos, R.B., Bales, K.R., Cummins, D.J., Paul, S.M. and Holtzman, D.M. (2002a). Brain to plasma amyloid-beta efflux: a measure of brain amyloid burden in a mouse model of Alzheimer's disease. *Science,* **295**, 2264–2267.

DeMattos, R.B., O'Dell, M.A., Parsadanian, M., Taylor, J.W., Harmony, J.A.K., Bales, K.R., Paul, S.M., Aronow, B.J. and Holtzman, D.M. (2002b). Clusterin promotes amyloid plaque formation and is critical for neuritic toxicity in a mouse model of Alzheimer's disease. *Proc Natl Acad Sci USA,* **99**(**16**), 10843–10848.

DeMattos, R.B., Cirrito, J.R., Parsadanian, M., May, P.C., O'Dell, M.A., Taylor, J.W., Harmony, J.A., Aronow, B.J., Bales, K.R., Paul, S.M. and Holtzman, D.M. (2004). ApoE and clusterin cooperatively suppress Abeta levels and deposition. Evidence that ApoE regulates extracellular Abeta metabolism *in vivo. Neuron,* **41**(2), 193–202.

Doan, A., Thinakaran, G., Borchelt, D.R., Slunt, H.H., Ratovitsky, T., Podlisny, M., Selkoe, D.J., Seeger, M., Gandy, S.E., Price, D.L. and Sisodia, S.S. (1996). Protein topology of presenilin 1. *Neuron,* **17**(5), 1023–1030.

Dodart, J.C., Bales, K.R., Gannon, K.S., Greene, S.J., DeMattos, R.B., Mathis, C., DeLong, C.A., Wu, S., Wu, X., Holtzman, D.M. and Paul, S. (2002). Immunization reverses memory deficits without reducing brain Abeta burden in Alzheimer's disease model. *Nat Neurosci,* **5**, 452–457.

Edbauer, D., Winkler, E., Haass, C. and Steiner, H. (2002). Presenilin and nicastrin regulate each other and determine amyloid beta- peptide production via complex formation. *Proc Natl Acad Sci USA,* **99**(**13**), 8666–8671.

Ertekin-Taner, N., Graff-Radford, N., Younkin, L.H., Eckman, C., Baker, M.G., Adamson, J., Ronald, J., Blangero, J., Hutton, M. and Younkin, S.G. (2000). Linkage of plasma Aβ42 to a quantitative locus on chromosome 10 in late-onset Alzheimer's disease pedigrees. *Science,* **290**, 2303–2304.

Esler, W.P., Kimberly, W.T., Ostaszewski, B.L., Diehl, T.S., Moore, C.L., Tsai, J.Y., Rahmati, T., Xia, W., Selkoe, D.J. and Wolfe, M.S. (2000). Transition-state analogue inhibitors of gamma-secretase bind directly to presenilin-1. *Nat Cell Biol,* **2**(7), 428–434.

Farris, W., Mansourian, S., Chang, Y., Lindsley, L., Eckman, E.A., Frosch, M.P., Eckman, C.B., Tanzi, R.E., Selkoe, D.J. and Guenette, S. (2003). Insulin-degrading enzyme regulates the levels of insulin, amyloid beta-protein, and the beta-amyloid precursor protein intracellular domain *in vivo. Proc Natl Acad Sci USA,* **100**(7), 4162–4167.

Farzan, M., Schnitzler, C.E., Vasilieva, N., Leung, D. and Choe, H. (2000). BACE2, a β-secretase homolog, cleaves at the β site and within the amyloid-β region of the amyloid-β precursor protein. *Proc Natl Acad Sci USA*, **97**, 9712–9717.

Feng, R., Rampon, C., Tang, Y.P., Shron, D., Jin, J., Kyin, M., Sopher, B., Martin, G., Kim, S.-H., Langdon, R., Sisodia, S. and Tsien, J.Z. (2001). Deficient neurogenesis in forebrain-specific presenilin-1 knockout mice is associated with reduced clearance of hippocampal memory traces. *Neuron*, **32**, 911–926.

Francis, R., McGrath, G., Zhang, J., Ruddy, D.A., Sym, M., Apfeld, J., Nicoll, M., Maxwell, M., Hai, B., Ellis, M.C., Parks, A.L., Xu, W., Li, J., Gurney, M., Myers, R.L., Himes, C.S., Hiebsch, R., Ruble, C., Nye, J.S. and Curtis, D. (2002). Aph-1 and pen-2 are required for Notch pathway signaling, gamma-secretase cleavage of beta APP, and presenilin protein accumulation. *Dev Cell*, **3**(**1**), 85–97.

Fukumoto, H., Cheung, B.S., Hyman, B.T. and Irizarry, M.C. (2002). Beta-secretase protein and activity are increased in the neocortex in Alzheimer disease. *Arch Neurol*, **59**(**9**), 1381–1389.

Gastard, M.C., Troncoso, J.C. and Koliatsos, V.E. (2003). Caspase activation in the limbic cortex of subjects with early Alzheimer's disease. *Ann Neurol*, **54**(**3**), 393–398.

Ghiso, J. and Wisniewski, T. (2004). An animal model of vascular amyloidosis. *Nat Neurosci*, **7**(**9**), 902–904.

Gomez-Isla, T., Price, J.L., McKeel Jr., D.W., Morris, J.C., Growdon, J.H. and Hyman, B.T. (1996). Profound loss of layer II entorhinal cortex neurons occurs in very mild Alzheimer's disease. *J Neurosci*, **16**(**14**), 4491–4500.

Gong, Y., Chang, L., Viola, K.L., Lacor, P.N., Lambert, M.P., Finch, C.E., Krafft, G.A. and Klein, W.L. (2003). Alzheimer's disease-affected brain: presence of oligomeric A beta ligands (ADDLs) suggests a molecular basis for reversible memory loss. *Proc Natl Acad Sci USA*, **100**(**18**), 10417–10422.

Götz, J., Chen, F., Barmettler, R. and Nitsch, R.M. (2001). Tau filament formation in transgenic mice expressing P301L tau. *J Biol Chem*, **276**, 529–534.

Gotz, J., Chen, F., Van Dorpe, J. and Nitsch, R.M. (2001). Formation of neurofibrillary tangles in P301l tau transgenic mice induced by Abeta fibrils. *Science*, **293**, 1491–1495.

Goutte, C., Tsunozaki, M., Hale, V.A. and Priess, J.R. (2002). APH-1 is a multipass membrane protein essential for the Notch signaling pathway in Caenorhabditis elegans embryos. *Proc Natl Acad Sci USA*, **99**(**2**), 775–779.

Haass, C. (2004). Take five-BACE and the gamma-secretase quartet conduct Alzheimer's amyloid beta-peptide generation. *EMBO J*, **23**(**3**), 483–488.

Hartley, D.M., Walsh, D.M., Ye, C.P., Diehl, T., Vasquez, S., Vassilev, P.M., Teplow, D.B. and Selkoe, D.J. (1999). Protofibrillar intermediates of amyloid beta-protein induce acute electrophysiological changes and progressive neurotoxicity in cortical neurons. *J Neurosci*, **19**(**20**), 8876–8884.

Heber, S., Herms, J., Gajic, V., Hainfellner, J., Aguzzi, A., Rulicke, T., von Kretzschmar, H., von Koch, C., Sisodia, S., Tremml, P., Lipp, H.P., Wolfer, D.P. and Muller, U. (2000). Mice with combined gene knock-outs reveal essential and partially redundant functions of amyloid precursor protein family members. *J Neurosci*, **20**(**21**), 7951–7963.

Herzig, M.C., Winkler, D.T., Burgermeister, P., Pfeifer, M., Kohler, E., Schmidt, S.D., Danner, S., Abramowski, D., Sturchler-Pierrat, C., Burki, K., van Duinen, S.G., Maat-Schieman, M.L., Staufenbiel, M., Mathews, P.M. and Jucker, M. (2004). Abeta is targeted to the vasculature in a mouse model of hereditary cerebral hemorrhage with amyloidosis. *Nat Neurosci*, **7**(**9**), 954–960.

Higuchi, M., Ishihara, T., Zhang, B., Hong, M., Andreadis, A., Trojanowski, J. and Lee, V.M. (2002). Transgenic mouse model of tauopathies with glial pathology and nervous system degeneration. *Neuron*, **35**(**3**), 433–446.

Hock, C., Konietzko, U., Streffer, J.R., Tracy, J., Signorell, A., Muller-Tillmanns, B., Lemke, U., Henke, K., Moritz, E., Garcia, E., Wollmer, M.A., Umbricht, D., de Quervain, D.J., Hofmann, M., Maddalena, A., Papassotiropoulos, A. and Nitsch, R.M. (2003). Antibodies against beta-amyloid slow cognitive decline in Alzheimer's disease. *Neuron*, **38**(**4**), 547–554.

Holtzman, D.M., Bales, K.R., Tenkova, T., Fagan, A.M., Parsadanian, M., Sartorius, L.J., Mackey, B., Olney, J., McKell, D., Wozniak, D. and Paul, S.M. (2000). Apolipoprotein E isoform-dependent amyloid deposition and neuritic degeneration in a mouse model of Alzheimer's disease. *Proc Natl Acad Sci USA*, **97**, 2892–2897.

Hsia, A.Y., Masliah, E., McConlogue, L., Yu, G.Q., Tatsuno, G., Hu, K., Kholodenko, D., Malenka, R.C., Nicoll, R.A. and Mucke, L. (1999). Plaque-independent disruption of neural circuits in Alzheimer's disease mouse models. *Proc Natl Acad Sci USA*, **96**, 3228–3233.

Huppert, S.S., Le, A., Schroeter, E.H., Mumm, J.S., Saxena, M.T., Milner, L.A. and Kopan, R. (2000). Embryonic lethality in mice homozygous for a processing-deficient allele of Notch1. *Nature*, **405**(**6789**), 966–970.

Hyman, B.T., Van Hoesen, G.W., Damasio, A.R. and Barnes, C.L. (1984). Alzheimer's disease: cell-specific pathology isolates the hippocampal formation. *Science*, **225**, 1168–1170.

Iwata, N., Tsubuki, S., Takaki, Y., Watanabe, K., Sekiguchi, M., Hosoki, E., Kawashima-Morishima, M., Lee, H.J., Hama, E.,

Sekine-Aizawa, Y. and Saido, T.C. (2000). Identification of the major Aβ_{1-42}-degrading catabolic pathway in brain parenchyma: supression leads to biochemical and pathological deposition. *Nat Med*, **2**, 143–150.

Iwata, N., Mizukami, H., Shirotani, K., Takaki, Y., Muramatsu, S., Lu, B., Gerard, N.P., Gerard, C., Ozawa, K. and Saido, T.C. (2004). Presynaptic localization of neprilysin contributes to efficient clearance of amyloid-beta peptide in mouse brain. *J Neurosci*, **24**(4), 991–998.

Iwatsubo, T. (2004). The gamma-secretase complex: machinery for intramembrane proteolysis. *Curr Opin Neurobiol*, **14**(3), 379–383.

Iwatsubo, T., Odaka, A., Suzuki, N., Mizusawa, H., Nukina, N. and Ihara, Y. (1994). Visualization of A beta 42(43) and A beta 40 in senile plaques with end-specific A beta monoclonals: evidence that an initially deposited species is A beta 42(43). *Neuron*, **13**(1), 45–53.

Jack Jr., C.R., Petersen, R.C., Xu, Y., O'Brien, P.C., Smith, G.E., Ivnik, R.J., Boeve, B.F., Tangalos, E.G. and Kokmen, E. (2000). Rates of hippocampal atrophy correlate with change in clinical status in aging and AD. *Neurology*, **55**(4), 484–489.

Jack Jr., C.R., Garwood, M., Wengenack, T.M., Borowski, B., Curran, G.L., Lin, J., Adriany, G., Grohn, O.H., Grimm, R. and Poduslo, J.F. (2004). *In vivo* visualization of Alzheimer's amyloid plaques by magnetic resonance imaging in transgenic mice without a contrast agent. *Magn Reson Med*, **52**(6), 1263–1271.

Kamenetz, F., Tomita, T., Hsieh, H., Seabrook, G., Borchelt, D., Iwatsubo, T., Sisodia, S. and Malinow, R. (2003). APP processing and synaptic function. *Neuron*, **37**(6), 925–937.

Killiany, R.J., Hyman, B.T., Gomez-Isla, T., Moss, M.B., Kikinis, R., Jolesz, F., Tanzi, R., Jones, K. and Albert, M.S. (2002). MRI measures of entorhinal cortex vs hippocampus in preclinical AD. *Neurology*, **58**(8), 1188–1196.

Klein, W.L., Krafft, G.A. and Finch, C.E. (2001). Targeting small Aβ oligomers: the solution to an Alzheimer's disease conundrum?. *Trend Neurosci*, **24**, 219–223.

Klunk, W.E., Engler, H., Nordberg, A., Wang, Y., Blomstrand, G., Holt, D.P., Bergstrom, M., Savitcheva, I., Huang, G.F., Estrada, S., Ausen, B., Debnath, M.L., Barletta, J., Price, J.C., Sandell, J., Lopresti, B.J., Wall, A., Koivisto, P., Antoni, G., Mathis, C.A. and Langstrom, B. (2004). Imaging brain amyloid in Alzheimer's disease using the novel positron emission tomography tracer, Pittsburgh compound-B. *Ann Neurol*, **55**, 1–14.

Koo, E.H. and Kopan, R. (2004). Potential role of presenilin-regulated signaling pathways in sporadic neurodegeneration. *Nat Med*, **10**(Suppl.), S26–S33.

Koo, E.H., Sisodia, S.S., Archer, D.R., Martin, L.J., Weidemann, A., Beyreuther, K.T., Fischer, P., Masters, C.L. and Price, D.L. (1990). Precursor of amyloid protein in Alzheimer disease undergoes fast anterograde axonal transport. *Proc Natl Acad Sci USA*, **87**, 1561–1565.

Kopan, R. and Goate, A. (2002). Aph-2/nicastrin: an essential component of gamma-secretase and regulator of notch signaling and presenilin localization. *Neuron*, **33**, 321–324.

Kotilinek, L.A., Bacskai, B.J., Westerman, M., Kawarabayashi, T., Younkin, L., Hyman, B.T., Younkin, S. and Ashe, K.H. (2002). Reversible memory loss in a mouse transgenic model of Alzheimer's disease. *J Neurosci*, **22**(15), 6331–6335.

Lambert, M.P., Barlow, A.K., Chromy, B.A., Edwards, C., Freed, R., Liosatos, M., Morgan, T.E., Rozovsky, I., Trommer, B., Viola, K.L., Wals, P., Zhang, C., Finch, C.E., Krafft, G.A. and Klein, W.L. (1998). Diffusible, nonfibrillar ligands derived from Abeta1–42 are potent central nervous system neurotoxins. *Proc Natl Acad Sci USA*, **95**(11), 6448–6453.

Lazarov, O., Lee, M., Peterson, D.A. and Sisodia, S.S. (2002). Evidence that synaptically released beta-amyloid accumulates as extracellular deposits in the hippocampus of transgenic mice. *J Neurosci*, **22**(22), 9785–9793.

Lee, V.M., Goedert, M. and Trojanowski, J.Q. (2001). Neurodegenerative tauopathies. *Annu Rev Neurosci*, **24**, 1121–1159.

Lesuisse, C., Xu, G., Anderson, J., Wong, M., Jankowsky, J., Holtz, G., Gonzalez, V., Wong, P.C.Y., Price, D.L., Tang, F., Wagner, S. and Borchelt, D.R. (2001). Hyper-expression of human apolipoprotein E4 in astroglia and neurons does not enhance amyloid deposition in transgenic mice. *Hum Mol Gen*, **10**, 2525–2537.

Lewis, J., McGowan, E., Rockwood, J., Melrose, H., Nacharaju, P., Van Slegtenhorst, M., Gwinn-Hardy, K., Paul, M.M., Baker, M.G., Yu, X., Duff, K., Hardy, J., Corral, A., Lin, W.L., Yen, S.H., Dickson, D.W., Davies, P. and Hutton, M. (2000). Neurofibrillary tangles, amyotrophy and progressive disturbance in mice expressing mutant (P301L) tau protein. *Nat Genet*, **25**, 402–405.

Lewis, J., Dickson, D.W., Lin, W.-L., Chisholm, L., Corral, A., Jones, G., Yen, S.-H., Sahara, N., Skipper, L., Yager, D., Eckman, C., Hardy, J., Hutton, M. and McGowan, E. (2001). Enhanced neurofibrillary degeneration in transgenic mice expressing mutat tau and APP. *Science*, **293**, 1487–1491.

Li, R., Lindholm, K., Yang, L.B., Yue, X., Citron, M., Yan, R., Beach, T.G., Sue, L., Sabbagh, M., Cai, H., Wong, P., Price, D. and Shen, Y. (2004). Amyloid beta peptide load is correlated with increased beta-secretase activity in sporadic Alzheimer's disease patients. *Proc Natl Acad Sci USA*, **101**(10), 3632–3637.

Li, T., Ma, G., Cai, H., Price, D.L. and Wong, P.C. (2003). Nicastrin is required for assembly of presenilin/gamma-secretase complexes to mediate notch signaling and for processing and trafficking of beta-amyloid precursor protein in mammals. *J Neurosci*, **23**(**8**), 3272–3277.

Li, T., Ma, G., Wen, H., Davenport, F., Price, D.L. and Wong, P.C. (2004). Mammalian APH-1 isoforms are functionally equivalent in regulated intramembrane proteolysis of Notch and APP. *Proc Natl Acad Sci USA* (submitted).

Li, Y.M., Lai, M.T., Xu, M., Huang, Q., DiMuzio-Mower, J., Sardana, M.K., Shi, X.P., Yin, K.C., Shafer, J.A. and Gardell, S.J. (2000a). Presenilin 1 is linked with gamma-secretase activity in the detergent solubilized state. *Proc Natl Acad Sci USA*, **97**(**11**), 6138–6143.

Li, Y.M., Xu, M., Lai, M.T., Huang, Q., Castro, J.L., DiMuzio-Mower, J., Harrison, T., Lellis, C., Nadin, A., Neduvelil, J.G., Register, R.B., Sardana, M.K., Shearman, M.S., Smith, A.L., Shi, X.P., Yin, K.C., Shafer, J.A. and Gardell, S.J. (2000b). Photoactivated gamma-secretase inhibitors directed to the active site covalently label presenilin 1. *Nature*, **405**(**6787**), 689–694.

Lim, G.P., Yang, F., Chu, T., Chen, P., Beech, W., Teter, B., Tran, T., Ubeda, O., Ashe, K.H., Frautschy, S.A. and Cole, G.M. (2000). Ibuprofen suppresses plaque pathology and inflammation in a mouse model for Alzheimer's disease. *J Neurosci*, **20**, 5709–5714.

Lue, L.F., Kuo, Y.M., Roher, A.E., Brachova, L., Shen, Y., Sue, L., Beach, T.G., Kurth, J.H., Rydel, R.E. and Rogers, J. (1999). Soluble amyloid beta peptide concentration as a predictor of synaptic change in Alzheimer's disease. *Am J Pathol*, **155**(**3**), 853–862.

Luo, Y., Bolon, B., Kahn, S., Bennett, B.D., Babu-Khan, S., Denis, P., Fan, W., Kha, H., Zhang, J., Gong, Y., Martin, L., Louis, J.C., Yan, Q., Richards, W.G., Citron, M. and Vassar, R. (2001). Mice deficient in BACE1, the Alzheimer's beta-secretase, have normal phenotype and abolished beta-amyloid generation. *Nat Neurosci*, **4**(**3**), 231–232.

Lyketsos, C.G., Lopez, O., Jones, B., Fitzpatrick, A.L., Breitner, J. and DeKosky, S. (2002). Prevalence of neuropsychiatric symptoms in dementia and mild cognitive impairment: results from the cardiovascular health study. *JAMA*, **288**(**12**), 1475–1483.

Ma, G., Li, T., Price, D.L. and Wong, P.C. (2004). APH-1a is the principal mammalian APH-1 isoform present in γ-secretase complexes during embryonic development. *J Neurosci* (in press).

Marjaux, E., Hartmann, D. and De Strooper, B. (2004). Presenilins in memory, Alzheimer's disease, and therapy. *Neuron*, **42**(**2**), 189–192.

Masliah, E., Mallory, M., Hansen, L., DeTeresa, R., Alford, M.F. and Terry, R. (1994). Synaptic and neuritic alterations during the progression of Alzheimer's disease. *Neurosci Lett*, **174**, 67–72.

Mattson, M. (2001). Apoptosis in neurodegenerative disorders. *Nature*, **1**, 120–129.

Mayeux, R. (2003). Epidemiology of neurodegeneration. *Annu Rev Neurosci*, **26**, 81–104.

McKhann, G., Drachman, D., Folstein, M., Katzman, R., Price, D. and Stadlan, E.M. (1984). Clinical diagnosis of Alzheimer's disease: report of the NINCDS-ADRDA Work Group under the auspices of the Department of Health and Human Services Task Force on Alzheimer's disease. *Neurology*, **34**, 939–944.

McLean, C.A., Cherny, R.A., Fraser, F.W., Fuller, S.J., Smith, M.J., Beyreuther, K.T., Bush, A.I. and Masters, C.L. (1999). Soluble pool of Abeta amyloid as a determinant of severity of neurodegeneration in Alzheimer's disease. *Ann Neurol*, **46**(**6**), 860–866.

Minger, S.L., Honer, W.G., Esiri, M.M., McDonald, B., Keene, J., Nicoll, J.A., Carter, J., Hope, T. and Francis, P.T. (2001). Synaptic pathology in prefrontal cortex is present only with severe dementia in Alzheimer disease. *J Neuropathol Exp Neurol*, **60**(**10**), 929–936.

Monsonego, A. and Weiner, H.L. (2003). Immunotherapeutic approaches to Alzheimer's disease. *Science*, **302**(**5646**), 834–838.

Morgan, D., Diamond, D.M., Gottschall, P.E., Ugen, K.E., Dickey, C., Hardy, J., Duff, K., Jantzen, P., DiCarlo, G., Wilcock, D., Connor, K., Hatcher, J., Hope, C., Gordon, M. and Arendash, G.W. (2000). Aβ peptide vaccination prevents memory loss in an animal model of Alzheimer's disease. *Nature*, **408**, 982–985.

Morris, J.C. and Price, J.L. (2001). Pathologic correlates of nondemented aging, mild cognitive impairment, and early-stage Alzheimer's disease. *J Mol Neurosci*, **17**(**2**), 101–118.

Morris, J.C., Storandt, M., Miller, J.P., McKeel, D.W., Price, J.L., Rubin, E.H. and Berg, L. (2001). Mild cognitive impairment represents early-stage Alzheimer disease. *Arch Neurol*, **58**(**3**), 397–405.

Mucke, L., Masliah, E., Yu, G.Q., Mallory, M., Rockenstein, E.M., Tatsuno, G., Hu, K., Kholodenko, D., Johnson-Wood, K. and McConlogue, L. (2000). High-level neuronal expression of Aβ$_{1–42}$ in wild-type human amyloid protein precursor transgenic mice: synaptotoxicity without plaque formation. *J Neurosci*, **20**, 4050–4058.

Myers, A., Holmans, P., Marshall, H., Kwon, J., Meyer, D., Ramic, D., Shears, S., Booth, J., DeVrieze, F.W., Crook, R., Hamshere, M., Abraham, R., Tunstall, N., Rice, F., Carty, S.,

Lillystone, S., Kehoe, P., Rudrasingham, V., Jones, L., Lovestone, S., Perez-Tur, J., Williams, J., Owen, M.J., Hardy, J. and Goate, A.M. (2000). Susceptibility locus for Alzheimer's disease on chromosome 10. *Science*, **290**, 2304–2305.

Naruse, S., Thinakaran, G., Luo, J.J., Kusiak, J.W., Tomita, T., Iwatsubo, T., Qian, X.Z., Ginty, D.D., Price, D.L., Borchelt, D.R., Wong, P.C. and Sisodia, S.S. (1998). Effects of PS1 deficiency on membrane protein trafficking in neurons. *Neuron*, **21**(**5**), 1213–1221.

Nestor, P.J., Scheltens, P. and Hodges, J.R. (2004). Advances in the early detection of Alzheimer's disease. *Nat Med*, **10**(**Suppl.**), S34–S41.

Nicoll, J.A., Wilkinson, D., Holmes, C., Steart, P., Markham, H. and Weller, R.O. (2003). Neuropathology of human Alzheimer disease after immunization with amyloid-beta peptide: a case report. *Nat Med*, **9**(**4**), 448–452.

Oddo, S., Caccamo, A., Shepherd, J.D., Murphy, M.P., Golde, T.E., Kayed, R., Metherate, R., Mattson, M.P., Akbari, Y. and LaFerla, F.M. (2003). Triple-transgenic model of Alzheimer's disease with plaques and tangles: intracellular Abeta and synaptic dysfunction. *Neuron*, **39**(**3**), 409–421.

Oddo, S., Billings, L., Kesslak, J.P., Cribbs, D.H. and LaFerla, F.M. (2004). Abeta immunotherapy leads to clearance of early, but not late, hyperphosphorylated tau aggregates via the proteasome. *Neuron*, **43**(**3**), 321–332.

Ohno, M., Sametsky, E.A., Younkin, L.H., Oakley, H., Younkin, S.G., Citron, M., Vassar, R. and Disterhoft, J.F. (2004). BACE1 deficiency rescues memory deficits and cholinergic dysfunction in a mouse model of Alzheimer's disease. *Neuron*, **41**(**1**), 27–33.

Petersen, R.C. (2003). Mild cognitive impairment clinical trials. *Nat Rev Drug Discov*, **2**(**8**), 646–653.

Petersen, R.C., Doody, R., Kurz, A., Mohs, R.C., Morris, J.C., Rabins, P.V., Ritchie, K., Rossor, M., Thal, L. and Winblad, B. (2001). Current concepts in mild cognitive impairment. *Arch Neurol*, **58**(**12**), 1985–1992.

Price, D.L. and Sisodia, S.S. (1998). Mutant genes in familial Alzheimer's disease and transgenic models. *Annu Rev Neurosci*, **21**, 479–505.

Price, J.L. and Morris, J.C. (1999). Tangles and plaques in non-demented aging and "preclinical" Alzheimer's disease. *Ann Neurol*, **45**(**3**), 358–368.

Price, D.L., Tanzi, R.E., Borchelt, D.R. and Sisodia, S.S. (1998). Alzheimer's disease: genetic studies and transgenic models. *Annu Rev Gen*, **32**, 461–493.

Savonenko, A.V., Xu, G.M., Price, D.L., Borchelt, D.R. and Markowska, A.L. (2003). Normal cognitive behavior in two distinct congenic lines of transgenic mice hyperexpressing mutant APPswe. *Neurobiol Dis*, **12**(**3**), 194–211.

Schenk, D., Barbour, R., Dunn, W., Gordon, G., Grajeda, H., Guido, T., Hu, K., Huang, J.P., Johnson-Wood, K., Khan, K., Kholodenko, D., Lee, M., Liao, Z.M., Lieberburg, I., Motter, R., Mutter, L., Soriano, F., Shopp, G., Vasquez, N., Vandevert, C., Walker, S., Wogulis, M., Yednock, T., Games, D. and Seubert, P. (1999). Immunization with amyloid-beta attenuates Alzheimer disease-like pathology in the PDAPP mouse. *Nature*, **400**(**6740**), 173–177.

Selkoe, D. and Kopan, R. (2003). Notch and presenilin: regulated intramembrane proteolysis links development and degeneration. *Annu Rev Neurosci*, **26**, 565–597.

Selkoe, D.J. and Schenk, D. (2003). Alzheimer's disease: molecular understanding predicts amyloid-based therapeutics. *Annu Rev Pharmacol Toxicol*, **43**, 545–584.

Shen, J., Bronson, R.T., Chen, D.F., Xia, W., Selkoe, D.J. and Tonegawa, S. (1997). Skeletal and CNS defects in presenilin-1-deficient mice. *Cell*, **89**(**4**), 629–639.

Sheng, J.G., Price, D.L. and Koliatsos, V.E. (2002). Disruption of corticocortical connections ameliorates amyloid burden in terminal fields in a transgenic model of Abeta amyloidosis. *J Neurosci*, **22**(**22**), 9794–9799.

Sheng, J.G., Price, D.L. and Koliatsos, V.E. (2004). Evidence that presenilin 1, and BACE1 are axonally transported to nerve terminals in the brain. *Exp Neurol* (submitted).

Sherrington, R., Rogaev, E.I., Liang, Y., Rogaeva, E.A., Levesque, G., Ikeda, M., Chi, H., Lin, C., Li, G., Holman, K., Tsuda, T., Mar, L., Foncin, J.-F., Bruni, A.C., Montesi, M.P., Sorbi, S., Rainero, I., Pinessi, L., Nee, L., Chumakov, I., Pollen, D., Brookes, A., Sanseau, P., Polinsky, R.J., Wasco, W., Da Silva, H.A.R., Haines, J.L., Pericak-Vance, M.A., Tanzi, R.E., Roses, A.D., Fraser, P.E., Rommens, J.M. and St George-Hyslop, P.H. (1995). Cloning of a gene bearing missense mutations in early-onset familial Alzheimer's disease. *Nature*, **375**, 754–760.

Silverman, D.H., Small, G.W., Chang, C.Y., Lu, C.S., Kung De Aburto, M.A., Chen, W., Czernin, J., Rapoport, S.I., Pietrini, P., Alexander, G.E., Schapiro, M.B., Jagust, W.J., Hoffman, J.M., Welsh-Bohmer, K.A., Alavi, A., Clark, C.M., Salmon, E., de Leon, M.J., Mielke, R., Cummings, J.L., Kowell, A.P., Gambhir, S.S., Hoh, C.K. and Phelps, M.E. (2001). Positron emission tomography in evaluation of dementia: regional brain metabolism and long-term outcome. *JAMA*, **286**(**17**), 2120–2127.

Sinha, S., Anderson, J.P., Barbour, R., Basl, G.S., Caccavello, R., Davis, D., Doan, M., Dovey, H.F., Frigon, N., Hong, J., Jacobson-Croak, K., Jewett, N., Kelm, P., Knops, J., Lleberburg, I., Power, M., Tan, H., Tatsuno, G., Tung, J., Schenk, D., Seubert, P., Suomensaari, S.M., Wang, S., Walker, D., Zhao, J., McConlogue, L. and John, V. (1999).

Purification and cloning of amyloid precursor protein beta-secretase from human brain. *Nature*, **402**, 537–540.

Sisodia, S.S. and George-Hyslop, P.H. (2002). Gamma-secretase, Notch, Abeta and Alzheimer's disease: where do the presenilins fit in?. *Nat Rev Neurosci*, **3**(4), 281–290.

Sisodia, S.S., Koo, E.H., Beyreuther, K.T., Unterbeck, A. and Price, D.L. (1990). Evidence that β-amyloid protein in Alzheimer's disease is not derived by normal processing. *Science*, **248**, 492–495.

Sisodia, S.S., Koo, E.H., Hoffman, P.N., Perry, G. and Price, D.L. (1993). Identification and transport of full-length amyloid precursor proteins in rat peripheral nervous system. *J Neurosci*, **13**, 3136–3142.

Steiner, H., Winkler, E., Edbauer, D., Prokop, S., Basset, G., Yamasaki, A., Kostka, M. and Haass, C. (2002). PEN-2 is an integral component of the gamma-secretase complex required for coordinated expression of presenilin and nicastrin. *J Biol Chem*, **277**(42), 39062–39065.

Strittmatter, W.J., Saunders, A.M., Schmechel, D., Pericak-Vance, M., Enghild, J., Salvesen, G.S. and Roses, A.D. (1993). Apolipoprotein E: high-avidity binding to β-amyloid and increased frequency of type 4 allele in late-onset familial Alzheimer disease. *Proc Natl Acad Sci USA*, **90**, 1977–1981.

Sturchler-Pierrat, C., Abramowski, D., Duke, M., Wiederhold, K.H., Mistl, C., Rothacher, S., Ledermann, B., Burki, K., Frey, P., Paganetti, P.A., Waridel, C., Calhoun, M.E., Jucker, M., Probst, A., Staufenbiel, M. and Sommer, B. (1997). Two amyloid precursor protein transgenic mouse models with Alzheimer disease-like pathology. *Proc Natl Acad Sci USA*, **94**, 13287–13292.

Sun, Y., Wu, S., Bu, G., Onifade, M.K., Patel, S.N., LaDu, M.J., Fagan, A.M. and Holtzman, D.M. (1998). Glial fibrillary acidic protein–apolipoprotein E (apoE) transgenic mice: astrocyte-specific expression and differing biological effects of astrocyte-secreted apoE3 and apoE4 lipoproteins. *J Neurosci*, **18**, 3261–3272.

Sunderland, T., Linker, G., Mirza, N., Putnam, K.T., Friedman, D.L., Kimmel, L.H., Bergeson, J., Manetti, G.J., Zimmermann, M., Tang, B., Bartko, J.J. and Cohen, R.M. (2003). Decreased beta-amyloid1–42 and increased tau levels in cerebrospinal fluid of patients with Alzheimer disease. *JAMA*, **289**(16), 2094–2103.

Sze, C.-I., Troncoso, J.C., Kawas, C.H., Mouton, P.R., Price, D.L. and Martin, L.J. (1997). Loss of the presynaptic vesicle protein synaptophysin in hippocampus correlates with early cognitive decline in aged humans. *J Neuropathol Exp Neurol*, **56**, 933–944.

Tanzi, R.E. and Bertram, L. (2001). New frontiers in Alzheimer's disease genetics. *Neuron*, **32**(2), 181–184.

Tanzi, R.E., Moir, R.D. and Wagner, S.L. (2004). Clearance of Alzheimer's Abeta peptide: the many roads to perdition. *Neuron*, **43**(5), 605–608.

Terry, R.D., Masliah, E., Salmon, D.P., Butters, N., DeTeresa, R., Hill, R., Hansen, L.A. and Katzman, R. (1991). Physical basis of cognitive alterations in Alzheimer's disease: synapse loss is the major correlate of cognitive impairment. *Ann Neurol*, **30**, 572–580.

Thinakaran, G., Harris, C.L., Ratovitski, T., Davenport, F., Slunt, H.H., Price, D.L., Borchelt, D.R. and Sisodia, S.S. (1997). Evidence that levels of presenilins (PS1 and PS2) are coordinately regulated by competition for limiting cellular factors. *J Biol Chem*, **272**, 28415–28422.

Vassar, R. and Citron, M. (2000). Aβ-generating enzymes: recent advances in β- and γ-secretase research. *Neuron*, **27**, 419–422.

Vassar, R., Bennett, B.D., Babu-Khan, S., Kahn, S., Mendiaz, E.A., Denis, P., Teplow, D.B., Ross, S., Amarante, P., Loeloff, R., Luo, L., Fisher, S., Fuller, J., Edenson, S., Lile, J., Jarosinski, M.A., Biere, A.L., Curran, E., Burgess, T., Louis, J.C., Collins, F., Treanor, J., Rogers, G. and Citron, M. (1999). β-secretase cleavage of Alzheimer's amyloid precursor protein by the transmembrane aspartic protease BACE. *Science*, **286**, 735–741.

Vekrellis, K., Ye, Z., Qiu, W.Q., Walsh, D., Hartley, D., Chesneau, V., Rosner, M.R. and Selkoe, D.J. (2000). Neurons regulate extracellular levels of amyloid α-protein via proteolysis by insulin-degrading enzyme. *J Neurosci*,. **20**, 1657–1665.

von Koch, C.S., Zheng, H., Chen, H., Trumbauer, M., Thinakaran, G., Van der Ploeg, L.H., Price, D.L. and Sisodia, S.S. (1997). Generation of APLP2 KO mice and early postnatal lethality in APLP2/APP double KO mice. *Neurobiol Aging*, **18**(6), 661–669.

Wadghiri, Y.Z., Sigurdsson, E.M., Sadowski, M., Elliott, J.I., Li, Y., Scholtzova, H., Tang, C.Y., Aguinaldo, G., Pappolla, M., Duff, K., Wisniewski, T. and Turnbull, D.H. (2003). Detection of Alzheimer's amyloid in transgenic mice using magnetic resonance microimaging. *Magn Reson Med*, **50**(2), 293–302.

Walsh, D.M. and Selkoe, D.J. (2004). Deciphering the molecular basis of memory failure in Alzheimer's disease. *Neuron*, **44**(1), 181–193.

Walsh, D.M., Hartley, D.M., Kusumoto, Y., Fezoui, Y., Condron, M.M., Lomakin, A., Benedek, G.B., Selkoe, D.J. and Teplow, D.B. (1999). Amyloid beta-protein fibrillogenesis. Structure and biological activity of protofibrillar intermediates. *J Biol Chem*, **274**(36), 25945–25952.

Walsh, D.M., Klyubin, I., Faden, A.I., Fadeeva, J.V., Cullen, W.K., Anwyl, R., Wolfe, M.S., Rowan, M.J. and Selkoe, D.J. (2002).

Naturally secreted oligomers of amyloid β-protein potently inhibit hippocampal LTP *in vivo*. *Nature*, **416**, 535–539.

Wang, H.W., Pasternak, J.F., Kuo, H., Ristic, H., Lambert, M.P., Chromy, B., Viola, K.L., Klein, W.L., Stine, W.B., Krafft, G.A. and Trommer, B.L. (2002). Soluble oligomers of beta amyloid (1–42) inhibit long-term potentiation but not long-term depression in rat dentate gyrus. *Brain Res*, **924**(2), 133–140.

Weggen, S., Eriksen, J.L., Das, P., Sagi, S.A., Wang, R., Pietrzik, C.U., Findlay, K.A., Smith, T.E., Murphy, M.P., Bulter, T., Kang, D.E., Marquez-Sterling, N., Golde, T.E. and Koo, E.H. (2001). A subset of NSAIDs lower amyloidogenic Aβ42 independently of cyclooxygenase activity. *Nature*, **414**, 212–216.

Whitehouse, P.J., Price, D.L., Clark, A.W., Coyle, J.T. and DeLong, M.R. (1981). Alzheimer disease: evidence for selective loss of cholinergic neurons in the nucleus basalis. *Ann Neurol*, **10**, 122–126.

Wolfe, M.S. (2002). Therapeutic strategies for Alzheimer's disease. *Nat Rev Drug Discov*, **1**(11), 859–866.

Wolfe, M.S., Xia, W., Ostaszewski, B.L., Diehl, T.S., Kimberly, W.T. and Selkoe, D.J. (1999). Two transmembrane aspartates in presenilin-1 required for presenilin endoproteolysis and gamma-secretase activity. *Nature*, **398**(6727), 513–517.

Wong, P.C., Zheng, H., Chen, H., Becher, M.W., Sirinathsinghji, D.J., Trumbauer, M.E., Chen, H.Y., Price, D.L., Van der Ploeg, L.H. and Sisodia, S.S. (1997). Presenilin 1 is required for Notch 1 and Dll1 expression in the paraxial mesoderm. *Nature*, **387**(6630), 288–292.

Wong, P.C., Price, D.L. and Cai, H. (2001). The brain's susceptibility to amyloid plaques. *Science*, **293**, 1434–1435.

Wong, P.C., Cai, H., Borchelt, D.R. and Price, D.L. (2002). Genetically engineered mouse models of neurodegenerative diseases. *Nat Neurosci*, **5**(7), 633–639.

Yan, X.X., Li, T., Rominger, C.M., Prakash, S.R., Wong, P.C., Olson, R.E., Zaczek, R. and Li, Y.W. (2004). Binding sites of gamma-secretase inhibitors in rodent brain: distribution, postnatal development, and effect of deafferentation. *J Neurosci*, **24**(12), 2942–2952.

Yang, L.B., Lindholm, K., Yan, R., Citron, M., Xia, W., Yang, X.L., Beach, T.G., Sue, L., Wong, P., Price, D., Li, R. and Shen, Y. (2003). Elevated beta-secretase expression and enzymatic activity detected in sporadic Alzheimer disease. *Nat Med*, **9**(1), 3–4.

Yu, G., Nishimura, M., Arawaka, S., Levitan, D., Zhang, L., Tandon, A., Song, Y.Q., Rogaeva, E., Chen, F., Kawarai, T., Supala, A., Levesque, L., Yu, H., Yang, D.S., Holmes, E., Milman, P., Liang, Y., Zhang, D.M., Xu, D.H., Sato, C., Rogaev, E., Smith, M., Janus, C., Zhang, Y., Aebersold, R., Farrer, L.S., Sorbi, S., Bruni, A., Fraser, P. and George-Hyslop, P. (2000). Nicastrin modulates presenilin-mediated notch/glp-1 signal transduction and beta APP processing. *Nature*, **407**(6800), 48–54.

Yu, H., Saura, C.A., Choi, S.-Y., Sun, L.D., Yang, X., Handler, M., Kawarabayashi, T., Younkin, L., Fedeles, B., Wilson, M.A., Younkin, S., Kandel, E.R., Kirkwood, A. and Shen, J. (2001). APP processing and synaptic plasticity in presenilin-1 conditional knockout mice. *Neuron*, **31**, 713–726.

Zhang, J., Yarowsky, P., Gordon, M.N., Di Carlo, G., Munireddy, S., van Zijl, P.C. and Mori, S. (2004). Detection of amyloid plaques in mouse models of Alzheimer's disease by magnetic resonance imaging. *Magn Reson Med.*, **51**(3), 452–457.

Zheng, H., Jiang, M.-H., Trumbauer, M.E., Sirinathsinghji, D.J.S., Hopkins, R., Smith, D.W., Heavens, R.P., Dawson, G.R., Boyce, S., Conner, M.W., Stevens, K.A., Slunt, H.H., Sisodia, S.S., Chen, H.Y. and Van der Ploeg, L.H.T. (1995). β-amyloid precursor protein-deficient mice show reactive gliosis and decreased locomotor activity. *Cell*, **81**, 525–531.

Biomimetic design of neural prostheses

Gerald E. Loeb and Cesar E. Blanco

Department of Biomedical Engineering and the A.E. Mann Institute for Biomedical Engineering,
University of Southern California, Los Angeles, CA, USA

32.1 Overview of human–machine interfaces for rehabilitation

As engineered devices and systems become more sophisticated and "intelligent" in their functionality, it is natural to apply them to the treatment of disabilities that arise through failure of their biological counterparts. It seems likely that one of the earliest tools fashioned by Homo sapiens would have been a walking stick or cane to compensate for an injured foot. The mechanical and materials science of the 18th and 19th centuries led to wheelchairs for invalids, cable-operated hooks for amputees and spectacles for myopes. These are all examples of interfaces that **augment** the otherwise reduced performance of a natural function.

The 20th century saw the rise of electronics, which can transduce energy between different forms, creating motion, light and sound where there was none. This led to attempts, mostly with limited success, to **substitute** one biological function for another (Marks, 1983; Kaczmarek et al., 1991), such as the Optacon tactile display of visual information (Hislop et al., 1983) and similar devices to represent sound (Reed et al., 1985; Tan et al., 1989; Waldstein and Boothroyd, 1995; Galvin et al., 1999), keyboard operated speech synthesizers (Carlson et al., 1981; Carlson, 1995; Flanagan, 1995; Liberman, 1995), voice-activated robots (Hammel et al., 1992; Van der Loos, 1995; Katevas et al., 1997; Burgar et al., 2000; Taylor et al., 2002) etc. Electronic communication systems use conversions from acoustic and light energy to electrical energy and back again. These technologies (which we mostly take for granted) effectively eliminate the need for a physical journey to achieve interpersonal communication. Thus hearing and vision substitute for locomotion, a great boon to patients with neuromuscular disabilities as well as a time-saver for us all.

This chapter is about neural prosthetic devices that **integrate** directly with the nervous system. In principle, this is an obvious strategy because of the inherent similarities between the nervous system and digital electronics. Both use pulsed electrical currents to represent all types of information and control signals. Only in the past 20 years, however, have we had the means to construct safe electronic human–machine interfaces and knowledge about how information is represented normally in different parts of the nervous system. The key word in the title of this chapter – **biomimetic** – summarizes a key realization that should enable dramatic improvements in rehabilitative technology in this new century: neural prostheses work best when their neural interfaces and internal processes mimic the signaling and computations that would have been performed by the intact nervous system.

32.2 Technology constraints

The individual computational elements of the nervous system – neurons – are physically small in diameter (a few microns), allowing them to be packed together into dense nerve tracts and nuclei. In order to achieve biomimetic function, it is desirable to exchange information with neurons on a similar spatial scale. Microelectronic technology is just starting to work comfortably at the micron scale, but it remains difficult to engineer interfaces between electronic and biological structures with such small dimensions.

Stimulation

Most neural prostheses work by applying electrical stimulation currents in the vicinity of neurons to recreate the temporospatial patterns of neural activity that represent the function to be replaced. Examples described below include stimulating motoneurons to reanimate paralyzed muscles and stimulating spiral ganglion cells to represent speech sounds to the brain. The nervous system differs from an electronic system in that it carries electrical currents by the flow of charged ions dissolved in water that is distributed everywhere in the body; electronic systems carry currents as the motion of electrons in metallic conductors that are usually well insulated from each other. This difference results in two fundamental problems for which solutions are still evolving:

- Electrical stimulation currents spread by volume conduction in all directions away from an electrode in the body, making it difficult to produce selective activation of specific neurons. This problem can be minimized by careful selection of an appropriate site in which to locate the neural prosthetic interface and by designing electrodes and stimulation parameters according to well-understood biophysical principles. For example, there are situations where relatively indiscriminate stimulation of large numbers of adjacent neurons is clinically effective. However, the fine scale of parallel information processing in the nervous system tends to push neural prosthetic design towards larger numbers of smaller electrodes.
- Passage of an electrical current from a metallic conductor into salt water usually results in corrosion of the metal and electrolysis of the solution, which would damage both a medical device and the patient in which it were implanted. The problem

can be avoided by judicious design of electrodes and stimulation parameters (reviewed in Loeb et al., 1982). This consideration tends to limit the design of small, dense electrode arrays because small electrodes may experience excessively high concentrations of electrical charge at their metal/electrolyte junctions.

Recording

Virtually all neural information processing involves bidirectional information transfers, for example, feedback from muscles to control systems or centrally initiated adjustments to the transmission of sound through the middle ear. Truly biomimetic systems should restore this two-way exchange by recording signals from the nervous system to produce natural and automatic control of the prosthesis. Unfortunately, the electrical signals generated by neurons are extremely weak and tend to be dispersed by the generally conductive media of the body fluids (Rall, 1962; Marks and Loeb, 1976). Adjacent neurons may carry quite different signals and may shift relative position over time, particularly as a consequence of wound healing and foreign body reaction following the insertion of an electrode (Beard et al., 1992; Schmidt et al., 1993; Grill and Mortimer, 1994; 2000; Williams et al., 1999; Stephan et al., 2001). This consideration pushes design towards large numbers of small, closely spaced electrodes; such arrays must be supported by even denser electronic circuits to amplify and interpret these weak and shifting signals. Technologies capable of deriving useful control signals from the nervous system while being deployed chronically in the body are just starting to be available (e.g., Rousche and Normann, 1998).

Packaging

The body is composed of warm saltwater that is constantly moving and rebuilding its structural elements. These are very hostile conditions for electronic devices, which work best when dry and stable. The first implanted electronic devices – cardiac pacemakers – relied on a simple interface (one electrode), bulky encapsulation and frequent replacement. Modern microelectronic technologies and packaging methods have allowed much greater functional complexity to be packed into much smaller packages that generally outlive the patient. Nevertheless, improving the biomimetic function of a neural prosthesis generally depends on packing yet more electrodes and signal processing functionality into ever-smaller places in the body from which they are not easily retrieved. The seemingly mundane requirements for packaging (and related functions such as flexible leads, hermetic feedthroughs, power and data transmission) are likely to remain limiting factors in the clinical performance of neural prostheses.

32.3 Goals and progress

Neuromodulation

Given the as yet limited technology at our disposal, it has been necessary to look for situations in which relatively crude interfaces happen to produce clinically useful effects. In general, these consist of pathologies in which neural function is altered rather than absent; neural prosthetic treatment then consists of crudely modulating the residual activity to achieve a net benefit.

Pain

Electrical stimulation to control chronic pain remains the largest market for neural prostheses (see Volume II, Chapters 9 and 15). The two basic approaches are transcutaneous electrical nerve stimulation (TENS; Fig. 32.1) and epidural spinal cord stimulation (SCS; Fig. 32.2). Both utilize the fact that signals from low-threshold cutaneous mechanoreceptors result in activation of inhibitory spinal interneurons; these reduce the excitability of the interneurons that normally transmit activity from nociceptive afferents (Melzack and Wall, 1965). There may also be indirect effects such as secretion of endogenous opiates such as endorphins (Wang et al., 1992), but see (Freeman et al., 1983).

Anyone who has ever rubbed the skin around an injured body part or used a counter-irritant such as a mentholated ointment is familiar with the ability of cutaneous stimulation to "gate" the perception of pain. Electrical stimulators to treat chronic pain mimic these behavioral strategies. As the responsible afferent axons are relatively large, they are readily excitable electrically, either at the peripheral nerves, the spinal roots or dorsal columns of the spinal cord. As the gating circuits are dermatomally organized, effective relief depends on spatial selectivity, which in turn depends on physically repositioning the electrode contacts (commonly used in TENS) or switching stimulation among multiple contacts (commonly used in SCS; North et al., 1991). Targeting information can be supplied by the patient, who generally perceives the stimulation as a buzz-like paresthesia overlapping the perceived location of the pain (North and Wetzel, 2002).

TENS and SCS are particularly effective for cutaneous pain and hypersensitivity syndromes arising from cutaneous lesions and neuromas (Cooney, 1997; Chabal et al., 1998; Lampl et al., 1998; North and Wetzel, 2002). They are much less effective for

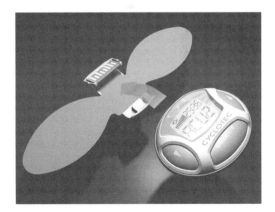

Figure 32.1. One of the TENS units manufactured by Cyclotec AMT for pain control. The compact stimulator design allows unit to be integrated with a variety of electrodes, eliminating the need for wires. Compact non-remote stimulator (compact TENS platform) is shown detached from electrodes configured for low back pain. (Diagrams courtesy of Cyclotec ©2004.)

deep myofascial pain (particularly low back pain) and visceral pain (Borjesson et al., 1998; Kruger et al., 1998; Borjesson, 1999; Brosseau et al., 2002). It is not clear whether this limitation arises from a fundamental difference in the interneuronal circuitry responsible for gating different types of pain or whether it reflects limitations in the currently available stimulation technology for targeting mechanoreceptors from those sites.

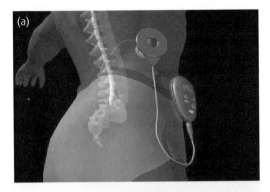

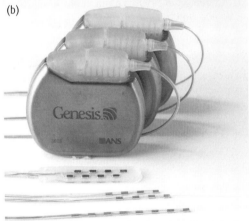

Figure 32.2. SCS unit manufacture by Advanced Neuromodulation Systems for the control of lower back pain. (a) Diagram depicting the deployment of the Genesys external controller and placement of electrodes in the spinal canal of the lumbar vertebrae. (b) Genesys external controller with several electrode designs for site-specific electrical stimulation of single or multiple spinal cord segments. (Diagram and photograph courtesy of Advanced Neuromodulation Systems.)

Disuse atrophy

Paralysis of muscles or just inability to exercise as a result of various diseases and trauma produces a relatively rapid loss of muscle mass, strength and fatigue-resistance (Peckham et al., 1976; Durand and Williams, 1990; Thomas et al., 1997; Felicetti et al., 1998). This disuse atrophy can itself result in morbidity that is distinct from the loss of movement produced by the muscles themselves (see Volume II, Chapter 21). At the least it leads to an extended rehabilitative period if and when the cause of the disuse is resolved (e.g., following surgical repair of bones, joints, ligaments and tendons). Loss of muscle padding can result in pressure points and breakdown of overlying soft tissues, forming pressure ulcers (Yarkony, 1994; Bouten et al., 2003). Loss of reserve muscle strength leads to increased stress on joints (e.g., quadriceps weakness correlated with progression of osteoarthritis of the knee (Slemenda et al., 1997; Brandt, 1998; 2003)). Atrophic muscles can become permanently shortened by contractures (e.g., flexion contractures of the hand in stroke patients (Pandyan et al., 1997; 2003)) or lengthened by unopposed passive stretch (e.g., shoulder subluxation in stroke patients (Ikai et al., 1998; Zorowitz, 2001)).

One relatively simple approach to preventing or reversing disuse atrophy is electrical stimulation to restore active contractile function to the paralyzed muscle (Baker et al., 2000). Muscle fibers respond readily to both normal exercise and electrically induced contraction; the latter can be used to produce specific patterns of activity that cannot be generated voluntarily (Sutherland et al., 2003). Electrical stimulation is generally feasible only if the muscle is still innervated by motoneurons because denervated muscle fibers are difficult to excite electrically (but see Kern et al., 2002). Transcutaneous electrical nerve stimulators (TENS) that can produce high-enough voltages and currents can be used for neuromuscular electrical stimulation (NMES), activating the terminal branches of the motoneurons within the target muscles (Vodovnik et al., 1988; Delitto and Snyder-Mackler, 1990; Kimberley et al., 2003). However, the high currents tend to produce noxious cutaneous sensations and may irritate or even burn the skin (Delitto et al., 1992; Yu et al., 2001). Placement of electrodes and adjustment of stimulation parameters usually requires a trained therapist, making it expensive and inconvenient for chronic use. Percutaneous wire electrodes injected into muscles are effective but unsuited for long-term use (Shimada et al., 1996; Agarwal et al., 2003). More recently, injectable stimulators called BIONs® (Loeb et al., 1991; Cameron et al., 1997) (Fig. 32.3) have been used successfully to prevent disuse atrophy in shoulder and quadriceps muscles (Dupont et al., 2001; 2004; Richmond et al., 2003), but they are not yet available commercially. Interestingly, unphysiologically low-stimulation rates (2–5 pps versus 5–30 pps for natural motoneuron activity) may be less fatiguing and more effective (Dupont Salter et al., 2003), perhaps acting through trophic mechanisms that depend on intermittent release of intracellular calcium rather than contractile force generation (Chin et al., 1998).

Movement disorders

Diseases of the basal ganglia, most notably Parkinson's disease, result in loss of signals that control the initiation and stabilization of voluntary movements through a complex series of inhibitory and excitatory interneurons projecting ultimately through the thalamus to the motor cortex. This gives rise to akinesia and dyskinesia such as tremor (Volume II, Chapter 35). Pharmacological augmentation of the native neurotransmitter dopamine is useful in the early stages but eventually loses efficacy and may produce side effects (Barone, 2003; Hershey et al., 2003; Nutt, 2003). Another effective approach is surgical ablation of regions in the basal ganglia that have lost normal inhibitory input and are excessively active (Takada et al., 2000; Ansari et al., 2002; Olanow 2002), but the sites are difficult to locate precisely and the intervention is irreversible. The treatment of choice now appears to be a multielectrode "deep brain stimulator" whose output can be tuned to produce relief of symptoms (Tasker, 1998; Benabid, 2003; Hariz, 2003; Mazzone, 2003). The temporospatial distribution of the neural excitation so achieved lacks

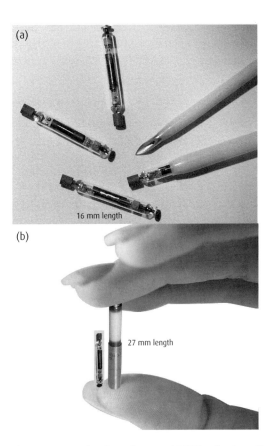

(a)

16 mm length

(b)

27 mm length

Figure 32.3. (a) Each inductively powered BION implant is small enough to inject into muscles or adjacent to nerves through a 12-G hypodermic needle. It receives power and digital command signals from an external coil that generates a radio frequency magnetic field. Multiple BIONs can be independently controlled by a single external coil worn on or near the body part where they are implanted. The glass hermetic package protects the electronics from body fluids; electrodes sealed into either end apply the stimulation pulses to the tissues to excite nearby nerve fibers (Cameron et al., 1997). Several clinical trials for various applications are underway (Dupont et al., 2004). (b) A battery-powered BION contains a rechargeable lithium ion cell that permits it to generate a preprogrammed sequence of stimulation pulses for several days before requiring recharging via an inductive link similar to the RF-powered BION. This device is being marketed in Europe to treat urinary urge incontinence by activating an inhibitory bladder reflex via afferents in the pudendal nerve. (Photo courtesy of manufacturer, Advanced Bionics Corporation.) An inductively powered BION was added to the image to allow direct size comparison.

most of the details of the normal circuitry, but it happens that even relatively crude biasing of this pathway can be remarkably effective clinically in these disorders (Benabid, 2003; Hamel et al., 2003).

Incontinence

Normal bladder and bowel function depend on primitive but complex circuits that are as yet poorly understood and difficult to access surgically or electrically (Shefchyk and Buss, 1998; see Volume II, Chapter 24). One such circuit that has proven useful is the inhibitory bladder reflex from cutaneous afferents in the clitoral or dorsal penile nerve (Nakamura and Sakurai, 1984). Patients with urinary urge incontinence have spastic bladders that tend to contract forcefully when distended by even a small volume of urine, resulting in discomfort and incontinence if they do not empty their bladders frequently (Herzog et al., 1988). Continuous stimulation of vaginal afferents blocks these reflexive contractions and provides substantial relief in many patients (Lindstrom et al., 1983). The Interstim® is a surgically implanted stimulator with electrodes in the sacral foramina, targeting the dorsal roots (Craggs and McFarlane, 1999). There are many different sensory pathways at this level, however, some of which produce uncomfortable sensations or may even increase bladder tone, so only about half of patients find this approach useful. More recently, a battery-powered version of the BION® (Fig. 32.3(b); Advanced Bionics Corp., Valencia, CA) has been injected near the pudendal nerve at the ischial notch, providing more selective stimulation of this same cutaneous pathway (Grill et al., 2001).

Most patients with spinal cord injury suffer from incontinence arising from a mechanism that is the converse of urge incontinence – overflow of the distended bladder because the descending pathways for initiating micturition have been interrupted. Researchers have been looking for an hypothesized "micturition center" in the spinal cord that could be stimulated electrically, but consistent effects have been elusive (Oliver et al., 1969; Birder et al., 1999). Electrical stimulation usually produces an unphysiological co-contraction of the bladder and the sphincter, preventing normal voiding (Grill et al.,

1999). The Vocare® stimulator for the sacral ventral roots can achieve urination in a series of spurts by taking advantage of the fact that the sphincter relaxes quickly when stimulation stops while the bladder contraction declines more slowly (Brindley and Rushton, 1990). However, it usually requires cutting some dorsal roots required for sexual function. More natural and complete micturition may be achievable by electrically stimulating the mechanoreceptors in the proximal urethra that normally detect flow of urine (Gustafson and Grill, 2001; Gustafson et al., 2003). Spinal reflexes from these afferents maintain bladder contraction while inhibiting the sphincter until the bladder is empty and flow ceases; however, a clinically suitable stimulation technology and surgical approach remain to be developed.

Sensory function

Cochlear implants

Cochlear implants remain the most sophisticated neural prosthesis to date and the only one that successfully replaces a completely absent sensory function. This is ironic because the initial success of cochlear implants was based on the unexpected result that an extremely primitive interface using only a single channel of stimulation could produce crude but useful percepts in profoundly deaf patients (Bilger, 1983). Modern cochlear implants (e.g., Fig. 32.4) have 8–20 separately controllable channels of information delivered via a delicate array of electrodes surgically implanted into the scala tympani (Loeb, 1985). An external microphone and speech processor continuously convert ambient acoustic information into a pattern of electrical stimulation pulses according to one of several different algorithms that have been developed (Wilson, 2000). This "speech-processing strategy" depends on a fairly large number of patient-specific parameters that are set during a "fitting session" in which the patient provides feedback on his/her percepts (posing a difficult problem for very young, pre-linguistically deaf patients; Loeb, 1989).

Performance of multichannel cochlear implants has been improving gradually and substantially for

(a)

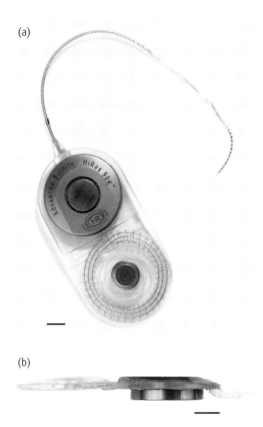

(b)

Figure 32.4. A modern cochlear implant consists of an electrode array (a) inserted into the scala tympani of the cochlea, a multichannel stimulation module (b) implanted in the temporal bone behind the ear, and an external speech-processing unit (not shown) that detects sound and converts it into a sequence of stimulation commands based on a program that is customized to the user. Calibration bar = 5 mm. (Photo courtesy of manufacturer, Advanced Bionics Corporation.)

the past 15 years. Most post-linguistically deafened adult recipients now use them to converse without lipreading, but there remains a substantial range in the rate of learning and ultimate performance levels for reasons that are not well understood (Loeb, 1989; Hughes et al., 2001; Miller et al., 2001; Svirsky, 2001). Congenitally and neonatally deafened children generally can participate in regular schools, particularly if they are implanted early in life when the nervous system seems most able to learn to hear (Kileny et al., 2001; Tobey and Geers, 2001). The variability in performance among recipients makes it difficult

to ascribe improved function to specific design and technology enhancements. In general, however, it appears to be related to improvements in the degree to which the temporospatial pattern of neural activation mimics the naturally occurring patterns in acoustic hearing. In addition, evidence suggested that plasticity in the auditory cortex helps to extract information from the reduced amount of signal complexity transmitted through the acoustic nerve (see Volume I, Chapter 10).

Visual prostheses

Prosthetic vision was one of the earliest goals for restoring neural function through biomimetic stimulation. Brindley and Lewin (1968) implanted an array of 85 electrodes and primitive radio receivers on the surface of the primary visual cortex of a blind volunteer and produced patterns of punctuate spots of light that they called "phosphenes". A commercial system based on such electrodes and a percutaneous connector has been tested recently (http://www.dobelle.com/), but high-stimulation thresholds and associated nonlinear interactions between electrode sites (Girvin, 1988) severely limit its functionality. That limitation appears to be overcome by microelectrodes implanted into the gray matter of the cortex (Bak et al., 1990; Schmidt et al., 1996), but the surgery and technology for a clinically useful system remain daunting challenges.

More recently, small arrays of 16 electrodes have been implanted onto the vitreous surface of the retina (Humayun et al., 2003), which could be useful in forms of blindness that leave the retinal ganglion cells intact (e.g., retinitis pigmentosa and macular degeneration but not glaucoma). It remains to be seen if this approach can be scaled up to the relatively large number of closely spaced stimulation channels that will be required to produce a usable image. Psychophysical studies suggest that this may require up to 1000 channels covering the central 30 degrees of vision (Cha et al., 1992a, b), a daunting task. Intraretinal arrays of microelectronic photocells have been suggested (Chow et al., 2001), but they do not seem capable of producing sufficient electrical power from incident photons to excite retinal neurons. It is difficult to anticipate the efficacy of a given technology, however, because retinal stimulation may work by modulating nonspiking neurons whose bias polarization is unknown and perhaps changing. Also it is unclear whether the technology can accommodate saccadic gaze shifts, which are an important aspect of normal visual function. The degree to which plasticity in visual cortex can enhance visual discrimination based on the limitations of retinal stimulation is unknown (see Volume I, Chapter 9).

Sensorimotor integration

Much of the effort over the past 35 years to develop technologies to electrically stimulate paralyzed muscles began with the goal of restoring locomotion to paraplegics. This has been an unexpectedly challenging and elusive goal, stemming from limitations in both the technology and basic understanding of normal biomechanics and sensorimotor control. Bipedal locomotion requires precise integration of visual, vestibular and proprioceptive feedback to modulate continuously the excitation of a large number of individual muscles distributed throughout both legs (Black et al., 1989; Jeka et al., 1998; Creath et al., 2002; Ferber et al., 2002; Kiemel et al., 2002; Lin and Woollacott, 2002; Oie et al., 2002; Peterka, 2002; Mergner et al., 2003; Peterka and Loughlin, 2004). In addition to many precisely controlled channels of stimulation, a biomimetic system would need many channels and several modalities of sensors to detect the voluntary intentions of the patient and provide feedback on the actual position and motion of the legs. The control system would have to integrate inputs and outputs to achieve the functionality of various parts of the brain and spinal cord whose underlying circuitry and computations are poorly understood. The isolated spinal cords of quadripedal mammals contain central pattern generators that can produce sequences of muscle activation and corrective reflexes associated with locomotion (Berkinblit et al., 1986; Volume I, Chapter 13), but the analogous circuits appear to be relatively weak and more difficult to activate and control in humans with spinal cord injuries (Calancie

et al., 1994; Volume II, Chapters 3 and 19). Current efforts to reanimate the legs tend to aim for simple standing; even so, achieving safe, stable and energetically efficient performance remains challenging (Bajd et al., 1999). Nevertheless, the spinal cord is capable of far more activity-dependent plasticity than previously recognized (see Volume I, Chapter 7) and this bodes well for ultimate success in developing neural prostheses for spinal cord injury.

Restoration of arm and hand function may offer a richer set of opportunities for functional electrical stimulation (FES). Patients present with a wide range of different disabilities, some of which are more likely to be suitable than others for a given technology. For many patients, even a modest increment in hand function could reduce reliance on expensive personal attendants (whereas locomotion can be more readily achieved by wheelchairs and accessible architectural design). The shortcomings of a primitive control system are less likely to result in physical injury in the arms than in the legs. An implanted eight-channel system called the Freehand® (Neural Control Corporation, Cleveland, OH) achieved useful assisted grasp function in C6–7 quadraplegics (Smith et al., 1998; Stroh et al., 1999) but was withdrawn from the market because of the complexity and cost of its surgical implantation and fitting procedures. It relied on a relatively simple but unnatural control strategy in which voluntary movement of the contralateral shoulder was used to trigger preprogrammed sequences of muscle stimulation.

The more severe the paralysis, the more difficult it is to find command signals under voluntary control of the patient and the more command information is needed to restore useful function. Command systems based on eye, head, tongue and breathing movements have been used to control powered wheelchairs and robotic manipulanda, but with limited user acceptance. One obvious solution is to record the electrical activity of the parts of the brain where motor command signals to the limbs normally originate. Electroencephalogram (EEG) signals are the most accessible source of such signals, but they have low spatial and temporal resolution and require a high degree of training and attention to produce data rates of only a few bits per minute (McFarland et al., 1998; Lauer et al., 1999). Similarly modest results were obtained by recording a couple of channels of data from cortical neurons (Kennedy, 1989; Kennedy et al., 1992). Such limited command signals may still be useful, however, to "locked in" patients suffering from pyramidal tract strokes and end-stage amyotrophic lateral sclerosis. Multichannel microelectrode recording systems have been used to record simultaneous unitary activity from scores of cortical cells in monkeys performing trained hand movements over many months (Donoghue et al., 1998; Maynard et al., 1999; Moran and Schwartz, 1999; Schwartz and Moran, 1999; 2000; Paninski et al., 2004; see Volume I, Chapter 8). Decoding algorithms can be trained to make reasonably accurate inferences about the hand movements associated with this activity (Hoffer et al., 1996; Schwartz et al., 2001). Monkeys have been trained to control computer cursors and simple robotic manipulanda by "thinking" without actually moving their arms (Taylor et al., 2002; Helms Tillery et al., 2003). Several research groups have started to tackle the formidable technical problems involved in converting such laboratory equipment into systems that could be implanted permanently into human research subjects (see Volume I, Chapter 33), but these are unlikely to be available clinically for many years.

32.4 Ultimate capabilities

Cognitive function

Many neurological deficits involve loss of function in central rather than peripheral pathways, such as inability to store or access information in various forms of dementia. In principle, a bidirectional prosthetic interface with the central nervous system could pick up the incoming signals to a defective portion of the brain such as the hippocampus, perform the missing computations in its circuitry, and inject the information back into the output neurons (Liaw and Berger, 1996; Iatrou et al., 1999; Alataris et al., 2000; Gholmieh et al., 2001). The feasibility of such an intervention depends on the sophistication

of the available interface technologies, which are still crude and difficult to deploy in deep, central structures. Research is underway to develop novel biomaterials that will not provoke even the "benign" foreign body reaction of present "biocompatible" materials so that electrode contacts can interact with individual neurons (Cyster et al., 2002; 2004; Shimono et al., 2002). It also depends on understanding the encoding and processing of information in brain centers responsible for clinical deficits. This has improved substantially as a result of experiments in animals with electrode arrays that might someday be adapted for chronic implantation in humans (see above). Sometimes relatively crude interventions can usefully improve function, particularly for patients with severe problems, as noted above for deep-brain stimulation and for early cochlear implants. Thus, it remains possible but not immediately likely that neural prosthetic technology will be used to augment and perhaps replace some cognitive function in patients.

Superhuman function

The word "bionic" was actually invented by a popular television show of the 1970s (The Six Million Dollar Man, MCA/Universal Studios). It was disdained by scientists for many years because of its original connotations of unrealistic superhuman performance. A web search of the term now produces >23,000 listings, including academicians who use the term to describe their research, companies that use the term in their corporate and product names, and patients and their caregivers who are desperate to find effective treatments for severe disabilities. It is a colorful past, a fanciful future but a sobering present.

Those who treat and advise patients and their families would do well to remember that medical technology moves like a glacier. Progress is slow but inexorable. Devices such as cochlear implants and deep-brain stimulators are now revolutionizing the treatment of disabilities such as deafness and tremor, but they took over a decade to achieve regulatory approval and insurance reimbursement *even after* their basic science and technologies were essentially in hand (a process that took about 20 years for each). Systems such as cortically controlled FES have already been in pre-clinical research for decades but are not yet ready for clinical trials. Patients still need to be persuaded to take full advantage of the conventional physical therapy and aids that are available now rather than waiting for an uncertain future. In at least some cases, that will be a necessary first step in preserving the body and the nervous system in order to be able to take advantage of neural prosthetic technology that is now in the pipeline. In most cases, this is just prudent medical care.

REFERENCES

Agarwal, S., Kobetic, R., Nandurkar, S. and Marsolais, E.B. (2003). Functional electrical stimulation for walking in paraplegia: 17-year follow-up of 2 cases. *J Spinal Cord Med*, **26**(1), 86–91.

Alataris, K., Berger, T.W. and Marmarelis, V.Z. (2000). A novel network for nonlinear modeling of neural systems with arbitrary point-process inputs. *Neural Netw*, **13**(2), 255–266.

Ansari, S.A., Nachanakian, A. and Biary, N.M. (2002). Current surgical treatment of Parkinsons disease. *Saudi Med J*, **23**(11), 1319–1323.

Bajd, T., Munih, M. and Kralj, A. (1999). Problems associated with FES-standing in paraplegia. *Technol Health Care*, **7**(4), 301–308.

Bak, M., Girvin, J.P., Hambrecht, F.T., Kufta, C.V., Loeb, G.E. and Schmidt, E.M. (1990). Visual sensations produced by intracortical microstimulation of the human occipital cortex. *Med Biol Eng Comput*, **28**(3), 257–259.

Baker, L.L., Wederich, C.L., McNeal, D.R., Newsam, C.J. and Waters, R.L. (2000). *NeuroMuscular Electrical Stimulation*, 4th edn Los Amigos Research and Education Institute, Inc., Downey, CA.

Barone, P. (2003). Clinical strategies to prevent and delay motor complications. *Neurology*, **61**(6 Suppl. 3), S12–S16.

Beard, R.B., Hung, B.N. and Schmukler, R. (1992). Biocompatibility considerations at stimulating electrode interfaces. *Ann Biomed Eng*, **20**(3), 395–410.

Benabid, A.L. (2003). Deep brain stimulation for Parkinson's disease. *Curr Opin Neurobiol*, **13**(6), 696–706.

Berkinblit, M.B., Feldman, A.G. and Fukson, O.I. (1986). Adaptability of innate motor patterns and motor control mechanisms. *Behav Brain Sci*, **9**, 585–638.

Bilger, R.C. (1983). Auditory results with single-channel implants. *Ann NY Acad Sci*, **405**, 337–342.

Birder, L.A., Roppolo, J.R., Erickson, V.L. and de Groat, W.C. (1999). Increased c-fos expression in spinal lumbosacral projection neurons and preganglionic neurons after irritation of the lower urinary tract in the rat. *Brain Res*, **834**(1–2), 55–65.

Black, F.O., Shupert, C.L., Peterka, R.J. and Nashner, L.M. (1989). Effects of unilateral loss of vestibular function on the vestibulo-ocular reflex and postural control. *Ann Otol Rhinol Laryngol*, **98**(11), 884–889.

Borjesson, M. (1999). Visceral chest pain in unstable angina pectoris and effects of transcutaneous electrical nerve stimulation (TENS). A review. *Herz*, **24**(2), 114–125.

Borjesson, M., Pilhall, M., Eliasson, T., Norssell, H., Mannheimer, C. and Rolny, P. (1998). Esophageal visceral pain sensitivity: effects of TENS and correlation with manometric findings. *Dig Dis Sci*, **43**(8), 1621–1628.

Bouten, C.V., Oomens, C.W., Baaijens, F.P. and Bader, D.L. (2003). The etiology of pressure ulcers: skin deep or muscle bound? *Arch Phys Med Rehabil*, **84**(4), 616–619.

Brandt, K.D. (1998). The importance of nonpharmacologic approaches in management of osteoarthritis. *Am J Med*, **105**(1B), 39S–44S.

Brandt, K.D. (2003). Response of joint structures to inactivity and to reloading after immobilization. *Arthritis Rheum*, **49**(2), 267–271.

Brindley, G.S. and Lewin, W.S. (1968). The sensations produced by electrical stimulation of the visual cortex. *J Physiol*, **196**, 479–493.

Brindley, G.S. and Rushton, D.N. (1990). Long-term follow-up of patients with sacral anterior root stimulator implants. *Paraplegia*, **28**, 469–475.

Brosseau, L., Milne, S., Robinson, V., Marchand, S., Shea, B., Wells, G. and Tugwell, P. (2002). Efficacy of the transcutaneous electrical nerve stimulation for the treatment of chronic low back pain: a meta-analysis. *Spine*, **27**(6), 596–603.

Burgar, C.G., Lum, P.S., Shor, P.C. and Van der Loos, H.F.M. (2000). Development of robots for rehabilitation therapy: the Palo Alto VA/Stanford experience. *J Rehab Res Dev*, **37**(6), 663–673.

Calancie, B., Needham-Shropshire, B., Jacobs, P., Willer, K., Zych, G. and Green, B.A. (1994). Involuntary stepping after chronic spinal cord injury. Evidence for a central rhythm generator for locomotion in man. *Brain*, **117**, 1143–1159.

Cameron, T., Liinamaa, T.L., Richmond, F.J.R. and Loeb, G.E. (1997). Muscle recruitment characteristics of an injectable miniature stimulator. *Proceedings of Canadian Medical Biological Engineering Society Annual Conference*.

Carlson, R. (1995). Models of speech synthesis. *Proc Natl Acad Sci USA*, **92**(**22**), 9932–9937.

Carlson, R., Galyas, K., Granstrom, B., Hunnicutt, S., Larsson, B. and Neovius, L. (1981). A multi-language, portable text-to-speech system for the disabled. *J Biomed Eng*, **3**(**4**), 285–288.

Cha, K., Horch, K. and Normann, R.A. (1992a). Mobility of performance with a pixelized vision system. *Vision Res*, **32**, 1367–1372.

Cha, K., Horch, K. and Normann, R.A. (1992b). Simulation of a phosphene-based visual field: visual acuity in a pixelized vision system. *Ann Biomed Eng*, **20**, 439–449.

Chabal, C., Fishbain, D.A., Weaver, M. and Heine, L.W. (1998). Long-term transcutaneous electrical nerve stimulation (TENS) use: impact on medication utilization and physical therapy costs. *Clin J Pain*, **14**(**1**), 66–73.

Chin, E.R., Olson, E.N., Richardson, J.A., Yang, Q., Humphries, C., Shelton, J.M., Wu, H., Zhu, W., Bassel-Duby, R. and Williams, R.S. (1998). A calcineurin-dependent transcriptional pathway controls skeletal muscle fiber type. *Gene Dev*, **12**, 2499–2509.

Chow, A.Y., Pardue, M.T., Chow, V.Y., Peyman, G.A., Liang, C., Perlman, J.I. and Peachey, N.S. (2001). Implantation of silicon chip microphotodiode arrays into the cat subretinal space. *IEEE Trans Neural Syst Rehabil Eng*, **9**(**1**), 86–95.

Cooney, W.P. (1997). Electrical stimulation and the treatment of complex regional pain syndromes of the upper extremity. *Hand Clin*, **13**(**3**), 519–526.

Craggs, M. and McFarlane, J. (1999). Neuromodulation of the lower urinary tract. *Exp Physiol*, **84**(**1**), 149–160.

Creath, R., Kiemel, T., Horak, F. and Jeka, J.J. (2002). Limited control strategies with the loss of vestibular function. *Exp Brain Res*, **145**(**3**), 323–333.

Cyster, L.A., Grant, D.M., Parker, K.G. and Parker, T.L. (2002). The effect of surface chemistry and structure of titanium nitride (TiN) films on primary hippocampal cells. *Biomol Eng*, **19**(**2–6**), 171–175.

Cyster, L.A., Parker, K.G., Parker, T.L. and Grant, D.M. (2004). The effect of surface chemistry and nanotopography of titanium nitride (TiN) films on primary hippocampal neurones. *Biomaterials*, **25**(**1**), 97–107.

Delitto, A. and Snyder-Mackler, L. (1990). Two theories of muscle strength augmentation using percutaneous electrical stimulation. *Phys Ther*, **70**(**3**), 158–164.

Delitto, A., Strube, M.J., Shulman, A.D. and Minor, S.D. (1992). A study of discomfort with electrical stimulation. *Phys Ther*, **72**(**6**), 410–421.

Donoghue, J.P., Sanes, J.N., Hatsopoulos, N.G. and Gaal, G. (1998). Neural discharge and local field potential oscilla-tions in primate motor cortex during voluntary move-ments. *J Neurophysiol*, **79**(**1**), 159–173.

Dupont, A.-C., Bagg, S.D., Creasy, J.L., Romano, C., Romano, D., Loeb, G.E. and Richmond, F.J.R. (2001). Clinical trials of BION™ injectable neuromuscular stimulators. *Proc IFESS*, **6**, 7–9.

Dupont, A.-C., Bagg, S.D., Creasy, J.L., Romano, C., Romano, D., Richmond, F.J.R. and Loeb, G.E. (2004). First patients with BION® implants for therapeutic electrical stimulation. *Neuromodulation*, **7**, 38–47.

Dupont Salter, A.-C., Richmond, F.J. and Loeb, G.E. (2003). Prevention of muscle disuse atrophy by low-frequency electrical stimulation in rats. *IEEE Trans Neural Syst Rehabil Eng*, **11**(**3**), 218–226.

Durand, D.L. and Williams, H.B. (1990). The prevention of mus-cle atrophy after peripheral motor nerve repair with an implantable electrical system. *Surg Forum*, **XLI**, 661–664.

Felicetti, G., Maini, M. and Rovescala, R. (1998). Disuse muscle atrophy in knee pathologies. In: *Advances Occupational Medicine and Rehabilitation* (eds Capodaglio, P. and Narici, M.V.), Vol. 4, Le Collane della Fondazione Salvatore Maugeri, Pavia, pp. 103–108.

Ferber, R., Osternig, L.R., Woollacott, M.H., Wasielewski, N.J. and Lee, J.H. (2002). Reactive balance adjustments to unex-pected perturbations during human walking. *Gait Posture*, **16**(**3**), 238–248.

Flanagan, J. (1995). Research in speech communication. *Proc Natl Acad Sci USA*, **92**(**22**), 9938–9945.

Freeman, T.B., Campbell, J.N. and Long, D.M. (1983). Naloxone does not affect pain relief induced by electrical stimulation in man. *Pain*, **17**(**2**), 189–195.

Galvin, K.L., Mavrias, G., Moore, A., Cowan, R.S., Blamey, P.J. and Clark, G.M. (1999). A comparison of Tactaid II−+ and Tactaid 7 use by adults with a profound hearing impair-ment. *Ear Hear*, **20**(**6**), 471–482.

Gholmieh, G., Soussou, W., Courellis, S., Marmarelis, V., Berger, T. and Baudry, M. (2001). A biosensor for detecting changes in cognitive processing based on nonlinear systems analysis. *Biosens Bioelectron*, **16**(**7–8**), 491–501.

Girvin, J.P. (1988). Current status of artificial vision by electro-cortical stimulation. *Neuroscience*, **15**, 58–62.

Grill, W.M. and Mortimer, J.T. (1994). Electrical properties of implant encapsulation tissue. *Ann Biomed Eng*, **22**(**1**), 23–33.

Grill, W.M. and Mortimer, J.T. (2000). Neural and connective tis-sue response to long-term implantation of multiple contact nerve cuff electrodes. *J Biomed Mater Res*, **50**(**2**), 215–226.

Grill, W.M., Bhadra, N. and Wang, B. (1999). Bladder and ure-thral pressures evoked by microstimulation of the sacral spinal cord in cats. *Brain Res*, **836**(**1–2**), 19–30.

Grill, W.M., Craggs, M.D., Foreman, R.D., Ludlow, C.L. and Buller, J.L. (2001). Emerging clinical applications of electrical stimulation: opportunities for restoration of function. *J Rehabil Res Dev*, **38**(**6**), 641–653.

Gustafson, K.J. and Grill, W.M. (2001). *Bladder Contractions Evoked by Electrical Stimulation of Pudendal Afferents in the Cat*, **6**, 16–18.

Gustafson, K.J., Creasey, G.H. and Grill, W.M. (2003). A catheter based method to activate urethral sensory nerve fibers. *J Urol*, **170**(**1**), 126–129.

Hamel, W., Fietzek, U., Morsnowski, A., Schrader, B., Herzog, J., Weinert, D., Pfister, G., Muller, D., Volkmann, J., Deuschl, G. and Mehdorn, H.M. (2003). Deep brain stimulation of the subthalamic nucleus in Parkinson's disease: evaluation of active electrode contacts. *J Neurol Neurosurg Psychiatr*, **74**(**8**), 1036–1046.

Hammel, J.M., Van der Loos, H.F. and Perkash, I. (1992). Evaluation of a vocational robot with a quadriplegic employee. *Arch Phys Med Rehabil*, **73**(**7**), 683–693.

Hariz, M.I. (2003). From functional neurosurgery to "interventional" neurology: survey of publications on thalamotomy, pallidotomy, and deep brain stimulation for Parkinson's disease from 1966 to 2001. *Mov Disord*, **18**(**8**), 845–853.

Helms Tillery, S.I., Taylor, D.M. and Schwartz, A.B. (2003). Training in cortical control of neuroprosthetic devices improves signal extraction from small neuronal ensembles. *Rev Neurosci*, **14**(**1–2**), 107–119.

Hershey, T., Black, K.J., Carl, J.L., McGee-Minnich, L., Snyder, A.Z. and Perlmutter, J.S. (2003). Long term treatment and disease severity change brain responses to levodopa in Parkinson's disease. *J Neurol Neurosurg Psychiatr*, **74**(**7**), 844–851.

Herzog, A.R., Fultz, N.H., Brock, B.M., Brown, M.B. and Diokno, A.C. (1988). Urinary incontinence and psychological distress among older adults. *Psychol Aging*, **3**(**2**), 115–121.

Hislop, D.W., Zuber, B.L. and Trimble, J.L. (1983). Characteristics of reading rate and manual scanning patterns of blind Optacon readers. *Hum Factors*, **25**(**4**), 379–389.

Hoffer, J.A., Stein, R.B., Haugland, M.K., Sinkjaer, T., Durfee, W.K., Schwartz, A.B., Loeb, G.E. and Kantor, C. (1996). Neural signals for command control and feedback in functional neuromuscular stimulation: a review. *J Rehabil Res Dev*, **33**(**2**), 145–157.

Hughes, M.L., Vander Werff, K.R., Brown, C.J., Abbas, P.J., Kelsay, D.M.R., Teagle, H.F.B. and Lowder, M.W. (2001). A longitudinal study of electrode impedance, the electrically evoked compound action potential, and behavioral measures in nucleus 24 cochlear implant users. *Ear Hear*, **22**(**6**), 471–486.

Humayun, M.S., Weiland, J.D., Fujii, G.Y., Greenberg, R., Williamson, R., Little, J., Mech, B., Cimmarusti, V., Van Boemel, G., Dagnelie, G. and de Juan, E. (2003). Visual perception in a blind subject with a chronic microelectronic retinal prosthesis. *Vision Res*, **43**(**24**), 2573–2581.

Iatrou, M., Berger, T.W. and Marmarelis, V.Z. (1999). Application of a novel modeling method to the nonstationary properties of potentiation in the rabbit hippocampus. *Ann Biomed Eng*, **27**(**5**), 581–591.

Ikai, T., Tei, K., Yoshida, K., Miyano, S. and Yonemoto, K. (1998). Evaluation and treatment of shoulder subluxation in hemiplegia: relationship between subluxation and pain. *Am J Phys Med Rehabil*, **77**(**5**), 421–426.

Jeka, J.J., Ribeiro, P., Oie, K. and Lackner, J.R. (1998). The structure of somatosensory information for human postural control. *Motor Control*, **2**(**1**), 13–33.

Kaczmarek, K.A., Webster, J.G., Rita, P. and Tompkins, W.J. (1991). Electrotactile and vibrotactile displays for sensory substitution systems. *IEEE Trans Biomed Eng*, **38**(**1**), 1–16.

Katevas, N.I., Sgouros, N.M., Tzafestas, S.G., Papakonstantinou, G., Beattie, P., Bishop, J.M., Tsanakas, P. and Koutsouris, D. (1997). The autonomous mobile robot SENARIO: a sensor aided intelligent navigation system for powered wheelchairs. *Robot Automat Mag, IEEE*, **4**, 60–70.

Kennedy, P.R. (1989). The cone electrode: a long-term electrode that records from neurites grown onto its recording surface. *J Neurosci Methods*, **29**(**3**), 181–193.

Kennedy, P.R., Mirra, S.S. and Bakay, R.A. (1992). The cone electrode: ultrastructural studies following long-term recording in rat and monkey cortex. *Neurosci Lett*, **142**(**1**), 89–94.

Kern, H., Hofer, C., Modlin, M., Forstner, C., Raschka-Hogler, D., Mayr, W. and Stohr, H. (2002). Denervated muscles in humans: limitations and problems of currently used functional electrical stimulation training protocols. *Artif Organs*, **26**(**3**), 216–218.

Kiemel, T., Oie, K.S. and Jeka, J.J. (2002). Multisensory fusion and the stochastic structure of postural sway. *Biol Cybern*, **87**(**4**), 262–277.

Kileny, P.R., Zwolan, T.A. and Ashbaugh, C. (2001). The influence of age at implantation on performance with a cochlear implant in children. *Otol Neurotol*, **22**(**1**), 42–46.

Kimberley, T.J., Lewis, S.M., Auerbach, E.J., Dorsey, L.L., Lojovich, J.M. and Carey, J.R. (2003). Electrical stimulation driving functional improvements and cortical changes in subjects with stroke. *Exp Brain Res*, **154**(**4**), 450–460.

Kruger, L.R., van der Linden, W.J. and Cleaton-Jones, P.E. (1998). Transcutaneous electrical nerve stimulation in the treatment of myofascial pain dysfunction. *S Afr J Surg*, **36**(**1**), 35–38.

Lampl, C., Kreczi, T. and Klingler, D. (1998). Transcutaneous electrical nerve stimulation in the treatment of chronic pain: predictive factors and evaluation of the method. *Clin J Pain*, **14**(2), 134–142.

Lauer, R.T., Peckham, P.H. and Kilgore, K.L. (1999). EEG-based control of a hand grasp neuroprosthesis. *NeuroReport*, **10**(8), 1767–1771.

Liaw, J.S. and Berger, T.W. (1996). Dynamic synapse: a new concept of neural representation and computation. *Hippocampus*, **6**(6), 591–600.

Liberman, M. (1995). Computer speech synthesis: its status and prospects. *Proc Natl Acad Sci USA*, **92**(22), 9928–9931.

Lin, S.I. and Woollacott, M.H. (2002). Postural muscle responses following changing balance threats in young, stable older, and unstable older adults. *J Mot Behav*, **34**(1), 37–44.

Lindstrom, S., Fall, M., Carlsson, C.A. and Erlandson, B.E. (1983). The neurophysiological basis of bladder inhibition in response to intravaginal electrical stimulation. *J Urol*, **129**(2), 405–410.

Loeb, G.E. (1985). The functional replacement of the ear. *Sci Am*, **252**(2), 104–111.

Loeb, G.E. (1989). Neural prosthetic strategies for young patients. In: *Cochlear Implants in Young Children* (eds Owens, E. and Kessler, D.), College-Hill Press, San Diego, pp. 137–152.

Loeb, G.E., McHardy, J. and Kelliher, E.M. (1982). Neural prosthesis. In: *Biocompatibility in Clinical Practice, Vol. II* (ed. Williams, D.F.), CRC Press, Inc., Boca Raton, 123–149.

Loeb, G.E., Zamin, C.J., Schulman, J.H. and Troyk, P.R. (1991). Injectable microstimulator for functional electrical stimulation. *Med Biol Eng Comput*, **29**(6), NS13–NS19.

Marks, L.E. (1983). Similarities and differences among the senses. *Int J Neurosci*, **19**(1–4), 1–11.

Marks, W.B. and Loeb, G.E. (1976). Action currents, internodal potentials, and extracellular records of myelinated mammalian nerve fibers derived from node potentials. *Biophys J*, **16**(6), 655–668.

Maynard, E.M., Hatsopoulos, N.G., Ojakangas, C.L., Acuna, B.D., Sanes, J.N., Normann, R.A. and Donoghue, J.P. (1999). Neuronal interactions improve cortical population coding of movement direction. *J Neurosci*, **19**(18), 8083–8093.

Mazzone, P. (2003). Deep brain stimulation in Parkinson's disease: bilateral implantation of globus pallidus and subthalamic nucleus. *J Neurosurg Sci*, **47**(1), 47–51.

McFarland, D.J., McCane, L.M. and Wolpaw, J.R. (1998). EEG-based communication and control: short-term role of feedback. *IEEE Trans Rehab Eng*, **6**(1), 7–11.

Melzack, R. and Wall, P.D. (1965). Pain mechanisms: a new theory. *Science*, **150**(699), 971–979.

Mergner, T., Maurer, C. and Peterka, R.J. (2003). A multisensory posture control model of human upright stance. *Prog Brain Res*, **142**, 189–201.

Miller, A.L., Arenberg, J.G., Middlebrooks, J.C. and Pfingst, B.E. (2001). Cochlear implant thresholds: comparison of middle latency responses with psychophysical and cortical-spike-activity thresholds. *Hear Res*, **152**, 55–66.

Moran, D.W. and Schwartz, A.B. (1999). Motor cortical representation of speed and direction during reaching. *J Neurophysiol*, **82**(5), 2676–2692.

Nakamura, M. and Sakurai, T. (1984). Bladder inhibition by penile electrical stimulation. *Br J Urol*, **56**(4), 413–415.

North, R.B. and Wetzel, F.T. (2002). Spinal cord stimulation for chronic pain of spinal origin: a valuable long-term solution. *Spine*, **27**(22), 2584–2591.

North, R.B., Ewend, M.G., Lawton, M.T. and Piantadosi, S. (1991). Spinal cord stimulation for chronic, intractable pain: superiority of "multi-channel" devices. *Pain*, **44**, 119–130.

Nutt, J.G. (2003). Long-term L-DOPA therapy: challenges to our understanding and for the care of people with Parkinson's disease. *Exp Neurol*, **184**(1), 9–13.

Oie, K.S., Kiemel, T. and Jeka, J.J. (2002). Multisensory fusion: simultaneous re-weighting of vision and touch for the control of human posture. *Brain Res Cogn Brain Res*, **14**(1), 164–176.

Olanow, C.W. (2002). Surgical therapy for Parkinson's disease. *Eur J Neurol*, **9**(**Suppl. 3**), 31–39.

Oliver, J., Bradley, W. and Fletcher, T. (1969). Spinal cord representation of the micturition reflex. *J Comp Neurol*, **137**, 329–346.

Pandyan, A.D., Granat, M.H. and Stott, D.J. (1997). Effects of electrical stimulation on flexion contractures in the hemiplegic wrist. *Clin Rehabil*, **11**(2), 123–130.

Pandyan, A.D., Cameron, M., Powell, J., Stott, D.J. and Granat, M.H. (2003). Contractures in the post-stroke wrist: a pilot study of its time course of development and its association with upper limb recovery. *Clin Rehabil*, **17**(1), 88–95.

Paninski, L., Fellows, M.R., Hatsopoulos, N.G. and Donoghue, J.P. (2004). Spatiotemporal tuning of motor cortical neurons for hand position and velocity. *J Neurophysiol*, **91**(1), 515–532.

Peckham, P.H., Mortimer, J.T. and Marsolais, E.B. (1976). Alteration in the force and fatigability of skeletal muscle in quadriplegic humans following exercise induced by chronic electrical stimulation. *Clin Orthop Relat Res*, **114**, 326–333.

Peterka, R.J. (2002). Sensorimotor integration in human postural control. *J Neurophysiol*, **88**(3), 1097–1118.

Peterka, R.J. and Loughlin, P.J. (2004). Dynamic regulation of sensorimotor integration in human postural control. *J Neurophysiol*, **91**(**1**), 410–423.

Rall, W. (1962). Electrophysiology of a dendritic neuron model. *Biophys J*, **2**, 145–167.

Reed, C.M., Rabinowitz, W.M., Durlach, N.I., Braida, L.D., Conway-Fithian, S. and Schultz, M.C. (1985). Research on the Tadoma method of speech communication. *J Acoust Soc Am*, **77**(**1**), 247–257.

Richmond, F.J.R., Dupont, A.-C., Tran, W.H., Stein, R.B., Romano, C. and Loeb, G.E. (2003). Tactical application of sensorimotor prosthetic technology. *Proceedings of the 25th Annual International Conference of the IEEE Engineering Medicine and Biological Society.*

Rousche, P.J. and Normann, R.A. (1998). Chronic recording capability of the Utah intracortical electrode array in cat sensory cortex. *J Neurosci Methods*, **82**(**1**), 1–15.

Schmidt, E.M., Bak, M.J., Hambrecht, F.T., Kufta, C.V., O'Rourke, D.K. and Vallabhanath, P. (1996). Feasibility of a visual prosthesis for the blind based on intracortical microstimulation of the visual cortex. *Brain*, **119**, 507–522.

Schmidt, S., Horch, K. and Normann, R. (1993). Biocompatibility of silicon-based electrode arrays implanted in feline cortical tissue. *J Biomed Mater Res*, **27**(**11**), 1393–1399.

Schwartz, A.B. and Moran, D.W. (1999). Motor cortical activity during drawing movements: population representation during lemniscate tracing. *J Neurophysiol*, **82**(**5**), 2705–2718.

Schwartz, A.B. and Moran, D.W. (2000). Arm trajectory and representation of movement processing in motor cortical activity. *Eur J Neurosci*, **12**(**6**), 1851–1856.

Schwartz, A.B., Taylor, D.M. and Tillery, S.I. (2001). Extraction algorithms for cortical control of arm prosthetics. *Curr Opin Neurobiol*, **11**(**6**), 701–707.

Shefchyk, S.J. and Buss, R.R. (1998). Urethral pudendal afferent-evoked bladder and sphincter reflexes in decerebrate and acute spinal cats. *Neurosci Lett*, **244**(**3**), 137–140.

Shimada, Y., Sato, K., Kagaya, H., Konishi, N., Miyamoto, S. and Matsunaga, T. (1996). Clinical use of percutaneous intramuscular electrodes for functional electrical stimulation. *Arch Phys Med Rehabil*, **77**(**10**), 1014–1018.

Shimono, K., Baudry, M., Ho, L., Taketani, M. and Lynch, G. (2002). Long-term recording of LTP in cultured hippocampal slices. *Neural Plast*, **9**(**4**), 249–254.

Slemenda, C., Brandt, K.D., Heilman, D.K., Mazzuca, S., Braunstein, E.M., Katz, B.P. and Wolinsky, F.D. (1997). Quadriceps weakness and osteoarthritis of the knee. *Ann Int Med*, **127**(**2**), 97–104.

Smith, B., Tang, Z., Johnson, M.W., Pourmehdi, S., Gazdik, M.M., Buckett, J.R. and Peckham, P.H. (1998). An externally powered, multichannel, implantable stimulator-telemeter for control of paralyzed muscle. *IEEE Trans Biomed Eng*, **45**(**4**), 463–475.

Stephan, C.L., Kepes, J.J., SantaCruz, K., Wilkinson, S.B., Fegley, B. and Osorio, I. (2001). Spectrum of clinical and histopathologic responses to intracranial electrodes: from multifocal aseptic meningitis to multifocal hypersensitivity-type meningovasculitis. *Epilepsia*, **42**(**7**), 895–901.

Stroh, W.K., Van Doren, C.L., Bryden, A.M., Peckham, P.H., Keith, M.W., Kilgore, K.L. and Grill, J.H. (1999). Satisfaction with and usage of a hand neuroprosthesis. *Arch Phys Med Rehabil*, **80**(**2**), 206–213.

Sutherland, H., Jarvis, J.C. and Salmons, S. (2003). Pattern dependence in the stimulation-induced type transformation of rabbit fast skeletal muscle. *Neuromodulation*, **6**, 176–189.

Svirsky, M.A. (2001). Auditory learning and adaptation after cochlear implantation: a preliminary study of discrimination and labeling of vowel sounds by cochlear implant users. *Acta Oto-Laryngol*, **121**(**2**), 262–265.

Takada, M., Matsumura, M., Kojima, J., Yamaji, Y., Inase, M., Tokuno, H., Nambu, A. and Imai, H. (2000). Protection against dopaminergic nigrostriatal cell death by excitatory input ablation. *Eur J Neurosci*, **12**(**5**), 1771–1780.

Tan, H.Z., Rabinowitz, W.M. and Durlach, N.I. (1989). Analysis of a synthetic Tadoma system as a multidimensional tactile display. *J Acoust Soc Am*, **86**(**3**), 981–988.

Tasker, R.R. (1998). Deep brain stimulation is preferable to thalamotomy for tremor suppression. *Surg Neurol*, **49**(**2**), 145–153.

Taylor, D.M., Tillery, S.I. and Schwartz, A.B. (2002). Direct cortical control of 3D neuroprosthetic devices. *Science*, **296**(**5574**), 1829–1832.

Thomas, C.K., Zaidner, E.Y., Calancie, B., Broton, J.G. and Bigland-Ritchie, B.R. (1997). Muscle weakness, paralysis, and atrophy after human cervical spinal cord injury. *Exp Neurol*, **148**(**2**), 414–423.

Tobey, E.A. and Geers, A. (2001). Harry Levitt legacies: studies of speech perception and intelligibility in children with cochlear implants. *J Acoust Soc Am*, **109**(**5**), 2354.

Van der Loos, H.F.M. (1995). VA/Stanford rehabilitation robotics research and development program: lessons learned in the application of robotics technology to the field of rehabilitation. *IEEE Trans Rehab Eng*, **3**(**1**), 46–55.

Vodovnik, L., Rebersek, S., Stefanovska, A., Zidar, J., Acimovic, R. and Gros, N. (1988). Electrical stimulation for control of paralysis and therapy of abnormal movements. *Scand J Rehabil Med Suppl*, **17**, 91–97.

Waldstein, R.S. and Boothroyd, A. (1995). Comparison of two multichannel tactile devices as supplements to speechreading in a postlingually deafened adult. *Ear Hear*, **16**(**2**), 198–208.

Wang, J.Q., Mao, L. and Han, J.S. (1992). Comparison of the antinociceptive effects induced by electroacupuncture and transcutaneous electrical nerve stimulation in the rat. *Int J Neurosci*, **65**(**1–4**), 117–129.

Williams, J.C., Rennaker, R.L. and Kipke, D.R. (1999). Long-term neural recording characteristics of wire microelectrode arrays implanted in cerebral cortex. *Brain Res Brain Res Protoc*, **4**(**3**), 303–313.

Wilson, B.S. (2000). Strategies for representing speech information with cochlear implants. In: *Cochlear Implants: Principles and Practices* (eds J.K. Niparko, et al.), Lipincott Williams and Wilkins, Philadelphia, PA, pp. 129–170.

Yarkony, G.M. (1994). Pressure ulcers: a review. *Arch Phys Med Rehabil*, **75**(**8**), 908–917.

Yu, D.T., Chae, J., Walker, M.E., Hart, R.L. and Petroski, G.F. (2001). Comparing stimulation-induced pain during percutaneous (intramuscular) and transcutaneous neuromuscular electric stimulation for treating shoulder subluxation in hemiplegia. *Arch Phys Med Rehabil*, **82**(**6**), 756–760.

Zorowitz, R.D. (2001). Recovery patterns of shoulder subluxation after stroke: a six-month follow-up study. *Top Stroke Rehabil*, **8**(**2**), 1–9.

Brain–computer interfaces for communication and control

Jonathan R. Wolpaw[1] and Niels Birbaumer[2]

[1]*Laboratory of Nervous System Disorders, Wadsworth Center, NYS Department of Health, Albany, NY, USA and*
[2]*Institute Behavioural Neuroscience, Eberhard-Karls-University, Tubingen, Germany*

33.1 Introduction

Early speculation

Electrical signals produced by brain activity were first recorded from the cortical surface in animals by Richard Caton in 1875 (Caton, 1875) and from the human scalp by Hans Berger in 1929 (Berger, 1929). In the 75 years since Berger's first report, electro-encephalographic (EEG) activity has been used mainly for clinical diagnosis and for exploring brain function. Nevertheless, throughout this period, scientists and others have speculated that the EEG or other measures of brain activity might serve an entirely different purpose, that they might provide the brain with another means of conveying messages and commands to the external world. While normal communication and control necessarily depend on peripheral nerves and muscles, brain signals such as the EEG suggested the possibility of non-muscular communication and control, achieved through a brain–computer interface (BCI).

Recent interest and activity

Despite long interest in this possibility, and despite isolated demonstrations (e.g., Vidal, 1973; 1977) it has only been in the past two decades that sustained research has begun, and only in the past 10 years that a recognizable field of BCI research, populated by a rapidly growing number of research groups, has developed (see Wolpaw et al. (2002) for review). This recent interest and activity reflect the confluence of four factors.

The first factor is the greatly increased appreciation of both the needs and the abilities of people severely affected by motor disorders such as cerebral palsy, spinal cord injury, brain stem stroke, amyotrophic lateral sclerosis (ALS), and muscular dystrophies. Modern life-support technology (e.g., home ventilators) now enables the most severely disabled people to survive for many years. Furthermore, it is now clear that even people who have little or no voluntary muscle control, who may be totally "locked-in" to their bodies, unable to communicate in any way, can lead lives that are enjoyable and productive if they can be provided with even the most minimal means of communication and control (Simmons et al., 2000; Maillot et al., 2001; Robbins et al., 2001).

The second factor is the greatly increased understanding of the nature and functional correlates of EEG and other measures of brain activity, understanding that has come from animal and human research. In tandem with this new knowledge have come better methods for recording these signals, both in the short and the long term. This new knowledge and technology are guiding and supporting increasingly sophisticated and effective BCI research and development.

The third factor is the availability of powerful low-cost computer hardware that allows complex real-time analyses of brain activity, which is essential for effective BCI operation. Much of the online signal processing used in present-day BCIs was impossible or prohibitively expensive until recently.

The fourth factor responsible for the recent surge in BCI research is new recognition of the remarkable adaptive capacities of the central nervous system (CNS), both in normal life and in response to damage or disease. This recognition has generated great excitement and interest in the possibility of engaging these adaptive capacities to establish new interactions between brain tissue and computer-based devices, interactions that can replace or augment the brain's normal neuromuscular interactions with the world.

33.2 What a BCI is, and what it is not

The definition of a BCI

A BCI is a communication and control system that does not depend in any way on the brain's normal neuromuscular output channels. The user's intent is conveyed by brain signals (such as EEG) rather than by peripheral nerves and muscles, and these brain signals do not depend for their generation on neuromuscular activity. (Thus, e.g., a device that uses visual evoked potentials to determine eye-gaze direction is not a true BCI, for it relies on neuromuscular control of eye position, and simply uses the EEG as a measure of that position.)

Furthermore, as a communication and control system, a BCI establishes a real-time interaction between the user and the outside world. The user receives feedback reflecting the outcome of the BC'Is operation, and that feedback can affect the user's subsequent intent and its expression in brain signals. For example, if a person uses a BCI to control the movements of a robotic arm, the arm's position after each movement is likely to affect the person's intent for the next movement and the brain signals that convey that intent. Thus, a system that simply records and analyzes brain signals, without providing the results of that analysis to the user in an online interactive fashion, is not a BCI. Figure 33.1 shows the basic design and operation of any BCI.

The fundamental principle of BCI operation

Much popular speculation and some scientific endeavors have been based on the fallacious assumption that BCIs are essentially "wire-tapping" or "mind-reading" technology, devices for listening in on the brain, detecting its intent, and then accomplishing that intent directly rather than through muscles. This misconception ignores the central feature of the brain's interactions with the external world: that the motor behaviors that achieve a person's intent, whether it be to walk in a certain direction, speak certain words, or play a certain piece on the piano, are acquired and maintained by initial and continuing *adaptive changes* in CNS function. During early development and throughout later life, CNS neurons and synapses continually change both to acquire new behaviors and to maintain those already acquired (Salmoni et al., 1984; Ghez and Krakauer, 2000). Such CNS plasticity underlies acquisition of standard skills such as locomotion and speech and more specialized skills as well, and it responds to and is guided by the results achieved. For example, as muscle strengths, limb lengths, and body weight change with growth and aging, the CNS adjusts its outputs so as to maintain the desired results.

This dependence on initial and continuing CNS adaptation is present whether the person's intent is accomplished in the normal fashion, that is, through peripheral nerves and muscles, or through an artificial interface, a BCI, that uses brain signals rather than nerves and muscles. BCI use depends on the interaction of two adaptive controllers: the user, who must generate brain signals that encode intent; and the BCI system, that must translate these signals into commands that accomplish the user's intent. Thus, BCI use is a skill that both user and system must acquire and maintain. The user must encode intent in signal features that the BCI system can measure; and the BCI system must measure these features and translate them into device commands. This dependence, both initially and continually, on the adaptation of user to system and system to user is the fundamental principle of BCI

BCI system

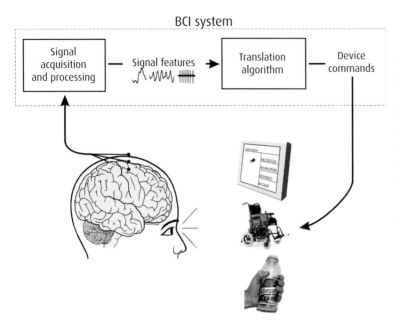

Figure 33.1. Design and operation of a BCI system (modified from Wolpaw et al., 2002; head image from www.BrainConnection. com). Electrophysiological signals reflecting brain activity are acquired from the scalp, from the cortical surface, or from within the brain and are processed to measure specific signal features (such as amplitudes of evoked potentials or EEG rhythms or firing rates of single neurons) that reflect the user's intent. These features are translated into commands that operate a device, such as a word-processing program, a wheelchair, or a neuroprosthesis.

operation; and its effective management is the principal challenge of BCI research and development.

33.3 Brain signals that can or might be used in a BCI

In theory, brain signals recorded by a variety of methodologies might be used in a BCI. These methodologies include: recording of electrical or magnetic fields; functional magnetic resonance imaging (fMRI); positron emission tomography (PET); and infrared (IR) imaging. In reality, however, most of these methods are at present not practical for clinical use due to their intricate technical demands, prohibitive expense, limited real-time capabilities, and/or early stage of development. Only electrical field recording is likely to be of significant practical value for clinical applications in the near future.

Alternative recording methods for electrical signals

The electrical fields produced by brain activity can be recorded from the scalp (EEG), from the cortical

surface (electrocorticographic activity (EcoG)), or from within the brain (local field potentials (LFPs)) or neuronal action potentials (spikes). These three alternatives are shown in Fig. 33.2. Each recording method has advantages and disadvantages. EEG recording is easy and non-invasive, but EEG has limited topographical resolution and frequency range and may be contaminated by artifacts such as electromyographic (EMG) activity from cranial muscles or electrooculographic (EOG) activity. ECoG has better topographical resolution and frequency range, but requires implantation of electrode arrays on the cortical surface, which has as yet been done only for short periods (e.g., a few days or weeks) in humans. Intracortical recording (or recording within other brain structures) provides the highest resolution signals, but requires insertion of multiple electrode arrays within brain tissue and faces as yet unresolved problems in minimizing tissue damage and scarring and ensuring long-term recording stability.

The ultimate practical value of each of these recording methods will depend on the range of communication and control applications it can support and the extent to which its limitations can be overcome.

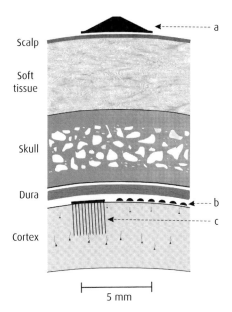

Scalp

Soft tissue

Skull

Dura

Cortex

5 mm

Figure 33.2. Recording sites for electrophysiological signals used by BCI systems. (a) EEG is recorded by electrodes on the scalp. (b) ECoG is recorded by electrodes on the cortical surface. (c) Action potentials from single neurons or LFPs are recorded by electrode arrays inserted into the cortex or other brain areas.

The issue of the relative value of non-invasive (i.e., EEG) methods, moderately invasive (e.g., ECoG) methods, and maximally invasive (e.g., intracortical) methods remains unresolved. On the one hand, stable, practical, and safe techniques for long-term recording within the brain may not prove that difficult to develop. On the other hand, despite expectations to the contrary (e.g., Donoghue, 2002), for actual practical applications, the information transfer rates possible with intracortical methods may turn out to be no greater than those achievable with less invasive methods (e.g., ECoG). Thorough evaluations of the characteristics and capacities of each recording method are needed.

33.4 Present-day BCIs

Human BCI experience to date has been confined almost entirely to EEG studies and short-term ECoG

studies. Intracortical BCI data come mainly from animals, primarily monkeys. The available human data indicate that EEG-based methods can certainly support simple applications and may be able to support more complex ones. Invasive methods appear able to support complex applications, but the issues of risk and long-term recording stability are not yet resolved.

EEG-based BCIs

Three different kinds of EEG-based BCIs have been tested in humans. They differ in the particular EEG features that serve to convey the user's intent. Figure 33.3(a) illustrates a P300-based BCI (Farwell and Donchin, 1988; Donchin et al., 2000). It uses the P300 component of the event-related brain potential, which appears in the centroparietal EEG about 300 ms after presentation of a salient or attended stimulus. The P300 BCI system described by Donchin's group flashes letters or other symbols in rapid succession. The letter or symbol that the user wants to select produces a P300 potential. By detecting this P300 potential, the BCI system can determine the user's choice. This BCI method appears able to support operation of a simple word-processing program that enables users to write words at a rate of one or a few letters per minute. Improvements in signal analysis may substantially increase its capacities. At the same time, the effects of long-term usage of a P300-based BCI on its communication performance remain to be determined: P300 size and reliability may improve with continued use so that performance improves, or P300 may habituate so that performance deteriorates.

Figure 33.3(b) illustrates a BCI based on slow cortical potentials (SCPs), which last from 300 ms to several seconds (Birbaumer et al., 1999; 2000; Kübler et al., 2001). In normal brain function, negative SCPs reflect preparatory depolarization of the underlying cortical network, while positive SCPs are usually interpreted as a sign of cortical disfacilitation or inhibition. Birbaumer and his colleagues have shown that, with appropriate training, people can learn to control SCPs so as to produce positive

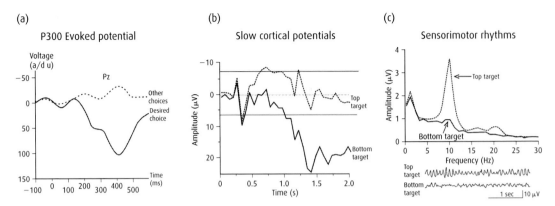

Figure 33.3. Non-invasive EEG-based BCI methods demonstrated in humans (modified from Kübler et al., 2001). These methods use EEG recorded from the scalp. (a) P300 evoked potential BCI (Farwell and Donchin, 1988; Donchin et al., 2000). A matrix of possible selections is shown on a screen. Scalp EEG is recorded over centroparietal cortex while these selections flash in succession. Only the selection desired by the user evokes a large P300 potential (i.e., a positive potential about 300ms after the flash). (b) Slow cortical potential BCI (Birbaumer et al., 1999; 2000; Kübler et al., 2001). Users learn to control SCPs to move a cursor to a target (e.g., a desired letter or icon) at the bottom (more positive SCP) or top (more negative SCP) of a computer screen. (c) Sensorimotor rhythm BCI (Wolpaw and McFarland, 1994; 2003; Wolpaw et al., 2002; 2003). Scalp EEG is recorded over sensorimotor cortex. Users control the amplitude of a 8–12Hz mu rhythm (or a 18–26 Hz beta rhythm) to move a cursor to a target at the top of the screen or to a target at the bottom (or to additional targets at intermediate locations). Frequency spectra (top) for top and bottom targets indicate that this user's control is clearly focused in the mu-rhythm frequency band. Sample EEG traces (bottom) also show that the mu rhythm is prominent with the top target and minimal with the bottom target. Trained users can also control movement in two dimensions.

or negative shifts. Furthermore, they can use this control to perform basic word-processing and other simple control tasks such as accessing the Internet. Most important, people who are severely disabled by ALS, and are otherwise unable to communicate, are capable of achieving SCP control and using it for effective communication.

Figure 33.3(c) illustrates a BCI based on sensori-motor rhythms (Wolpaw et al., 1991; 2003; Wolpaw and McFarland, 1994; 2003; Kostov and Polak, 2000; Roberts and Penny, 2000; Pfurtscheller et al., 2003a). Sensorimotor rhythms are 8–12 Hz (mu) and 18–26 Hz (beta) oscillations in the EEG recorded over sensori-motor cortices. In normal brain function, changes in mu and/or beta rhythm amplitudes are associ-ated with movement and sensation, and with motor imagery as well. Several laboratories have shown that people can learn to control mu or beta rhythm ampli-tudes in the absence of movement or sensation and

can use this control to move a cursor to select letters or icons on a screen or to operate a simple orthotic device. Both one- and two-dimensional control are possible. Like the P300- and SCP-based BCIs, sensorimotor rhythm-based BCIs can support basic word-processing or other simple functions. They may also support multi-dimensional control of a neuroprosthesis or other device such as a robotic arm.

These present-day BCI methods all rely on selec-tion protocols that begin at fixed times set by the sys-tem. However, in real-life applications, BCIs in which the onset and timing of operation are determined by the user may be preferable. Efforts to develop such user-initiated methods, based on detection of certain features in the ongoing EEG, have begun (Mason and Birch, 2000). Present-day BCIs also depend on visual stimuli. People who are severely disabled (e.g., locked-in) may not be able to follow such stimuli, especially if they change rapidly. In this case, BCI systems (e.g., P300-based) that use auditory rather than visual stimuli may prove effective.

ECoG-based BCIs

Figure 33.4(a) illustrates a BCI based on sensorimotor rhythms in ECoG recorded by electrode arrays placed on the cortical surface. ECoG has much higher spatial and temporal resolution than scalp-recorded EEG. It can resolve activity limited to a few mm^2 of cortical surface, and it includes not only mu and beta rhythms, but higher-frequency gamma (>30 Hz) rhythms, which are very small or absent in EEG. ECoG studies to date have been limited to short-term experiments in individuals temporarily implanted with electrode arrays prior to epilepsy surgery. They reveal sharply focused ECoG activity associated with movement and sensation and with motor imagery (Pfurtscheller et al., 2003b; Leuthardt et al., 2004). Furthermore, with only a few minutes of training, people can learn to use such imagery to control cursor movement (Fig. 33.4(a)) (Leuthardt et al., 2004).

The rapidity of this learning, which occurs much faster than that typically found with scalp-recorded sensorimotor rhythms, combined with the high topographical resolution and wide spectral range of ECoG and its freedom from artifacts such as EMG, suggests that ECoG-based BCIs might support communication and control superior to that possible with EEG-based BCIs. Their clinical use will depend on development of fully implanted systems (i.e., systems that do not require wires passing through the skin) and on strong evidence that they can provide safe and stable recording over periods of years.

Intracortical BCIs

Figure 33.4(b) shows data from a BCI based on the firing rates of a set of single cortical neurons recorded by a fine-wire array chronically implanted in monkey motor cortex. Intracortical BCIs studied to date have used such neuronal activity (Kennedy and Bakay, 1998; Chapin et al., 1999; Kennedy et al., 2000; Taylor et al., 2002; 2003; Serruya et al., 2002; Carmena et al., 2003; Musallam et al., 2004) and have shown that it can support rapid and accurate control of cursor movements in one, two, or even three dimensions. Related data suggest that LFPs, which can be recorded by the same electrode arrays and reflect nearby synaptic and neuronal activity, might also support BCI operation (Pesaran et al., 2002). The basic strategy in the single-neuron studies has been to define the neuronal activity associated with standardized limb movements, then to use this activity to simultaneously control comparable movements of a cursor, and finally to show that the neuronal activity can continue to control cursor movements in the absence of actual limb movements. In the most thorough and successful study to date (Taylor et al., 2002), in which neuronal control of three-dimensional cursor movement was observed over many sessions, neuronal activity was found to adapt over sessions so as to improve cursor control. Figure 33.4(b) illustrates this adaptation. Like the comparable adaptations seen with EEG- and ECoG-based BCIs, it reflects the fundamental BCI principle described above: dependence on initial and continuing adaptation of system to user and user to system.

The major issues that must be resolved prior to clinical use of intracortical BCIs include their long-term safety, the stability of their signals in the face of cortical tissue reactions to the implanted electrodes, and whether their capabilities in actual practical applications (e.g., in neuroprosthesis control) substantially exceed those of less invasive BCIs.

33.5 Signal processing

A BCI records brain signals and processes them to produce device commands. This signal processing has two stages. The first stage is feature extraction, the calculation of the values of specific features of the signals. These features may be relatively simple measures such as amplitudes or latencies of specific potentials (e.g., P300), amplitudes, or frequencies of specific rhythms (e.g., sensorimotor rhythms), or

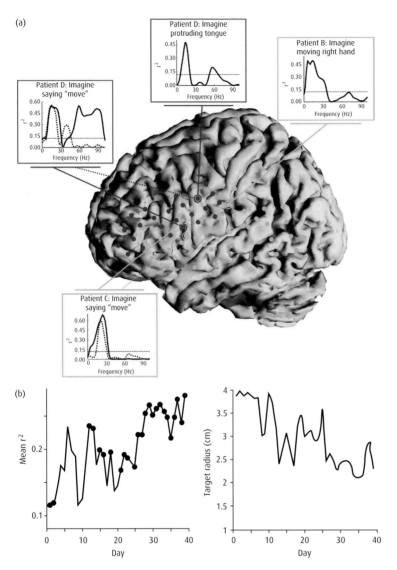

Figure 33.4. Invasive BCI methods. (a) Electrode arrays on the cortical surface. Human ECoG control of vertical cursor movement using specific motor imagery to move the cursor up and rest (i.e., no imagery) to move it down (from Leuthardt et al., 2004). The electrodes used for online control are circled and the spectral correlations of their ECoG activity with target location (i.e., top or bottom of screen) are shown. Electrode arrays for Patients B, C, and D are green, blue, and red, respectively. The particular imagined actions used are indicated. The substantial levels of control achieved with different types of imagery are evident. (The dashed lines indicate significance at the 0.01 level). For Patients C and D, the solid and dotted r^2 spectra correspond to the sites indicated by the dotted and solid line locators, respectively. (b) Control of three-dimensional cursor movements by single neurons in motor cortex of a monkey (from Taylor et al., 2003). The left graph shows the improvement over training sessions of the average correlation between the firing rate of an individual cortical neuron and target direction. The right graph shows the resulting improvement in performance (measured as the mean target radius needed to maintain a 70% target hit rate). As the firing rates of the neurons that are controlling cursor movement become more closely correlated with target direction, the size of the target can be steadily reduced.

firing rates of individual cortical neurons, or they may be more complex measures such as spectral coherences. To support effective BCI performance, the feature-extraction stage of signal processing must focus on features that encode the user's intent, and it must extract those features as accurately as possible.

The second stage is a translation algorithm that translates these features into device commands. Features such as rhythm amplitudes or neuronal firing rates are translated into commands that specify outputs such as cursor movements, icon selection, or prosthesis operation. Translation algorithms may be simple (e.g., linear equations), or more complex (e.g., neural networks, support vector machines) (Müller et al., 2003).

To be effective, a translation algorithm must ensure that the user's range of control of the chosen features allows selection of the full range of device commands. For example, suppose that the feature is the amplitude of a 8–12 Hz mu rhythm in the EEG over sensorimotor cortex; that the user can vary this feature over a range of 2–10 μV; and that the application is vertical cursor movement. In this case, the translation algorithm must ensure that the 2–10 μV range allows the user to move the cursor both up and down. Furthermore, the algorithm must accommodate spontaneous variations in the user's range of control (e.g., if diurnal change, fatigue, or another factor changes the available voltage range) (e.g., Ramoser et al., 1997). Finally the translation algorithm should have the capacity to at least accommodate, and at best encourage, improvements in the user's control. For example, if the user's range of control improves from 2–10 to 1–15 μV, the translation algorithm should take advantage of this improvement to increase the speed and/or precision of cursor movement control.

This need for continual adaptation of the translation algorithm to accommodate spontaneous and other changes in the signal features is in accord with the fundamental principle of BCI operation (i.e., the continuing dependence on system/user and user/system adaptation), and has important implications. First, it means that new algorithms cannot be adequately evaluated simply by offline analyses. They must also be tested online, so that the effects of their adaptive interactions with the user can be assessed. This testing should be long term as well as short term, for important adaptive interactions may develop gradually. Second, the need for continual adaptation means that simpler algorithms, for which adaptation is usually easier and more effective, have an inherent advantage. Simple algorithms (e.g., linear equations) should be abandoned for complex alternatives (e.g., neural networks) only when online as well as offline evaluations clearly show that the complex alternatives provide superior performance.

33.6 Potential users

In their present early state of development, BCIs are likely to be of practical value mainly for those with the most severe neuromuscular disabilities, people for whom conventional assistive communication technologies, all of which require some measure of voluntary muscle control, are not viable options. These include people with ALS who elect to accept artificial ventilation (rather than to die) as their disease progresses, children and adults with severe cerebral palsy who lack any useful muscle control, patients with brain stem strokes who are left only with minimal eye movement control, those with severe muscular dystrophies or chronic peripheral neuropathies, and possibly people with short-term disorders associated with extensive paralysis (such as Landry-Guillain-Barré syndrome). It is also possible that people with less severe disabilities, such as those with high-cervical spinal cord injuries, may find BCI technology preferable to conventional assistive communication methods that co-opt remaining voluntary muscle control (e.g., methods that depend on gaze direction or EMG of facial muscles). BCIs might eventually also prove useful for those with less severe motor disabilities. The eventual extent and impact of BCI applications will depend on the speed and precision of the control that can be achieved and on the reliability and convenience of their use.

People with disabilities of different origins are likely to differ in the BCI methods that are of most use to them. For some, the CNS deficits responsible for their disability may affect their ability to control particular brain signals and not others. For example, the motor cortex damage that can be associated with ALS or the subcortical damage of severe cerebral palsy may compromise generation or control of sensorimotor rhythms or neuronal activity. In such individuals, other brain signals, such as P300 potentials or neuronal activity from other brain regions, might provide viable alternatives.

Prosaic and even ostensibly trivial factors are also likely to play significant roles in the eventual practical success of BCI applications. Issues such as the steps involved in donning and doffing electrodes or in accessing a BCI application, or a person's appearance while using it, may greatly affect the number of people interested in the system and the extent to which they actually use it.

33.7 Applications

The range of possible applications

BCIs have a wide range of possible practical applications, from extremely simple to very complex. Simple BCI applications have already been demonstrated in the laboratory and in limited clinical use. They include systems for answering Yes/No questions, managing basic environmental control (e.g., lights, temperature), controlling a television, or opening and closing a hand orthosis (Miner et al., 1998; Birbaumer et al., 1999; Pfurtscheller et al., 2003a). Such simple systems can be configured for basic word-processing or for accessing the Internet (e.g., Mellinger et al., 2003). For people who are totally paralyzed (i.e., "locked-in") and thus cannot use conventional assistive communication devices (see Volume II, Chapter 22), these simple BCI applications may make possible lives that are pleasant and even productive. Indeed, several recent studies indicate that severely paralyzed people, if they have good supportive care and the capacity for basic

communication, may enjoy a reasonable quality of life and are only slightly more likely to be depressed than people without physical disabilities (Simmons et al., 2000; Maillot et al., 2001; Robbins et al., 2001). Thus, simple BCI applications appear to have a secure future in their potential to make a difference in the lives of extremely disabled people.

More complex BCI applications might support control of devices such as a motorized wheelchair, a robotic arm, or a neuroprosthesis that enables the multi-dimensional movements of a paralyzed limb. While most present efforts are focused on development of invasive BCI systems to support such applications, non-invasive EEG-based BCIs also appear to offer the possibility of such control (Wolpaw and McFarland, 1994; 2003). The ultimate practical importance of such BCI applications will depend on their capacities and reliability, on their acceptance by specific user population groups, and on whether they provide clear advantages over conventional methodologies.

Process control versus goal selection

Two alternative approaches underlie BCI applications: process control and goal selection. In the process-control approach, the BCI directly controls every aspect of device operation. This approach underlies most current efforts to develop intracortical BCI systems. For neuroprosthesis operation, this approach vests in a specific set of cortical neurons (and/or other brain neurons) ongoing interactive control of all the muscles that move a limb so as to carry out the user's intent. Thus, the approach requires that the BCI supports complex high-speed interactions; and it requires that cortical neurons assume functions normally performed by lower-level (e.g., spinal cord) neurons.

In the alternative approach of goal selection, the BCI simply determines the user's intent, which is then executed by the system. This approach underlies most efforts to develop non-invasive or minimally invasive BCI methods. While it has been most often used for simple applications (e.g., Yes/No), this approach can apply also to the most complex applications, such as multidimensional control of a neuroprosthesis. For example, the user might communicate the command: "pick up the book." The complex control of the shoulder, arm, and hand muscles that execute that command would then be orchestrated by a device that stimulates muscles and simultaneously monitors the resulting movements so as to accomplish the task. This design, in which task execution is delegated to lower-level structures, is similar in principle to normal motor control, in which subcortical and spinal areas play crucial parts, particularly in managing high-speed real-time interactions between the CNS and the limb it is controlling.

The process-control approach clearly requires that the BCI have information transfer rates and capacities for high-speed real-time interaction substantially greater than those required by the goal-selection approach. Which approach can ultimately provide the most flexible, effective, and natural movement control remains to be determined.

Establishing the practical value of BCI applications

The establishment of BCI applications as clinically valuable methods will require comprehensive clinical testing that demonstrates their long-term reliability and shows that people actually use the applications and that this use has beneficial effects on factors such as mood, quality of life, productivity, etc. Especially in the initial stages of their development, this will often entail configuring applications that match the unique needs, desires, and physical and social environments of each user. While the cost of BCI equipment is relatively modest, current systems require substantial and continuing expert oversight, which is extremely expensive and currently limited to a few research laboratories. As a result, these systems are not readily available to most potential users. Thus, the widespread clinical use of BCI applications will also depend on the extent to which the need for such oversight can be reduced. BCI systems must be easy to set up and easy to maintain if they are to have substantial practical impact.

33.8 Nature and needs of BCI research and development

BCI research and development is an inherently multidisciplinary task. It involves neuroscience, engineering, applied mathematics, computer science, psychology, and rehabilitation. BCI research is not merely a signal-processing problem, a neurobiological problem, or a human-factors problem, though it has often been viewed in each of these limited ways in the past. The need to select appropriate brain signals, to record them accurately and reliably, to analyze them appropriately in real time, to control devices that provide functions of practical value to people with severe disabilities, to manage the complex short-term and long-term adaptive interactions between user and system, and to integrate BCI applications into the lives of their users, means that the expertise and efforts of all these disciplines are critical for success. This reality requires either that each BCI research group incorporate all relevant disciplines, or that groups with different expertises collaborate closely. Such interactions have been encouraged and facilitated by recent meetings drawing BCI researchers from all relevant disciplines and from all over the world (Wolpaw et al., 2000; Vaughan et al., 2003), and by comprehensive sets of peer-reviewed BCI articles (see Wolpaw et al., 2000; Vaughan et al., 2003; Nicolelis et al., 2004 for review).

Up to now, BCI research has consisted primarily of demonstrations, of limited studies showing that a specific brain signal processed in a specific way by specific hardware and software and applied to a specific device can supply communication or control of a specific kind. Successful development and widespread clinical use depend on moving beyond demonstrations. They require effective and efficient techniques for comparing, combining, and evaluating alternative brain signals, analysis methods, and applications, and thereby optimizing BCIs and the usefulness of their applications. This requirement has been the impetus for the original and ongoing development of BCI2000, the first general-purpose BCI system (Schalk et al., 2004). Founded on a design made up of four modules (signal acquisition, signal processing, device control, and system operation), BCI2000 can accommodate a wide variety of alternative signals, processing methods, applications, and operating protocols. Thus, it greatly facilitates the comprehensive quantitative comparative studies critical for continued progress. BCI2000, with source code and documentation, is freely available to research laboratories (at http://www. bci2000.org) and is already in use by many laboratories throughout the world.

Summary

The possibility that EEG activity or other electrophysiological measures of brain function might provide new non-muscular channels for communication and control (i.e., BCIs) has been a topic of speculation for many years. Over the past 15 years, numerous productive BCI research and development programs have been initiated. These endeavors focus on developing new augmentative communication and control technology for those with severe neuromuscular disorders, such as ALS, brain stem stroke, and spinal cord injury. The immediate objective is to give these users, who may be totally paralyzed, or "locked-in," basic communication capabilities so that they can express their desires to caregivers or even operate word-processing programs or neuroprostheses. Current BCIs determine the intent of the user from electrophysiological signals recorded non-invasively from the scalp (EEG) or invasively from the cortical surface (ECoG) or from within the brain (neuronal action potentials). These signals are translated in real-time into commands that operate a computer display or other device. Successful operation requires that the user encode commands in these signals and that the BCI derive the commands from the signals. Thus, the user and the BCI system need to adapt to each other both initially and continually so as to ensure stable performance. This dependence on the mutual adaptation of user to system and system to user is the fundamental principle of BCI operation.

BCI research and development is an inherently interdisciplinary problem, involving neurobiology, psychology, engineering, mathematics, computer science, and clinical rehabilitation. Its future progress and eventual practical impact depend on a number of critical issues. The relative advantages and disadvantages of non-invasive and invasive methods remain to be determined. On the one hand, the full capacities of non-invasive methods are not clear; on the other hand, the long-term safety and stability of invasive methods are uncertain. The optimal signal processing techniques also remain to be determined. On the one hand, simple algorithms facilitate the continuing adaptation that is essential for effective BCI operation; on the other hand, more complex algorithms might provide better communication and control. Appropriate user groups and applications, and appropriate matches of one to the other, remain to be determined. Present BCIs, which have relatively limited capacities, may be most useful for those with the most severe disabilities. At the same time, the CNS deficits associated with some disorders may impair ability to use certain BCI methods. Widespread clinical use depends also on factors that affect the user acceptance and the practicality of augmentative technology, including ease of use, cosmesis, provision of those communication and control capacities that are most important to the user, and minimization of the need for continuing expert oversight. With proper recognition and effective engagement of all these issues, BCI systems could eventually be important new communication and control options for people with motor disabilities and might also provide to people without disabilities as a supplementary control channel or a control channel useful in special circumstances.

ACKNOWLEDGEMENTS

Drs. Dennis J. McFarland and Elizabeth Winter Wolpaw provided valuable comments on the manuscript, and Mr. Scott Parsons provided excellent assistance with illustrations. Work in the authors' laboratories has been supported by NIH (Grants HD30146 and EB00856), the James S. McDonnell Foundation, the ALS Hope Foundation, and the DFG (Grant SFB 550/B5).

REFERENCES

Berger, H. (1929). Über das electrenkephalogramm des menchen. *Archiv für Psychiatrie Nervenkrankheiten*, **87**, 527–570.

Birbaumer, N., Ghanayim, N., Hinterberger, T., Iversen, I., Kotchoubey, B., Kübler, A., Perelmouter, J., Taub, E. and Flor, H. (1999). A spelling device for the paralyzed. *Nature*, **398**, 297–298.

Birbaumer, N., Kübler, A., Ghanayim, N., Hinterberger, T., Perelmouter, J., Kaiser, J., Iversen, I., Kotchoubey, B., Neumann, N. and Flor, H. (2000). The thought translation device (TTD) for completely paralyzed patients. *IEEE Trans Rehabil Eng*, **8**, 190–193.

Birbaumer, N., Kübler, A., Ghanayim, N., Hinterberger, T., Perelmouter, J., Kaiser, J., Iversen, I., Kotchoubey, B., Neumann, N. and Flor, H. (2003). The thought translation device (TTD) for completely paralyzed patients. *IEEE Trans Rehabil Eng*, **8**, 190–192.

Carmena, J.M., Lebedev, M.A., Crist, R.E., O'Doherty, J.E., Santucci, D.M., Dimitrov, D.F., Patil, P.G., Henriquez, C.S. and Nicolelis, M.A. (2003). Learning to control a brain-machine interface for reaching and grasping by primates. *PLOS Biol*, **1**(**3**), Online.

Caton, R. (1875). The electric currents of the brain. *Br Med J*, **2**, 278.

Chapin, J.K., Moxon, K.A., Markowitz, R.S. and Nicolelis, M.A. (1999). Real-time control of a robot arm using simultaneously recorded neurons in the motor cortex. *Nat Neurosci*, **2**, 664–670.

Donchin, E., Spencer, K.M. and Wijesinghe, R. (2000). The mental prosthesis: assessing the speed of a P300-based brain-computer interface. *IEEE Trans Rehabil Eng*, **8**, 174–179.

Donoghue, J.P. (2002). Connecting cortex to machines: recent advances in brain interfaces. *Nat Neurosci*, **5**, 1085–1088.

Farwell, L.A. and Donchin, E. (1988). Talking off the top of your head: toward a mental prosthesis utilizing event-related brain potentials. *Electroencephalogr Clin Neurophysiol*, **70**, 510–523.

Ghez, C. and Krakauer, J. (2000). Voluntary movement. In: *Principles of Neural Science* (eds Kandel, E.R., Schwartz, J.H. and Jessell, T.M.), 4th edn, McGraw-Hill, NY, pp. 653–674.

Kennedy, P.R. and Bakay, R.A. (1998). Restoration of neural output from a paralyzed patient by a direct brain connection. *NeuroReport*, **9**, 1707–1711.

Kennedy, P.R., Bakay, R.A.E., Moore, M.M., Adams, K. and Goldwaithe, J. (2000). Direct control of a computer from the human central nervous system. *IEEE Trans Rehabil Eng*, **8**, 198–202.

Kostov, A. and Polak, M. (2000). Parallel man-machine training in development of EEG-based cursor control. *IEEE Trans Rehabil Eng*, **8**, 203–205.

Kübler, A., Kotchoubey, B., Kaiser, J., Wolpaw, J.R. and Birbaumer, N. (2001). Brain-computer communication: unlocking the locked in. *Psychol Bull*, **127**, 358–375.

Leuthardt, E.C., Schalk, G., Wolpaw, J.R., Ojemann, J.G. and Moran, D.W. (2004). A brain-computer interface using electrocorticographic signals in humans. *J Neural Eng*, **1**, 63–71.

Maillot, F., Laueriere, L., Hazouard, E., Giraudeau, B. and Corcia, P. (2001). Quality of life in ALS is maintained as physical function declines.(Correspondence), *Neurology*, **57**, 939.

Mason, S.G. and Birch, G.E. (2000). A brain-controlled switch for asynchronous control applications. *IEEE Trans Biomed Eng*, **47**, 1297–1307.

Mellinger, J., Hinterberger, T., Bensch, M., Schröder, M. and Birbaumer, N. (2003). Surfing the web with electrical brain signals: the brain web surfer (BSW) for the completely paralysed. In: *Proceedings of the 2nd World Congress International Society Physical and Rehabilitation Medicine – ISPRM* (eds Ring, H. and Soroker, N.), Monduzzi, Bologna, pp. 731–738.

Miner, L.A., McFarland, D.J. and Wolpaw, J.R. (1998). Answering questions with an EEG-based brain-computer interface (BCI). *Arch Phys Med Rehabil*, **79**, 1029–1033.

Müller, K.-R., Anderson, C.W. and Birch, G.E. (2003). Linear and nonlinear methods for brain-computer interfaces. *IEEE Trans Neural Sys Rehabil Eng*, **11**, 165–169.

Musallam, S., Corneil, B.D., Greger, B., Scherberger, H. and Andersen, R.A. (2004). Cognitive control signals for neural prosthetics. *Science*, **305**(**5681**), 258–262.

Nicolelis, M.A.L., Birbaumer, N., Müller, K.-R. (2004). Guest editorial (Brain-machine interfaces). *IEEE Trans Biomed Eng*, **51**, 877.

Pesaran, B., Pezaris, J.S., Sahani, M., Mitra, P.P. and Andersen, R.A. (2002). Temporal structure in neuronal activity during working memory in macaque parietal cortex. *Nat Neurosci*, **5**, 805–811.

Pfurtscheller, G., Neuper, C., Müller, G.R., Obermaier, B., Krausz, G., Schlögl, A., Scherer, R., Graimann, B., Keinrath, C., Skliris, D., Wörtz, M., Supp, G. and Schrank, C. (2003a).

Graz-BCI: state of the art and clinical applications. *IEEE Trans Neural Sys Rehabil Eng*, **11**, 177–180.

Pfurtscheller, G., Graimann, B., Huggins, J.E., Levine, S.P. and Schuh, L.A. (2003b). Spatiotemporal patterns of beta desynchronization and gamma synchronization in corticographic data during self-paced movement. *Clin Neurophysiol*, **114**, 1226–1236.

Ramoser, H., Wolpaw, J.R. and Pfurtscheller, G. (1997). EEG-based communication: evaluation of alternative signal prediction methods. *Biomedical Technik*, **42**, 226–233.

Robbins, R.A., Simmons, Z., Bremer, B.A., Walsh, S.M. and Fischer, S. (2001). Quality of life in ALS is maintained as physical function declines. *Neurology*, **56**, 442–444.

Roberts, S.J. and Penny, W.D. (2000). Real-time brain–computer interfacing: a preliminary study using Bayesian learning. *Med Biol Eng Comp*, **38**, 56–61.

Salmoni, A.R., Schmidt, R.A. and Walter, C.B. (1984). Knowledge of results and motor learning: a review and critical appraisal. *Psychol Bull*, **5**, 355–386.

Schalk, G., McFarland, D.J., Hinterberger, T., Birbaumer, N. and Wolpaw, J.R. (2004). BCI2000: a general-purpose brain–computer interface (BCI) system. *IEEE Trans Biomed Eng*, **51**, 1034–1043.

Serruya, M.D., Hatsopoulos, N.G., Paninski, L., Fellows, M.R. and Donoghue, J.P. (2002). Instant neural control of a movement signal. *Nature*, **416**, 141–142.

Simmons, Z., Bremer, B.A., Robbins, R.A., Walsh, S.M. and Fischer, S. (2000). Quality of life in ALS depends on factors other than strength and physical function. *Neurology*, **55**, 388–392.

Taylor, D.M., Tillery, S.I. and Schwartz, A.B. (2002). Direct cortical control of 3D neuroprosthetic devices. *Science*, **296**, 829–832.

Taylor, D.M., Helms Tillery, S.I. and Schwartz, A.B. (2003). Information conveyed through braincontrol: cursor versus robot. *IEEE Trans Neural Sys Rehabil Eng*, **11**(2), 195–199.

Vaughan, T.M., Heetderks, W.J., Trejo, L.J., Rymer, W.Z., Weinrich, M., Moore, M.M., Kübler, A., Dobkin, B.H., Birbaumer, N., Donchin, E., Wolpaw, E.W. and Wolpaw, J.R. (2003). Brain–computer interface technology: a review of the second international meeting. *IEEE Trans Neural Sys Rehabil Eng*, **11**, 94–109.

Vidal, J.J. (1973). Towards direct brain–computer communication. *Ann Rev of Biophy Bioeng*, **2**, 157–180.

Vidal, J.J. (1977). Real-time detection of brain events in EEG. *IEEE Proc Spl Issue Biol Signal Proc Anal*, **65**, 633–664.

Wolpaw, J.R. and McFarland, D.J. (1994). Multichannel EEG-based brain–computer communication. *Electroencephalogr Clinl Neurophy*, **90**, 444–449.

Wolpaw, J.R. and McFarland, D.J. (2003). Two-dimensional movement control by scalp-recorded sensorimotor rhythms in humans. Program No. 607.2. 2003 Abstract Viewer/Itinerary Planner. Society for Neuroscience, Online, Washington, DC.

Wolpaw, J.R., McFarland, D.J., Neat, G.W. and Forneris, C.A. (1991). An EEG-based braincomputer interface for cursor control. *Electroencephalogr Clin Neurophy*, **78**, 252–259.

Wolpaw, J.R., Birbaumer, N., Heetderks, W.J., McFarland, D.J., Peckham, P.H., Schalk, G., Donchin, E., Quatrano, L.A., Robinson, C.J. and Vaughan, T.M. (2000). Brain–computer interface technology: a review of the first international meeting. *IEEE Trans Rehabil Eng*, **8**, 164–173.

Wolpaw, J.R., Birbaumer, N., McFarland, D.J., Pfurtscheller, G. and Vaughan, T.M. (2002). Brain–computer interfaces for communication and control. *Clin Neurophysiol*, **113**, 767–791.

Wolpaw, J.R., McFarland, D.J., Vaughan, T.M. and Schalk, G. (2003). The Wadsworth center brain–computer interface research and development program. *IEEE Trans Neural Sys Rehabil Eng*, **11**, 204–207.

Status of neural repair clinical trials in brain diseases

Olle Lindvall[1] and Peter Hagell[1,2]

[1]Section of Restorative Neurology, Wallenberg Neuroscience Center, University Hospital and
[2]Department of Nursing, Lund University, Lund, Sweden

34.1 Introduction

The interest in neuronal replacement therapies for human brain disorders dates back to the late 1970s when it was demonstrated that intrastriatal grafts of embryonic mesencephalic tissue, rich in dopamine (DA) neurons, induced functional recovery in rats with neurotoxin-induced lesions of the nigrostriatal dopaminergic system (for references see, e.g., Brundin et al., 1994). These observations provided the first evidence that neurons implanted into the adult brain could reverse behavioral deficits in an animal model of a human neurological disorder, Parkinson's disease (PD). Based on a bulk of experimental data in rodents and non-human primates (Annett, 1994; Brundin et al., 1994), the first clinical trials with neural transplantation in PD were initiated in 1987. Successful studies in animal models of Huntington's disease (HD) (for references see, e.g., Dunnett et al., 2000) lead to the first attempts with embryonic striatal grafts implanted into the striatum of HD patients in the 1990s. In addition, neural transplantation has been applied, with varying degree of scientific foundation, also in patients with other disorders such as stroke and epilepsy. Although the clinical studies with primary embryonic tissue seem to provide proof-of-principle for the cell replacement strategy, at least in PD (see Volume II, Chapter 6), it is obvious that other sources of cells are needed if cell-based approaches should become clinically competitive.

Stem cells or their derivatives might be able to solve several of the problems associated with the use of embryonic tissue grafts, such as the poor availability and lack of standardization of the cell material. Stem cells can be defined as immature cells with prolonged self-renewal capacity and, depending on their origin, ability to differentiate into multiple cell types or all cells of the body. From stem cells it should be possible to produce virtually unlimited numbers of neurons with a specific phenotype, such as dopaminergic neurons, in preparations which are standardized and quality-controlled. Two recent scientific developments support the notion that neuronal replacement from stem cells could become a novel therapeutic strategy: (i) Functional neurons with specific phenotype can be generated from different types of stem cells *in vitro* and survive transplantation *in vivo* (for references see, e.g., Lindvall, 2003). (ii) Endogenous neural stem cells (NSCs) in the adult brain are recruited after damage and produce new neurons, which seem to replace those which have died (Arvidsson et al., 2002; Nakatomi et al., 2002; Parent et al., 2002).

In this chapter, we will review the clinical observations following neural transplantation in three major brain disorders, namely PD, HD, and stroke (for clinical discussions see Volume II, Chapters 35 and 36). We will also discuss the scientific advancements that will be needed for the further development of cell-based therapies. In each of the diseases considered here, a different spectrum of cell types is affected and, therefore, different types of neurons are required for replacement. We will consider, in particular, the future role of the stem cell technology for the generation of these neurons.

34.2 Clinical experiences in PD

Symptomatic effects of neural grafts

The main pathology underlying disease symptoms in PD is a rather selective degeneration of the nigrostriatal DA neuron system. An estimated number of 350 patients with PD have so far received intrastriatal implants of human embryonic mesencephalic tissue. The tissue has been taken from dead aborted human embryos, aged 6–9-week post-conception. Several open-label trials have reported clinical benefit associated with graft survival (Lindvall et al., 1990; 1992; 1994; Sawle et al., 1992; Peschanski et al., 1994; Freeman et al., 1995; Remy et al., 1995; Defer et al., 1996; Wenning et al., 1997; Hagell et al., 1999; Hauser et al., 1999; Brundin et al., 2000; Mendez et al., 2000; 2002; Cochen et al., 2003). In the most successful cases, patients have been able to withdraw L-dopa treatment during several years after transplantation (Wenning et al., 1997; Hagell et al., 1999; Piccini et al., 1999; Brundin et al., 2000). The magnitude of the overall clinical benefit at 10–24 months postoperatively in three open-label trials (Hagell et al., 1999; Hauser et al., 1999; Brundin et al., 2000) is summarized in Table 34.1. All patients were grafted bilaterally with tissue from about three to five donors into each putamen. In some cases, tissue was also implanted in the caudate nucleus. According to the Unified Parkinson's Disease Rating Scale (UPDRS) motor score during practically defined "off" (i.e., in the morning, at least 12 h after the last dose of antiparkinsonian medication), the overall symptomatic relief at 10–24 months post-operatively was between 30% and 40%. In addition, there was a decrease (by 43% to 59%) of the average daily time spent in the "off" phase. The mean daily L-dopa requirements were reduced by 16% to 45%. It is interesting to note that in these three studies, even if the patients showed increased uptake of [^{18}F] fluorodopa (FD) (by about 60%) in the putamen, assessed by positron emission tomography (PET), indicating graft survival (see below), the uptake after transplantation was still only about 50% of the normal mean. This probably explains, at least to some extent, the incomplete functional recovery and indicates that there is room for considerable improvement.

The first double-blind, sham surgery-controlled study (Freed et al., 2001) demonstrated a more modest clinical response with 18% reduction of UPDRS motor score in "off" at 12 months after bilateral putaminal grafts (Table 34.1), but no improvement in the sham-operated group. In patients younger than 60 years, the improvement of UPDRS was 34%. These data are important because they provide direct evidence of a specific graft-induced symptomatic improvement, distinguishable from a placebo effect. In this trial, less tissue was implanted as compared to the open-label trials and, in agreement, the increase of FD uptake was lower (only 40% as compared to 60%). In two patients who died after grafting, the number of dopaminergic neurons in each putamen was between 7000 and 40,000 (Freed et al., 2001), which was much lower than that found in two patients in one of the open-label trials (see below; Kordower et al., 1995; 1996; 1998). The low cell number is probably due to that tissue from only two donors was implanted in each putamen (compared to tissue from three to five donors in the open-label trials) and that the tissue was stored in cell culture for up to 4 weeks before implantation. Furthermore, no immunosuppressive treatment was given, which also may have compromised DA graft survival. In agreement, the postoperative clinical improvement was smaller as compared to what was reported in the other patient series. These findings provide further support for the notion that the number of viable implanted DA neurons is an important factor partly determining the magnitude of symptomatic relief (Hagell and Brundin, 2001).

In a second, sham surgery-controlled, double-blind randomized clinical trial (Olanow et al., 2003), solid pieces of human embryonic mesencephalic tissue from one or four donors were implanted in each post-commissural putamen. Immunosuppressive treatment with cyclosporine was given for 6 months after surgery and patients were followed for 2 years. The trial failed to meet its primary outcome, that is, change in UPDRS motor scores at 24 months compared to baseline (Table 34.1). However, in

Table 34.1. Amount of graft tissue and magnitude of postoperative changes of putaminal FD uptake and motor function in five series of patients with idiopathic PD at 10–24 months after bilateral intrastriatal implantation of human embryonic mesencephalic tissue.

	Hauser et al., 1999 ($n = 6$)	Hagell et al., 1999 ($n = 4^a$)	Brundin et al., 2000 ($n = 5$)	Freed et al., 2001; Nakamura et al., 2001 ($n = 19$)	Olanow et al., 2003 ($n = 11/12$)[b]
Number of ventral mesencephalon/putamen	3–4	4.9	2.8[c]	2	1/4
FD uptake (putamen)					
Preoperatively[d]	34%	31%	31%	39%	n.r.[e]
Postoperatively[d]	55%	52%	48%	55%	n.r.[e]
Δ	+61%	+69%	+55%	+40%	n.r.[e]
UPDRS motor score in "off" (Δ)[f]	−30%	−30%	−40%	−18%	+3.5%/−0.72%
Daily time in "off" phase (Δ)	−43%	−59%	−43%	n.r.	+7.8%/−0.9%
Daily L-dopa dose (Δ)	−16%	−37%	−45%	n.r.	−20%/−11%

[a] Exluding one patient with possible multiple system atrophy.

[b] One-/four-donor groups, respectively.

[c] The graft tissue was treated with the lazaroid tirilazad mesylate.

[d] Mean percent FD uptake compared to the normal mean as measured in healthy volunteers.

[e] Only change in uptake from baseline reported.

[f] As assessed during practically defined "off".

Δ: mean postoperative change (%) from baseline; n.r.: not reported.

resemblance with the open-label trials, the patients grafted with tissue from four donors showed progressive improvements up to between 6 and 9 months after surgery (but deteriorated thereafter). Putaminal FD uptake was significantly increased in grafted patients at 12 months, as compared to controls and non-grafted striatal areas, and remained largely stable at 2 years after transplantation.

Why was the functional improvement in this study so modest and clearly different from that in the open-label trials? The first hypothesis is that the patients had more pronounced degenerative changes and were more severely disabled at the time of transplantation. In support of this hypothesis, the patients in the study of Olanow et al. (2003) required clearly higher doses of antiparkinsonian medication as compared to the Lund patients (mean daily L-dopa equivalent dose 1363.3 versus 932.5 mg, respectively). Furthermore, when Olanow and co-workers (2003) analyzed their less severely disabled patients, they observed a significant difference

compared to sham-operated patients at 2 years. However, this difference was mainly due to deterioration in the placebo group rather than improvement in the grafted patients, who remained fairly stable throughout the trial (a mean change in UPDRS motor score of 1.5). In this context it should be emphasized that it is highly likely that the extent, degree, and rate of degeneration of the patient's own dopaminergic and non-dopaminergic neurons prior to and after transplantation will influence to what extent a dopaminergic graft can restore normal function (Fig. 34.1). For example, in a patient with a widespread denervation in several brain areas, such as putamen, caudate nucleus, ventral striatum, and cerebral cortex, a dopaminergic graft in the posterior putamen will conceivably give only modest clinical recovery. In contrast, a patient with a dopaminergic denervation largely restricted to the putamen is more likely to benefit substantially from an intraputaminal graft. The second hypothesis is that although the grafts survived in the study of Olanow et al.

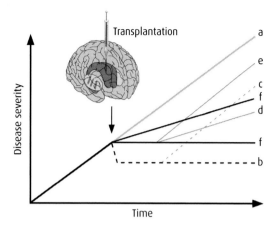

Figure 34.1. Schematic illustration of various hypothetical clinical courses following neural transplantation in chronic progressive brain disorders: (a) ineffective grafts with continuing natural disease progression; (b) long-lasting symptomatic effects; (c) transient symptomatic effect followed by a return to natural disease progression; (d) transient stabilizing effect followed by an improved clinical disease progression; (e) transient stabilizing effect followed by a return to natural disease progression; (f) lack of symptomatic effects but varying degrees of improved clinical disease progression. It should be noted that several of these developments could be presented in the same patient regarding various features of the disease, depending on patterns and rates of intrinsic cell degeneration and graft-induced reinnervation.

(2003), their function may have been impaired due to an immune reaction. Only short-term immunosuppression was given and cyclosporine levels were not monitored. Several open-label trials reporting clear clinical benefit have used strictly controlled multiple immunosuppressive regimens for at least 1–2 years after transplantation. The improvement compared to sham-operated patients up to between 6 and 9 months, and the deterioration thereafter in the study of Olanow and collaborators (2003) are consistent with an immune reaction after withdrawal of immunosuppression. Furthermore, in those patients who came to autopsy, the grafts were surrounded by activated microglia (Olanow et al., 2003), which is a hallmark of inflammation. For additional discussion of the sham surgery-controlled clinical trials see Volume II, Chapter 6.

When analyzing the modest results of the two sham surgery-controlled clinical trials, it is of course important to ask the question whether the symptomatic improvements in the open-label studies have been just placebo effects or observer bias. There are several arguments against such an interpretation:

(i)   Improvements after unilateral grafts have been predominantly contralateral, and in several patients their most parkinsonian side of the body has switched after transplantation.

(ii) Improvements have occurred gradually, starting after about 3 months and continuing up to 1–2 years after grafting.

(iii) Improvements have been detectable also with objective neurophysiological methods measuring arm and hand movements.

(iv) Some patients have improved to the extent that they have been able to return to work and withdraw L-dopa treatment for several years.

(v)   Improvements have been long-lasting, up to 10 years after transplantation.

(vi) Not only improvements but also deteriorations have been described in open-label trials.

(vii) Reported changes in motor function broadly correspond to the degree of graft survival and restoration of movement-related frontal cortical activation.

Mechanisms of action of neural grafts

It is well established that human embryonic mesencephalic DA neurons survive transplantation into the brain of PD patients. Significant increases of FD uptake in the grafted striatum have been shown in several studies (Lindvall et al., 1990; 1994; Sawle et al., 1992; Peschanski et al., 1994; Freeman et al., 1995; Remy et al., 1995; Wenning et al., 1997; Hagell et al., 1999; Hauser et al., 1999; Brundin et al., 2000; Mendez et al., 2000; 2002; Freed et al., 2001; Cochen et al., 2003; Olanow et al., 2003), and in one patient, the uptake was completely normalized after transplantation (Wenning et al., 1997; Piccini et al., 1999). FD-PET has also demonstrated that the grafts can survive for at least 10 years despite an ongoing disease process and continuous antiparkinsonian drug treatment (Piccini et al., 1999). Histopathological analyses have confirmed the survival of dopaminergic grafts and demonstrated their ability to reinnervate the striatum (Kordower et al., 1995; 1996; 1998). In two transplanted patients, between 80,000 and 135,000 dopaminergic neurons had survived on each side, with neuritic outgrowth from the grafted neurons extending up to approximately 7 mm within the putamen. Between 24% and 78% of the post-commissural putamen were reinnervated, and electron microscopy revealed synaptic connections between graft and host.

The grafts can also restore regulated release of DA in the striatum. Thus, in one patient who was transplanted unilaterally in the putamen, FD uptake in the grafted putamen was normal at 10 years postoperatively (Piccini et al., 1999). The uptake in the non-grafted putamen was only about 10% of normal level. DA release, quantified using [^{11}C] raclopride and PET, was normal in the grafted putamen both under basal conditions and following amphetamine administration. In contrast, the release in the contralateral, non-grafted putamen was very low. It seems highly likely that the efficient restoration of DA release in large parts of the grafted putamen underlies this patient's major clinical improvement.

Finally, the embryonic mesencephalic grafts can become functionally integrated into neural circuitries in the PD patient's brain. Normally, substantia nigra DA neurons are important regulators of cortico-striatal neurotransmission. Deficient striatal dopaminergic function as a consequence of the loss of substantia nigra neurons in PD leads to increased threshold for activation of the striato-pallido-thalamic output pathway. This causes impairment of the movement-related activation of frontal motor cortical areas, which is believed to underlie parkinsonian akinesia (Playford et al., 1992). Piccini and co-workers (2000) analyzed movement-related cortical activation, using PET and regional cerebral blood flow measurements, in four PD patients grafted bilaterally in the caudate nucleus and putamen. Postoperatively, there was a gradual restoration of the movement-related activation of frontal motor cortical areas which paralleled the time course of clinical improvement. These findings indicate that

successful grafts in patients with PD, by improving striatal dopaminergic neurotransmission, can restore movement-related cortical activation, which probably is necessary to induce substantial clinical improvement.

Adverse effects of neural grafts

The adverse events considered to have a possible or probable relationship with either the surgical procedure or the implanted tissue have generally been few, mild, and transient following neural transplantation in PD. In the recent double-blind clinical trial by Olanow et al. (2003), the overall rate of reported adverse events did not differ between either of the two grafted or the sham-operated groups of patients. In several studies, transient mental side effects, such as confusion, hallucination, disorientation, and frontal syndromes, have been observed during the immediate postoperative period (Defer et al., 1996; Hauser et al., 1999; Jaques et al., 1999; Brundin et al., 2000). These side effects have typically resolved spontaneously within the first month, and are likely to be related to the surgical trauma and subsequent edema along the trajectories. A few cases of postoperative seizures have been described (Hauser et al., 1999; Jaques et al., 1999); they have resolved without later reoccurrence either spontaneously or after anticonvulsive therapy. In the reported series of grafted PD patients, there has been a 4–5% incidence of intracerebral hemorrhage, of which one had a fatal outcome (Freed et al., 1994). Another serious adverse event is the introduction of non-neural tissue together with the graft, which can have disastrous consequences (Folkerth and Durso, 1996). Fortunately, this adverse event is rare but existing reports serve as an important reminder of the necessity of careful tissue dissection.

The most debated complication from current clinical transplantation protocols for PD is the occurrence of postoperative graft-induced dyskinesias (GID) (for detailed review, see Cenci and Hagell, 2004). Freed et al. (2001) reported that 15% of their grafted patients developed severe postoperative dyskinesias. Hagell et al. (2002) found that among 14 grafted PD patients, eight displayed postoperative "off"-phase dyskinesias that were mild and caused no distress or disability. In the remaining six patients, dyskinesias were of moderate severity and in one patient they constituted a clinical therapeutic problem. In the study of Olanow et al. (2003), 56.5% of the grafted patients developed postoperative "off"-phase dyskinesias, which consisted of stereotypic, rhythmic movements in the lower extremities. Dyskinesia severity appeared to be generally mild, as judged by mean scores of 3.2 and 2.7 out of a possible maximum score of 28 in the one- and four-donor group, respectively (no significant difference between groups), but were disabling and required surgery in three cases.

The mechanism(s) underlying GID is obscure (Cenci and Hagell, 2004). The first attempt to explain GID postulated excess DA due to continued fiber outgrowth from the grafts (Freed et al., 2001). However, several lines of evidence speak against this hypothesis. First, there is a lack of correlation between the magnitude of GID and that of the antiparkinsonian graft response (Hagell et al., 2002; Olanow et al., 2003). Second, the two have also displayed different temporal developments following transplantation (Freed et al., 2001; Hagell et al., 2002; Olanow et al., 2003). For example, in three bilaterally grafted patients reported by Hagell et al. (2002), dyskinesias reached their maximum at 24–48 months after transplantation, whereas the antiparkinsonian response developed during the first 12 months. Third, the occurrence of GID has not been associated with high postoperative striatal FD uptake or to the most pronounced graft-induced increases in striatal FD uptake (Hagell et al., 2002; Olanow et al., 2003). When comparing regional putaminal FD uptake in dyskinetic and non-dyskinetic grafted patients, Ma et al. (2002) found evidence of an imbalance between the dopaminergic innervation in the ventral and dorsal putamen in the dyskinetic cases. However, Olanow et al. (2003) reported no differences in either regional or global levels of striatal FD uptake between patients with and without GID. Finally, from a phenomenological point of view, GID have differed from L-dopa induced "on"-phase dyskinesias and instead been reminis-

cent of biphasic dyskinesias (Ma et al., 2002; Olanow et al., 2003; Cenci and Hagell, 2004), which could suggest intermediate (not excess) DA levels.

Observations in patients and experimental animals suggest several possible factors which may contribute to the development of GID (for detailed review and references, see Cenci and Hagell, 2004). First, failure of the grafts to restore a precise distribution of dopaminergic synaptic contacts on host neurons could result in an abnormal gating of cortico-striatal inputs, causing abnormal striatal signalling and synaptic plasticity. Second, GID might be due to small grafts giving rise to islands of reinnervation, surrounded by denervated striatal areas. Third, the underlying mechanism could be an unfavorable composition of the graft with respect to the predominant type of mesencephalic DA neuron from substantia nigra or ventral tegmental area, and proportion of non-dopaminergic cells. Several properties, for example, firing pattern, transmitter release, and axonal growth capacity, differ between the two types of mesencephalic DA neuron (Isacson et al., 2003). Finally, the occurrence of GID could be dependent on inflammatory and immune responses around the graft. In the study of Olanow et al. (2003), dyskinesias developed after discontinuation of immunosuppressive therapy, and there were signs of an inflammatory reaction around the graft in autopsied cases.

34.3 How shall cell therapy be developed in PD?

The clinical trials with embryonic mesencephalic grafts in PD patients have provided proof-of-principle that cell replacement can restore function in the parkinsonian brain. However, a clinically competitive cell therapy has to provide advantages over currently available treatments for alleviation of motor symptoms in PD patients. Cell-based approaches should thus give rise to long-lasting, major improvements of mobility and suppression of dyskinesias without the need for further therapeutic interventions. Alternatively, the cells should improve symptoms that are largely resistant to current treatments such as postural and non-motor disturbances. So far, the improvements after intrastriatal transplantation of DA neurons in patients (Lindvall and Hagell, 2000; Freed et al., 2001; Olanow et al., 2003) have not exceeded those found with subthalamic deep brain stimulation (Vitek, 2002), and there is no convincing evidence that drug-resistant symptoms are reversed by these grafts (Lindvall and Hagell, 2000). The incomplete recovery after transplantation could be due to that only part of the striatum has been reinnervated (Kordower et al., 1996; Lindvall and Hagell, 2000). However, also in animals with good reinnervation, improvements are only partial with intrastriatal embryonic mesencephalic grafts (Winkler et al., 2000), indicating that their ectopic placement and lack of appropriate regulatory input may be of crucial importance. Grafts implanted in the substantia nigra region give some improvements in animals (Winkler et al., 2000; Mukhida et al., 2001), and have also been tested clinically (Mendez et al., 2002). However, such grafts have not been able to significantly reconstruct the nigrostriatal pathway, or to induce clinical improvements that are appreciably different from those observed following intrastriatal transplantation.

It is unlikely that transplantation of human embryonic mesencephalic tissue will become routine treatment for PD due to problems with tissue availability and standardization of the grafts leading too much variation in functional outcome. Nevertheless, human embryonic mesencephalic grafts will most probably continue to be the "golden standard" in clinical cell therapy research for PD in the foreseeable future. However, for the development of a clinically competitive cell replacement therapy, four major scientific achievements have to be reached.

Generation of large numbers of DA neurons in standardized and quality-controlled preparations

For this purpose, other sources of cells, such as xenogeneic mesencephalic DA neurons (Barker, 2002), have to be considered. However, clinical trials

using intrastriatal transplantation of porcine embryonic mesencephalic tissue in patients with PD (Schumacher et al., 2000; Watts et al., 2001) have not provided any evidence of graft survival or unequivocal clinical benefits. The main interest is now instead focused on the production of DA neurons from stem cells in culture and subsequent transplantation (Fig. 34.2). These neurons have to work, at least, as well as the primary DA neurons in the embryonic mesencephalic grafts used so far in PD patients. Based on results obtained with such transplants in animals and in patients, a set of requirements can be identified which probably have to be fulfilled also by stem cell-derived cells in order to induce marked clinical improvement:

1 The cells should release DA in a regulated manner, and exhibit the molecular, morphological, and electrophysiological properties of substantia nigra neurons (Isacson et al., 2003).
2 The cells must be able to reverse motor deficits in animal models resembling the symptoms in patients.
3 The yield of cells should allow for 100,000 or more grafted DA neurons to survive long term in each human putamen (Hagell and Brundin, 2001).
4 The grafted DA neurons should reestablish a dense terminal network throughout the striatum.
5 The grafts have to become functionally integrated into host neural circuitries (Piccini et al., 2000).

Neurons with dopaminergic phenotype surviving transplantation in animal models of PD have been generated in culture from mouse and monkey embryonic stem (ES) cells, and from NSCs derived from the embryonic rodent and human brain (for review, see Lindvall, 2003; Lindvall et al., 2004). Currently, there is little evidence that DA neurons for grafting can be made from NSCs isolated from the adult brain, or from stem cells in other tissues. In most cases, it is unclear whether the stem cell-derived cells after transplantation to animal models can substantially reinnervate the striatum, restore DA release, and markedly improve deficits resembling the symptoms of the human disease

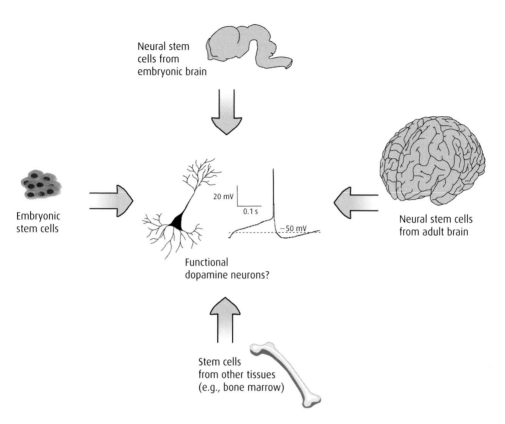

Figure 34.2. Possible sources of stem cells for the *in vitro* generation of functional DA neurons for cell therapy in PD.

(Table 34.2). The most promising results so far have been obtained using mouse ES cells (Kim et al., 2002). Preliminary data indicate that large numbers of DA neurons can be generated also when the ES cells are of human origin, which probably is necessary for a clinical application.

Improved patient selection

We must define better criteria for patient selection with respect to stage and type of disease, and we must know the preoperative degeneration pattern so that we can define what should be repaired. Dopaminergic cell therapy will most likely be successful only in those patients who can exhibit marked symptomatic benefit in response to L-dopa, and in whom the main pathology is a loss of DA neurons. Several debilitating

symptoms in PD and related disorders are probably also caused by pathological changes in non-dopaminergic systems. Until we know how to repair these systems, patients with such symptoms should not be subjected to cell therapy.

Improved functional efficacy of grafts

The transplantation procedure needs to be tailor-made with respect to the dose and location of grafted cells based on preoperative imaging so that the repair of the DA system will be as complete as possible in each patient's brain. There is no evidence that DA neurons, pre-differentiated from stem cells in culture, will be able to induce a more pronounced improvement as compared to primary DA neurons. One advantage with stem cells might be the

Table 34.2. Properties of stem/precursor cell grafts in animal models of PD.

Cell source	Striatal reinnervation	*In vivo* DA release	Improvement of Parkinson-like symptoms
Mouse ES cells	Partial	?	Significant
Monkey ES cells	Neurites	?	?
Human ES cells	?	?	?
Immortalized mouse embryonic cerebellar precursors	?	?	?
Rat embryonic VM-derived precursors	Partial	?	?
Rat or human embryonic VM-derived DA precursors	Fibers	?	?
Mouse bone marrow cells	?	?	?

For references, see Lindvall et al. (2004).

possibility for controlled genetic modification which, hypothetically, could be used to increase survival, migration, and function of their progeny. For a more complete reversal of PD symptoms, it may be necessary to develop tools to stimulate growth of axons from DA neuron grafts in the substantia nigra to the striatum, which probably will require modulation of host growth inhibitory mechanisms. It is currently unknown if immunosuppressive treatment will be needed in a clinical setting when the stem cells are of human origin. Results with allogenic embryonic mesencephalic grafts (Olanow et al., 2003) suggest, however, that effective immunosuppression, at least for 1 year after transplantation as used in several open-label trials, is necessary to optimize the functional outcome.

Strategies to avoid adverse effects

New animal models are needed to reveal the pathophysiological mechanisms of GID (Steece-Collier et al., 2003). The risk for teratoma from ES cells (Björklund et al., 2002), and the consequences of the introduction of new genes in stem cell-derived neurons should be carefully evaluated after transplantation in experimental animals. Current data with rodent ES cells indicate that the risk for teratoma is reduced if the cells are pre-differentiated *in vitro*.

34.4 Clinical experiences in HD

HD is a fatal disorder characterized by progressive dementia and choreic movements. Effective therapy is lacking. The main pathology is a massive loss of medium spiny projection neurons in the striatum due to a mutation in the huntingtin gene. Over the past decade, a number of groups have initiated transplantation trials in patients with HD. The available data on graft survival and clinical effects after neural transplantation in HD mainly emanate from two studies (Bachoud-Lévy et al., 2000; Hauser et al., 2002) and results from a third one are underway (Rosser et al., 2002; Watts et al., 2003). Bachoud-Lévy et al. (2000) described five patients with HD who received intrastriatal grafts bilaterally, with a year's interval between the two grafts. Striatal tissue from one or two 7–9-week-old-human embryos was injected into each caudate nucleus and putamen. Immunosuppressive therapy was given until 12 months after the second transplantation. Measurement of [18F] -fluorodeoxyglucose uptake using PET showed that, compared to preoperatively, three of the five patients had either increased or stable metabolic activity throughout the striatum, and higher activity in some small areas, at 1 year after the second graft. These data are consistent with the survival of metabolically active neural grafts.

A cohort of 22 patients with HD, who were assessed in parallel, showed worsening of chorea and performance in most neuropsychological tests. By contrast, the patients with presumed surviving grafts had stable or even improved neuropsychological test results, improvement in activities of daily living, and reductions in severity of chorea and bradykinesia. Two of these patients had improvements in somatosensory-evoked potentials, which were not found in the untreated patients. In support of the possibility that the survival of the grafts accounted for the observed clinical benefit in the three patients, the decreased metabolic activity in the striatum postoperatively in the other two patients was accompanied by deterioration of cognitive and motor function. Interestingly, clinical improvement was associated with reduction of striatal and cortical hypometabolism, suggesting that the grafts had restored function in striato-cortical neural loops (Gaura et al., 2004).

In a parallel study, Hauser et al. (2002) implanted human embryonic striatal tissue from 8- to 9-week-old donors bilaterally into the striatum in seven HD patients at two surgical sessions, up to 14 weeks apart. Subjects received tissue from 0 to 2 striata in each caudate nucleus and 2 to 6 striata in each putamen. Cyclosporine was given for 6 months after surgery. There was no significant improvement of either the Unified Huntington's Disease Rating Scale (UHDRS) motor scores or the rate of worsening at 12 months as compared to preoperatively for the whole group of patients. The authors also performed a post hoc analysis in which they excluded one patient who exhibited cognitive and motor deterioration after developing bilateral subdural hemorrhages. The remaining six patients showed significant (19%) improvement of UHDRS scores. The striatal fluorodeoxyglucose uptake was not significantly changed. However, Freeman et al. (2000) demonstrated, using histopathological techniques, surviving grafts with morphological features of developing striatum in one of the patients who died 18 months after transplantation. The striatum-like part of the grafted tissue, which occupied about 50% of the graft volume, was innervated by dopaminergic fibers from the host brain.

34.5 How shall cell therapy be developed in HD?

Whereas some investigators argue for a pause in clinical studies (Albin, 2002; Greenamyre and Shoulson, 2002), further evaluation of the safety and efficacy of embryonic striatal grafts in HD is planned in a European Multicenter Trial (Peschanski and Dunnett, 2002). The findings in the clinical trials seem encouraging and support the rationale for a cell replacement strategy in HD. However, it remains unclear whether cell therapy can be developed into a clinically useful treatment for HD patients. First, the effects of intrastriatal grafts on the course of the disease are unknown (Fig. 34.1). The ability of the graft to maintain a stable condition over a long time will be essential for its therapeutic value. Since follow-up data after bilateral transplantation thus far are limited to 1 year, it remains to be determined whether the striatal transplants can survive and function long enough to prevent further clinical deterioration. It is also unknown to what extent striatal transplants can counteract the concurrent degenerative processes in the host brain. Reconstruction of the striatal circuitry alone may be insufficient, since the progressive degeneration in the neocortex seen in patients with HD is unlikely to be caused by retrograde changes secondary to neuronal loss in the striatum. Second, since the primary mode of action of the grafts is to replace lost striatal neurons, the total number of surviving grafted striatal neurons is likely to be critical for the magnitude of the therapeutic effect. In the study of Bachoud-Lévy et al. (2000), it is not clear how much of the normal volume of the striatum was replaced by the grafts. In Freeman and colleagues' study (2000), the total volume of the surviving grafts corresponded to only 8–10% of the volume of the remaining caudate nucleus and putamen.

It is conceivable that substantial therapeutic benefit following cell therapy in HD will require many more surviving grafted striatal neurons. The generation of striatal GABAergic projection neurons from stem cells *in vitro* could dramatically increase the availability of such cells. Basic research should now explore how to generate and select striatal projection neurons from stem cells. Subsequently, it will be necessary to show that the neurons survive, become anatomically and functionally integrated, and improve motor and cognitive function after grafting in HD models.

34.6 Clinical experiences in stroke

In stroke, occlusion of a cerebral artery leads to focal ischemia in a restricted brain region. Many different types of neurons and glial cells die in stroke, leading to atrophy. It has not yet been convincingly demonstrated that neuronal replacement can induce symptomatic relief in stroke patients. In the only clinical trial reported so far, 12 patients with stroke affecting the basal ganglia received implants of neurons generated from the human teratocarcinoma cell line NTera-2 (NT-2) into the infarcted area (Kondziolka et al., 2000). This cell line gives rise to neurons after a complex induction process. Slight postoperative improvements were reported up to 12 months after surgery (Kondziolka et al., 2000; Meltzer et al., 2001). The improvements in some of the operated patients correlated with increased metabolic activity at the graft site (Meltzer et al., 2001). This finding could be interpreted as graft function but might as well reflect inflammation or increased activity in host neurons. Autopsy in one patient revealed a population of grafted cells expressing a neuronal marker at 2 years after surgery (Nelson et al., 2002).

34.7 How shall cell therapy be developed in stroke?

To repair the human brain after stroke may seem unrealistic because of atrophy and loss of many cell types. However, even reestablishment of only a fraction of damaged neuronal circuitries could have significant implications. Cells from different sources have been tested for their ability to reconstruct the forebrain and improve function after transplantation in animals subjected to stroke (for references see, e.g., Lindvall et al., 2004). The transplants including, for example, rat embryonic striatal and cortical tissue, a mouse neuroepithelial stem cell line, the human NT-2 cell line, and rat bone marrow cells, have been reported to partly reverse some behavioral deficits. However, in most cases, the underlying mechanisms are unclear and there is little evidence for neuronal replacement. Only few grafted cells have survived and they have not exhibited the phenotype of the dead neurons. Moreover, it is unknown, if the observed grafted cells are functional neurons and establish afferent and efferent connections with host neurons.

Recent findings in rodents suggest an alternative approach to cell therapy in stroke based on self-repair (Fig. 34.3; for references see Kokaia and Lindvall, 2003). Stroke leads to increased generation of neurons from NSCs in the subventricular zone (SVZ), lining the lateral ventricles. These immature neurons migrate into the damaged striatum, where they express markers of striatal medium spiny projection neurons. Thus, the new neurons seem to differentiate into the phenotype of most of the neurons destroyed by the ischemic lesion. Although there is currently a lot of enthusiasm about the therapeutic potential of endogenous neurogenesis in stroke (see Volume I, Chapter 18), it has to be underscored that we have very little knowledge about the importance of endogenous neurogenesis for brain repair. How the various steps of neurogenesis are regulated after stroke is virtually unknown. It is also unclear if the new neurons are functional neurons and become integrated into host neural circuitries. Finally, it should be emphasized that this endogenous repair mechanism is not effective in stroke. One major problem is that more than 80% of the new neurons die during the first weeks after stroke and therefore, they only replace a small fraction (about 0.2%) of the mature striatal neurons which have died. Importantly, several factors have now been identified which can increase neurogenesis by stimulating the formation and/or improving survival of the

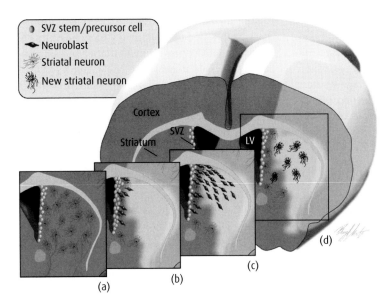

- SVZ stem/precursor cell
- Neuroblast
- Striatal neuron
- New striatal neuron

Cortex

SVZ

Striatum

LV

(a)

(b)

(c)

(d)

Figure 34.3. Generation of striatal neurons from endogenous stem cells in the adult brain after stroke. (a) Neural stem/precursor cells reside in the SVZ lining the lateral ventricle. (b) Stroke induced by middle cerebral artery occlusion, which leads to death of striatal and cortical neurons (white area), triggers increased proliferation of SVZ precursors. (c) The newly formed neurons migrate to the damaged part of the striatum. (d) After maturation, the new neurons express markers specific for striatal projection neurons or interneurons. From Lindvall et al. (2004).

new neurons (for references see, e.g., Kokaia and Lindvall, 2003).

The optimum strategy for neuronal replacement in stroke will probably be to combine transplantation of NSCs close to the damaged area with stimulation of neurogenesis from endogenous NSCs. This strategy requires that the largely unknown developmental mechanisms, instructing stem cells to differentiate into specific cell types, will work also in the patient's brain. Newly generated neurons are able to migrate towards the damage (Arvidsson et al., 2002; Parent et al., 2002) and, at least to some extent, adopt the phenotype of those cells which have died (Arvidsson et al., 2002; Modo et al., 2002; Parent et al., 2002). Available data provide evidence for a neurogenic potential also in the human brain. Neurogenesis from precursors in the SVZ has been demonstrated *in vivo* in humans (Eriksson et al., 1998) and precursors capable of forming neurons are found in human subcortical white matter (Nunes et al., 2003).

The inadequate blood supply to the ischemic core region will cause massive loss of newly formed neurons. If cells are implanted into the penumbra area (region-at-risk), they will probably be supported by collateral circulation. Adult hippocampal neurogenesis is closely associated with angiogenesis from endothelial cell precursors (Palmer et al., 2000). The creation of such a vascular niche and the stimulation of vascularization after stroke will be crucial for the survival of the new neurons. Administration of vascular endothelial growth factor promotes both neurogenesis in the SVZ and angiogenesis in the ischemic penumbra region following stroke (Sun et al., 2003). However, for efficient repair after stroke it may be necessary to provide the NSCs with a platform so that they can reform appropriate brain structure and connections. A study in neonatal mice (Park et al., 2002) shows that if NSCs are seeded on synthetic extracellular matrix, implanted into the ischemia-damaged area, new parenchyma comprising neurons and glia is formed and becomes vascularized.

In order to develop stem cell therapy towards clinical application in stroke, three different tasks should be accomplished: The *first task* is to obtain proof-of-principle that implanted stem cells, or neurons that are generated from endogenous NSCs, can survive in large numbers in animals subjected to stroke, migrate to appropriate locations, exhibit morphological and functional properties of those neurons which have died, and establish afferent and efferent synaptic interactions with neurons that survived the insult. Magnetic resonance imaging seems ideal for non-invasive imaging at high spatial and temporal resolution of the survival, migration and differentiation of grafted cells (Hoehn et al., 2002). The *second task* is to optimize the behavioral recovery induced by neuronal replacement in animal models. Strategies to improve survival, differentiation, and integration of endogenous and grafted stem cells will require detailed knowledge of how these processes are regulated. The time window after the insult when the generation of new neurons will lead to maximum restitution of neuronal circuitries and functional recovery should be determined. The *third task* is to define which patients are suitable for stem cell therapy based on findings in animal models regarding which cell types can be produced and replaced. The occurrence of striatal neurogenesis after stroke (Arvidsson et al., 2002; Parent et al., 2002) focuses the interest on patients with basal ganglia infarcts. If stem cells can generate also cortical neurons and repair axonal damage, patients with lesions in the cerebral cortex may be included. A strategy for repair of infarcted white matter was suggested recently by the observation that adult neurospheres injected intravenously or intraventricularly in mice (Pluchino et al., 2003) gave rise to cells which migrated to demyelinated areas, differentiated into oligodendrocyte progenitors, remyelinated axons, and improved function.

34.8 Conclusions

The development of cell-based therapies for human brain diseases is still at an early stage and, currently, there exists no clinically competitive cell therapy for any such disorder. However, we now know, primarily from the clinical trials with embryonic grafts in PD patients and to some extent also in HD patients, that function can be restored in the diseased human brain by neuronal replacement. Although human embryonic tissue will probably remain the golden standard in clinical cell therapy research for

a considerable time, other sources of cells will be needed if cell-based treatments should ever become available for large numbers of patients. Stem cell-based approaches seem to be the most promising alternative to the use of human embryonic tissue for cell replacement. Recent progress shows that specific types of neurons and glia cells suitable for transplantation can be generated from stem cells in culture. Also, that the adult brain produces new neurons from its own stem cells in response to stroke. Although these findings raise hope for the development of stem cell therapies for brain repair, many basic issues remain to be solved. We need to move forward with caution and avoid scientifically ill-founded trials in patients. Before clinical trials with stem cell-based approaches are initiated, we need to know much more regarding how to control stem cell proliferation and differentiation into specific phenotypes, induce their integration into existing neural and synaptic circuits, and optimize the functional recovery in animal models closely mimicking the human disease. These major scientific efforts seem clearly justified because for the first time, there is now real hope that we in the future can offer patients, with currently intractable brain diseases, effective cell-based treatments to restore brain function.

ACKNOWLEDGMENT

The authors' own work within this field has been supported by the Skane County Council Research and Development Foundation, the Swedish Medical Research Council, and the Kock, Wiberg, Söderberg, and King Gustav V and Queen Victoria Foundations.

REFERENCES

Albin, R.L. (2002). Fetal striatal transplantation in Huntington's disease: time for a pause. *J Neurol Neurosurg Psychiatr*, **73**, 612.

Annett, L.E. (1994). Functional studies of neural grafts in parkinsonian primates. In: *Functional Neural Transplantation* (eds Dunnett, S.B. and Björklund, A.), Raven Press, New York, pp. 71–102.

Arvidsson, A., Collin, T., Kirik, D., Kokaia, Z. and Lindvall, O. (2002). Neuronal replacement from endogenous precursors in the adult brain after stroke. *Nat Med*, **8**, 963–970.

Bachoud-Lévi, A.-C., Remy, P., Nguyen, J.P., Brugieres, P., Lefaucheur, J.P., Bourdet, C., Baudic, S., Gaura, V., Maison, P., Haddad, B., Boisse, M.F., Grandmougin, T., Jeny, R., Bartolomeo, P., Dalla Barba, G., Degos, J.D., Lisovoski, F., Ergis, A.M., Pailhous, E., Cesaro, P., Hantraye, P. and Peschanski, M. (2000). Motor and cognitive improvements in patients with Huntington's disease after neural transplantation. *Lancet*, **356**, 1975–1979.

Barker, R.A. (2002). Repairing the brain in Parkinson's disease: where next? *Movement Disord*, **17**, 233–241.

Björklund, L.M., Sanchez-Pernaute, R., Chung, S., Andersson, T., Chen, I.Y., McNaught, K.S., Brownell, A.L., Jenkins, B.G., Wahlestedt, C., Kim, K.S. and Isacson, O. (2002). Embryonic stem cells develop into functional dopaminergic neurons after transplantation in a Parkinson rat model. *Proc Natl Acad Sci USA*, **99**, 2344–2349.

Brundin, P., Duan, W.M. and Sauer, H. (1994). Functional effects of mesencephalic dopamine neurons and adrenal chromaffin cells grafted to the rodent striatum. In: *Functional Neural Transplantation* (eds Dunnett, S.B. and Björklund, A.), Raven Press, New York, pp. 9–46.

Brundin, P., Pogarell, O., Hagell, P., Piccini, P., Widner, H., Schrag, A., Kupsch, A., Crabb, L., Odin, P., Gustavii, B., Björklund, A., Brooks, D.J., Marsden, C.D., Oertel, W.H., Quinn, N.P., Rehncrona, S. and Lindvall, O. (2000). Bilateral caudate and putamen grafts of embryonic mesencephalic tissue treated with lazaroids in Parkinson's disease. *Brain*, **123**, 1380–1390.

Cenci, M.A. and Hagell, P. (2004). Dyskinesias and neural grafting in Parkinson's disease. In: *Restorative Therapies in Parkinson's Disease* (eds Olanow, C.W. and Brundin, P.), Kluwer Academic/Plenum Publishers, New York (in press).

Cochen, V., Ribeiro, M.J., Nguyen, J.P., Gurruchaga, J.M., Villafane, G., Loc'h, C., Defer, G., Samson, Y., Peschanski, M., Hantraye, P., Cesaro, P. and Remy, P. (2003). Transplantation in Parkinson's disease: PET changes correlate with the amount of grafted tissue. *Movement Disord*, **18**, 928–932.

Defer, G.L., Geny, C., Ricolfi, F., Fénelon, G., Monfort, J.C., Remy, P., Villafane, G., Jeny, R., Samson, Y., Kéravel, Y., Gaston, A., Degos, J.D., Peschanski, M., Cesaro, P. and Nguyen, J.P. (1996). Long-term outcome of unilaterally transplanted parkinsonian patients. I. Clinical approach. *Brain*, **119**, 41–50.

Dunnett, S.B., Nathwani, F. and Björklund, A. (2000). The integration and function of striatal grafts. *Prog Brain Res*, **127**, 345–380.

Eriksson, P.S., Perfilieva, E., Bjork-Eriksson, T., Alborn, A.M., Nordborg, C., Peterson, D.A. and Gage, F.H. (1998). Neurogenesis in the adult human hippocampus. *Nat Med*, **4**, 1313–1317.

Folkerth, R.D. and Durso, R. (1996). Survival and proliferation of nonneural tissues, with obstruction of cerebral ventricles, in a parkinsonian patient treated with fetal allografts. *Neurology*, **46**, 1219–1225.

Freed, C.R., Breeze, R.E., Schneck, S.A., O'Brien, C.F., Mazziotta, J.C., Hutchinson, M. and Ansari, A.A. (1994). Human fetal dopamine cells survive and develop processes after implantation into humans with Parkinson's disease. *Soc Neurosci Abstr*, **20**, 9.

Freed, C.R., Greene, P.E., Breeze, R.E., Tsai, W.-Y., DuMouchel, W., Kao, R., Dillon, S., Winfield, H., Culver, S., Trojanowski, J.Q., Eidelberg, D. and Fahn, S. (2001). Transplantation of embryonic dopamine neurons for severe Parkinson's disease. *New Engl J Med*, **344**, 710–719.

Freeman, T.B., Olanow, C.W., Hauser, R.A., Nauert, G.M., Smith, D.A., Borlongan, C.V., Sanberg, P.R., Holt, D.A., Kordower, J.H., Vingerhoets, F.J.G., Snow, B.J., Calne, D. and Gauger, L.L. (1995). Bilateral fetal nigral transplantation into the postcommissural putamen in Parkinson's disease. *Ann Neurol*, **38**, 379–388.

Freeman, T.B., Cicchetti, F., Hauser, R.A., Deacon, T.W., Li, X.-J., Hersch, S.M., Nauert, G.M., Sanberg, P.R., Kordower, J.H., Saporta, S. and Isacson, O. (2000). Transplanted fetal striatum in Huntington's disease: phenotypic development and lack of pathology. *Proc Natl Acad Sci USA*, **97**, 13877–13882.

Gaura, V., Bachoud-Lévi, A.-C., Ribeiro, M.-J., Nguyen, J.-P., Frouin, V., Baudic, S., Bruières, P., Mangin, J.-F., Boissé, M.-F., Palfi, S., Cesaro, P., Samson, Y., Hantraye, P., Peschanski, M. and Remy, P. (2004). *Brain*, **127**, 65–72.

Greenamyre, J.T. and Shoulson, I. (2002). We need something better, and we need it now: fetal striatal transplantation in Huntington's disease? *Neurology*, **58**, 675–676.

Hagell, P. and Brundin, P. (2001). Cell survival and clinical outcome following intrastriatal transplantation in Parkinson's disease. *J Neuropathol Exp Neurol*, **60**, 741–752.

Hagell, P., Schrag, A., Piccini, P., Jahanshahi, M., Brown, R., Rehncrona, S., Widner, H., Brundin, P., Rothwell, J.C., Odin, P., Wenning, G.K., Morrish, P., Gustavii, B., Björklund, A., Brooks, D.J., Marsden, C.D., Quinn, N.P. and Lindvall, O. (1999). Sequential bilateral transplantation in Parkinson's disease: effects of the second graft. *Brain*, **122**, 1121–1132.

Hagell, P., Piccini, P., Björklund, A., Brundin, P., Rehncrona, S., Widner, H., Crabb, L., Pavese, N., Oertel, W.H., Quinn, N., Brooks, D.J. and Lindvall, O. (2002). Dyskinesias following neural transplantation in Parkinson's disease. *Nat Neurosci*, **5**, 627–628.

Hauser, R.A., Freeman, T.B., Snow, B.J., Nauert, M., Gauger, L., Kordower, J.H. and Olanow, C.W. (1999) Long-term evaluation of bilateral fetal nigral transplantation in Parkinson disease. *Arch Neurol*, **56**, 179–187.

Hauser, R.A., Furtado, S., Cimino, C.R., Delgado, H., Eichler, S., Schwartz, S., Scott, D., Nauert, G.M., Soety, E., Sossi, V., Holt, D.A., Sanberg, P.R., Stoessl, A.J. and Freeman, T.B. (2002). Bilateral human fetal striatal transplantation in Huntington's disease. *Neurology*, **58**, 687–695.

Hoehn, M., Kustermann, E., Blunk, J., Wiedermann, D., Trapp, T., Wecker, S., Föcking, M., Arnold, H., Hescheler, J., Fleischmann, B.K., Schwindt, W. and Buhrle, C. (2002). Monitoring of implanted stem cell migration *in vivo*: a highly resolved *in vivo* magnetic resonance imaging investigation of experimental stroke in rat. *Proc Natl Acad Sci USA*, **99**, 16267–16272.

Isacson, O., Björklund, L. and Schumacher, J.M. (2003). Toward full restoration of synaptic and terminal function of the dopaminergic system in Parkinson's disease by stem cells. *Ann Neurol*, **53**(**Suppl. 3**), S315–S148.

Jacques, D., Kopyov, O., Eagle, K., Carter, T. and Lieberman, A. (1999). Outcomes and complications of fetal tissue transplantation in Parkinson's disease. *Movement Disord*, **72**, 219–224.

Kim, J.H., Auerbach, J.M., Rodriguez-Gomez, J.A., Velasco, I., Gavin, D., Lumelsky, N., Lee, S.H., Nguyen, J., Sanchez-Pernaute, R., Bankiewicz, K. and McKay, R. (2002). Dopamine neurons derived from embryonic stem cells function in an animal model of Parkinson's disease. *Nature*, **418**, 50–56.

Kokaia, Z. and Lindvall, O. (2003). Neurogenesis after ischaemic brain insults. *Curr Opin Neurobiol*, **13**, 127–132.

Kondziolka, D., Wechsler, L., Goldstein, S., Meltzer, C., Thulborn, K.R., Gebel, J., Janetta, P., DeCesare, S., Elder, E.M., McGrogan, M., Reitman, M.A. and Bynum, L. (2000). Transplantation of cultured human neuronal cells for patients with stroke. *Neurology*, **55**, 565–569.

Kordower, J.H., Freeman, T.B., Snow, B.J., Vingerhoets, F.J.G., Mufson, E.J., Sanberg, P.R., Hauser, R.A., Smith, D.A., Nauert, G.M., Perl, D.P. and Olanow, C.W. (1995). Neuropathological evidence of graft survival and striatal reinnervation after the transplantation of fetal mesencephalic tissue in a patient with Parkinson's disease. *New Engl J Med*, **332**, 1118–1124.

Kordower, J.H., Rosenstein, J.M., Collier, T.J., Burke, M.A., Chen, E.-Y., Li, J.M., Martel, L., Levey, A.E., Mufson, E.J., Freeman, T.B. and Olanow, C.W. (1996). Functional fetal nigral grafts in a patient with Parkinson's disease: chemoanatomic, ultrastructural, and metabolic studies. *J Comp Neurol*, **370**, 203–230.

Kordower, J.H., Freeman, T.B., Chen, E.Y., Mufson, E.J., Sanberg, P.R., Hauser, R.A., Snow, B.J. and Olanow, C.W. (1998). Fetal nigral grafts survive and mediate clinical benefit in a patient with Parkinson's disease. *Movement Disord*, **13**, 383–393.

Lindvall, O. (2003). Stem cells for cell therapy in Parkinson's disease. *Pharmacolog Res*, **47**, 279–287.

Lindvall, O. and Hagell, P. (2000). Clinical observations after neural transplantation in Parkinson's disease. *Prog Brain Res*, **127**, 299–320.

Lindvall, O., Brundin, P., Widner, H., Rehncrona, S., Gustavii, B., Frackowiak, R., Leenders, K.L., Sawle, G., Rothwell, J.C., Marsden, C.D. and Björklund, A. (1990). Grafts of fetal dopamine neurons survive and improve motor function in Parkinson's disease. *Science*, **247**, 574–577.

Lindvall, O., Widner, H., Rehncrona, S., Brundin, P., Odin, P., Gustavii, B., Frackowiak, R., Leenders, K.L., Sawle, G., Rothwell, J.C., Björklund, A. and Marsden, C.D. (1992). Transplantation of fetal dopamine neurons in Parkinson's disease: 1-year clinical and neurophysiological observations in two patients with putaminal implants. *Ann Neurol*, **31**, 155–165.

Lindvall, O., Sawle, G., Widner, H., Rothwell, J.C., Björklund, A., Brooks, D.J., Brundin, P., Frackowiak, R., Marsden, C.D., Odin, P. and Rehncrona, S. (1994). Evidence for long-term survival and function of dopaminergic grafts in progressive Parkinson's disease. *Ann Neurol*, **35**, 172–180.

Lindvall, O., Kokaia, Z. and Martinez-Serrano, A. (2004). Stem cell therapy for neurodegenerative disorders – how to make it work. *Nat Med* (provisionally accepted).

Ma, Y., Feigin, A., Dhawan, V., Fukuda, M., Shi, Q., Greene, P., Breeze, R., Fahn, S., Freed, C. and Eidelberg, D. (2002). Dyskinesia after fetal cell transplantation for parkinsonism: a PET study. *Ann Neurol*, **52**, 628–634.

Meltzer, C.C., Kondziolka, D., Villemagne, V.L., Wechsler, L., Goldstein, S., Thulborn, K.R., Gebel, J., Elder, E.M., DeCesare, S. and Jacobs, A. (2001). Serial [^{18}F]fluorodeoxyglucose positron emission tomography after human neuronal implantation for stroke. *Neurosurgery*, **49**, 586–592.

Mendez, I., Dagher, A., Hong, M., Hebb, A., Gaudet, P., Law, A., Weerasinghe, S., King, D., Desrosiers, J., Darvesh, S., Acorn, T. and Robertson, H. (2000). Enhancement of survival of stored dopaminergic cells and promotion of graft survival by exposure of human fetal nigral tissue to glial cell line-derived neurotrophic factor in patients with Parkinson's disease. *J Neurosurg*, **92**, 863–869.

Mendez, I., Dagher, A., Hong, M., Gaudet, P., Weerasinghe, S., McAlister, V., King, D., Desrosiers, J., Darvesh, S., Acorn, T. and Robertson, H. (2002). Simultaneous intrastriatal and intranigral fetal dopaminergic grafts in patients with Parkinson's disease: a pilot study. Report of three cases. *J Neurosurg*, **96**, 589–596.

Modo, M., Stroemer, R.P., Tang, E., Patel, S. and Hodges, H. (2002). Effects of implantation site of stem cell grafts on behavioral recovery from stroke damage. *Stroke*, **33**, 2270–2278.

Mukhida, K., Baker, K.A., Sadi, D. and Mendez, I. (2001). Enhancement of sensorimotor behavioral recovery in hemiparkinsonian rats with intrastriatal, intranigral, and intrasubthalamic nucleus dopaminergic transplants. *J Neurosci*, **21**, 3521–3530.

Nakatomi, H., Kariu, T., Okabe, S., Yuamamoto, S., Hatano, O., Kawahara, N., Tamura, A., Kirino, T. and Nakafuko, M. (2002). Regeneration of hippocampal pyramidal neurons after ischemic brain injury by recruitment of endogenous neural progenitors. *Cell*, **110**, 429–441.

Nelson, P.T., Kondziolka, D., Wechsler, L., Goldstein, S., Gebel, J., DeCesare, S., Elder, E.M., Zhang, P.J., Jacobs, A., McGrogan, M., Lee, V.M.-Y. and Trojanowski, J.Q. (2002). Clonal human (hNT) neuron grafts for stroke therapy. Neuropathology in a patient 27 months after implantation. *Am J Pathol*, **160**, 1201–1206.

Nunes, M., Roy, N.S., Keyoung, H.M., Goodman, R., McKann, G., Kang, J., Jiang, L., Nedergaard, M. and Goldman, S.A. (2003). Identification and isolation of multipotential neural progenitor cells from the subcortical white matter of the adult human brain. *Nat Med*, **9**, 439–447.

Olanow, C.W., Goetz, C.G., Kordower, J.H., Stoessl, A.J., Sossi, V., Brin, M.F., Shannon, K.M., Nauert, G.M., Perl, D.P., Godbold, J. and Freeman, T.B. (2003). A double-blind controlled trial of bilateral fetal nigral transplantation in Parkinson's disease. *Ann Neurol*, **54**, 403–414.

Palmer, T.D., Willhoite, A.R. and Gage, F.H. (2000). Vascular niche for adult hippocampal neurogenesis. *J Comp Neurol*, **425**, 479–494.

Parent, J.M., Vexler, Z.S., Gong, C., Derugin, N. and Ferriero, D.M. (2002). Rat forebrain neurogenesis and striatal neuron replacement after focal stroke. *Ann Neurol*, **52**, 802–813.

Park, K.I., Teng, Y.D. and Snyder, E.Y. (2002). The injured brain interacts reciprocally with neural stem cells supported by scaffolds to reconstitute lost tissue. *Nat Biotechnol*, **20**, 1111–1117.

Perrier, A.L., Tabar, V., Barberi, T., Rubio, M.E., Bruses, J., Topf, N., Harrison, N.L. and Studer, L. (2004). Derivation of midbrain dopamine neurons from human embryonic stem cells. *Proc Natl Acad Sci USA*, **101**, 12543–12548.

Peschanski, M. and Dunnett, S.B. (2002). Cell therapy for Huntington's disease, the next step forward. *Lancet Neurol*, **1**, 81.

Peschanski, M., Defer, G., N'Guyen, J.P., Ricolfi, F., Monfort, J.C., Remy, P., Geny, C., Samson, Y., Hantraye, P., Jeny, R., Gaston, A., Kéravel, Y., Degos, J.D. and Cesaro, P. (1994). Bilateral motor improvement and alteration of L-dopa effect in two patients with Parkinson's disease following intrastriatal transplantation of foetal ventral mesencephalon. *Brain*, **117**, 487–499.

Piccini, P., Brooks, D.J., Björklund, A., Gunn, R.N., Grasby, P.M., Rimoldi, O., Brundin, P., Hagell, P., Rehncrona, S., Widner, H. and Lindvall, O. (1999). Dopamine release from nigral transplants visualized *in vivo* in a Parkinson's patient. *Nat Neurosci*, **2**, 1137–1140.

Piccini, P., Lindvall, O., Björklund, A., Brundin, P., Hagell, P., Oertel, W., Quinn, N., Samuel, M., Ceravolo, R., Rehncrona, S., Widner, H. and Brooks, D.J. (2000) Delayed recovery of movement-related cortical function in Parkinson's disease after striatal dopaminergic grafts. *Ann Neurol*, **48**, 689–695.

Playford, E.D., Jenkins, I.H., Passingham, R.E., Nutt, J., Frackowiak, R.S. and Brooks, D.J. (1992). Impaired mesial frontal and putamen activation in Parkinson's disease: a positron emission tomographic study. *Ann Neurol*, **32**, 151–161.

Pluchino, S., Quattrini, A., Brambilla, E., Gritti, A., Salani, G., Dina, G., Galli, R., Del Carro, U., Amadio, S., Bergami, A., Furlan, R., Comi, G., Vescovi, A.L. and Martino, G. (2003). Injection of adult neurospheres induces recovery in a chronic model of multiple sclerosis. *Nature*, **422**, 688–694.

Remy, P., Samson, Y., Hantraye, P., Fontaine, A., Defer, G., Mangin, J.-F., Fénelon, G., Gény, C., Ricolfi, F., Frouin, V., N'Guyen, J.P., Jeny, R., Degos, J.D., Peschanski, M. and Cesaro, P. (1995). Clinical correlates of [18F]fluorodopa uptake in five grafted parkinsonian patients. *Ann Neurol*, **38**, 580–588.

Rosser, A.E., Barker, R.A., Harrower, T., Watts, C., Farrington, M., Ho, A.K., Burnstein, R.M., Menon, D.K., Gillard, J.H., Pickard, J., Dunnett, S.B. and NEST-UK. (2002). Unilateral transplantation of human primary fetal tissue in four patients with Huntington's disease: NEST-UK safety report ISRCTN no 36485475. *J Neurol Neurosurg Psychiatr*, **73**, 678–685.

Sawle, G.V., Bloomfield, P.M., Björklund, A., Brooks, D.J., Brundin, P., Leenders, K.L., Lindvall, O., Marsden, C.D., Rehncrona, S., Widner, H. and Frackowiak, R.S.J. (1992). Transplantation of fetal dopamine neurons in Parkinson's disease: PET [18F]6-L-fluorodopa studies in two patients with putaminal implants. *Ann Neurol*, **31**, 166–173.

Schumacher, J.M., Ellias, S.A., Palmer, E.P., Kott, H.S., Dinsmore, J., Dempsey, P.K., Fischman, A.J., Thomas, C., Feldman, R.G., Kassissieh, S., Raineri, R., Manhart, C., Penney, D., Fink, J.S. and Isacson, O. (2000). Transplantation of embryonic porcine mesencephalic tissue in patients with PD. *Neurology*, **54**, 1042–1050.

Steece-Collier, K., Collier, T.J., Danielson, P.D., Kurlan, R., Yurek, D.M. and Sladek Jr., J.R. (2003). Embryonic mesencephalic grafts increase levodopa-induced forelimb hyperkinesia in parkinsonian rats. *Movement Disord*, **18**, 1442–1454.

Sun, Y., Jin, K., Xie, L., Childs, J., Mao, X.O., Logvinove, A. and Greenberg, D.A. (2003). VEGF-induced neuroprotection, neurogenesis, and angiogenesis after focal cerebral ischemia. *J Clin Invest*, **111**, 1843–1851.

Vitek, J.L. (2002). Deep brain stimulation for Parkinson's disease. A critical reevaluation of STN versus GPi DBS. *Stereot Funct Neurosurg*, **78**, 119–131.

Watts, C., Donovan, T., Gillard, J.H., Antoun, N.M., Burnstein, R., Menon, D.K., Carpenter, T.A., Fryer, T., Thomas, D.G.T. and Pickard, J.D. (2003). Evaluation of an MRI-based protocol for cell implantation in four patients with Huntington's disease. *Cell Transplant*, **12**, 697–704.

Watts, R.L., Freeman, T.B., Hauser, R.A., Bakay, R.A., Ellias, S.A., Stoessl, A.J., Eidelberg, D. and Fink, J.S. (2001). A double-blind, randomized, controlled, multicenter clinical trial of the safety and efficacy of stereotoxic intrastriatal implantation of fetal porcine ventral mesencephalic tissue (Neurocell™-PD) vs imitation surgery in patients with Parkinson's disease (PD). *Parkinsonism Relat Disord*, **7**(**Suppl.**), S87.

Wenning, G.K., Odin, P., Morrish, P., Rehncrona, S., Widner, H., Brundin, P., Rothwell, J.C., Brown, R., Gustavii, B., Hagell, P., Jahanshahi, M., Sawle, G., Björklund, A., Brooks, D., Marsden, C.D., Quinn, N.P. and Lindvall, O. (1997). Short- and long-term survival and function of unilateral intrastriatal dopaminergic grafts in Parkinson's disease. *Ann Neurol*, **42**, 95–107.

Winkler, C., Kirik, D., Björklund, A. and Dunnett, S.B. (2000). Transplantation in the rat model of Parkinson's disease. Ectopic versus homotopic graft placement. *Prog Brain Res*, **127**, 233–265.

Index

Page numbers in **bold** refer to **Volume I** and otherwise to Volume II.

633

Page numbers in **bold** refer to **Volume I** and otherwise to Volume II.

Page numbers in **bold** refer to **Volume I** and otherwise to Volume II.

Page numbers in **bold** refer to **Volume I** and otherwise to Volume II.

Page numbers in **bold** refer to **Volume I** and otherwise to Volume II.

Page numbers in **bold** refer to **Volume I** and otherwise to Volume II.

Page numbers in **bold** refer to **Volume I** and otherwise to Volume II.

Page numbers in **bold** refer to **Volume I** and otherwise to Volume II.

Page numbers in **bold** refer to **Volume I** and otherwise to Volume II.

Page numbers in **bold** refer to **Volume I** and otherwise to Volume II.